VOLUME 4

3rd Edition

DIAGNOSIS OF BONE AND JOINT DISORDERS

Donald Resnick, M.D.

Professor of Radiology
University of California, San Diego
Chief of Osteoradiology Section
Veterans Administration Medical Center
San Diego, California

With the Editorial Assistance of Catherine F. Fix
With the Technical Assistance of Debra J. Trudell

W.B. SAUNDERS COMPANY
A Division of Harcourt Brace & Company
Philadelphia   London   Toronto   Montreal   Sydney   Tokyo

W.B. SAUNDERS COMPANY
A Division of
Harcourt Brace & Company

The Curtis Center
Independence Square West
Philadelphia, Pennsylvania 19106

Library of Congress Cataloging-in-Publication Data

Resnick, Donald

Diagnosis of bone and joint disorders / Donald Resnick.—3rd ed.

p.   cm.

Includes bibliographical references and indexes.

ISBN 0–7216–5066–X (set)

1. Musculoskeletal system—Diseases—Diagnosis.   2. Bones—Diseases—
   Diagnosis.   3. Joints—Diseases—Diagnosis.   4. Diagnostic
   imaging.   I. Title.

[DNLM: 1. Bone Diseases—diagnosis.   2. Joint Diseases—diagnosis.
3. Diagnosis Imaging.   WE 300 R434d 1995]

RC925.7.R47 1995

616.7′1075—dc20

DNLM/DLC   93–48321

Diagnosis of Bone and Joint Disorders, 3rd edition

Volume One	ISBN	0–7216–5067–8
Volume Two	ISBN	0–7216–5068–6
Volume Three	ISBN	0–7216–5069–4
Volume Four	ISBN	0–7216–5070–8
Volume Five	ISBN	0–7216–5071–6
Volume Six	ISBN	0–7216–5072–4
Six Volume Set	ISBN	0–7216–5066–X

Printed in the United States of America.

Last digit is the print number: 9   8   7   6   5   4   3   2   1

CONTENTS

▼

Contents   v

SECTION

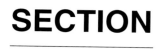

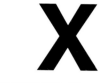

Metabolic Diseases

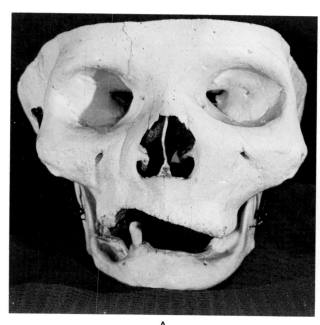

A

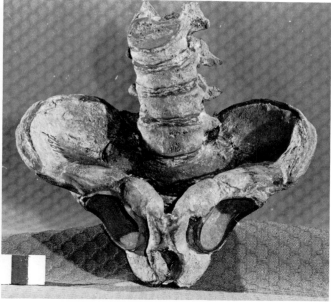

B

A Paget's Disease: The frontal view of the cranial vault shows diffuse hyperostosis of the facial bones with porous subperiosteal bone deposition.
B Osteomalacia: Typical pelvic deformity with cardboard-like bones is evident.
(From Ortner DJ, Putschar WGJ: Identification of Pathological Conditions in Human Skeletal Remains. Washington, DC, Smithsonian Institution Press, 1981.)

51

Osteoporosis

Donald Resnick, M.D., and Gen Niwayama, M.D.

Osteoporosis is the most frequent metabolic bone disease. In this disease, a generalized decrease in bone mass is seen. The remaining bone is normal structurally as determined by histologic and chemical analysis. The diagnosis of osteoporosis generally is made on the basis of characteristic radiographic abnormalities, although routine radio-graphic procedures are not very helpful in the early detection of this metabolic condition. It has been estimated that 30 to 50 per cent of skeletal calcium must be lost before a change appears on the radiographs.[1, 2] Because of this inadequacy, newer diagnostic techniques have been used for the earlier detection and the quantitation of osteoporosis. These techniques, which include photon absorptiometry,[3–6, 330–336] transaxial CT scanning,[7–11, 194, 195, 197, 336–348] dual-energy radiographic absorptiometry,[336, 348–353] and ultrasonography,[12, 13] are discussed elsewhere in this book.

In previous chapters, bone physiology and pathophysiology as well as morphology in metabolic and endocrine disorders have been discussed. The purpose of this chapter is to describe the radiographic approach to osteoporosis. The discussion will include the appropriate terminology, the various causes of generalized and regional osteoporosis, the fundamental radiologic and pathologic features, the abnormalities that are apparent at specific skeletal sites, and the findings with CT scanning and MR imaging.

TERMINOLOGY

The terms osteoporosis and osteomalacia were introduced by Pommer in 1885,[14, 15] who was able to distinguish between these two major conditions affecting the human skeleton. Osteoporosis was defined as a condition with decreased skeletal mass associated with increased porosity; osteomalacia was defined as a condition with decreased mineralization associated with the presence of nonmineralized osteoid seams. It was not until much later that the discovery was made that osteomalacia in adults, like rickets in children, was due to a deficiency of vitamin D.

Osteoporosis is characterized by qualitatively normal but quantitatively deficient bone (Fig. 51–1). The diagnosis of osteoporosis frequently is suggested by the radiologic examination. Radiographs in patients with osteoporosis reveal increased radiolucency of bone, a finding that is best termed osteopenia, meaning "poverty of bone." The discovery of osteopenia on a radiograph does not allow a precise diagnosis of osteoporosis, however, as this finding is present in a variety of conditions that lead to rarefied or radiolucent

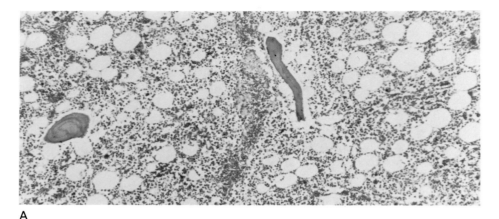

A

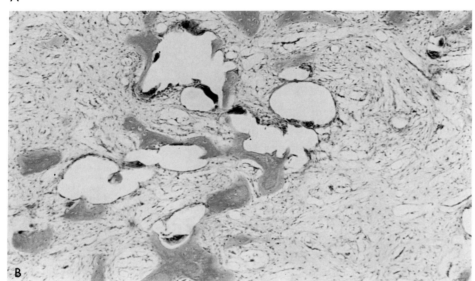

B

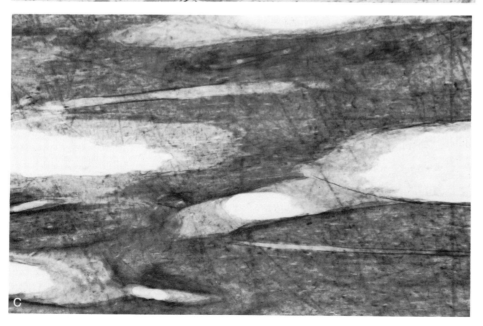

C

FIGURE 51–1. Osteoporosis: Pathologic abnormalities and differentiation from osteitis fibrosa cystica and osteomalacia.

A Osteoporosis. The bone is qualitatively normal but quantitatively deficient (100×). Osteoclastosis is not a significant feature.

B Osteitis fibrosa cystica (hyperparathyroidism). Diffuse fibrosis of the stroma of the bone marrow is associated with osteoclastic resorption and new bone formation (100×).

C Osteomalacia. Undecalcified section of bone stained for calcium reveals superficial osteoid tissue that is not so heavily stained as the calcified bone (86×).

bone. Rather, the use of this generic term rests on the frequent inability to distinguish among the various causes of osteopenia by gross radiographic appearances.[16] Other terms, such as "demineralization" and "undermineralization," are unacceptable as accurate descriptions of this radiographic finding: "Demineralization" implies a specific loss of mineral without concomitant loss of organic component of bone, a phenomenon called halisteresis, which is not prominent in osseous tissue; and "undermineralization" might be a term more accurately applied to osteomalacia, in which there is an inadequate secretion of mineral into osteoid matrix.[16] The term "deossification" implies abnormal loss of bone occurring as a result of accelerated bone resorption. In fact, some types of osteoporosis are associated with increased rates of resorption, although others are characterized by normal rates of resorption. Thus, osteoporosis and deossification are not equivalent terms.

At present, osteopenia is the most suitable term to describe increased radiolucency of bone. Osteopenia occurs when bone resorption exceeds bone formation no matter what the specific pathogenesis (Table 51–1). Diffuse osteopenia is found in osteoporosis, osteomalacia, hyperparathyroidism, neoplasm, and a variety of other conditions. Once osteopenia is discovered, radiographs must be searched carefully for additional and more specific abnormalities; for example, osteomalacia can lead to characteristic linear radiolucent areas termed Looser's zones; hyperparathyroidism can produce aggressive subperiosteal and subchondral resorption of bone; and neoplasms, such as plasma cell myeloma, can be associated with focal skeletal radiolucent lesions. Osteoporosis, too, can lead to additional radiographic findings, but, in general, these findings are not specific. Thus, the accurate diagnosis of osteoporosis rests on the radiologic findings of osteopenia coupled with typical clinical and histologic features. The inclusion of the clinical and histologic features in the definition of osteoporosis is required owing to the loss of bone that occurs normally in all persons as they age, a process that is more prominent in women than in men. Osteoporosis is established when the decrease in bone mass is greater than that expected for a person of a given age, sex, and race, and when it results in structural bone failure manifested by fractures.[200] These fractures are most typical in the spine, proximal portion of the femur, and distal portion of the radius; they are produced by trabecular or cortical bone loss, or both, depending on the site of involvement.[200–204] The magnitude of the problem becomes apparent considering the estimates that osteoporosis affects approximately 15 to 20 million people in the United States[354] and that of the 1 million fractures occurring annually in the United States in women older than 45 years of age, 350,000 could be prevented by the elimination of osteoporosis.[200]

ETIOLOGY

Osteoporosis can be classified as generalized (involving the major portion of the skeleton, particularly its axial component), regional (involving one segment of the skeleton), or localized (single or multiple focal areas of osteoporosis). There are many causes of generalized, regional, and localized osteoporosis. Some of the diseases that are associated with generalized or regional osteoporosis are discussed here. Localized osteoporosis may accompany focal skeletal lesions such as arthritis, infection, and neoplasm, and it often is overshadowed by the radiographic features of the primary process itself.

Generalized Osteoporosis

The osseous manifestations of conditions leading to generalized osteoporosis predominate in the axial skeleton and proximal portions of the long bones of the appendicular skeleton. Abnormalities of the spine are particularly prominent, leading not only to osteopenia but also to changes in vertebral contour characterized by biconcave vertebral bodies ("fish vertebrae") and collapse. Changes in the pelvis include osteopenia and a coarsened trabecular pattern. Trabecular resorption occurs in certain areas of the appendicular skeleton, such as in the femoral necks. In both the axial and the appendicular skeleton, the decrease in radiodensity usually is uniform, particularly in those conditions with slowly progressive and long-standing osteoporosis. Although some differences are apparent in the distribution and appearance of osteopenia among the various diseases that produce generalized osteoporosis (Table 51–2), the previously mentioned characteristics are most typical.

Senile and Postmenopausal Osteoporosis (Fig. 51–2). Senescent osteoporosis and postmenopausal osteoporosis constitute the most common causes of generalized osteoporosis. The reported frequency of osteoporosis in older

TABLE 51–1. Major Causes of Diffuse Osteopenia

Osteoporosis
Osteomalacia
Hyperparathyroidism
Neoplasm

TABLE 51–2. Major Causes of Generalized Osteoporosis

Senile and postmenopausal states
Medication
Steroids
Heparin
Endocrine states
Hyperthyroidism
Hyperparathyroidism
Cushing's disease
Acromegaly
Pregnancy
Diabetes mellitus
Hypogonadism
Deficiency states
Scurvy
Malnutrition
Calcium deficiency
Alcoholism
Chronic liver disease
Anemic states
Osteogenesis imperfecta
Idiopathic condition

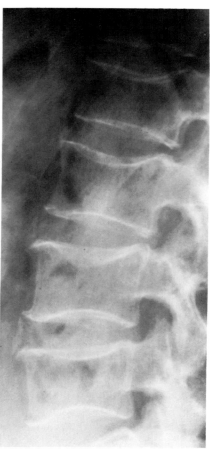

FIGURE 51–2. Senile and postmenopausal osteoporosis. In this elderly woman, a lateral radiograph of the lumbar spine outlines increased lucency and biconcave deformity (fish vertebra) of multiple vertebral bodies.

persons has varied, influenced considerably by a number of factors, including the diagnostic method used to detect osteoporosis and the person's sex, hormone balance, skeletal size, level of exercise or activity, and nutritional status. Using either morphometry or osteodensitometry, Meema and collaborators[17] estimated that 50 per cent of women over the age of 60 years have significantly less bone than expected. In another series, the frequency of radiographically demonstrable osteoporosis of the spine in ambulatory women between 45 and 79 years of age was reported as 29 per cent.[18] In this latter series, 4.6 per cent of the women revealed wedge-shaped vertebrae or compression fractures of one or more vertebral bodies. In a different report, 20 per cent of men and 29 per cent of women between the ages of 63 and 95 years showed compression fractures of the vertebral bodies.[19]

Evidence exists that peak bone mass occurs in the second decade of life, although heredity and environmental factors may influence this timing. The peak bone mass is approximately 20 per cent greater in men than in women and is greater in black than in white persons.[358] In general, a gradual loss of skeletal mass occurs beginning in the fifth or sixth decade of life in men and in the fourth decade in women. After the age of about 50 years, bone loss takes place at a rate of 0.4 per cent each year in men; after the

age of approximately 35 years, women lose bone at a yearly rate of 0.75 to 1 per cent, which increases to a rate of 2 to 3 per cent after the menopause.[201, 205, 206] Up to the age of 80 years, women appear to be affected four times more frequently than men. After this age, there is no sex difference in the frequency of osteoporosis.[20] Although loss of both compact and trabecular bone occurs in older men and women, the magnitude of the loss of compact bone in women after the menopause is much greater than that in men.[207] The endosteal diameter of the bone increases more rapidly than the periosteal diameter, leading to an expansion of the medullary cavity at the expense of the cortex.[208] This finding, combined with progressive trabeculation of the cortex,[208] is responsible for a net loss of cortical bone.[202] Concomitant reduction of trabecular bone is evident,[209] and the resulting diminution of bone mass produces a decrease in strength and a propensity to fracture. The importance of loss of trabecular bone in the production of fractures in postmenopausal women has been emphasized in numerous publications, although the precise contribution of trabecular versus cortical weakening to fracture occurrence is difficult to define.[207, 322]

Patients with senile or postmenopausal osteoporosis may be entirely asymptomatic, although significant loss of bone mass may be accompanied by various clinical findings. Bone pain, particularly in the back, may be associated with loss of height owing to vertebral compression.[21] Increased thoracic kyphosis is apparent. Neurologic complications are unusual.[2] Generally (but not uniformly[322]) it is reported that patients with osteoporosis in the vertebral column have a high frequency of femoral fracture, particularly in the transcervical and subtrochanteric regions of the femoral neck. The rate of occurrence of osteoporosis in older patients with such fractures has been estimated at 75 to 85 per cent.[22–24] These fractures occur spontaneously or after minor trauma and may be accompanied by fractures of the ribs, humerus, or radius.

Laboratory analysis generally yields unremarkable results (Table 51–3). Levels of serum and urinary calcium and phosphorus, as well as of serum alkaline and acid phosphatase, are normal. Urinary hydroxyproline levels may be elevated.

The pathogenesis of postmenopausal and senile osteoporosis is not clear. For many years this variety of osteoporosis was considered to be due primarily to a failure of bone formation; bone resorption was not thought to be a prominent factor. This concept was strengthened by the lack of histologic evidence of excessive osteoclastic activity. A defect in the production of collagen and nitrogenous matrix of bone was suspected, which might be influenced by hormonal imbalance[193]; a loss of estrogenic steroids in postmenopausal women was regarded as an important factor. More recently, application of newer techniques, such as radioactive calcium kinetic analysis and microradiography, has indicated that bone formation is normal in this condition.[2, 25–27] The results regarding bone resorption have been conflicting. Calcium kinetic studies have indicated that absolute bone resorption rates are not increased over the rates in normal adults corrected for body size,[28, 29] although resorption might exceed formation by 50 to 100 mg per day,[27] a loss that could explain the development of osteoporosis over several years. Microradiographic analysis has

TABLE 51–3. Laboratory Diagnosis of Metabolic Bone Disease*†

	Serum Levels					Urine Levels		
	Ca	P	AP	Urea or Creatinine	PTH	Ca	Tubular Resorption of Phosphate	Hydroxy-proline
Senile and postmenopausal osteoporosis	N	N	N	N	N	N	N	N; I
Osteogenesis imperfecta	N	N	N	N	N	N	N	N
Hyperthyroidism	N; I	N	N	N	N; D	I	N	I
Primary	I	D	N; I	N; I	I	N; I	D	I
Secondary	N; D	I	I	I	I	D	D	I
"Tertiary"	I	N; D	N; I	N; I	I	N; I	D	I
Hypoparathyroidism	D	I	N	N	D	D	I	N
Pseudohypoparathyroidism	D	I	N	N	N; I	D	I	N
Pseudopseudohypoparathyroidism	N	N	N	N	N	N	N	N
Paget's disease	N	N	I	N	N	N	N	I
Rickets or osteomalacia								
Vitamin D deficiency	D	D	I	N	I	D	D	N
Vitamin D refractory	N	D	I	N; I	N; I	D	D	N
Hypophosphatasia	N; I	N	D	N	?	N; I	N	D

*After Goldsmith RS: Orthop Clin North Am 3:545, 1972.
†N, Normal; I, increased; D, decreased; Ca, calcium; P, phosphorus; AP, alkaline phosphatase; PTH, parathyroid hormone.

shown a striking increase in the resorptive surface, suggesting that excessive bone resorption is the fundamental abnormality in postmenopausal and senile osteoporosis.[25] Even more recently, morphometric methods based on tetracycline-estimated rates of apposition have revealed impaired bone formation in many patients with osteoporosis.[1]

The possibility that different cellular mechanisms are at work in patients with postmenopausal or senile osteoporosis (and other forms of osteoporosis) is supported by evidence of heterogeneity in the histologic findings. Some persons demonstrate marked suppression of the dynamics of bone remodeling (inactive or low-turnover osteoporosis) whereas others show increased bone remodeling (active or high-turnover osteoporosis).[357] In low-turnover osteoporosis, which is characteristic of aging, deposition of new bone by osteoblasts in resorptive cavities of normal, decreased, or increased depth may be deficient; in high-turnover osteoporosis, the bone may have an elevated number of osteoclasts and empty Howship's lacunae.[359, 360] Involutional bone loss in men appears to be associated with an age-related reduction in osteoblast function, possibly due to decreased osteoblast longevity or impaired regulation of osteoblast activity and recruitment.[359] A decrease in hematopoietic osteoblast progenitor cells owing to an increase in marrow fat may be a contributory factor.[361]

The importance of loss of ovarian function in the evolution of postmenopausal osteoporosis was first emphasized by Albright and collaborators in 1940.[210] Estrogen deficiency resulting from menopause (or oophorectomy) has been implicated in the pathogenesis of such osteoporosis. The negative calcium balance relates principally to an increase in bone resorption and a reduction in the efficiency of calcium absorption.[211] The mechanism that accounts for bone loss is not entirely clear, although parathyroid hormone, 1,25-dihydroxyvitamin D, and calcitonin are potential mediators.[212] One model for postmenopausal bone loss[213] is based on the assumption that estrogen antagonizes the effect of parathyroid hormone on bone but not the effect of parathyroid hormone on 1,25-dihydroxyvitamin D synthesis; estrogen withdrawal increases bone resorption, infusing calcium into the extracellular fluid and reducing the secretion of parathyroid hormone, resulting in a reduction in the synthesis of 1,25-dihydroxyvitamin D and in calcium absorption.[211] Evidence supporting the role of calcitonin deficiency in producing or aggravating postmenopausal osteoporosis has been inconsistent.[214, 355] Whatever the precise mechanism, the apparent relationship between loss of ovarian function and osteoporosis after the menopause—a relationship that is supported by the occurrence of osteoporosis in young oophorectomized women, in female athletes with secondary amenorrhea,[216, 356, 357] in women with hyperprolactinemia,[217] and in patients with Turner's syndrome—has led to preventive and therapeutic use of estrogen. Recommendations regarding timing and length of therapy vary, however.[215] Estrogens are known to inhibit bone resorption, although the precise mechanism of this effect is not clear.

Obviously many questions regarding the pathogenesis of osteoporosis in older persons remain unanswered. The possibility exists that osteoporosis is a general involutional process of aging. It is well known that osteoblastic activity produces the organic matrix of osseous tissue. In older patients, involution of osteoblasts may occur. Furthermore, osteocytes, which arise from osteoblasts that are trapped in the mineralized bony matrix, also may be altered in the aging skeleton. Thus, diminished osteoblastic and osteocytic activity could dramatically influence the composition of bone and lead to postmenopausal and senile osteoporosis. Although this scheme emphasizes the involutional characteristics of osteoporosis in older persons, a variety of dietary and hormonal factors may contribute to an acceleration of this process. Calcium deficiency, fluctuating levels of adrenocortical and gonadal steroids, and activity of parathyroid hormone, calcitonin, thyroid hormone, and growth hormone are influential factors.

Hyperparathyroidism. Osteoporosis may occur during the course of hyperparathyroidism.[30] The characteristic skeletal changes in this disease relate to increased rates of both bone resorption and bone formation.[25] Superimposed on osteoporosis are the typical findings of osteitis fibrosa cystica (see Chapter 57).

Steroid-Induced Osteoporosis (Fig. 51–3). Osteoporosis occurring during the course of either Cushing's syndrome or exogenous (iatrogenic) hypercortisolism is well known. Histologic studies have revealed decreased bone formation and increased bone resorption, the latter being manifested as increased osteoclastic cell numbers, activity, and resorption sites.[31, 32, 218] The decrease in rate of bone formation has been attributed to direct corticosteroid inhibition of osteoblast formation. Moderate doses of steroids decrease the synthesis of bone collagen by preexisting osteoblasts and the conversion of precursor cells to functioning osteoblasts.[31-33] Increased bone resorption rates have been attributed variously to either direct stimulation of osteoclastic activity or increased parathyroid hormone secretion.[34, 35] This latter effect may relate, at least in part, to a decrease in intestinal absorption of calcium induced by corticosteroid administration[36, 37] although direct stimulation of the parathyroid glands by cortisol has been observed experimentally.[218]

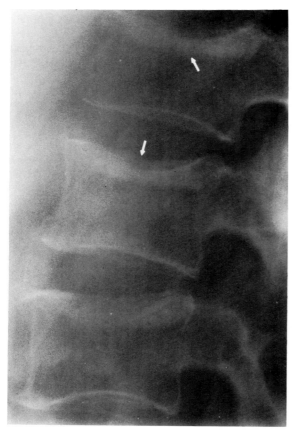

FIGURE 51–3. Steroid-induced osteoporosis. A lateral radiograph of the lumbar spine outlines osteoporosis and compressed vertebral bodies with peripheral condensation of bone (arrows). This latter feature, which leads to radiodense superior and inferior vertebral margins, is characteristic of exogenous or endogenous hypercortisolism.

Laboratory analysis reveals negative calcium balance and hypercalciuria. Although serum levels of calcium, phosphorus, and alkaline phosphatase usually are normal, they may be elevated in severe forms of the disease. Radiographic evaluation indicates the usual findings of osteoporosis, although peculiar condensation of bone at the margins of the vertebral bodies and involvement of extraspinal sites may be encountered. Furthermore, as discussed in Chapter 74 and illustrated later in the present chapter, insufficiency fractures in the axial (pelvis) and appendicular skeleton are characteristic and easily overlooked.

Hyperthyroidism. Osteoporosis in hyperthyroidism is associated with an increase in both bone resorption and bone formation.[25, 38] Osteoblastic and osteoclastic hyperactivity is apparent on bone biopsy. Hypercalcemia, hypercalciuria, hyperphosphatemia, and elevation of serum levels of alkaline phosphatase can occur.[38] Radiologic findings are typical of osteoporosis, although rapid progression prior to treatment and rapid improvement after therapy can be evident (see Chapter 56).

Acromegaly. Osteoporosis can occur in acromegaly associated with other forms of endocrine dysfunction or in acromegaly unaccompanied by such dysfunction.[27] A negative calcium, phosphorus, and nitrogen balance is seen (see Chapter 55).[39]

Pregnancy and Related Conditions. Although uncommon, osteoporosis may be observed in childbearing women.[40] Documentation of its cause in this clinical setting has not occurred, although possible factors include vitamin D and calcium deficiencies and secondary hyperparathyroidism. A study of young black women who were using certain oral contraceptives has revealed higher concentrations of bone mineral than in nonusers.[41] In the same study, women who had lactated tended to have poorly mineralized bones. Osteoporosis appearing in association with pregnancy or lactation is accompanied by normal results on histologic and serum and urinary laboratory analysis.[219]

Heparin-Induced Osteoporosis (Fig. 51–4). The development of osteoporosis has been documented in patients who are receiving large doses of heparin (greater than 15,000 units per day).[42, 220] The changes may be reversible with cessation of therapy. The mechanism of osteoporosis in these patients is not known. Heparin has inhibited bone formation in animals.[43] In tissue culture, heparin may promote bone resorption,[44] perhaps related to an increase in collagenolytic activity.[45, 46] Although a definite decrease in bone collagen has been verified in animals,[47] it is not clear whether this is due to decreased synthesis or increased breakdown of collagen. Heparin also may potentiate the effects of parathyroid hormone.[44] The activity of mast cells (which store heparin) may be an important factor in heparin-induced osteoporosis, and osteopenia is a recognized feature of mastocytosis.[221] The pathologic[48] and radiologic[49] features of heparin-induced osteoporosis have been described. Typical radiographic findings in the spine include osteopenia and vertebral compression.[192]

Alcoholism. Alcoholic patients reveal a reduced bone mass compared with controls[50-53] and increased bone fragility manifested as a high rate of occurrence of fractures.[54] The cause of this loss in bone mineral is not known. A relationship between bone mass and variables such as physical activity,[51] nutrition,[55] and gastric surgery for peptic

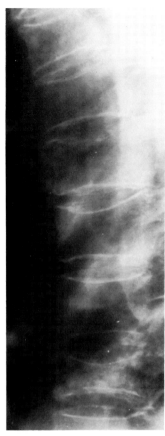

FIGURE 51–4. Heparin-induced osteoporosis. Osteoporotic and collapsed thoracic vertebral bodies in this patient may have been related to prolonged administration of heparin.

ulcer disease[52] may be operational in alcoholic persons; however, data exist that indicate a direct effect of alcohol on bone leading to a profound decrease in bone turnover.[222–224] Alcohol consumption appears to depress bone formation, with much less effect on bone resorption.[465]

Idiopathic Juvenile Osteoporosis (Fig. 51–5). Idiopathic juvenile osteoporosis is an uncommon, self-limited disease of childhood.[56–59, 225–227, 466] Clinically affected children come to medical attention about 2 years before puberty with spinal and extraspinal symptoms, which may simulate those of an arthritis. Less typically, younger children are affected.[225] On radiographic examination, osteoporosis of the spine, particularly in the thoracic and lumbar regions, may be combined with vertebral collapse.[228] Kyphosis represents the characteristic spinal complication, although progressive scoliosis has been observed in some cases.[229] Although transverse and oblique fractures in the bones of the peripheral skeleton may occur, a more typical feature appears to be metaphyseal injury, especially about the knees and ankles, a finding that is less common in osteogenesis imperfecta, the disease that is most likely to be confused with idiopathic juvenile osteoporosis.[59] The peculiar vulnerability of the metaphysis in this condition may be due to bony abnormality that is occurring as bone is being formed at the physeal growth plate. Metaphyseal lucent lesions may lead to complete fractures with subsequent deformities; fractures of the diaphyses generally heal well, although delayed union or pseudarthrosis can become apparent. In other patients, no permanent sequelae are apparent in the metaphyses or diaphyses of the tubular bones or the spine.

The pathologic aberrations in idiopathic juvenile osteoporosis include a quantitative rather than a qualitative change in bone characterized by an increase in bone resorption surface.[60] Although defective osteoblastic function may be present in this condition,[359] increased osteoclastic activity also may be operational and may lead to excessive resorption (however, this latter finding is not uniformly present). Despite this possible increase in osteoclastosis, most laboratory parameters are normal; serum calcium, phosphorus, and alkaline phosphatase levels are not abnormal. Hypercalciuria occasionally is evident.

The major problem in differential diagnosis is distinguishing idiopathic juvenile osteoporosis from osteogenesis imperfecta (Fig. 51–6). Osteogenesis imperfecta congenita appears in early infancy with distinctive features. Osteogenesis imperfecta tarda forms may not produce abnormalities until later childhood or adolescence. Osteogenesis imperfecta (see Chapter 87) may be associated with blue sclerae, progressive cranial, facial, and pelvic deformities, and a qualitative abnormality of bone on histologic examination, findings not evident in idiopathic juvenile osteoporosis. In osteogenesis imperfecta, thin cortices of the diaphyses lead to characteristic fractures of the shaft. Other childhood disorders, such as leukemia, homocystinuria, Cushing's disease, and juvenile chronic arthritis, usually are easily differentiated from idiopathic juvenile osteoporosis.

The osteoporosis pseudoglioma syndrome, although leading to osteoporosis in children, is more likely to be confused with osteogenesis imperfecta than with idiopathic juvenile osteoporosis. This syndrome is a rare, genetically determined disorder that leads to developmental abnormalities of the skeleton and eyes.[362, 363] Of autosomal recessive inheritance, the osteoporosis pseudoglioma syndrome is characterized by severe ocular abnormalities occurring early in life and associated with calcifications, ligament laxity, generalized osteoporosis with bowing deformities of tubular bones and fractures of spinal and extraspinal sites,[467] frequent mental retardation, and the absence of blue sclerae, dental abnormalities, and deafness. Blindness also is characteristic. Osteoporosis pseudoglioma syndrome can be differentiated from osteogenesis imperfecta by means of examination of a biopsy specimen of the iliac crest.[467]

Other Disorders. Generalized osteoporosis may accompany plasma cell myeloma, Gaucher's disease and glycogen storage disease, anemias, nutritional deficiencies,[230, 231, 315, 327] diabetes mellitus, immunodeficiency states,[232] and chronic liver disease[2, 27, 61, 233, 364] (Fig. 51–7). In some of these disorders (plasma cell myeloma, storage diseases), the primary disease process involves the bone directly; in others (sickle cell anemia, neoplasms), the bone is altered as a complication of the primary disease.

Bone mass and strength are dependent on adequate nutrition and exercise. Dietary inadequacy and physical inactivity lead to deficiencies in both the amount and integrity of bone.[365] Immobilization or disuse, or insufficient calcium or protein intake, each can lead to osteoporosis. As an example, early and significant deficits of bone mass occur in anorexia nervosa.[231, 315, 327, 366] Pathologic fractures may result. Estrogen deficiency, glucocorticoid excess, malnutrition, and low calcium intake have been proposed as contributory factors.[366]

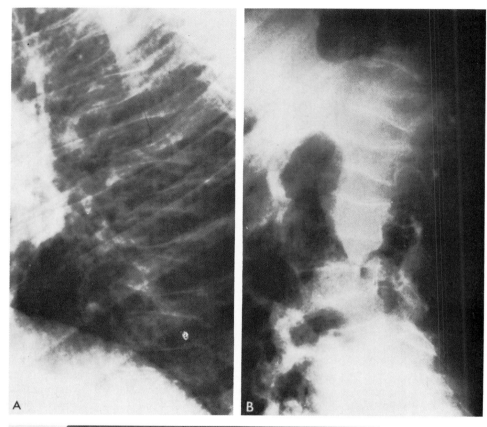

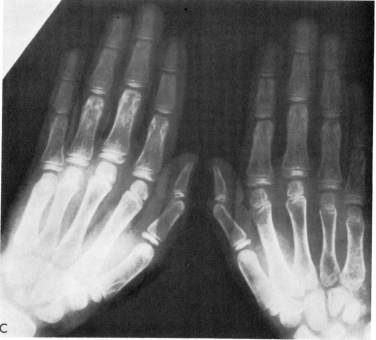

FIGURE 51–5. Idiopathic juvenile osteoporosis. This 11 year old girl developed progressive osteoporosis in the appendicular and axial skeleton. There was no clinical evidence of blue sclerae or deafness. Laboratory evaluation was unremarkable. Family history was noncontributory.

A A lateral radiograph of the thoracic spine reveals severe compression and collapse of multiple radiolucent vertebral bodies. The disc spaces appear ballooned.

B In the lumbar spine, similar alterations are evident. Observe the severe osteoporosis of the vertebral bodies. Biconcave deformities and anterior wedging are evident.

C A radiograph of the hands outlines osteopenic bones with thinned cortices.

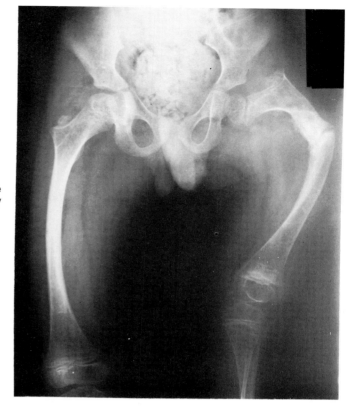

FIGURE 51–6. Osteogenesis imperfecta. In a child, observe the generalized osteoporosis, cortical diminution, and osseous deformity and fracture.

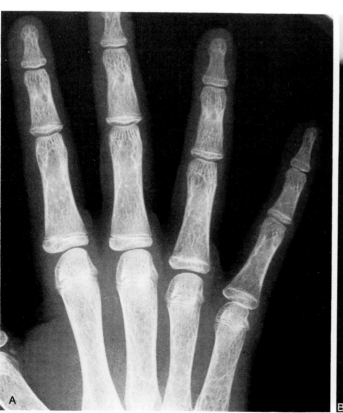

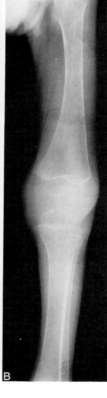

FIGURE 51–7. Additional causes of generalized osteoporosis.

A Thalassemia. Severe osteoporosis in the metacarpals and phalanges is associated with a reticulated and cystic appearance. These findings are characteristic.

B Marasmic protein-calorie malnutrition (kwashiorkor). Observe extensive osteopenia with marked diminution in the cortical thickness. Soft tissue atrophy also is apparent in this 6 year old African boy.

(**B**, Courtesy of B. J. Cremin, M.D., Cape Town, Republic of South Africa.)

Long-standing testosterone deficiency appears to be an important causative factor in men with spinal osteoporosis.[367] The typical age of clinical presentation is the sixth decade of life in patients who have had hypogonadal symptoms for more than 20 years.[359] Causes of hypogonadism in osteoporotic men include Klinefelter's syndrome, hyperprolactinemia, hemochromatosis, anorexia nervosa, hypothalamic-pituitary dysfunction, and idiopathic hypogonadotropic hypogonadism.[359]

Differential Diagnosis. The differentiation between generalized osteoporosis and osteomalacia, especially in adults, may be extremely difficult on the basis of radiographic abnormalities and, ultimately, may require histologic evaluation of skeletal tissue (see Chapter 53). In infants and children, the presence of rickets with its characteristic metaphyseal changes represents a valuable diagnostic clue. Accurate diagnosis becomes important in infants, particularly those receiving long-term intravenous hyperalimentation, in whom the development of rickets may lead to multiple fractures that contribute to an erroneous diagnosis of osteogenesis imperfecta, the child abuse syndrome, or copper deficiency[305, 306] (Fig. 51–8). Unfortunately, typical rachitic changes are not present universally, so that the discovery of fractures of the ribs or tubular bones in infants receiving such hyperalimentation should raise the possibility of rickets.[306]

In adults with osteomalacia, diffuse osteopenia simulates generalized osteoporosis. In some cases, additional radiographic abnormalities allow differentiation of the two disorders; in osteomalacia, trabeculae may appear indistinct and the interface of cortical and medullary bone may be obscured. These features, however, often are subtle and require magnification techniques. More helpful is the identification of osseous deformity (such as acetabular protrusion and a bell-shaped thorax) and insufficiency fractures (pseudofractures), which are most frequent in the pubic

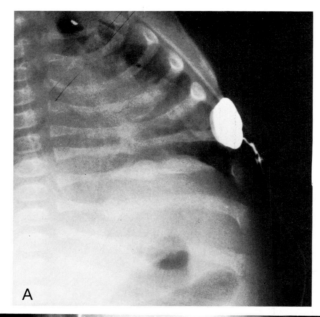

A

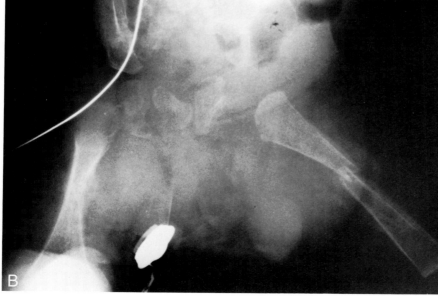

B

FIGURE 51–8. Rickets secondary to intravenous hyperalimentation. In this infant multiple fractures of the ribs and femora simulate those seen in the child abuse syndrome. (Courtesy of M. Dalinka, M.D., Philadelphia, Pennsylvania.)

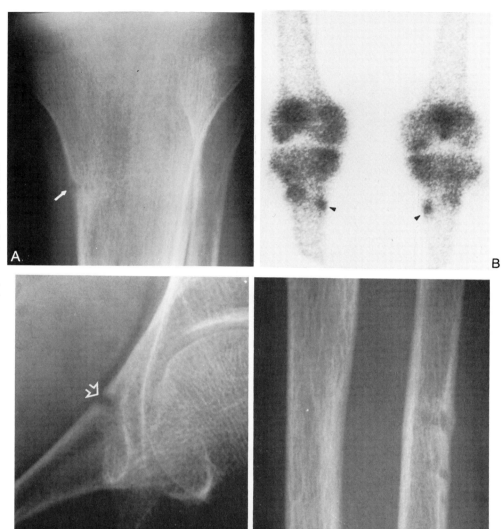

FIGURE 51–9. Osteomalacia.

A, B This 36 year old man with chronic renal disease was treated with hemodialysis and phosphate-binding medications. A biopsy confirmed the presence of osteomalacia and hyperparathyroidism. Observe an insufficiency fracture in the medial aspect of the left tibial metaphysis (arrow), which, along with a similar alteration on the opposite side, accumulates the bone-seeking radiopharmaceutical agent (arrowheads). Additional fractures were evident in the ribs related to an upper respiratory infection with excessive coughing. (Courtesy of G. Greenway, M.D., Dallas, Texas.)

C, D In another patient, typical insufficiency fractures involve the iliopubic column (open arrow) and ulna.

rami, medial portion of the femoral neck, axillary margins of the ribs, scapula, and, occasionally, tubular bones (Fig. 51–9). In some forms of osteomalacia, additional distinctive alterations are apparent (see Chapter 53). X-linked hypophosphatemic osteomalacia (or rickets) is associated with a generalized enthesopathy in which bone proliferation at sites of tendon and ligament attachment and tendinous, ligamentous, and capsular calcification become evident; calcification of cartilage and small ossicles also may be noted[307] (Fig. 51–10). Atypical axial osteomalacia[308–310] is characterized by involvement of the spine and pelvis, a coarsened trabecular pattern (particularly in the cervical region), normal or near-normal laboratory values, and osteomalacia on histologic analysis. Adults of both sexes are affected, and a family history of the disease sometimes is encountered.

Primary or secondary hyperparathyroidism generally leads to diagnostic abnormalities in addition to osteopenia; aggressive bone resorption occurs in subperiosteal, intracortical, endosteal, subligamentous, and subchondral locations. In patients with renal osteodystrophy, these changes are accompanied by osteosclerosis, osteomalacia, and vascular, soft tissue, and periarticular calcification (see Chapter 57).

Fibrogenesis imperfecta ossium is a rare disorder of bone characterized by the formation of abnormal collagen fibers in osteoid that are not birefringent when examined under polarized light[311–314, 328] (see Chapter 87). The age of onset of disease varies from childhood to adulthood, although an onset in the fifth decade of life is most typical. The disorder is progressive, leading to crippling deformity and death. A consistent biochemical abnormality is elevation of serum levels of alkaline phosphatase. Radiographic alterations include amorphous sclerosis of the medullary cavity, obscuring the trabecular pattern, or a fish-net or basket-weave appearance, with sparsely distributed trabeculae[313, 314] (Figs. 51–11 and 51–12). Osseous protuberances, especially in the pelvis, scapula, and proximal portion of the femur, are characteristic. Pathologic fractures in the axial and appendicular bones are frequent.

Regional Osteoporosis

Osteoporosis confined to a region or segment of the body is associated with disorders of the appendicular skeleton. The classic example of such a disorder is osteoporosis associated with disuse or immobilization of a limb or portion

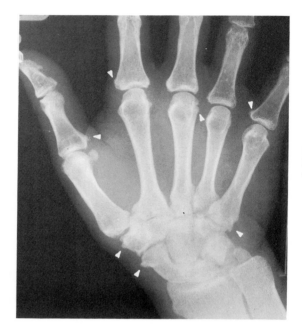

FIGURE 51–10. X-linked hypophosphatemic osteomalacia. Observe a generalized enthesopathy characterized by osseous protuberances in the carpus, metacarpals, and phalanges (arrowheads).

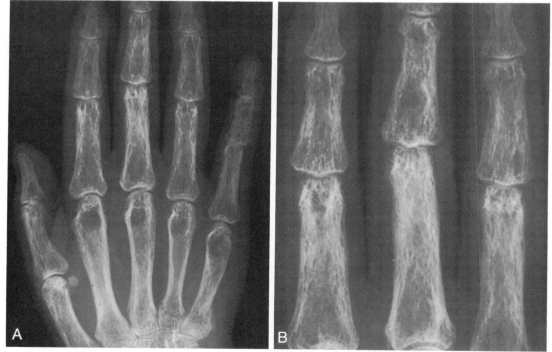

FIGURE 51–11. Fibrogenesis imperfecta ossium. In this 44 year old woman, note osteopenia and a coarsened trabecular pattern in the metacarpal bones and phalanges. The interface between the cortex and the medullary canal is obliterated, and there is no evidence of subperiosteal resorption. (Courtesy of P. Kline, M.D., San Antonio, Texas.)

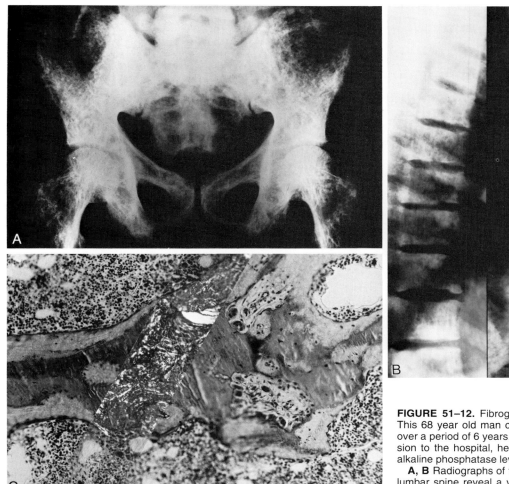

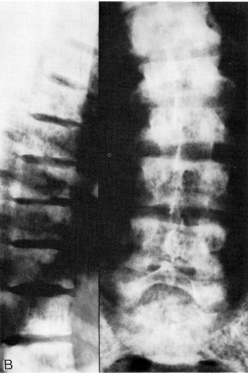

FIGURE 51–12. Fibrogenesis imperfecta ossium. This 68 year old man complained of skeletal pain over a period of 6 years. One month prior to admission to the hospital, he fractured his ulna. Serum alkaline phosphatase level was elevated.

A, B Radiographs of the pelvis and thoracic and lumbar spine reveal a very coarse trabecular pattern simulating that of renal osteodystrophy or Paget's disease. The overall density of the bone appears to be increased, but the trabecular alterations predominate. Similar changes were evident in the appendicular skeleton.

C A photomicrograph (75×) in ordinary light with an inset in polarized light of an undercalcified section of the biopsied iliac crest reveals wide and extensively distributed osteoid. With polarized light, deficient and disorganized collagen is seen.

(**A, C**, Courtesy of D. Stoker, M.D., and P.D. Byers, M.D., London, England; **B**, From Byers, PD, et al: Skel Radiol *13*:72, 1985.)

of a limb. Other examples include reflex sympathetic dystrophy (RSD) and transient regional osteoporosis (Table 51–4).

As opposed to the uniform increase in skeletal radiolucency that is most typical of generalized osteoporosis, the radiographic patterns of regional osteoporosis are more variable. Uniform osteopenia may accompany regional osteoporosis of long duration, such as that associated with chronic disuse in patients who are paralyzed or who have undergone amputation. Bandlike osteopenia (in the subchondral or metaphyseal regions) and patchy osteopenia (particularly in the epiphyses) may indicate a more acutely developing osteoporosis, such as that occurring in RSD. In

TABLE 51–4. Major Causes of Regional Osteoporosis

Immobilization and disuse
Reflex sympathetic dystrophy
Transient regional osteoporosis
  Transient osteoporosis of the hip
  Regional migratory osteoporosis

acute osteoporosis, both cortical and spongy bone can show dramatic alterations. The cortical abnormalities, which include subperiosteal, intracortical, and endosteal erosion, may require high quality radiography for their detection.

Osteoporosis of Immobilization and Disuse (Figs. 51–13 and 51–14). This type of osteoporosis occurs most characteristically in the immobilized regions of patients with fractures, motor paralysis due to central nervous system disease or trauma, and bone and joint inflammation. Experimentally it can be produced in animals by transection of tendons and nerves and by use of casts.[62–67, 234]

In humans, disuse osteoporosis is associated with a negative calcium balance, as evidenced by an increase in urinary and fecal calcium excretion, which is sustained through the period of immobilization.[68] The source of this calcium is the skeleton. As a result, osteoporosis develops in paralyzed or immobilized patients. The radiographic appearance of osteoporosis depends on many factors, including the age of the patient (osteoporosis appears sooner in younger persons) and the extent and duration of the negative calcium balance (osteoporosis is more severe when calcium loss is more prominent). After paralysis, osteopo-

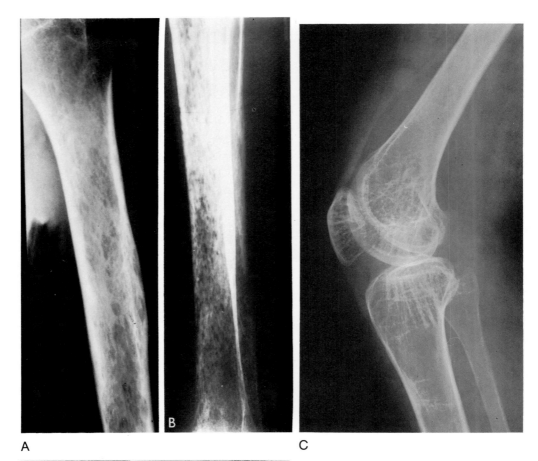

A   C

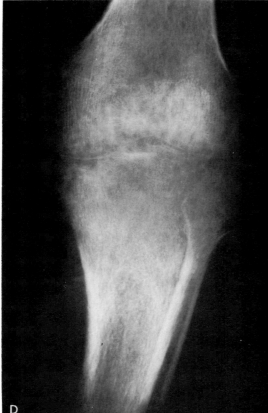

D

FIGURE 51–13. Osteoporosis of immobilization and disuse.

A–C Neurologic injuries. As a result of disuse due to neurologic abnormality, variable patterns of bone resorption can be observed, which may appear highly aggressive. In the upper humeral shaft **(A)**, scalloping of the endosteal surface of the cortex simulates the findings of plasma cell myeloma. Intracortical lucent areas also are observed. In the tibia and fibula in a different patient **(B)**, a permeative pattern of bone destruction simulates the appearance of neoplasm or infection. In a patient **(C)** who had had poliomyelitis as a child, diffuse osteoporosis with periarticular accentuation is evident.

D Amputation. After a below-the-knee amputation for osteomyelitis in this diabetic patient, patchy or spotty osteoporosis is evident, particularly in periarticular areas. The joint space is poorly evaluated because of knee flexion.

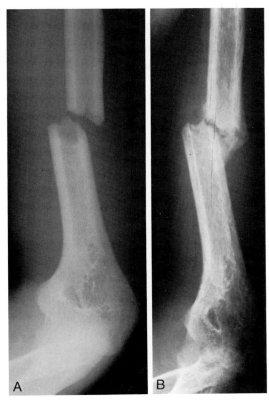

FIGURE 51–14. Osteoporosis of immobilization and disuse: Fracture. In this 28 year old woman, radiographs obtained immediately after a fracture of the humeral shaft **(A)** and two months later **(B)** are shown. Observe in **B** the extent of the osteopenia both above and below the healing fracture. Note intracortical radiolucent lines.

rosis generally appears within 2 or 3 months[69]; the findings initially appear in the appendicular skeleton, although the pelvis subsequently may become abnormal. Spinal abnormalities are not prominent. The radiographic features of osteoporosis occurring after immobilization of fractures generally are similar to those seen after paralysis.[70] The appearance of significant osteoporosis is more common after 8 weeks of immobilization, although it may occur before this, particularly in patients younger than 20 years or older than 50 years.[70] The radiographic patterns associated with osteoporosis of immobilization are uniform osteoporosis (most common type), speckled or spotty osteoporosis (characterized by small, spheroid lucent areas most frequently in periarticular regions and in the carpal and tarsal areas), bandlike osteoporosis (in the subchondral or metaphyseal regions), and cortical lamellation or scalloping (translucency of the outer or inner aspects of the cortex).[69, 70] These radiographic appearances may simulate those of malignancy.[71] Furthermore, insufficiency type of stress fractures or true fractures may occur in bones that have been rendered osteoporotic by immobilization.[468]

In association with osteoporosis of disuse, patients may reveal hypercalcemia (which usually is transient, occurring in the early weeks of immobilization) and hypercalciuria (which may lead to renal or ureteral calculi).[72, 368] Serum phosphorus levels also may be elevated during disuse.

The pathogenesis of disuse osteoporosis is debated. Microradiographic studies have emphasized the traditional view that the principal abnormality is reduction in bone formation[25]; other studies have revealed an increase in bone resorption.[1] Heaney[73] has demonstrated that both bone resorption and bone formation are increased after paralysis, but resorption more than formation. It now is clear that immobilization (or paralysis) is associated with a rapid and significant increase in bone resorption[69]; bone formation may be increased slightly[69] or decreased.[235, 236] Thus, osteoporosis of immobilization is a high-turnover osteoporosis characterized by urinary loss of calcium and phosphorus without a compensatory increase in intestinal calcium absorption. The process may be self-limited and somewhat reversible,[74, 196] although the period of recovery is several times longer than the period of bone loss, and the degree of recovery shows wide individual variation.[236] An eventual decrease in bone turnover appears to be related to the extent of paralysis rather than to the restoration of passive physical activity.[75] Weight-bearing and positive stress maneuvers do not completely suppress the excessive bone resorption, which subsides gradually and spontaneously in the extensively paralyzed patient after 1 or 2 years and sooner in the patient who recovers partially or completely.[69] Additional factors in the development of disuse osteoporosis may include vascular stasis and neurologic and humoral factors.[75, 76]

Intra-articular complications of disuse also are well known. Restricted motion is the sequela of capsular and pericapsular contractures and the concomitant encroachment on or obliteration of the joint by intra-articular fibrofatty connective tissue.[77–79] Cartilage fibrillation, erosion, denudation, and atrophy and subchondral bone abnormalities, including cysts, are additional recognized findings. Rarely, intra-articular bony ankylosis can be seen.[185] These articular alterations are discussed elsewhere in this book.

Finally, it should be recognized that although a regional distribution is the hallmark of disuse osteoporosis, generalized or scattered patterns may be observed in unusual circumstances. This phenomenon has been noted in quadriplegic persons and may be observed in astronauts as a result of weightlessness owing to lack of gravitational force.[80, 81] In the latter situation, slight bone loss in the calcaneus and phalanges of the hands may be prevented, in part, by an adequate exercise program. Experimentally, significant mineral loss in the axial skeleton of immobilized monkeys has been delineated with CT scanning, and the results have suggested that long-term effects of immobilization may be more severe in the axial skeleton than in the appendicular skeleton.[197]

Reflex Sympathetic Dystrophy (Fig. 51–15). Reflex sympathetic dystrophy (RSD) is a distinct entity that was first described in detail by Mitchell and his colleagues in 1864.[82] It is produced in a variety of clinical situations, which has led to confusion of terminology. Some of the many terms applied to RSD are causalgia,[83] acute bony atrophy,[84] Sudeck's atrophy or osteodystrophy,[85] posttraumatic osteoporosis,[86] traumatic angiospasm or vasospasm,[87, 88] algodystrophy, reflex dystrophy of the extremities,[89] minor causalgia,[90] postinfarctional sclerodactyly,[91] shoulder-hand syndrome,[92] reflex neurovascular dystrophy,[93] and the reflex sympathetic dystrophy syndrome.[95–97, 178] Currently RSD appears to be the most appropriate name for this entity.[94, 369]

Any neurally related visceral, musculoskeletal, neurologic, or vascular condition is a potential source for RSD,

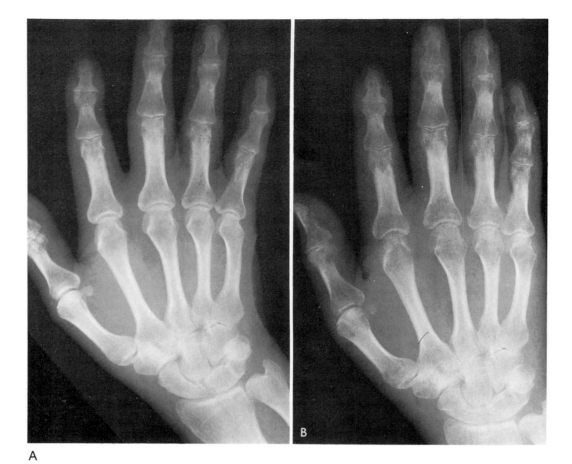

A

B

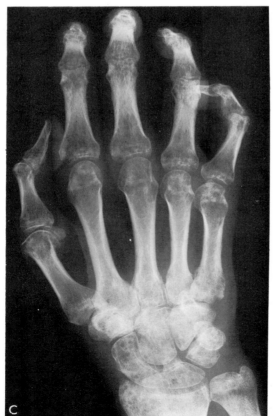

C

FIGURE 51–15. Reflex sympathetic dystrophy: Radiographic abnormalities.

A, B A 65 year old man developed pain and swelling after a minor injury to the hand. An initial film **(A)** outlines mild periarticular osteoporosis and soft tissue swelling. Six weeks later **(B)**, osteoporosis is much more exaggerated. The periarticular osteoporosis simulates the appearance of rheumatoid arthritis.

C In another patient, spotty osteoporosis with predilection for periarticular regions is evident.

Illustration continued on opposite page

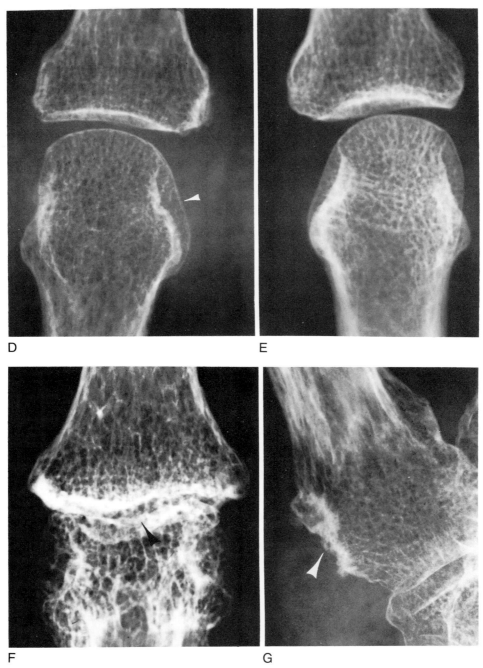

FIGURE 51–15 *Continued* **D–G** Fine-detail radiography in three different patients with RSD delineates periarticular abnormalities. In a metacarpophalangeal joint **(D)**, observe soft tissue swelling and thinning of the subchondral bone plate (arrowhead) with disruption of the osseous line. Compare with the normal side **(E)**. At a proximal interphalangeal joint **(F)**, an irregular and ragged surface of the phalangeal bone is associated with collapse and eburnation (arrowhead). At a first carpometacarpal joint **(G)**, an irregular osseous surface with bone proliferation is seen (arrowhead). (From Genant H, et al: Radiology *117*:21, 1975.)

although an incipient cause frequently is not identifiable. The most common initiating event appears to be trauma; estimates suggest that RSD may occur in as many as 5 per cent of patients with traumatic injuries.[371] RSD develops in fewer than 1 per cent to approximately 20 per cent of patients with Colles' fractures.[372] It occurs in 1 per cent to 20 per cent of patients with myocardial infarction[369, 371] and in 12 to 20 per cent of those with hemiplegia.[371] Other reported associated conditions have included cerebrovascular disorders, degenerative disease of the cervical spine, discal herniation,[237] polymyalgia rheumatica,[238] postsurgical[470] and postinfectious states, calcific tendinitis, treatment with certain drugs (antituberculous and anticonvulsant drugs and cyclosporine[373]), some forms of osteomalacia,[374] hyperparathyroidism,[376] osteoporosis,[375] osteogenesis imperfecta,[469] vasculitis, and neoplasm.[369] With regard to the last category, malignant tumors associated with RSD have arisen in the brain, lung, ovary, breast, pancreas, bladder, or other sites.[239–241, 316, 377, 378] In the presence of serious conditions, the findings of RSD can be obscured by or, at other times, may themselves obscure the underlying disorder. Incipient reflex neurovascular reactions may resolve unnoticed. RSD is less frequent in children than in adults. In the former group of patients, RSD is more common in girls than in boys, more often involves the lower extremity, has unique radionuclide features, generally follows a physical injury, and is self-limited and benign, with no clinical residua.[242, 243, 379–381, 477]

The pathogenesis of RSD is not entirely clear. The most widely held theory is that of the ''internuncial pool''[98] in which it is assumed that an injury or lesion produces painful impulses that travel via afferent pathways to the spinal cord, where a series of reflexes are initiated that spread via the interconnecting pool of neurons. These latter reflexes stimulate the lateral and anterior tracts, provoking efferent pathways that travel to the peripheral nerves, producing the local findings of the RSD. Doupe and coworkers[99] suggested that the causalgic pain in this syndrome resulted from activation of sensory fibers by sympathetic impulses. Physiologic studies using oscillography,[89, 100] plethysmography,[100, 101] skin temperature measurements,[88, 89, 100] and venous blood gas determinations[101] have demonstrated increased blood flow and increased venous oxygen saturation in the affected extremity, data that support the suggestion that RSD can be related to overactivity of the sympathetic nervous system. The importance of the sympathetic nervous system in the pathogenesis of RSD is further supported by the identification of nerve fibers in the periosteum that are sympathetic in origin and contain vasoactive intestinal peptide, a substance that dramatically stimulates bone resorption,[323] and by the significant effect on distal blood flow that accompanies sympathectomy.[382]

Clinical symptoms and signs are variable.[369, 371, 387] They may be evident in any involved site, although the characteristic distribution is the shoulder and hand. Rarely, multiple extremities are affected.[471] Both men and women are affected with shoulder and hand lesions, with approximately equal frequency, usually after 50 years of age. Initially (at any site), stiffness, pain, tenderness, and weakness may be associated with swelling, vasomotor changes, hyperesthesia, and disability. As it applies to the shoulder, the resulting clinical picture can be divided into three stages[102]: In the first stage, shoulder and hand involvement is appar-

ent, lasting 3 to 6 months; in the second stage, resolution of the swelling, vasospasm, or vasodilation is noted in association with early trophic skin changes (skin atrophy, pigmentary abnormality, hypertrichosis, hyperhidrosis, nail changes) and contracture; in the final stage, tenderness and vasomotor disturbance have disappeared, but increased prominence of trophic skin changes is evident. These three stages are not always clearly separable or, for that matter, clearly evident in all patients. The duration of the RSD varies, and, in some cases, findings may persist for years, becoming irreversible. In those cases that do resolve, recurrent clinical manifestations may occur weeks or months later.[370]

The diagnosis of this syndrome relies not only on the clinical evaluation but also on the radiographic examination.[69] Soft tissue swelling and regional osteoporosis are the most important radiographic findings. Fine-detail radiography has revealed five types of bone resorption[97]: Resorption of cancellous or trabecular bone in the metaphyseal region, which may be especially prominent in children,[251] leads to bandlike, patchy, or periarticular osteoporosis; subperiosteal bone resorption is similar to that occurring in cases of hyperparathyroidism (findings that support the concept that parathyroid hormone is fundamental in mediating the resorptive changes of this syndrome)[65]; intracortical bone resorption produces excessive striation or tunneling in cortices[179]; endosteal bone resorption, which is the region of greatest bone mineral loss in this condition, causes initial excavation and scalloping of the endosteal surface, with subsequent uniform remodeling of the endosteum and widening of the medullary canal; and subchondral and juxta-articular erosion may lead to small periarticular erosions and intra-articular gaps in the subchondral bone.[383] Because of the widespread nature and severity of bone resorption in RSD, the radiographs may reveal rapid and severe osteopenia, particularly in periarticular regions, which simulates the appearance of primary articular disorders.[198] The absence of significant intra-articular erosions and joint space loss usually allows accurate differentiation of RSD from these various arthritides. The preservation of joint space cannot be overemphasized as a characteristic finding in this syndrome, although articular space loss and focal bony ankylosis have been noted in some cases, presumably owing to immobilization.[180, 185, 189] In rare instances, RSD has been accompanied by insufficiency fractures.[388]

Bone and joint scintigraphy also demonstrates typical abnormalities in RSD, which may antedate clinical and radiographic changes.[95–97, 103, 182, 188, 252–255] Joint imaging with ^{99m}Tc-pertechnetate reveals increased radionuclide accumulation in articular regions. This finding appears to be related to increased vascularity of the synovial membrane, as a similar increase of uptake of radionuclide agents has been described in a variety of articular disorders characterized by synovial inflammation and hyperemia.[104] Bone-seeking agents, such as technetium-tagged polyphosphate and pyrophosphate, reveal a similar increased accumulation in involved bones in RSD (Fig. 51–16). This, too, appears to be related to increased blood flow as the mechanism of uptake is the result of rapid ion exchange at highly vascularized bone surfaces.[105] The uptake of the bone-seeking radiopharmaceutical agent tends to be diffuse, with accentuation of tracer accumulation in periarticular regions.[396] With three-phase bone scanning, the delayed images appear to deline-

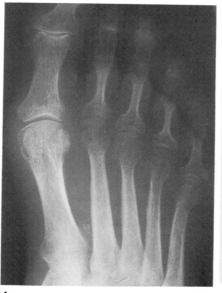

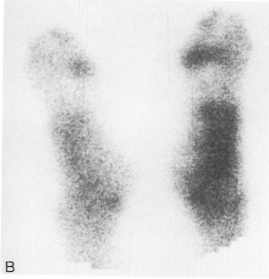

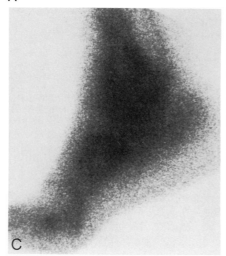

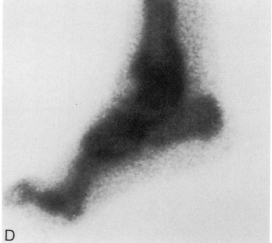

FIGURE 51–16. Reflex sympathetic dystrophy: Scintigraphic abnormalities.

A, B In this 55 year old woman who developed symptoms and signs of RSD after a burn, a radiograph **(A)** reveals diffuse and periarticular osteopenia. A delayed image during a bone scan **(B)** shows abnormal uptake of the radionuclide in the midfoot and forefoot on the left side with similar but mild changes in the opposite foot.

C, D In a 34 year old woman who also was burned (in areas other than the foot and ankle), an early (blood pool or tissue phase) image (lateral view of ankle and foot) during a bone scan **(C)** demonstrates diffuse radionuclide activity. The delayed image **(D)** documents the intense radionuclide accumulation in the bones about the ankle and in the midfoot and forefoot.

ate this pattern most frequently, although scintigraphic abnormalities also occur during the angiographic and blood-pool stages of the study.[396] Bone scans obtained at different times in a single patient may reveal migration of scintigraphic abnormality from one side of a joint to another.[397] Rarely, decreased or normal accumulation of the radionuclide on bone scans is observed, a finding that may be more frequent in children.[256, 257, 390–395] Scintigraphic assessment of patients with RSD who are being treated with corticosteroids may reveal decreasing radionuclide accumulation, which correlates with clinical improvement.[182, 252]

Quantitative bone mineral analysis has confirmed progressive bone mineral loss in involved skeletal sites due to increased porosity and thinning of cortical bone and loss of intramedullary trabecular bone.[97, 478]

Radiographic, scintigraphic, and quantitative bone mineral analyses all have revealed that RSD is a bilateral process[95–97, 244]; the abnormalities are much more marked on one side than on the other. This bilateral distribution has been recorded in 25 to 50 per cent of patients with the shoulder-hand syndrome,[93, 106, 107] although sophisticated diagnostic techniques may indicate bilateral alterations in all patients

with this syndrome.[95] Almost universally, an entire extremity distal to an affected site is altered, although the changes on the less involved extremity may appear patchy in distribution. Rarely, a segmental pattern affecting only a portion of an extremity may be encountered, a distribution that is consistent with a neurally mediated bony response.[187] This localized form of RSD (a form that also is evident in some patients with transient regional osteoporosis) may lead to involvement of one joint in an extremity, of one or several digits of the hand or foot, or of a portion of an articular surface (e.g., patella, femoral condyle)[245–247, 329, 384] (Fig. 51–17). A more generalized form of RSD also has been emphasized, although it is not well documented. Indeed, some investigators believe that RSD may lead to osteopenia and decreased bone strength in the axial skeleton.[375] Vertebral crush fractures may be preceded by the RSD syndrome.[389] Delayed posttraumatic vertebral collapse, Kümmell's phenomenon, may represent an example of this type of occurrence.

Synovial biopsies in symptomatic joints demonstrate edema, proliferation, and disarray of synovial lining cells, capillary proliferative changes, fibrosis of the subsynovium,

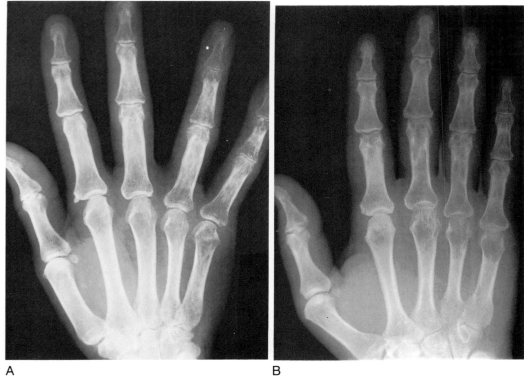

A   B

FIGURE 51–17. Reflex sympathetic dystrophy: Partial or localized form.
   A In this 71 year old woman, involvement was localized to the ulnar aspect of the hand. Note osteopenia affecting all of the bones of the fourth and fifth digits and, to a lesser extent, the third digit. (Courtesy of J. Mink, M.D., Los Angeles, California.)
   B In a different patient, osteopenia involves the bones of the third, fourth, and fifth digits. The thumb and index finger are spared.

and slight perivascular infiltration with chronic inflammatory cells (chiefly lymphocytes).[95] Cartilage abnormalities, observed predominantly in the knee, have consisted of fibrosis in the superficial areas.[248] Histologic examination of the skin and subcutaneous and muscle tissues in RSD indicates no abnormalities or nonspecific changes, whereas evaluation of the fascia of affected hands reveals similar alterations to those that occur in Dupuytren's contracture. In affected bone, increased vascularity, osteocytic degeneration, and prominent osteoclastic activity are observed[84, 85, 89, 100, 249] (Fig. 51–18).

These histologic aberrations resemble the reported findings accompanying immobilization of limbs[108] or direct irritation of the stellate ganglion[109] in animals. As pointed out by Kozin and coworkers,[95] these histologic findings combined with abnormalities detected on other studies (radiographic, scintigraphic, blood flow measurement, oxygen saturation) suggest a prominent pathogenetic role of local hyperemia in RSD, a role that explains the severe regional osteoporosis with periarticular accentuation that is observed in this condition.[250]

Transient Regional Osteoporosis. Transient regional osteoporosis[69] is a term applied to conditions that share certain features: rapidly developing osteoporosis affecting periarticular bone; self-limited and reversible nature; and the absence of clear-cut evidence of inciting events, such as trauma and immobilization. There are two important diseases (which are probably related[258]) that fall into this category: transient osteoporosis of the hip and regional migratory osteoporosis. They possess similar clinical, radiologic, and pathologic characteristics.

Difficulties arise with regard to the nomenclature used for these diseases, however. First, it is possible, if not likely, that both disorders are related in some fashion to RSD and, as such, are not distinct diseases. Second, cases seemingly falling into one category subsequently may reveal characteristics typical of the other. Third, and perhaps most importantly, the names used for these disorders imply the diagnostic requirement of radiographically evident osteoporosis. Although this requirement appears to be fulfilled in most cases of either disorder, it has become apparent in recent years, through the application of MR imaging, that patients with similar or identical clinical manifestations may show no radiographic evidence of osteoporosis. Rather, the main associated imaging abnormalities are seen with MR imaging and consist of distinctive alterations in signal intensity in the bone marrow consistent with edema. This has led to the introduction of the term transient bone marrow edema.[398] Finally, owing to an overlap in their patterns of abnormality with MR imaging, the interface between transient bone marrow edema (or transient regional osteoporosis) and osteonecrosis has become less distinct. These issues are addressed in this section and later in this chapter in the discussion dealing with MR imaging.

Transient Osteoporosis of the Hip (Figs. 51–19 and 51–20). In 1959, Curtiss and Kincaid[110] described a peculiar pattern of regional osteoporosis of the hip occurring in women in the third trimester of pregnancy. Other reports of this disease confirmed its occurrence during late pregnancy.[111–114] The patients complained of joint pain, an antalgic limp, and limited hip motion. Radiographic changes included osteoporosis of periarticular bone. Involvement

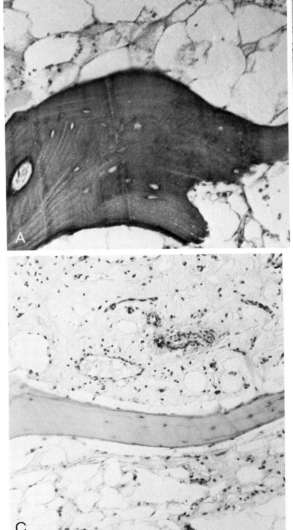

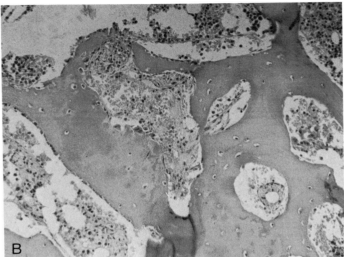

FIGURE 51–18. Reflex sympathetic dystrophy: Histologic abnormalities in bone. Observations are based on biopsies of affected tissues in several patients with this syndrome.

A Three weeks after the onset of clinical manifestations, spongy trabeculae show necrosis and vacant lacunae.

B Four weeks after the clinical onset of the disorder, bone remodeling is seen. Observe osteoblasts in epithelioid formation and numerous osteoclasts at the surface of the trabeculae.

C Four months after the onset of clinical manifestations, the bone marrow contains fibroadipose tissue, the blood vessels have a slightly thickened wall, and the trabeculum is thin.

(From Basle MF, et al: Metab Bone Dis Rel Res 4:305, 1983.)

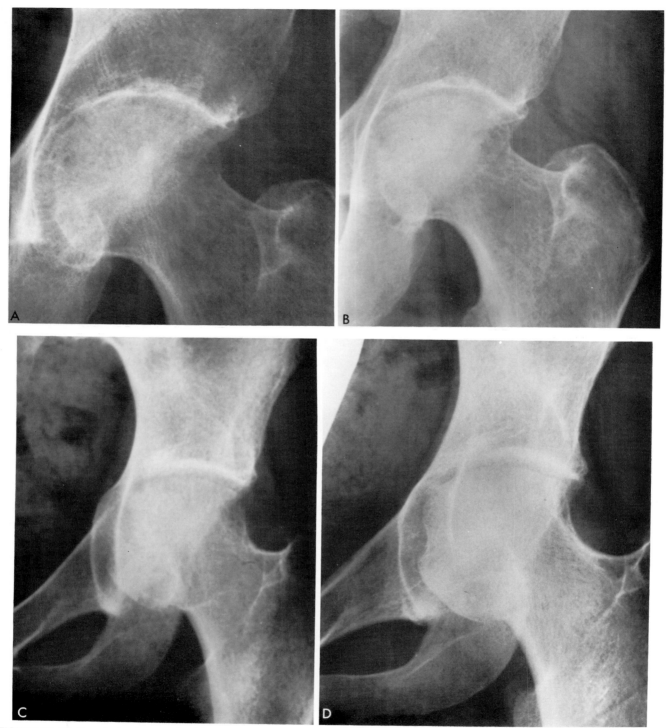

FIGURE 51–19. Transient osteoporosis of the hip.

A, B A 49 year old lawyer complained of progressive pain in his hip. Joint aspiration was unrewarding. The initial radiograph **(A)** outlines periarticular osteoporosis, particularly of the femoral head, with thinning and obscuration of the subchondral bone plate. The articular space is relatively normal, and there is no osseous collapse. Two months later **(B)**, without institution of specific therapy, the osteoporosis is less striking. The joint space still is maintained.

C, D A 23 year old woman developed rapid onset of hip pain. Laboratory values were unremarkable with the exception of mild elevation of the erythrocyte sedimentation rate. Aspiration of the hip demonstrated no growth of organisms after appropriate culture. On the initial radiograph **(C)**, there is marked osteopenia of the femoral head with loss of definition of the subchondral bone plate. The joint space is relatively preserved. Acetabular protrusion was evident bilaterally. Ten weeks later **(D)**, without specific therapy, osteoporosis largely has disappeared.

(C, D, Courtesy of R. Richley, M.D., San Diego, California.)

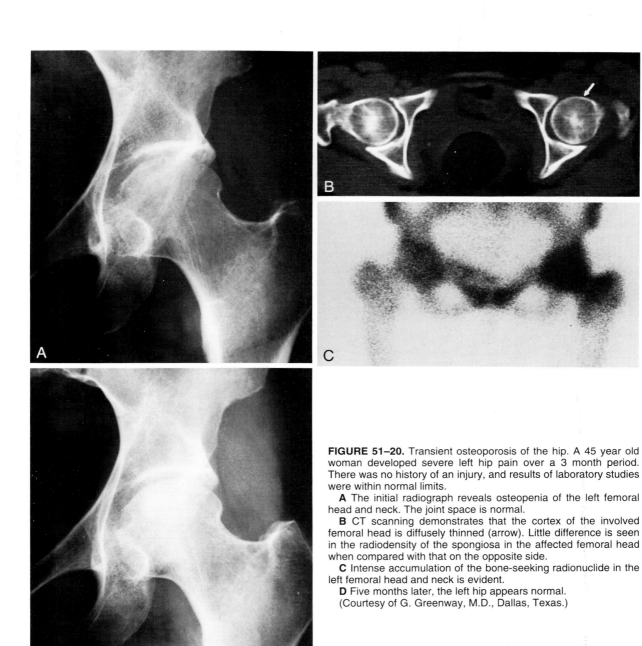

FIGURE 51–20. Transient osteoporosis of the hip. A 45 year old woman developed severe left hip pain over a 3 month period. There was no history of an injury, and results of laboratory studies were within normal limits.

A The initial radiograph reveals osteopenia of the left femoral head and neck. The joint space is normal.

B CT scanning demonstrates that the cortex of the involved femoral head is diffusely thinned (arrow). Little difference is seen in the radiodensity of the spongiosa in the affected femoral head when compared with that on the opposite side.

C Intense accumulation of the bone-seeking radionuclide in the left femoral head and neck is evident.

D Five months later, the left hip appears normal.

(Courtesy of G. Greenway, M.D., Dallas, Texas.)

was usually although not invariably unilateral in distribution. Laboratory data were normal except for mild elevation of the erythrocyte sedimentation rate in some patients. The clinical course was self-limited, full recovery being evident in 3 months to 1 year. Subsequently, it became apparent that a similar disorder could be observed in nonpregnant women and in men.[115-119, 259, 264] The clinical, laboratory, and radiologic findings were identical and, in most persons, a history of significant trauma was lacking.

It now is known that this condition typically is seen in young and middle-aged adults, particularly men. In male patients, either hip may be involved, whereas in female patients, the left hip is affected almost exclusively. Rarely, familial cases[260] and presentation in childhood[261, 401] occur. Hip pain begins spontaneously, without an antecedent history of trauma or infection. Pain may be rapid or gradual in onset and is aggravated by weight-bearing. It usually progresses within a few weeks, becoming severe enough to produce a limp. Joint motion may be slightly restricted. The clinical findings regress in 2 to 6 months without permanent sequelae; the limp disappears and joint motion is completely restored.

Joint fluid may be increased in quantity, and synovial biopsy either yields normal results or shows mild chronic inflammatory changes.[69] Bone biopsy may indicate necrosis and an increase in resorption and new bone surface.[111] Furthermore, such biopsy may reveal edema of the bone marrow.[479]

Radiographic findings are characteristic. Progressive and marked osteoporosis of the femoral head, which begins several weeks after the onset of clinical abnormalities, is associated with less extensive involvement of the femoral neck and acetabulum. The femoral subchondral bone plate is thin but otherwise intact. The joint space is not diminished in size. Incomplete or complete fractures of the femoral neck may occur[120, 400, 403] (Fig. 51–21). In children, osseous enlargement is encountered.[261] Restoration of normal radiographic density of the bone takes place rapidly. Radionuclide studies using bone-seeking agents reveal abnormal accumulation of isotope prior to radiographically demonstrable osteoporosis.[119, 190, 191] CT scanning reveals osteopenia with cortical thinning[262] but generally is not required for accurate diagnosis. MR imaging may show altered signal intensity of the bone marrow in affected sites (see discussion later in this chapter).

The cause of this condition is unknown. Initial reports of its occurrence in pregnancy suggested several possible factors that might be important in the pathogenesis of this condition: increased demand for protein and mineral in the pregnant woman; endocrine dysfunction during pregnancy; and local compression of vessels and nerves by the enlarging fetus. The discovery of this same syndrome in early pregnancy[120, 402] and in nonpregnant women and men and of involvement in pregnancy of joints other than the hip[404] made questionable most of these factors. Although the condition has been regarded as a self-limited ischemic necrosis of bone,[263] its similarity to RSD suggests a related neurogenic pathogenesis. Of particular interest was the observation that transient osteoporosis of the hip could occasionally be bilateral in distribution, with simultaneous or successive involvement of the joints (Fig. 51–22), or involve other articulations (Fig. 51–23), suggesting a relationship with regional migratory osteoporosis.[113, 121, 258, 399, 403]

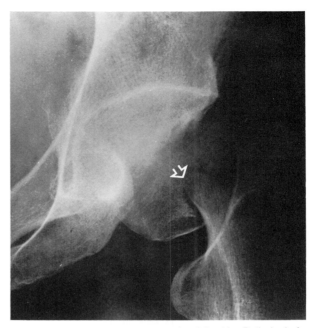

FIGURE 51–21. Transient osteoporosis of the hip: Pathologic fracture of the femoral neck. An intracapsular fracture of the femoral neck (open arrow) has occurred as a complication of transient osteoporosis of the hip in a young woman in the postpartum period. (Courtesy of A. G. Bergman, M.D., Stanford, California.)

Regional Migratory Osteoporosis (Figs. 51–24 and 51–25). The second form of transient osteoporosis is migratory in nature. Abnormalities of the hip are less frequent than abnormalities in other areas, particularly the knee, the ankle, and the foot.[122] This entity most frequently is termed regional migratory osteoporosis,[123-125, 265] although it also is referred to as transient "painful" osteoporosis of the lower extremity.[121, 126-128, 266] It occurs in men more frequently than in women and usually becomes evident in the fourth or fifth decade of life. The disorder is characterized by local pain and swelling, particularly in the lower extremity, which develop rapidly, last up to 9 months, and then diminish and disappear. Subsequent involvement occurs in other regions of the same or opposite extremity. Several recurrences can occur successively within 2 years or be separated by 2 years or a longer period of time.[69] Radiographic evidence of osteoporosis becomes apparent within weeks or months of the onset of clinical findings. It too progresses rapidly, diminishes subsequently, and appears at other sites. In extreme cases, periarticular osteoporosis extends for a considerable distance into the adjacent bone. The joint space is not narrowed, nor is there evidence of intra-articular erosion, although the subchondral bone plate may be thinned to such an extent that it is difficult to detect. Wavy periosteal bone formation may be evident along the shaft of the tubular bones.[123] Bone scanning reveals increased activity in involved areas.[129, 181, 183, 186] MR imaging shows alterations of signal intensity in the bone marrow (see discussion later in this chapter). Laboratory analysis may document an increase in the urinary excretion of calcium, hydroxyproline, and fluoride.[266] Furthermore, hypophosphatemia with elevated alkaline phosphatase activity also has been observed in some patients with this syndrome.[324]

The migratory nature of the syndrome is the major feature that differentiates this condition from transient osteo-

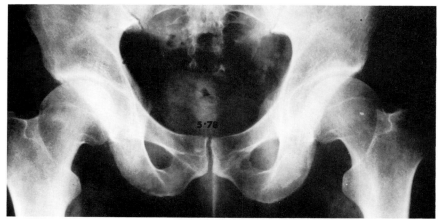

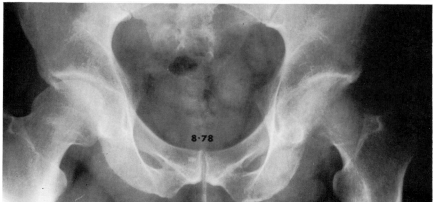

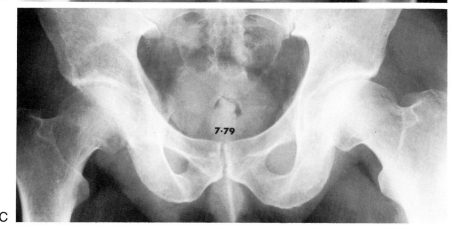

FIGURE 51–22. Transient osteoporosis of the hip: Bilateral involvement. An initial radiograph **(A)** is essentially normal. Three months later **(B)**, observe osteoporosis involving the left hip. At this time, joint aspiration was unremarkable. Eleven months later **(C)**, the left hip has returned to normal and osteoporosis has become evident in the right hip. The radiographic findings were accompanied by clinical abnormalities, including pain and restricted motion in the corresponding locations. With disappearance of the osteoporosis, the clinical manifestations disappeared. Cases such as this support a hypothesis of a common pathogenesis for regional migratory osteoporosis and transient osteoporosis of the hip.

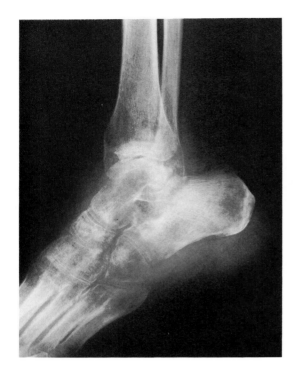

FIGURE 51–23. Transient osteoporosis of the ankle. A 39 year old woman developed the onset of pain and swelling in the right foot at the beginning of the third trimester of pregnancy. One month before a normal term delivery, her symptoms abruptly worsened. A radiograph reveals considerable osteopenia in the foot and distal portions of the tibia and fibula. During the first 4 months post partum, the clinical findings resolved. (Courtesy of L. Rogers, M.D., Chicago, Illinois.)

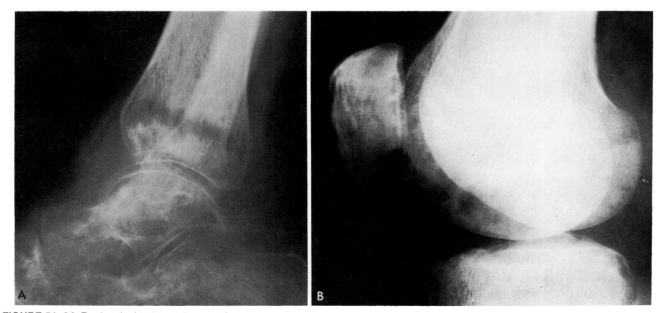

FIGURE 51–24. Regional migratory osteoporosis.
A, B Typical in this condition is transient pain and swelling of one joint associated with periarticular osteoporosis, followed by spontaneous improvement and involvement of an adjacent joint. Observe the soft tissue swelling and bandlike osteopenia of the tibia and talus **(A)** and the spotty osteoporosis of the distal portion of the femur and patella **(B)**.

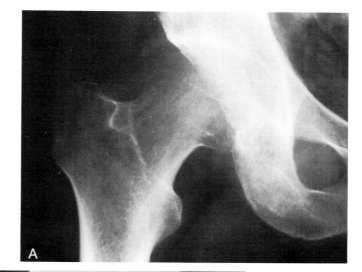

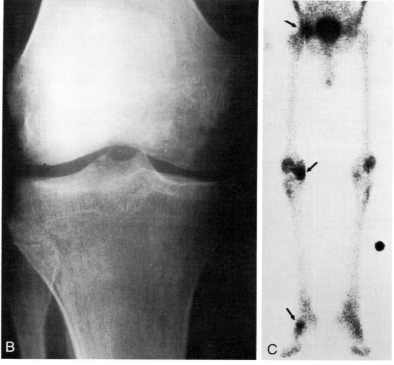

FIGURE 51–25. Regional migratory osteoporosis. This 58 year old man first developed pain in his right groin, which was exacerbated by motion or weight-bearing. He had had two previous episodes of left knee pain.

A A radiograph of the right hip reveals mild osteopenia in the femoral head. Intense accumulation of a bone-seeking radionuclide about this hip was documented (not shown).

B Two months later, the pain in the right hip had diminished only slightly, and more intense discomfort occurred in the right knee. Palpation revealed exquisite tenderness over the medial condyle of the right femur. A radiograph of this knee shows moderate osteopenia, especially in the medial femoral condyle.

C A bone scan at this time demonstrates increased uptake of the radionuclide in the femoral head, medial femoral condyle, and midfoot, all on the right side (arrows). The patient's subsequent course included increasing pain in the right ankle and midfoot with osteopenia in these regions demonstrated by radiography and, 2 months later, a decrease in clinical manifestations in the hip and knee. The findings are compatible with regional migratory osteoporosis.

porosis of the hip. Usually the joint nearest to the diseased one is the next to be involved. The clinical features may overlap so that more than one joint can be symptomatic at any given time. In fact, three or four joints can demonstrate manifestations at the same time.[122, 123] Rarely, cases demonstrating similar clinical and radiographic features remain isolated in a single articulation. In the hip, this results in the transient osteoporosis that already has been described. Osteoporosis limited to the knee also has been recorded.[130, 131, 245, 405] In this location, a similar appearance may follow meniscectomy.[178, 184]

Lequesne and coworkers[132] delineated a variant of this syndrome termed partial transient osteoporosis, in which a portion of a joint was involved. In the radial type of partial transient osteoporosis (Fig. 51–26), one or two rays of a hand or foot are affected. Changes may extend from the carpus through the metacarpus to the phalanges of the hand, or from the tarsus through the metatarsus to the phalanges of the foot. In the zonal type of partial transient osteoporosis (Fig. 51–27), involvement of the knee is characterized by abnormality of the medial or lateral condyle of the femur, and involvement of the hip is characterized by abnormality of a single quadrant of the femoral head. Migration to the entire region or to another joint in the radial form of the disease is not common; migration in the zonal form resembles that observed in the classic type of regional migratory osteoporosis. Spontaneous recovery occurs in both the radial and the zonal forms of the disease.

Although regional migratory osteoporosis traditionally has been considered to be a disease of the extremities, recent reports have emphasized the occurrence of spinal osteoporosis in this condition.[406–408] Such osteoporosis can be severe, accompanied by vertebral collapse. Hypercalciuria may be an associated laboratory finding. Verification

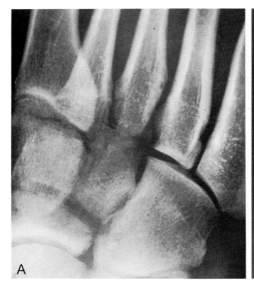
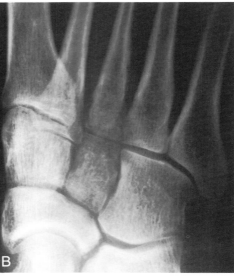

FIGURE 51–26. Partial transient osteoporosis: Radial type. Two examples are shown.

A In this 21 year old man, note osteopenia involving principally the second and third metatarsal bases, adjacent cuneiforms, and a portion of the tarsal navicular. (Courtesy of M. Dalinka, M.D., Philadelphia, Pennsylvania.)

B In a 41 year old man, a similar pattern of osteopenia affects the third metatarsal, the second metatarsal (to a lesser extent), the lateral cuneiform bone, and the distal portion of the tarsal navicular. (From Lequesne M, et al: Skel Radiol *2*:1, 1977.)

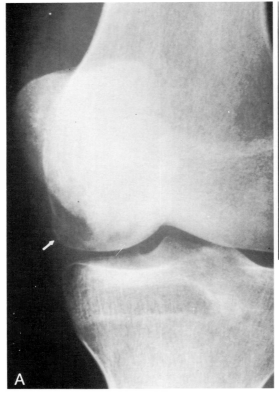
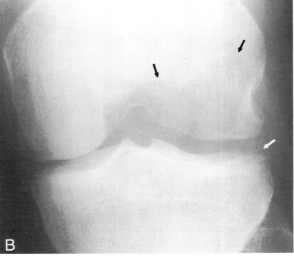

FIGURE 51–27. Partial transient osteoporosis: Zonal type. Two examples are shown.

A In this 45 year old male radiologist with a painful knee, a radiograph reveals osteopenia in the medial aspect of the medial femoral condyle (arrow). (Courtesy of A. D'Abreu, M.D., Porto Alegre, Brazil.)

B In a 40 year old man, a similar pattern of osteopenia involves the lateral femoral condyle and, to a lesser extent, the lateral tibial plateau (arrows). (From Lequesne M, et al: Skel Radiol *2*:1, 1977.)

of an association between vertebral osteoporosis and regional migratory osteoporosis, as in the case of RSD,[375, 389] awaits the results of further investigations.

Histologic evaluation of synovium in regional migratory osteoporosis delineates thickened tissue with chronic inflammatory cellular reaction.[265] The bone itself is osteoporotic, with increased numbers of osteoblasts and osteoclasts, but it otherwise is normal.[123]

The pathogenesis of this condition is not known. Electromyographic studies in some patients have revealed denervation patterns coincident with time and location of each acute attack.[125] The observed pattern has suggested a combination of a local inflammatory reaction of the nerve endings and a more central nerve entrapment, such as a radiculopathy. The findings are compatible with ischemic events in small vessels supplying proximal nerve roots.

A body of evidence exists suggesting that regional migratory osteoporosis and RSD are closely related or identical diseases: (1) trauma appears to be an important precipitating event in both disorders; (2) RSD may precede the clinical onset of regional migratory osteoporosis; (3) the pattern of osteoporosis, as seen radiographically, is similar in the two disorders; (4) as in regional migratory osteoporosis, bilateral involvement and spread from one part of a joint to another occur in RSD; (5) scintigraphic abnormalities are identical in the two disorders; (6) in both diseases, clinical improvement may occur with sympathetic blocks; and (7) blood flow to affected areas is increased in both conditions.[409] Similarly, transient osteoporosis of the hip appears to be closely related or identical to the two other diseases. Any separation of these diseases has been clouded

by reports of "transient osteoporosis of the hip" migrating to the opposite hip or other joints, "regional migratory osteoporosis" beginning in the knee or foot and never affecting additional articulations, and all three conditions occurring after trauma in complete or partial forms. Furthermore, it appears that characteristic and similar abnormalities on MR images occur in these disorders, particularly transient osteoporosis of the hip and regional migratory osteoporosis, and that a common denominator may be a painful and transient type of bone marrow edema (see discussion later in this chapter).

Differential Diagnosis. The accurate diagnosis of regional osteoporosis associated with disuse is not difficult. That associated with RSD, transient osteoporosis of the hip, and regional migratory osteoporosis may simulate other conditions. Septic arthritis can lead to regional osteoporosis (Fig. 51–28); however, joint space narrowing and osseous erosion eventually are observed in infection, whereas in regional osteoporosis, these findings are not apparent. Similarly, in rheumatoid arthritis, intense synovial inflammation can produce significant cartilaginous and osseous destruction. In addition, symmetric involvement of multiple joints is characteristic of rheumatoid arthritis. Monoarticular processes such as pigmented villonodular synovitis and idiopathic synovial osteochondromatosis may lead to clinical and radiographic findings that simulate those of regional osteoporosis (Fig. 51–29). In both pigmented villonodular synovitis and idiopathic synovial osteochondromatosis, osteoporosis generally is not striking and, when present, occurs late in the course of the articular disease. Osseous erosions may be apparent in both of these latter disorders.

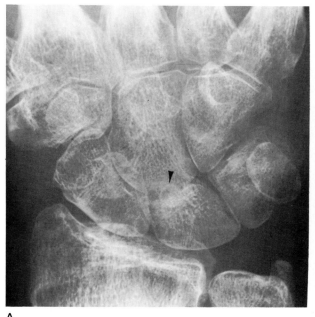
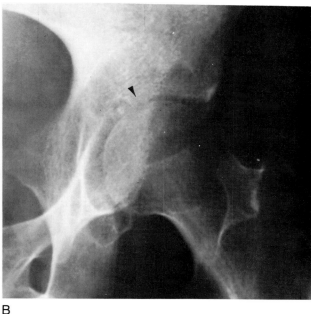

A   B

FIGURE 51–28. Osteomyelitis and septic arthritis.

A, Although the radiograph of this patient with infection of the wrist reveals osteoporosis similar to that in disuse or RSD, the presence of midcarpal joint space narrowing, particularly between lunate and capitate (arrowhead), indicates cartilaginous destruction, a finding not evident in uncomplicated osteoporosis.

B This 23 year old Mexican woman developed progressive hip pain over a 1 year period. The appearance of osteoporosis in the femoral head and the acetabulum resembles transient osteoporosis of the hip. The presence of joint space narrowing (arrowhead), however, signifies cartilaginous destruction, in this case related to tuberculosis.

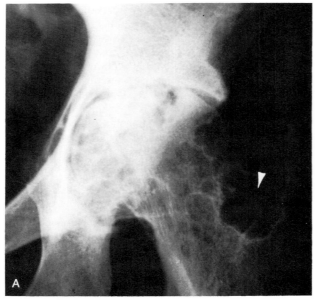

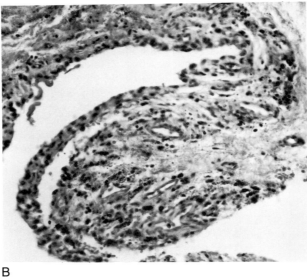

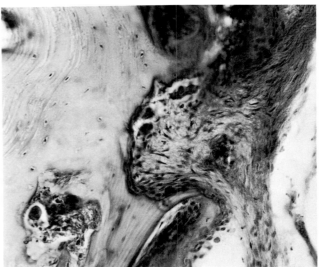

FIGURE 51–29. Pigmented villonodular synovitis. Monoarticular disease characterizes pigmented villonodular synovitis. Osteoporosis and joint space narrowing generally are not prominent in this disorder, although in this patient, the degree of articular space loss is marked.

A Typical of pigmented villonodular synovitis in the hip is the presence of cystic erosions in the acetabulum and, especially, the femoral neck (arrowhead).

B Microscopic examination shows villous proliferation of the synovial membrane (250×). Elsewhere, giant cells and hemosiderin deposition were evident.

C In another specimen, observe synovial tissue invading the femoral head.

In idiopathic synovial osteochondromatosis, intra-articular calcification may be encountered. Arthrography in either pigmented villonodular synovitis or idiopathic synovial osteochondromatosis can delineate multiple intra-articular filling defects, and MR imaging shows characteristic findings in both of these disorders.

Monoarticular involvement of the hip or other joints is not infrequent in osteonecrosis (Fig. 51–30). In osteonecrosis, the presence of osteoporosis on radiographic examination, increased radionuclide accumulation on scintigraphic examination, and the absence of articular space narrowing are findings that are identical to those in regional osteoporosis. Furthermore, there is an overlap in the MR imaging features of certain types of regional osteoporosis and of ischemic necrosis of bone. Although one condition certainly can occur without the other, a meaningful association may exist of the two (see discussion later in this chapter).

RADIOGRAPHIC-PATHOLOGIC CORRELATION

General Distribution of Abnormalities

Generalized osteoporosis is most prominent in the axial skeleton, particularly the vertebral column, the pelvis, the ribs, and the sternum (Fig. 51–31). Eventually, less extensive changes may become evident in the long and short tubular bones of the appendicular skeleton. Cranial vault alterations usually are mild, although in some disorders, such as hyperthyroidism and Cushing's disease, they can be impressive. In regional osteoporosis, alterations in the appendicular skeleton predominate over those in the axial skeleton. Depending on the exact cause of the osteoporosis, either the upper extremity or the lower extremity may be affected.

The radiologic and pathologic findings depend on the specific site of involvement.[133, 134, 410] In the pelvis and

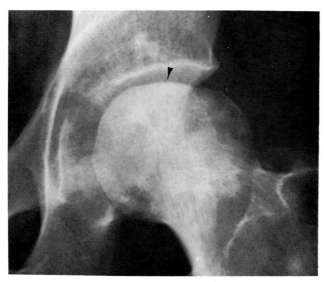

FIGURE 51–30. Osteonecrosis. The diagnosis is established by the depression of the articular surface of the femoral head (arrowhead), which is associated with patchy lucent areas and sclerosis.

thorax, osteoporosis is manifested radiographically as increased radiolucency of bone, abnormality of trabecular structure, and cortical thinning; pathologically osteoporosis leads to thin and sparse trabeculae in the spongiosa bone and porosity and diminution of the cortex. It is in the vertebral column of the axial skeleton, in the proximal portion of the femur, and in the small tubular bones of the appendicular skeleton that the most characteristic radiographic and pathologic findings become apparent.

Spine

The diagnosis of osteoporosis of the spine is made on the basis of changes in radiolucency of the bone, in trabecular pattern, and in shape of the vertebral bodies.[135, 267]

Change in Radiolucency (Fig. 51–32). Osteoporosis produces increased radiolucency of vertebral bone. It must be realized, however, that approximately 30 to 80 per cent of bone tissue must be lost before a recognizable abnormality can be detected on spinal radiographs[439, 440] and that lesions less than 2 cm may escape detection.[136] Also, variability in technical factors used to obtain the radiograph in addition to variations in the extent and content of overlying soft tissues may increase the difficulty in assessing early changes in vertebral density. Furthermore, associated vertebral compression can lead to increase in bone density owing to compaction of trabeculae and callus formation.[268] Despite these diagnostic difficulties, some investigators report success with regard to the assessment of vertebral bone density with routine radiography.[472] For example, Michel and coworkers[411] compared findings on plain films of the lumbar spine with the bone mineral content of the first lumbar vertebra assessed by quantitative CT in 80 healthy subjects with a mean age of 60 years. Using a bone mineral content of 110 mg/cm^3 as the value separating the osteoporotic and nonosteoporotic groups, these investigators found three radiographic criteria to be helpful in determining whether an individual patient's bone mineral content fell

above or below this value: the apparent density of the vertebral body compared with that of the adjacent soft tissue; the "amount of trabeculations"; and an overall estimate of vertebral osteopenia.

Although these results are encouraging, most investigators share the view that the radiographic diagnosis of mild to moderate osteoporosis remains difficult. With increasing severity of osteoporosis, however, typical radiographic changes appear, with a relative lucency of the central portion of the vertebral bodies compared with the radiodensity of the subchondral bone plates at the superior and inferior margins of the vertebrae.

Change in Trabecular Pattern (Fig. 51–32). In osteoporosis, individual trabeculae are thinned, and some are lost. The changes are more prominent in the horizontal trabeculae than in the vertical trabeculae. In fact, relative accentuation of the vertical trabeculae leads to vertical radiodense striations (bars), which simulate the appearance of a hemangioma (Fig. 51–33). The discrepancy in resorption of horizontal and vertical trabeculae may be related to biomechanical or bioelectric effects of loading in compression.[135] Furthermore, in osteoporosis, a distinct but thinned subchondral bone plate becomes evident in the superior and inferior portions of the vertebral body. These typical changes of trabecular structure in osteoporosis are different from those in osteomalacia. In osteomalacia, individual trabeculae appear indistinct or fuzzy, producing a coarsened or spongy pattern. In some instances of osteomalacia, the density of the bone actually is increased.[135] Endplate sclerosis as seen in renal osteodystrophy, which leads to the rugger-jersey spine, likewise is not a feature of osteoporosis.

Change in Shape of the Vertebral Bodies (Table 51–5). Characteristic abnormalities of vertebral shape are observed in osteoporosis, which must be distinguished from normal variations of vertebral contour as well as from artifacts produced by improper radiographic examination (Fig. 51–34). Poor technique during lateral radiography in normal persons can result in an oblique projection of the vertebral endplates, causing a false impression of discal ballooning and vertebral compression.[137] In addition, the posterior and anterior heights of an individual vertebral body are not identical. This normal difference in height should not be misinterpreted as a compressive or wedge-shaped deformity. The posterior heights of the thoracic vertebrae often measure 1 to 3 mm more than the anterior heights, a difference that is caused by a slight prominence just anterior to the superior rib facet.[137] The prominence levels off abruptly, and from this area the superior and inferior surfaces of the vertebral body usually are parallel. If the normal prominence of the posterior surface of the vertebral body is taken into account, a difference in vertical height of 4 mm or more between the anterior and posterior surfaces should be considered a true vertebral compression; if this normal prominence is not used in the measurement, a difference of 2 mm or more in vertical height is indicative of abnormality.[137] The same criteria that are used to measure thoracic vertebrae can be applied to measurement of lumbar vertebrae, although the vertical heights of the anterior borders of the third to fifth lumbar vertebral bodies normally may be slightly less than the posterior heights of these vertebral bodies.

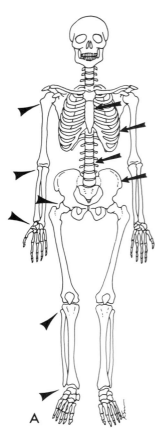

A

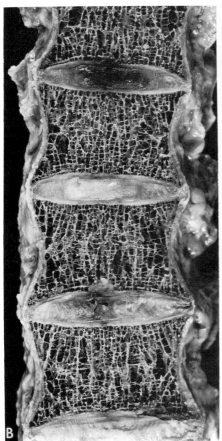

B

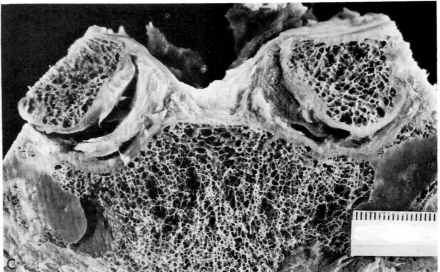

C

FIGURE 51–31. Osteoporosis: Distribution of abnormalities.

A Generalized versus regional osteoporosis. In generalized osteoporosis (arrows, on right half of diagram), the spine, the pelvis, the ribs, and the sternum are affected most commonly. In regional osteoporosis (arrowheads, on left half), the appendicular skeleton is the predominant site of alterations, particularly in periarticular regions.

B, C Generalized osteoporosis. Findings predominate in the spine **(B)**, sternum **(C)**, and pelvis. Note sparse trabeculae about the sternum and sternoclavicular joints and in the vertebral bodies (in association with a cartilaginous node on the inferior surface of one of the vertebral bodies).

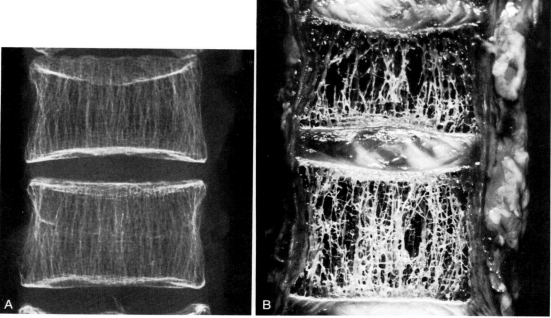

FIGURE 51–32. Osteoporosis: Spine—changes in radiolucency and trabecular pattern. In two different cadaveric spines, observe accentuation of the vertical trabeculae with preferential resorption of horizontal trabeculae. Additional findings characteristic of osteoporosis are the depression of the superior margin of the vertebral body and a distinct but thinned bone plate at the superior and inferior surfaces of the vertebral bodies.

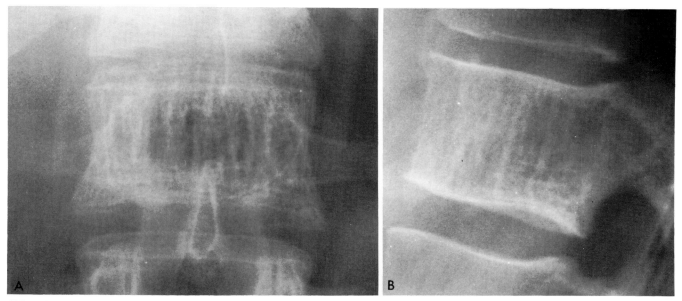

FIGURE 51–33. Hemangioma. Frontal and lateral radiographs demonstrate the typical characteristics of a hemangioma of a vertebral body: increased radiolucency and coarse vertical trabeculae producing a spongy appearance.

TABLE 51-5. Abnormalities of Vertebral Body Shape

Abnormality	Common Causes	Characteristics
Biconcave (fish) vertebrae	Osteoporosis Osteomalacia Paget's disease Hyperparathyroidism	Archlike contour defects of superior and inferior vertebral surfaces, particularly in the lower thoracic and lumbar areas
Cupid's bow vertebrae	Normal	Parasagittal concavities on the inferior surface of the lower lumbar vertebrae
Butterfly vertebrae	Congenital	Funnel-like defect through vertebra dividing it into right and left halves
Cartilaginous nodes	Scheuermann's disease Trauma Hyperparathyroidism Intervertebral osteochondrosis	Depression and discontinuity of the vertebral endplate with intraosseous lucent area and surrounding sclerosis
H vertebrae	Sickle cell anemia Gaucher's disease	Steplike central depression of the vertebral endplates

On the basis of these criteria and others, different alterations of vertebral shape have been identified: *wedge-shaped* vertebrae, with a reduced anterior border but normal posterior border; and *compression*, in which the central portion of the vertebral body alone, both the anterior and central portions of the vertebral body, or the anterior, central and posterior portions of the vertebral body are decreased. If the degree of compression is severe and uniform, a *pancake* vertebral body is present. In osteoporosis, any or all of these deformities may be evident. In the discussion that follows, four important alterations in the shape of the osteoporotic vertebral body are considered (i.e., wedge-shaped vertebral body, compressed vertebral body, fish vertebrae, and cartilaginous nodes). Owing to newer concepts of spinal stability that emphasize the existence of three vertebral columns (anterior, middle, and posterior) (see Chapter 69), compressed vertebral bodies in osteoporosis can be classified further as simple compressions and those with middle column involvement.

Wedged-shaped and Compressed Vertebrae (Fig. 51–35). Both wedging and compression in osteoporosis indicate a fracture of the vertebral body.[138] The particular pattern of altered vertebral shape is influenced by the specific spinal segment that is affected, the type and amount of stress placed on the spine, and the degree of osteoporosis. For example, wedge-shaped vertebral bodies are particularly common in the thoracic region, owing to the normal thoracic kyphosis, as the vertebra is strengthened posteriorly by the neural arch and paravertebral muscles. In some instances, however, compressed or pancake vertebral bodies also are evident in this region,[413] perhaps related, in part, to muscle atrophy that accompanies spinal osteoporosis.[412]

The different patterns of vertebral compression have led to difficulties in terminology. A compression fracture of the vertebral body typically is thought of as one in which the posterior portion of the vertebral body (the middle column of the spine) is not affected; a burst fracture of the vertebral body commonly is defined as one that affects both the anterior and the posterior portions of the vertebral body (the anterior and the middle columns). Using these definitions, both compression and burst fractures of the vertebral bodies can occur spontaneously in patients with osteoporosis. The burst fractures can be stable, without neurologic compromise (the designation of compression fractures with middle column involvement could be used in such cases), or unstable, with neurologic compromise (a more typical burst fracture).[414] Unstable burst fractures in osteoporosis generally occur in the lower thoracic spine and in the lumbar spine; stable burst fractures (compression fractures with middle column involvement) have a similar distribution; typical compression fractures (with an intact middle col-

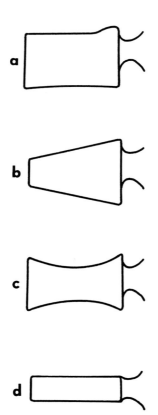

FIGURE 51–34. Osteoporosis: Spine—changes in vertebral shape. a, In the normal situation, the superior and inferior vertebral outlines are relatively parallel, although a slight elevation or protuberance can be seen at the posterosuperior aspect of the vertebral bodies. b, Wedge-shaped vertebrae relate to collapse of the anterior aspect of the vertebral body. c, Biconcave or fish vertebrae are characterized by bioconcave deformity of the superior and inferior surfaces of the vertebral body. d, Flattened or pancake vertebrae are associated with compression of the entire vertebral surface.

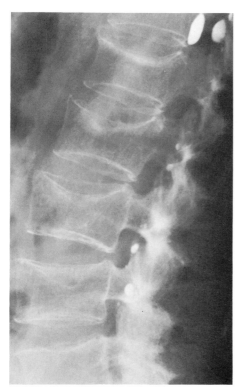

FIGURE 51–35. Osteoporosis: Vertebral compression. A lateral radiograph of the lumbar spine in this 68 year old woman shows multiple compression fractures of the vertebral bodies. Note that the osseous depressions involve mainly the central portion of the superior bone plate and are accompanied by an increase in radiodensity at the fracture site in the first and second lumbar vertebral bodies. Acutely, such radiodense areas may represent compression of trabeculae; subacutely or chronically, they may indicate new bone formation at the site of fracture. In this case, the posterior surface of the vertebral body (the middle column) is not affected. Slight loss of height of the anterior vertebral surface is seen in the first lumbar vertebral body.

umn) occur predominantly in the lumbar spine; and vertebral wedge fractures (anterior column involvement) are most common in the midthoracic region and thoracolumbar junction.[415, 416, 426] Any of these fractures are rare cephalad to the seventh thoracic vertebra, so that fractures above this spinal level, even in patients with severe osteoporosis, should raise the suspicion of another underlying disease process.[415] Furthermore, although exaggerated thoracic kyphosis may accompany multiple wedged vertebral bodies in the osteoporotic thoracic spine, such kyphosis may occur in the absence of wedge fractures, reflecting the presence of another condition, such as senile kyphosis (see Chapter 40).

The occurrence of typical compression fractures in the lumbar spine, as opposed to other regions of the spine, probably relates to several factors. Their most common sites of involvement, between the first and fourth lumbar levels, correspond in position to an area of the spine that is straight or exhibits some degree of lordosis. Axial forces placed on this vertebral region might be expected to affect predominantly the central portion of the vertebral body. Furthermore, the thicker cortex of the lumbar vertebral bodies may resist anterior wedging.[415] Compression fractures of the vertebral bodies may occur as a complication of a single traumatic event, a few separate traumatic events, or a slow structural remodeling from chronic microfractures.[415]

In the last of these complications, particularly in instances in which the compression is confined to the central portion of the vertebral body with an intact anterior margin of the vertebral body, the designation ''fish vertebrae'' commonly is employed (see following discussion).

Fish Vertebrae. Increased concavity of the vertebral bodies in osteoporosis produces typical fish vertebrae.[269] The precise origin of this term frequently is debated; some observers contend that the altered vertebral body resembles the shape of a fish, but others find a similarity of the resulting biconvexity of the adjacent intervertebral discs to the shape of a fish mouth. On radiographs of the spine of normal fish, a series of biconcave vertebral bodies is revealed, indicating a more logical explanation for the designation fish vertebrae (Fig. 51–36). What is normal in fish is considered abnormal in humans. An assessment of the degree of biconcave deformity can be obtained by expressing the shortest vertical distance between the endplates as a fraction of the height of the posterior vertebral wall.[139] This exaggerated concavity, which should not be mistaken for a normal concavity as may be seen particularly on the inferior surface of the lower lumbar vertebrae,[140] can be associated with intra-osseous discal displacements (cartilaginous or Schmorl's nodes). An understanding of the pathogenesis of fish vertebrae and cartilaginous nodes requires a thorough knowledge of the normal anatomy of the discovertebral junction.

In the normal development of the spine, the chorda dorsalis passes as a rodlike structure through the cartilaginous anlage of the vertebral body and intervertebral disc[141] (Fig. 51–37). With the onset of ossification in the vertebral body, the chorda dorsalis regresses at the level of the vertebra.[325] Eventually it disappears within the vertebral body, although a remnant may remain in the intervertebral disc. A broad cartilaginous surface covers the vertebral body during its

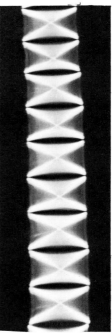

FIGURE 51–36. Fish vertebrae: Origin of the term. A radiograph of the spine of a normal fish reveals depressions in the superior and inferior surfaces of each vertebral body.

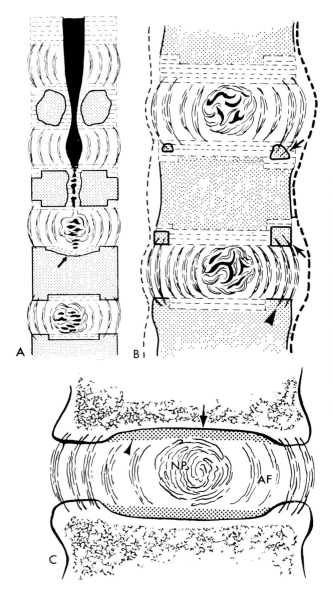

FIGURE 51–37. Normal development of the spine.

A Involution of the chorda dorsalis. The chorda dorsalis (in black) extends as a tube through the cartilaginous anlage of the vertebral body. The chorda disappears with vertebral ossification, although some cells may remain in the area of the nucleus pulposus. If the area of penetration of the cartilaginous plate (dashed area) by the chorda dorsalis is not closed completely, an indentation remains (arrow).

B Ossification centers (arrows) form within the cartilaginous plate and eventually unite with the vertebral body, appearing as an elevated bony rim along the edge of the vertebra. Finally, the cartilaginous plate covers the inner portion of the vertebral plate. Note the presence of fibers (arrowhead), which connect the anulus fibrosus and ossification centers.

C The fully developed discovertebral junction exists between the intervertebral disc (NP, central nucleus pulposus; AF, peripheral anulus fibrosus) and vertebral body. A central depression of the vertebral surface is covered with a cartilaginous endplate (arrowhead), beneath which is a subchondral bone plate (arrow).

(**A, B,** From Schmorl G, Junghanns H: The Human Spine in Health and Disease. 2nd American Ed. New York, Grune & Stratton, 1971. Courtesy of Georg Thieme Verlag.)

development. Ossification centers (vertebral body epiphyses) appear within the cartilaginous rims. They grow and ultimately fuse with the vertebral body. The fully developed discovertebral junction exists as an interface between the intervertebral disc and the vertebral body. Discal material is adherent to thin layers of hyaline cartilage, which cover the superior and inferior surfaces of the vertebral body. These layers are called cartilaginous endplates; beneath them are subchondral bone plates of variable thickness.

Gradually developing biconcave deformities of the vertebral bodies (fish vertebrae) are characteristic of disorders in which there is diffuse weakening of the bone (Fig. 51–38). One such disorder is osteoporosis, although similar abnormalities may be seen in osteomalacia, Paget's disease, hyperparathyroidism, and neoplasm. In all of these diseases, osseous deformity results from the expansile pressure of the adjacent intervertebral discs. This pressure produces arch-like indentations on the bony outline. Commonly, these indentations occur on both the superior and the inferior margins of the vertebral bodies, although the extent of involvement may not be identical on the two margins. Patho-

logic examinations of most fish vertebrae reveal thinning and stretching of the cartilaginous endplates without disruption. In patients with advanced disease, particularly when associated with trauma, focal disruption of the cartilaginous endplate may be observed, allowing displacement of discal material into the vertebral body (cartilaginous or Schmorl's nodes). In these instances, the smooth indentation of a disc on the vertebral outline may become more angular, with focal areas of radiolucency corresponding to intraosseous sites of discal tissue.

Fish vertebrae are particularly common in the lower thoracic and upper lumbar spine. At these sites, the pressure of the disc on the weakened vertebral body occurs opposite the nucleus pulposus in the approximate midportion of the vertebra. The edges of the vertebral body, the bony rim, are more resistant to such pressure. As indicated earlier, in the middle and upper thoracic spine, a normal dorsal kyphosis exists, with maximum pressure on the anterior surface of the vertebra. In this region, osseous weakening leads to anterior wedging of the vertebral body, with increasing kyphosis.

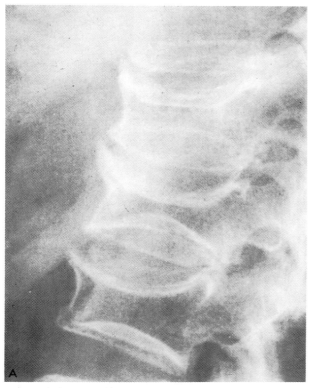
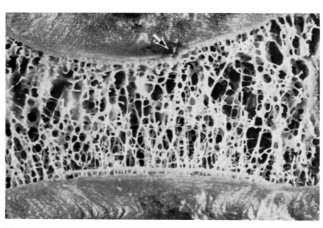
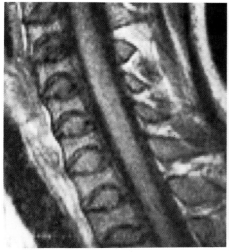
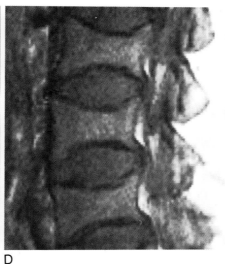

FIGURE 51–38. Osteoporosis: Fish vertebrae.

A A lateral radiograph of the lumbar spine reveals severe osteoporosis with multiple fish vertebrae. Note that the superior and inferior surfaces of the vertebral bodies are not involved to the same extent. Note also that the subchondral bone plates appear dense compared with the lucent central portion of the vertebral bodies. In this case, the anterior and posterior surfaces of multiple vertebral bodies are decreased in height.

B A photograph of a coronal section of the vertebral body outlines a fish vertebra in osteoporosis. Although the indentations appear relatively smooth, the superior and inferior surfaces of the vertebral body are not involved to the same extent. A small cartilaginous node also is apparent (arrow).

(**B** From Resnick D, Niwayama G: Radiology *126*:57, 1978.)

C, D Sagittal MR images (TR/TE, 200/26) in a 22 year old woman reveal biconcave vertebral bodies in the cervical (**C**) and lumbar (**D**) segments. Of interest, the precise cause of the vertebral abnormalities was not clear in this patient, as extensive clinical evaluation failed to reveal evidence of an underlying disorder. As a child, however, this patient had received corticosteroid medication for several months in a dosage sufficient to lead to Cushing-like features.

(**C, D**, Courtesy of G. Greenway, M.D., Dallas, Texas.)

These typical spinal deformities depend on the relative integrity of the nucleus pulposus. This integrity is required if an expansile pressure of the disc is to be of sufficient magnitude to create osseous contour defects. If the nucleus pulposus is abnormal, fish vertebrae do not develop, but diffuse flattening of the vertebral body is noted.

Fish vertebrae complicating osteoporosis must be differentiated from fish vertebrae in other metabolic disorders as well as from certain normal and abnormal changes in vertebral shape. In osteomalacia, biconcave vertebral deformities have been reported to be smoother than those in osteoporosis and to involve superior and inferior margins of the vertebral body with equal severity[135] (Fig. 51–39). In addition, wedging and compression fractures of vertebrae are unusual. In osteoporosis, the weakened and brittle bone leads to more irregular collapse, and the upper and lower margins of the vertebrae are not involved to similar degrees. In osteomalacia, adjacent vertebrae are affected to the same extent, although the lumbar spine may be involved more severely than the thoracic spine[142]; in osteoporosis, abnormalities of vertebral shape may be distributed unevenly throughout the spine, and several affected vertebrae may be separated by relatively normal vertebrae.[135] It should be emphasized that these differentiating characteristics regarding fish vertebrae in osteoporosis and osteomalacia are only guidelines, as exceptions to these rules are frequent. In many instances, differentiation of osteoporosis and osteomalacia on the basis of changes in vertebral shape is not possible. Fish vertebrae in Paget's disease, hyperparathyroidism, renal osteodystrophy, and neoplasm also resemble those in osteoporosis, although additional characteristics of the underlying disease process usually are discernible.

Cupid's-bow contour is a name applied to a normal concavity on the inferior aspect of the third, fourth, and fifth lumbar vertebral bodies, which may resemble the biconcave changes of fish vertebrae[140] (Fig. 51–40). When viewed from the front, parasagittal concavities on the undersurface of the vertebrae resemble a bow, pointing cephalad, with the spinous processes representing the arrows. On lateral views, these vertebral depressions are located posteriorly. With CT scanning, transaxial images reveal two areas of circular radiolucency, termed "owl's eyes," in the posterior regions of the vertebral body just above the discovertebral junction.[270, 271] The Cupid's-bow appearance also is well

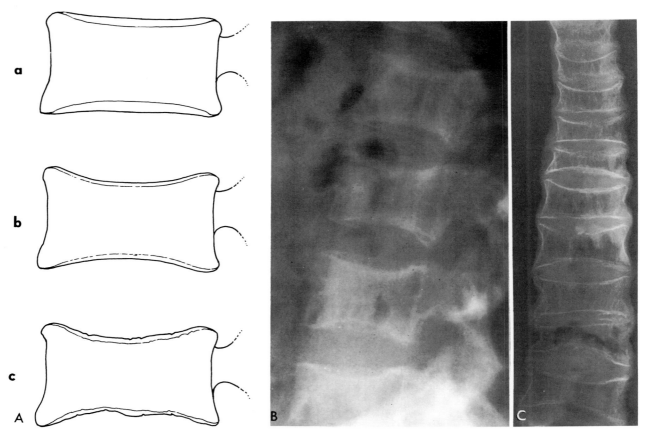

FIGURE 51–39. Fish vertebrae: Differential diagnosis of osteoporosis and osteomalacia.

A The normal vertebra (a) becomes biconcave in outline in both osteomalacia (b) and osteoporosis (c). In osteomalacia, however, the indentation of the osseous surface is smooth, and both superior and inferior borders are involved to approximately the same degree. In osteoporosis, the depression is more angular or irregular, and superior and inferior surfaces of the vertebral body are frequently involved to different degrees.

B Osteomalacia. On a lateral radiograph of the lumbar spine, observe the smooth biconcave deformities (fish vertebrae) of the vertebral bodies and the poorly defined trabeculae. Vertical trabeculae are not accentuated.

C Osteoporosis. On a radiograph of a coronal section of an involved spine, osteopenia and biconcave deformities are evident in most of the vertebrae. The subchondral bone plates are distinct and the superior and inferior surfaces of the vertebral bodies are not involved to the same extent.

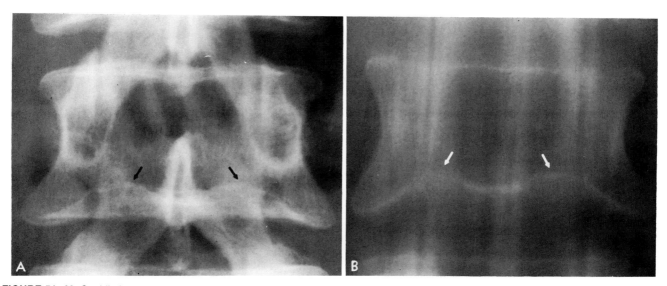

FIGURE 51–40. Cupid's-bow contour.
A frontal radiograph **(A)** and conventional tomogram **(B)** of a lower lumbar vertebral body reveal a normal variation of vertebral outline, the Cupid's-bow contour. Observe smooth parasagittal concavities on the inferior surface of the vertebral body (arrows).

shown with MR imaging. The precise cause of the Cupid's-bow contour is not known, although it may be related to nuclear expansion produced by the turgor of the nucleus pulposus.[143] This contour is more frequent in men than in women and in tall persons.[317]

Abnormalities of vertebral shape other than fish vertebrae can accompany many diseases. Incomplete embryologic regression of the chorda dorsalis alters vertebral contour and can lead to sagittal clefts in the vertebral body, producing a distinctive butterfly configuration (Fig. 51–41). The superior and inferior surfaces of the divided vertebral body are depressed and assume a funnel-shaped defect through which two adjacent discs are connected; the lateral aspects of the vertebral bodies appear broadened. Extensive osseous destruction in neoplasm and infection can lead to irregular vertebral collapse. In these instances, the pattern of bony lysis differs from that of osteoporosis, and osteosclerosis also may be evident. Furthermore, in infection, discal destruction with disc space narrowing is characteristic.

Cartilaginous (Schmorl's) Nodes. In addition to

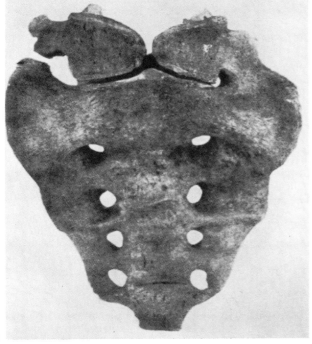

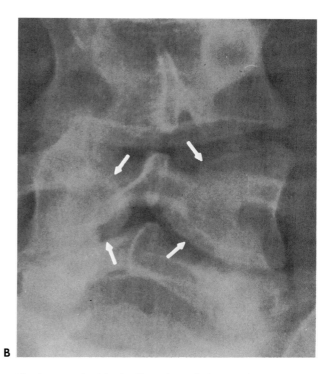

A

B

FIGURE 51–41. Butterfly vertebrae.
A This photograph reveals a sagittal cleft in a transitional type lowest lumbar vertebral body. Note the cylindrical defect dividing the vertebrae into right and left sides. (From Schmorl G, Junghanns H: The Human Spine in Health and Disease. 2nd American Ed. New York, Grune & Stratton, 1971. Courtesy of Georg Thieme Verlag.)
B Among the spinal anomalies present in this patient, observe a typical butterfly vertebra (arrows).

wedged-shaped, compressed, and fish vertebrae, another contour defect can be apparent in many metabolic disorders, including osteoporosis, which can be attributed to displacement of a portion of the intervertebral disc into the vertebral body[144] (Fig. 51–42). These discal displacements are termed cartilaginous or Schmorl's nodes. They occur when the cartilaginous plate of the vertebral body has been disrupted. Such disruption can be produced by an intrinsic abnormality of the plate itself or by alterations in the subchondral bone of the vertebral body. Potential weak areas in the cartilaginous plate include indentation sites left during the regression of the chorda dorsalis, ossification gaps, and previous vascular channels.[143, 145] The subchondral bone may be altered by numerous local and systemic processes. Whatever the cause of the damage to the cartilaginous endplate or the subchondral bone of the vertebral body, or to both structures, a weakened area is created that no longer can resist the expansive pressure of the adjacent nucleus pulposus.[146] As this pressure is greater in young persons owing to the turgor present within the nucleus pulposus, cartilaginous node formation in these persons may be rapid. In older people, this turgor decreases owing to loss of fluid in the nucleus pulposus, and displacement occurs more gradually.

This pathogenetic scheme explains the appearance of cartilaginous nodes in such diverse osseous processes as osteoporosis, osteomalacia, Paget's disease, hyperparathyroidism, infection, and neoplasm, and such cartilaginous processes as degenerative disc disease (intervertebral [osteo]chondrosis), infection, and juvenile kyphosis (Scheuermann's disease). It also explains the common occurrence of cartilaginous nodes that has been noted in previous reports: Schmorl observed that cartilaginous nodes occurred in 38 per cent of all the vertebral columns that he examined[141]; Batts[147] found cartilaginous nodes that were visible to the naked eye in 20 per cent of his gross specimens; Coventry and coworkers,[146] in an investigation of specimens of the lumbosacral region, found that 2 per cent had cartilaginous nodes visible on specimen radiographs, 5 per cent had cartilaginous nodes found on gross examination of the microscopic slides, and a majority demonstrated microscopic cartilaginous nodes; and Hilton and associates,[148] studying slab radiographs of the spine below the ninth thoracic vertebral body, noted that 76 per cent of 50 patients had cartilaginous nodes. This variability in the reported frequency of cartilaginous nodes obviously is related to the method used for investigation, the age of the patient population, and the presence or absence of underlying disease processes. The ability to detect cartilaginous nodes on patient radiographs depends on several factors, including the size of the patient, the quality of the radiographs, the location and the size of the cartilaginous nodes, and the degree of surrounding bone sclerosis.

Metabolic disorders produce cartilaginous nodes by diffusely weakening the osseous structure of the vertebral body. With subchondral bone destruction, a portion of the cartilaginous endplate becomes depressed into the subjacent bone. Cartilaginous nodes certainly are encountered in osteoporosis,[144, 149, 272] although some investigators have discounted any causal relationship.[150] In the authors' experience, cartilaginous nodes in osteoporosis generally are small and usually are associated with biconcave deformities

of the involved vertebral bodies. They are more common in the lower cartilaginous plate than in the upper one.

The radiographic evidence of cartilaginous node formation is based on the presence of a break in the subchondral bone plate (corresponding to the site of discal displacement), a lucent area of varying size bordering on the intervertebral disc (corresponding to the site and variable amount of protruded disc material), and a small degree of surrounding bone sclerosis (corresponding to trabecular condensation and thickening).

Proximal Portion of the Femur

In 1970, Singh and coworkers[151] emphasized the usefulness of analysis of the trabecular pattern of the upper end of the femur as an index of osteoporosis (Fig. 51–43). In this region, five anatomic groups of trabeculae can be identified:

1. *Principal compressive group.* This group comprises the uppermost compression trabeculae, which extend from the medial cortex of the femoral neck to the upper portion of the femoral head in slightly curved radial lines. It contains the thickest and most densely packed trabeculae in the region.

2. *Secondary compressive group.* Those trabeculae that arise from the medial cortex of the shaft below the principal compressive group form this group. They curve upward and slightly laterally toward the greater trochanter and the upper portion of the femoral neck. These trabeculae are thin and widely spaced.

3. *Greater trochanter group.* This group is composed of slender and poorly defined tensile trabeculae, which arise laterally below the greater trochanter and extend upward to terminate near its superior surface.

4. *Principal tensile group.* The trabeculae that arise from the lateral cortex below the greater trochanter and extend in a curvilinear fashion superiorly and medially across the femoral neck, ending in the inferior portion of the femoral head, form the thickest tensile trabeculae.

5. *Secondary tensile group.* These trabeculae arise from the lateral cortex below the principal tensile group. They extend superiorly and medially to terminate after crossing the middle of the femoral neck.

In the femoral neck, a triangular area, Ward's triangle, contains thin and loosely arranged trabeculae. This area is enclosed by trabeculae from the principal compressive, secondary compressive, and tensile groups.[326]

Singh and coworkers[151] correlated patterns of trabecular loss with increasing severity of osteoporosis (Fig. 51–44). With early trabecular resorption, they noted accentuation of the structure of the principal compressive and principal tensile trabecular groups. The secondary compressive trabeculae were no longer demarcated clearly, and Ward's triangle became more prominent. The prominence of the principal trabeculae was related to resorption of the thin trabeculae, which were obscuring their detail.[152]

With an increased degree of trabecular resorption, tensile trabeculae were reduced in number. Principal tensile trabeculae could be traced from the lateral cortex for a variable distance, although their medial limit was obscured. The

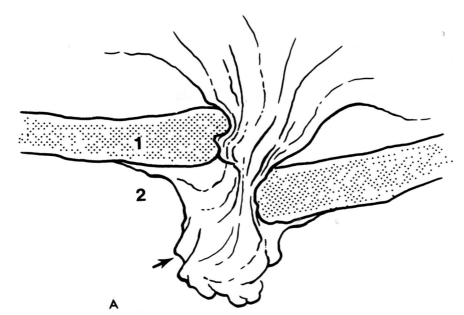

FIGURE 51–42. Osteoporosis: Cartilaginous (Schmorl's) nodes.

A Cartilaginous (Schmorl's) nodes occur when a portion of the intervertebal disc protrudes into the vertebral body (arrow) through a gap in the cartilaginous endplate (1) and subchondral bone plate (2).

B, C A photograph and radiograph of a coronal section reveal depression of the subchondral bone (arrowheads). A cartilaginous node (arrows) has resulted from disruption of the cartilaginous and bony plates. It has created a radiolucent defect within the bone with a small rim of sclerosis. A small cartilaginous node is noted on the opposite side of the vertebral body.

(**B, C**, From Resnick D, Niwayama G: Radiology *126*:57, 1978.)

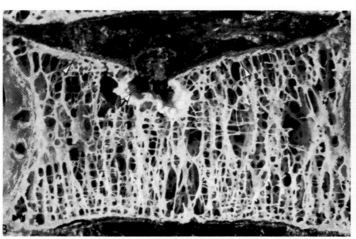

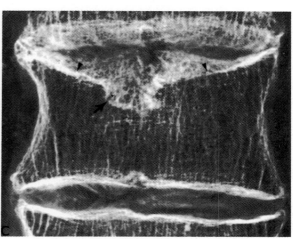

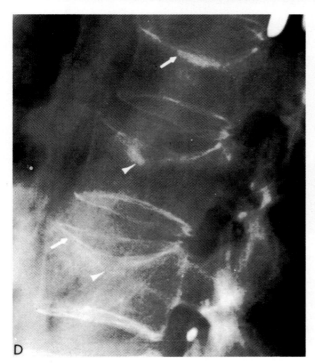

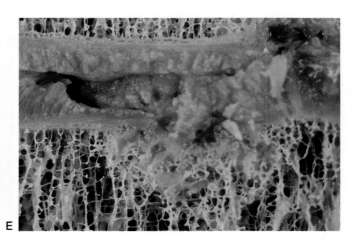

D On a lateral radiograph of the lumbar spine in a patient with osteoporosis, biconcave (fish) vertebrae, compression fractures (arrows), and cartilaginous (Schmorl's) nodes (arrowheads) are evident. A previous myelogram had been accomplished.

E In this coronal section of an osteoporotic lumbar spine, note the prominent cartilaginous node on the superior surface of the involved vertebral body with surrounding sclerosis.

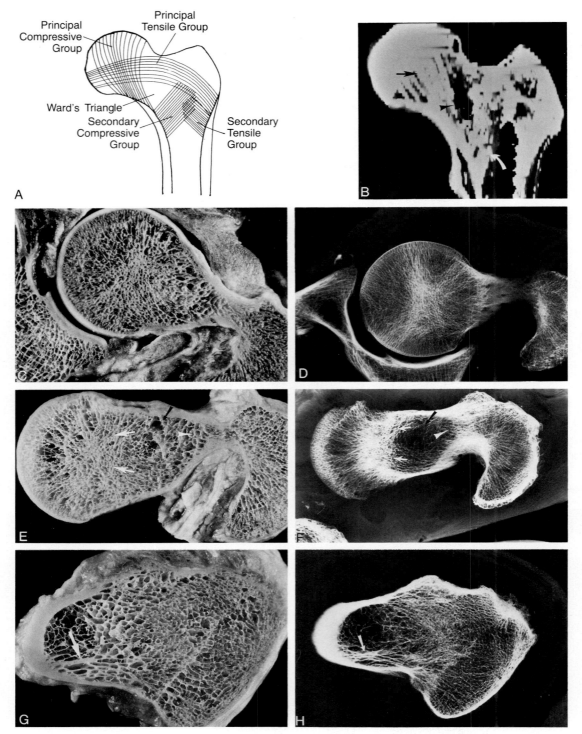

FIGURE 51–43. Proximal portion of the femur: Normal trabecular pattern.

A Four of the five anatomic groups of trabeculae are indicated in this schematic diagram. Ward's triangle lies within the neutral axis wherein compressive and tensile forces balance one another and contains thin, widely spaced trabeculae.

B A midcoronal three-dimensional CT section of a normal macerated specimen demonstrates primary compressive trabeculae (arrow), secondary compressive trabeculae (curved arrow), and Ward's triangle (arrowhead).

C, D A specimen photograph and radiograph of a transaxial section through the femoral head reveal thick, closely packed primary compressive trabeculae radiating from the center in the pattern of an asterisk or stylized star.

E, F A specimen photograph and radiograph of a transaxial section through the femoral neck reveal Ward's triangle (black arrows) as an area of relative paucity of trabeculae, bordered medially by primary compressive trabeculae (white arrows) and laterally by primary tensile and secondary compressive trabeculae (arrowheads).

G, H A specimen photograph and radiograph of a transaxial section through the intertrochanteric region demonstrate the superior portion of the calcar femorale (arrows) arising from the posteromedial cortex.

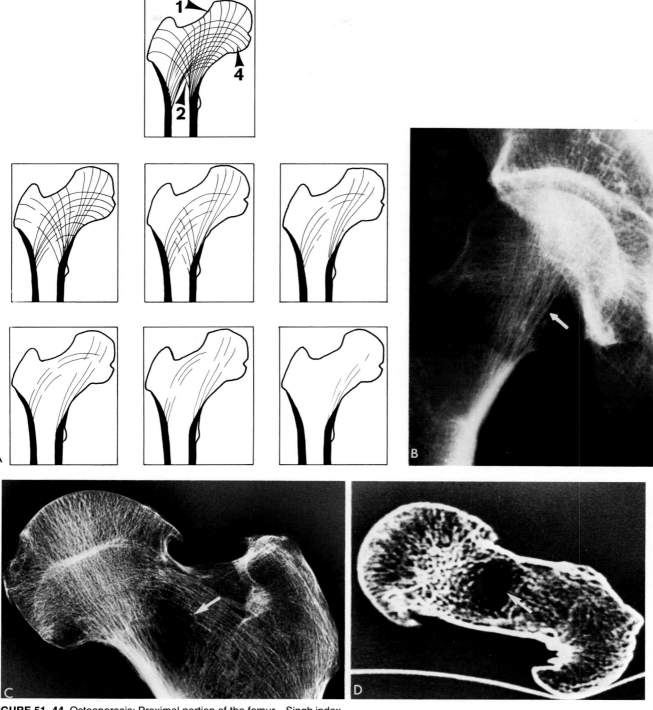

FIGURE 51–44. Osteoporosis: Proximal portion of the femur—Singh index.

A, B In the proximal portion of the femur are five groups of osseous trabeculae. In the normal situation, frequently it is difficult to identify all of these groups, but with increasing osteoporosis, they initially may be identifiable and subsequently may be resorbed. In the top drawing, three groups can be well seen: the principal compressive group (1); the secondary compressive group (2); and the principal tensile group (4). In the subsequent drawings, increasing degrees of osteoporosis lead to trabecular resorption. The principal compressive group is the last to be obliterated (arrow, **B**).

C, D A frontal radiograph and a transaxial CT section of a macerated specimen with bone resorption demonstrate increased trabecular spacing and enlargement of Ward's triangle (arrows).

secondary tensile group was completely resorbed so that Ward's triangle opened up laterally.

With further increase in trabecular resorption, the outer portion of the principal tensile trabeculae opposite the greater trochanter disappeared. These investigators concluded that persons demonstrating this trabecular pattern indeed were osteoporotic.

As osteoporosis increased in severity, resorption of all trabecular groups occurred, with the exception of bony trabeculae in the principal compressive group. With severe osteoporosis, even these latter trabeculae were partially or completely obliterated.

On the basis of these observations and additional ones that correlated the degree of trabecular resorption with the risk of femoral neck fracture and the presence of histologic evidence of osteoporosis, the authors concluded that classification of trabeculae in the femoral neck was a useful technique in evaluating osteoporotic patients.

Subsequent to this initial report, other investigations of the femoral trabecular index have been recorded.[153-155, 273-277, 318, 417, 418, 473, 480] In some, good correlation was detected between this index and the amount of trabecular bone in the proximal portion of the femur and vertebrae as well as the frequency of compressive fractures of the spine[153, 275] and the risk of fracture of the femoral neck,[274] although fractures could develop without any change in the index.[135, 154, 155, 276, 278] The index correlated poorly with the cortical thickness in the lower portion of the femoral neck,[417] as well as with the mineral content of the radius determined by photon absorptiometry.[156, 157] These results probably reflect the inadequacy of cortical bone in the extremities as a guide to trabecular bone in the spine,[158] although the radial cortical bone may correlate well with the bone mineral content of the femoral neck,[158] which itself may correlate well with the mechanical strength of the femoral neck.[159] A further deficiency of the Singh index is unacceptably high interobserver variation in its application.[418]

Attempts to use trabecular patterns at other sites, such as the calcaneus,[286, 287] as an indicator of the presence and severity of osteoporosis have met with mixed success.

Currently, owing to the availability of a number of quantitative techniques, including dual energy photon absorptiometry,[419, 420] CT,[340] dual energy radiographic absorptiometry,[349] and others,[421] which can be applied to the analysis of the bone mineral content in the proximal femur and other appendicular skeletal sites, the role of the Singh index and other radiographic indices in such analysis appears to be limited.

From a diagnostic standpoint, crossing trabeculae in the proximal portion of the femur detected with routine radiography and CT in normal persons and those with osteoporosis (or osteoarthritis) may lead to radiodense regions that simulate the findings of an enchondroma or bone infarct.[422]

Cortex of the Tubular Bones

In recent years, close evaluation of cortical bone loss in metabolic bone disease has been accomplished.[160-167, 279, 280, 423, 424] Although this evaluation can be applied to various sites in the skeleton, it is the tubular bones of the hand that usually are investigated. Newer methods of radiographic analysis have been used in this investigation. These methods require high quality radiographs and application of op-

tical and radiographic magnification. Interpretation of the films is based on the envelope theory of bone resorption.[168, 280]

There are three specific sites at which osseous resorption of bone cortices may become apparent (Table 51-6) (Fig. 51-45). A cellular, vascularized membrane covering the endosteal surface of the cortex may be designated the endosteal envelope; an intracortical (haversian) envelope constitutes the surfaces within the cortical bone (haversian and Volkmann's canals); and a periosteal envelope covers the surface of the cortex. The response to stimuli induced by various endocrine and metabolic disorders is not always identical in these three bone envelopes.[160, 165] It is for this reason that careful investigation of cortical bone in the hand may provide important differential diagnostic clues even though the bone, because of the great mass of compact trabeculae, may appear normal on casual inspection. The cortices can be evaluated using optical or radiographic magnification techniques in combination with fine-grain films (microradioscopy). In this manner, early resorptive changes can be visualized and cortical dimensions can be calculated (radiographic morphometry).

Endosteal resorption produces scalloped concavities on the inner margin of the cortex, enlarging the marrow cavity. Interpretation of subtle changes at the endosteal envelope is difficult because normal remodeling changes, which include both bone resorption and bone formation, occur in the endosteal zone. Progressive irregularities of the endosteal surface are indicative of a pathologic process.

Intracortical resorption is characterized by the appearance of prominent longitudinal striations within the cortex. Changes may appear throughout the cortex, although they usually predominate in the subendosteal zone. Histologically, resorption is characterized by the appearance of a small osteoclastic focus within the compact bone. With further osteoclastic proliferation, a resorptive tunnel is created, which is associated with mesenchymal cell proliferation, leading to an increased amount of connective tissue and blood vessels.[165, 169] This resorptive phase may be followed by a reparative phase, which begins with osteoblastic accumulation, osteoid production, and osteoid calcification. In normal persons, bone resorption and bone formation proceed in an equal fashion; in patients with certain metabolic disorders, high bone turnover is associated with osteoclastic activity that predominates over osteoblastic activity, leading to an increase in the number of resorptive tunnels

TABLE 51-6. Patterns of Osseous Resorption in Tubular Bones

Site	Pattern
Cortex:	
Endosteal	Diffuse cortical thinning or scalloped erosions
Intracortical	Cortical radiolucent areas or striations
Periosteal	Subperiosteal erosions
Spongiosa:	
Subchondral	Linear, bandlike, or spotty radiolucent areas
Metaphyseal	Bandlike radiolucent areas
Diffuse	Homogeneous or spotty radiolucent areas

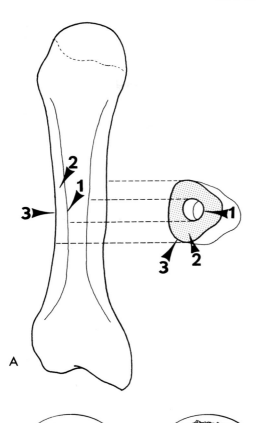

A

FIGURE 51–45. Cortex of tubular bones: Sites of osseous resorption.

  A Three envelopes exist at which cortical resorption may occur. These are the endosteal envelope (1), intracortical (haversian) envelope (2), and periosteal envelope (3).

  B Diagram indicates the normal situation (top left), endosteal resorption (top right), intracortical resorption (bottom left), and subperiosteal resorption (bottom right).

  C Magnification radiograph of a phalanx in a patient with RSD reveals endosteal (arrowhead) and intracortical (arrow) resorption.

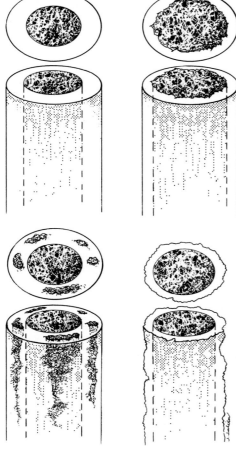

B

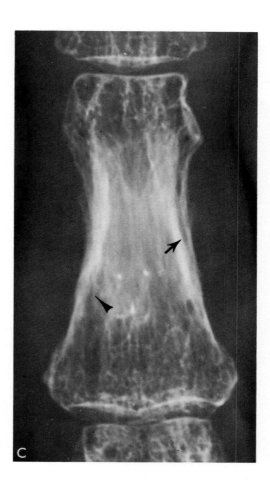

C

in cortical bone.[170, 179] These tunnels measure approximately 200 to 300 μm in diameter and therefore are not clearly visible during routine radiography, although they may become evident with magnification techniques. Their appearance and number can be graded using the second metacarpal shaft as a reference point.[165, 281] The detection of several radiolucent striae deep within a localized portion of the cortex can be a normal finding. An increased number of striae with wider distribution is indicative of an abnormal situation. In some instances, abnormal linear resorption may localize to the outer cortical area, simulating subperiosteal bone resorption or even periosteal bone formation—pseudoperiostitis.[171] Abnormal linear radiolucent areas within the cortex can be detected in such disorders as hyperparathyroidism, hyperthyroidism, acromegaly, osteomalacia, renal osteodystrophy, disuse osteoporosis, and RSD. Cortical lucent lesions generally are not apparent in low bone turnover states, such as senile or postmenopausal osteoporosis and Cushing's disease.

Subperiosteal resorption produces irregularity and poor definition of the outer surface of the cortex. It becomes prominent in diseases of rapid bone turnover, particularly hyperparathyroidism. Moderate to severe subperiosteal resorption is virtually specific for this condition, although mild subperiosteal changes may be apparent in other diseases, such as RSD. As indicated previously, peripheral intracortical resorption (or juxtaperiosteal resorption) in hyperthyroidism, acromegaly, and additional conditions leads to linear radiolucency of the superficial aspect of the cortex, which resembles the findings of subperiosteal resorption.

Cortical resorption, which can be detected using magnification radiography, can be quantitated with radiographic morphometry. This procedure consists of measuring cortical dimensions on a routine radiographic film with a suitable caliper. Although it is applicable to various sites,[199] including the humerus,[282] clavicle,[283] radius, femur, and mandible,[284, 285] radiographic morphometry usually is accomplished in the hands using the shaft of a metacarpal bone, particularly the second[162, 165, 172, 173, 281] (Fig. 51–46). The basic measurements that are obtained are the outer diameter of the bone, the width of the medullary canal, and the width of the cortex. The most widely used measurement is the combined cortical thickness (CCT). To obtain this measurement, the midportion of the second metacarpal shaft is determined by dividing in half the length between the most distal part of the base of the bone and the most distal part of its head. Next, the outer diameter *(W)* and marrow cavity *(m)* widths are determined. The CCT represents the difference between these two measurements *(CCT = W − m)*. The measured CCT value then must be compared to normal values, which can be found in certain references.[165, 174, 175] If the measured CCT value is below the

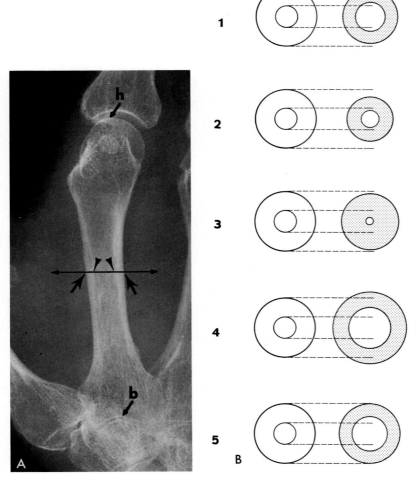

FIGURE 51–46. Cortex of tubular bones: Radiographic morphometry.

A Normal measurements. The length of the metacarpal is measured from the most distal point of its base (b) to the most distal point of its head (h). The midpoint is found and a line can be drawn across the shaft. Measurements then are made of the outer diameter or width (*W*—between arrows), the marrow cavity width (*m*—between arrowheads), and the combined cortical thickness *(CCT = W − m)*.

B Five abnormal situations are depicted. In each state, an initial normal representation of the tubular bone is indicated on the left side and the abnormal representation is indicated on the right side. 1, Decreased bone formation and increased bone loss (decrease in *W*; increase in *m*; decrease in *CCT*). 2, Decreased bone formation and slight decreased bone loss (decrease in *W*; decrease in *m*; decrease in *CCT*). 3, Decreased bone formation and marked decreased bone loss (decrease in *W*; marked decrease in *m*; increase in *CCT*). 4, Increased bone formation and increased bone loss (increase in *W*; marked increase in *m*; decrease in *CCT*). 5, Normal bone formation and increased bone loss (no change in *W*; increase in *m*; decrease in *CCT*).

(From Garn SM, et al: Radiology *100*:509, 1971.)

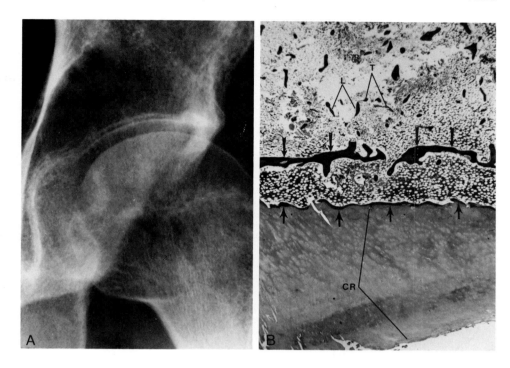

FIGURE 51-47. Subchondral bone plate of flat bone: Sites of osseous resorption.

A In a patient who had been paraplegic for 9 months, a curvilinear radiolucent area is identified in the subchondral bone plate of the acetabulum.

B Histologic study of this area in a cadaver of a patient with similar paraplegia reveals acetabular cartilage *(CR)*, two parallel layers of compact bone (arrows) with intervening bone marrow (reflecting the cause of the radiolucent area in **A**), and remnants of transverse *(T)* and longitudinal *(L)* trabeculae.

(Reproduced with permission from Yagan R, et al: Radiology *165*:171, 1987.)

normal range for the 20 to 50 year old age groups, endosteal bone loss has been confirmed; in this age group, the cause of the bone loss may include metabolic abnormalities and immobilization.[165] After the age of 50 years, a low CCT value usually is indicative of postmenopausal or senile osteoporosis. In equivocal cases, an additional measurement, the percentage of cortical area *(CA)*, can be calculated. This measurement can be obtained using the following formula:
% $CA = (W^2 - m^2/w^2) \times 100$.

Although measurement of the CCT usually is applied to the appraisal of endosteal resorption, it, along with other measurements (total width, medullary canal width, CA), may allow distinction among a variety of metabolic diseases.[160] With these measurements, it is possible to divide disorders into those characterized by decreased bone formation and increased bone loss (e.g., Turner's syndrome), decreased bone formation and decreased bone loss (e.g., osteogenesis imperfecta), increased bone formation and increased bone loss (e.g., cerebral gigantism), and normal bone formation and increased bone loss (e.g., gastrectomy).[160]

From this description, it is evident that the envelope theory of bone resorption emphasizes three potential sites of cortical lysis: endosteal, intracortical, and subperiosteal. Endosteal erosion is the least specific; it occurs in any metabolic disease, including osteoporosis, and may accompany certain neoplasms, such as plasma cell myeloma. Intracortical erosion is more specific; excessive tunneling is seen in disease states characterized by rapid bone turnover, including disuse osteoporosis and RSD. Subperiosteal resorption is the most specific; when extensive, it is pathognomonic of hyperparathyroidism, although lesser degrees of subperiosteal resorption may be seen with other causes of rapid bone turnover, such as RSD. Although all types of cortical resorption generally are observed in the tubular bones, similar patterns may be apparent as well in the flat and irregular bones, in both the axial and the appendicular

skeleton. As an example, the subchondral bone plate of the acetabulum, a region of compact bone, may reveal an internal radiolucent area, designated the "double cortical line," in patients with osteoporosis[425] (Fig. 51–47).

Spongiosa in the Appendicular Skeleton

The spongy bone undergoes early and significant changes in osteoporosis and related metabolic conditions (Table 51–6). Several radiographic patterns can be distinguished in the tubular bones and the carpal and tarsal areas: diffuse or homogeneous osteoporosis; speckled or spotty osteoporosis, which is particularly prominent in periarticular areas; and linear and bandlike osteoporosis in subchondral and metaphyseal areas (Figs. 51–48 and 51–49). Although all of these different patterns may be detectable in a single patient with osteoporosis, one or two may predominate. In postmenopausal or senile osteoporosis, diffuse osteoporosis is most characteristic; in RSD and immobilization states, speckled, linear, or bandlike patterns may become prominent. In children, extensive metaphyseal osteopenia can simulate the appearance of an infection.

The periarticular distribution of bone resorption, which is evident in the speckled or bandlike pattern, is not surprising. Cancellous bone in this area is highly vascularized and thereby susceptible to such resorption.[176, 250] In subchondral locations, linear radiolucent bands produce thinning of the overlying bone plate, linear or curvilinear radiolucent regions within the bone plate (the "double cortical line," as described previously) (see Fig. 51–47), and small areas of osseous disruption. These last-mentioned bony defects can occur centrally or at the margins of the joint. Marginally, they can simulate the erosions of rheumatoid arthritis and related diseases, whereas centrally, they may resemble the subchondral fractures of osteonecrosis. The absence of large gaps in the subchondral bone plate and of joint space narrowing allows differentiation from rheumatoid arthritis;

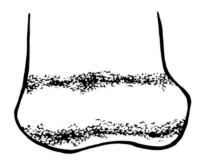
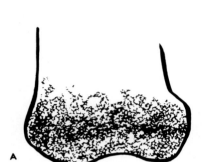

FIGURE 51–48. Spongiosa of tubular bones: Sites of osseous resorption.

A Patterns of bone loss include bandlike radiolucent areas in the metaphysis or subchondral bone (top drawing) and homogeneous periarticular radiolucent areas (bottom drawing).

B Bandlike resorption: Metaphyseal and subchondral linear radiolucent areas are evident.

C Spotty resorption: A cystic pattern is apparent.

D, E Subchondral erosions: Severe resorption in periarticular regions can lead to small gaps in cartilage and bone simulating erosions of inflammatory arthritis. On the radiograph **(D)** defects in the subchondral bone plate of multiple metacarpal heads (arrows) are apparent in this patient with RSD. On a coronal section of the metacarpal heads **(E)**, thinning or disruption of the cartilage and bone plate is evident (arrows).

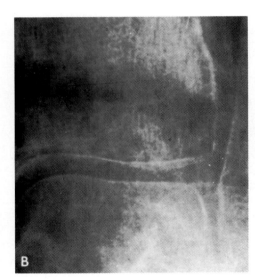
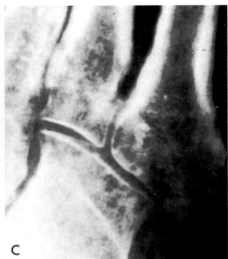
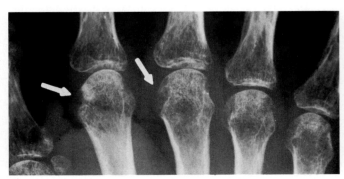
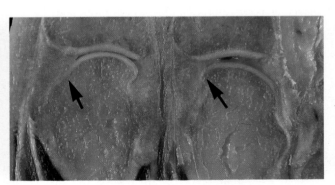

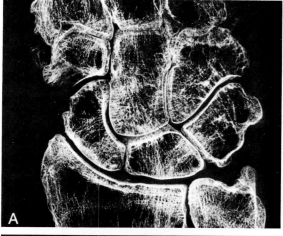
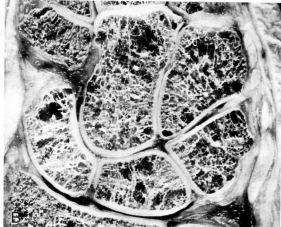
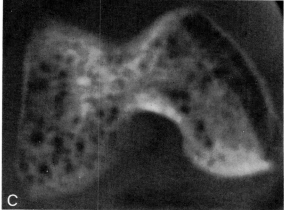

FIGURE 51–49. Spongiosa of tubular bone: Spotty osteoporosis.

A, B In a cadaveric wrist, cystic lesions in the carpal bones represent one characteristic pattern of regional osteoporosis.

C A transaxial CT scan at the level of the femoral condyles reveals cystic osteoporosis simulating plasma cell myeloma.

the absence of significant bony collapse facilitates differentiation from osteonecrosis. It must be emphasized, however, that the degree of periarticular bone resorption in osteoporosis can become striking, producing an alarming radiographic picture that will test the diagnostic acumen of the observer. Casual inspection of the radiographs may lead to an erroneous diagnosis of arthritis, infection, or even neoplastic disease.[319] These radiographic changes of aggressive bone resorption in osteoporosis may be altered with time; over a period of years, a pattern of homogeneous or diffuse osteoporosis and cortical thinning can appear identical to that in postmenopausal or senile states.[16] Pathologically an initial highly aggressive type of osteoclastic bone resorption may be transformed into a less aggressive, low remodeling state.

Additional Skeletal Manifestations of Osteoporosis

Fractures. Acute fractures are an important complication of osteoporosis[177]; the most common sites of such fractures are the vertebral bodies, the neck and intertrochanteric region of the femur, the distal portion of the radius, and the humeral neck. The prevalence of this complication, however, is not clear. Although it has been estimated that spinal compression fractures will occur in approximately 50 per cent of American women by the age of 75 years,[427] this figure requires clarification. As some studies have indicated that vertebral wedge fractures occur frequently in patients

with no reduction in bone mass, their inclusion in the assessment of the prevalence of osteoporotic spinal fractures may not be correct.[428] In an analysis of the risk of fractures in patients with osteoporosis, Meuleman[428] indicated that the prevalence of vertebral crush fractures (as distinct from vertebral wedge fractures) among women in the eighth decade of life was 5 to 10 per cent; the lifetime risk of a hip fracture in women was 15 per cent; and the risk of any osteoporotic fracture by the age of 75 years in white women was approximately 25 per cent. Most investigators indicate that fractures of the vertebral body predominate over those at other sites in patients with osteoporosis. Fractures of the proximal portion of the femur, however, are more significant clinically in these patients, leading in some instances to permanent disability or even death.[354] Fractures at both these sites, as well as in other locations, are not unique to postmenopausal or senile osteoporosis; rather, they also may accompany other forms of osteoporosis and additional metabolic diseases.[429]

Although attempts have been made to define the importance of trabecular bone loss or cortical bone loss, or both, as factors contributing to such fractures, there is no uniform agreement on the subject. In general, it appears that trabecular bone loss is more significant than cortical bone loss in the pathogenesis of fractures in the spine[431] and distal portion of the radius.[320, 321] Indeed, the loss of horizontal plates of trabeculae leads to the vertical striations seen radiographically in the osteoporotic vertebral body.[431] Certainly, loss of cortical bone must be considered, however, especially in the femur,[322] and other factors probably are important. As an example, in the femur, it has been suggested that the relatively increased frequency of femoral neck fractures compared with that of the shaft is related to an increase in mechanical rigidity in the latter area as a consequence of progressive circumferential enlargement of bone. This increased shaft rigidity transfers stress to the proximal part of the femur, leading to fracture. Although it has been emphasized repeatedly in the literature that osteoporosis increases the likelihood of such fractures of the femoral neck, some studies have indicated that the increased risk of fracture in this location in osteoporotic patients compared with controls is not very dramatic, suggesting that factors other than bone mass, such as a tendency to fall, are important determinants of which elderly persons will have fractures.[288, 289] Diseases other than osteoporosis lead to similar femoral fractures. Pathologic fractures of the femoral neck are particularly frequent in skeletal metastasis, whereas pathologic fractures of the femoral shaft usually are secondary to skeletal metastasis or Paget's disease.[177] The prevalence of osteomalacia among elderly patients with fractures of the femoral neck apparently is low.[430]

The existence of osteoporosis does not appear to alter healing time of the fracture. The cortical bone is porous in this condition, and its vascularity is excellent. Prompt healing is expected.

Subchondral resorption of bone in osteoporosis leads to mechanical weakening and conceivably could be associated with epiphyseal collapse. Although this complication is recognized in hyperparathyroidism and steroid-induced osteoporosis, generally it is not observed in other varieties of osteoporosis.

The insufficiency type of stress fracture may appear in patients with osteoporosis. The typical sites of involvement are the symphysis pubis (Figs. 51–50 and 51–51) and pubic rami,[290–292] sacrum (Fig. 51–52),[293–295, 432, 433, 481] supra-acetabular area,[296] other regions of the bony pelvis,[293] femoral neck,[297, 482] proximal and distal portions of the tibia,[298, 299]

and sternum[300, 434–436] (Fig. 51–53). Potential contributing factors include rheumatoid arthritis and corticosteroid or radiation therapy. Accurate radiologic diagnosis in all of these locations may be difficult owing to the presence of osteopenia and the subtle finding of patchy osteosclerosis. Scintigraphy represents a useful initial screening examination and should be supplemented with conventional tomography, CT scanning, or MR imaging (see later discussion) when necessary.

Insufficiency fractures of the pubic rami may be accompanied by considerable osteolysis and fragmentation of bone, findings that simulate a malignant tumor. Those of the sacrum are associated with hip, back or buttock pain and with a characteristic scintigraphic pattern in which vertical and horizontal regions of increased accumulation of the bone-seeking radiopharmaceutical agent produce a configuration that is referred to as the "H pattern." Typical MR imaging abnormalities also occur (see later discussion). Insufficiency fractures of the supra-acetabular bone produce poorly defined zones of increased radiodensity of variable size. All of these pelvic fractures may occur in isolation but often are observed in various combinations. Similar fractures of the tibial plateau resemble osteoarthritis or spontaneous osteonecrosis. Those of the sternum may occur with or without progressive thoracic kyphosis in the osteoporotic thoracic spine. In this last location, displaced or nondisplaced linear fractures, sternomanubrial joint separation, or sternal buckling may be apparent, and associated osteolysis and soft tissue swelling simulate the findings of an aggressive neoplasm. Such sternal abnormalities also may occur in patients with renal osteodystrophy or multiple myeloma and, in all instances, accompanying pain may lead to an erroneous diagnosis of myocardial infarction[437] or pulmonary embolism.[438]

Reinforcement Lines (Bone Bars). In patients with chronic osteopenia, usually related to osteoporosis associated with disuse mandated by neurologic injury, physical trauma, surgical amputation, or debilitating illness, radiographs of the tubular bones, particularly the femur and tibia, commonly reveal strands of trabeculae of variable thickness, extending partially or completely across the marrow cavity (Fig. 51–54). They frequently branch and are oriented at right angles to the cortex in the diaphysis or in an oblique fashion in the metaphysis (Fig. 51–55). These strands, which are referred to as reinforcement lines or bone bars, are evident in both adults and children. Their linear nature readily is apparent when they are viewed en face; punctate or short linear dense foci, simulating bone infarction or cartilaginous tumor, are evident when they are seen in profile (Fig. 51–56). Histologic examination confirms the existence of mature lamellar bone without evidence of recent bone deposition (Fig. 51–57).

Although the precise pathogenesis of bone bars is not clear, several possibilities exist. It might be suggested that they are a normal variation in trabecular pattern. Although in certain locations, such as the humerus (Fig. 51–58) or femoral neck, prominent trabeculae commonly are apparent, bone bars occur in other sites, such as the distal portion of the femur and the proximal portion of the tibia, where prominent trabeculae normally are not encountered. Rather, the coexistence of bone bars and chronic osteopenia raises the possibility of three major pathogenetic occurrences: (1) such structures are formed during skeletal growth, remain

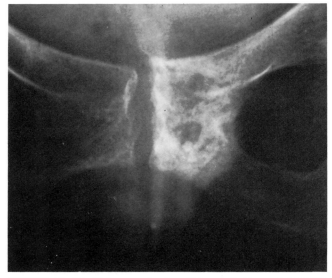

FIGURE 51–50. Osteoporosis: Insufficiency fracture—symphysis pubis. The radiographic appearance of such fractures includes irregular osteolysis and osteosclerosis simulating a malignant neoplasm. (Courtesy of V. Vint, M.D., San Diego, California.)

Text continued on page 1837

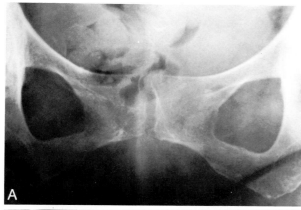

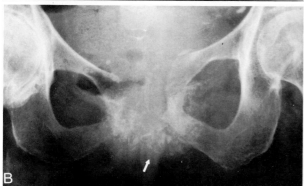
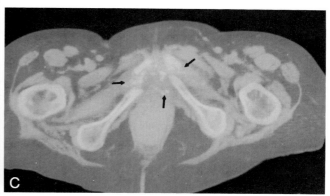

FIGURE 51–51. Osteoporosis: Insufficiency fracture—symphysis pubis. A 72 year old woman with rheumatoid arthritis received corticosteroid therapy. She developed progressive pain and tenderness about the symphysis pubis.

A An initial radiograph reveals subtle irregularity in parasymphyseal bone but otherwise is normal.

B, C Several weeks later, considerable bone fragmentation and subluxation are evident (arrows). The findings again are diagnostic of an insufficiency fracture, although they easily are misinterpreted as evidence of a malignant neoplasm.

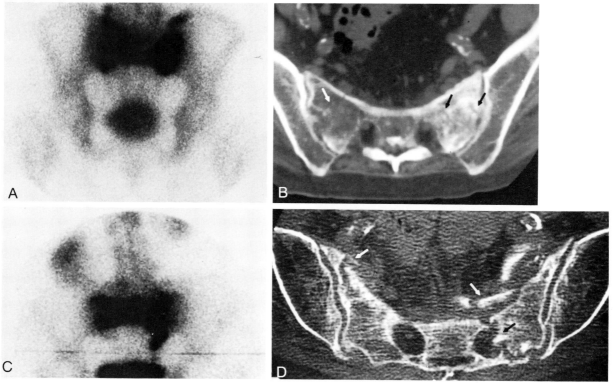

FIGURE 51–52. Osteoporosis: Insufficiency fracture—sacrum.

A, B In an 80 year old woman with osteoporosis, the spontaneous onset of low back pain occurred. Routine radiographs were interpreted as normal. The bone scan **(A)** reveals intense accumulation of the radiopharmaceutical agent in the sacrum. CT scan **(B)** shows sacral fractures (arrows) and bone sclerosis. The sacral foramen on the left is involved.

C, D In a 74 year old woman in a nursing home, a similar history was obtained. Accumulation of the bone-seeking radionuclide **(C)** is evident in the sacrum. CT scan **(D)** documents fractures with extensive fragmentation (arrows). Note disruption of the sacral foramen.

(Courtesy of T. Goergen, M.D., San Diego, California.)

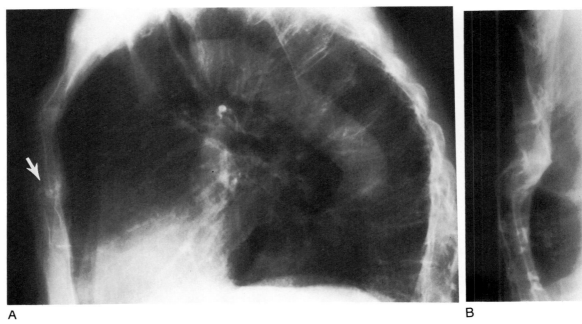

A   **B**

FIGURE 51–53. Osteoporosis: Insufficiency fracture—sternum.

A In association with progressive kyphosis in the thoracic spine, a fracture of the sternum (arrow) has occurred. (Courtesy of P. Kaplan, M.D., Charlottesville, Virginia.)

B In another patient, a lateral view of the sternum shows a buckling fracture. The patient denied a history of trauma or chest pain. Exaggerated thoracic kyphosis attributable to multiple vertebral compression fractures was evident on a chest radiograph.

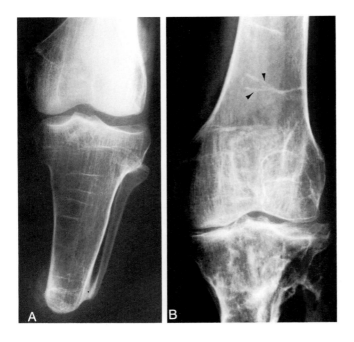

FIGURE 51–54. Reinforcement lines (bone bars): Radiographic abnormalities—association with chronic osteoporosis.

A Observe numerous thick bone bars in the metaphysis and diaphysis of the tibia in association with diffuse osteopenia in a patient who had had his leg amputated many years previously. In large part, the bars extend completely across the medullary canal. (Courtesy of P. Kaplan, M.D., Charlottesville, Virginia.)

B In a different patient with a remote history of a tibial and fibular fracture, diffuse osteopenia is accompanied by horizontally and obliquely oriented bone bars in the femoral metaphysis and diaphysis. One of these is branching (arrowheads).

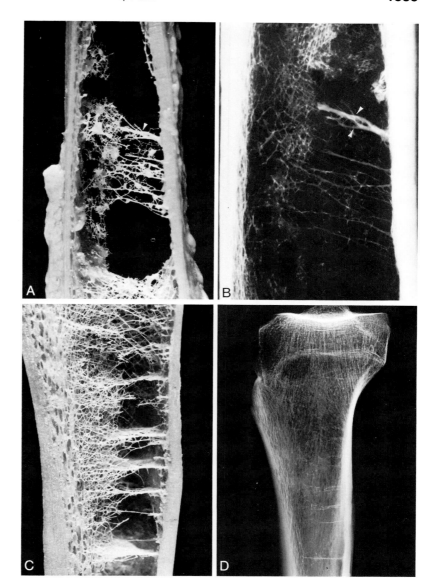

FIGURE 51–55. Reinforcement lines (bone bars): Radiographic-pathologic correlation.

A, B A photograph and magnification radiograph of a macerated midsagittal section of the femur show a branching bone bar (arrowheads) extending incompletely across the distal portion of the diaphysis. It is oriented at approximately 75 degrees to the cortex. Numerous similar but thinner bars are evident distally, some extending across the entire medullary canal.

C, D In this tibia, which has been sectioned in the sagittal plane, numerous parallel bars arise from the posterior surface of the bone. They are oriented at approximately 90 degrees to the cortex and extend almost entirely across the medullary canal.

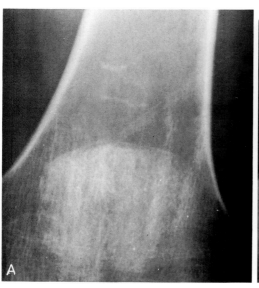
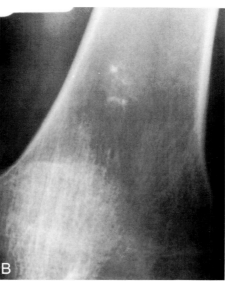

FIGURE 51–56. Reinforcement lines (bone bars): Radiographic abnormalities simulating enchondroma. Radiographs obtained in an anteroposterior **(A)** and oblique **(B)** position show how the configuration of the bone bars can change from punctate to linear radiodense shadows.

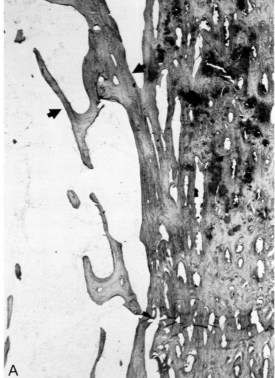

FIGURE 51–57. Reinforcement lines (bone bars): Histologic abnormalities.

A Low power photomicrograph. Emanating from the femoral metaphyseal cortex is a thick, branching trabecula (between arrows) projecting obliquely into the medullary cavity. (Hematoxylin and eosin stain, 4×).

B Higher magnification of the bone bar reveals a few osteons and the lamellar nature of the bone. Note that the bone tissue closer to the medullary cavity and farther from the cortex shows an irregular but well-defined line of demarcation resembling a reversal line (arrows). This bone also is lamellar and shows a very small, poorly formed osteon. The morphology suggests that it was added to the bone attached to the inner cortex. The total width of the bar is 0.9 mm. (Hematoxylin and eosin stain, 16×.)

C, The bone bar viewed under polarized light reveals a lamellar configuration. (Hematoxylin and eosin stain, 16×.)

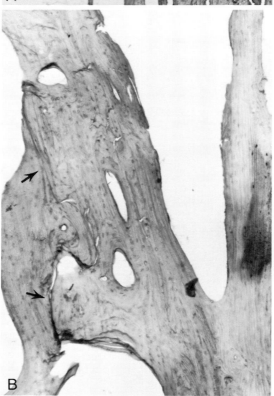

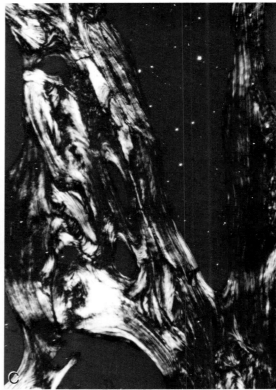

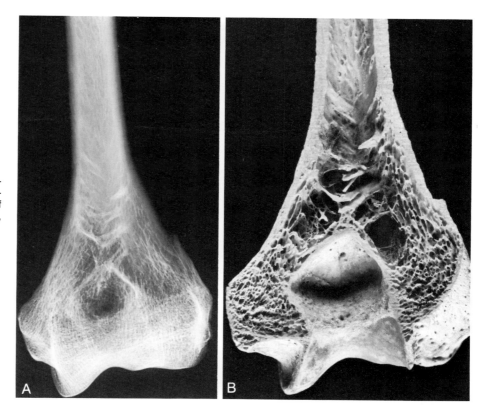

FIGURE 51–58. Normal prominent trabeculae: Humerus. These obliquely oriented trabeculae in the distal portion of the humerus, termed the chevron sign, are normal.

hidden in the normal skeleton and are unmasked by osseous resorption; (2) bone bars initially are formed in part or in totality in the osteopenic skeleton as a response to biomechanical stress; or (3) both mechanisms are at work.

Evidence exists that supports the importance of biomechanical principles in the causation of bone bars. The structure of human bone is closely adapted to the mechanical stresses that exist at every point in each bone.[301, 302] Many of the bone bars correspond in position and in curvature to the lines of maximum compressive stress, whereas others obey biomechanical principles that state that a long, slender column braced at frequent intervals acts as effectively as a short column whose height is the distance between the braces. These observations support the concept that some of the bars of bone in the osteopenic skeleton are the body's attempt at reinforcement as a response to normal stresses. This remodeling process occurs through a sequence of resorption and production of lamellar bone, a sequence that results in reversal zones in which irregular cement lines are deposited.[303] These zones are apparent in histologic examination of bone bars.

Bone bars are not a prominent feature in diseases associated with rapid osteopenia, such as RSD and acute neurologic injury. They appear to represent a response to prolonged stress in which existing normal trabeculae within the medullary canal are reinforced by the slow deposition of new bone. Such bars also are apparent about stable or slowly developing lesions or in areas of osseous deformity.

A question arises concerning the contribution of growth recovery lines of the immature skeleton to the bone bars of the osteopenic mature skeleton. The work of Garn and his associates[304] demonstrated that growth recovery lines may be found in the metaphyses and diaphyses of older children and, probably, adolescents and adults as well. It is conceiv-

able that some of the bone bars represent residual growth recovery lines that are unmasked by chronic osteopenia or that these recovery lines represent the template on which the new bone is formed. Some evidence, however, suggests that many of these bars are unrelated to growth recovery lines: They initially may appear in the adult, even when acute osteopenia is apparent on earlier radiographs (Fig. 51–59); their position correlates with that of normal trabeculae; they may branch or extend across the entire width of the bone, findings generally inconsistent with growth recovery lines; they commonly are thicker than diaphyseal recovery lines; and they may be asymmetric or unilateral in distribution, influenced by the cause of the chronic osteopenia.

MAGNETIC RESONANCE IMAGING ABNORMALITIES

Generalized Osteoporosis

Potential applications of MR imaging in patients with generalized osteoporosis include the assessment of vertebral body fractures; the analysis of extraspinal sites of insufficiency fractures; and the evaluation of bone mass and strength.

Vertebral Body Fractures. The common occurrence of both osteoporosis and fractures of the vertebral body in postmenopausal women and in elderly men and women presents an immediate diagnostic challenge, particularly in those persons with a known extraosseous malignant neoplasm. Is the vertebral collapse related to osteoporosis alone or does it indicate that the vertebral body contains metastatic foci? Although routine radiography may be helpful in addressing this question, the results of the routine radio-

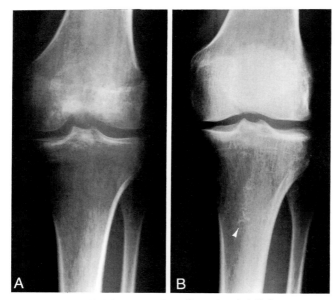

FIGURE 51–59. Reinforcement lines (bone bars): Initial appearance in the mature skeleton. This patient developed acute osteopenia after an injury to the knee.

A A radiograph of the knee shortly after the injury demonstrates patchy osteopenia in the femur, tibia, and fibula.

B Two years later, typical bone bars (arrowhead) are present in the proximal portion of the tibia.

graphic examination may not be conclusive. The absence of osteolytic or osteosclerotic foci in the vertebral body, of pediculate destruction, of cortical disruption, or of an adjacent soft tissue mass is reassuring evidence that tumor is absent, but unfortunately does not eliminate altogether the possibility of a pathologic (tumorous) fracture. The known insensitivity of routine radiography to the detection of medullary lesions within the vertebral body contributes to this diagnostic uncertainty.[440, 441] Radionuclide scintigraphy also may provide findings that lack specificity in this regard. The detection of multiple regions of abnormal activity on the bone scan is strong evidence that skeletal metastases are present, but scintigraphic abnormality confined to a single vertebra remains nondiagnostic. Furthermore, a normal examination with bone scintigraphy occasionally is encountered in patients with osseous metastatic deposits, particularly those patients who are debilitated and in whom a highly aggressive tumor is accompanied by little or no bone remodeling. A similar situation with negative results on scintigraphy can occur in patients with plasma cell myeloma. CT scanning represents a third imaging method that can be used to assess vertebral collapse. Morphologic characteristics of the involved vertebral body may allow documentation that a tumor is present, but the absence of these characteristics frequently leads again to diagnostic uncertainty.

MR imaging can be used effectively in this clinical setting if certain diagnostic pitfalls are taken into account (also see Chapter 85). The potential value of this technique relies on alterations in the signal intensity of the bone marrow in the involved vertebral body that allow differentiation of a tumorous process from that accompanying osteoporosis alone. In theory, this method seems attractive, but in practice, difficulties arise owing to variations in signal intensity of normal bone marrow as well as of bone marrow that has been injured.

The basic microstructure of bone marrow consists of a trabecular framework that houses fat cells covered with hematopoietic cells, both supported by a system of reticulum cells, nerves, and vascular sinusoids coursing among them.[441] In adults, the normal vertebral column is composed primarily of hematopoietic bone marrow that contains a significant amount of fat, ranging from 25 to 50 per cent and increasing with age.[442] Some variations in the rate and extent of this age-related physiologic conversion from cellular to fatty marrow are encountered, however, and regional differences in this conversion in various segments of the spine have been documented.[443] In middle-aged and elderly persons, in whom the differentiation of "benign" versus "malignant" osteoporotic vertebral body fractures most commonly is required, the MR imaging signal intensity of the normal vertebral marrow generally is dominated by its fatty content. Therefore, with standard spin echo technique, high signal intensity on T1-weighted images and intermediate signal intensity on T2-weighted images in the normal marrow of the vertebral body is expected. In the presence of tumor or any other condition in which replacement of marrow fat has occurred, a decreased signal intensity is seen in the marrow on T1-weighted images, and T2-weighted images show either low or high signal, depending on the specific pathologic process that is present.[442] With most tumors, foci of increased signal intensity are noted on T2-weighted spin echo images.

The documentation of the presence of tumor within a collapsed vertebral body with MR imaging is based on the identification of such areas of altered signal intensity. Baker and coworkers[442] noted that pathologic fractures of the vertebral body (defined as fractures related to skeletal metastasis) resulted in homogeneous replacement of vertebral marrow, producing low signal intensity on T1-weighted spin echo images and high signal intensity on T2-weighted sequences. The diffuse nature of the signal alterations was emphasized in this report. Furthermore, these investigators used both chemical shift and short tau inversion recovery (STIR) imaging techniques to evaluate these fractures. The chemical shift method, using a presaturation technique, provided images in which the lipid signal was suppressed ("water" images) and those in which the water signal was suppressed ("fat" images). Fat images in instances of pathologic fracture were characterized by complete replacement of normal fatty marrow, shown as absent signal intensity in the involved vertebral body; water and STIR images (in which normal fat signal is suppressed) in the same instances showed diffuse high signal intensity in the affected vertebral body, with the STIR images revealing the highest contrast between regions of abnormal and normal marrow.

The benefit that any or all of these MR imaging methods bring in allowing discrimination between "pathologic" and "benign" osteoporotic fractures of the vertebral body depends on the existence of different signal intensity characteristics in the two types of fractures (Fig. 51–60). Herein lie some of the limitations of MR imaging in this clinical setting. The MR imaging findings of a so-called benign fracture, in common with the scintigraphic abnormalities, are dependent in part on the age of the fracture. Hemor-

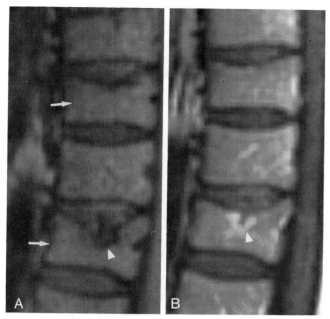

FIGURE 51–60. Vertebral body fractures: Value of MR imaging. In this postmenopausal woman with multiple osteoporotic compression fractures of the thoracic spine, a sagittal T1-weighted (TR/TE, 600/20) spin echo MR image **(A)** shows compression fractures of two thoracic vertebral bodies (arrows). The signal of the bone marrow in the involved vertebral bodies is identical in intensity to that in the uninvolved vertebrae. In one of the collapsed vertebrae, a localized Schmorl's node (arrowhead) is apparent. After the intravenous injection of gadolinium contrast agent, a similar MR image (TR/TE, 600/20) **(B)** shows enhancement of signal intensity only in the area of the Schmorl's node (arrowhead) and basivertebral veins. (Courtesy of P. Chu, M.D., San Diego, California.)

rhage and edema initially occurring after a vertebral fracture would be expected to resolve over a period of time, although the precise length of time required for complete resolution is not clear and, in fact, may be variable. With bone scintigraphy, the abnormal accumulation of the radionuclide at the site of fracture (which usually is apparent within 48 hours of fracture) may diminish progressively and disappear altogether over a period of 1 or 2 years,[483] but this time course is variable and, in some cases, abnormal scintigraphic activity persists for many years or even indefinitely.[444]

Baker and associates[442] included benign vertebral body fractures in their previously cited MR imaging study. The ages of these fractures at the time of MR imaging varied from 2 days to 17 years. In those persons with long-standing or chronic benign fractures, isointense marrow signal comparable with that of normal vertebral bodies was evident on all of the MR sequences that were employed. In those persons with more acute benign fractures, high signal intensity in the bone marrow of the affected vertebral body was evident on T2-weighted spin echo images, STIR images, and "water" images using chemical shift imaging, although the MR signal intensity pattern generally was more inhomogeneous and less pronounced than that observed in cases of pathologic fracture. "Fat" images in patients with acute benign fractures generally showed only partial replacement of the signal of normal fatty marrow by signal of low intensity, in contrast to the complete absence

of normal marrow signal typical of pathologic fractures. These investigators estimated that the MR imaging characteristics of the bone marrow in instances of acute compression fractures converted to a normal pattern in 1 to 3 months.

Although other investigators have found it difficult to differentiate between osteoporotic and neoplastic fractures of the vertebral body with MR imaging,[445] Yuh and collaborators[446] reported results that were far more favorable; in 64 patients with 109 vertebral compression fractures, they found that MR imaging allowed such differentiation in 94 per cent of fractures. Standard T1- and T2-weighted spin echo sequences were the dominant methods used. Three categories of MR imaging abnormality were found: complete replacement of normal MR signal in the vertebral body; incomplete replacement with some residual normal bone marrow signal; and complete preservation of normal marrow signal in the deformed vertebral body. Most of the vertebral fractures resulting from metastatic involvement were associated with bone marrow replacement on T1-weighted images (seen as foci of decreased signal intensity), and in 88 per cent of such fractures, the replacement was total. Conversely, with most benign fractures (defined as those in which subsequent radiography performed at least 16 months later showed no change in vertebral appearance) in patients without a history of injury (such fractures then were considered osteoporotic in nature), normal bone marrow signal was preserved throughout the vertebral body on both T1- and T2-weighted spin echo images. The authors postulated that in cases of tumor, vertebral compression occurs only when the entire bone marrow in the vertebral body is replaced and, in cases of osteoporosis alone, the bone marrow in the vertebral body remains relatively intact and is displaced in accordance with the vector of the compression force. Thus, Yuh and coworkers[446] observed that even in instances in which incomplete replacement of marrow signal was evident (category 2), areas of such replacement were poorly defined and irregular in cases of tumor and smooth in cases of osteoporosis alone. As in the study of Baker and associates,[442] some diagnostic problems occurred, however, in Yuh and coworkers'[446] analysis of MR imaging patterns in patients with acute non-neoplastic fractures of the vertebral body. Furthermore, common to both studies was the assumption that the abnormal MR imaging signal associated with such acute fractures would convert to normal over a period of time, allowing their differentiation from tumoral fractures, in which signal aberrations would be persistent and progressive.

The initial experience exploring the diagnostic role of MR imaging in the assessment of vertebral compression fractures has been encouraging, but the preliminary nature of the data must be recognized, as must the need for other studies, prospective in nature, employing greater numbers of patients.

Insufficiency Fractures of Extraspinal Sites. As discussed earlier in this chapter and in Chapter 67, the insufficiency type of stress fracture represents an important consequence of generalized osteoporosis. Normal or abnormal amounts of stress placed on bones that are structurally weak lead (gradually or acutely) to osseous failure. Involvement of pelvic sites carries with it a risk both for missed diagnosis and for misdiagnosis. With regard to the latter, osteolysis and bone fragmentation accompanying insufficiency fractures in such locations as parasymphyseal bone are not dissimilar to findings of skeletal malignant tumors. With regard to missed diagnosis, bowel gas and soft tissues overlying these pelvic fractures lead to diagnostic inadequacy of routine radiography. Additional imaging methods, including bone scintigraphy and CT, as indicated earlier in this chapter, provide increased sensitivity and specificity over routine radiography in this clinical setting. MR imaging, also, has superior sensitivity and specificity in the analysis of insufficiency fractures of the pelvic bones.

The sensitivity of the MR examination in this situation relates to the occurrence of bone marrow edema as an early manifestation of the fracture. In common with edema from other causes and with other processes in which bone marrow is replaced or modified, the MR imaging characteristics of traumatic edema include decreased signal intensity on T1-weighted spin echo images and increased signal inten-

sity on T2-weighted spin echo images. The application of additional MR imaging methods, such as chemical shift and STIR imaging techniques, increases the sensitivity of the examination; in both of these methods, the suppression of the signal derived from normal fat aids in the detection of the increased signal intensity occurring in areas of edematous marrow.

The specificity of the MR examination relies, in large part, on the morphology and distribution of the abnormal foci. Involvement of that portion of the sacrum that is located just medial to the sacroiliac joint in a unilateral or bilateral distribution, of that portion of the symphysis pubis that abuts on the fibrocartilaginous disc, of the inner contour of the ilium, and of supra-acetabular bone is most characteristic of insufficiency fractures of the pelvis[464, 481] (Figs. 51–61 and 51–62). With regard to the sacral fractures, linear regions of altered signal intensity may parallel the margin of the sacroiliac joint, and involvement of the

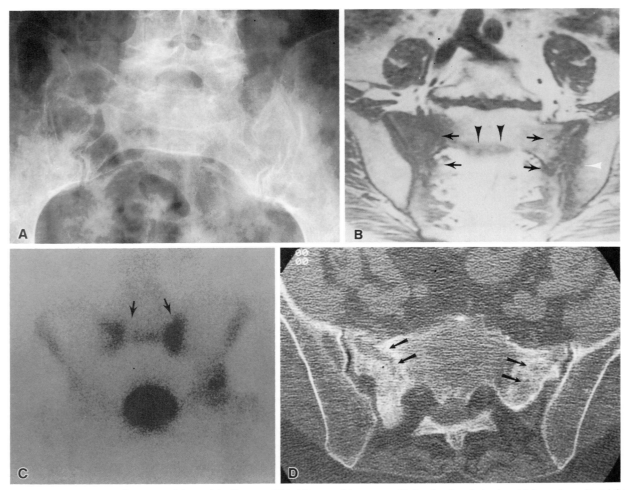

FIGURE 51–61. Insufficiency fractures of the pelvis: Sacrum. This 70 year old woman with low back pain had no history of previous injury to this area.

   A The routine radiograph reveals osteopenia.

   B A coronal T1-weighted (TR/TE, 650/20) MR image shows bands of decreased signal intensity paralleling both sacroiliac joints (arrows) and extending across the body of the sacrum (black arrowheads). Decreased signal intensity also is seen along the iliac side of the joint (white arrowhead).

   C Bone scintigraphy shows accumulation of the radionuclide within the sacral alae and body (arrows). Note the classic H-shaped appearance of the scintigraphic activity.

   D Transaxial CT scan delineates the fracture lines (arrows) in the sacrum.

   (From Brahme SK, et al: Skel Radiol *19*:489, 1990.)

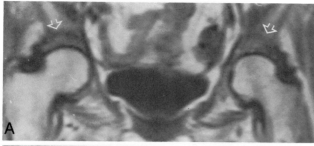

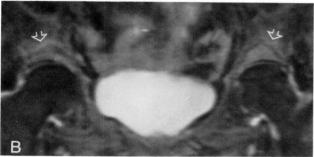

FIGURE 51–62. Insufficiency fractures of the pelvis: Supra-acetabular bone. This 64 year old woman developed bilateral groin pain.

A On a coronal T1-weighted (TR/TE, 650/20) spin echo MR image, abnormal regions of low signal intensity in the ilia, above the acetabuli, are evident (open arrows). That on the right side has a linear configuration.

B With STIR imaging (TR/TE, 2500/40; inversion time, 160 msecs), these areas show increased signal intensity (open arrows), although a region of persistent low signal intensity is seen on the right. Bilateral hip effusions are present.

adjacent portion of the ilium also may be observed. Most importantly, however, in the accurate assessment of the MR imaging findings is the identification of multiple pelvic insufficiency fractures in the same person.

Some diagnostic pitfalls exist when MR imaging is used in the analysis of pelvic insufficiency fractures. First, the pelvis also is a frequent site of skeletal metastasis, and the resulting altered signal intensity is similar to that seen in instances of fracture. Second, cortical disruption and fragmentation accompanying insufficiency fractures, when detected on the MR examination (as well as on the routine radiograph and CT examination), resemble findings of an aggressive tumor. Discrete soft tissue masses, however, generally do not occur in cases of insufficiency fracture. Third, the conversion of hematopoietic marrow to fatty marrow in normal persons is not so complete in the pelvis as in other extraspinal locations; a relatively large proportion of the marrow remains hematopoietic, even in older persons, although scattered fatty foci may be identified, especially about the acetabulum.[443] Therefore, reliance on T1-weighted spin echo images alone for the detection of insufficiency fractures of the pelvis may lead to missed diagnosis owing to the difficulty encountered in distinguishing between the decreased signal intensity of such a fracture and the decreased signal intensity in areas of hematopoietic marrow. The same diagnostic difficulty, of course, arises in the detection of skeletal metastasis in the pelvis (or spine).

A word of caution also must be included with regard to the MR imaging diagnosis of insufficiency fractures of the femoral neck and intertrochanteric region. Although the conversion of red to yellow marrow in this anatomic site is

well documented and may be almost complete,[443] linear and curvilinear regions of low signal intensity on T1-weighted images may be identified in normal persons. These areas correspond in position to the trabecular groups described previously in this chapter, and the regions of low signal intensity in the femoral neck may become prominent in patients with osteoporosis. Their differentiation from insufficiency fractures of the femoral neck relies first on characteristic patterns of distribution; insufficiency fractures tend to course horizontally, across the femoral neck, at angles almost perpendicular to those of some of the trabecular groups (Fig. 51–63). Furthermore, the low signal intensity of (normal or abnormal) trabeculae persists on T2-weighted spin echo images, whereas high signal intensity accompanies an insufficiency fracture on such images. Similar analysis allows differentiation between insufficiency fractures and osteophytes of the femoral neck.

Bone Mass and Strength. Although quantitative assessment of bone mineral content is discussed more fully in Chapter 52, a brief description of the potential of MR imaging in the analysis of bone mass and strength is included here.

Wehrli and coworkers[447] proposed a method of MR interferometry to evaluate the trabecular structure of vertebrae. Their technique was based on the hypothesis that the presence of two physical phases—bone and bone marrow—causes magnetic field distribution across the imaging voxel. As described by these investigators, the resulting spread in resonance frequency produces line broadening. This is measured as the decay rate of the signal intensity in the region of interest. The resulting interferogram relates to chemical shifting of the two principal components of bone marrow, fat and water. These components get in and out of phase with one another, the signals from both being attenuated by T2* (effective transverse relaxation time) effects from the distribution of the magnetic field within the meas-

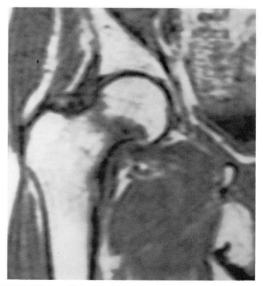

FIGURE 51–63. Insufficiency fracture of the femoral neck. In this 75 year old woman, a fracture of the right femoral neck occurred spontaneously. A routine radiograph (not shown) was interpreted as negative. The T1-weighted (TR/TE, 600/20) coronal spin echo MR image reveals the characteristic, serpentine region of low signal intensity in the subcapital region of the right femoral neck.

uring volume. The T2* values differ in healthy patients and in those with osteoporosis; in osteoporotic persons, a prolonged T2* value may arise from an increase in intertrabecular space. Basically, the effect on the T2* value is consistent with an expected increase in local magnetic field homogeneity that is secondary to a decrease in trabecular density occurring in osteoporotic bone.[447, 448]

Although this is but one MR imaging method that might be used to study skeletal structure, the basic concept probably will be expanded to allow for other techniques of MR imaging analysis. The matrix of trabecular bone has a significant influence on the signal intensity derived from bone marrow. As the compositions of trabecular bone and the adjacent bone marrow differ considerably, their magnetic properties also differ. Such differences in magnetic properties lead to local distortions of the magnetic lines of force and, thus, to an inhomogeneous magnetic field.[348] With gradient echo imaging, these inhomogeneities affect the apparent transverse relaxation time, or T2*. Analysis of changes in T2* provides information regarding the density and geometry of the trabecular network.[348] T2* shortening would be expected to be more pronounced in the presence of rarefied osteoporotic trabeculae. This effect has been confirmed not only in the work of Wehrli and associates[447] but also in a number of in vitro and in vivo experiments.[449–451, 474]

Regional Osteoporosis

Transient Bone Marrow Edema. In 1988, Wilson and associates[398] introduced the concept of transient bone marrow edema in an analysis of 10 patients with debilitating hip or knee pain who were examined with MR imaging. Although routine radiographs in some of these patients were normal, the clinical manifestations were identical to those of transient osteoporosis of the hip or regional migratory osteoporosis. The MR imaging findings were uniform, both in the patients without osteoporosis and in those with osteoporosis. In each case, a decrease in signal intensity was noted in the bone marrow on T1-weighted spin echo images and an increase in signal intensity on T2-weighted spin echo images. In four patients in whom biopsy was performed, no evidence of tumor or osteonecrosis was found, and the clinical manifestations resolved spontaneously in all 10 patients. The authors speculated that the MR imaging findings were consistent with a transient increase in the water content of the bone marrow and the entity termed transient bone marrow edema was born (Fig. 51–64).

One earlier report[452] and many subsequent ones[453–459, 475, 476, 479] have confirmed the occurrence of MR imaging abnormalities in patients with transient osteoporosis of the hip, and similar abnormalities have been reported in patients, including children, whose routine radiographs of the hip were normal.[401] In most of these studies, spin echo MR imaging sequences were employed, and a relatively homogeneous area of the femoral head and neck was affected. Decreased signal intensity in this area on T1-weighted sequences and increased signal intensity in the corresponding region on T2-weighted sequences typically were observed (Fig. 51–65). Associated joint effusions in the affected hip were common. The MR imaging findings, along with the

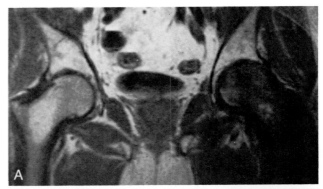
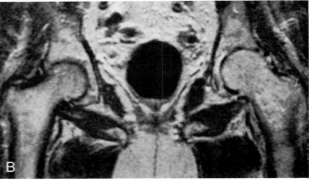

FIGURE 51–64. Transient bone marrow edema. This patient complained of left hip pain of several months' duration. Routine radiographs were normal, and bone scintigraphy was not performed.
A A coronal T1-weighted (TR/TE, 930/26) spin echo MR image reveals low signal intensity replacing the normal signal of the bone marrow in the left femoral head and neck. The acetabulum appears normal, as does the opposite hip.
B A coronal T2-weighted (TR/TE, 2000/80) spin echo MR image reveals increased signal intensity in the left femoral head and neck. The signal intensity is slightly greater than that on the opposite side. A very small joint effusion is present. The pain and MR imaging abnormalities diminished over a period of 3 months.

clinical manifestations, regressed partially or completely over a period of months. Repeatedly in these articles, the more diffuse nature of the MR imaging abnormalities was used to differentiate the findings from those of osteonecrosis. In some cases, more than one hip or a region other than a hip was affected.

The use of chemical shift, fat suppression imaging, and STIR imaging can be effective in the detection of transient bone marrow edema. As in other disease processes in which normal bone marrow is replaced, these methods, by suppressing the signal of normal fatty marrow, are accompanied by alterations in marrow signal intensity that are more exaggerated than those seen with standard spin echo techniques (Fig. 51–66). The inversion recovery method is one of the simplest to use, differing from a standard spin echo sequence only through the application of an initial 180 degree radiofrequency pulse that is used to invert the longitudinal magnetization. With a selection of a short inversion time, one that corresponds to the time when the recovering longitudinal magnetization of fat is zero or at its null point, fat suppression is achieved. STIR imaging, however, employs relatively long repetition times (TR), on the order of 1800 to 2000 ms, suppresses tissues other than fat that possess similar inversion times, and is incompatible with the effective use of intravenous administration of gad-

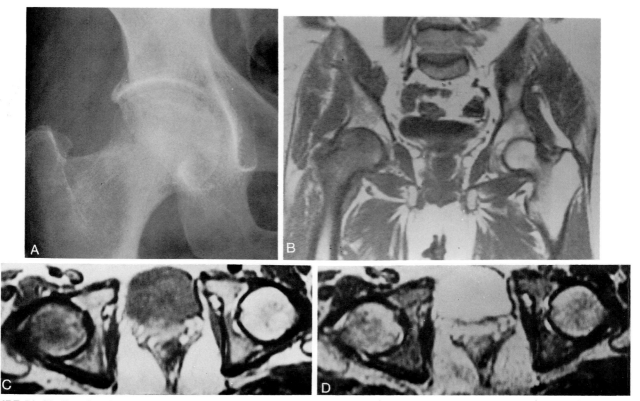

FIGURE 51–65. Transient bone marrow edema in association with transient osteoporosis of the hip. Pain in the right hip occurred in this young man.

A A radiograph reveals mild osteopenia of the femoral head. The joint space is preserved, and no collapse of the subchondral bone is evident.

B A coronal T1-weighted (TR/TE, 600/20) spin echo MR image shows diminished signal intensity of the bone marrow throughout the right femoral head and neck. The opposite side is normal.

C, D Transaxial proton density (TR/TE, 2000/20) **(C)** and T2-weighted (TR/TE, 2000/80) **(D)** spin echo MR images show abnormal marrow signal intensity in the right femoral head. Considerable brightening of signal intensity is noted in **D**. A joint effusion is seen on the right, with a smaller one noted in the left hip.

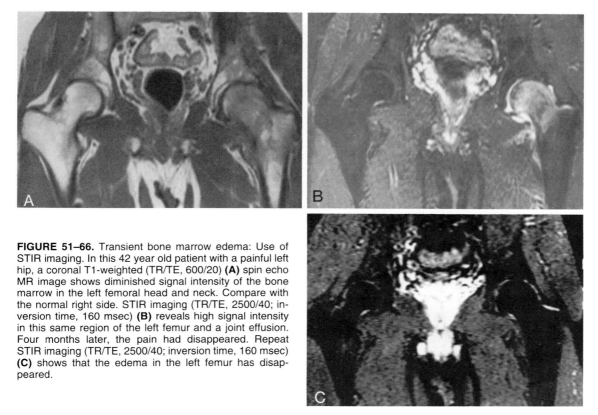

FIGURE 51–66. Transient bone marrow edema: Use of STIR imaging. In this 42 year old patient with a painful left hip, a coronal T1-weighted (TR/TE, 600/20) **(A)** spin echo MR image shows diminished signal intensity of the bone marrow in the left femoral head and neck. Compare with the normal right side. STIR imaging (TR/TE, 2500/40; inversion time, 160 msec) **(B)** reveals high signal intensity in this same region of the left femur and a joint effusion. Four months later, the pain had disappeared. Repeat STIR imaging (TR/TE, 2500/40; inversion time, 160 msec) **(C)** shows that the edema in the left femur has disappeared.

olinium-based contrast agent. Fat suppression with STIR imaging is not influenced by magnetic inhomogeneity, and, as an added benefit, the contrast effects of T1 recovery and T2 decay are additive. Furthermore, the recent introduction of fast STIR imaging allows the examination to be accomplished in a shorter period of time. Chemical presaturation techniques also can be employed in such a fashion as to suppress the signal of fat alone, and these techniques can be coupled with intravenous administration of a gadolinium-based contrast agent. To work effectively, however, a very homogeneous static magnetic field is required, and small to moderately sized fields of view should be employed. Longer minimum TR times and fewer available slices also characterize the chemical presaturation techniques.

Several questions regarding transient bone marrow edema require clarification. First, what is its relationship to transient osteoporosis of the hip? Certainly, on the basis of observed clinical manifestations, these disorders are closely related or identical. Both involve the hip, lead to pain and disability, and resolve spontaneously. Both diseases affect both men and women and predominate in young and middle-aged persons. The major difference between the two, the presence (by definition) of osteoporosis in transient osteoporosis of the hip and its possible absence in transient bone marrow edema, may indicate only that routine radiography is an insensitive technique for the detection of osteoporosis. The quantitative assessment of bone mineral content in the femoral head, through the application of CT, dual-energy photon absorptiometry, or dual-energy radiographic absorptiometry, might indicate a decreased value in all patients with transient bone marrow edema. Even if this were not the case, the absence of osteoporosis in cases of transient bone marrow edema may indicate a lesser degree of involvement and not a true qualitative difference between the two disorders. Documentation that transient bone marrow edema can involve both hips and other joints, with abnormalities moving from one location to another, suggests that this disorder is related to regional migratory osteoporosis as well (Fig. 51–67). Furthermore, partial types of bone marrow edema, with distribution patterns similar to those seen in regional osteoporosis, may be observed (Fig. 51–68).

A second question relates to the specificity of the MR imaging findings in transient bone marrow edema. The MR imaging pattern that is observed most frequently in this condition indicates involvement of both the femoral head and the femoral neck. A similar distribution may characterize the MR imaging appearance of femoral involvement in a number of infectious or neoplastic processes, including skeletal metastasis and lymphoma. This distribution differs from that typically seen in cases of osteonecrosis of the femoral head (see later discussion). In transient bone marrow edema, the description of a migrating MR imaging pattern, with abnormalities appearing first in the anterior portions of the femoral head and neck and then being seen in the posterior portions,[457] is interesting, but requires further documentation (Fig. 51–69).

A third (and perhaps most important) question regarding transient bone marrow edema is concerned with its relationship to ischemic necrosis of bone. Relevant to this question are the data contained in a recent report by Turner and coworkers.[460] MR imaging was used by these investigators to evaluate six painful hips in five patients, and diffuse signal intensity abnormalities were observed in the marrow of the femoral head and neck in all hips, which extended into the intertrochanteric area in five hips. The MR imaging findings, which were characterized by low signal intensity on T1-weighted images and isointensity or hyperintensity of signal on T2-weighted images, were identical to those reported in cases of transient bone marrow edema. Osteonecrosis of the femoral head subsequently was diagnosed in all hips owing either to characteristic histologic changes in specimens derived from core biopsy (three hips) or to the development of focal MR imaging alterations reported to be highly specific for osteonecrosis (three hips). These results appear to indicate that a subgroup of patients who have bone marrow edema in the femoral head subsequently will develop osteonecrosis at this site. This complication is not entirely surprising, as vascular congestion and edema of the bone marrow are thought to occur early in the course of ischemic necrosis of bone.[461, 462] Indeed, such congestion and edema may be accompanied by necrotic and reparative processes involving bone and marrow similar to those of early osteonecrosis.[479] It is not clear, however, what percentage of patients with transient bone marrow edema will develop osteonecrosis, what factors are responsible for this occurrence in some patients and not in others, and how this complication can be predicted on the basis of the initial MR imaging pattern that indicates only bone marrow edema. Furthermore, it is not clear how often osteonecrosis of the femoral head is accompanied by a diffuse rather than a focal pattern of MR imaging abnormality and how often segmental collapse of a femoral head in cases of transient bone marrow edema reflects compression of weakened bone rather than osteonecrosis. A role of MR imaging, combined with intravenous administration of gadolinium compounds, in allowing differentiation of transient bone marrow edema and the edema pattern of osteonecrosis has been suggested.[476]

Reflex Sympathetic Dystrophy. Little data have been accumulated with regard to the MR imaging findings in RSD. Koch and coworkers,[463] in examining 17 patients with RSD of the extremities, employed both T1-weighted and T2-weighted spin echo MR imaging sequences. The diagnosis of RSD in these patients was based on typical clinical and scintigraphic abnormalities. In 10 of the 17 patients, the MR images were interpreted as completely normal. Nonspecific soft tissue changes were observed on MR imaging in three patients; these changes consisted of edema (one patient) and muscle atrophy (two patients). The bone marrow signal was interpreted as abnormal in three patients, two of whom had had a fracture. In the third of these three patients, an MR imaging pattern consistent with that of edema was observed. Adjacent joint effusions were evident in two patients.

The paucity of MR imaging findings in this report is surprising in view of the commonly held belief that RSD is closely linked to other causes of regional osteoporosis. It is possible that the degree of bone marrow edema accompanying RSD is less prominent than that in transient osteoporosis of the hip or that anatomic differences between the hip and other regions of the extremities influence the MR imaging pattern in RSD.[463]

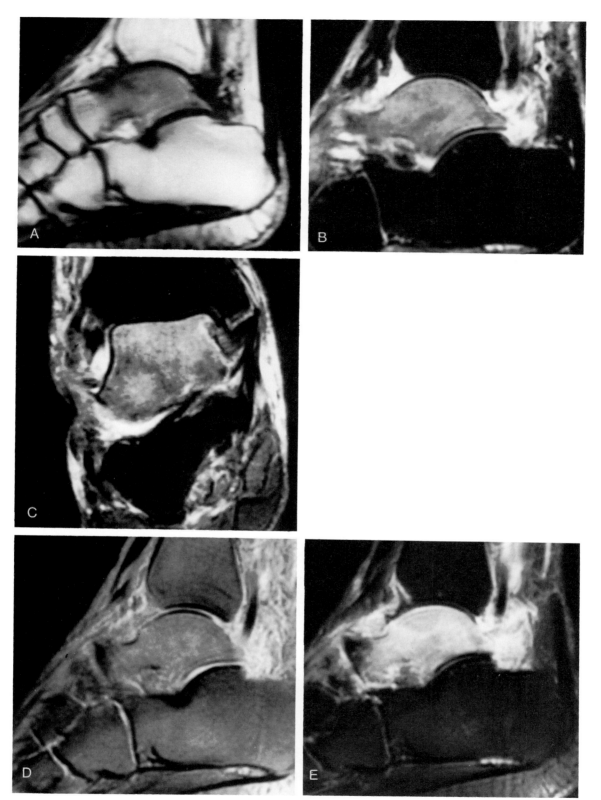

FIGURE 51-67. Transient bone marrow edema: Involvement of the talus. This 61 year old man had had an injury to the left ankle. He then developed RSD mainly on the injured side. This syndrome then cleared, and symptoms, including pain, developed in the right ankle.

   A A sagittal T1-weighted (TR/TE, 367/16) spin echo MR image shows diminished signal intensity in a portion of the talus. The other tarsal bones appear normal.

   B A sagittal STIR image (TR/TE, 3000/27; inversion time, 160 msec) reveals increased signal intensity in the talus, with an associated joint effusion of both the ankle and posterior subtalar joint. Note the edematous soft tissues.

   C A coronal T2-weighted (TR/TE, 2500/76) spin echo MR image with chemical shift imaging (used for fat presaturation) demonstrates the high signal intensity of the edematous bone marrow in the talus. Joint fluid is seen in the ankle and posterior subtalar joint.

   D A sagittal T1-weighted (TR/TE, 650/19) spin echo MR image with fat presaturation (chemical shift imaging) reveals only slightly increased signal intensity in the marrow of the talus.

   E With the same imaging parameters as in **D**, the intravenous administration of gadolinium contrast agent leads to an accentuation of the signal intensity in the edematous marrow of the talus.

   (**A-E**, Courtesy of S. Eilenberg, M.D., San Diego, California.)

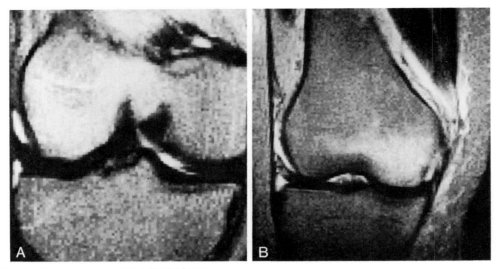

FIGURE 51–68. Transient bone marrow edema: Partial forms.
  A Nontraumatic bone marrow edema. On a proton density weighted (TR/TE, 3240/30) coronal spin echo MR image, edema resulting in high signal intensity is confined to the lateral femoral condyle. A small joint effusion also is seen.
  B Traumatic bone marrow edema. On a similar proton density weighted (TR/TE, 3240/30) MR image in a patient who had had an injury to the knee, high signal intensity, representing a bone "bruise," is confined to the medial femoral condyle. The medial collateral ligament was injured in this patient; note the presence of edema in the medial soft tissues.
  (**A, B**, Courtesy of Y. Dirheimer, M.D., Strasbourg, France.)

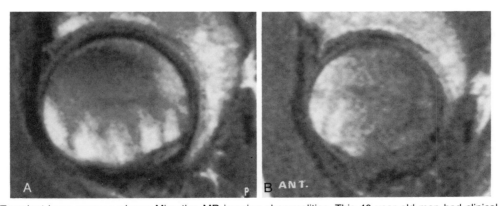

FIGURE 51–69. Transient bone marrow edema: Migrating MR imaging abnormalities. This 46 year old man had clinical and radiographic evidence of transient osteoporosis of the hip.
  A A sagittal T1-weighted (TR/TE, 475/20) spin echo MR image obtained 2 months after the onset of pain shows a decrease in signal intensity in the anterior and superior portions of the femoral head (*A*, anterior; *P*, posterior).
  B Three months later, a similar sagittal spin echo MR image (TR/TE, 475/20) now reveals that the region of low signal intensity is located in the posterior part of the femoral head (*ANT*, anterior).
  (From Hauzeur JP, et al: J Rheumatol *18*:1211, 1991.)

SUMMARY

Osteoporosis is an extremely common metabolic disorder that can accompany a variety of disease processes. It can be divided conveniently into generalized, regional, and localized types. Localized osteoporosis commonly is associated with focal skeletal lesions, such as neoplasm and infection.

Generalized osteoporosis accompanies senile and postmenopausal states, endocrine disorders such as acromegaly, hyperthyroidism, hyperparathyroidism, and Cushing's disease, pregnancy, heparin administration, and alcoholism. This type of osteoporosis, which must be distinguished from other metabolic disorders such as osteomalacia and hyperparathyroidism (osteitis fibrosa cystica), predominates in the axial skeleton, with major effect on the vertebrae; abnormalities of the appendicular skeleton are mild, consisting of uniform loss of osseous density (osteopenia). In the vertebral bodies, characteristic changes in radiolucency, trabecular pattern, and osseous contour are encountered.

Regional osteoporosis accompanies disuse or immobilization, RSD, and transient regional osteoporosis. Changes predominate in the appendicular skeleton. A more aggressive type of bone resorption in these conditions can lead to cortical bone changes at endosteal, intracortical, and subperiosteal bony envelopes and to spongy bone changes at subchondral and metaphyseal locations. Differential diagnosis is facilitated by application of magnification radiography and radiographic morphometry.

Additional manifestations of osteoporosis include acute and insufficiency stress fractures and bone bars (reinforcement lines).

The application of MR imaging shows promise in the assessment of some forms of regional osteoporosis and of complications associated with generalized osteoporosis. In the future, this technique may be applied to the quantitative analysis of skeletal architecture and bone mass.

References

1. Harris WH, Heaney RP: Skeletal renewal and metabolic bone disease. N Engl J Med 280:193, 1969.
2. Lutwak L, Whedon GD: Osteoporosis. DM, p 1, April 1963.
3. Griffiths HJ, Zimmerman RE: The clinical application of bone mineral analysis. Skel Radiol 3:1, 1978.
4. Wahner HW, Riggs BL, Beabout JW: Diagnosis of osteoporosis: Usefulness of photon absorptiometry at the radius. J Nucl Med 18:432, 1977.
5. Cameron JR, Sorenson J: Measurement of bone mineral in vivo. An improved method. Science 142:230, 1963.
6. Cameron JR, Mazess RB, Sorenson JA: Precision and accuracy of bone mineral determination by direct photon absorptiometry. Invest Radiol 3:141, 1968.
7. Genant HK, Boyd D: Quantitative bone mineral analysis using dual energy computed tomography. Invest Radiol 12:545, 1977.
8. Reich NE, Seidelmann FE, Tubbs RR, et al: Determination of bone mineral content using CT scanning. AJR 127:593, 1976.
9. Posner I, Griffiths HJ: Comparison of CT scanning with photon absorptiometric measurement of bone mineral content in the appendicular skeleton. Invest Radiol 12:542, 1977.
10. Ruegsegger P, Elsasser U, Anliker M, et al: Quantification of bone mineralization using computed tomography. Radiology 121:93, 1976.
11. Bradley JG, Huang HK, Ledley RS: Evaluation of calcium concentration in bones from CT scans. Radiology 128:103, 1978.
12. Smith RW, Keiper DA: Dynamic measurement of the viscoelastic properties of bone. Am J Med Electron 4:156, 1965.
13. Selle WA, Jurist JM: Acoustical detection of senile osteoporosis. Proc Soc Exp Biol 121:150, 1966.
14. Lang FJ: Arthritis deformans und spondylitis deformans. In O Lubarsch, F Henke (Eds.): Handbuch der Spezieller Pathologischen Anatomie und Histologie. Berlin, Springer-Verlag, 1934.
15. Trueta J: Studies of the Development and Decay of the Human Frame. Philadelphia, WB Saunders Co, 1968, p 316.
16. Genant H: Osteoporosis. Bone Disease (Third Series) Syllabus. Chicago, American College of Radiology, 1980.
17. Meema S, Bunker ML, Meema HE: Preventive effect of estrogen on postmenopausal bone loss. Arch Intern Med 135:1436, 1975.
18. Smith RW Jr, Eyler WR, Mellinger RC: On the incidence of senile osteoporosis. Ann Intern Med 52:773, 1960.
19. Gershon-Cohen J, Rechtman AM, Shraer H, et al: Asymptomatic fractures in osteoporotic spines of the aged. JAMA 153:625, 1953.
20. Bernstein DS, Sadowsky N, Hegsted DM, et al: Prevalence of osteoporosis in high and low fluoride areas of North Dakota. JAMA 198:499, 1966.
21. Dunn AW: Senile osteoporosis. Geriatrics 22:175, 1967.
22. Urist MR, Zaccalini PS, MacDonald NS, et al: New approaches to the problem of osteoporosis. J Bone Joint Surg [Br] 44:464, 1962.
23. Stevens J, Freeman PA, Nordin BEC, et al: The incidence of osteoporosis in patients with femoral neck fracture. J Bone Joint Surg [Br] 44:520, 1962.
24. Stevens J, Abrami G: Osteoporosis in patients with femoral neck fractures. A follow-up study. J Bone Joint Surg [Br] 46:24, 1964.
25. Jowsey J: Quantitative microradiography. A new approach in the evaluation of metabolic bone disease. Am J Med 40:485, 1966.
26. Klein L, Lafferty FW, Pearson OH, et al: Correlation of urinary hydroxyproline, serum alkaline phosphatase and skeletal calcium turnover. Metabolism 13:272, 1964.
27. Potts JT Jr, Deftos LJ: Parathyroid hormone, calcitonin, vitamin D, bone and bone mineral metabolism. In PK Bondy, LE Rosenberg (Eds): Duncan's Diseases of Metabolism. Endocrinology. 7th Ed. Philadelphia, WB Saunders Co, 1974, p 1375.
28. Luckert BP, Bolinger RE, Meek JC: Acute effect of fluoride on 45-calcium dynamics in osteoporosis. J Clin Endocrinol Metab 27:828, 1967.
29. Avioli LV, McDonald JE, Lee SW: The influence of age on the intestinal absorption of ^{47}Ca in women and its relation to ^{47}Ca absorption in postmenopausal osteoporosis. J Clin Invest 44:1960, 1965.
30. Follis RH: Skeletal changes associated with hyperthyroidism. Bull Johns Hopkins Hosp 92:405, 1953.
31. Jowsey J, Riggs BL: Bone formation in hypercortisonism. Acta Endocrinol 63:21, 1970.
32. Frost HM, Villanueva AR: Human osteoblastic activity. III. The effect of cortisone on lamellar osteoblastic activity. Henry Ford Hosp Med Bull 9:97, 1961.
33. Thompson JS, Palmieri GMA, Crawford RL: The effect of porcine calcitonin on osteoporosis induced by adrenal cortical steroids. J Bone Joint Surg [Am] 54:1490, 1972.
34. Fucik RF, Kukreja SC, Hargis GK, et al: Effect of glucocorticoids on function of the parathyroid glands in man. J Clin Endocrinol Metab 40:152, 1975.
35. Hahn BH, Hahn TJ: Reduction of steroid osteopenia by treatment with 25-OH vitamin D and calcium (Abstr). Arthritis Rheum 19:800, 1976.
36. Collins EJ, Garrett ER, Johnston RL: Effect of adrenal steroids on radiocalcium metabolism in dogs. Metabolism 11:716, 1962.
37. Wajchenberg BL, Periera VG, Kieffer J, et al: Effect of dexamethasone on calcium metabolism and ^{47}Ca kinetics in normal subjects. Acta Endocrinol 61:173, 1969.
38. Krane SM, Brownell GL, Stanbury JB, et al: Effect of thyroid disease on calcium metabolism in man. J Clin Invest 35:874, 1956.
39. Bell NH, Bartter FC: Studies of ^{47}Ca metabolism in acromegaly. J Clin Endocrinol Metab 27:178, 1967.
40. Nordin BEC, Roper A: Post-pregnancy osteoporosis, a syndrome? Lancet 1:431, 1955.
41. Goldsmith NF, Johnston JO: Bone mineral: Effects of oral contraceptives, pregnancy and lactation. J Bone Joint Surg [Am] 57:657, 1975.
42. Griffith CC, Nichols G, Asher JD, et al: Heparin osteoporosis. JAMA 193:91, 1965.
43. Stinchfield FE, SanKaran B, Samilson R: Effect of anticoagulant therapy on bone repair. J Bone Joint Surg [Am] 38:270, 1956.
44. Goldhaber P: Heparin enhancement of factors stimulating bone resorption in tissue culture. Science 147:407, 1965.
45. Asher JD, Nichols G: Heparin stimulation of bone collagenase activity. Fed Proc 24:211, 1965.
46. Woods JF, Nichols G: Intracellular location of bone collagenase. Fed Proc 24:211, 1964.
47. Thompson RC Jr: Heparin osteoporosis. An experimental model using rats. J Bone Joint Surg [Am] 55:606, 1973.
48. Schuster J, Meier-Ruge W, Egli F: Zur Pathologie der Osteopathie nach Heparin behandlung. Dtsch Med Wochenschr 94:2334, 1969.
49. Sackler JP, Liu L: Heparin-induced osteoporosis. Br J Radiol 46:548, 1973.
50. Saville PD: Changes in bone mass with age and alcoholism. J Bone Joint Surg [Am] 47:492, 1965.
51. Dalen N, Feldreich AL: Osteopenia in alcoholism. Clin Orthop 99:201, 1974.
52. Nilsson BE, Westlin NE: Change in bone mass in alcoholics. Clin Orthop 90:229, 1973.
53. Dalen N, Lamke B: Bone mineral losses in alcoholics. Acta Orthop Scand 47:469, 1976.
54. Nilsson BE: Conditions contributing to fracture of the femoral neck. Acta Chir Scand 136:383, 1970.
55. Lowe WC, Labbate VA: The osteoporosis of cirrhosis. Clin Res 18:366, 1970.
56. Schippers JC: "Spontaneous" generalized osteoporosis in a girl 10 years old. Maandschr Kindergeneesk 8:108, 1938.
57. Berglund G, Lindquist B: Osteopenia in adolescence. Clin Orthop 17:259, 1960.

58. Dent CE, Friedman M: Idiopathic juvenile osteoporosis. Q J Med 34:177, 1965.
59. Houang MTW, Brenton DP, Renton P, et al: Idiopathic juvenile osteoporosis. Skel Radiol 3:17, 1978.
60. Jowsey J, Johnson KA: Juvenile osteoporosis: Bone findings in seven patients. J Pediatr 81:511, 1972.
61. Tseng CT, Daeschner CW, Singleton EB, et al: Liver diseases and osteoporosis in children. I. Clinical observations. J Pediatr 59:684, 1961.
62. Pottorf JL: An experimental study of bone growth in the dog. Anat Rec 10:234, 1916.
63. Armstrong WD: Bone growth in paralyzed limbs. Proc Soc Exp Biol Med 61:358, 1946.
64. Allison N, Brooks B: Bone atrophy. An experimental and clinical study of the changes in bone which result from non-use. Surg Gynaecol Obstet 33:250, 1921.
65. Burkhart JM, Jowsey J: Parathyroid and thyroid hormones in the development of immobilization osteoporosis. Endocrinology 81:1053, 1967.
66. Delling G, Schafer A, Schleicher HJ, et al: The effect of calcitonin on disuse atrophy of bone in the rat. Calcif Tissue Res 6:143, 1970.
67. Pennock J, Kalu DN, Clark MB, et al: Hypoplasia of bone induced by immobilization. Br J Radiol 45:641, 1972.
68. Whedon DG: Osteoporosis: Atrophy of disuse. In K Rodahl, et al (Eds): Bone as a Tissue. New York, McGraw-Hill Book Co, 1960.
69. Arnstein AR: Regional osteoporosis. Orthop Clin North Am 3:585, 1972.
70. Jones G: Radiological appearances of disuse osteoporosis. Clin Radiol 20:345, 1969.
71. Keats TE, Harrison RB: A pattern of post-traumatic demineralization of bone simulating permeative neoplastic replacement: A potential source of misinterpretation. Skel Radiol 3:113, 1978.
72. Bunts RC: Management of urologic complications in 1000 paraplegics. J Urol 79:733, 1958.
73. Heaney RP: Radiocalcium metabolism in disuse osteoporosis in man. Am J Med 33:188, 1962.
74. Mattsson S: The reversibility of disuse osteoporosis. Experimental studies in the adult rat. Acta Orthop Scand Suppl 144:5, 1972.
75. Dunning MF, Plum F: Hypercalciuria following poliomyelitis. Its relationship to site and degree of paralysis. Arch Intern Med 99:716, 1958.
76. Geiser M, Trueta J: Muscle action, bone rarefaction and bone formation. J Bone Joint Surg [Br] 40:282, 1958.
77. Evans EB, Eggers GWN, Butler JK, et al: Experimental immobilization and remobilization of rat knee joints. J Bone Joint Surg [Am] 42:737, 1960.
78. Hall MC: Cartilage changes after experimental immobilization of the knee joint of the young rat. J Bone Joint Surg [Am] 45:36, 1963.
79. Enneking WF, Horowitz M: The intra-articular effects of immobilization on the human knee. J Bone Joint Surg [Am] 54:973, 1972.
80. Mack PB, LaChance PA, Vose GP, et al: Bone demineralization of foot and hand of Gemini-Titan IV, V and VII astronauts during orbital flight. AJR 100:503, 1967.
81. Vose GP: Review of roentgenographic bone demineralization studies of the Gemini space flights. AJR 121:1, 1974.
82. Mitchell SW, Morehouse GR, Keen WW: Gunshot Wounds and Other Injuries of Nerves. Philadelphia, JB Lippincott, 1864.
83. Mitchell SW: Injuries of Nerves and Their Consequences. Philadelphia, JB Lippincott, 1872.
84. Sudeck P: Uber die akute (reflectorische) Knochenatrophie nach Entzundungen und Verletzungen an den Extremitaten und ihre Klinische Erscheinungen. ROFO 5:277, 1901–1902.
85. Lenggenhager K: Sudeck's osteodystrophy: Its pathogenesis, prophylaxis and therapy. Minn Med 54:967, 1971.
86. Fontaine R, Herrmann L: Post-traumatic painful osteoporosis. Ann Surg 97:26, 1933.
87. Morton JJ, Scott WJM: Some angiospastic syndromes in the extremities. Ann Surg 94:839, 1931.
88. Lehman EJP: Traumatic vasospasm: A study of 4 cases of vasospasm in the upper extremity. Arch Surg 29:92, 1934.
89. DeTakats G: Reflex dystrophy of the extremities. Arch Surg 34:939, 1937.
90. Homans J: Minor causalgia: A hyperesthetic neurovascular syndrome. N Engl J Med 222:870, 1940.
91. Johnson AC: Disabling changes in the hands resembling sclerodactylia following myocardial infarctions. Ann Intern Med 19:433, 1943.
92. Steinbrocker O: The shoulder-hand syndrome. Am J Med 3:403, 1947.
93. Steinbrocker O, Spitzer N, Friedman H: The shoulder-hand syndrome in reflex dystrophy of the upper extremity. Ann Intern Med 29:22, 1948.
94. Evans JA: Reflex sympathetic dystrophy: A report on 57 cases. Ann Intern Med 26:417, 1947.
95. Kozin F, McCarty DJ, Simms J, et al: The reflex sympathetic dystrophy syndrome. I. Clinical and histologic studies: Evidence for bilaterality, response to corticosteroids and articular involvement. Am J Med 60:321, 1976.
96. Kozin F, Genant H, Bekerman C, et al: The reflex sympathetic dystrophy syndrome. II. Roentgenographic and scintigraphic evidence of bilaterality and of peri-articular accentuation. Am J Med 60:332, 1976.
97. Genant HK, Kozin F, Bekerman C, et al: The reflex sympathetic dystrophy syndrome. A comprehensive analysis using fine-detail radiography, photon absorptiometry and bone and joint scintigraphy. Radiology 117:21, 1975.
98. Lorente de No R: Analysis of the activity of the chains of internuncial neurons. J Neurophysiol 1:207, 1938.
99. Doupe J, Cullen CH, Chance CQ: Post-traumatic pain and causalgic syndrome. J Neurol Neurosurg Psychiatry 7:33, 1944.
100. Miller DS, DeTakats G: Post-traumatic dystrophy of the extremities: Sudeck's atrophy. Surg Gynecol Obstet 75:558, 1942.
101. Stolte BH, Stolte JB, Leyten JF: De pathofysiologie van het schouderhandsyndroom. Nederl T Geneesk 114:1208, 1970.
102. Steinbrocker O: The painful shoulder. In JL Hollander, DJ McCarty Jr (Eds): Arthritis and Allied Conditions. 8th Ed. Philadelphia, Lea & Febiger, 1972, p 1461.
103. Kutzner J, Hahn K, Grimm W, et al: Skelettszintigraphische Untersuchungen bei der Sudeckschen Knochendystrophie. ROFO 121:361, 1974.
104. McCarty DJ, Polcyn RE, Collins PA, et al: 99mTechnetium scintiphotography in arthritis. I. Technique and interpretation. Arthritis Rheum 13:11, 1970.
105. Genant HK, Bautovich GJ, Singh M, et al: Bone-seeking radionuclides: An in vivo study of factors affecting skeletal uptake. Radiology 113:373, 1974.
106. Rosen PS, Graham W: The shoulder-hand syndrome: Historical review with observations on 73 patients. Can Med Assoc J 77:86, 1957.
107. Thompson M: The shoulder-hand syndrome. Proc Roy Soc Med 54:679, 1961.
108. Finsterbush A, Friedman B: Early changes in immobilized rabbit knee joints: A light and electron microscopic study. Clin Orthop 92:305, 1973.
109. Folkerts JF, Wiertz-Hoessels ELMJ, Krediet P, et al: Reflex sympathetic dystrophy: A clinical, histological, histochemical, and experimental study. Confin Neurol 31:145, 1969.
110. Curtiss PH Jr, Kincaid WE: Transitory demineralization of the hip in pregnancy. J Bone Joint Surg [Am] 41:1327, 1959.
111. Hunder GG, Kelly PJ: Roentgenologic transient osteoporosis of the hip. A clinical syndrome? Ann Intern Med 68:539, 1968.
112. Longstreth PL, Malinak LR, Hill CS: Transient osteoporosis of the hip in pregnancy. Obstet Gynecol 41:563, 1973.
113. Rosen RA: Transitory demineralization of the femoral head. Radiology 94:509, 1970.
114. Beaulieu JG, Razzano D, Levine RB: Transient osteoporosis of the hip in pregnancy. Review of the literature and a case report. Clin Orthop 115:165, 1976.
115. Pantazopoulos T, Exarchou E, Hartofilikidis-Garofalidis G: Idiopathic transient osteoporosis of the hip. J Bone Joint Surg [Am] 55:315, 1973.
116. DeMarchi E, Santacroce A, Solarino GB: Su di una peculiare artropatia rarefacente dell'anca. Arch Putti Chir Organi Mov 21:62, 1966.
117. Lequesne M: L'algodystrophie de la hanche. Presse Med 76:793, 1968.
118. Lequesne M: Transient osteoporosis of the hip. A nontraumatic variety of Sudeck's atrophy. Ann Rheum Dis 27:463, 1968.
119. Valenzuela F, Aris H, Jacobelli S: Transient osteoporosis of the hip. J Rheumatol 4:59, 1977.
120. Karasick D, Edeiken J: Case report 19. Skel Radiol 1:181, 1977.
121. Swezey RL: Transient osteoporosis of the hip, foot and knee. Arthritis Rheum 13:858, 1970.
122. Duncan H, Frame B, Frost H, et al: Regional migratory osteoporosis. South Med J 62:41, 1969.
123. Steiner RM, McKeever C: Regional migratory osteoporosis. J Can Assoc Radiol 24:70, 1973.
124. Gupta RC, Popovtzer MM, Huffer WE, et al: Regional migratory osteoporosis. Arthritis Rheum 16:363, 1973.
125. McCord WC, Nies KM, Campion DS, et al: Regional migratory osteoporosis. A denervation disease. Arthritis Rheum 21:834, 1978.
126. Langloh ND, Hunder GG, Riggs BL, et al: Transient painful osteoporosis of the lower extremities. J Bone Joint Surg [Am] 55:1188, 1973.
127. Durivage J, Levesque H-P: L'osteoporose douloureuse transitoire. Union Med Can 105:562, 1976.
128. Levy D, Hinterbuckner C: Transient or migratory osteoporosis of lower extremity. NY State J Med 76:739, 1976.
129. O'Mara RE, Pinals RS: Bone scanning in regional migratory osteoporosis. Case report. Radiology 97:579, 1970.
130. Renier JC: Les algodystrophies du membre inférieur et leur traitement. Rev Practicien 8:3835, 1958.
131. Corbett M, Colston JR, Tucker AK: Pain in the knee associated with osteoporosis of the patella. Ann Rheum Dis 36:188, 1977.
132. Lequesne M, Kerboull M, Bensasson M, et al: Partial transient osteoporosis. Skel Radiol 2:1, 1977.
133. Reynolds WA, Karo JJ: Radiologic diagnosis of metabolic bone disease. Orthop Clin North Am 3:521, 1972.
134. Steinbach HL: The roentgen appearance of osteoporosis. Radiol Clin North Am 2:191, 1964.
135. Parfitt AM, Duncan H: Metabolic bone disease affecting the spine. In RH Rothman, FA Simeone (Eds): The Spine. Philadelphia, WB Saunders Co, 1975, p 599.
136. Ardran GM: Bone destruction not demonstrable by radiography. Br J Radiol 24:107, 1951.
137. Hurxthal LM: Measurement of anterior vertebral compressions and biconcave vertebrae. AJR 103:635, 1968.
138. Brandner ME: Normal values of the vertebral body and intervertebral disc index in adults. AJR 114:411, 1972.
139. Barnett E, Nordin BEC: The radiologic diagnosis of osteoporosis: A new approach. Clin Radiol 11:166, 1960.
140. Dietz GW, Christensen EE: Normal "cupid's bow" contour of the lower lumbar vertebrae. Radiology 121:577, 1976.

141. Schmorl G, Junghanns H: The Human Spine in Health and Disease. 2nd Ed. New York, Grune & Stratton, 1971, pp 2, 158.
142. Chalmers J: Osteomalacia. J R Coll Surg Edinb 13:255, 1968.
143. Coventry MB, Ghormley RK, Kernohan JW: Intervertebral disc; its microscopic anatomy and pathology. Changes in the intervertebral disc concomitant with age. J Bone Joint Surg 27:233, 1945.
144. Resnick D, Niwayama G: Intravertebral disk herniations: Cartilaginous (Schmorl's) nodes. Radiology 126:57, 1978.
145. Hassler O: The human intervertebral disc. A microangiographical study on its vascular supply at various stages. Acta Orthop Scand 40:765, 1970.
146. Coventry MB, Ghormley RK, Kernohan JW: Intervertebral disc; its microscopic anatomy and pathology; pathological changes in the intervertebral disc. J Bone Joint Surg 27:460, 1945.
147. Batts M Jr: Rupture of the nucleus pulposus: An anatomical study. J Bone Joint Surg 21:121, 1939.
148. Hilton RC, Ball J, Benn RT: Vertebral end-plate lesions (Schmorl's nodes) in the dorsolumbar spine. Ann Rheum Dis 35:127, 1976.
149. Geist ES: The intervertebral disc. JAMA 96:1696, 1931.
150. Boukhris R, Becker KL: Schmorl's nodes and osteoporosis. Clin Orthop 104:275, 1974.
151. Singh M, Nagrath AR, Maini PS: Changes in trabecular pattern of the upper end of the femur as an index of osteoporosis. J Bone Joint Surg [Am] 52:457, 1970.
152. Siffert RS: Trabecular patterns in bone. AJR 99:746, 1967.
153. Singh M, Riggs B, Beabout JW, et al: Femoral trabecular pattern index for evaluation of spinal osteoporosis. Ann Intern Med 77:63, 1972.
154. Dequeker J, Gautama K, Roh YS: Femoral trabecular patterns in asymptomatic spinal osteoporosis and femoral neck fracture. Clin Radiol 25:243, 1974.
155. Roh YS, Dequeker J, Mulier JC: Trabecular pattern of the upper end of the femur in primary osteoarthrosis and in symptomatic osteoporosis. J Belge Radiol 57:89, 1974.
156. Kranendonk DH, Jurist JM, Lee HG: Femoral trabecular patterns and bone mineral content. J Bone Joint Surg [Am] 54:1472, 1972.
157. Khairi MRA, Cronin JH, Robb JA, et al: Femoral trabecular pattern index and bone mineral content measurement by photon absorption in senile osteoporosis. J Bone Joint Surg [Am] 58:221, 1976.
158. Wilson CR: Bone-mineral content of the femoral neck and spine versus the radius or ulna. J Bone Joint Surg [Am] 59:665, 1977.
159. Dalen N, Lars-Gosta H, Jacobson B: Bone mineral content and mechanical strength of the femoral neck. Acta Orthop Scand 47:503, 1976.
160. Garn SM, Poznanski AK, Nagy JM: Bone measurement in the differential diagnosis of osteopenia and osteoporosis. Radiology 100:509, 1971.
161. Evans RA, McDonnell GD, Schieb M: Metacarpal cortical area as an index of bone mass. Br J Radiol 51:428, 1978.
162. Dequeker J: Quantitative radiology: Radiogrammetry of cortical bone. Br J Radiol 49:912, 1976.
163. Robertson A: A look at bone. Australas Radiol 20:346, 1976.
164. Meema HE: Radiology of osteoporosis. Ther Umsch 34:628, 1977.
165. Meema HE: Recognition of cortical bone resorption in metabolic bone disease in vivo. Skel Radiol 2:11, 1977.
166. Meema HE, Meema S: Comparison of microradioscopic and morphometric findings in the hand bones with densitometric findings in the proximal radius in thyrotoxicosis and in renal osteodystrophy. Invest Radiol 7:88, 1972.
167. Meema HE, Meema S: Improved roentgenologic diagnosis of osteomalacia by microradioscopy of hand bones. AJR 125:925, 1975.
168. Frost HM: Bone Remodelling and Its Relationship to Metabolic Bone Diseases. Springfield, Ill, Charles C Thomas, 1973.
169. Jaworski ZF, Lok E: The rate of osteosclerosis bone erosion in haversian remodelling sites of adult dog's rib. Calcif Tissue Res 10:103, 1972.
170. Villaneuva AR, Ilnicki L, Duncan J, et al: Bone and cell dynamics in the osteoporoses: A review of measurements by tetracycline bone-labelling. Clin Orthop 49:135, 1966.
171. Forrester DM, Kirkpatrick J: Periostitis and pseudoperiostitis. Radiology 118:597, 1976.
172. Dequeker J: Bone Loss in Normal and Pathological Conditions. Leuven, University Press, 1972.
173. Garn SM: Earlier Gain and Later Loss of Cortical Bone. Springfield, Ill, Charles C Thomas, 1970.
174. Lusted LB, Keats TE: Atlas of Roentgenographic Measurement. 3rd Ed. Chicago, Year Book Medical Publishers, 1972, p 138.
175. Steinbach HL, Gold RH, Preger L: Roentgen Appearance of the Hand in Diffuse Disease. Chicago, Year Book Medical Publishers, 1975, p 32.
176. Schworer I, Schmidtkunz U: Die bandformige Osteoporose. ROFO 128:264, 1978.
177. Mitchell DC: Fractures in brittle bone diseases. Orthop Clin North Am 3:787, 1972.
178. Kim JH, Kozin F, Johnson RP, et al: Reflex sympathetic dystrophy syndrome of the knee following meniscectomy. Report of three cases. Arthritis Rheum 22:177, 1979.
179. Wilson JS, Genant HK: In vivo assessment of bone metabolism using the cortical striation index. Invest Radiol 14:131, 1979.
180. Lagier R, Van Linthoudt D: Dystrophie de Sudeck de l'arriere-pied. Confrontation anatomo-radiologique. Ann Radiol 21:539, 1978.
181. Strashun A, Chayes Z: Migratory osteolysis. J Nucl Med 20:129, 1979.
182. Ryan LM, Carrera GF, Soin JS, et al: Radiographic and scintigraphic changes in patients with the reflex sympathetic dystrophy syndrome (Abstr). Arthritis Rheum 23:741, 1980.
183. Tannenbaum H, Esdaile J, Rosenthal L: Joint imaging in regional migratory osteoporosis (Abstr). Arthritis Rheum 23:754, 1980.
184. Martin VM: Reflex sympathetic dystrophy syndrome of the knee after meniscectomy. Arthritis Rheum 23:780, 1980.
185. Louis DS, Hartwig RH, Poznanski AK: Case report 116. Skel Radiol 5:127, 1980.
186. Tannenbaum H, Esdaile J, Rosenthall L: Joint imaging in regional migratory osteoporosis. J Rheumatol 7:237, 1980.
187. Helms CA, O'Brien ET, Katzberg RW: Segmental reflex sympathetic dystrophy syndrome. Radiology 135:67, 1980.
188. Simon H, Carlson DH: The use of bone scanning in the diagnosis of reflex sympathetic dystrophy. Clin Nucl Med 5:116, 1980.
189. Lagier R, Van Linthoudt D: Articular changes due to disuse in Sudeck's atrophy. Int Orthop (SICOT) 3:1, 1979.
190. Gaucher A, Colomb J-N, Naoun AR, et al: The diagnostic value of 99mTc-diphosphonate bone imaging in transient osteoporosis of the hip. J Rheumatol 6:574, 1979.
191. Bray ST, Partain L, Teates CD, et al: The value of the bone scan in idiopathic regional migratory osteoporosis. J Nucl Med 20:1268, 1979.
192. Squires JW, Pinch LW: Heparin-induced spinal fracture. JAMA 241:2417, 1979.
193. Rico H, Del Rio A, Vila T, et al: The role of growth hormone in the pathogenesis of postmenopausal osteoporosis. Arch Intern Med 139:1263, 1979.
194. Jensen PS, Orphanoudakis SC, Rauschkolb EN, et al: Assessment of bone mass in the radius by computed tomography. AJR 134:285, 1980.
195. Elsasser U, Ruegsegger P, Anliker M, et al: Loss and recovery of trabecular bone in the distal radius following fracture—immobilization of the upper limb in children. Klin Wochenschr 57:763, 1979.
196. Jaworski ZFG, Liskova-Kiar M, Uhthoff HK: Effect of long-term immobilization on the pattern of bone loss in older dogs. J Bone Joint Surg [Br] 62:104, 1980.
197. Cann CE, Genant HK, Young DR: Comparison of vertebral and peripheral mineral losses in disuse osteoporosis in monkeys. Radiology 134:525, 1980.
198. Doherty M, Watt I, Dieppe P: Apparent bone erosions in painful regional osteoporosis. Rheumatol Rehabil 19:95, 1980.
199. Bloom RA: A comparative estimation of the combined cortical thickness of various bone sites. Skel Radiol 5:167, 1980.
200. Lukert BP: Osteoporosis—a review and update. Arch Phys Med Rehabil 63:480, 1982.
201. Einhorn TA: Osteoporosis and metabolic bone disease. Adv Orthop Surg, 1984, p 175.
202. Lane JM, Vigorita VJ: Osteoporosis. J Bone Joint Surg [Am] 65:274, 1983.
203. Lane JM, Vigorita VJ: Osteoporosis. Orthop Clin North Am 15:711, 1984.
204. Lindsay R, Dempster DW: Osteoporosis: Current concepts. Bull NY Acad Med 61:307, 1985.
205. Smith E: Exercise for prevention for osteoporosis: A review. Phys Sports Med 10:72, 1982.
206. Mazess RB: Measurement of skeletal status by noninvasive methods. Calcif Tissue Int 28:89, 1979.
207. Mazess RB: On aging bone loss. Clin Orthop 165:239, 1982.
208. Keshawarz NM, Recker RR: Expansion of the medullary cavity at the expense of cortex in postmenopausal osteoporosis. Metab Bone Dis Rel Res 5:223, 1984.
209. Ruegsegger P, Dambacher MA, Ruegsegger E, et al: Bone loss in premenopausal and postmenopausal women. J Bone Joint Surg [Am] 66:1015, 1984.
210. Albright F, Bloomberg E, Smith PH: Post-menopausal osteoporosis. Trans Assoc Am Physicians 55:298, 1940.
211. Aloia JF, Vaswani AN, Yeh JK, et al: Determinants of bone mass in postmenopausal women. Arch Intern Med 143:1700, 1983.
212. Genant HK, Cann CE, Ettinger B, et al: Quantitative computed tomography of vertebral spongiosa: A sensitive method for detecting early bone loss after oophorectomy. Ann Intern Med 97:699, 1982.
213. Heaney RP: Calcium metabolic changes at menopause—their possible relationship to post-menopausal osteoporosis. In US Barzel (Ed): Osteoporosis II. New York, Grune & Stratton, 1979, p 101.
214. Tiegs RD, Body JJ, Wahner HW, et al: Calcitonin secretion in postmenopausal osteoporosis. N Engl J Med 312:1097, 1985.
215. Specht EE: Hip fracture, skeletal fragility, osteoporosis and hormonal deprivation in elderly women. West J Med 133:297, 1980.
216. Marcus R, Cann C, Madvig P, et al: Menstrual function and bone mass in elite women distance runners. Endocrine and metabolic features. Ann Intern Med 102:158, 1985.
217. Cann CE, Martin MC, Genant HK, et al: Decreased spinal mineral content in amenorrheic women. JAMA 251:626, 1984.
218. Hahn TJ: Drug-induced disorders of vitamin D and mineral metabolism. Clin Endocrinol Metab 9:107, 1980.
219. Gruber HE, Gutteridge DH, Baylink DJ: Osteoporosis associated with pregnancy and lactation: Bone biopsy and skeletal features in three patients. Metab Bone Dis Rel Res 5:159, 1984.
220. Megard M, Cuche M, Grapeloux A, et al: Ostéoporose de l'héparinotherapie. Nouv Presse Med 11:261, 1982.
221. Rafii M, Firooznia H, Golimbu C, et al: Pathologic fracture in systemic mastocytosis. Radiographic spectrum and review of the literature. Clin Orthop 180:260, 1983.

222. Bikle DD, Genant HK, Cann C, et al: Bone disease in alcohol abuse. Ann Intern Med 103:42, 1985.
223. De Vernejoul MC, Bielakoff J, Herve M, et al: Evidence for defective osteoblastic function. A role for alcohol and tobacco consumption in osteoporosis in middle-aged men. Clin Orthop 179:107, 1983.
224. Johnell O, Nilsson BE, Wiklund PE: Bone morphometry in alcoholics. Clin Orthop 165:253, 1982.
225. Exner GU, Prader A, Elsasser U, et al: Idiopathic osteoporosis in a three-year old girl. Helv Paediatr Acta 39:517, 1984.
226. Smith R: Idiopathic osteoporosis in the young. J Bone Joint Surg [Br] 62:417, 1980.
227. Towbin R, Dunbar JS: Generalized osteoporosis with multiple fractures in an adolescent. Invest Radiol 16:171, 1981.
228. Jones ET, Hensinger RN: Spinal deformity in idiopathic juvenile osteoporosis. Spine 6:1, 1981.
229. Bartal E, Gage JR: Idiopathic juvenile osteoporosis and scoliosis. J Pediatr Orthop 2:295, 1982.
230. Chase HP, Kumar V, Caldwell RT, et al: Kwashiorkor in the United States. Pediatrics 66:972, 1980.
231. Rigotti NA, Nussbaum SR, Herzog DB, et al: Osteoporosis in women with anorexia nervosa. N Engl J Med 311:1601, 1984.
232. Kirchner SG, Sivit DJ, Wright PF: Hyperimmunoglobulinemia E syndrome: Association with osteoporosis and recurrent fractures. Radiology 156:362, 1985.
233. Kato Y, Epstein O, Dick R, et al: Radiological patterns of cortical bone modelling in women with chronic liver disease. Clin Radiol 33:313, 1982.
234. Wronski TJ, Morey ER: Inhibition of cortical and trabecular bone formation in the long bones of immobilized monkeys. Clin Orthop 181:269, 1983.
235. Minaire P, Meunier P, Edouard C, et al: Histomorphometric study of acute osteoporosis in paraplegic patients. Paraplegia 20:281, 1982.
236. Mazess RB, Whedon GD: Immobilization and bone. Calcif Tissue Int 35:265, 1983.
237. Bernini PM, Simeone FA: Reflex sympathetic dystrophy associated with low lumbar disc herniation. Spine 6:180, 1981.
238. Wysenbeek AJ, Calabrese LH, Scherbel AL: Reflex sympathetic dystrophy syndrome complicating polymyalgia rheumatica. Arthritis Rheum 24:863, 1981.
239. Michaels RM, Sorber JA: Reflex sympathetic dystrophy as a probable paraneoplastic syndrome: Case report and literature review. Arthritis Rheum 27:1183, 1984.
240. Taggart AJ, Iveson JMI, Wright V: Shoulder-hand syndrome and symmetrical arthralgia in patients with tubo-ovarian carcinoma. Ann Rheum Dis 43:391, 1984.
241. Medsger TA Jr, Dixon JA, Garwood VF: Palmar fasciitis and polyarthritis associated with ovarian carcinoma. Ann Intern Med 96:424, 1982.
242. Ruggeri SB, Athreya BH, Doughty R, et al: Reflex sympathetic dystrophy in children. Clin Orthop 163:225, 1982.
243. Rush PJ, Wilmot D, Saunders N, et al: Severe reflex neurovascular dystrophy in childhood. Arthritis Rheum 28:952, 1985.
244. Karasick S, Karasick D: Case report 193. Skel Radiol 8:151, 1982.
245. Lagier R: Partial algodystrophy of the knee. An anatomico-radiological study of one case. J Rheumatol 10:255, 1983.
246. Doury P: Les formes atypiques partielles, parcellaires et infraradiologiques des algodystrophies. Rev Rhum Mal Osteoartic 49:781, 1982.
247. Lagier R: Post-traumatic Sudeck's dystrophy localized in the metatarsophalangeal region. ROFO 138:496, 1983.
248. Arlet J, Ficat P, Durroux R, et al: The histopathology of bone and cartilaginous lesions in reflex sympathetic dystrophy (RSD) of the knee. Sixteen cases. Rev Rhum Mal Osteoartic 49:208, 1982.
249. Basle MF, Rebel A, Renier JC: Bone tissue in reflex sympathetic dystrophy syndrome—Sudeck's atrophy; structural and ultrastructural studies. Metab Bone Dis Rel Res 4:305, 1983.
250. Brower AC, Allman RM: Vascular influence on patterns of deossification. Arthritis Rheum 25:333, 1982.
251. Betend B, Lebacq E, Kohler R, et al: Osteolyse metaphysaire. Aspect inhabituel de l'algodystrophie reflexe de l'enfant. Arch Fr Pediatr 38:121, 1981.
252. Kozin F, Soin JS, Ryan LM, et al: Bone scintigraphy in the reflex sympathetic dystrophy syndrome. Radiology 138:437, 1981.
253. Gaucher A, Raul P, Wiederkehr P, et al: Bone scan study of reflex sympathetic dystrophy. Rev Rhum Mal Osteoartic 50:409, 1983.
254. Mackinnon SE, Holder LE: The use of three-phase radionuclide bone scanning in the diagnosis of reflex sympathetic dystrophy. J Hand Surg [Am] 9:556, 1984.
255. Holder LE, Mackinnon SE: Reflex sympathetic dystrophy in the hands: clinical and scintigraphic criteria. Radiology 152:517, 1984.
256. Laxer RM, Allen RC, Malleson PN, et al: Technetium-99m methylene diphosphonate bone scans in children with reflex neurovascular dystrophy. J Pediatr 106:437, 1985.
257. Doury P, Granier R, Pattin S, et al: Algodystrophie avec hypofixation à la scintigraphie osseuse par les pyrophosphates de technetium-99m. Sem Hop Paris 57:1325, 1981.
258. Naides S, Resnick D, Zvaifler N: Idiopathic regional osteoporosis. J Rheumatol 12:763, 1985.
259. Lequesne M, Mauger M: 100 cases of transient osteoporosis of the hip in 74 patients. Rev Rhum Mal Osteoartic 50:401, 1983.
260. Albert J, Ott H: Three brothers with algodystrophy of the hip. Ann Rheum Dis 42:411, 1983.
261. Nicol RO, Williams PF, Hill DJ: Transient osteopaenia of the hip in children. J Pediatr Orthop 4:590, 1984.
262. Dihlmann W, Thomas W: Diagnostischer Algorithmus für die transitorische Hüftosteoporose—unter Einbeziehung der Computertomographie. ROFO 138:214, 1983.
263. Dihlmann W, Delling G: Ist die transitorische Huftosteoporose eine transitorische Osteonekrose? Z Rheumatol 44:82, 1985.
264. Kaplan SS, Stegman CJ: Transient osteoporosis of the hip. A case report and review of the literature. J Bone Joint Surg [Am] 67:490, 1985.
265. Byrd JW, Ricciardi JM, Jung BI: Regional migratory osteoporosis and tarsal tunnel syndrome. Clin Orthop 157:164, 1981.
266. Jacox RF, Waterhouse C, Taves DR: Transient painful osteolysis—a metabolic study. J Rheumatol 9:279, 1982.
267. Pitt M: Osteopenic bone disease. Orthop Clin North Am 14:65, 1983.
268. Hansson T, Roos B: Microcalluses of the trabeculae in lumbar vertebrae and their relation to the bone mineral content. Spine 6:375, 1981.
269. Resnick DL: Fish vertebrae. Arthritis Rheum 25:1073, 1982.
270. Ramirez H Jr, Navarro JE, Bennett WF: "Cupid's bow" contour of the lumbar vertebral endplates detected by computed tomography. J Comput Assist Tomogr 8:121, 1984.
271. Firooznia H, Tyler I, Golimbu C, et al: Computerized tomography of the cupid's bow contour of the lumbar spine. Comput Radiol 7:347, 1983.
272. Hansson T, Roos B: The amount of bone mineral and Schmorl's nodes in lumbar vertebrae. Spine 8:266, 1983.
273. Osborne D, Effmann E: Disturbances of trabecular architecture in the upper end of the femur in childhood. Skel Radiol 6:165, 1981.
274. Horsman A, Nordin C, Simpson M, et al: Cortical and trabecular bone status in elderly women with femoral neck fracture. Clin Orthop 166:143, 1982.
275. Seror P, Sebert JL, Rouleau L, et al: L'indice fémoral de Singh dans l'ostéoporose vertébrale. Sem Hop Paris 58:2315, 1982.
276. Wicks M, Garrett R, Vernon-Roberts B, et al: Absence of metabolic bone disease in the proximal femur in patients with fracture of the femoral neck. J Bone Joint Surg [Br] 64:319, 1982.
277. Kovarik J, Kuster W, Seidl G, et al: Clinical relevance of radiologic examination of the skeleton and bone density measurements in osteoporosis of old age. Skel Radiol 7:37, 1981.
278. Pogrund H, Rigal WM, Makin M, et al: Determination of osteoporosis in patients with fractured femoral neck using the Singh index: A Jerusalem study. Clin Orthop 156:189, 1981.
279. Frost HM: The osteoporoses in the late 1980's: A field in flux. IM 3:65, 1982.
280. Courpron P: Bone tissue mechanisms underlying osteoporoses. Orthop Clin North Am 12:513, 1981.
281. Bloom RA, Pogrund H, Libson E: Radiogrammetry of the metacarpal: A critical reappraisal. Skel Radiol 10:5, 1981.
282. Bloom RA, Pogrund H: Humeral cortical thickness in female Bantu—its relationship to the incidence of femoral neck fracture. Skel Radiol 8:59, 1982.
283. Hermanutz KD, Ehlenz P, Verburg B: Morphometrie und Bestimmung kortikodiaphyser Indizes Klavikula im konventionellen Thoraxröntgenbild bei Gesunden und Knockenerkrankungen. ROFO 137:281, 1982.
284. Bras J, Van Ooij CP, Abraham-Inpijn L, et al: Radiographic interpretation of the mandibular angular cortex: A diagnostic tool in metabolic bone loss. Part I. Normal state. Oral Surg Oral Med Oral Pathol 53:541, 1982.
285. Bras J, Van Ooij CP, Abraham-Inpijn L, et al: Radiographic interpretation of the mandibular angular cortex: A diagnostic tool in metabolic bone loss. Part II. Renal osteodystrophy. Oral Surg Oral Med Oral Pathol 53:647, 1982.
286. Jhamaria NL, Lal KB, Udawat M, et al: The trabecular pattern of the calcaneum as an index of osteoporosis. J Bone Joint Surg [Br] 65:195, 1983.
287. Cockshott WP, Occleshaw CJ, Webber C, et al: Can a calcaneal morphologic index determine the degree of osteoporosis? Skel Radiol 12:119, 1984.
288. Cummings SR: Are patients with hip fractures more osteoporotic? Review of the evidence. Am J Med 78:487, 1985.
289. Evans RA, Ashwell JR, Dunstan CR: Lack of metabolic bone disease in patients with fracture of the femoral neck. Aust NZ J Med 11:158, 1981.
290. De Smet AA, Neff JR: Pubic and sacral insufficiency fractures: clinical course and radiologic findings. AJR 145:601, 1985.
291. Staple TW: Postfracture pubic osteolysis simulating malignancy. AJR 143:433, 1984.
292. Casey D, Mirra J, Staple TW: Parasymphyseal insufficiency fractures of the os pubis. AJR 142:581, 1984.
293. Cooper KL, Beabout JW, Swee RG: Insufficiency fractures of the sacrum. Radiology 156:15, 1985.
294. Lourie H: Spontaneous osteoporotic fracture of the sacrum. An unrecognized syndrome of the elderly. JAMA 248:715, 1982.
295. Schneider R, Yacovone J, Ghelman B: Unsuspected sacral fractures: Detection by radionuclide bone scanning. AJR 144:337, 1985.
296. Cooper KL, Beabout JW, McLeod RA: Supraacetabular insufficiency fractures. Radiology 157:15, 1985.
297. Dorne HL, Lander PH: Spontaneous stress fracture of the femoral neck. AJR 144:343, 1985.
298. Bauer G, Gustafsson M, Mortensson W, et al: Insufficiency fractures in the tibial condyles in elderly individuals. Acta Radiol (Diagn) 22:619, 1981.
299. Manco LG, Schneider R, Pavlov H: Insufficiency fractures of the tibial plateau. AJR 140:1211, 1983.
300. Itani M, Evans GA, Park WM: Spontaneous sternal collapse. J Bone Joint Surg [Br] 64:432, 1982.
301. Koch JG: The laws of bone architecture. Am J Anat 21:177, 1917.

302. Pugh JW, Rose RM, Radin EL: Elastic and viscoelastic properties of trabecular bone: Dependence on structure. J Biomech 6:475, 1973.

303. Jee WSS: The skeletal tissues. *In* L Weiss (Ed): Histology: Cell and Tissue Biology. The Skeletal Tissues. New York: Elsevier Biomedical, 1983, p 200.

304. Garn SM, Silverman FN, Hertzog KP, et al: Lines and bands of increased density. Med Radiogr Photogr 44:58, 1968.

305. Levy J, Berdon WE, Abramson SJ: Epiphyseal separation simulating pyarthrosis, secondary to copper deficiency, in an infant receiving total parenteral nutrition. Br J Radiol 57:636, 1984.

306. Gefter WB, Epstein DM, Anday EK, et al: Rickets presenting as multiple fractures in premature infants on hyperalimentation. Radiology 142:371, 1982.

307. Polisson RP, Martinez S, Khoury M, et al: Calcification of entheses associated with X-linked hypophosphatemic osteomalacia. N Engl J Med 313:1, 1985.

308. Frame B, Frost HM, Ormond RS, et al: Atypical osteomalacia involving the axial skeleton. Ann Intern Med 55:632, 1961.

309. Whyte MP, Fallon MD, Murphy WA, et al: Axial osteomalacia. Clinical, laboratory and genetic investigation of an affected mother and son. Am J Med 71:1041, 1981.

310. Nelson AM, Riggs BL, Jowsey JO: Atypical axial osteomalacia. Report of four cases with two having features of ankylosing spondylitis. Arthritis Rheum 21:715, 1978.

311. Baker SL, Dent CE, Friedman M, et al: Fibrogenesis imperfecta ossium. J Bone Joint Surg [Br] 48:804, 1966.

312. Golding FC: Fibrogenesis imperfecta. J Bone Joint Surg [Br] 50:619, 1968.

313. Stoddart PGP, Wickrematchi T, Hollingworth P, et al: Fibrogenesis imperfecta ossium. Br J Radiol 57:744, 1984.

314. Byers PD, Stamp TCB, Stoker DJ: Case report 296. Skel Radiol 13:72, 1985.

315. Crosby LO, Kaplan FS, Pertschuk MJ, et al: The effect of anorexia nervosa on bone morphometry in young women. Clin Orthop 201:271, 1985.

316. Goldberg E, Dobransky R, Gill R: Reflex sympathetic dystrophy associated with malignancy. Arthritis Rheum 26:1079, 1985.

317. Tsuji H, Yoshioka T, Sainoh H: Developmental balloon disc of the lumbar spine in healthy subjects. Spine 10:907, 1986.

318. Cooper C, Barker DJP, Hall AJ: Evaluation of the Singh index and femoral calcar width as epidemiological methods for measuring bone mass in the femoral neck. Clin Radiol 37:123, 1986.

319. Joyce JM, Keats TE: Disuse osteoporosis: Mimic of neoplastic disease. Skel Radiol 15:129, 1986.

320. Härmä M, Karjalainen P: Trabecular osteopenia in Colles' fracture. Acta Orthop Scand 57:38, 1986.

321. Härmä M, Karjalainen P, Hoikka V, et al: Bone density in women with spinal and hip fractures. Acta Orthop Scand 56:380, 1985.

322. Firooznia H, Rafii M, Golimbu C, et al: Trabecular mineral content of the spine in women with hip fracture: CT measurement. Radiology 159:737, 1986.

323. Hohmann EL, Elde RP, Rysavy JA, et al: Innervation of periosteum and bone by sympathetic vasoactive intestinal peptide–containing nerve fibers. Science 232:868, 1986.

324. Gerster J-C, Jaeger P, Gobelet C, et al: Adult sporadic hypophosphatemic osteomalacia presenting as regional migratory osteoporosis. Arthritis Rheum 29:688, 1986.

325. Goto S, Uhthoff HK: Notochord action on spinal development. A histologic and morphometric investigation. Acta Orthop Scand 57:85, 1985.

326. Kerr R, Resnick D, Sartoris DJ, et al: Computed tomography of proximal femoral trabecular patterns. J Orthop Res 4:45, 1986.

327. Kaplan FS, Pertschuk M, Fallon M, et al: Osteoporosis and hip fracture in a young woman with anorexia nervosa. Clin Orthop 212:250, 1986.

328. Lang R, Vignery AMC, Jensen PS: Fibrogenesis imperfecta ossium with early onset: Observations after 20 years of illness. Bone 7:237, 1986.

329. Tietjen R: Reflex sympathetic dystrophy of the knee. Clin Orthop 209:234, 1986.

330. Ross PD, Wasnich RD, Vogel JM: Precision error in dual-photon absorptiometry related to source age. Radiology 166:523, 1988.

331. Glüer C-C, Steiger P, Genant H: Validity of dual-photon absorptiometry. Radiology 166:574, 1988.

332. Bohr HH, Schaadt O: Mineral content of upper tibia assessed by dual photon densitometry. Acta Orthop Scand 58:557, 1987.

333. Bilbrey GL, Weix J, Kaplan GD: Value of single photon absorptiometry in osteoporosis screening. Clin Nucl Med 13:7, 1988.

334. Eriksson S, Isberg B, Lindgren U: Vertebral bone mineral measurement using dual photon absorptiometry and computed tomography. Acta Radiol 29:89, 1988.

335. Mazess RB, Barden HS, Ettinger M: Radial and spinal bone mineral density in a patient population. Arthritis Rheum 31:891, 1988.

336. Lang P, Steiger P, Faulkner K, et al: Osteoporosis. Current techniques and recent developments in quantitative bone densitometry. Radiol Clin North Am 29:49, 1991.

337. Lambiase R, Sartoris DJ, Fellingham L, et al: Vertebral mineral status: Assessment with single- versus multi-section CT. Radiology 164:231, 1987.

338. Kalender WA, Klotz E, Suess C: Vertebral bone mineral analysis: An integrated approach with CT. Radiology 164:419, 1987.

339. Goodsitt MM, Rosenthal DI: Quantitative computed tomography scanning for measurement of bone and bone marrow fat content. Invest Radiol 22:799, 1987.

340. Bhasin S, Sartoris DJ, Fellingham L, et al: Three-dimensional quantitative CT of the proximal femur: Relationship to vertebral trabecular bone density in postmenopausal women. Radiology 167:145, 1988.

341. Kalender WA, Brestowsky H, Felsenberg D: Bone mineral measurement: Automated determination of midvertebral CT section. Radiology 168:219, 1988.

342. Nickoloff EL, Feldman F, Atherton JV: Bone mineral assessment: New dual-energy CT approach. Radiology 168:223, 1988.

343. Biggemann M, Hilweg D, Brinckmann P: Prediction of the compressive strength of vertebral bodies of the lumbar spine by quantitative computed tomography. Skel Radiol 17:264, 1988.

344. Cann CE: Quantitative CT for determination of bone mineral density: A review. Radiology 166:509, 1988.

345. Lang SM, Moyle DD, Berg EW, et al: Correlation of mechanical properties of vertebral trabecular bone with equivalent mineral density as measured by computed tomography. J Bone Joint Surg [Am] 70:1531, 1988.

346. Steiger P, Block JE, Steiger S, et al: Spinal bone mineral density measured with quantitative CT: Effect of region of interest, vertebral level, and technique. Radiology 175:537, 1990.

347. Steenbeek JCM, van Kuijk C, Grashuis JL: Influence of calibration materials in single- and dual-energy quantitative CT. Radiology 183:849, 1992.

348. Faulkner KG, Glüer C-C, Majumdar S, et al: Noninvasive measurements of bone mass, structure, and strength: Current methods and experimental techniques. AJR 157:1229, 1991.

349. Sartoris DJ, Resnick D: Dual-energy radiographic absorptiometry for bone densitometry: Current status and perspective. AJR 152:241, 1989.

350. Borders J, Kerr E, Sartoris DJ, et al: Quantitative dual-energy radiographic absorptiometry of the lumbar spine: In vivo comparison with dual-photon absorptiometry. Radiology 170:129, 1989.

351. Gundry CR, Miller CW, Ramos E, et al: Dual-energy radiographic absorptiometry of the lumbar spine: Clinical experience with two different systems. Radiology 174:539, 1990.

352. Ho CP, Kim RW, Schaffler MB, et al: Accuracy of dual-energy radiographic absorptiometry of the lumbar spine: Cadaver study. Radiology 176:171, 1990.

353. Southard RN, Morris JD, Mahan JD, et al: Bone mass in healthy children: Measurement with quantitative DXA. Radiology 179:735, 1991.

354. Wasserman SHS, Barzel US: Osteoporosis: The state of the art in 1987: A review. Semin Nucl Med 17:283, 1987.

355. Hurley DL, Tiegs RD, Wahner HW, et al: Axial and appendicular bone mineral density in patients with long-term deficiency or excess of calcitonin. N Engl J Med 317:537, 1987.

356. Lindberg JS, Powell MR, Hunt MM, et al: Increased vertebral bone mineral in response to reduced exercise in amenorrheic runners. West J Med 146:39, 1987.

357. Wolman RL: Bone mineral density levels in elite female athletes. Ann Rheum Dis 49:1013, 1990.

358. Gillespy T III, Gillespy MP: Osteoporosis. Radiol Clin North Am 29:77, 1991.

359. Jackson JA, Kleerekoper M: Osteoporosis in men: Diagnosis, pathophysiology, and prevention. Medicine 69:137, 1990.

360. Rosenberg AE: The pathology of metabolic bone disease. Radiol Clin North Am 29:19, 1991.

361. Centrella M, Canalis E: Local regulators of skeletal growth: A perspective. Endocr Rev 6:544, 1985.

362. Swoboda W, Grill F: The osteoporosis pseudoglioma syndrome: Update and report on two affected siblings. Pediatr Radiol 18:399, 1988.

363. Spriggs DW: Case report 613. Skel Radiol 19:302, 1990.

364. Sezai S, Hirano M, Iwase T: Osteodystrophy in liver cirrhosis: Detection and treatment evaluation using ^{99}Tc^m methylene diphosphonate bone scintigraphy. Clin Radiol 43:32, 1991.

365. Santora AC II: Role of nutrition and exercise in osteoporosis. Am J Med 82:73, 1987.

366. Bachrach LK, Guido D, Katzman D, et al: Decreased bone density in adolescent girls with anorexia nervosa. Pediatrics 86:440, 1990.

367. Jackson JA, Kleerekoper M, Parfitt AM, et al: Bone histomorphometry in hypogonadal and eugonadal men with spinal osteoporosis. J Clin Endocrinol Metab 65:53, 1987.

368. Clouston WM, Lloyd HM: Immobilization-induced hypercalcemia and regional osteoporosis. Clin Orthop 216:247, 1987.

369. Schwartzman RJ, McLellan TL: Reflex sympathetic dystrophy. A review. Arch Neurol 44:555, 1987.

370. Learmonth DJA, Eyres KS, Harding ML: Reflex sympathetic dystrophy of the knee: The need for early diagnosis. J Orthop Rheumatol 5:63, 1992.

371. Kozin F: Reflex sympathetic dystrophy syndrome. Bull Rheum Dis 36:1, 1986.

372. Atkins RM, Duckworth T, Kanis JA: Algodystrophy following Colles' fracture. J Hand Surg [Br] 14:161, 1989.

373. Munoz-Gomez J, Collado A, Gratacos J, et al: Reflex sympathetic dystrophy syndrome of the lower limbs in renal transplant patients treated with cyclosporin A. Arthritis Rheum 34:625, 1991.

374. Huaux JP, Malghem J, Maldaque B, et al: Reflex sympathetic syndrome: An unusual mode of presentation of osteomalacia. Arthritis Rheum 29:918, 1986.

375. Franck JL, Arlet P, Mazières B, et al: Algodystrophie au cours des déminéralisations diffuses. Rev Rhum Mal Osteoartic 49:803, 1982.

376. Laroche C, Cremer G, Sereni D: Association d'une algodystrophie sévère et d'une hyperparathyroïdie primitive. Rev Med Interne 1:91, 1980.

377. Prowse M, Higgs CMB, Forrester-Wood C, et al: Reflex sympathetic dystrophy associated with squamous cell carcinoma of the lung. Ann Rheum Dis 48:339, 1989.

378. Ameratunga R, Daly M, Caughey DE: Metastatic malignancy associated with reflex sympathetic dystrophy. J Rheumatol 16:406, 1989.

379. Goldsmith DP, Vivino FB, Eichenfield AH, et al: Nuclear imaging and clinical

features of childhood reflex neurovascular dystrophy: Comparison with adults. Arthritis Rheum 32:480, 1989.

380. Dietz FR, Mathews KD, Montgomery WJ: Reflex sympathetic dystrophy in children. Clin Orthop 258:225, 1990.

381. Wilder RT, Berde CB, Wolohan M, et al: Reflex sympathetic dystrophy in children. Clinical characteristics and follow-up of seventy patients. J Bone Joint Surg [Am] 74:910, 1992.

382. Davis RF, Jones LC, Hungerford DS: The effect of sympathectomy on blood flow in bone. Regional distribution and effect over time. J Bone Joint Surg [Am] 69:1384, 1987.

383. Griffiths HJ, Virtama P: Juxta-articular erosions in reflex sympathetic dystrophy. Acta Radiol 29:183, 1988.

384. Laukaitas JP, Varma VM, Borenstein DG: Reflex sympathetic dystrophy localized to a single digit. J Rheumatol 16:402, 1989.

385. Katz MM, Hungerford DS: Reflex sympathetic dystrophy affecting the knee. J Bone Joint Surg [Br] 69:797, 1987.

386. Ogilvie-Harris DJ, Roscoe M: Reflex sympathetic dystrophy of the knee. J Bone Joint Surg [Br] 69:804, 1977.

387. Malkin LH: Reflex sympathetic dystrophy syndrome following trauma to the foot. Orthopedics 13:851, 1990.

388. Doury P, Pattin S, Eulry F, et al: Fractures de fatigue du col fémoral suivies d'algodystrophie. Rev Rhum Mal Osteoartic 54:425, 1987.

389. Dequeker J, Geusens P, Verstaeten A, et al: Vertebral crush fracture syndrome and reflex sympathetic dystrophy. Bone 7:89, 1986.

390. Doury P, Pattin S, Eulry F, et al: Algodystrophie de l'enfant et de l'adulte jeune avec hypofixation osseuse isotopique. Med Chir Pied 8:121, 1986.

391. Lemahieu R-A, Van Laere C, Verbruggen LA: Reflex sympathetic dystrophy: An underreported syndrome in children? Eur J Pediatr 147:47, 1988.

392. Doury P, Wendling D, Pattin S, et al: L'hypofixation osseuse isotopique dans les algodystrophies. Sem Hôp Paris 64:1287, 1988.

393. Labenne M, Bertrand AM, Wendling D, et al: L'algodystrophie, une affection peu connue chez l'enfant. Ann Pédiatr 34:603, 1987.

394. Doury P, Pattin S, Gaillard F, et al: L'algodystrophie de l'enfant. Ann Pédiatr 35:469, 1988.

395. Heck LL: Recognition of atypical reflex sympathetic dystrophy. Clin Nucl Med 12:925, 1987.

396. Holder LE, Cole LA, Myerson MS: Reflex sympathetic dystrophy in the foot: Clinical and scintigraphic criteria. Radiology 184:531, 1992.

397. Hauzeur J-P: Epiphyseal migration of abnormalities in algodystrophy: The role of bone scintigraphy. J Rheumatol 19:1486, 1992.

398. Wilson AJ, Murphy WA, Hardy DC, et al: Transient osteoporosis: Transient bone marrow edema? Radiology 167:757, 1988.

399. Bramlett KW, Killian JT, Nasca RJ, et al: Transient osteoporosis. Clin Orthop 222:197, 1987.

400. Brodell JD, Burns JE Jr, Heiple KG: Transient osteoporosis of the hip of pregnancy. Two cases complicated by pathological fracture. J Bone Joint Surg [Am] 71:1252, 1989.

401. Pay NT, Singer WS, Bartal E: Hip pain in three children accompanied by transient abnormal findings on MR images. Radiology 171:147, 1989.

402. Chigara M, Watanabe H, Udagawa E: Transient osteoporosis of the hip in the first trimester of pregnancy. A case report and review of Japanese literature. Arch Orthop Trauma Surg 107:178, 1988.

403. Shifrin LZ, Reis ND, Zinman H, et al: Idiopathic transient osteoporosis of the hip. J Bone Joint Surg [Br] 69:769, 1987.

404. Wurnig CH, Kotz R: Algodystrophie in der Schwangerschaft. Z Orthop 129:146, 1991.

405. Lechevalier D, Eulry F, Crozes P, et al: Les algodystrophies du genou migratrices in situ. Intérêt de l'imagerie moderne. Rev Rhum Mal Ostéoartic 59:29, 1992.

406. Mavichak V, Murray TM, Hodsman AB, et al: Regional migratory osteoporosis of the lower extremities with vertebral osteoporosis. Bone 7:343, 1986.

407. Shier CK, Ellis BI, Kleerekoper M, et al: Disseminated migratory osteoporosis: An unusual pattern of osteoporosis. J Can Assoc Radiol 38:56, 1987.

408. Banas MP, Kaplan FS, Fallon MD, et al: Regional migratory osteoporosis. A case report and review of the literature. Clin Orthop 250:303, 1990.

409. Mailis A, Inman R, Pham D: Transient migratory osteoporosis: A variant of reflex sympathetic dystrophy? Report of 3 cases and literature review. J Rheumatol 19:758, 1992.

410. Mayo-Smith W, Rosenthal DI: Radiographic appearance of osteopenia. Radiol Clin North Am 29:37, 1991.

411. Michel BA, Lane NE, Jones HH, et al: Plain radiographs can be useful in estimating lumbar bone density. J Rheumatol 17:528, 1990.

412. Pogrund H, Bloom RA, Weinberg H: Relationship of psoas width to osteoporosis. Acta Orthop Scand 57:208, 1986.

413. Salomon C, Chopin D, Benoist M: Spinal cord compression: An exceptional complication of spinal osteoporosis. Spine 13:222, 1988.

414. Kaplan PA, Orton DF, Asleson RJ: Osteoporosis with vertebral compression fractures, retropulsed fragments, and neurologic compromise. Radiology 165:533, 1987.

415. DeSmet AA, Robinson RG, Johnson BE, et al: Spinal compression fractures in osteoporotic women: Patterns and relationship to hyperkyphosis. Radiology 166:497, 1988.

416. Lafforgue P, Daumen-Legre V, Schiano A, et al: Les complications neurologiques des tassements vertébraux ostéoporotiques. Rev Rhum Mal Osteoartic 57:619, 1990.

417. Griffiths HJ, Virtama P: Cortical thickness and trabecular pattern of the femoral neck as a measure of osteopenia. Invest Radiol 25:1116, 1990.

418. Kawashima T, Uhthoff HK: Patterns of bone loss of the proximal femur: A radiologic, densitometric, and histomorphometric study. J Orthop Res 9:634, 1990.

419. Balseiro J, Fahey FH, Zeissman HH, et al: Comparison of bone mineral density in both hips. Radiology 167:151, 1988.

420. Seldwin DW, Esser PD, Alderson PO: Comparison of bone different measurements from different skeletal sites. J Nucl Med 29:168, 1988.

421. Shukla SS, Krutoff B, Koutouratsas L, et al: Measurement of trabecular bone mineral density in the femur in vitro by using the coherent to Compton scatter ratio. Invest Radiol 23:305, 1988.

422. Kerr R, Resnick D, Pineda C: CT analysis of proximal femoral trabecular pattern simulating skeletal pathology. J Comput Assist Tomogr 12:227, 1988.

423. Meema HE: Radiologic study of endosteal, intracortical, and periosteal surfaces of hand bones in metabolic bone diseases. Hand Clin 7:37, 1991.

424. Meema HE, Meema S: Longitudinal microradioscopic comparisons on endosteal and juxtaendosteal bone loss in premenopausal and postmenopausal women, and in those with end-stage renal disease. Bone 8:343, 1988.

425. Yagan R, Radivoyevitch M, Khan MA: Double cortical line in the acetabular roof: A sign of disuse osteoporosis. Radiology 165:171, 1987.

426. Arciero RA, Leung KYK, Pierce JH: Spontaneous unstable burst fracture of the thoracolumbar spine in osteoporosis. A report of two cases. Spine 14:114, 1989.

427. Lane JM, Vigorita VJ: Osteoporosis. Orthop Clin North Am 15:711, 1984.

428. Meuleman J: Beliefs about osteoporosis. A critical appraisal. Arch Intern Med 147:762, 1987.

429. Buchanan JR, Myers CA, Greer RB III: A comparison of the risk of vertebral fracture in menopausal osteoporosis and other metabolic disturbances. J Bone Joint Surg [Am] 70:704, 1988.

430. Wilton TJ, Hosking DJ, Pawley E, et al: Osteomalacia and femoral neck fractures in the elderly patient. J Bone Joint Surg [Br] 69:388, 1987.

431. Parfitt AM: Trabecular bone architecture in the pathogenesis and prevention of fracture. Am J Med 82:68, 1987.

432. Rawlings CE III, Wilkins RH, Martinez S, et al: Osteoporotic sacral fractures: A clinical study. Neurosurgery 22:72, 1988.

433. Marx MV, Panzer FD: Recurrent radiculopathy in an elderly woman. Invest Radiol 23:147, 1988.

434. Kuhlencordt F, Kruse H-P: Case report 422. Skel Radiol 16:407, 1987.

435. Cooper KL: Insufficiency fractures of the sternum: A consequence of thoracic kyphosis? Radiology 167:471, 1988.

436. Chen C, Chandnani V, Kang HS, et al: Insufficiency fracture of the sternum caused by osteopenia: Plain film findings in seven patients. AJR 154:1025, 1990.

437. Rutledge DI: Spontaneous fractures of the sternum simulating myocardial infarction. Postgrad Med 32:502, 1962.

438. Vassalo L: Spontaneous fracture of the sternum simulating pulmonary embolism. Br J Clin Pract 23:288, 1969.

439. Haller J, André MP, Resnick D, et al: Detection of thoracolumbar vertebral body destruction with lateral spine radiography. Part I. Investigation in cadavers. Invest Radiol 25:517, 1990.

440. Haller J, André MP, Resnick D, et al: Detection of thoracolumbar vertebral body destruction with lateral spine radiography. Part II. Clinical investigation with computed tomography. Invest Radiol 25:523, 1990.

441. Vogler JB III, Murphy WA: Bone marrow imaging. Radiology 168:679, 1988.

442. Baker LL, Goodman SB, Perkash I, et al: Benign versus pathologic compression fractures of vertebral bodies: Assessment with conventional spin-echo, chemical-shift, and STIR MR imaging. Radiology 174:495, 1990.

443. Ricci C, Cova M, Kang YS, et al: Normal age-related patterns of cellular and fatty bone marrow distribution in the axial skeleton: MR imaging study. Radiology 177:83, 1990.

444. Kim H, Thrall JH, Keyes JW Jr: Skeletal scintigraphy following incidental trauma. Radiology 130:447, 1979.

445. Frager D, Elkin C, Swerdlow M, et al: Subacute osteoporotic compression fracture: Misleading magnetic resonance appearance. Skel Radiol 17:123, 1988.

446. Yuh WTC, Zachar CZ, Barloon TJ, et al: Vertebral compression fractures: Distinction between benign and malignant causes with MR imaging. Radiology 172:215, 1989.

447. Wehrli FW, Ford JC, Attie M, et al: Trabecular structure: Preliminary application of MR interferometry. Radiology 179:615, 1991.

448. Cann CE: Skeletal structure—function revisited. Radiology 179:607, 1991.

449. Rosenthal H, Thulborn KR, Rosenthal D, et al: Magnetic susceptibility effects of trabecular bone on magnetic resonance bone marrow imaging. Invest Radiol 25:173, 1990.

450. Sebag GH, Moore SG: Effect of trabecular bone on the appearance of marrow in gradient-echo imaging of the appendicular skeleton. Radiology 174:855, 1990.

451. Ford JC, Wehrli FW, Gusnard DA: Quantification of the intrinsic magnetic field inhomogeneity of trabecular bone. Magn Reson Imaging 851:37, 1990.

452. Alarcón GS, Sanders C, Daniel WW: Transient osteoporosis of the hip: Magnetic resonance imaging. J Rheumatol 14:1184, 1987.

453. Bloem JL: Transient osteoporosis of the hip: MR imaging. Radiology 167:753, 1988.

454. Leonidas JC: MR imaging of transient osteoporosis. Radiology 170:281, 1989.

455. Urbanski SR, de Lange EE, Eschenroeder HC Jr, et al: Magnetic resonance

imaging of transient osteoporosis of the hip. A case report. J Bone Joint Surg [Am] *73*:451, 1991.

456. Takatori Y, Kokubu T, Ninomiya S, et al: Transient osteoporosis of the hip. Magnetic resonance imaging. Clin Orthop *271*:190, 1991.

457. Hauzeur JP, Hanquinet S, Gevenois PA, et al: Study of magnetic resonance imaging in transient osteoporosis of the hip. J Rheumatol *18*:1211, 1991.

458. Grimm J, Higer HP, Benning R, et al: MRI of transient osteoporosis of the hip. Arch Orthop Trauma Surg *110*:98, 1991.

459. Potter H, Moran M, Schneider R, et al: Magnetic resonance imaging in diagnosis of transient osteoporosis of hip. Clin Orthop *280*:223, 1992.

460. Turner DA, Templeton AC, Selzer PM, et al: Femoral capital osteonecrosis: MR findings of diffuse marrow abnormalities without focal lesions. Radiology *171*:135, 1989.

461. Hungerford DS: Pathogenetic considerations in ischemic necrosis of bone. Can J Surg *24*:583, 1981.

462. Ficat RP: Idiopathic bone necrosis of the femoral head: Early diagnosis and treatment. J Bone Joint Surg [Br] *67*:3, 1985.

463. Koch E, Hofer HO, Sialer G, et al: Failure of MR imaging to detect reflex sympathetic dystrophy of the extremities. AJR *156*:113, 1991.

464. Brahme SK, Cervilla V, Vint V, et al: Magnetic resonance appearance of sacral insufficiency fractures. Skel Radiol *19*:489, 1990.

465. Chon KS, Sartoris DJ, Brown SA, et al: Alcoholism-associated spinal and femoral bone loss in abstinent male alcoholics, as measured by dual x-ray absorptiometry. Skel Radiol *21*:431, 1992.

466. Marhaug G: Idiopathic juvenile osteoporosis. Scand J Rheumatol *22*:45, 1993.

467. McDowell CL, Moore JD: Multiple fractures in a child: The osteoporosis pseudoglioma syndrome. J Bone Joint Surg [Am] *74*:1247, 1992.

468. Sarangi PP, Ward AJ, Atkins RM: Fractures after regional disuse osteoporosis. J Orthop Rheumatol *5*:233, 1992.

469. Karras D, Karargiris G, Vassilopoulos D, et al: Reflex sympathetic dystrophy syndrome and osteogenesis imperfecta. A report and review of the literature. J Rheumatol *20*:162, 1993.

470. Sachs BL, Zindrick MR, Beasley RD: Reflex sympathetic dystrophy after operative procedures on the lumbar spine. J Bone Joint Surg [Am] *75*:721, 1993.

471. Schiffenbauer J, Fagien M: Reflex sympathetic dystrophy involving multiple extremities. J Rheumatol *20*:165, 1993.

472. Michel BA, Bjorkengren AG, Lambert E, et al: Estimating lumbar bone mineral density from routine radiographs of the lumbar spine. Clin Rheumatol *12*:49, 1993.

473. Smith MD, Cody DD, Goldstein SA, et al: Proximal femoral bone density and its correlation to fracture load and hip-screw penetration load. Clin Orthop *283*:244, 1992.

474. Sugimoto H, Kimura T, Ohsawa T: Susceptibility effects of bone trabeculae. Quantification in vivo using an asymmetric spin-echo technique. Invest Radiol *28*:208, 1993.

475. Daniel WW, Sanders PC, Alarcón GS: The early diagnosis of transient osteoporosis by magnetic resonance imaging. A case report. J Bone Joint Surg [Am] *74*:1262, 1992.

476. Vande Berg BE, Malghem JJ, Labaisse MA, et al: MR imaging of avascular necrosis and transient marrow edema of the femoral head. RadioGraphics *13*:501, 1993.

477. Stanton RP, Malcolm JR, Wesdock KA, et al: Reflex sympathetic dystrophy in children: An orthopedic perspective. Orthopedics *16*:773, 1993.

478. Arriagada M, Arinoviche R: X-ray bone densitometry in the diagnosis and followup of reflex sympathetic dystrophy syndrome. J Rheumatol *21*:498, 1994.

479. Hofmann S, Engel A, Neuhold A, et al: Bone-marrow oedema syndrome and transient osteoporosis of the hip. An MRI-controlled study of treatment by core decompression. J Bone Joint Surg [Br] *75*:210, 1993.

480. Saitoh S, Nakatsuchi Y, Latta L, et al: An absence of structural changes in the proximal femur with osteoporosis. Skel Radiol *22*:425, 1993.

481. Leroux JL, Denat B, Thomas E, et al: Sacral insufficiency fractures presenting as acute low-back pain. Biomechanical aspects. Spine *18*:2502, 1993.

482. Schwappach JR, Murphey MD, Kokmeyer SF, et al: Subcapital fractures of the femoral neck: Prevalence and cause of radiographic appearance simulating pathologic fracture. AJR *162*:651, 1994.

483. Ryan PJ, Fogelman I: Osteoporotic vertebral fractures: Diagnosis with radiography and bone scintigraphy. Radiology *190*:669, 1994.

52

Quantitative Bone Mineral Analysis

Michael Jergas, M.D., and Harry K. Genant, M.D.

Osteoporosis is a common disorder affecting large numbers of adults and resulting in considerable morbidity, mortality, and public health expenditure. In the United States more than 25 million people are afflicted, particularly women. Many of them suffer from disabling fractures, with the spine being the earliest and most common site of involvement. Osteoporosis is believed to be responsible for about 1.3 million fractures annually, including more than 500,000 spine, 250,000 hip, and 240,000 wrist fractures.[1] Up to 30 per cent of elderly people with hip fracture die within 6 months of their injury.[2, 3] The difference in sex distribution in osteoporosis is especially significant as women who are 65 years of age or older represent the fastest growing segment of the population in the United States. The worldwide increase in life expectancy will most likely result in a concomitant rise in the prevalence of osteoporotic fractures of all kinds over the next decades (Fig. 52–1).[4]

During the past decades, osteoporosis, called the ''silent epidemic'' by the popular press, has gained increasing at-tention. The involvement chiefly of women and the insidious loss of bone manifested primarily as crush fractures of the spine, hip, and wrist are widely known facts. Public awareness of this disorder also has been heightened by the resulting increase in health care expenditure that currently is estimated to be in excess of $7 billion.[5, 6] The growing importance of osteoporosis is emphasized by many official and private initiatives with the objective to explore the epidemiology and the underlying causes of the disease, to investigate new ways for diagnosis, prophylaxis, and treatment, and to find appropriate ways to counter its sequelae.

OVERVIEW

In recent years considerable effort has been expended in the development of methods for assessing the skeleton quantitatively so that osteoporosis could be detected early or its progression and response to therapy could be moni-

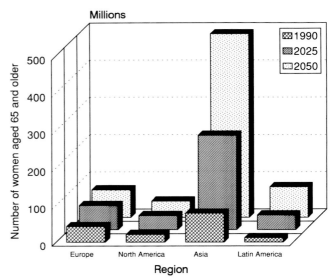

FIGURE 52–1. Estimated female population aged 65 years and older in four different regions of the world. (Data from Cooper and associates.[4])

TABLE 52–1. Comparison of Cortical and Trabecular Bone

Bone Tissue	Total Volume	Surface-to-Volume Ratio	Bone Turnover Ratio
	Relative Amounts		
Cortical (compact)	4	1	1
Trabecular (cancellous)	1	4	8

tored reliably; however, a consensus has not yet been reached regarding which methods are most efficacious in the diagnosis and serial assessment of osteoporosis in an individual patient or in diagnostic screening of large populations. In this regard, the selection of anatomic sites and methods for quantifying skeletal mass is of considerable importance. The skeleton as a whole is composed of about 80 per cent cortical (compact) bone and 20 per cent trabecular (cancellous) bone (Table 52–1). The appendicular skeleton is composed predominantly of cortical bone, whereas the spine contains a combination of cancellous bone (mainly in the vertebral bodies) and compact bone (particularly in the dense vertebral endplates and posterior osseous elements). Trabecular bone has a turnover rate that is approximately eight times that of compact bone, owing in part to its high surface-to-volume ratio.[7] This high turnover rate makes trabecular bone a sensitive measuring site that is highly responsive to metabolic stimuli, which probably ac-

counts for the clinical observation that osteoporotic fractures occur first in the vertebral bodies or distal portion of the radius, areas composed predominantly of trabecular bone.[8]

Numerous methods have been used for quantitative assessment of the skeleton in osteoporosis, with variable precision (deviation based on multiple measurements, often represented on a percentage basis as coefficient of variation), accuracy (reliability or assurance that the measured value reflects true mineral content), and sensitivity (capacity to readily separate an abnormal state from the normal in a population or to readily detect changes over time in a patient or in a population). The requirements for a clinically useful measurement of bone mineral differ, depending on the specific clinical problem under investigation. For serial determination in a given patient, precision and sensitivity are critical. When used as a diagnostic procedure to identify a patient with osteoporosis, accuracy and sensitivity are required. Accuracy, precision, and radiation dose for commonly used bone densitometry techniques are given in Table 52–2.

The pattern and rate of bone loss in the peripheral skeleton versus the axial skeleton or in compact bone versus cancellous bone may vary appreciably in different disease states and therapeutic interventions. Therefore, the variations in sensitivity observed for bone mineral measurements made at different anatomic sites not only are a function of systematic errors found with each technique but also are complicated by the physiologic variation occurring natu-

TABLE 52–2. Comparison of Precision, Accuracy Error, and Radiation Dose of Currently Used Techniques for Bone Mineral Measurement

Technique	Precision (%)	Accuracy Error (%)	Effective Dose Equivalent (μSv)*
Conventional Radiograph			
Lumbar spine (anteroposterior)			~550
Lumbar spine (lateral)			~450
Photodensitometry	1–3.5	5–10	1
SPA	1–2	4–6	<1
DPA			
Lumbar spine	2–3	2–11	5
Proximal portion of femur	2–5		3
DXA			
Posteroanterior lumbar spine	1	1–10	1
Lateral lumbar spine			
Decubitus position	2–6	8–10	3
Supine position	1–2		3
Proximal portion of femur	1–2		1
Forearm	~1		<1
Whole body	1		3
Quantitative CT			
Single energy quantitative CT	1.5–4	5–15	50
Dual energy quantitative CT	4–6	3–6	100
pQCT	0.5–1	2–8	<1
Quantitative Ultrasound			
Speed of sound	0.3–1.2	?†	0
Broadband ultrasound attenuation	1.3–3.8	?†	0
Quantitative MR Imaging	?‡	?†	0

*The effective dose equivalent, introduced by the International Commission on Radiological Protection in 1977, allows comparison of estimates of the radiologic risk of partial body radiation exposures to whole body radiation exposure.[163, 306, 307] For perspective, the effective dose equivalent for a posteroanterior chest film is 50 μSv and annual background irradiation amounts to 2400 μSv.

†Influenced by bone mineral density and bone structure.

‡Early state of development; unknown.

SPA, Single photon absorptiometry; DPA, dual photon absorptiometry; DXA, dual x-ray absorptiometry.

rally in different regions of the body. Additionally, a comparison of the sensitivity of these techniques is complicated by the problem of defining clinically "normal" and "diseased" populations. For example, by all methods of measurement of age-related bone loss, overlap occurs between osteoporotic patients and age-matched controls, and, in general, the difference between the two groups is on the order of one standard deviation. Osteoporotic patients in this setting generally are defined as those persons who sustain vertebral fractures, the so-called vertebral crush syndrome. It is clear, however, that some osteoporotic patients do not have fractures of the spine, whereas others with relatively minor osteopenia reveal such fractures. Additionally, evidence exists that patients with femoral neck fractures may differ in some respects from those with vertebral fractures, although both types of patients frequently are osteoporotic. Thus, these biologic discrepancies in combination with technical errors lessen the discriminatory capability or diagnostic potential of any given technique.

The first quantitative bone mineral methods to be developed were radiogrammetry and photodensitometry, which measure primarily the cortical bone of the appendicular skeleton. Depending on the precise site of measurement, with trabecular and cortical bone contributing in distinct patterns, single photon absorptiometry measures the sum of both cortical and trabecular bone in the appendicular skeleton. In recent years, techniques have become available that can quantify bone mineral content in the spine, a site of early osteoporosis. Dual photon and x-ray absorptiometry measure the sum of compact and cancellous bone in the axial, appendicular, or entire skeleton, whereas quantitative computed tomography (CT) provides a measure of purely trabecular bone in the vertebral spongiosa or other sites. Quantitative ultrasonographic methods may become the first radiation-free approach for the assessment of osteoporosis. Sonographic measurements also may depend on bone properties other than density. To the extent that newly developed methods for the determination of bone mineral density provided ease of use, high diagnostic standards, and wide availability, they have tended to replace older methods that required greater expenditure or that were associated with a significant radiation exposure of the patient (e.g., neutron activation analysis or Compton scattering); the older methods have lost their clinical importance.[9] Terminology and units that are used commonly with the various bone densitometry techniques are listed in Table 52–3.

APPENDICULAR BONE MEASUREMENTS

Measurements of appendicular mineral content are relatively easy to perform by techniques that are generally available. They have provided important population-based information of skeletal mass (e.g., the bone density of whites is lower than that of blacks at all ages; in many ethnic groups, men have a higher bone density than women; both sexes lose bone with aging; and accelerated bone loss occurs after menopause). During the last years appendicular bone mass measurements have been supplemented by a number of improvements of established methods or new developments such as peripheral quantitative CT. Enhanced precision and ease of use of these methods have stirred up the discussion on the ideal site for bone density measurements.[10–14]

RADIOGRAMMETRY

Radiogrammetry, a simple measurement of cortical thickness of virtually every long bone, is easy to perform with a caliper or with a graduated magnifying glass. Simple cortical measurements may be represented in several ways: One method involves summing the thickness of both cortices as an index of bone mass; another method uses the combined cortical thickness divided by the total bone width as a measure of density; finally, a circular cross section of bone is taken as a given with the measurements of bone width and cortical thickness converted to cortical areas that parallel actual physical mass more closely (Fig. 52–2). These methods have proved to be reproducible within 5 to 10 per cent depending on the specific site that is measured.[15–17] Radiogrammetry is applied most often to the metacarpal bones. Rico and Hernandez[18] reported an intraobserver precision of about 2 per cent using a magnifying glass, compared to 2.8 to 4.3 per cent when a caliper was used. The interobserver precision in this study was about 5 per cent, versus 6.5 per cent for each of the methods, respectively. Using a digitization technique rather than the caliper measurement, Kalla and associates[19] reported a precision of better than 5 per cent for intraobserver reproducibility for the combined cortical thickness at single metacarpal bones. The interobserver reproducibility error was 5 to 8.5 per cent.[19] Horsman and Simpson reported a precision of 1.5 per cent when using combined radiogrammetry of six metacarpal bones.[20]

TABLE 52–3. Terminology and Units Used in Bone Densitometry

Terminology	Unit	Technique
Combined cortical thickness	cm	Radiogrammetry
Cortical area	cm^2	Radiogrammetry
Specific bone mass, composite volume density	mm Al (Eq/mm^3)	Photodensitometry
Bone mineral content, bone mass	g	SPA, SXA, DPA, DXA
Linear density	g/cm	SPA, SXA
Bone mineral density (area)	g/cm^2	SPA, SXA, DPA, DXA
"Standardized" bone mineral density (but also bone mineral density)	mg/cm^2	DXA
		SPA, SXA
Bone mineral density (true volumetric)	g/cm^3 or mg/cm^3	Quantitative CT, DXA*
Ultrasound transmission velocity	m/sec	Quantitative ultrasound
Broadband ultrasound attenuation	dB/MHz	Quantitative ultrasound

*DXA allows for a width-adjusted estimate of the volumetric density of the vertebral body.

Abbreviations: g, gram; cm, centimeter; mm, millimeter; Al, aluminum; Eq, equivalent; dB, decibel; MHz, megahertz; SPA, single photon absorptiometry; SXA, single x-ray absorptiometry; DPA, dual photon absorptiometry; DXA, dual x-ray absorptiometry.

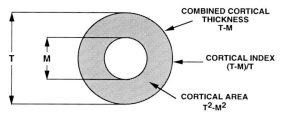

FIGURE 52–2. Schematic representation of a cross section of a tubular bone, showing several parameters determined by radiogrammetry.

Systematic errors are introduced by variations in soft tissue thickness and in radiographic geometry. As a consequence of these inaccuracies and the imprecision of the measurements, the values for compact bone area derived from radiogrammetry at different skeletal locations are intercorrelated only moderately ($r = 0.5$ to 0.7), whereas intercorrelation between right- and left-sided bones is higher ($r = 0.75$ to 0.9).[21, 22] Although Meema and Meindok[23] reported a good correlation between radiogrammetric measurements and dual photon absorptiometry of the spine, other studies suggest only a poor to moderate correlation with other methods of bone mineral measurements, such as single and dual photon absorptiometry at various sites.[23–25]

Simple cortical measurements, particularly when obtained at several anatomic sites, provide information that is more useful in clinical research than in individual patient management. For example, extensive data on metacarpal changes in populations show a loss with aging in the area of compact bone on the order of 0.9 per cent per year in women and of 0.4 per cent per year in men in the age range from 50 to 80 years.[16, 24, 26, 27] Falch and Sandvik described a premenopausal annual decrease in the combined cortical width of 0.4 per cent compared to a postmenopausal annual decrease of 1.3 per cent.[28] Meema and Meema found radiogrammetry to be a good discriminator between postmenopausal women with and without vertebral fractures.[29, 30] Studies of patients with primary hyperparathyroidism, rheumatoid arthritis, and systemic lupus erythematosus have revealed substantial reductions of the combined cortical thickness in comparison to normal controls (Fig. 52–3).[31, 32]

One major limitation leading to the potential insensitivity of radiogrammetry is related to the failure to measure intracortical resorption or porosity and irregular endosteal scalloping or erosion. As intracortical resorption and trabecular bone resorption (Fig. 52–4) are important indicators of high bone turnover states, the fact that they are not measured by this technique is significant. Despite its shortcomings when applied to individual patients, radiogrammetry remains an important research tool, especially to study changes in cortical bone.[33–35]

PHOTODENSITOMETRY

It has been known for many years that the photographic density on a film is roughly proportional to the mass of bone located in the x-ray beam. A relatively large change in bone mineral content (25 to 50 per cent) must occur, however, before it can be detected with visual observation of radiographs.[36, 37] In an effort to quantitate bone mass, a number of investigators have measured the optical density

of bone contained in radiographs in which both the anatomic part to be studied and a reference wedge are included in the exposure area (Fig. 52–5).[38–40] The simultaneous exposure of a reference system (normally a wedge or step wedge consisting of aluminum or hydroxyapatite) allows for a reproducible determination of bone density with an appropriate exposure technique. After the film processing, bone and reference wedge are evaluated using a photodensitometer. In its long history, many names have been assigned to this technique, such as radiographic photodensitometry, radiographic absorptiometry, quantitative Röntgen microdensitometry, and even digital image processing. However, all of these names denote basically the same technique using more or less sophisticated approaches.

Photodensitometry is a low dose and low cost technique, which measures integral bone (trabecular and cortical). Moreover, it is easy to perform. Multiple technical problems arise, however, such as nonuniformity of x-ray inten-

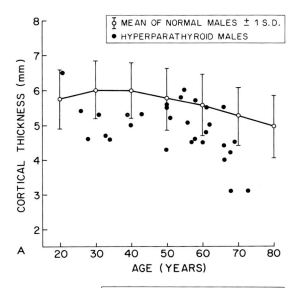

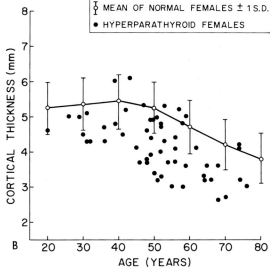

FIGURE 52–3. The combined cortical thickness of the second metacarpal bone is plotted versus age for a normal population and for hyperparathyroid men **(A)** and women **(B).** (From Genant HK, et al: Proceedings of the International Conference on Bone Mineral Measurement. Washington, DC, National Institute of Arthritis, Metabolism, and Digestive Diseases, 1974.)

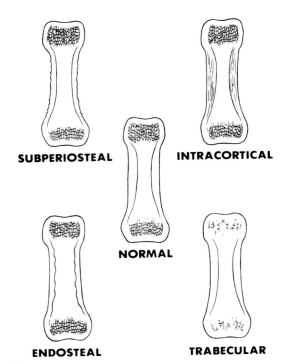

FIGURE 52–4. Schematic representation of four forms of bone resorption. Intracortical resorption and trabecular bone resorption are not measured by radiogrammetry.

sity, beam hardening due to the polychromatic radiation source, and variation in film sensitivity related to processing. Because of soft tissue inhomogeneities, the application of photodensitometry is limited to the peripheral skeleton. Various measurement sites in the upper and lower extremities are reported in the literature. Metacarpal or phalangeal bones are preferred sites for this technique. Heuck and Schmidt reported an accuracy of 5 to 10 per cent for photodensitometry of the femoral neck and the calcaneus.[38] Hagiwara and associates found the correlation coefficient between photodensitometry of the metacarpal bones and their ash density to be $r = 0.95$ (coefficient of variation = 3.4 per cent).[41] Results using newer photodensitometric techniques suggest that precision of between 1 and 3.5 per cent is possible for photodensitometry of the phalangeal or metacarpal bones.[42–44]

Population studies in which photodensitometry was used have documented a fundamental sexual dimorphism in cortical bone mass. The early investigations of Meema and Meema[45] showed that, at all ages, women have less cortical bone than men and that age-related bone loss starts earlier, proceeds more rapidly, and results in a much greater depletion of the skeleton in women than in men. With regard to the radius, men first show significant loss of cortical bone by the age of 60 or 70 years. At this same time, as detected by photodensitometry, women have been found to have a reduced hydroxyapatite content of the radius with a decrease from 700 mg/cm^2 to 350 mg/cm^2 (Fig. 52–6).[45] More recent cross-sectional and longitudinal studies confirmed the accelerated bone loss in the early menopause that also was seen with other densitometric techniques.[43, 46] Results derived from photodensitometry of the hand compared significantly with other bone density measurements in vivo.

Correlation coefficients from $r = 0.6$ to $r = 0.7$ for spinal bone mineral density using a dual photon absorptiometry technique and photodensitometry of the hand were reported. The correlation with other measurement sites was found to be of the same order.[47]

Numerous physical factors influencing the radiographic image also may affect photodensitometry adversely. Nevertheless, its cost effectiveness, ease of use, and theoretically ubiquitous availability make this technique a continuously interesting option for the assessment of bone mass.

SINGLE PHOTON AND X-RAY ABSORPTIOMETRY

Single photon absorptiometry (SPA) was introduced in the 1960s.[48, 49] With this method, a quantitative assessment of the bone mineral content at a peripheral site of the skeleton (e.g., distal or ultradistal portion of the radius, calcaneus) is possible. The measurement of the attenuation (or absorption) of a monoenergetic beam that is derived from a single energy source (iodine-125, 27.5 keV, or americium-241, 59.4 keV) gave this method its name. The measured attenuation is converted to bone mineral content or bone mineral density using a known standard. For an accurate measurement, SPA requires a constant soft tissue thickness. Figure 52–7 demonstrates the influence of soft tissue on the attenuation profile. Soft tissue contributes critically to the measured absorption, and the introduction of a water bath in which the measured body part is immersed, or a water bag that surrounds the measured site, may correct for the inconstant path length caused by the soft tissue.

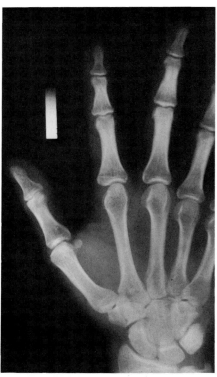

FIGURE 52–5. The simultaneous exposure of an aluminum wedge on a hand radiograph allows for a reproducible determination of bone density with an appropriate exposure technique.

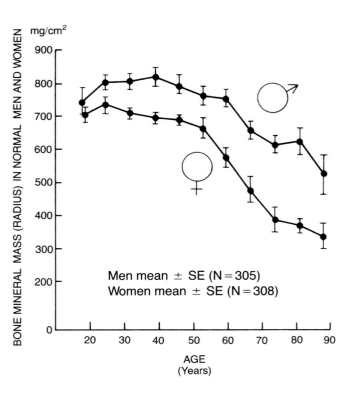

FIGURE 52–6. Hydroxyapatite content of the radius by photodensitometry in 305 normal white men and 308 normal white women. The bars indicate the standard error of the mean. (From Meema S, Meema HE: Isr J Med Sci *12:*601, 1976.)

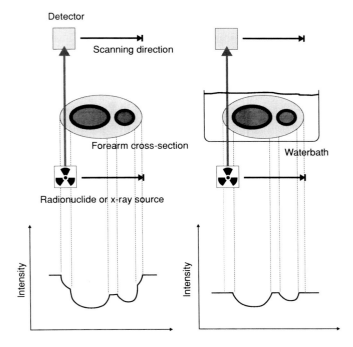

FIGURE 52–7. Soft tissue contributes critically to the measured absorption in SPA. The introduction of a water bath in which the measured body part is immersed corrects for the inconstant path length that is caused by the soft tissue, as illustrated by the intensity profiles at the bottom of the figure.

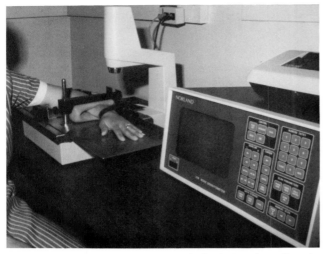

FIGURE 52–8. The Norland-Cameron single photon absorptiometry scanner was widely used in the 1970s and 1980s for bone mass measurements of the forearm. Note that the measured forearm is surrounded by a water bag to correct for the soft tissue component.

Many SPA devices have been developed since the method's inception, of which the Norland-Cameron absorptiometer was the most widely accepted and clinically applied device in the 1970s and early 1980s. These devices measure the radial shaft using an ^{125}I source that is interfaced with a sodium iodide scintillation detector (Fig. 52–8). The forearm is surrounded by a water bag or placed in a water bath, and a baseline measurement is obtained in the region of the interosseous membrane. The gamma ray source and detector then are moved across the forearm, and changes in beam intensity are measured continuously. The average attenuation of the ^{125}I beam by the bone is calculated and then compared with data contained in a standard curve derived from a potassium phosphate (K_2HPO_4) reference. With the Norland-Cameron method, the number of grams of bone mineral contained in a 1 cm wide path through the radius is indicated in grams per centimeter. Bone width also is determined automatically, and the amount of bone mineral contained in a uniform area is calculated (g/cm^2). Two sites in the radius commonly are measured with these devices: the middiaphysis, which consists of about 95 per cent cortical bone, and the distal radial metaphysis, which contains about 75 per cent cortical bone and 25 per cent trabecular bone.[50–52]

SPA overcomes some of the technical problems of photodensitometry. However, the major limitation of the early standard SPA techniques is that they reflected primarily the status of the cortex in the peripheral tubular bones. These methods are less reliable in the assessment of the overall skeletal status in an individual patient and, therefore, are of restricted diagnostic value in many metabolic diseases.[10] As accumulating evidence has suggested that metabolic processes occur more rapidly in cancellous bone, modifications in SPA have been introduced to provide raster or rectilinear scanning (Fig. 52–9) of the more distal portion of the radius or of the calcaneus, as well as to provide a higher precision than has been possible previously.[53–56] At the distal end of the radius, a site referred to as the "ultradistal" radius, the percentage of trabecular bone is similar to that found in the lumbar spine.[51, 53, 54] However, a major difficulty in studying this portion of the radius is the large change in bone mineral content that occurs over a short distance. Furthermore, methods that depend on palpation of osseous landmarks, such as the ulnar styloid process, do not permit precise relocation of the scanning site. Several approaches were made to define a distal scanning site that met the criteria of good reproducibility and assessment of trabecular bone at the same time. Nilas and collaborators[54] scanned the radius and ulna and then used a computer-based edge detection program to determine the site at which the gap between the two bones was 8 mm. From this point, four scans were made in a distal direction at 2 mm increments.[54] Awbrey and coworkers also used the gap between the radius and the

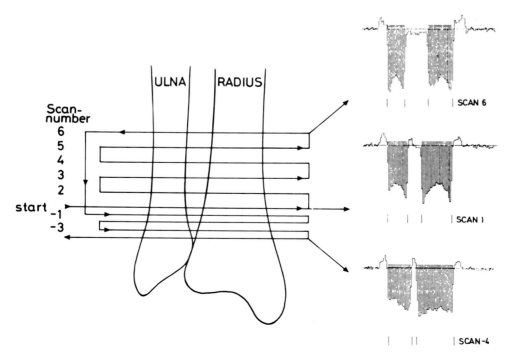

FIGURE 52–9. Rectilinear scanning of the distal end of the forearm using the Molsgaard single photon absorptiometry system. (From Wilas L, et al: J Nucl Med *26*:1257, 1985.)

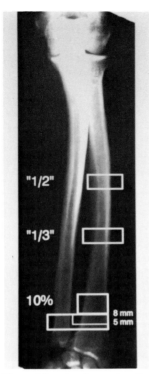

FIGURE 52–10. Sites of forearm bone density measurements by SPA. The midshaft ("1/2"), "1/3", and 10 per cent sites commonly were used.[10] The distances are related to the ulnar length. Nilas and associates measured a distal site beginning where the gap between radius and ulna is 8 mm and then extending for a distance of 8 mm.[54] Awbrey and coworkers made one measurement where the radius-ulna gap is 5 mm.[53]

ulna to permit similar positioning on each examination and obtained a single scan where this gap measured 5 mm.[53] In Figure 52–10 the measurement sites commonly used in the radius are shown.

Grubb and coworkers and Nilas and associates reported correlation coefficients of 0.52 and 0.64, respectively, between the bone density of the ultradistal radius and that of the lumbar spine.[57, 58] These correlation coefficients are statistically significant but are inadequate in terms of extrapolating lumbar spine density from the density of the ultradistal radius for an individual person and are similar to results obtained when predicting lumbar spine density from the patient's age alone. Wahner and coworkers noted further that in cross-sectional studies of bone density in the ultradistal radius, no decline was found in women until after the menopause.[51] The pattern of postmenopausal bone loss was found to be comparable in the axial and appendicular skeleton in several studies. However, findings are contradictory in premenopausal women. Whereas Nilas and associates reported a premenopausal bone loss in the spine and the distal portion of the radius, Aloia and colleagues found a premenopausal decline of bone mineral density only in the axial skeleton, indicating a differential behavior of these two sites.[58, 59] On the basis of these investigations and others, it still is uncertain whether the rates of bone mineral density loss in the distal portion of the radius and in the axial skeleton are similar.[10, 53, 60, 61]

The measurements obtained by SPA correlate with the weight of the individual bone, the mass at other skeletal sites, the weight of other long bones, the total skeletal weight, and the total body calcium.[59, 62] Wilson has shown that measurements of the diaphyses of the radius and ulna correlated highly ($r = 0.85$) with the bone mineral content of the femoral neck and less well ($r = 0.7$) with the bone mineral content in the spine.[63] Other investigators have indicated, generally, lower degrees of correlation.[14, 59]

In studies of bone mineral content in the radius, values in persons with osteoporosis have been shown to be approximately one standard deviation (in this case, 15 per cent) below those in age-matched controls and two standard deviations (or 30 per cent) below levels in young adults. However, considerable overlap occurs in the bone mineral content of normal and osteoporotic persons as determined by this method as well as by iliac crest biopsy and trabecular bone volume determination.[64, 65]

The rectilinear, area scanning approach also has been applied to measurement of the calcaneus as a convenient appendicular site containing almost purely trabecular bone. The SPA technique applied to the calcaneus is similar to that used in the SPA devices described earlier. Using a rectilinear scanner, a large volume of the calcaneus can be assessed. The central portion of the calcaneus corresponds to the area that normally represents the least bone mineral content. The ability to obtain a permanent scanning record of the bone profiles ensures that comparable sampling sites will be present in each examination, which is essential to maintain high precision.[50, 56, 66] Using this approach Wasnich and coworkers reported a precision of 0.9 per cent for embedded calcanei and an in vivo short-term coefficient of variation of 1.2 per cent.[67]

Results of population studies have shown that such measurements in the calcaneus are related significantly to the person's body weight and height and the level of exercise.[50, 68] Calcaneal bone mineral content correlates moderately with bone mineral density measurements at the lumbar spine ($r = 0.77$) and the distal end of the radius ($r = 0.71$). Vogel also reported a comparable reduction of bone mineral content in the lumbar spine and in the calcaneus with age in pre- and postmenopausal women.[50] Bone mass measurements of the calcaneus provide information regarding the risk of spinal fractures comparable to that obtained by measurements of the radius. Studies also have suggested that the calcaneal measurement may be a good indicator of the risk of fractures (other than vertebral fractures) and is comparable or even superior to bone mineral density measurements of other skeletal sites.[69–72]

The radionuclide source has now been replaced by an x-ray tube in some SPA systems. Analogously to SPA, this method is called single x-ray absorptiometry, widely referred to as SXA. Using an x-ray tube rather than a radionuclide source eliminates the need for replacing the source and thereby reduces radioactive waste. Furthermore, extensive quality control measures to compensate for radioactive decay do not apply. However, the operator may have to correct for beam hardening due to the polychromatic spectrum of the x-ray source.

Bone mineral density measurements of the appendicular skeleton have been adapted to dual photon and x-ray absorptiometry on the basis of the experiences with SPA and SXA. Designated software already exists for forearm measurements and is used widely in clinical densitometry, and several groups have reported on the possibility of measuring calcaneal bone mineral density.[73, 74] The enormous versatility of dual x-ray absorptiometry that allows for an application of this technique at virtually any skeletal site contributes to the dwindling usage of SPA in bone densitometry.

NEUTRON ACTIVATION ANALYSIS AND COMPTON SCATTERING TECHNIQUES

With neutron activation analysis, neutrons are used to bombard a small fraction of the total calcium-48 contained in the human body, producing [44]Ca (with a half-life of 8.8 min), which then is counted with external detectors. The neutrons (with energies of 1 to 15 MeV) are derived from accelerators, reactors, or alpha neutron sources.[75, 76] The technique provides an estimate of bone mineral content because, at least in the skeleton, calcium makes up a constant fraction (0.395) of the mineral. The radiation dose for such measurements ranges from 200 to 3000 microsieverts (μSv), depending on the neutron energy and the detector efficiency. Several studies suggest a precision and accuracy on the order of 2 to 5 per cent.[77]

A total body calcium measurement by neutron activation analysis reflects primarily compact bone, which constitutes approximately 80 per cent of the total skeletal mass and, therefore, correlates closely with other measurements of cortical bone. Total body calcium measurements obtained by neutron activation analysis have been compared with results obtained by peripheral SPA; correlation coefficients of approximately 0.9 were obtained.[78–81] Processes occurring initially or predominantly in cancellous bone may not be detected as readily with this technique. For example, in osteoporotic patients, the correlation between peripheral measurements by photon absorptiometry and total body neutron activation analysis is not ideal. Heterotopic calcification, such as vascular and costochondral calcification, or heterotopic ossification, such as osteophytosis and myositis ossificans, will cause inaccuracies in the estimation of skeletal calcium by neutron activation analysis. Nevertheless, Cohn and collaborators reported that total body neutron activation analysis allowed for a better discrimination between osteoporotic and nonosteoporotic subjects than did photon absorptiometry of the radius and the lumbar spine.[82]

In an attempt to measure predominantly cancellous bone, methods have been developed for partial body neutron activation in which areas of the trunk (e.g., pelvis, spine, and rib cage) are measured.[83] Precision and dosages for these local measurements are comparable to those obtained with the total body activation techniques.

Compton scattering techniques have been used to estimate the density of selected volumes of bone.[84–89] These methods make use of the information extracted primarily from the scattered beam, not from the transmitted beam. The electron density of a tissue volume is estimated by the extent of Compton scattering produced by incident radiation. Such radiation generally is of relatively high photon energy, on the order of 100 to 500 keV, emanating from a monoenergetic isotope source. A highly collimated gamma ray source and a highly collimated detector are positioned such that their "sensitive areas" project pathways that intersect perpendicularly to each other within the object and that define the volume to be measured (Fig. 52–11). The technique measures a composite of all the medullary com-

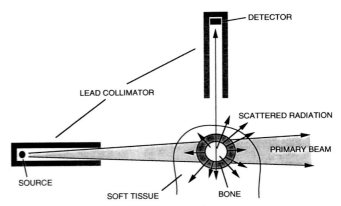

FIGURE 52–11. Schematic representation of the source and the scatter for Compton scatter densitometry.

ponents producing the scatter, not simply the density of bone mineral. The detected scatter is proportional to the electron density, independent of atomic number z. For this reason, the method is somewhat less sensitive to the calcium level than is SPA applied at low energies.[88] The precision of the method is 2 to 5 per cent. Its accuracy is affected by photon attenuation in tissues outside the region of interest. The use of high photon energy diminishes these problems at the expense of an increased radiation dose.[90–93] No studies have been published on the effective dose equivalent of Compton scattering. When applied to the appendicular skeleton, however, the radiation dose should be small.

A variant of the foregoing scattered photon technique is coherent scattering as proposed by Puumalainen and colleagues. With this method, both Compton scattering and coherent scattering of photons are determined in a particular volume of tissue, such as cancellous bone. This is made possible by the use of a solid state detector, which provides good discrimination. Coherent scattering, like photoelectric absorption, depends on the cube of the atomic number (z^3), and thus the ratio of coherent to Compton scattered photons is a measure of the effective atomic number, independent of density. A decreased ratio, therefore, may be observed in osteopenic diseases. Likewise, the ratio is unaffected by scatter outside the region of interest, so that complicated corrections for this potential inaccuracy are not necessary.

Only few clinical studies exist using either neutron activation analysis or Compton scattering techniques.[59, 79, 82, 94–96] Their extreme technical requirements, the relatively high radiation dose for neutron activation analysis, and the development of competitive methods with comparable or higher precision and easier applicability all have made these methods nearly obsolete in bone densitometry. Today neutron activation analysis and Compton scattering are regarded as investigational techniques with negligible clinical impact.

DUAL PHOTON AND X-RAY ABSORPTIOMETRY

Dual photon absorptiometry (DPA) has been studied extensively as a technique to measure the mineral content in the spine and hip; it also was used through the 1980s to measure total bone mineral content in the whole body.[10, 97–102] This approach uses a radionuclide source at two effective

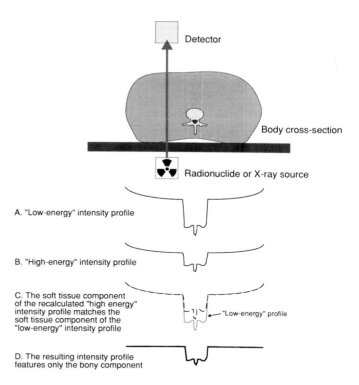

FIGURE 52-12. Principle of DPA and DXA. Radiation of distinct energies is attenuated by tissues to different extents. In both soft tissue and bone, a low energy beam is attenuated to a greater degree than a high energy beam. In bone, this attenuation occurs to a much greater extent than in soft tissue. By entering the attenuation profiles for a low and a high energy beam into a mathematical equation system, an attenuation profile of the bony components may be calculated.

discrete energy levels. The principle of DPA is based on the fact that radiation of distinct energies is attenuated by tissues to different extents. In both soft tissue and bone, a low energy beam is attenuated to a greater degree than a high energy beam. Because this attenuation occurs in bone to a much greater extent than in soft tissue, the contrast in attenuation between bone and soft tissue is greater for the low energy beam than for the high energy beam. Entering both attenuation profiles into a mathematical equation system, an attenuation profile of the bony components may be calculated (Fig. 52–12). The application of this technique eliminates the need for a constant path length.

When DPA was first employed, the radionuclide source consisted of radionuclide combinations such as ^{125}I and [241]Am. The dual emitter gadolinium-153 (with photons at energy levels of predominantly 44 and 100 KeV) was introduced in the early 1970s and became the standard radionuclide source for DPA in conjunction with a rectilinear scanner.[103] Bone mass is expressed quantitatively in grams per square centimeter, reflecting an area rather than a volumetric measurement. This measurement assesses the sum or integral of all mineral within the scan path, which includes not only the predominantly trabecular bone of the vertebral bodies but also the vertebral endplates and posterior elements, with their greater percentage of compact bone (Fig. 52–13).

Vertebral compression fractures, kyphoscoliosis, articular facet hypertrophy, discogenic bone sclerosis, marginal osteophytes, and extraosseous calcification (such as in the aorta) also are included in this integral spinal measurement and may result in inaccurate and poorly reproducible vertebral measurements, especially in elderly subjects.[104–109] In healthy persons, the precision of DPA measurements of the lumbar spine is approximately 2 to 3 per cent. The accuracy of this technique when applied to reference models, or

phantoms, is 1 to 2 per cent; when applied to vertebral specimens, DPA has an accuracy of 2 to 11 per cent.[64, 100, 110–114] In such experimental situations, DPA appears to indicate bone mass and density accurately, and it is affected only slightly by either surrounding soft tissue or fat within the bone marrow.

Dual x-ray absorptiometry (DXA), based on the method of x-ray spectrophotometry, was introduced commercially as the direct successor to DPA in 1987.[115, 116] Using the principles of DPA, the radionuclide source is replaced by an x-ray tube in DXA. Depending on the manufacturer, two distinct energy level beams are either generated by the x-ray generator or filtered from an x-ray spectrum. Using a bone and a soft tissue standard for internal calibration, the method allows direct assessment of both bone mineral and soft tissue composition. The main advantages of an x-ray system over a DPA radionuclide system are the shortened examination time, due to an increased photon flux of the x-ray tube, and a greater accuracy and precision, due to higher resolution and the lack of radionuclide decay.[117–120] Of course, the exchange of a radionuclide source does not apply to DXA. DXA has taken the place of DPA, thereby reaching great acceptance in clinical medicine and research. A multitude of synonyms exist for DXA, such as DEXA (dual energy x-ray absorptiometry), DER (dual energy radiography), DEPR (dual energy projection radiography), QDR (quantitative digital radiography), and DPX (dual photon x-ray absorptiometry). Some of these acronyms are linked to tradenames of manufacturers. To avoid favoring a particular manufacturer and because DXA is derived from DPA, DXA has been suggested as an acronym for this technique.[121, 122]

The preferred anatomic sites for DXA measurement of bone mineral content or density include the lumbar spine, proximal portion of the femur, forearm, and whole body,

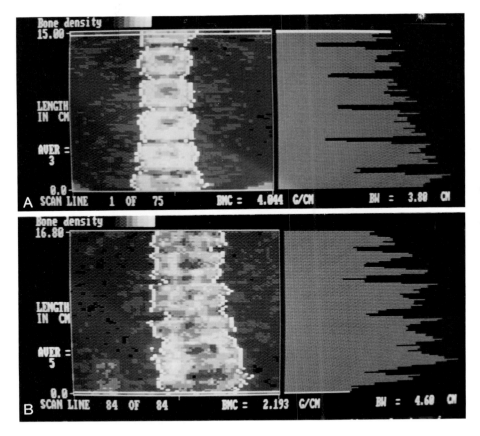

FIGURE 52–13. Video displays of a normal **(A)** and an osteoporotic **(B)** spine measured by DPA. Notice the poorly defined bone edges in the osteoporotic spine.

but virtually all parts of the body, such as the calcaneus, also can be scanned (Figs. 52–14 and 52–15). The digital image resulting from the measurement allows a gross survey of the region examined. The software of all DXA devices allows the radiologist to identify regions of interest with distinct compositions of trabecular and cortical bone, such as the femoral neck and Ward's triangle, and the ultradistal site of the radius. In contrast to SPA, the ultradistal site of the radius in DXA is defined as a region 1 cm wide located directly adjacent to the cortical endplate of the radius. The image quality of DXA and the availability of sophisticated software for scan analysis definitely contribute to the excellent precision of DXA (e.g., a direct comparison of baseline and follow-up scans on the screen allows the regions of interest on the follow-up scan to be aligned with those of the baseline analysis). Owing to distinct subregion specifications among the manufacturers, measurements of some subregions, such as the Ward's triangle, that were obtained on machines of different manufacturers cannot be compared easily.

The examination procedure with the initial devices required 6 to 15 min; newly developed devices using higher power generators or a fan beam instead of a pencil beam x-ray source make the process even faster, shortening the examination time to 2 min or even less.[123] Studies comparing results derived from a pencil beam device with those of a fan beam device showed that area and bone mineral content data are affected significantly by this change; however, the effect on bone mineral density is negligible, and bone mineral density data show excellent correlations.[124, 125] The in vivo precision of the posteroanterior DXA exami-

nation of the lumbar spine is 0.5 to 1.5 per cent with an accuracy error of 1 to 10 per cent.[117, 119, 126–128]

DXA has become the most widely used method to assess bone mineral density. Important features of DXA that made it popular were ease of use, high precision, and low radiation exposure to the patient. DXA measurements have been used in a multitude of clinical and experimental studies to assess risk factors of osteoporosis, such as alcoholism, thyroid or corticosteroid medication, and the effect of exercise on bone mineral density.[129–134] The noninvasive measurement of bone mass in the rat using DXA has proved to be accurate and precise, and DXA has become a primary research tool for the assessment of bone mineral density in an experimental environment.[135] These developments also have inspired a multitude of clinical studies with serial bone mineral density assessment using DXA measurements to assess the efficacy of the study medication in preserving or gaining bone mass.

Some of the limitations that apply to the DPA measurement of the spine also apply to DXA measurements. Osteophytes, aortic calcifications, degenerative hypertrophy of the articular facets, and intervertebral disc space narrowing in degenerative disc disease may increase the measured bone mineral density artificially in the posteroanterior measurement of the lumbar spine.[105–108, 136] This is an important drawback of this method, especially in elderly patients. Furthermore, the area projectional measurement includes substantial portions of cortical bone, thereby reducing discrimination between osteoporotic and nonosteoporotic subjects. A lateral examination of the lumbar spine makes possible an evaluation of the vertebral body, with almost

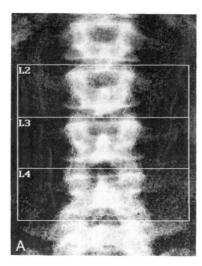

Region	Est.Area (cm2)	Est.BMC (grams)	BMD (gms/cm2)
L2	13.70	11.38	0.831
L3	15.06	12.75	0.847
L4	16.53	12.79	0.774
TOTAL	45.29	36.92	0.815

FIGURE 52–14. Lumbar spine **(A)**, hip **(B)**, and forearm **(C)** as they are depicted by DXA. These are the typical anatomic sites that are used for the application of DXA. Compared to DPA (Fig. 52–13) DXA has a superior resolution, allowing a more detailed depiction of the measured site. UD, Ultradistal radius. Troch, trochanter; Inter, intertrochanteric region; Ward's, Ward's triangle. BMC, Bone mineral content. BMD, Bone mineral density.

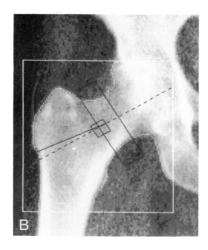

Region	Area (cm2)	BMC (grams)	BMD (gms/cm2)
Neck	5.53	2.94	0.532
Troch	12.74	6.28	0.493
Inter	20.42	17.40	0.852
TOTAL	38.69	26.62	0.688
Ward's	0.99	0.35	0.354

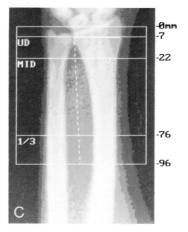

RADIUS	Area (cm2)	BMC (grams)	BMD (gms/cm2)
UD	3.86	1.22	0.316
MID	8.19	3.43	0.419
1/3	2.78	1.42	0.509
TOTAL	14.84	6.07	0.409

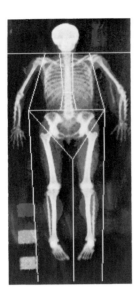

Region	Area (cm2)	BMC (grams)	BMD (gms/cm2)
L Arm	245.12	165.17	0.674
R Arm	242.74	170.71	0.703
L Ribs	109.25	63.09	0.577
R Ribs	119.19	73.26	0.615
T Spine	148.58	124.12	0.835
L Spine	58.00	55.55	0.958
Pelvis	217.31	263.42	1.212
L Leg	416.75	495.85	1.190
R Leg	419.53	480.31	1.145
SubTot	1976.49	1891.48	0.957
Head	245.12	485.73	1.982
TOTAL	2221.61	2377.21	1.070

F.S.   68.00%   0(10.00)%
Head assumes 17.0% brain fat
LBM 73.2% water

Region	Fat (grams)	Lean+BMC (grams)	% Fat (%)
L Arm	3646.6	1594.1	69.6
R Arm	3071.2	1445.0	68.0
Trunk	12280.3	23134.9	34.7
L Leg	6648.4	6081.0	52.2
R Leg	7796.0	6590.7	54.2
SubTot	33442.5	38845.7	46.3
Head	793.2	3479.2	18.6
TOTAL	34235.7	42324.9	44.7

FIGURE 52–15. DXA of the whole body allows for a measurement of bone density of selected skeletal sites as well as for an estimate of the soft tissue composition. BMC, bone mineral content. BMD, bone mineral density.

exclusive measurement of the trabecular bone.[137, 138] Therefore, the correlation between lateral examinations with DXA and quantitative CT, which measure the vertebral body, have been found to be greater than that of posteroanterior examinations with DXA and quantitative CT.[139] The lateral DXA method can reduce some of the errors mentioned previously; however, owing to overlap of the vertebrae by the ribs and iliac crest, the number of vertebrae that can be evaluated is limited to two—L3 and L4.[140] Furthermore, the reproducibility of the lateral DXA measurement is poorer primarily because the patient usually is examined in the lateral decubitus position.[141] Modern scanning devices use a C-arm, so that a lateral spine examination can be obtained with the patient supine, a technique that reduces the amount of spinal overlap by the ribs and innominate bone and, thereby, improves in vivo reproducibility.[142]

Although excellent correlations exist between the measurements made on machines of the different manufacturers of DXA devices, comparison of results is not easy, as manufacturers all use different standards to determine the bone mineral content of a given object and different algorithms for edge-detection and thresholding. These technical variations result in considerable differences in the absolute bone mineral density values for the individual patient that are dependent on which machine is used.[143–145] In an effort to standardize bone mineral density measurements, representatives of the major DXA manufacturers agreed to standardize their bone mineral density results on the bases of (1) in vivo measurements, and (2) in vitro measurements using a European spine phantom that was engineered with the intention of intercomparing bone density results independently of the device being used.[146] Bone density also may be expressed as standardized bone mineral density in milligrams per square centimeter. A major advantage of this new unit is that distinct reference populations that exist for one scanner may be transferred to another. However, owing to software specifications that are unique to each manufacturer, it still may not be advisable to employ more

than one type of scanner for serial assessment of bone density in the individual patient.

Results of projectional posteroanterior examinations of the spine with DXA may be misleading because of the variability in bone size (especially thickness). To correct for this deficiency, Carter and collaborators, using a mathematical model, calculated a bone mineral apparent density in grams per cubic centimeter that was independent of subject height and weight, and further, an index that potentially represented bone strength, expressed as g^2/cm^4.[147] The practical clinical usefulness of this approach still has to be determined. Using synchronized DXA measurements of the spine in the posteroanterior and lateral projections, a calculation of an estimated width-adjusted (volumetric) density of the vertebral bodies is possible (Fig. 52–16). This approach to DXA measurements aims to provide results that are comparable to those obtained with quantitative CT measurements of the lumbar spine and requires further evaluation.[148]

Owing to the relatively high resolution of DXA scanners (although the resolution is far inferior to that of conventional x-ray), anatomic details of the examined region are depicted clearly with the resulting digital images. Using DXA for obtaining lateral images of the lumbar spine offers the advantage that the scanning beam, in contrast to conventional cone beam radiography, always is parallel to the vertebral endplates. This may improve the definition of vertebral dimensions for morphometric analysis. This method, based on DXA, has been referred to as morphometric x-ray absorptiometry (MXA) (Fig. 52–17).[149] Overlying osseous structures, including the ribs or the iliac crest, however, may have an adverse effect on the morphometric analysis. To enhance the accuracy of morphometric x-ray absorptiometry, technical modifications of the x-ray tube and the detector system may provide images with higher resolution and, thus, enhance the analysis of vertebral deformities. The disadvantage of such technical modifications, when compared to regular DXA, is higher radiation dose applied to the patient. Although MXA is in an early devel-

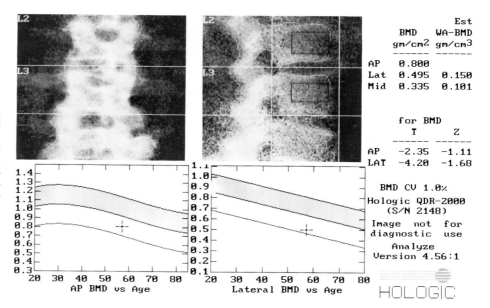

		BMD gm/cm2	Est WA-BMD gm/cm3
AP		0.800	
Lat		0.495	0.150
Mid		0.335	0.101

for BMD

	T	Z
AP	-2.35	-1.11
LAT	-4.20	-1.68

BMD CV 1.0%

Hologic QDR-2000
(S/N 2148)

Image not for
diagnostic use

Analyze
Version 4.56:1

HOLOGIC

FIGURE 52–16. Synchronized postero-anterior and lateral measurement of bone mineral density (BMD) of the lumbar spine. For comparison with young normal and an age-matched population, the results also are given as T- and Z-scores. The synchronized acquisition allows for a width-adjusted estimate of volumetric bone density (WA-BMD).

opmental stage, if it is proved suitable for the diagnosis of vertebral fractures, MXA eventually may replace conventional spine radiography, offering low radiation exposure and simultaneous measurements of bone density.

QUANTITATIVE COMPUTED TOMOGRAPHY

Computed tomography (CT) has been widely investigated in recent years as a means for noninvasive quantitative determination of bone mineral content. The usefulness of CT for measurement of bone mineral lies in its ability to provide a quantitative image and, thereby, measure trabecular, cortical, or integral bone in the central or peripheral skeleton. For measurements in the spine, the potential advantages of quantitative CT over DPA or DXA are its

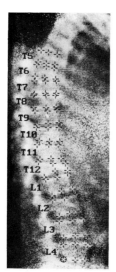

SD:	1mm PH (mm)	1mm MH (mm)	1mm AH (mm)	0.05 WEDGE	0.05 MWEDGE
T5	17.1	16.1	15.2	0.89	0.94
T6	17.5	15.9	16.4	0.94	0.91
T7	18.8	17.8	18.3	0.97	0.95
T8	17.3	17.8	16.4	0.94	1.03
T9	19.4	18.3	19.4	1.00	0.94
T10	19.6	20.4	19.3	0.99	1.04
T11	21.6	20.0	20.1	0.93	0.93
T12	22.5	11.2	10.1	0.45	0.50
L1	24.6	20.5	23.6	0.96	0.83
L2	24.4	23.6	25.2	1.03	0.97
L3	24.0	22.6	23.7	0.99	0.94
L4	21.8	23.3	24.0	1.10	1.07

FIGURE 52–17. Morphometric x-ray absorptiometry (MXA) of the spine. Anterior, middle, and posterior vertebral heights are determined using a semiautomated procedure. Several models can be applied to the resulting vertebral heights and their ratios for the determination of vertebral deformities. This example illustrates the detection of an anterior wedge deformity of T12 by MXA. PH, Posterior height. MH, Middle height. AH, Anterior height.

capability for both precise three-dimensional anatomic localization, providing a direct density measurement, and spatial separation of highly responsive cancellous bone from less responsive cortical bone.[150–153] The lumbar vertebrae contain substantial amounts of compact bone, with only part of the spinal mineral being high turnover trabecular bone. The sensitivity of a technique measuring an integral of compact and cancellous bone may be low compared with quantitative CT, owing to the inclusion of low turnover compact bone and extraosseous abnormalities, such as osteophytes and aortic calcification. Quantitative CT has been shown to measure changes in trabecular mineral content in the spine as well as the radius and tibia with great sensitivity and precision. Conventional CT scanners may be used for most applications; however, the extraction of quantitative information from the CT image requires sophisticated calibration and positioning techniques and careful technical monitoring. Specifically designed, small scale CT scanners using isotope or x-ray sources also have been developed and applied both on a research basis and in a clinical environment, principally for measurement of the trabecular and cortical bone in the appendicular skeleton.[153–155]

The principle of quantitative evaluations using CT is based on the fact that the CT image is a display of a map of x-ray attenuation coefficients of volume elements (voxels) in which average attenuation values of certain objects of interest can be determined. Attenuation values in CT are given in Hounsfield units. Using a mineral reference standard of a material that mimics bone, a bone mineral equivalent value of a given region of interest in a CT image can be calculated (Fig. 52–18). Common reference standards consist of either different solutions of K_2HPO_4 in water (liquid phantom, e.g., Cann-Genant phantom) or calcium hydroxyapatite ($Ca_5[PO_4]_3OH$) in a water equivalent plastic (solid state phantom).[152, 156] Solid state phantoms have proved to be stable in terms of their attenuation characteristics, unlike liquid phantoms that tend to produce air bubbles and need refills. Therefore, in the last years liquid phantoms have been replaced widely by solid state phantoms. For clinical practice, it is important to notice that quantitative CT measurements with solid state phantoms

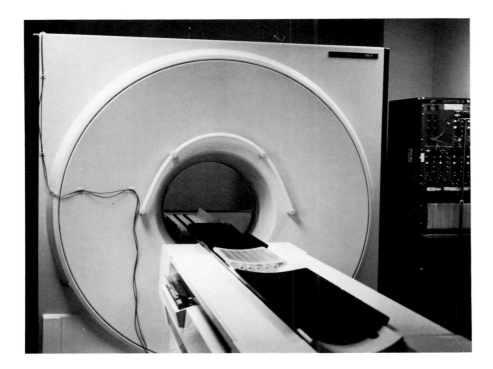

FIGURE 52–18. For simultaneous calibration, a phantom is placed under the patient during scanning.

yield 10 to 15 per cent higher results than with liquid phantoms. This fact has to be considered when comparing the results in an individual patient to normative data, or when assessing the longitudinal changes in bone mineral density in cases in which the calibration standard has changed.[157–159]

Typically, quantitative CT measurements of the axial skeleton are performed as single energy quantitative CT (using only one energy) of three to four consecutive lumbar vertebrae (Fig. 52–19). A digital computed radiograph (scout view, topogram) is obtained for localization of the slices at the midvertebral level. Depending on the manufacturer and the available software, the selection of these slices is done either manually by the CT operator or automatically. The use of automatic selection of midvertebral slices has proved to improve the reproducibility of quantitative CT.[160, 161] The slice thickness typically used is 8 to 10 mm. Quantitative image analysis of the CT slices includes two steps. First, the mean Hounsfield units of the mineral standards are determined. The values for the mineral standards are plotted against their respective mineral equivalent value, and a linear regression analysis is computed. Then, a representative volume of purely trabecular bone is selected as the region of interest, and the mean Hounsfield unit of this region is converted to a mineral equivalent value using the regression equation. For simultaneous calibration, in which the reference standard is placed directly underneath the specific region of interest (e.g., the patient's back), this procedure has to be repeated for each vertebral level. Nonsimultaneous calibration involves the measurement of a quasi-anthropomorphic phantom before or after a patient measurement, and therefore, the calculation of a regression equation is required only once, and all vertebral levels then are calculated using one equation. However, although simultaneous calibration allows correction of short-term instabilities in the measurement, nonsimultaneous calibration does not.[162]

A single energy quantitative CT examination as just described takes 5 to 10 min, and the radiation exposure is approximately 50 μSv, approximately 10 per cent of the radiation dose of a routine CT study (Table 52–2).[163] The radiation exposure may be greater when certain CT systems are used in which the manufacturers have restricted the capability for reducing kVp or mAs settings and is about two times greater when dual energy quantitative CT is used.

Although, classically, an elliptical region of interest placed in the anterior part of the vertebral body is used, the flexibility of the CT software permits the use of a region of interest of almost any shape, size, and location. This apparent advantage (i.e., customizing the region of interest for the corresponding clinical or research application) in actuality may be a disadvantage because it makes the manual evaluation of a quantitative CT scan highly operator dependent, thereby decreasing the reproducibility of serial examinations obtained over a substantial period of time. Kalender and associates and Steiger and coworkers independently proposed methods for an automated definition of the region of interest (Fig. 52–20).[164, 165] Using an automated definition of the region of interest, a short-term precision of 2 per cent or better can be reached.[164, 166] Both approaches allow the operator to obtain various regions of interest of which a peeled region of interest includes a maximum of trabecular bone of the vertebral body with exclusion of the retrovertebral plexus. Regions of interest that include purely cortical bone or an integral of cortical and trabecular bone can be defined.

The possibility of studying cortical and trabecular bone reproducibly has initiated studies on the differential behavior of bone loss of trabecular and cortical bone as it occurs in the spine. Cortical bone mineral density in the lumbar

FIGURE 52–19. Quantitative CT. The lateral scout view **(A)** provides a rapid and simple method to define the midplane of four vertebral bodies **(A)**, and a single 8 to 10 mm thick section is obtained at each level **(B)**. The classic oval region of interest is placed anteriorly in the middle of the vertebral body of three to four consecutive lumbar vertebrae and contains purely trabecular bone **(C)**. For reference, regions of interest also are placed in the compartments of the calibration standards that contain distinct solutions of K_2HPO_4 **(D)**.

spine was found to decrease at a slower rate than trabecular bone mineral density.[167, 168] However, these results have to be judged with caution, as analysis of the relatively small cortical rim may be influenced substantially by partial volume effects, and thinning of the cortical rim may amplify this effect. The assessment of cortical bone density is of some interest because, in vertebral bodies with decreasing trabecular bone density, the cortical rim appears to contribute substantially to vertebral strength.

The accuracy of single energy quantitative CT is 1 to 2 per cent for K_2HPO_4 solutions and 5 to 15 per cent for

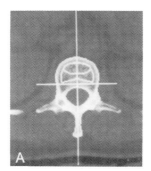
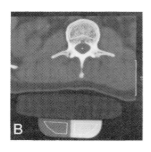

FIGURE 52–20. Automated detection of the regions of interest in a lumbar vertebra using the methods by Steiger and coworkers[164] **(A)** and Kalender and associates[165] **(B)**. The peeled region of interest that is depicted in both figures contains a maximum of trabecular bone under exclusion of the retrovertebral venous plexus. A solid state calibration phantom is depicted under the patient's back in **B**.

human vertebral specimens derived from cadavers of highly variable ages.[169–171] The accuracy of quantitative CT (and DPA or DXA), however, can be reduced in an elderly osteoporotic population. With regard to quantitative CT, the sources of error are partially correctable. The density of yellow marrow is less than that of red marrow because of the presence of fat, which falsely reduces the measured spinal mineral value (by 7 mg per 10 per cent fat by volume at 80 kVp), and can result in inaccuracies (in this case underestimation of the real bone mineral density) of 20 to 30 per cent in elderly patients with osteoporosis.[172, 173]

Dual energy quantitative CT which is offered by several equipment manufacturers, can reduce the magnitude of this error (in an aged population) to approximately 5 per cent but at the expense of reduced precision and higher radiation exposure (Fig. 52–21).[174–176] With dual energy quantitative CT, two slices at two distinct energy levels (e.g., 80 and 140 kVp) are obtained, and bone mineral density values are calculated numerically either from regular CT images at both energy levels (postacquisition processing technique) or from a calcium-equivalent density image using the principle of basis material decomposition (preprocessing technique).[150, 177–179] The images may be obtained as two successively acquired back-to-back slices or, with certain scanners, within one acquisition using fast kVp switching. The latter technique reduces artifacts and measurement errors produced by patient movement between the two scans. Reinbold and associates reported an accuracy error of only 1.4 per cent for specimens derived from vertebral bone

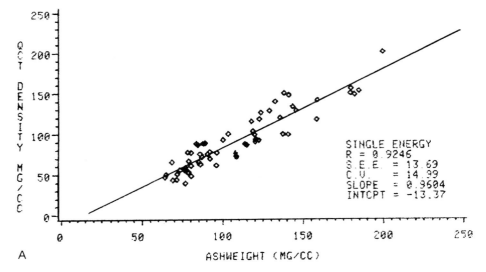

A

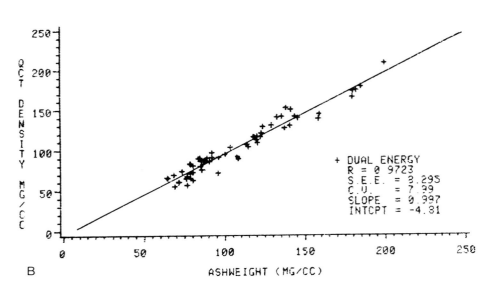

B

FIGURE 52–21. Accuracy of quantitative CT. **A,** The accuracy of single energy quantitative CT is shown for fresh vertebral specimens (derived from 62 samples) from 28 cadavers (20 men and 8 women with a mean age of 60 years) with a predictive error of 13 mg/ml. **B,** Accuracy is improved with dual energy quantitative CT.

using a dual energy quantitative CT technique.[174] Dual energy quantitative CT is considered unnecessary for most clinical applications. However, when highly accurate measurements are needed, as in special research endeavors, both single and dual energy quantitative CT can be performed initially as a baseline study, after which single energy quantitative CT alone can be applied for longitudinal follow-up examinations. Furthermore, the fat-related uncertainty of single energy quantitative CT is far lower than the biologic variation that is to be expected in a normal population, and it is reduced further by the fact that the normal data are based on single energy quantitative CT data that account for most of the variability of marrow fat with age. The selection of a tube voltage for single energy quantitative CT that is as low as possible (e.g., 80 kVp) also will help to minimize the fat-induced underestimation of the real bone mineral density.[169, 180]

Quantitative CT has made it possible to obtain a multitude of clinical observations on age-related trabecular bone loss and the effects of menopause and estrogen replace-

ment.[169, 181, 182] The rate of spinal trabecular bone loss due to abrupt cessation of ovarian function after surgical menopause (oophorectomy) was found to be even more excessive compared to the bone loss after natural menopause.[151] With respect to these studies, the evidence linking estrogen to maintenance of skeletal mass in women is convincing. The rates of postmenopausal spinal trabecular bone loss as observed with quantitative CT were found to be greater than those observed by dual photon or x-ray absorptiometry of the spine.[10, 183]

Rapid technologic advances in CT ensure that most CT scanners may be modified inexpensively for quantitative CT measurements. Reductions in patient scanning time and radiation exposure make this an attractive technique for noninvasive measurement of bone mass. With a careful cross-calibration that takes the different fat-sensitivities of CT scanners and the used calibration standards into account, and sound longitudinal quality assurance (e.g., daily phantom scans), quantitative CT measurements are relatively independent of the CT scanner type that is being

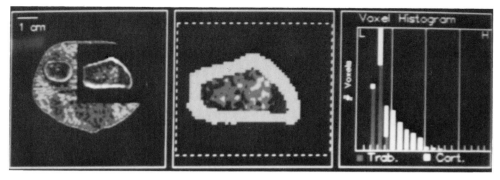

FIGURE 52–22. Peripheral quantitative CT of the forearm. Cortical and trabecular bone are identified in the distal portion of the radius, and bone density is determined for each compartment separately.

used, and comparison of results between scanners is possible.[158, 159, 184] Indeed, normative data and clinical results obtained using a CT scanner at one site may be extrapolated to those obtained at a different location. However, normative data derived from one population may not necessarily be correct for other populations, or specifically for different ethnic groups.[185] Quantitative CT vertebral mineral determination by this approach has been implemented at many sites worldwide using a multitude of different commercial scanners. However, the lack of designated quantitative CT scanners is a major limitation of this technique.

The principle of quantitative CT has been applied to measurements of the appendicular skeleton using a special purpose peripheral quantitative CT (pQCT) scanner. Initially, a radionuclide source (preferably ^{125}I) was used in most pQCT devices; however, it has now been replaced by an x-ray source.[55, 186–188] The preferred anatomic site for analysis with this technique is the ultradistal radius (Fig. 52–22). Modern pQCT scanners using a multislice technique offer short examination times, small precision error, and small radiation doses.[189, 190] Using a high resolution pQCT scanner Rüegsegger and coworkers found that, in contrast to trabecular bone mineral density of the radius, which declined with age, cortical bone density in this site remained constant between the age of 20 and 70 years.[191] Ease of use and the possibility of assessing trabecular bone alone make this method an interesting alternative to other techniques. However, because the relation between peripheral and axial bone density remains controversial, further evaluation of this method is required.

Boden and collaborators reported an approach for spinal quantitative CT without the use of an external calibration phantom.[192] Instead, paraspinal muscle and subcutaneous fat are used as internal reference standards for the calculation of bone mineral density, based on the concept that muscle and fat have known linear attenuation coefficients and therefore can be used to correct the CT numbers that are measured in every slice. Although initial results indicated a good reproducibility of this technique and its possible diagnostic potential, a careful evaluation of this method in comparison to established quantitative CT methods still is required.[193] In its present form, this method cannot be recommended for routine clinical applications.

QUANTITATIVE ULTRASONOGRAPHY

Ultrasonographic techniques used to assess material properties are well known in industrial testing. The first experiments to determine material properties of bone using

ultrasound transmission velocity were performed in the 1960s.[194, 195] Although these experiments showed promising results, sonographic techniques for the detection of osteoporosis were not employed widely until recent years. Owing to developments in hardware and software that have resulted in enhanced precision and ease of use, these techniques have reemerged as a promising option for the assessment of the material properties of the bone.

The ultrasound transmission velocity (UTV), or speed of sound, is calculated as the quotient of the transit time of an ultrasound wave through bone and the width or diameter of this bone (Fig. 52–23). This velocity is expressed in meters per second. UTV is a function of mass density and elastic modulus, which may be influenced by bone mass, distribu-

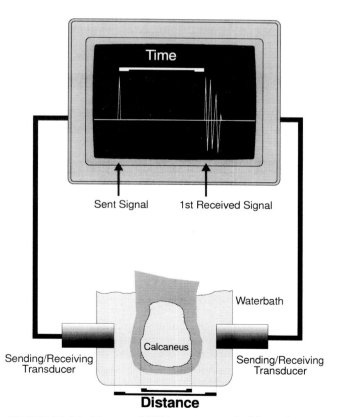

FIGURE 52–23. Diagram of UTV measurement of the calcaneus. The velocity is calculated as the quotient of the known distance between the ultrasound transducers or a diameter of the measured bone and the time between when the signal is sent and when it is first received. The UTV is expressed as meters per second.

tion of trabecular and cortical bone, trabecular orientation, composition of organic and inorganic components, and fatigue damage of bone. Accordingly, bone mass and other characteristics of bone contribute to UTV. Abendschein and Hyatt found a significant correlation between UTV and elastic modulus ($r = 0.855$) and between UTV and physical density ($r = 0.866$).[194] Tavakoli and Evans reported a correlation of 0.97 for UTV and bone mineral content of cancellous bone.[196] Other results indicate that structural properties may have an even greater influence on UTV than bone mass. The velocities measured in vitro have a wide range from 1400 to 2300 m/sec for cancellous bone to 3000 to 3600 m/sec for cortical bone.[194, 197, 198]

Only a few in vivo studies have been performed to examine the diagnostic value of UTV for the detection of osteoporosis. Jergas and associates found a significant difference in the UTV in osteoporotic and nonosteoporotic women as measured in the proximal phalanges of the second and third fingers.[199] Heaney and coworkers indicated that UTV measurements of the patella allow a discrimination between normal and osteoporotic women that equals that provided by bone densitometry of the axial skeleton.[200] Brandenburger and collaborators reported that subjects with a UTV value for the calcaneus of one standard deviation or more below normal had a three to five times increased risk for vertebral crush fractures in the following 2 years than subjects with normal results.[201] Schott and coinvestigators described a continuous decline of UTV as measured in the calcaneus with advancing age starting at the age of 20 years.[202]

Data concerning correlations between UTV and bone mineral density measurements at various skeletal sites are controversial. Depending on the positioning of the ultrasound transducers, Zagzebski and coworkers reported a correlation of $r = 0.51$ to 0.72 between UTV and bone mineral density measurements of the calcaneus.[203] Herd and associates reported a relatively poor correlation of $r = 0.55$ between UTV measurements of the calcaneus and bone mineral density measurements of the lumbar spine.[204] Correlation coefficients of this magnitude also were observed in other studies involving UTV and bone mineral density measurements of various other skeletal sites.[199, 202, 205]

Antich and coworkers have reported on a sonographic reflection technique in which the ultrasound velocity is measured at a "critical angle" at which the amplitude reflected from the bone surface is maximal.[206, 207] Excellent to good correlations were found between UTV and ultrasound reflection velocities (URV) for isotropic materials and cortical bone samples. No significant change in URV was noticed after removal of soft tissue in vitro. In vivo results were obtained at the ulnar head (cancellous site) and the ulnar shaft (cortical site). For the cancellous site, an inverse correlation of URV with age was found. A significantly lower URV also was demonstrated for postmenopausal compared to premenopausal women at this site, and a significant longitudinal increase for cancellous URV was seen prospectively in patients treated with sodium fluoride and calcium citrate. The cortical site showed similar trends that were not statistically significant.

Attenuation measurements of ultrasound waves in humans were performed in the 1970s. The purpose of these early experiments was to establish a method for a cranial diagnostic ultrasonographic image comparable to the CT

scan.[208] Reflection and absorption are the main components that contribute to the attenuation of the ultrasound wave penetrating a material. In addition, attenuation strongly depends on the frequency of the ultrasound wave that is employed. With the use of a low frequency range (approximately 200 to 600 kHz) the attenuation is an almost linear function of frequency. With higher frequencies the attenuation increases in a nonlinear fashion. In quantitative ultrasonography the attenuation of the ultrasound wave is measured using the low frequency range (e.g., 200 to 600 kHz). This technique is called broadband ultrasound attenuation (BUA). The slope of the resulting regression line is the BUA value and is given in units of decibels per megahertz (dB/MHz) (Fig. 52–24).

In vitro studies show significant correlations between physical density and BUA.[209] Agren and coworkers were able to demonstrate a high correlation between BUA and trabecular bone volume.[210] Glüer and colleagues demonstrated a significant impact of trabecular orientation on BUA measurements, thus revealing the ability of BUA measurements to detect structural changes of the bone.[211]

Clinical studies using BUA measurements have concentrated mainly on the calcaneus as a measurement site. BUA was found to be correlated significantly with age in postmenopausal women in one study. In contrast to UTV, however, no significant age-related decrease of BUA was seen in premenopausal women.[202] In a prospective study Porter and associates demonstrated a significant association of low BUA with an increased prevalence of hip fractures.[212] Baran and colleagues compared calcaneal BUA with DPA measurements of vertebral bodies and femoral neck and found a significant decrease of BUA values in women with low bone mass. The diagnostic sensitivity and specificity of BUA measurements were found to be about 80 per cent. For patients with a femoral neck fracture, sensitivity and specificity were even higher.[213] Glüer and coworkers compared SXA of the calcaneus with BUA measurements of this site and found an overall correlation of $r = 0.58$ for a mixed population, and for a subgroup of only women the

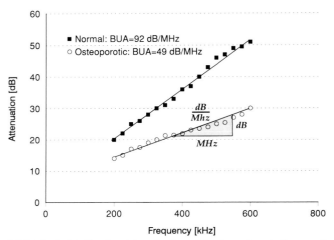

FIGURE 52–24. For the determination of the broadband ultrasound attenuation (BUA), the attenuation of the ultrasound wave at a series of frequencies, commonly between 200 and 600 kHz, is measured. A linear regression of the curve is calculated. The slope of this regression line is the BUA value, expressed as decibels per megahertz.

correlation was 0.72, leaving about 50 per cent of unexplained variability. The authors drew the conclusion that the 50 per cent that were unexplained may relate to properties of the bone other than density.[214] Numerous studies have been published that examine the relationship between calcaneal BUA and bone mineral density at various sites. Massie and associates examined 1000 women using DXA of hip and spine and calcaneal BUA. For all results, the best numerical correlation was found between trochanteric bone mineral density and BUA ($r = 0.354$, $p < 0.001$). However, the subgroup of postmenopausal women yielded better correlations.[215] These results partly contradict the findings of Schott and colleagues, who found better correlations in a group that included younger women than in a group that included older women.[202] Truscott and coworkers reported correlation coefficients ranging from 0.49 to 0.62 (all $p < 0.001$) for spinal, femoral, whole body, and forearm bone mineral density and calcaneal BUA.[216]

Comparing UTV and BUA, Ramalingham and coworkers found a correlation of $r = 0.81$.[217] Using a system with direct coupling of the ultrasound transmitters to the heel rather than a measurement in a water bath, Herd and associates found a comparable correlation of 0.75.[218] The correlation between BUA values using two devices of different manufacturers was 0.83.[217] Statements concerning the reproducibility of UTV and BUA measurements depend strongly on the devices used. The precision error for calcaneus measurements using the most common devices is reported to be between 1 and 4 per cent for BUA measurements and between 0.15 to 1.2 per cent for measurements of the UTV.[202, 214, 218] Antich and colleagues reported a precision of 1.8 per cent for the in vivo measurement of URV at the ulnar head.[207]

A main advantage of ultrasonographic examination is the complete absence of radiation and low cost of the equipment; however, a multitude of questions need to be answered. The relationship between bone mass, elastic properties of the bone, and ultrasound waves, is uncertain; in addition other issues, such as the influence of surrounding soft tissue, the path of the ultrasound wave through the bone, and the effect of physical activity, still need to be addressed.[197, 209, 219–222] Although a significant number of ultrasound devices already have been distributed, the ability of such devices to allow monitoring of the course of disease in patients with osteoporosis and to allow prediction of the likelihood of subsequent fractures will have to be determined to clarify the clinical applicability of quantitative ultrasonography as a routine diagnostic tool.

QUANTITATIVE MAGNETIC RESONANCE IMAGING

Age- and sex-dependent changes in the depiction of bone marrow have been noticed with MR imaging. The influence of sex and age on T1 and T2 relaxation time measurements was first reported by Dooms and associates.[223] Using a region of interest in the central part of the first and second lumbar vertebral bodies in the sagittal plane, these authors found a decrease of the bone marrow T1 relaxation times with age in both sexes. However, although T2 relaxation time decreased in the male patient group with age, no significant decrease was found for the female patients. These results could be explained in part by the replacement of

hematopoietic marrow by fatty marrow. The authors suggested that the absence of a decline in the T2 relaxation time of the vertebral marrow in women may be explained by a disproportionally higher loss of bone mineral density and trabecular structures in aging women than in men. Comparable results for T1 measurements at several anatomic locations also were reported by Richards and associates.[224] Women using oral contraceptives were found to have a slightly but not significantly increased T1 bone marrow relaxation time than those who did not use oral contraceptives, and T1 relaxation times were higher in men than in women. In contrast to these reports, Jenkins and coworkers did not see age- or sex-related changes in T1 or T2 relaxation times and reported a great variation of the bone marrow relaxation times.[225] LeBlanc and colleagues found a decrease of T2 of bone marrow in the spine and in the lower limb after 5 weeks of bed rest.[226, 227] The data, however, also showed great variation. The small magnetic field strengths that were used in the aforementioned studies may not provide an assessment of bone mineral density or susceptibility effects of the bone marrow interface in a sufficient way, however.

Davis and coinvestigators studied the spin-lattice relaxation times (T1) and the effective spin-spin relaxation times (T2*, a parameter distinct from the spin-spin relaxation time or T2) of water, acetone, and cottonseed oil in the presence of different concentrations of bone powder. Although bone contributed significantly to the local magnetic inhomogeneity as evidenced by shortened T2* values for all solutions, the relaxation time T1 did not change significantly in the presence of bone.[228] Using an asymmetric spin echo technique, Rosenthal and associates confirmed these results at a lower field strength (0.6 Tesla) with specimens of trabecular bone that were immersed in water.[229] Ito and colleagues recently examined the relationship between T1 relaxation time and bone mineral density at 1.5 Tesla using a spin echo technique. The addition of cottonseed oil to solutions of $CaCO_3$ in various concentrations diminished the differences among the T1 relaxation times of the original solutions so that the different concentrations of $CaCO_3$ could not be identified reliably on the bases of T1 measurements. The relationship between T1 relaxation times as determined by MR imaging and bone mineral density as measured by dual energy and single energy quantitative CT in excised vertebrae was only moderate.[230]

T1 and T2 relaxation times as derived from spin echo techniques may not be sufficient to describe properties of bone marrow that relate to bone mineral density. However, the in vitro studies have demonstrated an effect of bone on the transverse relaxation time, T2*. This effect is related to variations in magnetic susceptibility at the interface of solid particles and surrounding protons. Magnetic susceptibility describes the magnetic response of a material to an applied magnetic field. The effects of magnetic susceptibility of bone marrow are illustrated impressively by the image obtained with a gradient echo sequence in Figure 52–25.[231] Here, the differences in magnetic susceptibility between bone marrow and trabecular bone result in a distortion in the lines of force, causing strong local inhomogeneities. Such magnetic field inhomogeneities result in a dephasing of the transverse magnetization in marrow tissue with a decrease in the marrow transverse relaxation time (T2*) and, consequently, a reduction of signal intensity. The num-

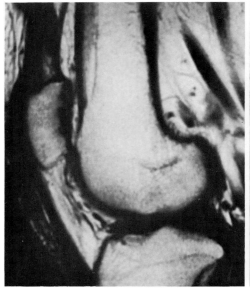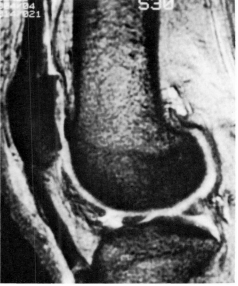

FIGURE 52–25. Sagittal spin echo (left) and gradient echo (right) MR images of the knee. Whereas in the spin echo sequence, bone marrow gives a nearly homogeneous bright signal, on gradient echo sequences the bone marrow appears inhomogeneous owing to susceptibility effects between trabeculae and the marrow space. Note the differences in the signal intensity of the bone marrow in the distal portion of the femur. The higher the signal intensity of the bone marrow, the lower is the density of the trabecular network.

ber and thickness of trabecular elements in a defined volume supposedly are major factors accounting for changes in bone marrow T2*; as the number of particles in a defined volume increases, T2* decreases (Fig. 52–26). Numerous factors, besides the number of particles within a magnetic field, such as geometric shape and spatial arrangement, may influence magnetic susceptibility. These considerations suggest that T2* measurements of bone marrow depend mostly on structural variations that in turn relate to bone density.

Experimentally, a relationship between T2* and bone density has been verified by Majumdar and associates, who showed modifications in the T2* of saline solutions containing variable amounts of trabecular bone at 1.5 Tesla.[232] Although T1 and T2 measurements did not show any sig-

nificant relationship to bone density, the transverse relaxation rate 1/T2* increased with bone mineral density at a rate of $0.2\ \mathrm{sec^{-1}/mg/cm^3}$. Variations in signal intensity also were demonstrated in vivo, and in a later study Majumdar and Genant demonstrated the relatively good correlation between 1/T2* and bone mineral density in the appendicular skeleton.[233] The relationship between T2* and trabecular plate density also was confirmed by the results of Ford and Wehrli, who used MR interferometry and localized spectroscopy in an evaluation of the distal femur.[234] Wehrli and coworkers also applied MR interferometry to the lumbar spine in vivo, and they found that T2* increases slightly with age in healthy subjects and is prolonged significantly in osteoporotic subjects in comparison to healthy volun-

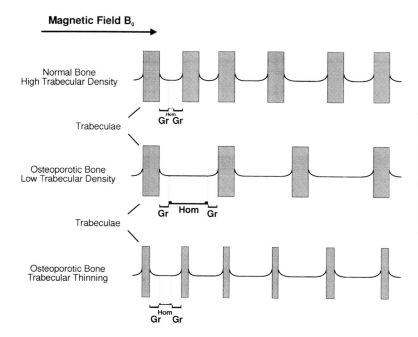

FIGURE 52–26. Effects of magnetic susceptibility. In this figure, low trabecular density and trabecular thinning as it can be seen in osteoporotic bone cause an increase of regions of homogeneous fields (Hom), whereas in normal bone more regions with nonlinear gradient fields (Gr) are present. Regions that are characterized by strong nonlinear gradients (high trabecular density) cause phase dispersion and consequently signal loss and a decrease in the transverse relaxation time (T2*). This effect is illustrated in the gradient echo image in Figure 52–25. (Adapted in part from Wehrli FW, et al: Radiology *179:*615, 1991.)

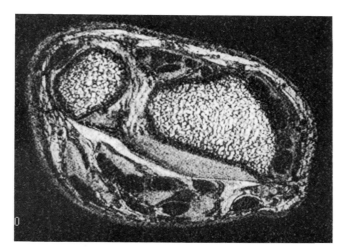

FIGURE 52–27. High resolution MR image of the forearm. The radius and ulna are depicted in the transaxial plane. Note the trabecular structure with low signal intensity surrounded by marrow space of high signal intensity. The in-plane resolution of this image is 156 μm.

teers.[235] A positive correlation ($r = 0.59$) between bone density and 1/T2* at the lumbar spine in vivo also was reported by Sugimoto and coworkers.[236]

Few reports exist on the application of MR spectroscopy to the evaluation of bone mineral density. One technique was described by Brown and associates, who used a 0.4 Tesla permanent magnet design.[237, 238] The bone mineral content of a bone sample was determined from its ^{31}P nuclear magnetic resonance (NMR) spectrum relative to that of potassium hexafluorophosphate (KPF_6), which served as a reference standard. The authors found that the weight of hydroxyapatite could be measured directly from the peak area of its ^{31}P NMR spectrum. The degree of inaccuracy of the method in vivo strongly depended on the site measured and was found to be on the order of 15 per cent for the bones in the human hand related to spectral contributions from dissolved cytosolic metabolites. The reproducible localization of a defined volume appears to be difficult, as is the interpretation of the ^{31}P spectrum, and the use of this technique subsequently has not been evaluated.

The development of new image sequences allows high resolution MR images of the appendicular skeleton to be obtained in vivo. Several studies reported a resolution of better than 100 μm and slice thickness on the order of 300 μm (Fig. 52–27). Obtaining images with such resolution makes the assessment of trabecular changes possible, and some studies on structural analysis of bone have been performed on the basis of these techniques.[239–241] The development of refined techniques for structural assessment of trabecular bone using MR imaging is a research field that may add defined structural qualitative parameters to the predominantly quantitative field of bone densitometry.[242]

STRUCTURAL ANALYSIS OF BONE

Coincident developments that include the availability of highly sophisticated imaging techniques such as MR imaging and CT scanning, advances in computer and programming technology, and the identification of new therapeutic agents all have supported an increased effort to obtain in-

formation regarding structural changes in bone. A guideline, and at the same time a standard, for all applied methods is given by the morphologic analysis of bone biopsies.[243–247]

Several studies have dealt with the application of methods for structural analysis to conventional radiographs. Geraets and coworkers found only poor correlations when they compared various trabecular pattern parameters, derived from a texture analysis of a radiograph of the distal portion of the radius, with bone mineral density measured by DPA of the spine.[248] Caligiuri and associates reported preliminary results of a texture analysis of vertebral bodies analyzing the power spectrum of a selected region of interest on a digitized radiograph. Although the correlations between bone mineral density obtained with spinal DPA and the first moment of power or root mean square values were poor, first moment of power and root square mean allowed for better discrimination between those patients with fractures and those without fractures than did measurements of bone mineral density.[249] However, these results await confirmation in a greater number of patients.

In addition to supplying the information regarding bone mineral density, quantitative CT is an imaging technique that can provide structural information for the regions examined. The use of high resolution CT scanning can be regarded as a basis for future structural analysis, thereby offering the chance of quantifying architectural changes in trabecular bone in vivo. Chevalier and collaborators applied an adaptive thresholding technique to high resolution CT images of the lumbar spine and calculated a "trabecular fragmentation index" (TFI) using a ratio of length of trabecular network and number of discontinuities found in the image. The correlation coefficient found between TFI and bone mineral density as measured by quantitative CT was -0.6. However, for women with vertebral density below normal, the TFI could distinguish those who had no fractures from those with vertebral fractures.[250] A gray level run-length method was applied to high resolution pQCT images of normal volunteers and osteoporotic patients after thresholding, and histomorphometric parameters were calculated.[251] Significant differences were found for the trabecular bone volume in osteoporotic persons and normal controls. A methodologic limitation is that a relatively subjective selection of threshold values separating trabeculae from intertrabecular space is required. This must be regarded critically and may make interindividual comparisons difficult. A possible alternative to thresholding is the application of a ridge-valley detection method that was introduced by Haralick.[252] The technical limitations of all these techniques are defined by the high demands upon image quality and resolution. However, the greatest challenge of all seems to be the three-dimensional assessment of structural parameters. Three-dimensional information may be essential for the determination of structural parameters, such as trabecular connectivity, as they cannot be determined readily from two-dimensional information alone.[253, 254]

The application of fractal geometry for the analysis of bone structure is based on the assumption that trabecular network may be characterized as an object with a typical fractal dimension. Fractal geometry is used to describe complicated structures, such as many naturally occurring objects (e.g., coastlines, clouds) that cannot be described easily using the tools of euclidean geometry. Majumdar and coworkers found that the fractal dimension was related to the variations of histomorphometric parameters of the trabecular network in high resolution MR images and photomicrographs of iliac crest biopsies.[241, 255] In certain limits, this approach appeared to be relatively insensitive to changes in image acquisition, resolution, and thresholding. Ruttimann and associates applied this method to intraoral radiographs of peridental alveolar bones and found that the fractal dimension was significantly higher in postmenopausal than in premenopausal women. This group also reported that the fractal dimension of bone radiographs increased after acid-induced demineralization.[256] Samarabandu and associates applied fractal analysis to radiographs of rat femurs and demonstrated a significant decrease in the fractal dimension of immobilized limbs from that in normal limbs.[257]

A method that combines the results of assessment of both density and morphology is the finite element analysis. Faulkner and coworkers used images derived from quantitative CT to calculate a finite element model of the vertebra and the femur.[258, 259] Principally a research tool, this technique may help to elucidate mechanisms of bone fragility in osteoporotic patients with respect to the interplay of bone density and bone structure.[260]

CLINICAL BONE DENSITOMETRY

Clinical Indications. In their present state the various methods of bone mineral density measurement appear more complementary than competitive. For clinical practice the choice of the technique depends on the specific disorder being evaluated and the availability of reliable measurement technology. In 1989 the Scientific Advisory Board of the National Osteoporosis Foundation published recommendations for the clinical use of bone densitometry.[261] In this publication three indications and a number of potential indications are listed. Although the monitoring of bone mass to assess the efficacy of therapy is mentioned only as a potential indication for bone mass measurements in these recommendations, the authors of this chapter believe that recent advances in bone densitometry, which lead to higher precision, make serial assessment of changes of bone mineral density feasible. They therefore advocate inclusion of serial assessment of bone mineral density during therapy in the list of indications for bone mass measurements with the understanding that therapeutic decisions may be affected (Table 52–4).[262] Other potential indications proposed by the

TABLE 52–4. Indications for Bone Densitometry

I	Patients receiving long-term glucocorticoid therapy,* patients with primary asymptomatic hyperparathyroidism,* or other patients at high risk for osteoporosis, such as amenorrheic women, anorexia nervosa, alcoholism, patients with atraumatic fractures, disuse atrophy, and similar conditions†
II	Assessment of early postmenopausal bone loss as an indication to initiate estrogen replacement therapy*
III	Diagnosis of osteoporosis suspected from radiographic findings or from clinical risk factors*
IV	Serial assessment of bone density (e.g., during treatment for osteoporosis or in anticipation of rapid bone loss)†

*Indication for bone mass measurements as outlined by the Scientific Advisory Board of the National Osteoporosis Foundation.[261]

†Potential indication for bone mass measurements as outlined by the Scientific Advisory Board of the National Osteoporosis Foundation.[261]

National Osteoporosis Foundation, such as the universal screening for osteoporosis prophylaxis and the identification of "fast losers," remain controversial. Radiation-free methods (e.g., ultrasonography) will, if proved feasible and economical, again raise the question of widespread screening to identify patients with potential for osteoporosis. The assessment of patients at high risk, outlined as another potential indication by the National Osteoporosis Foundation, also may be regarded as a clear indication, considering the enhanced diagnostic capabilities of densitometric methods and new options of therapeutic intervention. In the following sections the clinical indications for bone densitometry are outlined briefly.

Assessment of the Skeletal Status of Patients with Metabolic Diseases or Other Risk Factors Known to Affect the Skeleton. A variety of metabolic disorders such as hyperparathyroidism, renal insufficiency, Cushing's syndrome, and amenorrhea in premenopausal women, as well as chronic immobilization and chronic steroid or thyroid therapy, are known to influence calcium metabolism and may affect the skeleton adversely. The effects on bone mineral density have been reported in several studies.[31, 134, 138, 263–269] Some of these secondary forms of osteoporosis, such as that in Cushing's syndrome, preferentially affect the trabecular bone, with relative sparing of cortical bone.[170] Diseases such as renal osteodystrophy may cause dramatic cortical demineralization whereas spinal trabecular density may be low, normal, or even high owing to sclerotic changes. These typical changes may be proved by quantitative CT, as a differential assessment of trabecular and integral bone density is possible. Therefore, assessment with a combination of techniques may be appropriate in some instances.[269] In these cases of secondary osteoporosis, bone density measurements are of particular importance because they may prompt therapeutic decisions such as a reduction in corticosteroid dose, the choice of subtotal parathyroidectomy in hyperparathyroidism, or the initiation of estrogen replacement therapy in premenopausal amenorrheic women.

Initiation of Estrogen Replacement or Therapy in Postmenopausal Women. Bone turnover increases significantly at menopause, with a greater increase in bone resorption than bone formation, resulting in an accelerated loss of bone.[151, 270] This finding has led some investigators to differentiate between a type 1 form of osteoporosis (representing the accelerated bone loss related to postmenopausal low estrogen levels), and a type 2 form (representing relatively slower, age-related bone loss).[271] Although this distinction is disputable, one third or one half of the bone loss in women may be attributable to the loss of ovarian function. Several studies have established the bone mass–preserving effect of estrogen therapy if begun soon after menopause, thereby reducing the subsequent rate of vertebral fractures by half.[272] Discontinuation of therapy results in resumption of normal postmenopausal bone loss.[273, 274] Studies show that estrogen therapy still is effective at a later postmenopausal age and in women with established osteoporosis, increasing the spinal bone density by more than 5 per cent per year.[275, 276] The benefits derived from estrogen therapy clearly seem to outweigh its adverse effects. However, estrogen therapy still is unacceptable for many women, and the compliance may be enhanced by quantitative information concerning fracture risk and therapeutic efficacy. In this context, the absolute level of bone mineral density at the menopause and the magnitude of subsequent loss are important considerations in assessing the future risk of fracture, and a decision to begin prophylaxis can be based on such considerations.

Establishing a Diagnosis of Osteoporosis. Bone density should be measured if factors predisposing to secondary forms of osteoporosis are found. However, risk factors based on history (e.g., low calcium intake, caffeine intake, smoking, family history of osteoporosis, petite frame), taken either alone or in combination, have limited predictive value for fracture risk or for bone density in the individual patient.[277] Similarly, conventional spinal radiography is neither highly sensitive nor specific for detecting osteoporosis, particularly in its early stages.[278–280] Furthermore, even the presence of osteoporotic fracture may confer variable or uncertain risk for future fracture, and biochemical analyses, although helpful in excluding secondary forms of osteoporosis, are of limited value in diagnosing osteoporosis or assessing its severity. Considering the predictive value of bone density, it should be recommended that measurements of bone mass be performed in persons in whom osteoporosis is suspected from the presence of an atraumatic fracture or on the basis of radiographic findings. Bone density measurements in persons with known clinical risk factors or who are concerned about their current skeletal status remain disputable. General recommendations cannot be given, and these decisions must be made individually.

Serial Assessment of Bone Density During Treatment or in the Course of Osteoporosis. The large precision errors of previous densitometric techniques have been overcome by new software and hardware developments as well as insights in quality control measures that allow serial changes in bone mineral density to be assessed with high reliability. Detailed analyses were made by several authors on the amount of bone that must be lost to be statistically significant.[262, 281, 282] Table 52–5 illustrates the differences in the required change for two-point serial measurements using a one- or a two-tailed approach for determining confidence intervals. The authors believe that the one-tailed approach may be adequate for the clinical practice. Short- and long-term variations of the machine as well as biologic variations contribute to the imprecision of bone density measurements.[283, 284] Using replicate measurements may help to reduce uncertainty due to short-term technical errors substantially. The degree of uncertainty is inversely proportional to the length of follow-up (i.e., the reliability of the bone loss rate improves with the length of the time period between the scans). Verheij and associates found, assuming a linear rate of bone mass changes, that measurements at the beginning and the end of an observation period were

the best estimate of actual changes in bone mass.[285] Considering the precision of DXA, these authors recommended a follow-up of patients with yearly duplicate measurements. In general, yearly duplicate measurements or measurements every 2 years appear to be a useful guideline. For clinical practice, however, the method used, the disease state, the expected rates of change, and the presence and type of therapeutic intervention will have a considerable impact on the required frequency of follow-up measurements.

Numerous studies have shown that large annual losses of bone from sites rich in trabecular bone can be observed in women undergoing natural or surgical menopause, in patients undergoing high dose steroid treatment, and in immobilized persons. Similarly, large annual gains of bone have been observed in osteoporotic patients receiving treatment with a variety of therapeutic agents, such as calcitonin, fluoride, bisphosphonates, or parathyroid hormone.[286–292] Given the marked effect of some types of intervention, the magnitude of postmenopausal loss of bone, and the continued improvements in measurement precision, it is difficult to pose arguments against serial assessment of bone mineral density for evaluation of therapeutic efficacy.

Which Site to Measure? "To diagnose spinal osteoporosis . . . a patient should have a measurement of bone mass at the spine."[261] This statement reflects the widespread opinion that the biologic variations between measurement sites hardly allow for a prediction of bone density at one site by measurement at another site. This impression is based, in part, on studies comparing sites in the peripheral and axial skeleton with only moderate correlation between the measurement sites.[14, 57–59] However, several studies show that bone mineral density as measured in the peripheral skeleton and bone mineral density derived from measurements of the axial skeleton may have comparable results in discriminating osteoporotic from nonosteoporotic women, and that differences between the techniques are marginal.[13, 65, 293, 294] Comparable results have been found for the capabilities of the various methods to predict fractures prospectively.[70, 295] This applies at least to most of the projectional techniques. A major difference among techniques is their capability to measure predominantly metabolically active trabecular bone. In this situation, quantitative CT proved to be superior, in several studies, in its discriminatory ability to identify patients with osteoporotic fractures of the spine (Table 52–6).[65, 293, 294, 296] It is well known that degenerative changes of the aging spine and the inclusion of cortical bone contribute to the relative insensitivity of projectional techniques applied to the lumbar spine to discriminate between osteoporotic and nonosteoporotic patients. Experience using lateral DXA in this respect is limited, and further study is required. The usefulness of hip measurements in addition to DXA of the spine has been discussed.[297] Soda and associates found that substantial bone loss in the hip lasted longer than that of the lumbar spine in postmenopausal women, potentially indicating the onset of spinal degenerative changes.[298] Ryan and collaborators found in a cross-sectional study that a number of patients with osteoporotic fractures and a low femoral bone mineral density could not be identified by vertebral bone mineral density measurements using DXA and vice versa.[299] Pouilles and colleagues described different rates of

TABLE 52–5. Required Changes in Bone Mineral Density to be Significant in a Two-Point Serial Measurement Using a Two-tailed and a One-tailed Estimation of the Confidence Limit[262, 281]

Precision Error (%)	90% Two-tailed Confidence Limit (%)	90% One-tailed Confidence Limit (%)
1	±2.3	1.8
2	±4.7	3.6
3	±7.0	5.4

TABLE 52–6. Comparison of Quantitative CT (QCT), Dual Photon or X-ray Absorptiometry (DPA/DXA), and Single Photon Absorptiometry (SPA) in Normal Subjects and Osteoporotic Persons with Vertebral Fractures

	QCT (mg/cm³)	DPA/DXA (g/cm²)*	SPA (g/cm)†
Reinbold et al.[293]			
Normal subjects	118.7 ± 24.2	1.067 ± 0.17	0.846 ± 0.119
Osteoporotic subjects	76.4 ± 19.7	0.921 ± 0.13	0.731 ± 0.112
Decrement	35.6%	13.7%	13.8%
Ott et al.[294]			
Normal subjects	92.6 ± 36.0	4.37 ± 0.86	0.779 ± 0.142
Osteoporotic subjects	59.0 ± 25.7	3.75 ± 0.82	0.658 ± 0.134
Decrement	44%	35%	36%
Van Berkum et al.[65]			
Normal subjects	81.1 ± 27.4	0.82 ± 0.10	0.89 ± 0.18
Osteoporotic subjects	40.3 ± 19.4	0.66 ± 0.11	0.78 ± 0.13
Decrement	50.3%	19.5%	12.4%
Pacifici et al.[296]			
Normal subjects	94.5 ± 27.5	0.81 ± 0.16	
Osteoporotic subjects	59.3 ± 21.5	0.68 ± 0.14	
Decrement	37.3%	14.8%	

*For Ott et al. Results are given in g/cm.
†For Van Berkum et al. Results are given in U/cm².

bone loss in the lumbar spine and the hip in individual patients, indicating that an evaluation of several sites may be useful to identify patients at risk for osteoporosis.[300]

In addition to fracture discrimination or assessment of postmenopausal bone loss, attention also must be given to the evaluation of therapeutic intervention. The efficacy of estrogen therapy in prevention of bone loss was demonstrated for appendicular and spinal measurements.[14] However, therapy with sodium fluoride underscores the differences in bone density changes in the appendicular and axial skeleton related to the differing composition of cortical and trabecular bone in these sites. Riggs and associates, in a prospective study, found that in the fluoride-treated patients the increase in bone mineral density was 7.8 per cent per year in the lumbar spine, 2.6 per cent per year in the femoral neck, and −1.4 per cent per year in the radial shaft in comparison to a placebo group.[291] Considering all results, the choice of an appropriate site for bone mass measurements remains controversial, and it appears that the established methods are complementary rather than competitive. Besides the measurement site, the composition of the bone measured and the technique (projectional [area] or true volumetric density) play a major role in the assessment and monitoring of bone density.

Interpretation of Densitometry Results. Changes in bone mineral density are observed with aging, and differences exist between sexes and ethnic groups. Therefore, bone mineral density results must be compared with those of age-, sex-, and race-matched controls. The use of T- and Z-scores has become an important concept for the interpretation of bone mineral density measurements. The Z-score gives the patient's result as the deviation from the mean of age-matched controls divided by the standard deviation of this mean, which is an indication of biologic variability. The T-score is referenced to the peak bone mass of young normal adults and calculated similarly to the Z-score. A T-score of −2 standard deviations is commonly used as a diagnostic criterion for osteopenia, a concept that originated from the idea of a "fracture threshold."[301, 302] However,

densitometric results indicate only a low bone mass (i.e., these results are relatively nonspecific). The diagnosis of osteoporosis requires a thorough diagnostic work-up of the patient to exclude other diseases that may be accompanied by demineralization of bone (e.g., atypical presentations of multiple myeloma may be associated with bone loss prior to the appearance of other characteristics of the disease).[303]

Furthermore, a gain in bone mass as seen during drug therapy for osteoporosis is not always equal to a gain in bone quality or bone strength. Despite the finding of a gain of bone mineral density in the lumbar spine, Riggs and associates did not find a significant difference in vertebral fracture rates between patients treated with sodium fluoride and those receiving placebo.[291] The results from this and other studies have questioned whether therapeutic intervention can restore mechanical competence of the bone and, from the perspective of bone densitometry, whether bone properties can be measured adequately.

Fracture Threshold and Gradient of Risk. The term "fracture threshold" was derived from epidemiologic studies that showed that the prevalence of fractures increases sharply below a certain value for bone mineral density, usually a relatively arbitrary level set as 2 standard deviations below the mean of that in a young normal population.[301, 302] From a clinical perspective, this concept offers significant guidance for therapeutic and diagnostic procedures. On the other hand, the term "fracture threshold" in its literal sense may be misleading because of the substantial overlap in bone mineral density in patients with and without fractures (Fig. 52–28). In terms of bone mass, an absolute discrimination between these groups is not possible. Furthermore, this discrimination is not the reason why bone mass measurements are obtained. Rather such measurements should be used as an estimate of the risk of future fractures. Osteoporosis should be understood as the lower part of a continuum of bone density, with the greatest risk of fracture occurring among those subjects with lowest absolute bone mineral density values (gradient of risk).[262, 304] Meanwhile, several prospective studies have assessed the

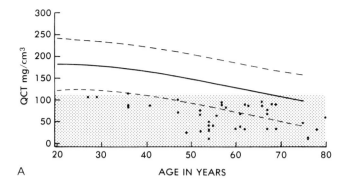

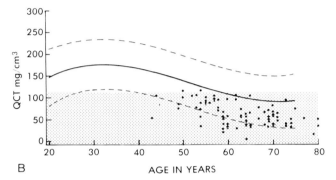

FIGURE 52–28. Fracture threshold. The graphs shows values derived from quantitative CT in men **(A)** and women **(B)** with vertebral fractures (solid circles). The values are compared to the regression curves of a normal population. For both sexes, a fracture threshold of 110 mg/cm³ is observed in this series, but it is evident that a great overlap exists in these values between persons without fractures and those with fractures.

predictive value of bone mineral measurements for future fractures. In a group of 1076 Swedish women followed for 13 years, forearm bone mass was a good predictor for vertebral crush fractures and hip fractures.[305] Black and coworkers concluded from a study of 8134 women aged 65 years or older that the inverse relationship between bone mass and the relative risk of extraspinal fractures is similar for absorptiometric measurements made at the hip, spine, calcaneus, and radius.[69] Cummings and associates found low bone density about the hip to be the strongest predictor of femoral neck fractures.[295] However, a low bone mineral density does not account entirely for an increased risk of fracture. Other factors, such as an increased risk of falling and bone properties other than density, also are significant.

SUMMARY

Osteoporosis is a common disorder with considerable health risk and medical care cost. Bone mineral density has been found to be a major determinant of the fracture risk that is associated with this disease. This chapter reviews a number of established and developing techniques that allow determination of bone density and structure, and addresses the specific advantages and limitations of each. Accuracy, sensitivity, and precision of any individual method play an important role in its clinical application. Projectional techniques such as DXA are influenced by overlying structures with a possible substantial impact on accuracy, especially in older patients. Despite its lower accuracy quantitative

CT, when compared to all standard methods, seems to be best in discriminating spinal osteoporosis. SXA, DXA, and pQCT measurements offer high precision and reasonably low radiation dose. However, the application of SXA and pQCT is restricted to measurement sites in the peripheral skeleton, and the relationship between serial bone mineral density changes in the peripheral and axial skeleton still is controversial. Currently, the various methods of BMD measurement appear complementary rather than competitive. For clinical practice the choice of an appropriate technique will depend on the specific disorder being evaluated and the availability of reliable measurement technology. Methods such as quantitative ultrasonography, quantitative MR imaging, and techniques of structural analysis require further study before they can be regarded as useful clinically.

References

1. Consensus Development Conference: Diagnosis, prophylaxis, and treatment of osteoporosis. Am J Med 94:646, 1993.
2. Cummings SR, Kelsey JL, Nevitt MC, et al: Epidemiology of osteoporosis and osteoporotic fractures. Epidemiol Rev 7:178, 1985.
3. Keene GS, Parker MJ, Pryor GA: Mortality and morbidity after hip fractures. Br Med J 307:1248, 1993.
4. Cooper C, Campion G, Melton LJ III: Hip fractures in the elderly: A wordwide projection. Osteoporosis Int 2:285, 1992.
5. Norris RJ: Medical costs of osteoporosis. Bone 13:S11, 1992.
6. Lindsay R: The growing problem of osteoporosis. Osteoporosis Int 2:267, 1992.
7. Frost HM: Dynamics of bone remodelling. In HM Frost (Ed): Bone Biodynamics. Boston, Little Brown, 1964, p 315.
8. Jones CD, Laval-Jeantet AM, Laval-Jeantet MH, et al: Importance of measurement of spongious vertebral bone mineral density in the assessment of osteoporosis. Bone 8:201, 1987.
9. Jergas M, Grampp S, Hagiwara S, et al: Perspectives on bone densitometry: Past/present/future. J Bone Miner Metal 11(Suppl 1):S7, 1993.
10. Riggs BL, Wahner HW, Dunn WL, et al: Differential changes in bone mineral density of the appendicular and axial skeleton with aging. J Clin Invest 67:328, 1981.
11. Slemenda CW, Johnston CC: Bone mass measurement: Which site to measure? Am J Med 84:643, 1988.
12. Need AG, Nordin BEC: Which bone to measure? Osteoporosis Int 1:3, 1990.
13. Nordin BEC, Wishart JM, Horowitz M, et al: The relation between forearm and vertebral mineral density and fractures in postmenopausal women. Bone Miner 5:21, 1988.
14. Riis BJ, Christiansen C: Measurement of spinal or peripheral bone mass to estimate early postmenopausal bone loss? Am J Med 84:646, 1988.
15. Virtama P, Helela T: Radiographic measurements of cortical bone. Acta Radiol (Stockh), Suppl 293, 1969.
16. Dequeker J: Quantitative radiology: Radiogrammetry of cortical bone. Br J Radiol 49:912, 1976.
17. Garn SM, Poznanski AK, Nagy JM: Bone measurement in the differential diagnosis of osteopenia and osteoporosis. Radiology 100:509, 1971.
18. Rico H, Hernandez ER: Bone radiogrametry: Caliper versus magnifying glass. Calcif Tissue Int 45:285, 1989.
19. Kalla AA, Meyers OL, Parkyn ND, et al: Osteoporosis screening—radiogrammetry revisited. Br J Rheumatol 28:511, 1989.
20. Horsman A, Simpson M: The measurement of sequential changes in cortical bone geometry. Br J Radiol 48:471, 1975.
21. Helela T, Virtama P: Cortical thickness of long bones in different age groups. Symposium Ossium. London, Churchill Livingstone, 1970, p 238.
22. Bloom RA: A comparative estimation of the combined cortical thickness of various bone sites. Skel Radiol 5:167, 1980.
23. Meema HE, Meindok H: Advantages of peripheral radiogrametry over dual-photon absorptiometry of the spine in the assessment of prevalence of osteoporotic vertebral fractures in women. J Bone Miner Res 7:897, 1992.
24. Geusens P, Dequeker J, Verstraeten A, et al: Age-, sex-, and menopause-related changes of vertebral and peripheral bone: Population study using dual and single photon absorptiometry and radiogrammetry. J Nucl Med 27:1540, 1986.
25. Rosenthal DI, Gregg GA, Slovik DM, et al: A comparison of quantitative computed tomography to four techniques of upper extremity bone mass measurement. In HK Genant (Ed): Osteoporosis Update 1987. San Francisco, Radiology Research and Education Foundation, 1987, p 87.
26. Evans RA, McDonell GD, Schieb M: Metacarpal cortical area as an index of bone mass. Br J Radiol 51:428, 1978.
27. Garn SM, Rohmann CG, Wagner B: Bone loss as a general phenomenon of man. Fed Proc 26:1729, 1967.
28. Falch JA, Sandvik L: Perimenopausal appendicular bone loss: A 10-year prospective study. Bone 11:425, 1990.

29. Meema HE: Improved vertebral fracture threshold in postmenopausal osteoporosis by radiographic measurements: Its usefulness in selection for preventative therapy. J Bone Miner Res 6:9, 1991.

30. Meema HE, Meema S: Postmenopausal osteoporosis: Simple screening method for diagnosis before structural failure. Radiology 164:405, 1987.

31. Genant HK, Heck LL, Lanzl LH, et al: Primary hyperparathyroidism. A comprehensive study of clinical, biochemical and radiographic manifestations. Radiology 109:513, 1973.

32. Kalla AA, Kotze TJvW, Meyers OL: Metacarpal bone mass in systemic lupus erythematosus. Clin Rheumatol 11:475, 1992.

33. Danielsen CC, Mosekilde L, Svenstrup B: Cortical bone mass, composition, and mechanical properties in female rats in relation to age, long-term ovariectomy, and estrogen substitution. Calcif Tissue Int 52:26, 1993.

34. Gallagher JC, Kable WT, Goldgar D: Effect of progestin therapy on cortical and trabecular bone: Comparison with estrogen. Am J Med 90:171, 1991.

35. Geusens P, Dequeker J, Nijs J, et al: Prevention and treatment of osteopenia in the ovariectomized rat: Effect of combined therapy with estrogens, 1-alpha vitamin D, and prednisolone. Calcif Tissue Int 48:127, 1991.

36. Lachmann E, Whelan M: The roentgen diagnosis of osteoporosis and its limitations. Radiology 26:165, 1936.

37. Virtama P: Uneven distribution of bone mineral and covering effect of non-mineralized tissue as reasons for impaired detectability of bone density from roentgenograms. Ann Med Int Fenn 49:57, 1960.

38. Heuck F, Schmidt E: Die quantitative Bestimmung des Mineralgehaltes des Knochens aus dem Röntgenbild. ROFO 93:523, 1960.

39. Steinbach HL: The roentgen appearance of osteoporosis. Radiol Clin North Am 2:191, 1964.

40. Mack PB, Vose GP, Nelson JD: New developments in equipment for the roentgenographic measurement of bone density. AJR 82:303, 1959.

41. Hagiwara S, Yang S-O, Dhillon MS, et al: Precision and accuracy of photodensitometry of metacarpal bone (digital image processing). J Bone Miner Res 8(Suppl 1): S346, 1993.

42. Hayashi Y, Yamamoto K, Fukunaga M, et al: Assessment of bone mass by image analysis of metacarpal bone roentgenograms: A quantitative digital image processing (DIP) method. Radiat Med 8:173, 1990.

43. Trouerbach WT, Birkenhäger JC, Collette BJA, et al: A study on the phalanx bone mineral content in 273 normal pre- and post-menopausal females (transverse study of age-dependent bone loss). Bone Miner 3:53, 1987.

44. Meema HE, Meema S: Cortical bone mineral density versus cortical thickness in the diagnosis of osteoporosis: A roentgenologic densitometric study. J Am Geriat Soc 17:120, 1969.

45. Meema S, Meema HE: Menopausal bone loss and estrogen replacement. Isr J Med Sci 12:601, 1976.

46. Trouerbach WT, Vecht-Hart CM, Collette HJA, et al: Cross-sectional and longitudinal study of age-related phalangeal bone loss in adult females. J Bone Miner Res 8:685, 1993.

47. Cosman F, Herrington B, Himmelstein S, et al: Radiographic absorptiometry: A simple method for determination of bone mass. Osteoporosis Int 2:34, 1991.

48. Cameron JR, Sorenson JA: Measurement of bone mineral in vivo: An improved method. Science 142:230, 1963.

49. Cameron JR, Mazess RB, Sorenson MS: Precision and accuracy of bone mineral determination by direct photon absorptiometry. Invest Radiol 3:141, 1968.

50. Vogel JM: Application principles and technical considerations in SPA. In HK Genant (Ed): Osteoporosis Update 1987. San Francisco, Radiology Research and Education Foundation, 1987, p 219.

51. Wahner HW, Eastell R, Riggs BL: Bone mineral density of the radius: Where do we stand? J Nucl Med 26:1339, 1985.

52. Schlenker RA, Von Seggen WW: The distribution of cortical and trabecular bone mass along the lengths of the radius and ulna and the implications for in vivo bone mass measurements. Calcif Tissue Res 20:41, 1976.

53. Awbrey BJ, Jacobson PC, Grubb SA, et al: Bone density in women: A modified procedure for measurement of distal radial density. J Orthop Res 2:314, 1984.

54. Nilas L, Borg J, Gotfredsen A, et al: Comparison of single- and dual-photon absorptiometry in postmenopausal bone mineral loss. J Nucl Med 26:1257, 1985.

55. Rüegsegger P, Dambacher MA, Rüegsegger MS, et al: Bone loss in premenopausal and postmenopausal women. J Bone Joint Surg [Am] 66:1015, 1984.

56. Vogel JM, Wasnich RD, Ross PD: The clinical relevance of calcaneus bone mineral measurements: A review. Bone Mineral 5:35, 1988.

57. Grubb SA, Jacobson PC, Awbrey BJ, et al: Comparison of single and dual photon absorptiometry in postmenopausal bone mineral loss. J Nucl Med 26:1257, 1984.

58. Nilas L, Gotriedsen A, Hadberg A, et al: Age-related bone loss in women evaluated by the single and dual photon technique. Bone Miner 4:95, 1988.

59. Aloia JF, Vaswani A, Ross P, et al: Aging bone loss from the femur, spine, radius, and total skeleton. Metabolism 39:1144, 1990.

60. Krølner B, Nielsen SP: Bone mineral content of the lumbar spine in normal and osteoporotic women: Cross-sectional and longitudinal studies. Clin Sci 62:329, 1982.

61. Nordin BEC, Chatterton BE, Steurer TA, et al: Forearm bone mineral content does not decline with age on premenopausal women. Clin Orthop 211:252, 1986.

62. Mazess RB: Non-invasive measurement of bone. In AS Barzel (Ed): Osteoporosis II. New-York, Grune and Stratton, 1979, p 5.

63. Wilson CR: Bone mineral content of the femoral neck and spine versus the radius or ulna. J Bone Joint Surg [Am] 59:665, 1977.

64. Christiansen C, Riis BJ: Comparison of noninvasive measurements of bone mass in postmenopausal women. In HK Genant (Ed): Osteoporosis Update 1987. San Francisco, Radiology Research and Education Foundation, 1987, p 81.

65. Van Berkum FNR, Birkenhäger JC, Van Veen LCP, et al: Noninvasive axial and peripheral assessment of bone mineral content: A comparison between osteoporotic women and normal subjects. J Bone Miner Res 5:679, 1989.

66. Vogel JM, Whittle MW: Bone mineral changes; the second Skylab mission. Aviat Space Environ Med 47:396, 1976.

67. Wasnich RD, Ross PD, Heilbrun LK, et al: Selection of the optimal site for fracture risk prediction. Clin Orthop 216:262, 1987.

68. Williams JA, Wagner J, Wasnich R, et al: The effect of long-distance running upon appendicular bone mineral content. Med Sci Sports Exerc 16:223, 1984.

69. Black D, Cummings SR, Melton LJ: Appendicular bone mineral and a woman's lifetime risk of hip fracture. J Bone Miner Res 7:639, 1992.

70. Black D, Cummings SR, Genant HK, et al: Axial and appendicular bone density predict fractures in older women. J Bone Miner Res 7:633, 1992.

71. Cummings SR, Black DM, Nevitt MC, et al: Appendicular bone density and age predict hip fracture in women. JAMA 263:665, 1990.

72. Wasnich RD, Ross PD, Heilbrun LK, et al: Prediction of postmenopausal fracture risk with use of bone mineral measurements. Am J Obstet Gynecol 153:745, 1985.

73. Szücs J, Jonson R, Granhed H, et al: Accuracy, precision, and homogeneity effects in the determination of the bone mineral content with dual photon absorptiometry in the heel bone. Bone 13:179, 1992.

74. Yamada M, Ito M, Hayashi K, et al: Calcaneus as a site for assessment of bone mineral density: Evaluation in cadavers and healthy volunteers. AJR 161:621, 1993.

75. Cohn SH: In-vivo neutron activation analysis: State of the art and future prospects. Med Phys 8:145, 1981.

76. Chamberlain MJ, Fremlin JH, Holloway I, et al: Use of the cyclotron for whole body neutron activation analysis: Theoretical and practical considerations. Int J Appl Radiat Isotop 21:725, 1970.

77. Williams ED, Boddy K, Harvey I, et al: Calibration and evaluation of a system for total body in vivo activation analysis using 14 MeV neutrons. Phys Med Biol 23:405, 1978.

78. Cohn SH, Yasumura AS, Zanzi AI, et al: Comparative skeletal mass and radial bone mineral content in black and white women. Metabolism 26:171, 1977.

79. Cohn SH, Ellis KJ, Wallach S, et al: Absolute and relative deficit in total-skeletal calcium and radial bone mineral in osteoporosis. J Nucl Med 15:428, 1974.

80. Aloia JF, Vaswani A, Atkins H, et al: Radiographic morphometry and osteopenia in spinal osteoporosis. J Nucl Med 18:425, 1977.

81. Manzke E, Chestnut CH III, Wergedal JE, et al: Relationship between local and total bone mass in osteoporosis. Metabolism 24:605, 1975.

82. Cohn SH, Aloia JF, Vaswani AN, et al: Women at risk for developing osteoporosis: Determination by total body neutron activation analysis and photon absorptiometry. Calcif Tissue Int 38:9, 1986.

83. McNeill KG, Thomas BJ, Sturtridge WC, et al: In vivo neutron activation analysis for calcium in man. J Nucl Med 14:502, 1973.

84. Clarke RL, Van Dyk G: A new method for measurement of bone mineral content using both transmitted and scattered beams of gamma-rays. Phys Med Biol 18:532, 1973.

85. Garnett ES, Kennett TJ, Kenyon DB, et al: A photon scattering technique for the measurement of absolute bone density in man. Radiology 106:209, 1973.

86. Kennett TJ, Garnett ES, Webber CE: An in vivo measurement of absolute bone density. J Can Assoc Radiol 23:168, 1972.

87. Webber CE, Kennett TJ: Bone density measured by photon scattering. I. A system for clinical use. Phys Med Biol 21:760, 1976.

88. Olkkonen H, Karjalainen P: A ^{170}Tm gamma scattering technique for the determination of absolute bone density. Br J Radiol 48:594, 1975.

89. Reiss KH, Steinle B: Medical application of the Compton effect. Siemens Forsch Entwickl Ber 2:16, 1973.

90. Battista JJ, Bronskill MR: Compton-scatter tissue densitometry: Calculation of single and multiple scatter photon fluences. Phys Med Biol 23:1, 1978.

91. Battista JJ, Bronskill MR: Compton-scatter imaging of transverse sections: Corrections for multiple scatter and attenuations. Phys Med Biol 22:229, 1977.

92. Kennett TJ, Webber CE: Bone density measured by photon scattering. II. Inherent sources of error. Phys Med Biol 21:770, 1976.

93. Hazan G, Leichter I, Loewinger E, et al: The early detection of osteoporosis by Compton gamma ray spectroscopy. Phys Med Biol 22:1073, 1977.

94. Ott SM, Murano R, Lewellen TK, et al: Total body calcium by neutron activation analysis in normals and osteoporotic populations: A discriminator of significant bone loss. J Lab Clin Med 102:637, 1983.

95. Cohn SH, Vaswani AN, Zanzi I, et al: Effect of aging on bone mass in adult women. Am J Physiol 230:143, 1976.

96. Roberts JG, DiTomasso E, Webber CE: Photon scattering measurements of calcaneal bone density: Results of in vivo cross-sectional studies. Invest Radiol 17:20, 1982.

97. Peppler WW, Mazess RB: Total body bone mineral and lean body mass by dual photon absorptiometry. I. Theory and measurement procedure. Calcif Tissue Int 33:353, 1981.

98. Roos B, Skoldborn H: Dual-photon absorptiometry in lumbar vertebrae. I. Theory and method. Acta Radiol 13:1, 1974.

99. Wahner HW, Dunn WL, Mazess RB, et al: Dual-photon Gd-153 absorptiometry of bone. Radiology 156:203, 1985.

100. Dunn WL, Wahner HW, Riggs BL: Measurement of bone mineral content in human vertebrae and hip by dual photon absorptiometry. Radiology 136:485, 1980.
101. Krølner B, Pors Nielsen S: Measurement of bone mineral content (BMC) of the lumbar spine. I. Theory and application of a new two-dimensional dual photon attenuation method. Scand J Clin Lab Invest 40:653, 1980.
102. Nord R: Technical considerations in DPA. In HK Genant (Ed): Osteoporosis Update 1987. San Francisco, Radiology Research and Education Foundation, 1987, p 203.
103. Mazess RB, Barden HS: Single- and dual photon absorptiometry for bone measurement in osteoporosis. In HK Genant (Ed): Osteoporosis Update 1987. San Francisco, Radiology Research and Education Foundation, 1987, p 73.
104. Frohn J, Wilken T, Falk S, et al: Effect of aortic sclerosis on bone mineral measurements by dual-photon absorptiometry. J Nucl Med 32:259, 1991.
105. Frye MA, Melton III LJ, Bryant SC, et al: Osteoporosis and calcification of the aorta. Bone Miner 19:185, 1992.
106. Drinka PJ, DeSmet AA, Bauwens SF, et al: The effect of overlying calcification on lumbar bone densitometry. Calcif Tissue Int 50:507, 1992.
107. Masud T, Langley S, Wiltshire P, et al: Effect of spinal osteophytosis on bone mineral density measurements in vertebral osteoporosis. Br Med J 307:172, 1993.
108. Ryan PJ, Evans P, Blake GM, et al: The effect of vertebral collapse on spinal bone mineral density measurements in osteoporosis. Bone Miner 18:267, 1992.
109. Ross PD, Wasnich RD, Vogel JM: Sources of accuracy and precision errors in dual photon absorptiometry. 6th International Workshop on Bone and Soft Tissue Densitometry, Buxton, England, 1987.
110. Dunn WL, Kan SH, Wahner HW: Errors in longitudinal measurements of bone mineral: Effect of source strength in single and dual photon absorptiometry. J Nucl Med 28:1751, 1987.
111. Kelly TL, Slovik DM, Neer RM: Calibration and standardization of bone mineral densitometers. J Bone Min Res 4:663, 1989.
112. Nilas L, Hassager C, Christiansen C: Long-term precision of dual-photon absorptiometry in the lumbar spine in clinical settings. Bone Miner 3:305, 1988.
113. Glüer CC, Steiger P, Genant HK: Validity of dual-photon absorptiometry. Radiology 166:574, 1988.
114. Reginster JY, Geusens P, Nijs J, et al: In vivo long-term precision of spinal bone mass measurement by dual photon absorptiometry. Bone Miner 6:225, 1989.
115. Gustavson L, Jacobson B, Kusoffsky L: X-ray spectrophotometry for bone mineral determinations. Med Biol Eng Comput 12:113, 1974.
116. Jacobson B: X-ray spectrophotometry in vivo. AJR 91:202, 1964.
117. Wahner HW, Dunn WL, Brown ML, et al: Comparison of dual-energy x-ray absorptiometry and dual photon absorptiometry for bone mineral measurements of the lumbar spine. Mayo Clin Proc 63:1075, 1988.
118. Kelly T, Slovick D, Schoenfield D, et al: Quantitative digital radiography versus dual photon absorptiometry of the lumbar spine. J Clin Endocr Metab 67:839, 1988.
119. Glüer CC, Steiger P, Selvidge R, et al: Comparative assessment of dual-photon-absorptiometry and dual-energy-radiography. Radiology 174:223, 1990.
120. Lees B, Stevenson JC: An evaluation of dual energy x-ray absorptiometry and comparison with dual-photon absorptiometry. Osteoporosis Int 2:146, 1992.
121. Wilson CR, Collier BD, Carrera GF, et al: Acronym for dual-energy x-ray absorptiometry. Radiology 176:875, 1990.
122. Glüer CC, Steiger P, Genant HK: Acronym for dual-energy x-ray absorptiometry. Radiology 176:875, 1990.
123. Mazess R, Chesnut CH III, McClung M, et al: Enhanced precision with dual-energy x-ray absorptiometry. Calcif Tissue Int 51:14, 1992.
124. Blake GM, Parker JC, Buxton FMA, et al: Dual x-ray absorptiometry: A comparison between fan beam and pencil beam scans. Br J Radiol 66:902, 1993.
125. Faulkner K, Glüer C, Estilo M, et al: Cross-calibration of DXA equipment: Upgrading from a Hologic QDR 1000/W to a QDR 2000. Calcif Tissue Int 52:79, 1993.
126. Ho CP, Kim RW, Schaffler MB, et al: Accuracy of dual-energy radiographic absorptiometry of the lumbar spine: Cadaver study. Radiology 176:171, 1990.
127. Lilley J, Walters BG, Heath DA, et al: In vivo and in vitro precision of bone density measured by dual-energy x-ray absorption. Osteoporosis Int 1:141, 1991.
128. Orwoll ES, Oviatt SK: Longitudinal precision of dual-energy x-ray absorptiometry in a multicenter study. J Bone Miner Res 6:191, 1991.
129. Hatori M, Hasegawa A, Adachi H, et al: The effects of walking at the anaerobic threshold level on vertebral bone loss in postmenopausal women. Calcif Tissue Int 52:411, 1993.
130. Karlsson MK, Johnell O, Obrant KJ: Bone mineral density in weight lifters. Calcif Tissue Int 52:212, 1993.
131. Ooms ME, Lips P, Van Lingen A, Valkenburg HA: Determinants of bone mineral density and risk factors for osteoporosis in healthy elderly women. J Bone Miner Res 8:669, 1993.
132. Chon KS, Sartoris DJ, Brown SA, et al: Alcoholism-associated spinal and femoral bone loss in abstinent male alcoholics, as measured by dual x-ray absorptiometry. Skeletal Radiol 21:431, 1992.
133. Ross DS: Bone density is not reduced during short-term administration of levothyroxine to postmenopausal women with sublinical hypothyroidism: A randomized, prospective study. Am J Med 95:385, 1993.
134. Campos-Pastor MM, Muñoz-Torrez M, Escobar-Jiménez F, et al: Bone mass in females with different thyroid disorders: Influence of menopausal status. Bone Miner 21:1, 1993.
135. Hagiwara S, Lane N, Engelke K, et al: Precision and accuracy for rat whole body and femur bone mineral determination with dual x-ray absorptiometry. Bone Miner 22:57, 1993.
136. Whitehouse RW, Karantanas A, Adams JE: Discrepancies in spinal bone mass measured by QCT and DXA. In EFG Ring (Ed): Current Research in Osteoporosis and Bone Mineral Measurement II: 1992. Bath, England, 1992, p 26.
137. Uebelhart D, Duboeuf F, Meunier PJ, et al: Lateral dual-photon absorptiometry: A new technique to measure the bone mineral density at the lumbar spine. J Bone Miner Res 5:525, 1990.
138. Reid IR, Evans MC, Stapleton J: Lateral spine densitometry is a more sensitive indicator of glucocorticoid-induced bone loss. J Bone Miner Res 7:221, 1992.
139. Lang P, Steiger P, Faulkner KG, et al: Osteoporosis: Current techniques and recent developments in quantitative bone densitometry. Radiol Clin North Am 29:49, 1991.
140. Rupich RC, Griffin MG, Pacifici R, et al: Lateral dual-energy radiography: Artifact error from rib and pelvic bone. J Bone Miner Res 7:97, 1992.
141. Larnach TA, Boyd SJ, Smart RC, et al: Reproducibility of lateral spine scans using dual energy x-ray absorptiometry. Calcif Tissue Int 51:255, 1992.
142. Steiger P, von Stetten E, Weiss H, et al: Paired AP and lateral supine dual x-ray absorptiometry of the spine: Initial results with a 32 detector system. Osteoporosis Int 1:190, 1991.
143. Arai H, Ito K, Nagao K, et al: The evaluation of three different bone densitometry systems: XR-26, QDR-1000, and DPX. Image Technology Information Display 22:1, 1990.
144. Lai KC, Goodsitt MM, Murano R, et al: A comparison of two dual-energy x-ray absorptiometry systems for spinal bone mineral measurement. Calcif Tissue Int 50:203, 1992.
145. Pocock NA, Sambrook PN, Nguyen T, et al: Assessment of spinal and femoral bone density by dual x-ray absorptiometry: Comparison of lunar and hologic instruments. J Bone Miner Res 7:1081, 1992.
146. Nord RH: Work in progress: A cross-correlation study on four DXA instruments designed to culminate in inter-manufacturer standardization. Osteoporosis Int 2:210, 1992.
147. Carter DR, Bouxsein ML, Marcus R: New approaches for interpreting projected bone densitometry data. J Bone Miner Res 7:137, 1992.
148. Duboeuf F, Pommet R, Meunier PJ, et al: Evaluation of the volumetric bone mineral density by lateral dual energy absorptiometry of the lumbar spine. Osteoporosis Int (in press).
149. Steiger P, Cummings SR, Genant HK, et al: Morphometric x-ray absorptiometry of the spine: Correlation in-vivo with morphometric radiography. In C Christiansen (Ed): 4th International Symposium on Osteoporosis and Consensus Development Conference, Hong Kong, 1993, p 18.
150. Genant HK, Boyd DP: Quantitative bone mineral analysis using dual energy computed tomography. Invest Radiol 12:545, 1977.
151. Genant HK, Cann CE, Ettinger B, et al: Quantitative computed tomography of vertebral spongiosa: A sensitive method for detecting early bone loss after oophorectomy. Ann Intern Med 97:699, 1982.
152. Cann CE, Genant HK: Precise measurement of vertebral mineral content using computed tomography. J Comput Assist Tomogr 4:493, 1980.
153. Rüegsegger P, Elsasser U, Anliker M, et al: Quantification of bone mineralization using computed tomography. Radiology 121:93, 1976.
154. Hangartner TN, Battista JJ, Overton TR: Performance evaluation of density measurements of axial and peripheral bone with x-ray and gamma-ray computed tomography. Phys Med Biol 32:1393, 1987.
155. Hosie CJ, Smith DA, Deacon AD, et al: Comparison of broadband ultrasonic attenuation of the os calcis and quantitative computed tomography of the distal radius. Clin Phys Physiol Meas 8:303, 1987.
156. Kalender WA, Süss C: A new calibration phantom for quantitative computed tomography. Med Phys 9:816, 1987.
157. Goodsitt MM: Conversion relations for quantitative CT bone mineral density measured with solid and liquid calibration standards. Bone Mineral 19:145, 1992.
158. Faulkner KG, Glüer CC, Grampp S, et al: Cross calibration of liquid and solid QCT calibration standards: Corrections to the UCSF normative data. Osteoporosis Int 3:36, 1993.
159. Glüer CC, Engelke K, Jergas M, et al: Changes in calibration standards for quantitative computed tomography: Recommendations for clinical practice. Osteoporosis Int 3:36, 1993.
160. Kalender WA, Brestowsky H, Felsenberg D: Bone mineral measurements: Automated determination of the midvertebral CT section. Radiology 168:219, 1988.
161. Louis O, Luypaert R, Kalender W, et al: Reproducibility of CT bone densitometry: Operator-made versus automated ROI definition. Eur J Radiol 8:70, 1988.
162. Cann CE: Quantitative CT for determination of bone mineral density: A review. Radiology 166:509, 1988.
163. Kalender WA: Effective dose values in bone mineral measurements by photon absorptiometry and computed tomography. Osteoporosis Int 2:82, 1992.
164. Kalender WA, Klotz E, Süss C: Vertebral bone mineral analysis: An integrated approach. Radiology 164:419, 1987.
165. Steiger P, Steiger S, Ruegsegger P, et al: Two- and three-dimensional quantitative image evaluation techniques for densitometry and volumetrics in longitudinal studies. In HK Genant (Ed): Osteoporosis Update 1987. San Francisco, University of California Printing Services, 1987, p 171.

166. Steiger P, Block JE, Steiger S, et al: Spinal bone mineral density by quantitative computed tomography: Effect of region of interest, vertebral level, and technique. Radiology 175:537, 1990.
167. Kalender WA, Felsenberg D, Louis O, et al: Reference values for trabecular and cortical vertebral bone density in single and dual-energy quantitative computed tomography. Eur J Radiol 9:75, 1989.
168. Pacifici R, Rupich RC, Avioli LV: Vertebral cortical bone mass measurement by a new quantitative computer tomography method: Correlations with vertebral trabecular bone measurements. Calcif Tissue Int 47:215, 1990.
169. Genant HK, Cann CE, Ettinger B, et al: Quantitative computed tomography for spinal mineral assessment: Current status. J Comput Assist Tomogr 9:602, 1985.
170. Richardson M, Genant HK, Cann CE: Assessment of metabolic bone disease by quantitative computed tomography. Clin Orthop 185:224, 1985.
171. Rohloff R, Hitzler H, Arndt W, et al: Experimentelle Untersuchungen zur Genauigkeit der Mineralsalzgehaltsbestimmung spongiöser Knochen mit Hilfe der quantitativen CT (Einenergiemessung). ROFO 143:692, 1985.
172. Mazess RB: Errors in measuring trabecular bone by computed tomography due to marrow and bone composition. Calcif Tissue Int 35:148, 1983.
173. Glüer CC, Genant HK: Impact of marrow fat on accuracy of quantitative CT. J Comput Assist Tomogr 13:1023, 1989.
174. Reinbold WD, Adler CP, Kalender WA, et al: Accuracy of vertebral mineral determination by dual-energy quantitative computed tomography. Skeletal Radiol 20:25, 1991.
175. Glüer CC, Reiser UJ, Davis CA, et al: Vertebral mineral determination by quantitative computed tomography (QCT): Accuracy of single and dual energy measurements. J Comput Assist Tomogr 12:242, 1988.
176. Laval-Jeantet AM, Laval-Jeantet M, Roger B, et al: Interét et limites de la mésure tomodensitométrique de la minéralisation vertebrale. J Radiol 65:151, 1984.
177. Alvarez RE, Macovski A: Energy-selective reconstructions in x-ray computerized tomography. Phys Med Biol 21:733, 1976.
178. Kalender WA, Perman WH, Vetter JR, et al: Evaluation of a prototype dual-energy computed tomographic apparatus. I. Phantom studies. Med Phys 13:334, 1986.
179. Vetter JR, Kalender WA, Mazess RB, et al: Evaluation of a prototype dual-energy computed tomographic apparatus. II. Determination of vertebral bone mineral content. Med Phys 13:340, 1986.
180. Genant HK, Cann CE, Pozzi-Mucelli RS, et al: Vertebral mineral determination by quantitative computed tomography: Clinical feasibility and normative data. J Comput Assist Tomogr 7:554, 1983.
181. Cann CE, Genant HK: Single versus dual-energy CT for vertebral mineral quantification. J Comp Assist Tomogr 7:551, 1983.
182. Ettinger B, Genant HK, Cann C: Menopausal bone loss can be prevented by low dose estrogen with calcium supplements. J Comput Assist Tomogr 9:633, 1985.
183. Steiger P, Cummings SR, Black DM, et al: Age-related decrements in bone mineral density in women over 65. J Bone Miner Res 7:625, 1992.
184. Glüer CC, Faulkner KG, Estilo MJ, et al: Quality assurance for bone densitometry research studies: Concept and impact. Osteoporosis Int 3:227, 1993.
185. Montag M, Dören M, Meyer-Galander HM, et al: Computertomographisch bestimmter Mineralgehalt in der LWS-Spongiosa. Radiologe 28:161, 1988.
186. Hangartner TN, Overton TR: Quantitative assessment of bone density using gamma-ray computed tomography. J Comput Assist Tomogr 6:1156, 1982.
187. Hosie CJ, Smith DA: Precision of measurement of bone density with a special purpose computed tomography scanner. Br J Radiol 59:345, 1986.
188. Schneider P, Börner W: Periphere quantitative Computertomographie zur Knochenmineralmessung mit einem neuen speziellen QCT-Scanner. ROFO 154:292, 1991.
189. Müller A, Rüegsegger E, Rüegsegger P: Peripheral QCT: A low risk procedure to identify women predisposed to osteoporosis. Phys Med Biol 34:741, 1989.
190. Rüegsegger P, Durand E, Dambacher MA: Localization of regional forearm bone loss from high resolution computed tomographic images. Osteoporosis Int 1:76, 1991.
191. Rüegsegger P, Durand E, Dambacher MA: Differential effect of aging and disease on trabecular and compact bone density of the radius. Bone 12:99, 1991.
192. Boden SD, Goodenough DJ, Stockham CD, et al: Precise measurement of vertebra bone density using computed tomography without the use of an external reference phantom. J Digital Imaging 2:31, 1989.
193. Gudmundsdottir H, Jonsdottir B, Kristinsson S, et al: Vertebral bone density in Icelandic women using quantitative computed tomography without an external reference phantom. Osteoporosis Int 3:84, 1993.
194. Abendschein W, Hyatt GW: Ultrasonics and selected physical properties of bone. Clin Orthop 69:294, 1970.
195. Floriani L, Debevoise N, Hyatt G: Mechanical properties of healing by the use of ultrasound. Surg Forum 18:468, 1967.
196. Tavakoli MB, Evans JA: Dependence of the velocity and attenuation of ultrasound in bone on the mineral content. Phys Med Biol 36:1529, 1991.
197. McCartney R, Jeffcott L: Combined 2.25 Mhz ultrasound velocity and bone mineral density measurements in the equine metacarpus and their in vivo applications. Med Biol Eng Comput 25:620, 1987.
198. Turner CH, Eich M: Ultrasonic velocity as a predictor of strength in bovine cancellous bone. Calcif Tissue Int 49:116, 1991.
199. Jergas M, Uffmann M, Müller P, Ultraschallgeschwindigkeitsmessungen zur Diagnose der postmenopausalen Osteoporose. ROFO 158:207, 1993.
200. Heaney RP, Avioli LV, Chestnut CH, et al: Osteoporotic bone fragility: Detection by ultrasound transmission velocity. JAMA 261:2986, 1989.
201. Brandenburger GH, Kwon S, McDougall SW: Preliminary results from a longitudinal clinical study of ultrasound velocity. In C Christiansen and K Overgaard (Eds): Third International Symposium on Osteoporosis. Copenhagen, 1991, p 199.
202. Schott AM, Hans D, Sornay-Rendu E, et al: Ultrasound measurements on os calcis: Precision and age-related changes in a normal female population. Osteoporosis Int 3:249, 1993.
203. Zagzebski JA, Rossmann PJ, Mesina C, et al: Ultrasound transmission measurements through the os calcis. Calcif Tissue Int 49:107, 1991.
204. Herd RJM, Blake GM, Miller CG, et al: Can ultrasonic measurements in the calcaneus predict osteopenia in the axial skeleton? In EFG Ring (Ed): Current Research in Osteoporosis and Bone Mineral Measurement II: 1992. Bath, England, 1992, p 45.
205. Klein K, Allolio B: A health promotion project "osteoporosis"—in cooperation with the insurance company "Deutsche Bank AG." In EFG Ring (Ed): Current Research in Osteoporosis and Bone Mineral Measurement II: 1992. Bath, England, 1992, p 97.
206. Antich PP, Anderson JA, Ashman RB: Measurement of mechanical properties of bone material in vitro by ultrasound reflection: Methodology and comparison with ultrasound transmission. J Bone Miner Res 6:417, 1991.
207. Antich PP, Pak CYC, Gonzales J, et al: Measurement of intrinsic bone quality in vivo by reflection ultrasound: Correction of impaired quality with slow-release sodium fluoride and calcium citrate. J Bone Miner Res 8:301, 1993.
208. Fry FJ, Barger JE: Acoustical properties of the human skull. J Acous Soc Am 63:1576, 1978.
209. McCloskey EV, Murray SA, Charlesworth D, et al: Assessment of broadband ultrasound attenuation in the os calcis in vitro. Clin Sci 78:221, 1990.
210. Agren M, Karellas A, Leahey D, et al: Ultrasound attenuation of the calcaneus: A sensitive and specific discriminator of osteopenia in postmenopausal women. Calcif Tissue Int 48:240, 1991.
211. Glüer CC, Wu CY, Genant HK: Broadband ultrasound attenuation signals depend on trabecular orientation: An in-vitro study. Osteoporosis Int 3:185, 1993.
212. Porter R, Miller C, Grainger D, et al: Prediction of hip fracture in elderly women: A prospective study. Br Med J 301:638, 1990.
213. Baran DT, Kelly AM, Karellas A, et al: Ultrasound attenuation of the os calcis in women with osteoporosis and hip fractures. Calcif Tissue Int 43:138, 1988.
214. Glüer CC, Vahlensieck M, Faulkner KG, et al: Site-matched calcaneal measurements of broadband ultrasound attenuation and single x-ray absorptiometry: Do they measure different skeletal properties? J Bone Miner Res 7:1071, 1992.
215. Massie A, Reid DM, Porter RW: Screening for osteoporosis: Comparison between dual energy x-ray absorptiometry and broadband ultrasound attenuation in 1000 perimenopausal women. Osteoporosis Int 3:107, 1993.
216. Truscott JG, Simpson M, Stewart SP, et al: Bone ultrasonic attenuation in women: Reproducibility, normal variation and comparison with photon absorptiometry. Calcif Tissue Int 49:112, 1992.
217. Ramalingham T, Herd RJM, Blake GM, et al: Ultrasonic measurements in the calcaneus: A comparison of two commercial scanners. In EFG Ring (Ed): Current Research in Osteoporosis and Bone Mineral Measurement II: 1992. Bath, England, 1992, p 44.
218. Herd RJM, Blake GM, Ramalingam T, et al: Measurements of postmenopausal bone loss with a new contact ultrasound system. Calcif Tissue Int 53:153, 1993.
219. Rubin C, Pratt G, Porter A, et al: The use of ultrasound in vivo to determine acute change in the mechanical properties of bone following intense physical activity. J Biomechanics 20:723, 1987.
220. Jergas M, Uffmann M, Wittenberg R, et al: Ultraschallgeschwindigkeitsmessungen an belastungstragenden und nicht-belastungstragenden Stellen des peripheren Skeletts. Der Einfluss körperlicher Aktivität bei Fussballspielern. ROFO 157:420, 1992.
221. Langton CM, Riggs CM, Evans GP: Pathway of ultrasound waves in the equine third metacarpal bone. J Biomed Eng 13:113, 1991.
222. Jones PRM, Hardmann AE, Hudson A, et al: Influence of brisk walking on the ultrasonic attenuation of the calcaneus in previously sedentary women aged 30–61 years. Calcif Tissue Int 49:112, 1991.
223. Dooms GC, Fisher MR, Hricak H, et al: Bone marrow imaging: Magnetic resonance studies related to age and sex. Radiology 155:429, 1985.
224. Richards MA, Webb JAW, Jewell SE, et al: In-vivo measurement of spin lattice relaxation time (T1) of bone marrow in healthy volunteers: The effects of age and sex. Br J Radiol 61:30, 1988.
225. Jenkins JPR, Stehling M, Sivewright G, et al: Quantitative magnetic resonance imaging of vertebral bodies: A T1 and T2 study. Magn Res Imaging 7:17, 1989.
226. LeBlanc A, Evans H, Schonfeld E, et al: Changes in nuclear magnetic resonance (T2) relaxation of limb tissue with bed rest. Magn Reson Med 4:487, 1987.
227. LeBlanc AD, Schonfeld E, Schneider VS, et al: The spine: Changes in T2 relaxation times from disuse. Radiology 169:105, 1988.
228. Davis CA, Genant HK, Dunham JS: The effects of bone on proton NMR relaxation times of surrounding liquids. Invest Radiol 21:472, 1986.
229. Rosenthal H, Thulborn KR, Rosenthal DI, et al: Magnetic susceptibility effects of trabecular bone on magnetic resonance bone marrow imaging. Invest Radiol 25:173, 1990.
230. Ito M, Hayashi K, Uetani M, et al: Bone mineral and other bone components in vertebrae evaluated by QCT and MRI. Skeletal Radiol 22:109, 1993.

231. Sebag GH, Moore SG: Effect of trabecular bone on the appearance of marrow in gradient-echo imaging of the appendicular skeleton. Radiology *174:*855, 1990.
232. Majumdar S, Thomasson D, Shimakawa A, et al: Quantitation of the susceptibility difference between trabecular bone and bone marrow: Experimental studies. Magn Reson Med *22:*111, 1991.
233. Majumdar S, Genant H: In vivo relationship between marrow T2* and trabecular bone density determined with a chemical shift-selective asymmetric spin-echo sequence. J Magn Reson Imaging *2:*209, 1992.
234. Ford JC, Wehrli FW: In vivo quantitative characterization of trabecular bone by NMR interferometry and localized proton spectroscopy. Magn Reson Med *17:*543, 1991.
235. Wehrli FW, Ford JC, Attie M, et al: Trabecular structure: Preliminary application of MR interferometry. Radiology *179:*615, 1991.
236. Sugimoto H, Kimura T, Ohsawa T: Susceptibility effects of bone trabeculae. Quantification in vivo using an asymmetric spin-echo technique. Invest Radiol *28:*208, 1993.
237. Brown CE, Allaway JR, Brown KL, et al: Noninvasive evaluation of mineral content of bone without use of ionizing radiation. Clin Chem *33:*227, 1987.
238. Brown CE, Battocletti JH, Shrinivasan R, et al: In vivo ^{31}P nuclear resonance spectroscopy of bone mineral for evaluation of osteoporosis. Clin Chem *34:*1431, 1988.
239. Chen Y, Dougherty ER, Totterman SM, et al: Classification of trabecular structure in magnetic resonance images based on morphological granulometries. Magn Reson Med *29:*358, 1993.
240. Jara H, Wehrli FW, Chung H, et al: High-resolution variable flip angle 3D MR imaging of trabecular microstructure in vivo. Magn Reson Med *29:*528, 1993.
241. Majumdar S, Genant HK, Jergas M, et al: Fractal analysis of high resolution MR images. 8th European Congress of Radiology, Vienna, 1993.
242. Wehrli FW, Ford JC, Chung H-W, et al: Potential role of nuclear magnetic resonance for the evaluation of trabecular bone quality. Calcif Tissue Int *53*(Suppl 1):S162, 1993.
243. Recker RR: Architecture and vertebral fracture. Calcif Tissue Int *53*(Suppl 1):S139, 1993.
244. Dempster DW, Ferguson-Pell MW, Mellish RWE, et al: Relationships between bone structure in the iliac crest and bone structure and strength in the lumbar spine. Osteoporosis Int *3:*90, 1993.
245. Parfitt AM: Trabecular bone architecture in the pathogenesis and prevention of fracture. Am J Med *82*(Suppl 1B):68, 1987.
246. Vogel M, Hahn M, Delling G: Relation between 2- and 3-dimensional architecture of trabecular bone in the human spine. Bone *14:*199, 1993.
247. Vesterby A: Marrow space star volume can reveal change of trabecular connectivity. Bone *14:*193, 1993.
248. Geraets WGM, VanDer Stelt PF, Netelenbos CJ, et al: A new method for automatic recognition of the radiographic trabecular pattern. J Bone Miner Res *5:*227, 1990.
249. Caligiuri P, Giger ML, Favus MJ, et al: Computerized radiographic analysis of osteoporosis: preliminary evaluation. Radiology *186:*471, 1993.
250. Chevalier F, Laval-Jeantet AM, Laval-Jeantet M, et al: CT image analysis of the vertebral trabecular network in vivo. Calcif Tissue Int *51:*8, 1992.
251. Durand EP, Rüegsegger P: Cancellous bone structure: Analysis of high-resolution CT images with the run-length method. J Comput Assist Tomogr *15:*133, 1991.
252. Haralick RM: Ridges and valleys on digital images. Computer Vision Graphics Image Processing *22:*28, 1983.
253. Goldstein SA, Goulet R, McCubbrey D: Measurement and significance of three-dimensional architecture to the mechanical integrity of trabecular bone. Calcif Tissue Int *53*(Suppl 1):S127, 1993.
254. Odgaard A, Gundersen HJG: Quantification of connectivity in cancellous bone, with special emphasis on 3D reconstructions. Bone *14:*173, 1993.
255. Majumdar S, Weinstein RS, Prasad RR: Application of fractal geometry techniques to the study of trabecular bone. Med Phys *20:*1611, 1993.
256. Ruttimann UE, Webber RL, Hazelrig JB: Fractal dimension from radiographs of peridental alveolar bone. A possible diagnostic indicator of osteoporosis. Oral Surg *74:*98, 1992.
257. Samarabandu J, Acharya R, Hausmann E, et al: Analysis of bone x-rays using morphological fractals. IEEE Trans Med Imaging *12:*466, 1993.
258. Faulkner KG, Cann CE, Hasegawa BH: Effect of bone distribution on vertebral strength: Assessment with patient-specific nonlinear finite element analysis. Radiology *179:*669, 1991.
259. Faulkner KG, Grampp S, Glüer C-C, et al: Patient specific finite element analysis of the proximal femur: Comparison with compression tests in-vitro. J Bone Miner Res *6:*344, 1991.
260. Mizrahi J, Silva MJ, Eng M, et al: Finite-element stress analysis of the normal and osteoporotic lumbar vertebral body. Spine *18:*2088, 1993.
261. Johnston CC Jr, Melton LJ III, Lindsay R, et al: Clinical indications for bone mass measurements. J Bone Miner Res *4:*1, 1989.
262. Genant HK, Block JE, Steiger P, et al: Appropriate use of bone densitometry. Radiology *170:*817, 1989.
263. Schlechte J, El-Khoury G, Kathol M, et al: Forearm and vertebral bone mineral in treated and untreated hyperprolactinemic amenorrhoea. J Clin Endocrinol Metabol *64:*1021, 1987.
264. Prezelj J, Kocijancic A: Bone mineral density in hyperandrogenic amenorrhoea. Calcif Tissue Int *52:*422, 1993.
265. Drinkwater BL, Nilson K, Chestnut CH, et al: Bone mineral content of amenorrheic and eumenorrheic athletes. N Engl J Med *311:*277, 1984.
266. Adinoff AD, Hollister JR: Steroid-induced fractures and bone loss in patients with asthma. N Engl J Med *309:*265, 1983.
267. Herzog W, Minne H, Deter C, et al: Outcome of bone mineral density in anorexia nervosa patients 11.7 years after first admission. J Bone Miner Res *8:*597, 1993.
268. Richardson ML, Pozzi-Mucelli RS, Kanter AS, et al: Bone mineral changes in primary hyperparathyroidism. Skel Radiol *15:*85, 1986.
269. Funke M, Mäurer J, Grabbe E, et al: Vergleichende Untersuchungen mit der quantitativen Computertomographie und der Dual-Energy-X-Ray-Absorptiometrie zur Knochendichte be renaler Osteopathie. ROFO *157:*145, 1993.
270. Pouilles JM, Tremollieres F, Ribot C: The effects of menopause on longitudinal bone loss from the spine. Calcif Tissue Int *52:*340, 1992.
271. Riggs BL, Melton LJ: Evidence for two distinct syndromes of involutional osteoporosis. Am J Med *75:*899, 1983.
272. Ettinger B, Genant HK, Cann CE: Long-term estrogen replacement therapy prevents bone loss and fractures. Ann Intern Med *102:*319, 1985.
273. Felson DT, Zhang Y, Hannan MT, et al: The effect of postmenopausal estrogen therapy on bone density in elderly women. New Engl J Med *329:*1141, 1993.
274. Heaney RP: Estrogen-calcium interactions in the postmenopause: A quantitative description. Bone Miner *11:*67, 1990.
275. Lindsay R, Tohme JF: Estrogen treatment of patients with established osteoporosis. Obstet Gynecol *76:*290, 1990.
276. Marx CW, Dailey GE III, Cheney C, et al: Do estrogens improve bone mineral density in osteoporotic women over age 65? J Bone Miner Res *7:*1275, 1992.
277. Citron JT, Ettinger B, Genant HK: Prediction of peak premenopausal bone mass using a scale of weighted clinical variables. *In* Christiansen, et al (Eds): Osteoporosis 1987: Proceedings of the International Symposium on Osteoporosis. Copenhagen, Osteopress, 1987, p 146.
278. Doyle FH, Gutteridge DH, Joplin GF, et al: An assessment of radiological criteria used in the study of spinal osteoporosis. Br J Radiol *40:*241, 1967.
279. Michel BA, Lane NE, Jones HH, et al: Plain radiographs can be useful in estimating lumbar bone density. J Rheumatol *17:*528, 1990.
280. Jergas M, Uffmann M, Escher H, et al: Interobserver variation in the detection of osteopenia by radiography and comparison with dual x-ray absorptiometry (DXA) of the lumbar spine. Skel Radiol (in press).
281. Cummings SR, Black D: Should perimenopausal women be screened for osteoporosis? Ann Int Med *104:*817, 1986.
282. Heaney RP: En recherche de la difference (P < 0.05). Bone Miner *1:*99, 1986.
283. Ross PD, Davis JW, Wasnich RD, et al: The clinical application of serial bone mass measurements. Bone Miner *12:*189, 1991.
284. He Y-F, Davis JW, Ross PD, et al: Declining bone loss rate variability with increasing follow-up time. Bone Miner *21:*119, 1993.
285. Verheij LF, Blokland AK, Papapoulos SE, et al: Optimization of follow-up measurements of bone mass. J Nucl Med *33:*1406, 1992.
286. Overgaard K, Riis BJ, Christiansen C, et al: Effect of salcatonin given intranasally on early postmenopausal bone loss. Br Med J *299:*477, 1989.
287. Reginster JY, Denis D, Albert A, et al: 1-Year controlled randomised trial of prevention of early postmenopausal bone loss by intranasal calcitonin. Lancet *2:*1481, 1987.
288. Storm T, Thamsborg G, Steiniche T, et al: Effect of intermittent cyclical etidronate therapy on bone mass and fracture rate in women with postmenopausal osteoporosis. N Engl J Med *322:*1265, 1990.
289. Watts NB, Harris ST, Genant HK, et al: Intermittent cyclical etidronate treatment of postmenopausal osteoporosis. N Engl J Med *323:*73, 1990.
290. Harris ST, Gertz BJ, Genant HK, et al: The effect of short-term treatment with alendronate on vertebral density and biochemical markers of bone remodeling on early postmenopausal women. J Clin Endocrin Metab *76:*1399, 1993.
291. Riggs BL, Hodgson SF, O'Fallon WM, et al: Effect of fluoride treatment on the fracture rate in postmenopausal women with osteoporosis. N Engl J Med *322:*802, 1990.
292. Slovik DM, Neer RM, Potts JT Jr: Short-term effects of synthetic human parathyroid hormone-(1–34) administration on bone mineral metabolism in osteoporotic patients. J Clin Invest *68:*1261, 1981.
293. Reinbold WD, Genant HK, Reiser UJ, et al: Bone mineral content in early-postmenopausal osteoporotic women and postmenopausal women: Comparison of measurement methods. Radiology *160:*469, 1986.
294. Ott S, Kilcoyne R, Chesnut C III: Ability of four different techniques of measuring bone mass to diagnose vertebral fractures in postmenopausal women. J Bone Miner Res *2:*201, 1987.
295. Cummings SR, Black DM, Nevitt MC, et al: Bone density at various sites for prediction of hip fractures: The study of osteoporotic fractures. Lancet *341:*72, 1993.
296. Pacifici R, Rupich R, Griffin M, et al: Dual energy radiography versus quantitative computer tomography for the diagnosis of osteoporosis. J Clin Endocrinol Metab *70:*705, 1990.
297. Lai K, Rencken M, Drinkwater BL, et al: Site of bone density measurement may affect therapy decision. Calcif Tissue Int *53:*225, 1993.
298. Soda M-Y, Mizunuma H, Honjo SI, et al: Pre- and postmenopausal bone mineral density of the spine and proximal femur in Japanese women assessed by dual-energy x-ray absorptiometry: A cross-sectional study. J Bone Miner Res *8:*183, 1993.
299. Ryan PJ, Blake GM, Herd R, et al: Spine and femur BMD by DXA in patients with varying severity spinal osteoporosis. Calcif Tissue Int *52:*263, 1993.
300. Pouilles JM, Tremollieres F, Ribot C: Spine and femur densitometry at the menopause: Are both sites necessary in the assessment of the risk of osteoporosis? Calcif Tissue Int *52:*344, 1993.

301. Nordin BEC: The definition and diagnosis of osteoporosis. Calcif Tissue Int *40:*57, 1987.

302. Wahner HW: Single- and dual-photon absorptiometry in osteoporosis and osteomalacia. Semin Nucl Med *17:*305, 1987.

303. Heider A, Niederle N, Ringe JD, et al: Verzögerung der Plasmozytomdiagnose durch führende Osteoporosesymptome. Osteologie *2:*80, 1993.

304. Wasnich R: Fracture prediction with bone mass measurements. *In* HK Genant (Ed): Osteoporosis Update 1987. San Francisco, Radiology Research and Education Foundation, 1987, p 95.

305. Gärdsell P, Johnell O, Nilsson BE, et al: Predicting various fragility fractures in women by forearm bone densitometry: A follow-up study. Calcif Tissue Int *52:*348, 1993.

306. Huda W, Bissessur K: Effective dose equivalents, H_E, in diagnostic radiology. Med Phys *17:*998, 1990.

307. ICRP: Recommendations of the International Commission on Radiation Protection (ICRP). ICRP Publication 26. Oxford, Pergamon Press, 1977.

308. Genant HK, Vander Horst J, Lanzl LH, et al: Skeletal demineralization in primary hyperparathyroidism. *In* RB Mazess (Ed): Proceedings of International Conference on Bone Mineral Measurement. Washington, DC, National Institute of Arthritis, Metabolism, and Digestive Diseases, 1974, p 177.

53

Rickets and Osteomalacia

Michael J. Pitt, M.D.

The terms rickets and osteomalacia describe a group of diseases demonstrating similar gross pathologic, radiologic, and histologic abnormalities. The pathologic changes result from inadequate or delayed mineralization of osteoid in mature cortical and spongy bone (osteomalacia) and an interruption in orderly development and mineralization of the growth plate (rickets). Therefore, prior to growth plate fusion, rickets and osteomalacia coexist.

The radiologic findings in affected bones and cartilage reflect the gross pathologic and histologic abnormalities. Although the general radiographic findings are similar in all of the rachitic and osteomalacic syndromes, some distinctive features may be of help in sorting out the various disease entities.

The etiologic factors vary and include ionic or hormonal aberrations, or both. The significant advances in the understanding of vitamin D metabolism over the past decade have provided new insights into the rachitic and osteomalacic syndromes. It has been established that "vitamin D" is a prohormone that requires two additional sequential hydroxylations before the active hormonal form, 1,25-dihydroxyvitamin D$_3$, is produced. The pertinent biochemistry is discussed in this chapter and the information applied to the various rachitic and osteomalacic syndromes.

Rickets was recognized in antiquity and was one of the earliest syndromes to be described clinically.[232, 387] The origin of the word remains in doubt.[182, 387, 443] It is one of the best known medical diseases; the name is familiar to laymen and health scientists alike.

The clinical presentations and medical conceptions of the disease have changed markedly in the past century as a result of research efforts in multiple scientific disciplines.[566] It is difficult today to appreciate the prevalence of the disorder and the paucity of medical information regarding pathogenesis and treatment that existed prior to the early part of this century[94, 269, 387]; Dent and Stamp described it as the "scourge of mankind."[94] As an example, Morse, reporting in the *Journal of the American Medical Association* in 1900, found evidence of rickets in approximately 80 per cent of infants under 2 years of age in Boston and its vicinity.[251] A history of rickets may be found in the reports by Dent,[95] Harris,[145] Loomis,[219] and Mankin[232]; Weick discussed the history of the disease in the United States.[387]

Little progress in the understanding of rickets was made from the time of Glisson's classic description in 1650[129] until the early part of the twentieth century. The studies of Mellanby in 1919[242] and 1925[243] were pivotal in directing scientific attention to a deficiency state. Mellanby, a British nutritionalist who was stimulated by the success of cod liver oil in the correction of rickets,[163] claimed further support for a dietary cause of rickets by producing the disease in puppies fed a variety of "rachitic diets." His concept of rickets as a dietary deficiency disease was in keeping with the newly proposed vitamin theories of that time and received the support of the influential British Medical Research Council.[219] Although the causative agent was originally considered to be vitamin A, in 1922 McCollum and associates[240, 567] established the separate identity of the "antirachitic factor" (isolated from cod liver oil) and suggested the term "vitamin D." Because the rachitic curing factor had been accepted as a vitamin and rickets had been produced by dietary manipulation, the inclusion of rickets in the classification of vitamin deficiency diseases at that time was logical. Although Mellanby's work may be criticized scientifically in retrospect,[219] his studies stimulated new clinical approaches and research. Much of the subsequent research focused on the relationship of rickets to a dietary deficiency. Treatment with synthetic vitamin D cured the majority of patients with rickets but unmasked a smaller group, who, although their conditions resembled usual rickets biochemically and radiologically, were refractory to the usual therapeutic doses of vitamin D. These disorders were noted by Bloomberg[29] in 1927 and were elaborated on by Albright and associates in 1937 as "rickets resistant to vitamin D therapy."[7] This group of vitamin D refractory disorders has been expanded to include acquired and congenital diseases marked by rickets, such as the Fanconi group of renal tubular dysfunctions.

We now know that so-called vitamin D is not a vitamin[219] and recognize the basic role of ultraviolet light in the prevention of usual rickets. Because of long and widespread use of this term, however, "vitamin D" will be used throughout this chapter to refer to the antirachitic factor. Although the vitamin theory generally was endorsed, substantial early evidence suggested the importance of ultraviolet light.[199, 219, 232, 267] Seasonal correlation of rickets reflecting the availability of ultraviolet light was indicated by several authors. In Germany, Kasowitz (1884) noted the development of this disease in children after the long indoor periods of the winter months.[219] Schmorl's 1909 autopsy series recorded rickets in over 80 per cent of the children examined in the winter, whereas autopsies conducted in summer demonstrated rickets in fewer than 50 per cent of cadavers.[331] In 1917 Hess and Unger remarked on the decreased frequency of rickets in the summer months and the increased frequency among the dark-skinned populations who were shielded from the solar rays.[163] In 1919 Huldschinsky used ultraviolet light from a mercury vapor quartz lamp to reverse rachitic changes in four children with advanced rickets.[180]

BIOCHEMISTRY OF VITAMIN D

Probably no disease has been subjected to more intensive research than rickets during the last twenty years, and in no disease has the method of attack shifted with such rapidity from morbid anatomy to dietetics, to biochemistry, spectroscopy, and the culminating artificial synthesis of the antirachitic vitamin D which is held by most people to be the substance, deficiency of which produces rickets.[145]

This statement was made in 1933 by Harris; with minor alterations it would appropriately describe the current activities in this field. Progress in the understanding of vitamin D metabolism has occurred at an exponentially rapid pace in the past 25 years, resulting in basic modifications of long-standing views.[568, 572] Until recently the general assumption was that vitamin D was a vitamin and was unaltered metabolically prior to discharging its physiologic function. Biochemical advances were delayed by the inability to synthesize a radioactively labeled molecule of vitamin D with a high specific activity. In 1966, Neville and DeLuca at the University of Wisconsin succeeded in preparing a vitamin D molecule, $1,2(^3H)$ vitamin D_3, with a sufficiently high specific activity to permit experimentation in the physiologic dose range.[257] After administration of this radioactive vitamin D to rats, these investigators noted an early accumulation of radioactivity in the liver, which then declined rapidly. Skeletal tissue, intestine, and to a lesser extent muscle and kidney subsequently demonstrated the major accumulation of radioactivity with a delay in maximum uptake of 4 to 9 hours. One explanation for the delay was possible metabolic conversion of vitamin D to more active forms,[257] a theory that had been discounted by earlier workers.[198, 199] This contention was supported, however, when Lund and DeLuca[224] showed that radioactive metabolites recovered from bone, blood, and liver after administration of the new high specific activity $1,2 (^3H)$ vitamin D_3 were effective in curing rickets in rats. The metabolite recovered in the greatest amount was found to be as active as the parent compound, vitamin D, in its antirachitic properties and was identified chemically by Blunt and coworkers in 1968 as 25-hydroxyvitamin D (25-OH-D_3).[30] The hydroxylation at the carbon 25 position was demonstrated to occur primarily in the liver.[292] During this same period, Haussler and associates[157] and Kodicek[199] identified an additional active metabolite of vitamin D,[152] which was found to be even more potent and more rapidly acting than 25-OH-D_3.[154, 260] In 1971, Holick and coworkers[172] identified this compound structurally as 1,25-dihydroxyvitamin D_3 $(1,25[OH]_2D_3)$.

Under physiologic conditions, the hydroxylation at the carbon 1 position occurs exclusively in the kidney. This important determination was first reported by Fraser and Kodicek in 1970.[119] The central, unique importance of the kidney in the scheme of vitamin D metabolism was confirmed rapidly by other investigators. Boyle and associates[37] demonstrated that decreased $1,25(OH)_2D$ production resulted from lack of renal tissue and not from a simple uremic state. Intestinal calcium transport was measured after 25-OH-D_3 administration to two groups of uremic animals. Animals with uremia secondary to nephrectomy did not show intestinal calcium transport, whereas animals with uremia after ureteral ligation exhibited expected intestinal calcium absorption.[37] Wong and coworkers[391] used biosynthetically prepared 1,25(OH)₂D₃ and obtained similar results. After nephrectomy, 1,25(OH)₂D₃ but not vitamin D₃ or 25-OH-D₃ produced intestinal calcium absorption. Holick and associates[171] showed that nephrectomy completely prevented the bone calcium mobilization response to 25-OH-D₃ but did not prevent a calcium mobilizing response to 1,25(OH)₂D₃.

Although the kidney is the major site of formation and regulation of 1,25(OH)₂D under *physiologic* conditions, extrarenal formation of 1,25(OH)₂D also has been demonstrated.[398] Production of 1,25(OH)₂D by the placenta (which also produces other hormones) probably plays a direct role in fetal bone and mineral metabolism. Turner and collaborators have shown in vitro formation of 1,25(OH)₂D in bone,[403] an intriguing finding, suggesting that 1,25(OH)₂D also may be produced at its major target site.

Extrarenal synthesis of 1,25(OH)₂D also has been confirmed in pathologic conditions. Up to 10 per cent of patients with sarcoidosis show hypercalcemia. A number of investigations have shown that this complication of sarcoidosis is associated with increased serum levels of 1,25(OH)₂D[399, 400–402] without elevations of serum 25-OH-D or parathyroid hormone.[399] Evidence that the generation of 1,25(OH)₂D in sarcoidosis is extrarenal is supported by the continued elevation of 1,25(OH)₂D following nephrectomy in a patient with sarcoidosis[400] and by the in vitro production of 1,25(OH)₂D from cultures of pulmonary alveolar macrophages from patients with active sarcoidosis[446] and from sarcoid tissue homogenates.[404]

Extrarenal production of 1,25(OH)₂D has been reported in association with lymphoma, both non-Hodgkin's and Hodgkin's types.[405, 406, 572] Hypercalcemia may occur in patients with lymphoma, particularly the T cell variety.[450, 451]

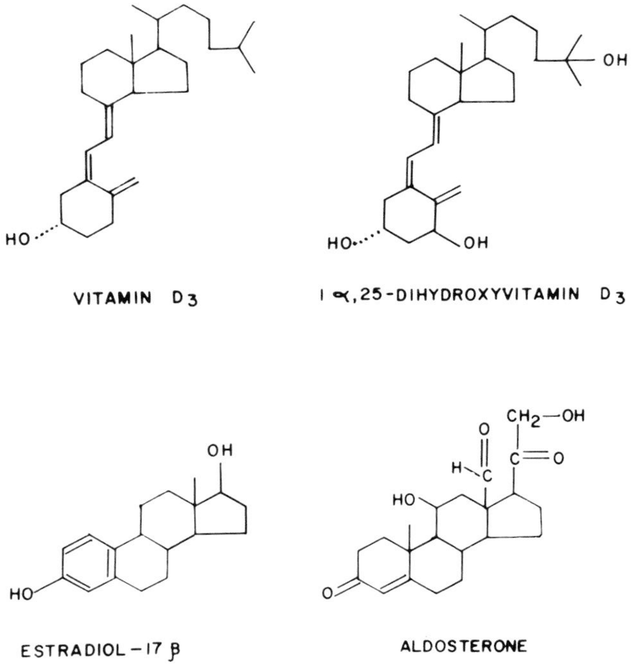

In some of the hypercalcemic patients there has been an associated elevation of 1,25(OH)₂D levels. Production of 1,25(OH)₂D in these patients appears to be poorly regulated and increases with concomitant increases in serum 25-OH-D.[405] After reduction of the lymphoma tissue mass by surgery[406] or medical therapy,[405, 406] both the serum calcium and the 1,25(OH)₂D levels have returned to normal, suggesting that 1,25(OH)₂D is produced in the lymphoma tissue mass.[405, 406]

Examination of the chemical structure of 1,25(OH)₂D and its precursors discloses a close resemblance to the classic steroidal hormones (Fig. 53–1). Vitamin D metabolites show an open B ring, but other structural features are similar to those of steroids. The positioning of functional hydroxyl groups at opposing ends of the molecule is especially pertinent in this regard. The existence of key hydroxyl groups separated by a complex ring structure is a universal feature of physiologically important steroids. The similar hydroxyl group arrangement in 1,25(OH)₂D provides impetus for including this substance in the general classification of steroid hormones. As will be noted later in this chapter, the biochemical mechanism of 1,25(OH)₂D action also is steroidal in nature.[508]

Physiologic Considerations

Two prohormonal forms of 1,25(OH)₂D are found in humans: vitamin D₃ and vitamin D₂. Vitamin D₃ is the natural, endogenously produced compound resulting from interaction of ultraviolet light with a cholesterol derivative, 7-dehydrocholesterol, in the deeper layers of the skin.[170, 299, 570] Small amounts of exogenous vitamin D₃ may be derived from dietary sources, such as dairy products and fish liver oils. Vitamin D₂ is prepared artificially by irradiation of ergosterol obtained from yeast or fungi[299] and is the compound used for food supplementation and pharmaceutical preparations.[220] Although quite similar structurally, vitamin D₂ is differentiated from vitamin D₃ by the presence of an additional methyl group at the 24 position and a double bond between carbons 22 and 23.[317]

Both vitamin D₃ and vitamin D₂ are hydroxylated at the carbon 25 position to form 25-OH-D₃ and 25-OH-D₂, respectively. This occurs predominantly in the liver, where the responsible enzyme, vitamin D–25-hydroxylase, is found mainly in the endoplasmic reticulum (microsomes) fraction of hepatic cells.[93, 292, 373] Hydroxylation at carbon 25 also has been noted in extrahepatic sites, such as the intestine and kidney,[373] but the importance of extrahepatic hydroxylation in humans is not known.[89] When both vitamin D₃ and vitamin D₂ are available in adequate amounts, the major portion of the circulating 25-hydroxylated form is 25-OH-D₃.[138] 25-OH-D₃ circulates bound to a specific binding protein,[169] which differs in various species.[317] In humans, the vitamin D binding protein is strikingly undersaturated (fewer than 1 per cent of binding sites occupied[35]) and the concentration far exceeds requirements for transport of 25-OH-D under normal circumstances. Similar findings of gross undersaturation have been found in the rat.[321] In addition, no reciprocal influence appears to exist between metabolism or concentration of 25-OH-D and vitamin D protein binding levels. Various assay techniques have used this binding protein to measure 25-OH-D₃ levels.[298, 299]

25-Hydroxyvitamin D is further hydroxylated at the 1α

FIGURE 53–1. Chemical structures of vitamin D₃ and the active hormonal form, 1,25(OH)₂D₃. Note the structural similarities to other steroid hormones. (From Pitt MJ, Haussler MR: Skel Radiol *1*:191, 1977.)

position, producing the active form of the hormone, 1,25-OH$_2$D$_3$. As noted, the 1α hydroxylating enzyme (25-OH-D-1α hydroxylase) is found exclusively in renal tissue[199, 244] and is located in the mitochondria.[152, 199, 244] The production of 1,25(OH)$_2$D$_3$ is related directly to body needs[183, 226] and is closely regulated by multiple factors, which may be integrated into classic hormonal feedback loops. In comparison to 25-OH-D, the serum levels of 1,25(OH)$_2$D$_3$ are relatively low. 1,25(OH)$_2$D$_3$ is produced and metabolized rapidly and, unlike 25-OH-D, has no significant tissue stores.[134]

At present, there is general agreement that 1,25(OH)$_2$D$_3$ represents the physiologically active form of the hormone.[88, 91, 123, 152, 220, 259, 290] The distinction between physiologic and pharmacologic levels of active vitamin D metabolites should be appreciated, however. For example, it has been shown that large or pharmacologic doses of 25-OH-D can stimulate intestinal absorption of calcium in humans[140] and cause calcium mobilization from bone in anephric rats.[281]

In addition to 1α-hydroxylation producing 1,25(OH)$_2$D, 25-OH-D also can be hydroxylated at carbons number 24 or 26 to produce dihydroxylated vitamin D compounds. 24,25(OH)$_2$D is produced by renal hydroxylation and is the major metabolite of 25-OH-D found under conditions of normal calcium concentration or hypercalcemia.[365] It is not believed to be active in bone metabolism.[151] 24,25(OH)$_2$D can be further hydroxylated to form 1,24,25(OH)$_3$D$_3$. At present, little is known about the significance of 26-hydroxylated D vitamins; they are not found in the main target organs (bone and intestine) after administration of labeled vitamin D to rachitic chicks.[158] All of the 24-hydroxylated forms of vitamin D are less active than the non-24-hydroxylated precursors.[89] It is probable that 24- and 26-hydroxylations of 25-OH-D represent inactivation and excretory pathways.[89, 90]

Action of Vitamin D

The long recognized functions of vitamin D are the homeostatic maintenance of serum calcium and phosphorus levels[92] and the mineralization of bone.[88, 267] The physiologic form of the vitamin, 1,25(OH)$_2$D$_3$, acts on two main target organs—the intestine and bone. The kidney and the parathyroid glands also have been identified as sites of action.

Before discussing the results of 1,25(OH)$_2$D$_3$ action on the intestine and bone, it is useful to appreciate the important distinction between calcium and phosphorus mineral homeostasis and skeletal homeostasis, as emphasized by Rasmussen and coworkers.[306] Common regulators with overlapping functions influence both of these areas. Extraosseous calcium and phosphorus homeostasis requires mediation by three different hormones: parathyroid hormone, 1,25(OH)$_2$D$_3$, and calcitonin[11, 261] (Fig. 53–2). These hormones interact at three main target organs: bone, kidney, and intestine. The skeleton serves as the major endogenous reservoir for calcium and phosphorus. Skeletal homeostasis requires maintenance of a skeletal mass capable of providing adequate structural support.[306] This involves a continual process of remodeling with breakdown of old bone and new reconstruction.

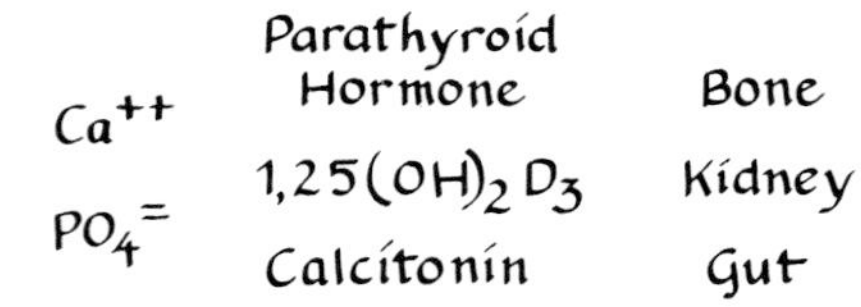

$$Ca^{++}$$
$$PO_4^{=}$$

Parathyroid Hormone — Bone
1,25(OH)$_2$D$_3$ — Kidney
Calcitonin — Gut

FIGURE 53–2. The hormones responsible for calcium and phosphate mineral metabolism are parathyroid hormone, 1,25(OH)$_2$D$_3$, and calcitonin. These hormones operate on and interact with the target tissues bone, kidney, and gut. (From Pitt MJ, et al: Crit Rev Radiol Sci 10:133, 1977.)

Intestines. The effect of 1,25(OH)$_2$D on the intestine is to increase the absorption of calcium[569] and phosphorus.[88, 91, 152, 199, 396] The mechanism at the intestinal cell level is similar to that of other steroid hormones, such as estrogen. 1,25(OH)$_2$D$_3$ enters the cell and joins a specific cytosol receptor. This hormone receptor complex migrates to the cell nucleus, where interaction with nuclear chromatin occurs.[49, 152, 157] By yet undetermined mechanisms, the hormone receptor complex opens a section(s) of the DNA helix of the chromatin. DNA-dependent RNA polymerases[397] operate at these "open" areas on the DNA helix, with template formation of a new RNA, which is termed messenger RNA (mRNA). Messenger RNA leaves the cell nucleus and is translated on the polyribosomes into a new protein, designated calcium-binding protein (CaBP).[199, 383, 385] This CaBP or "calcium carrier" becomes localized in the periodic acid-Schiff (PAS)-positive goblet cells and surface coat (microvillar membrane),[366] where it participates in the transfer of calcium from the intestinal lumen into the mucosal cells. Additional biochemical aspects of this process and the conveyance of calcium from the mucosal cell to the serum have not been well characterized[283]; other, as yet unidentified vitamin D–dependent factors could play a role.[396]

Vitamin D–dependent CaBP formation has been identified in the parathyroid glands and kidneys[265, 367]; the protein has properties similar to those of intestinal CaBP. Other organs demonstrating a high calcium flux, such as the eggshell gland of laying hens, also have been associated with CaBP. Therefore, the formation of a CaBP may be the common biochemical denominator in 1,25(OH)$_2$D function.

Although it has been well established that 1,25(OH)$_2$D increases intestinal calcium transport, its influence on phosphate absorption from the intestine has been defined only recently. In addition to passive absorption of phosphorus in conjunction with the active intestinal transport of calcium,[267] active phosphate transporting mechanisms reflecting vitamin D activity have been demonstrated.[148, 384]

Bone. In the skeleton, 1,25(OH)$_2$D has two actions, which initially appear to be diametrically opposed: mobilization of calcium and phosphorus from previously formed bone and promotion of maturation[57] and mineralization of organic matrix.[88, 267, 306]

1,25(OH)$_2$D mobilizes calcium and phosphorus from previously formed bone by stimulating osteocytic osteolysis[306] and in this way participates in the breakdown process occurring as part of skeletal homeostasis. The process requires the presence of both 1,25(OH)$_2$D and parathyroid hormone.[88, 126, 307] (As a corollary, parathyroid hormone probably requires an active form of vitamin D to accomplish its well-known deossifying role.[249, 306])

The presence of vitamin D clearly is essential for adequate deposition of bone mineral. Two hormonal roles are possible: the maintenance of adequate serum calcium and phosphorus levels or a direct effect on skeletal tissue (or both). The role of vitamin D in the preservation of normal serum levels of calcium and phosphorus has been established firmly. In fact, many investigators have considered this to be the major concern of vitamin D in mineralization.[88, 153, 185, 267] Undoubtedly, low levels of serum calcium or phosphorus (or both), regardless of cause (e.g., deficiency of 1,25[OH]$_2$D, diet, renal loss, and so forth) are important factors in the development of rickets and osteomalacia.[83, 156] Clinical experience shows a poor correlation between the serum calcium and phosphorus concentrations and the severity of rachitic and osteomalacic states, however.[188, 306] Administration of vitamin D in these conditions can result in a positive bone mineralization response, which precedes correction of the serum calcium and phosphorus levels.[188, 306] Therefore, the distinct possibility that vitamin D metabolites have a direct effect on bone cells and matrix during the process of mineralization must be considered.[306, 363, 386] Canas and associates showed an increased rate of tritiated proline incorporation into bone collagen after vitamin D supplementation to rachitic chicks compared with normal controls.[57] Incorporation of radioactive proline into bone collagen occurred before changes in serum calcium levels were noted. A concomitant increase in radioactive proline content in the skin of rachitic chicks was not noted. Favus and Wezeman have provided evidence that 1,25(OH)$_2$D (or a metabolite) localizes in bone and cartilage.[114]

Kidneys and Parathyroid Glands. Although the intestine and skeleton are the major targets of 1,25(OH)$_2$D$_3$ action, the kidney and parathyroid glands also are target organs affected by vitamin D. Action on the kidney was first suggested by Harrison and Harrison in 1941.[150] Administration of vitamin D to dogs resulted in increased renal tubular resorption of phosphate. These animals had intact parathyroid glands, however, and critics point out that parathyroid hormone suppression due to serum calcium elevation (resulting from vitamin D action on the gut or skeleton[267] or a direct suppressive effect of vitamin D on the parathyroid gland, or both)[53, 160, 207] may have caused the increased tubular resorption of phosphate. Puschett and associates provided additional evidence indicating a direct effect of vitamin D on proximal renal tubular function.[301] In their study, they eliminated the influence of parathyroid hormone by thyroparathyroidectomy. A significant depression in the percentage of filtered phosphate excreted by the kidney was noted following the administration of vitamin D$_3$ or 25-OH-D$_3$. Popovtzer and associates have demonstrated enhancement of tubular resorption of phosphate after 25-OH-D$_3$ administration.[293, 294] Their studies were performed on parathyroidectomized rats: The effect of 25-OH-D on phosphate resorption occurred only after administration of parathyroid hormone, suggesting a parathyroid-dependent mechanism of 25-OH-D action on the kidney.

Direct action of 1,25(OH)$_2$D$_3$ on the parathyroid glands has been demonstrated,[53, 160, 265] with resulting suppression of parathyroid hormone secretion.[64] In vitamin D–deficient

animals, 1,25(OH)$_2$D$_3$ localized in the parathyroid glands,[160] combining with specific intracellular receptors located in both the nucleus and the cytoplasm.[53] It has been shown that this reaction can cause formation of a calcium binding protein[265]; the similar mechanism of 1,25(OH)$_2$D$_3$ action on the intestine (and kidney) should be recognized.[367] It may be postulated that the calcium binding protein raises the calcium environment in the parathyroid gland. Regardless of exact mechanism, Chertow and associates[64] have found a decrease in parathyroid hormone secretion after 1,25(OH)$_2$D$_3$ administration that was independent of serum calcium levels. It should be noted, however, that several workers have failed to show that 1,25(OH)$_2$D$_3$ suppresses parathyroid hormone secretion in in vitro systems of humans and several animals.[266]

Assays for Vitamin D Metabolites

Sensitive biochemical assays for 25-OH-D have been employed by a number of researchers. These assays are all competitive binding methods, based on high affinity association of labeled 25-OH-D$_3$ with various specific binding proteins. An unknown concentration of 25-OH-D in plasma samples is quantitated by virtue of its competition with labeled 25-OH-D$_3$. Haddad and Chyu used a 25-OH-D binding protein, found in the cytoplasmic fraction of all nucleated cells, to devise a 25-OH-D assay.[137] Belsey and coworkers developed a similar competitive binding assay using a serum protein from rats, which binds 25-OH-D with high affinity.[23] Hughes and associates have used the 1,25(OH)$_2$D$_3$ receptor system from chick intestine to quantitate 25-OH-D by its ability to displace labeled 1,25(OH)$_2$D$_3$ from this protein.[183] All assays for 25-OH-D have yielded normal plasma concentrations of 10 to 80 ng/ml (2.5 × 10^{-8} to 2 × 10^{-7} M), depending on diet and degree of sunlight exposure.

Brumbaugh and associates,[51, 52] Haussler and coworkers,[153] and Hughes and coauthors[183] have developed a radioligand receptor assay for 1,25(OH)$_2$D$_3$ that is based on competition between unlabeled hormone from plasma and radioactive 1,25(OH)$_2$D$_3$ for the chick intestinal receptor system. This receptor system consists of a two-step binding process, initially binding the hormone to a high affinity cytoplasmic receptor protein and subsequently binding the hormone receptor complexes to chromatin with isolation by filtration. The assay is more complicated than standard competitive protein binding methods in that it requires detailed technical knowledge and skill to use the receptor system, as well as extensive purification of the plasma 1,25(OH)$_2$D$_3$ by chromatography of each sample (20 ml plasma for triplicate assay) on three successive columns.[52] Studies in normal humans indicate that the level of 1,25(OH)$_2$D is 2.1 to 4.5 ng/100 ml plasma on sunlight exposure. This level has been confirmed independently by the bioassay of Hill and coworkers[164] using vitamin D–deficient rats. This bioassay requires 100 to 200 ml of plasma from each patient, however; therefore, it will probably not be useful as a clinical tool. An independent competitive protein binding assay for 1,25(OH)$_2$D$_3$ has been developed by Eisman and colleagues.[110] This assay uses the same receptor protein discovered by Brumbaugh and Haussler,[50] but it includes a new procedure for separating bound from free hormone and requires only 5 ml of plasma for a triplicate assay. The normal circulating human level of 1,25(OH)$_2$D measured by this assay is very similar to that measured by the other assay procedures.

Regulators of 1,25(OH)$_2$D$_3$ Production

Considerable evidence has justified the designation of vitamin D as a hormone.[14, 17, 91, 93, 125, 134, 153, 161, 199, 261, 267, 299, 571] As with other hormones, only one specific organ, the kidney, produces the substance using the substrates formed in extrarenal sites. 1,25(OH)$_2$D$_3$ is secreted and transported to target organs, where it has an intranuclear mechanism of action resembling that of other steroid hormones. The renal production of 1,25(OH)$_2$D$_3$ is closely supervised by several factors that may be integrated into classic endocrine loops with typical feedback features. The established regulators are the levels of serum calcium, parathyroid hormone, and serum phosphate. Less certain are the roles of 1,25(OH)$_2$D itself, calcitonin,[221, 308] corticosteroids,[65, 139, 195, 222] sex hormones,[362] thyroid hormone,[375] and growth hormones.

Calcium and Parathyroid Hormone. Although calcium and parathyroid hormone exert a significant regulatory influence on 1,25(OH)$_2$D formation, the issues of how this is accomplished and the importance of parathyroid hormone control remain to be defined more completely. 1,25(OH)$_2$D formation correlates with the levels of serum calcium.[83, 88, 93] Low intake of dietary calcium with subsequent hypocalcemia is associated with increased levels of 1,25(OH)$_2$D and increased absorption of calcium from the gut; high dietary calcium intake has the opposite effect, with depression of 1,25(OH)$_2$D levels and diminished intestinal absorption of calcium.[51, 83, 88] The increase in 1,25(OH)$_2$D$_3$ production elicited by hypocalcemia is thought by many to be mediated via the parathyroid glands. Boyle and coworkers have shown that when the plasma calcium concentration in vitamin D–deficient rats is low, the rate of conversion of 25-OH-D to 1,25(OH)$_2$D$_3$ in vivo is increased.[36] Garabedian and coworkers[126] demonstrated that the stimulation of 1,25(OH)$_2$D$_3$ production by hypocalcemia was greatly diminished after thyroparathyroidectomy. Administration of exogenous parathyroid hormone to these same hypocalcemic animals stimulated the production of 1,25(OH)$_2$D$_3$, which could not be attributed to changes in serum calcium or phosphorus levels. Similar results were obtained by Hughes and associates.[184] Direct measurements of 1,25(OH)$_2$D$_3$ showed a fivefold increase of this hormone in rats maintained on low calcium or low phosphate diets. After thyroparathyroidectomy, the increase in 1,25(OH)$_2$D$_3$ was greatly diminished in response to the low calcium diet. Rasmussen and collaborators[308] have shown in vitro that parathyroid hormone and cyclic adenosine monophosphate (cAMP) stimulate isolated renal tubules to convert 25-OH-D$_3$ to 1,25(OH)$_2$D$_3$, whereas low calcium levels do not stimulate this reaction. Chase and coworkers[60–62] have shown that the renal tubular response to parathyroid hormone is mediated through stimulation of the adenyl cyclase system with production of cyclic adenosine-3′,5′ monophosphate (see discussion on parathyroid gland abnormalities later in this chapter). Direct measurement of the renal enzyme responsible for 1,25(OH)$_2$D formation (25-OH-D-1α hydroxylase) showed a significant decrease in enzyme activity after thyroparathyroidectomy, with the decrease oc-

curring within 24 hours.[161] Clinically, Bilezikian and associates[25] produced hypocalcemia in eight patients with Paget's disease by administration of mithramycin, an osteoclast inhibitor. Parathyroid hormone levels promptly increased, whereas serum phosphate levels decreased; these changes were followed within 12 to 24 hours by elevation of the serum 1,25(OH)$_2$D concentration. The time course is consistent with regulation by parathyroid hormone. Haussler and associates have demonstrated increased levels of 1,25(OH)$_2$D$_3$ in patients with primary hyperparathyroidism and reduced levels of 1,25(OH)$_2$D$_3$ in patients with hypoparathyroidism and pseudohypoparathyroidism (Albright's hereditary osteodystrophy).[153, 155] Therefore, besides the recognized effect of depressing renal tubular phosphate resorption, considerable evidence exists suggesting that parathyroid hormone also serves as a trophic factor in the renal production of the hormone 1,25(OH)$_2$D$_3$.

Although the data presented previously indicate that the increase in 1,25(OH)$_2$D$_3$ elicited by low serum calcium levels is mediated primarily by the parathyroid hormone, the necessity and importance of parathyroid hormone in this loop have been questioned. Favus and coworkers have shown that thyroparathyroidectomized rats can adapt to a low calcium diet with increased intestinal absorption of calcium.[113] Although plasma levels of 1,25(OH)$_2$D$_3$ were reduced in the thyroparathyroidectomized animals compared with sham operated controls, the accumulation of this hormone in the intestinal mucosa of both groups was identical. These authors suggest that a reduced but continued level of 1,25(OH)$_2$D$_3$ production continues after thyroparathyroidectomy, with probable selective accumulation in the intestinal mucosa (high affinity binding sites), which can account for the adaptation to low calcium diets. Some direct influence of low calcium may be present. Hughes and associates[184] demonstrated a twofold increase in 1,25(OH)$_2$D$_3$ levels in thyroparathyroidectomized animals when normal calcium diets were replaced by low calcium diets. Larkins and coworkers also believe that an increase in 1,25(OH)$_2$D$_3$ levels is a direct consequence of low serum calcium level.[206]

The conflicting information regarding the importance of parathyroid hormone in the regulation of 1,25(OH)$_2$D production might be somewhat resolved if the results are interpreted in terms of acuteness and chronicity. The consensus is that under acute conditions stimulation of 1,25(OH)$_2$D production by signals stemming from low calcium levels is mediated primarily by parathyroid hormone. Physiologically, in the absence of parathyroid hormone deficient or resistant states, this is most likely the important operative mechanism. In situations in which chronic parathyroid hormone deficiency or resistance exists, the body apparently has the adaptive capacity to produce 1,25(OH)$_2$D$_3$ in response to low serum calcium levels.

Phosphate. Dietary and serum inorganic phosphorus levels significantly influence and regulate 1,25(OH)$_2$D$_3$ formation. Vitamin D research has been relatively inattentive to this ion in comparison to calcium.[93, 363] Hypophosphatemia frequently is noted in the deficiency rachitic states, however, and is probably the primary factor in the development of rickets and osteomalacia in the syndromes associated with renal tubular phosphate loss (e.g., X-linked hypophosphatemia and Fanconi syndromes). Indeed, as suggested in 1921 by Howland and Kramer[175] and more recently by Tanaka and DeLuca,[363] depression of serum phosphate level may be of more importance than low calcium levels in the development of rickets and osteomalacia. Low dietary phosphate is associated with increased levels of 25-OH-D-1α hydroxylase activity[83, 156] and increased serum levels of 1,25(OH)$_2$D$_3$.[184] Studies by several groups indicate that hypophosphatemia stimulates 1,25(OH)$_2$D$_3$ production[83, 88, 93, 153, 156] directly; in contrast to the acute hypocalcemic signal, this effect is independent of parathyroid hormone.[184, 364] Tanaka and DeLuca showed that rats fed a low phosphate diet exhibited marked synthesis of 1,25(OH)$_2$D$_3$.[364] Thyroparathyroidectomy did not prevent this response. Hughes and coworkers demonstrated a fivefold increase in 1,25(OH)$_2$D from normal levels in rats fed low calcium and low phosphate diets.[184] After thyroparathyroidectomy, the same low phosphate diets provoked a comparable increase in 1,25(OH)$_2$D$_3$ levels; the low calcium diets elicited only a minimal increase in 1,25(OH)$_2$D$_3$. Similar results also were obtained in pigs.[156] Tanaka and DeLuca[364] noted a close correlation between reduced inorganic phosphorus levels in the renal cortex and the synthesis of 1,25(OH)$_2$D$_3$. They have suggested that the inorganic phosphorus level of the renal cells underlies the regulation of 1,25(OH)$_2$D synthesis and is the common denominator in the formation of 1,25(OH)$_2$D stimulated by parathyroid hormone and low phosphorus.[364]

Although it is clear that inorganic phosphorus plays a highly significant role in the regulation of 1,25(OH)$_2$D formation, direct measurements of the renal enzyme 25-OH-D-1α hydroxylase in response to a hypophosphatemic signal have produced conflicting results. Henry and associates found no relationship between enzyme activity and serum levels of phosphate.[161] This contrasts with the study by Baxter and DeLuca,[20] who demonstrated increased enzyme activity in response to low phosphate levels.

1,25(OH)$_2$D$_3$ (a Self-Regulator). 1,25-(OH)$_2$D$_3$ affects its own production by both direct and indirect means. The indirect influence occurs through suppression of parathyroid hormone secretion and is discussed earlier in this chapter in the section on action of vitamin D.

A direct negative feedback effect of 1,25(OH)$_2$D$_3$ on its own production has been demonstrated in vitro by Larkins and coworkers.[207] Suppression of enzymatic conversion of 25-OH-D$_3$ to 1,25(OH)$_2$D$_3$ in isolated renal tubules occurred in the presence of 1,25(OH)$_2$D$_3$. These workers proposed an intranuclear mechanism of action for this suppression analogous to the other steroidal modes of action of vitamin D. It is known that a vitamin D–dependent calcium binding protein is formed in the kidney.[367] This calcium binding protein, produced in response to the renal action of 1,25(OH)$_2$D$_3$, could raise the renal cellular calcium levels. Elevations of serum calcium have been shown to suppress the 25-OH-D-1α hydroxylase system.[74]

Calcitonin. There is little information concerning the effect of calcitonin on vitamin D metabolism. Although in vitro studies by Rasmussen and associates[308] demonstrated inhibition of 25-OH-D conversion to 1,25(OH)$_2$D$_3$, in vivo work by Lorenc and colleagues indicates that calcitonin does not affect vitamin D directly.[221] In rats, increases in serum levels of 1,25(OH)$_2$D$_3$ recorded after administration of calcitonin were not noted after thyroparathyroidectomy. The results indicate that the effect of calcitonin on 1,25(OH)$_2$D$_3$ is mediated by the parathyroid glands.[221]

Summary of Regulatory Controls. Two main regula-

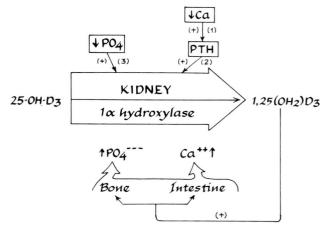

FIGURE 53–3. 25-OH-D is converted in the kidney to 1,25(OH)$_2$D by the action of the renal enzyme 1α-hydroxylase. This reaction is regulated by serum phosphate (3) and parathyroid hormone (2). Serum calcium (1) influences the reaction indirectly through its effect on the parathyroid glands. The two main target organs of 1,25(OH)$_2$D action, bone and intestine, are depicted. A plus (+) indicates a stimulatory effect. (From Pitt MJ, et al: Crit Rev Radiol Sci *10*:135, 1977.)

tory loops initiated by low serum calcium and low serum phosphate levels, respectively, may be postulated (Fig. 53–3). Acute depressions of serum calcium level signal the production of parathyroid hormone, which in turn stimulates 1,25(OH)$_2$D$_3$ production. Serum calcium and phosphate levels rise owing to the subsequent action of 1,25(OH)$_2$D$_3$ on the intestine and to the combined effects of parathyroid hormone and 1,25(OH)$_2$D$_3$ on bone, causing calcium and phosphate mobilization. The elevation of serum phosphate concentration is negated by increased renal excretion of phosphate from parathyroid action on the renal tubules. The net result is an increase in serum calcium levels.

The hypophosphatemic signal stimulates 1,25(OH)$_2$D production directly. Elevation of serum phosphate and calcium results from 1,25(OH)$_2$D action on the intestine, bone, and kidney. Subsequent suppression of parathyroid hormone secretion, resulting from the 1,25(OH)$_2$D-induced elevation of serum calcium level and the direct suppressive effect of 1,25(OH)$_2$D on the parathyroid glands, together with the hypercalcemia, leads to an increase in urinary calcium excretion but a decrease in urinary phosphate excretion. 1,25(OH)$_2$D also may increase serum phosphate concentration by mobilization of phosphate from soft tissue stores.[93] The total sequence accounts for a net increase in serum phosphate level.

1,25(OH)$_2$D acts to close each of these controlling loops by (directly and indirectly) depressing its own formation. The role of calcitonin and other hormones awaits further investigation.

STRUCTURAL PATHOANATOMY OF RICKETS AND OSTEOMALACIA

Gross Pathology and Histology

Regardless of their causes, the rachitic and osteomalacic syndromes display remarkably similar histologic and radiographic features. The characteristic changes of rickets are identified in the growth plates prior to closure; abnormalities of osteomalacia are seen in mature areas of trabecular and cortical bone. Because rickets and osteomalacia result from the same pathophysiologic mechanisms, findings representative of both lesions are present in persons affected prior to growth plate fusion.[272, 333, 350] Although rickets and osteomalacia may coexist, it is convenient and classic to describe each separately.

The structure of the normal growth plate must be understood before the changes of rickets may be appreciated. The typical growth plate, a complex structure composed of fibrous, cartilaginous, and osseous tissues, is located at the ends of long bones and situated between the epiphysis and the metaphysis. Although the growth plate is in apposition to the epiphysis, functionally it is part of the shaft. Therefore, the commonly used term "epiphyseal plate" is inaccurate.[304] The usual growth plate is discoid in configuration, but variations are present depending on the specific anatomic location. For example, the growth plate of the proximal portion of the femur is elongated and extends to the greater trochanteric region. Growth plates of the vertebral bodies are similar in organization to those of long bones but lack an overlying epiphysis. Small bones of the hands and feet have only one growth plate.

Histologically, the cellular arrangement of the normal growth plate is characterized by *order*. From epiphyseal to metaphyseal side, a progressive increase occurs in the number and size of cartilage cells and a development of cell columns aligned with the long axis of the shaft. Zones of development may be identified that have been described by various names.[3, 186, 232, 304] The review of this subject by Brighton is recommended.[46]

The following terminology may be applied:

1. The *reserve zone* (also termed resting or germinal zone) is subjacent to the epiphysis. The cartilage cells are few in number, are randomly situated either singly or in pairs, and are spherical. They are not resting, are not germinal cells, and are not small in comparison with cells in the proliferative zone.[46] Their function may be nutritional as they store various materials, particularly lipids.[46]

2. The *proliferating zone* is where the chondrocytes become flattened and arranged into longitudinal, parallel columns. These are the only cells in the cartilaginous portion of the growth plate that actively divide.[46] The function of this zone is matrix production and cellular proliferation.

3. The *hypertrophic zone* is a region that may be subdivided further into zones of *maturation, degeneration,* and *provisional calcification.* The change in cell morphology from the proliferative to the hypertrophic zones usually is abrupt and marked by sphericity and progressive enlargement. Cells nearing the metaphyseal side of the growth plate become quite large and vacuolated, with the last cells in the column becoming nonviable.[46] The upper portions of this zone are active metabolically, and calcification of intervening cartilage matrix occurs.

4. The *zones of primary* and *secondary spongiosa* are located in the metaphysis immediately subjacent to the growth plate. Cartilage bars are partially or completely calcified and become ensheathed with osteoblasts, which produce layers of osteoid. Bone is produced by endochondral ossification.[46]

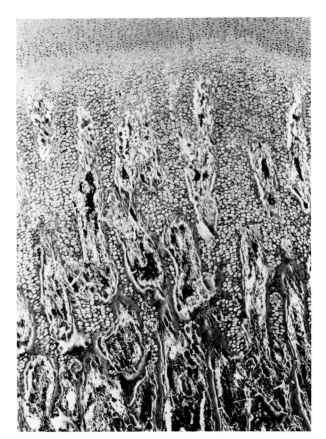

FIGURE 53–4. Normal chick growth plate with zone of proliferation at top. Observe orderly cartilaginous cell columns with zone of primary spongiosa at bottom. (Hematoxylin and eosin stain, 200×.) (From Pitt MJ, et al: Crit Rev Radiol Sci *10*:140, 1977.)

The rachitic lesion displays disorganization in the growth plate and subjacent metaphysis. The resting and proliferative zones of the cartilaginous growth plate are not altered significantly from the normal pattern. The zone of maturation is grossly abnormal, however, with a disorganized increase in the number of cells and a loss of normal columnar pattern. This cell mass results in an increase in length and width of the growth plate. Concomitantly, vascular intrusion from the metaphysis and subsequent calcification of the intervening cartilaginous bars are decreased and grossly disordered. Defective mineralization in the zone of primary spongiosa and a lack of proper formation of bone lamellae and haversian systems occur.[275] Figures 53–4 and 53–5 compare the growth plate of a normal control with an experimentally produced rachitic lesion in 6 week old chicks.

Osteomalacia is characterized by abnormal quantities of osteoid (inadequately mineralized bone matrix) coating the surfaces of trabeculae and lining the haversian canals in the cortex ("osteoid seams"). Excessive accumulations of osteoid also may be deposited in subperiosteal areas (see Fig. 53–10). Trabeculae become thin and decrease in number.[99] In the cortex, the haversian systems become irregular and large channels develop. Osteoid seams are not pathognomonic for osteomalacia and may be found in other states of high bone turnover. In osteomalacia, however, these osteoid seams increase in both number and width.[146, 188] Looser's lines or Milkman's pseudofractures[245, 246], which strongly

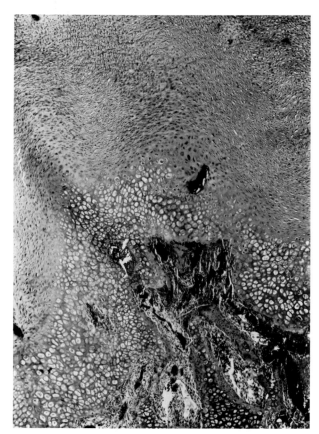

FIGURE 53–5. Rachitic chick growth plate with thick disordered hypertrophic zone virtually filling the field. Epiphyseal side appears at top. (Hematoxylin and eosin stain, 200×.) (From Pitt MJ, et al: Crit Rev Radiol Sci *10*:140, 1977.)

suggest the radiographic diagnoses of osteomalacia (but are *not* pathognomonic[499]), are composed of focal accumulations of osteoid.[186] Osteitis fibrosa cystica frequently is superimposed on the lesions of rickets and osteomalacia, reflecting hyperparathyroidism[186] (secondary to the low serum calcium level). This feature is particularly prominent in renal osteodystrophy.[270] Figures 53–6 and 53–7 demonstrate the typical appearance of osteomalacia in the subcortical spongy bone in a vitamin D–deficient chick and in a normal, age-matched control.

Radiologic Diagnosis of Rickets and Osteomalacia

Before discussing the characteristic radiographic features of osteomalacia and rickets, a few general remarks are in order. Rachitic changes will be more obvious in regions of the most active growth.[55, 276, 315, 359] Therefore, in order of decreasing sensitivity, the sites of highest radiographic yield would be the costochondral junctions of middle ribs, the distal part of the femur, the proximal portion of the humerus, both ends of the tibia, and the distal ends of ulna and radius.[276] Signs of rickets may be masked by systemic malnutrition,[277, 327, 315] with retardation of bone growth resulting from underproduction of (nonmineralized) osseous matrix. This accounts for earlier observations of accelerated rachitic changes developing after restoration of adequate general nutrition in vitamin D–deprived children. Acceler-

ated bone age during recovery from rickets also may be observed.[3]

Rickets. Nonspecific radiographic features include a general retardation in body growth[83, 176, 191] and osteopenia. Characteristic changes appear at the growth plate. These reflect the disordered increase in cell growth in the zone of hypertrophy, coupled with the deficient mineralization of the zone of provisional calcification.[232] Slight axial widening at the growth plate represents the earliest specific radiographic change.[359] This is followed by a decrease in density at the zone of provisional calcification (on the metaphyseal side of the growth plate). As the disease progresses, further widening of the growth plate occurs, and the zone of provisional calcification becomes irregular.[55] Disorganization and "fraying" of the spongy bone occur in the metaphyseal region. Widening and cupping of the metaphysis can be explained by the chaotic cartilage cell growth in the zone of maturation, which deposits an increased cell mass in both the longitudinal and the latitudinal axes; this bulky mass places abnormal stress on the growth plate with inward protrusion on the more central areas of the metaphysis. The vector forces have been compared to a piston-type mechanism.[232] On occasion, a thin bony margin is seen extending from the peripheral portions of the metaphysis surrounding the uncalcified cartilage mass (see Fig. 53–10). This probably results from periosteal intramembranous new bone,

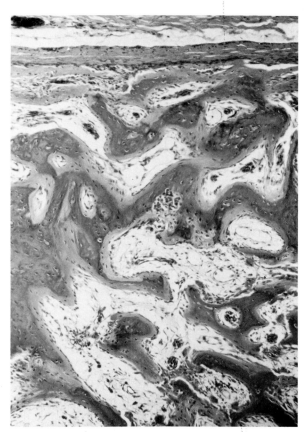

FIGURE 53–6. Osteomalacic cortex and subcortical spongy bone from metaphyseal region of a vitamin D–deficient chick. Trabeculae are thinned and irregular in shape and distribution. Sheaths of lightly stained osteoid almost equal the girth of bone in the trabeculae. Interspicular tissue is loosely fibrocartilaginous. (Hematoxylin and eosin stain, 500×.) (From Pitt MJ, et al: Crit Rev Radiol Sci *10:* 141, 1977.)

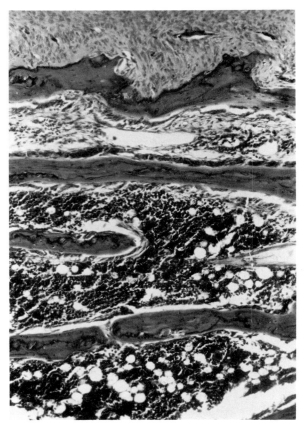

FIGURE 53–7. Normal cortex of chick metaphysis obtained at similar level to that in Figure 53–6. Periosteum is at top. (Hematoxylin and eosin stain, 500×.) (From Pitt MJ, et al: Crit Rev Radiol Sci *10*:141, 1977.)

the first months of life. During this period, the skull must accommodate to the most rapidly growing organ, the brain.[3] The rapid accommodation by the skull is associated with excess osteoid formation, particularly at the central margins and outer table. Resorption at the inner table continues. The thin calvarium is subject to supine postural influences, resulting in posterior flattening. Continued accumulation of osteoid in the frontal and parietal regions results in the squared configuration known as craniotabes.

During infancy and early childhood, the long bones show the greatest deformity, both at the cartilage-shaft junctions and in the diaphyses. The characteristic bowing deformities of the arms and legs can be related to the sitting position assumed by the infant and child. "The infant with severe rickets often sits all day long for months with legs crossed, tailor-fashion, leaning slightly forward and supporting the body on the outstretched hands."[276] Bowing also is a result of displacement of the growth centers owing to asymmetric musculotendinous pulls on the weakened growth plate. For example, the saber shin deformity of the tibia results from the strong posterior pull of the Achilles tendon on the calcaneus.

With increasing age the effects of weight-bearing become prominent. Scoliosis frequently develops and, coupled with bending deformities of long bones, results in an overall decrease in height. In severe cases, the external appearance suggests a dwarfing syndrome. In the spine, the

which is relatively less affected by the rachitic process than the endochondral bone in the cartilaginous portion of the growth plate. Figures 53–8 to 53–10 demonstrate a radiographic spectrum of rachitic changes.

Conceptually, the ossified center of the epiphysis is surrounded by cartilage cells, which are organized in a similar fashion to the growth plate. The peripheral rim of the ossified epiphyseal nucleus is analogous to the zone of provisional calcification. Changes similar to those seen in the growth plate are present, consisting of deossification and unsharpness of the ossified periphery.

The bulky growth plates at the shaft bone-cartilage junctions of long bones and ribs explain some of the characteristic physical findings of rickets. Swelling about joints is typical and a "rachitic rosary" develops at the costochondral junctions of the middle ribs. These latter areas are weakened and, influenced by the negative intrathoracic pressures developed during respiration, frequently are depressed. An additional semicoronal impression may be found at the costal attachment of the diaphragm (Harrison's groove).[176]

The deformities caused by rickets exhibit different patterns, depending on the child's age when the disease develops. Park described these patterns and the age relationship of the deformities.[276] He noted that stress and strain were applied differently as the posture and activity changed with increasing age. The head was particularly affected during

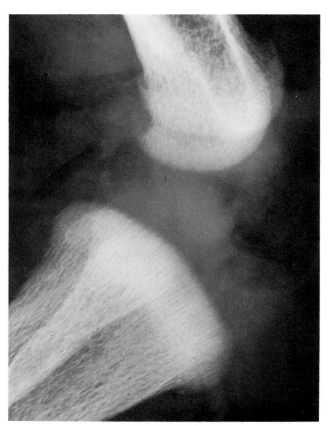

FIGURE 53–8. Normal knee radiograph of a 6 week old chick. Compare with Figures 53–9 and 53–10. Note the well-mineralized, organized zone of provisional calcification and the primary spongiosa in the metaphyseal regions of the femur and tibia. Cortical and trabecular bony margins are well defined, with sharp margins.

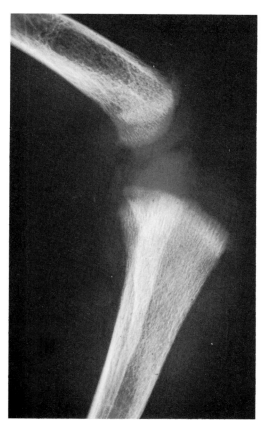

FIGURE 53–9. Knee radiograph of 6 week old chick demonstrating mild dietary deficiency rickets. Note the decreased mineralization and early disorganization in the zones of provisional calcification and primary spongiosa. (From Pitt MJ, et al: Crit Rev Radiol Sci *10*:143, 1977.)

intervertebral discs expand, producing concave impressions on the vertebral endplates. In contrast to osteoporosis, most vertebral bodies are involved to a similar degree. The skull shows basilar invagination, and intrusion of the hip and spine into the soft pelvis produces a triradiate configuration. The sacral orientation becomes more horizontal. Pelvic deformity may cause considerable difficulty during parturition.

Osteomalacia. The radiographic confirmation of osteomalacia is difficult. Many changes, such as osteopenia, are nonspecific. Gross deformities of the long bones, spine, pelvis, and skull have been discussed in the previous section on rickets. Areas of spongy bone show a decrease in the total number of trabeculae, owing to a loss of secondary trabeculae. The remaining trabeculae appear prominent and project a "coarsened" pattern; careful attention to their margins reveals an unsharpness reflecting the inadequately mineralized coats of osteoid. Lucent sites in the cortex reflect accumulations of osteoid and widened, irregular haversian canals.

Osteoid may be deposited in excessive amounts at various sites, particularly in the spine and pelvis. Thickening of long bones may result from subperiosteal osteoid deposition.[277] This is demonstrated in the posterior aspect of the femoral cortices in Figure 53–10. Subsequent mineralization of these areas may occur. Although this osteoid remains relatively mineral deficient per unit area, the exces-

sive total amount of osteoid can result in areas of increased density. This is particularly true in renal osteodystrophy.

Looser's zones or pseudofractures, usually appearing later in the clinical course of osteomalacia, may precede other radiographic changes.[359, 499] These lucent areas are oriented at right angles to the cortex and incompletely span the diameter of the bone. They tend to occur in characteristic sites, such as the axillary margins of the scapula, ribs, superior and inferior pubic rami, inner margins of the proximal ends of the femora, and posterior margins of the proximal portions of the ulnae[358] (Fig. 53–11). Pseudofractures typically are bilateral and symmetric.[358] Sclerosis often demarcates the intraosseous margins; new bone on the periosteal aspect suggests callus. True fractures can occur through these weakened areas.

Looser's zones are considered to be a form of insufficiency type of stress fracture.[499] In contrast to fatigue type stress fractures, pseudofractures do not necessarily involve weight-bearing bones and may remain unaltered over long periods of observation.[461] In addition, Looser's zones appear as broad radiolucent bands, perpendicular to the cortical surface, with defined, parallel margins showing mild to moderate sclerosis and, generally, with an absence of cal-

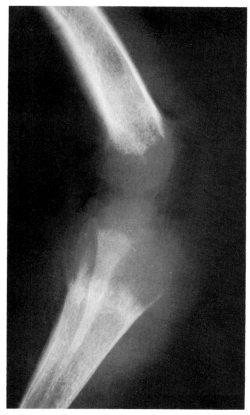

FIGURE 53–10. Knee radiograph of 6 week old chick showing advanced dietary deficiency rickets. Compare with Figures 53–8 and 53–9 and observe the advanced demineralization and disorganization in the metaphysis subjacent to the enlarged (unmineralized) growth plates. On occasion, as seen in the proximal part of the tibia in this specimen, a thin rim of circumferential new bone may be seen surrounding the rachitic growth plate. Also note the thickened, blunted posterior femoral cortex representing an increase in inadequately mineralized osteoid. (From Pitt MJ, et al: Crit Rev Radiol Sci *10*:144, 1977.)

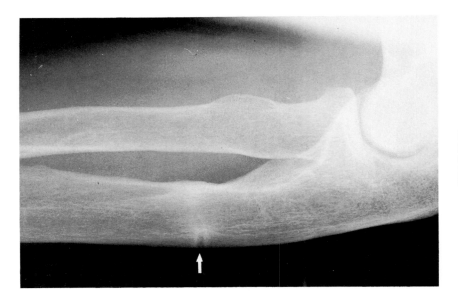

FIGURE 53–11. Pseudofracture (arrow) in adult patient with X-linked hypophosphatemic osteomalacia occurring in characteristic location in proximal ulna. Note bowing of ulna. (From Pitt MJ, et al: Crit Rev Radiol Sci *10*:145, 1977.)

lus.[499] The bilateral, symmetric pattern of pseudofractures also is a distinguishing feature. No preceding traumatic event has occurred. Radiolucent areas similar to pseudofractures may be found in bones affected by Paget's disease and fibrous dysplasia. The radiolucent zones in these diseases, however, are confined to the affected bone and, unlike pseudofractures, are not generalized. Looser's zones form at sites of increased stress and therefore accelerated bone turnover. The osteoid laid down in this normal bone replacement process is inadequately mineralized, which is responsible for the lucent radiographic appearance.

Although the presence of typical pseudofractures has been considered to be pathognomonic for the presence of osteomalacia, patients have been reported who had "typical" pseudofractures but did not show evidence of osteomalacia on bone biopsy.[461, 499]

Hypervitaminosis D results in a high bone turnover state. Infants and children may develop radiodense metaphyseal bands.[573] Cortical thickening, due to periosteal apposition, occurs at some sites, whereas cortical thinning is present at other locations.[573] Adults may show focal or diffuse deossification.[573]

CLINICAL SYNDROMES

As indicated in earlier sections of this chapter, the terms rickets and osteomalacia encompass a group of disorders with similar gross pathologic, histologic, radiologic, and biochemical findings but diverse causes. Well over 60 causes or associated diseases have been identified.[94] An association with a dietary deficiency of "vitamin D" was identified by Mellanby in 1919.[242] The subsequent synthesis of vitamin D and its use in persons with rickets provided a cure for the majority of patients. The concept of rickets as a simple deficiency disease, however, was expanded by the recognition of forms resistant or refractory to simple vitamin D dietary supplementation.[7, 29, 278, 279] These resistant (refractory) forms of both congenital and acquired origin now are the main foci of clinical concern.[500] Biochemical advances in vitamin D metabolism have explained many of

the resistant states and have indicated that the mechanism for resistance is variable; aberrations of vitamin D metabolism are not always present. In fact, some diseases that are rachitic in nature, such as hypophosphatasia or metaphyseal chondrodysplasia, have no known abnormalities of calcium, phosphorus, or vitamin D metabolism. In addition, the biochemical advances in vitamin D metabolism have provided new understanding of parathyroid gland disorders.

In the following sections, an etiologic approach to the rachitic and osteomalacic disorders will be considered, as organized in Figure 53–12:

1. Abnormalities of vitamin D metabolism:
   Abnormalities in prohormone vitamin D
   Abnormalities in 25-OH-D
   Abnormalities in 1,25(OH)$_2$D
2. Rachitic and osteomalacic syndromes resulting primarily from renal tubular *phosphate loss.*
3. Rachitic and osteomalacic syndromes that do not show abnormalities of vitamin D metabolism or aberrations of calcium or phosphorus metabolism.

The discussion is conceptually oriented and is not meant to be totally comprehensive. It should be appreciated that, as is often the case with disease, several contributing factors frequently are present.

Vitamin D Deficiency

Classic vitamin D deficiency rickets is encountered uncommonly in the United States today owing to the widespread addition of synthetic vitamin D$_2$ to foods, notably dairy products and bread.[14, 149] Between 1956 and 1960, a review by the American Academy of Pediatrics of 266 teaching hospitals disclosed a frequency of less than 0.4 cases of nutritional rickets per 100,000 pediatric admissions[75] (some of these cases may not have been nutritional in origin).

As noted in earlier sections of this chapter, the natural source of vitamin D for humans is not dietary.[149, 220, 255, 267

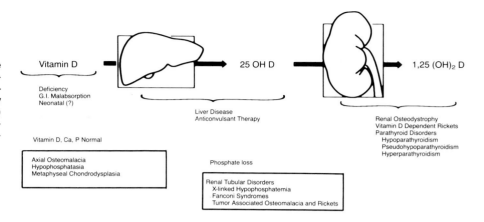

FIGURE 53–12. Etiologic approach to the rachitic and osteomalacic syndromes organized in a framework of (1) abnormalities of vitamin D; (2) syndromes secondary to renal tubular loss of phosphate; and (3) syndromes in which there is no known abnormality of vitamin D metabolism or calcium-phosphorus homeostasis.

Although small amounts of vitamin D_3 are found in eggs, milk, liver, and oily fishes such as tuna, mackerel, sardine, and salmon,[340] humans depend mainly on the ultraviolet rays of the sun for endogenous conversion of 7-dehydrocholesterol in the skin to the prohormone vitamin D_3 (cholecalciferol). Therefore, prior to the synthesis of vitamin D_3 in 1922,[240] people were dependent (like plants) on the sun for their health.[219, 220] The natural production of vitamin D_3 is quite efficient. It is estimated that 1 cm^2 of human skin exposed to sunlight produces 6 IU of vitamin D_3 per hour[22] (as quoted by Rab and Baseer[303]). A reasonable degree of exposure to the sun should prevent the development of rickets and osteomalacia in the normal person whose diet contains adequate amounts of calcium and phosphorus.[72, 261, 300]

Historically the frequency of rickets increased commensurately with the spread of sunless, crowded urban centers that developed as part of the industrial revolution.[219, 220] In fact, rickets may be the first example of an air pollution disease,[219] because factory-produced smog filters and further decreases the available ultraviolet light.

The importance of ultraviolet light exposure is demonstrated by the significant seasonal variations that have been recorded in 25-OH-D levels.[1, 19, 264, 355] Levels are lowest in the spring after the decrease in sun exposure during the cold, inclement months of winter, and are highest in the autumn.[355] A similar, corresponding seasonal variation also has been reported in the frequency of osteomalacia (by iliac crest biopsy) in older persons.[1] A study of elderly patients from Leeds, England, with fractures of the femoral neck showed significantly lower levels of 25-OH-D (and considerably less sunlight exposure) than in similar age-matched controls.[19] Studies of 25-OH-D levels in Danish patients with femoral neck fractures did not show seasonal variations.[225] This most likely reflects the vitamin D supplementation of milk in Denmark in contrast to the lack of supplementation in England,[95, 225] rather than a difference in sunlight exposure. In a South African report, 25-OH-D levels correlated with environmental temperature rather than with mean levels of daily sunshine; 25-OH-D levels were higher in the warmer months, commensurate with outdoor activity.[284]

In worldwide perspective, deficiency rickets and osteomalacia still represent a health problem.[14, 82, 289, 355] In the United Kingdom, the occurrence of rickets and osteomalacia among the immigrant Indian and Pakistani population is significant.[94, 132, 288, 316, 354] Although most of these patients are asymptomatic,[111] as many as 30 per cent show biochemical abnormalities (decreased serum calcium, increased serum alkaline phosphatase, and increased serum parathyroid hormone levels) consistent with rickets and osteomalacia.[111, 173] These abnormalities are particularly evident during pregnancy.[174, 303] This might be anticipated, as 25-OH-D levels also have been shown to be depressed during pregnancy, unrelated to dietary intake.[182] As expected, radiographic identification of rickets is less common. A report from Glasgow, Scotland, which was one of the early urban pockets of rickets, demonstrated radiographic findings of rickets in 9 per cent of young children.[316] Cooke and associates found a 4 per cent frequency of radiographically identified rickets in schoolchildren 14 to 17 years of age.[81]

The factors contributing to the development of rickets and osteomalacia in the British Asian population are multiple. Levels of 25-OH-D are low but are not related to primary impairment of intestinal absorption of vitamin D or rapid clearance of 25-OH-D from the plasma; ethnic traditions and dietary patterns are most contributory. The custom of Asian girls and women to remain indoors and wear traditional dress limits endogenous production of vitamin D by decreasing exposure to the sun.[173, 181] Chupatti flour, a dietary staple in this group, also is an important factor.[288, 312] The high phytate content in the wheat fiber binds to calcium and zinc and results in increased fecal loss. In addition, lignin, a component of the wheat fiber, binds to bile acids and increases their fecal excretion.[107] Vitamin D may combine with this fiber–bile acid complex and be unavailable for absorption.[107, 312] Removal of chupatti flour from the diet corrects the biochemical abnormalities characteristic of rickets.[312] Addition of vitamin D_2 to chupatti flour or separate supplementation with vitamin D successfully raised 25-OH-D levels to a normal range in a group of Asians from Glasgow.[288]

Deficiency rickets and osteomalacia have been reported even in sun-rich areas. Again, custom and diet are major factors. In Ethiopia, for example, classic vitamin D deficiency rickets is common; about 30 per cent of the children seen at the Ethio-Swedish Pediatric Clinic in Addis Ababa have clinically detectable rickets.[234] Review of infants with advanced rickets disclosed they had received no dietary supplementation with vitamin D and had had minimal periods of breastfeeding. In spite of adequate available sunshine, their exposure was reduced because of fear of the "evil eye" and their mothers' reluctance to allow their children's skin to become darker.[234]

In Nigeria, deficiency rickets is reported to be prevalent.[204] The custom of purdah, in which mothers and their children were exposed inadequately to the sun, may be causative.[204] Reports from Iran also indicate that rickets is a common disease.[8, 327] In children less than 1 year of age among the poorer classes of Tehran, general malnutrition frequently masked the clinical and biochemical signs of rickets. These children usually are kept indoors for most of the first year of life[327] and are wrapped up (swaddled) when they are taken outside[8]; sunlight is avoided. The high phytate content in their diet also binds calcium,[8, 312, 327] similar to the case with chupatti flour.

The osteomalacia that develops in Negev Desert Bedouin women of childbearing age also is related to eating raghif, an unleavened bread rich in phytates.[340] Levels of 25-OH-D in these women are within normal limits.[340]

In sunny Riyadh, the capital of Saudi Arabia, vitamin D deficiency rickets is not uncommon, occurring mainly among breast-fed infants.[433] Measured levels of 25-OH-D are low in both the rachitic children and their mothers, consequences of a Saudi Arabian custom of avoiding the hot sunshine, the design of urban housing, which does not provide the privacy necessary for the women to expose even their faces and hands to the sun, the custom of almost complete wrapping of the infants, and the low vitamin D content of the Saudian diet, which is not supplemented with vitamin D.

In the United States, where food cults and food faddists are more numerous than ever before,[112] reports of rickets in children on vegetarian diets have appeared.[106, 116, 440] Vegetarianism is practiced to varying degrees by members of such groups as Yoga, Seventh Day Adventists, the New Vrindaban International Society for Krishna Consciousness, the Zen Macrobiotic Movement, and Veganism.[112] The nutritional adequacy varies not only among groups but also within the individual sects.[116] Malnutrition may be a problem,[307] particularly in children less than 2 years of age, in whom low growth velocity compared with normals has been recorded.[330]

In developed countries, it is important to appreciate the occurrence of osteomalacia in the elderly.[94] This segment of the population perhaps constitutes the largest group subject to development of osteomalacia,[10, 355] particularly those patients who are house-bound or institutionalized for long periods.[441] Although decreased exposure to the sun is a prime cause, other postulated factors include deficient intake of oral vitamin D_2,[442] intestinal malabsorption of the elderly, and lower vitamin D hydroxylase activity in the liver and kidney.[10, 84, 94, 355] Even elderly patients who have a normal caloric intake may have insufficient amounts of various vitamin supplements.[94] 25-OH-D levels in long-term institutionalized geriatric patients not receiving vitamin D supplementation were low.[84] Dietary vitamin D supplementation restores these levels to the normal range.[226] As indicated previously, osteomalacia is a contributing factor in the genesis of femoral neck fractures in the elderly.[1]

"Deficiency" rickets (and osteomalacia) usually connotes a lack of vitamin D; insufficiencies of calcium or phosphorus, or both, should also be considered.[47] Rickets secondary to phosphorus deficiency usually is a result of congenital or acquired renal disease. Proximal renal tubular dysfunction with defective absorption of phosphorus, as seen in X-linked hypophosphatemia and Fanconi syndromes (to be considered later in this chapter), is the most common example of this group. Phosphate loss also may complicate hemodialysis,[286] cadaveric renal transplantation,[247] or excessive ingestion of aluminum hydroxide, which binds phosphate in the gut.[28, 494-496] An adequate amount of phosphorus usually is provided in the normal diet.[47]

Rickets secondary to insufficient calcium in the diet is rare. Reported cases are few and have been iatrogenic.[136, 201, 229] Humans show considerable adaptation to dietary variations of calcium through appropriate elicitation of $1,25(OH)_2D_3$ production in the kidney.[51, 83, 88] Low calcium diets appear to result in relative increases in calcium absorption with decreased elimination in the gut. For example, the malnutrition accompanying World War II situations was not associated with an increase in the frequency of rickets.[380] No good evidence exists that a diet chronically low in calcium is deleterious to humans (or that an increase in calcium intake would be beneficial in preventing bone disease).[381]

Gastrointestinal Malabsorption

Disorders of the small bowel, hepatobiliary system, and pancreas associated with intestinal malabsorption are the most common causes of vitamin D deficiency in the United States.[72] Vitamin D loss in malabsorption syndromes includes not only orally administered vitamin D but also endogenously produced substances.[78, 250]

Rickets and osteomalacia may develop in many small bowel malabsorptive states, including sprue, gluten-sensitive enteropathy (celiac disease)[279] (Fig. 53–13), regional enteritis, scleroderma,[188, 231, 347] and even unusual conditions such as multiple jejunal diverticula[190] or stagnant (blind) loop syndromes.[230] Decreased absorption and excessive fecal loss of both vitamin D and (probably) calcium are contributory.[197, 347] As stressed by Dent and Stamp, mild chronic malabsorption, as measured biochemically, may lead to severe osteomalacia.[94]

Small intestinal bypass surgery, performed for intractable morbid obesity, has been associated with multiple complications, such as diarrhea, electrolyte imbalance, liver disease, nephrocalcinosis and nephrolithiasis (oxalate),[93] and an arthritis syndrome resembling rheumatoid arthritis,[322, 339] in addition to the postoperative morbidity related to obesity.[56] Osteomalacia now has been recognized to be an additional common complication.[77, 168, 274, 347, 368] Although bone pain, tenderness, and proximal myopathy develop in the minority of these patients,[77, 274] disability from bone disease may be significant.[168] Histologic evidence of osteomalacia was identified in 25 per cent of intestinal bypass patients in one British study.[77] Radiographic findings of osteomalacia are much less common.[77, 274]

Reports of vitamin D status after small bowel resection vary. Low levels of plasma 25-OH-D have been recorded in the majority of intestinal bypass patients.[76, 368] Compston and Creamer[76] have demonstrated a reduced intestinal absorption of 25-OH-D. With time and adaptation, the levels of 25-OH-D return to normal.[368]

Preece and Valman[300] found that resection of large portions of the ileum did not cause rickets or produce abnor-

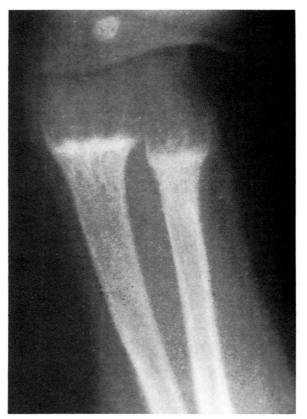

FIGURE 53–13. Rickets in a 4 month old Mexican infant with celiac disease. The metaphysis is demineralized and disorganized. Metaphyseal widening reflects the enlarged growth plate.

malities of vitamin D status. The authors noted normal levels of 25-OH-D in these patients and attributed these normal values to sufficient sun exposure with endogenous production of adequate amounts of vitamin D in the skin. The fact that vitamin D is absorbed chiefly in the proximal three fourths of the small bowel offers an additional explanation. Schachter and coworkers found a maximum vitamin D absorption in the midjejunum, with minimal absorption in the terminal ileum.[328]

Osteomalacia is a well-recognized complication of partial gastrectomy (usually Billroth II procedures), but the reported prevalence of skeletal disease varies considerably.[71, 109, 248, 370, 395] Eddy's study of postgastrectomy patients in the United States (Texas) indicated that osteomalacia was present in 25 per cent of patients.[109] Radiographic evaluation in this study, which compared postgastrectomy patients with a group of nonsurgical patients with peptic ulcer disease, showed that the former group had a significant decrease in thoracolumbar mineralization, a 2.4 per cent frequency of pseudofractures, and a 5.8 per cent frequency of pathologic fractures.[109] Zanzi and colleagues, using neutron activation analysis to measure total body calcium in a group of 18 unselected postgastrectomy patients, found that one third had a significant decrease in bone mineral[395]; spinal radiographs suggested osteopenia in only two of these patients.

The pathogenesis of postgastrectomy skeletal disease is not understood fully, but altered vitamin D metabolism is contributory. Although serum levels of 25-OH-D are depressed,[127, 213] Gertner and coworkers[127] found that ab-

sorption of 25-OH-D was normal. Their findings suggest that oral intake of vitamin D may be inadequate; in addition, decreased exposure to the sun existed in many of these patients. Other pathogenic factors that were suggested include postgastrectomy steatorrhea (which is not always present[71]) and reduced absorption of calcium.

Malabsorption associated with pancreatic insufficiency, even when pronounced, is associated with osteomalacia infrequently.[94] Children with cystic fibrosis, in contrast to other malabsorptive diseases, seldom develop rickets.[94, 144, 334] Studies of 25-OH-D levels in cystic fibrosis are conflicting: Hubbard and associates found normal levels,[177] whereas Hahn and coworkers found significant reductions.[144] The latter group also noted intestinal calcium malabsorption with slight hypocalcemia, secondary hypoparathyroidism, and a 14 per cent decrease in bone mass measured by photon absorption techniques.[144]

Previous studies have indicated a significant enterohepatic circulation of 25-OH-D,[13, 78] suggesting a functional conservation mechanism for vitamin D analogous to the enterohepatic circulation of bile salts. It was postulated that interference with the enterohepatic circulation of 25-OH-D was the important common denominator in vitamin D deficiency associated with gastrointestinal malabsorptive and hepatobiliary diseases. More recent work by Clements and coworkers[462] has shown that the enterohepatic circulation of 25-OH-D is negligible; therefore, interference with enterohepatic circulation of 25-OH-D cannot be a significant cause of the vitamin D deficiency associated with gastrointestinal malabsorption or hepatobiliary diseases.

Rickets Associated with Prematurity (Neonatal Rickets; Metabolic Bone Disease of Prematurity)

Abnormal mineral homeostasis with low serum levels of calcium and phosphorus is a well-recognized complication in low birth weight premature infants.[526, 528, 529] Hypocalcemia frequently occurs during the first days of life, and in very low birth weight infants it is practically the rule.[529] Metabolic bone disease is common. The radiographic identification of rickets (and osteomalacia in the long bones) may be more frequent than generally is appreciated[128, 135, 166, 369, 374, 438, 524, 527]; for example, a study by Lyon and coworkers showed a prevalence of 54 per cent.[525] Although the radiographic changes of rickets (and osteomalacia) usually are nonspecific, Thomas and coworkers have called attention to the "mandibular mantle" resulting from periosteal new bone formation paralleling the mandible.[369]

Affected infants usually weigh less than 1000 gm at birth or are of less than 28 weeks' gestation.[436] Although bone disease usually appears at about 12 weeks of age,[166] it may develop later, particularly in situations in which prolonged parenteral nutrition is required, such as in necrotizing enterocolitis[136] or in the neonatal respiratory distress syndrome (Fig. 53–14). In fact, patients with rachitic weakening of the thorax may have respiratory distress as their presenting clinical feature.[128, 369] As a corollary, the neonatal respiratory distress syndrome may be further complicated by rachitic involvement of the thorax.

The pathogenesis of the bone disease in prematurity is multifactorial[526, 528] and can be related to a combination of nutritional,[128] metabolic,[524] and sometimes iatrogenic fac-

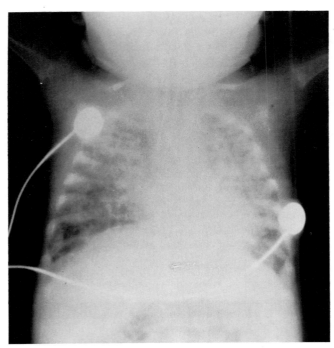

FIGURE 53–14. Four month old infant with generalized rachitic changes. Observe demineralization and disorganization of proximal humeral metaphyses. Respiratory distress syndrome developed after premature birth, with subsequent development of bronchopulmonary dysplasia. Parenteral nutrition provided inadequate amounts of vitamin D and calcium.

tors,[136, 209, 323] the last relating to a lack of appreciation or inattention to the requirements for supplementations of calcium, phosphorus, and vitamin D. Skeletal development is occurring at a very rapid rate during the last trimester of pregnancy. Eighty per cent of bone mineralization occurs during this period.[323] Therefore, the premature infant's requirements for calcium, phosphorus, and vitamin D[166] are greater than those of the infant born at term. This increased need may not be provided for in the diet.[374, 437, 438] The problem is compounded by the smaller feeding portions premature infants are able to take, which results in quantitative deficiencies of multiple types. Human milk and standard infant formulas, which are adequate for the term baby, have insufficient amounts of vitamin D,[434, 435] phosphorus,[323] and probably calcium[342] for the premature infant. The absolute requirement for vitamin D in premature infants is increased and may be three to six times greater than for the full term infant.[166] Vitamin D metabolism in newborn and preterm infants has been shown to be normal.[529, 530] Low levels of 25-OH-D demonstrated in many of these premature infants[165, 166, 437, 438] may relate to low maternal stores of vitamin D. Activation of the vitamin D hormonal sequence is operative within 24 hours after birth.[529] A study by Hillman and collaborators[459] found that 1,25(OH)₂D levels were normal or elevated in a group of premature infants and that the mean concentration of 1,25(OH)₂D increased with age. Their study also suggested that premature infants regulate 1,25(OH)₂D production in a manner similar to that of more mature infants and children. Hillman and colleagues found that ''independent of (1) birth weight and gestation, (2) mineral availability, and (3) ability to attain or maintain a

normal 25-OH-D serum concentration, an improvement in mineralization and an increase in serum calcium and phosphorus are seen as the premature infant reaches postconceptional maturity.''[437, 459] The postulation that the rickets of prematurity is related to immaturity of 1,25(OH)₂D receptors in the intestine, bone, and other tissues rather than to the deficiency in 1,25(OH)₂D[439, 459, 460] does not appear to be valid. The pathogenesis of hypomineralization in the premature term infant seems to be due largely to the low intake of calcium or phosphorus or to poor absorption of calcium in the case of vitamin D deficiency, or to both factors.[530]

Rickets and osteomalacia developing in these premature infants lead to significant morbidity from fractures, respiratory distress, and skeletal deformity. Koo and associates[531] followed a group of these patients with serial radiographs. At 6 months after birth, these infants showed complete resolution of rickets, healing of fractures, and no residual skeletal deformities. These authors suggest conservative management of the skeletal deformities.[531]

Liver Disease

Metabolic bone disease, termed hepatic osteodystrophy, is a well-recognized complication of chronic biliary ductal and hepatocellular disorders.[4, 140, 217, 218, 347, 463–465] Both osteoporosis and osteomalacia are found histologically.[340, 390] Although many patients are asymptomatic, morbidity relating to bone pain, tenderness, and fractures may be significant, particularly in patients with primary biliary cirrhosis and other chronic cholestatic diseases.[4, 465]

When present, radiologic changes usually are those of nonspecific osteopenia. Pseudofractures indicate the presence of osteomalacia. Hypertrophic osteoarthropathy has been reported but is not common.[54, 262] Marx and O'Connell have reported an erosive, asymmetric, nondeforming arthritis of the hands in patients with primary biliary cirrhosis.[235, 262]

Like renal osteodystrophy, the cause of hepatic osteodystrophy is multifactorial.[140, 464] Decreased levels of 25-OH-D commonly are found in patients with a variety of liver diseases, including chronic alcoholic hepatitis, cirrhosis, chronic active hepatitis, symptomatic biliary cirrhosis, and acute and chronic biliary disease.[78, 162, 168, 217, 348, 379, 464, 465] Because the liver is the major site for the initial hydroxylation of vitamin D, abnormalities in vitamin D metabolism might be expected. 25-Hydroxylation activity of the liver appears to be almost normal,[463] however, and 25-OH-D levels usually can be corrected with vitamin D supplementation.[464] The low serum levels of 25-OH-D are more likely a reflection of inadequate amounts of prohormone resulting from decreased exposure to ultraviolet light, decreased vitamin D supplementation, and—particularly if steatorrhea is present—malabsorption of vitamin D.

Long and associates found that although 25-OH-D levels were depressed significantly in the majority of patients with untreated liver disease, those who had been exposed to the sun adequately had normal levels.[217] Chronic depletion of vitamin D also is suggested by Skinner and coworkers' study of untreated patients with primary biliary cirrhosis.[348] After a single injection of vitamin D, serum 25-OH-D levels did not change significantly after 12 days, in contrast to a significant increase in 25-OH-D levels in normal controls and in patients with nutritional osteomalacia. 25-OH-D levels returned to normal with long-term administration of vitamin D, however.

Impaired intestinal absorption of vitamin D also may be present in liver disease. Compston and Thompson found a significant reduction of 25-OH-D intestinal absorption in a group of patients with primary biliary cirrhosis.[78] They pointed out that treatment with cholestyramine, a drug that binds bile acids in the intestine, may add considerably to the risk of osteomalacia. In fact, the frequency of osteomalacia in their patients correlated more closely with long-term cholestyramine administration than with the severity of liver disease.[78] Studies of patients with alcoholic liver disease did not show defective vitamin D absorption.[352]

Certain aspects of vitamin D metabolism in patients with liver disease remain perplexing. For example, although 25-OH-D levels generally are low, correlation between measured levels and histologic osteomalacia is poor.[218, 394] In some patients, bone pain may persist despite adequate vitamin D therapy; in some of these patients, calcium infusions have been shown to have an ameliorative effect.[4] Because the normal circulating level of 25-OH-D is much greater than the level of the physiologic form, $1,25(OH)_2D_3$, direct measurements of the latter will be helpful in evaluating the clinical significance of depressed 25-OH-D levels in patients with liver disease.

Rickets developing in four patients with neonatal hepatitis was reported by Yu and colleagues and may be more common than is generally appreciated.[394] This study showed no correlation between the development of rickets and the severity of the hepatitis as evaluated by clinical, biochemical, and histologic parameters. The rickets developed despite routine vitamin D supplementation of 300 to 400 IU per day; healing occurred after therapeutic doses of 2000 to 10,000 IU per day.[394] Rickets resulting from cirrhotic liver disease in childhood is uncommon.[372]

Because bile salts are necessary for the absorption of vitamin D,[300, 328] biliary duct obstruction, such as that which occurs in congenital biliary atresia (usually extrahepatic duct involvement), may be associated with typical rachitic changes, which may appear before 6 months of age (Fig. 53–15). In a study of five patients with extrahepatic biliary atresia, Daum and associates[87] found serum levels of 25-OH-D to be distinctly low. Healing of skeletal rickets in their patients was noted after only moderate doses of daily oral 25-OH-D.

Anticonvulsant Drug–Related Rickets and Osteomalacia

Rickets and osteomalacia may be seen both histologically and radiographically in patients receiving anticonvulsant drug therapy, particularly phenobarbital and phenytoin (Dilantin). The reported prevalence of clinical bone disease and abnormal radiographic changes in these patients varies, but it probably is low. The mechanisms responsible for the production of rickets and osteomalacia are incompletely understood, and conflicting data are found in the literature (see later discussion). Consideration must be given to the specific drug or drug combinations administered, the amount of drug and duration of treatment, the diet, the patient's general physical activity, whether or not the patient is institutionalized, and the amount of sunlight exposure.

Biochemical abnormalities reflecting abnormal bone and mineral metabolism frequently have been reported in patients receiving anticonvulsant drug therapy.[388] An increase in serum alkaline phosphatase level during anticonvulsant therapy was noted first in 1965 by Wright,[392] although the correlation with metabolic bone disease was not recognized. Subsequent studies have shown that elevations of serum alkaline phosphatase level occur early during the course of anticonvulsant therapy[210] and frequently are present.[68, 70, 142, 211, 302, 353, 392] Elevations have been found in as many as 42 per cent of patients.[85] The source has been both bone and liver. Reduced serum ionized calcium levels may be found in from 20 to 48 per cent of patients.[34, 68, 70, 142, 211, 353, 392, 444, 449] Although some patients will have marked hypocalcemia, the usual presentation is more subtle, and the reduced levels may be unsuspected clinically.[444] Decreased intestinal absorption of calcium, which is noted early in the course of drug therapy,[58] probably is a contributing cause of the hypocalcemia.

Interference with vitamin D metabolism related to anticonvulsant drugs has been implicated as a cause of the mineral and bone abnormalities. Decreased serum levels of 25-OH-D have been recorded by many investigators.[34, 141, 142, 163, 193, 252, 388, 444, 449] Gastrointestinal absorption of vitamin D is normal[239, 329]; hepatic conversion of vitamin D to 25-OH-D actually is increased.[239, 371, 445] Initially, serum levels of 25-OH-D may be elevated, with concomitant increases

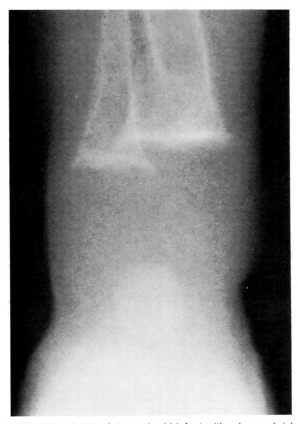

FIGURE 53–15. Ankle of 4 month old infant with advanced rickets secondary to extrahepatic biliary ductal atresia. Generalized demineralization is present, with disorganization and widening of the areas subjacent to the growth plate. The soft tissues at the ankle are prominent, reflecting the latitudinal widening of the bulky growth plate. A pathologic fracture is present in the distal end of the tibia.

in serum calcium levels.[445] A study in rats showed that the 25-OH-D levels declined to subnormal concentrations 21 days after initiation of anticonvulsive drug therapy.[445] Hahn and coworkers[143] and Hoffbrand[167] have related the decrease in 25-OH-D to an increase in hepatic microsomal hydroxylase activity resulting in an increase in inactive multihydroxylated vitamin D metabolites.[141] The frequently found decrease in serum 25-OH-D levels, however, cannot explain the severity of the bone and mineral abnormalities[448]; levels of $1,25(OH)_2D$ in these patients have been found to be within normal limits.[192, 444] A relative lack of correlation also exists between the presence and severity of bone abnormalities and the reduced levels of 25-OH-D.[252] Also, in contrast to simple deficiency forms of rickets and osteomalacia, the improvement in biochemical abnormalities associated with anticonvulsant drug therapy differs with the form of vitamin D administered. Rodbro and Christiansen found that administration of vitamin D_2 (ergosterol) produced an increase in bone mineral content but did not raise the serum calcium level.[320] Vitamin D_3 and 25-OH-D_3 produced increases in the serum calcium level but did not improve the bone mineral content.[67]

Data relating the development of biochemical and structural bony abnormalities to the duration of treatment and drug dose are conflicting. Crosley and coworkers' study of outpatient children on long-term anticonvulsant therapy,[85] which showed a high frequency of elevated alkaline phosphatase levels and an 8 per cent frequency of rickets radiographically (although the method used for the radiographic confirmation might be criticized), found a lack of correlation of the duration of treatment and drug dose with the degree of elevation of alkaline phosphatase level or the severity of radiographic changes. This contrasts with the findings of Tolman and associates, who found that duration of anticonvulsant drug therapy was the most important contributing factor to the development of osteomalacia in institutionalized patients.[371] Animal studies of rachitic changes occurring after phenytoin (Dilantin) administration showed direct correlations of the degree of rachitic change with the drug dose administered.[377]

The mechanism of action of the various anticonvulsant drugs differs with regard to the development of bone disease. Although both phenytoin and phenobarbital induce hepatic hydroxylase activity,[143, 167] Dilantin, but not phenobarbital,[196] also decreases intestinal absorption of calcium,[196, 377, 378] apparently by decreasing the activity of vitamin D–dependent calcium binding protein.[331, 377] These findings may implicate Dilantin as the most important anticonvulsant drug in the development of osteomalacia. This impression is supported by Koch and others, who noted that most epileptic patients demonstrating abnormalities of calcium or bone metabolism have received Dilantin either alone or in combination with other drugs, which did not always include phenobarbital.[196] Of tangential interest is the observation that Dilantin, while contributing to bone mineral loss, also has been found to enhance fracture healing.[124] This is believed to result from a general stimulatory effect on collagen synthesis.[124]

In another study of patients receiving various anticonvulsant drugs, firm evidence of vitamin D deficiency occurred only in those patients receiving primidone.[388] Acetazolamide-induced acceleration of osteomalacia also has been reported.[227]

Bone mineral content has been reduced significantly, as measured by photon absorption techniques[34, 66, 142, 444] and by neutron activation analysis.[302] Christiansen and collaborators[68] found that 20 per cent of patients receiving anticonvulsant drug therapy had subnormal bone mineral content.[68] The degree of mineral loss correlated with the total drug dose and duration of therapy. These authors also noted a fairly rapid decrease in bone mineral content, which developed within a few months after therapy.[70]

Radiographic changes of rickets and osteomalacia in association with anticonvulsant drug therapy were reported first by Kruse in 1968.[203] The reported frequency of radiographic changes varies: Livingston and coworkers failed to identify radiographic (or biochemical) evidence suggesting rickets or osteomalacia in a review of 15,000 patients seen at the Johns Hopkins Epilepsy Clinic during a 36 year period,[215] whereas Lifshitz and Maclaren found positive radiographic changes in up to 22 per cent of patients receiving long-term anticonvulsant treatment.[211, 212] When present, the radiographic changes are nonspecific and cannot be differentiated from those of rickets or osteomalacia resulting from other causes. Changes of osteomalacia may be quite severe, particularly in nonambulatory, long-term institutionalized patients.[343] Pierides and associates have reported a significant increase in pathologic fractures and histologic osteomalacia in both hemodialysis and post–renal transplant patients receiving phenobarbital.[287] Long-term Dilantin therapy, in addition to producing radiographic evidence of rickets, also may be associated with diffuse calvarial thickening, dental root abnormalities varying from widespread resorption to stumpy shortening, cleft palate, and occasional syndactyly.[447]

Patients on long-term anticonvulsant drug therapy show improvement in biochemical and radiologic abnormalities and a decrease in the prevalence of osteopenic fractures[343] when modest supplementation of vitamin D[34, 69, 70, 142, 210, 211, 320] in the range of 5000[69, 264] to 10,000 IU[142] per week is provided.

The introduction of newer anticonvulsant drugs such as carbamazepine (Tegretol) and valproic acid derivatives such as Depakote most likely will replace Dilantin and phenobarbital in the future treatment of epilepsy. Many epileptic patients whose disorder is well controlled on Dilantin and phenobarbital no doubt will continue to take these drugs. Also, Dilantin may be combined with the newer drugs for refractory epilepsy. At this time, it is not known whether the newer drugs will cause complications such as osteomalacia and rickets.

Renal Osteodystrophy (Uremic Osteopathy)

The bone disease associated with chronic renal failure results from multiple complex factors.[17, 21, 115, 189, 223, 319, 344, 349] Although the pathogenesis remains incompletely explained, two main mechanisms (probably acting in concert) are responsible: secondary hyperparathyroidism and abnormal vitamin D metabolism.

Secondary Hyperparathyroidism. Secondary hyperparathyroidism is noted consistently in untreated uremia occurring early in the course of the disease.[17, 40, 189, 238] Parathyroid hormone levels may be increased significantly and frequently are higher than the levels reached in primary hyperparathyroidism.[191] The secondary hyperparathyroidism is provoked by hypocalcemia, which results from several different mechanisms; phosphate retention is the major factor.[40, 189, 236, 238, 349] It is postulated that, in *early* renal failure, transient elevations of serum phosphate levels depress serum calcium levels indirectly by inhibiting synthesis of $1,25(OH)_2D$[238] (see Fig. 53–3). The lower $1,25(OH)_2D$ levels result in decreased intestinal absorption of calcium, lowering serum calcium levels. (Low levels of $1,25[OH]_2D$ in *early* renal failure have not been recorded definitely, however.[349]) Phosphate retention becomes more constant with moderate to advanced renal failure, and the elevated serum phosphate concentration reciprocally depresses the serum calcium level (calcium $\times$ phosphorus ion product).

Another important cause of hypocalcemia in patients with renal failure may be the skeletal resistance to the calcium-mobilizing action of parathyroid hormone, which has been noted by Massry and others.[216, 237, 238] This phenomenon may be seen in mild uremia and has been detected within 3 hours after induction of acute uremia in experimental animals.[351] Lower levels of serum calcium would result from a relative ineffectiveness of parathyroid hormone action on bone. Although depressed levels of $1,25(OH)_2D$ (or vitamin D metabolites) are believed to influence the skeletal resistance to parathyroid hormone,[73, 238, 349] their role is controversial.[351]

Other factors also contribute to the development of secondary hyperparathyroidism. Low levels of $1,25(OH)_2D$ in more advanced uremia account for increased parathyroid hormone levels by decreasing the negative feedback suppression on the parathyroid glands.[53, 64, 160] (See section on biochemistry.) Decreased renal degradation of parathyroid hormone also may result in higher levels.[238, 349]

Abnormal Vitamin D Metabolism. The singular importance of the kidney as the only organ capable of producing the physiologically active form of vitamin D, $1,25(OH)_2D$, was emphasized earlier in this chapter. It also has been noted that impaired conversion of 25-OH-D to $1,25(OH)_2D$ in renal disease reflects a decrease in kidney cell mass rather than a simple loss of renal function.[17, 37, 133] Loss of renal tissue in acquired renal disease therefore would be expected to be associated with low levels of $1,25(OH)_2D$. The hyperphosphatemia of renal failure also inhibits $1,25(OH)_2D$ production (see Fig. 53–3).

Decreased amounts of $1,25(OH)_2D$ in early renal failure have not yet been demonstrated[349]; measurements in patients with moderate to advanced renal failure have shown depressed or absent levels.[152, 153] Clinically these effects of decreased $1,25(OH)_2D$ production are not recognized until the glomerular filtration rate has been reduced to 25 to 30 ml/min.[223] Even in advanced uremia it is likely that the kidney continues to produce a small amount of $1,25(OH)_2D$. After nephrectomy in uremic patients, Oettinger and coworkers[263] found further reduction of already low intestinal calcium absorption. Resistance to administration of pharmacologic doses of vitamin D[17, 356] becomes more severe as the renal disease progresses and relates to the loss of renal 25-OH-D-1α hydroxylase. Therapy with low doses (physiologic range) of $1,25(OH)_2D$ has improved the metabolic and osseous aberrations[41, 43, 45, 159, 346] in many but not all patients.[115] After renal transplantation, $1,25(OH)_2D$ levels rapidly return to the normal range.[152, 285]

Histology and Radiology. The histologic and radiographic findings in chronic renal failure reflect hyperparathyroidism and deficiency of $1,25(OH)_2D$. The major abnormalities are osteitis fibrosa cystica, osteomalacia or rickets (or both), osteosclerosis (representing areas of increased bone volume), and osteoporosis[31–33, 179, 228, 319, 341, 349] (see also Chapter 57). The reported predominance of these features varies[32, 108, 223, 356] and does not correlate well with clinical or laboratory signs.[31] The clinical presentation is influenced by the patient's age at onset of renal failure, the cause of the renal disease, the dietary content of protein, phosphate, and calcium, the geographic differences in vitamin D availability, and the various forms of treatment.[31, 223, 270, 296, 356]

Histologic evidence of secondary hyperparathyroidism invariably is present[384] and usually is the dominant finding.[228] The extent of bone resorption depends on the duration and degree of parathyroid hormone elevation.[228]

Osteomalacia or rickets, or both, is present in variable degrees and in several patterns. An increase in the number of osteoid borders or seams surrounding trabecular bone frequently is present but may result from either parathyroid hormone excess or vitamin D deficiency. An increase in the thickness of the seams, in addition to an increase in number, indicates vitamin D deficiency. In addition, focal accumulations of osteoid are found often. Osteomalacia is a comparatively infrequent finding.[73] Kanis and associates, in a study of patients with end-stage renal disease, identified osteomalacia in 16 per cent of iliac crest biopsies.[194] Bordier and coworkers[33] found no evidence of osteomalacia in eight of nine patients who underwent serial biopsies after bilateral nephrectomy and maintenance hemodialysis. All of these patients demonstrated osteitis fibrosa cystica, however. An iatrogenic increase in the frequency of osteomalacia or rickets may result from treatment regimens that decrease serum phosphate levels to subnormal values.[32] These complications of treatment include excessive ingestion of oral phosphate binders,[310] dialysis problems,[26, 286] and sequelae of renal transplantation.[247]

Radiographic abnormalities in chronic renal disease are found in both the bones and the soft tissues. Bone changes reflect the abnormal histologic pattern and display secondary hyperparathyroidism (Fig. 53–16), rickets or osteomalacia (or both), and osteosclerosis (Fig. 53–17).[18, 273] A combination of these abnormalities frequently is present.[367]

Rickets may be the presenting feature and the first indication of chronic renal disease in children.[282] Although rickets usually is the predominant feature, osteitis fibrosa cystica also may be conspicuous. General retardation of growth is noted as the disease progresses.

In adults, the earliest radiographic changes usually are found in the hands. Subperiosteal resorption of bone on the radial aspects of the middle phalanges of the index and long fingers is identified radiographically by an unsharp, "lacy" outline of the cortex. A similar lack of definition may be seen in the cortex of the distal phalangeal tufts. Various radiologic techniques, using microfocal spot tubes, fine detail film, and direct magnification, aid considerably in the early identification of these abnormalities. With more advanced disease, other bones show evidence of subperiosteal resorption in concave areas ("cutback zones"), such as the medial margins of the femoral necks and inner aspects of the proximal tibiae. Widening of various joints, such as the acromioclavicular and sacroiliac joints and symphysis

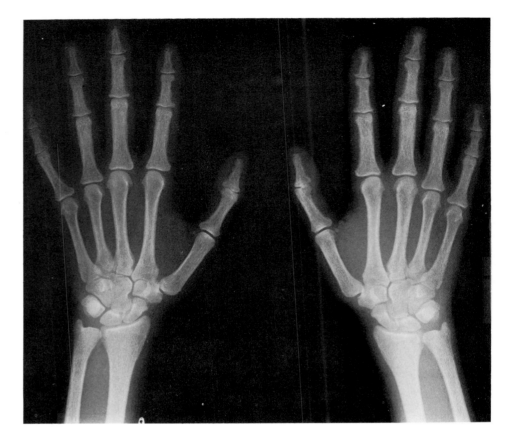

FIGURE 53–16. Long-standing renal failure in a 20 year old woman. Note resorption of the distal phalangeal tufts and the characteristic subperiosteal resorption identified on the radial aspects of the proximal and middle phalanges of the index and long fingers bilaterally. A generalized deossified pattern of osteitis fibrosa cystica is present. (From Pitt MJ, et al: Crit Rev Radiol Sci *10*:151, 1977.)

pubis, may occur secondary to subchondral resorption of bone and replacement fibrosis.[314] Brown tumors, previously thought to be unusual in uremic osteopathy, are being seen and reported with increasing frequency.

Areas of increased density (osteosclerosis) are seen frequently in uremic osteopathy[18] and histologically represent accumulations of excessive osteoid; these accumulations, although deficiently mineralized per unit area, appear to be of increased density because of increased volume. These areas are characteristic in the spine, subjacent to the cartilaginous plates, and account for the characteristic rugger-jersey appearance (Fig. 53–17). Areas of increased sclerosis also are noted in the pelvis and metaphyses of long bones. Subperiosteal new bone in the pelvis and paralleling the shafts of long bones (i.e., periosteal neostosis) likewise has been reported.[241, 258, 318]

After renal transplantation, further osteopenia resulting from steroid therapy and continued secondary hyperparathyroidism[178, 189] (sometimes resulting in tertiary hyperparathyroidism) may appear, in addition to steroid-related ischemic necrosis of the femoral heads.[268]

Soft tissue calcifications in uremia may be visceral or nonvisceral.[160, 271, 273] Visceral calcifications occur in the heart, lungs, skeletal muscle, stomach, and kidneys.[80] With the exception of the kidneys and lungs, these changes rarely are detected radiographically. Nonvisceral calcification occurs in the eyes, skin, periarticular areas, and arteries.[80, 271] The calcium deposition in visceral areas is amorphous; nonvisceral calcified areas demonstrate a hydroxyapatite composition almost identical to that of uremic bone.[80] Vascular

calcification is of the Mönckeberg type and probably is a reflection of hyperphosphatemia.[271, 273, 376] Accumulations of amorphous calcium in periarticular regions also are a reflection of increased serum phosphate levels. These deposits can become quite large; they may be single or multiple and appear multiloculated, containing a high calcium content (Fig. 53–18).[271] These masses may be painful, and often they drain spontaneously through the skin. Some of these patients have been shown to have elevated levels of $1,25(OH)_2D$, probably the result of extrarenal production.[565] Periarticular calcification in the capsule and tendons of both large and small joints is not uncommon.[341] Chondrocalcinosis, a feature of primary hyperparathyroidism, is less common in advanced renal failure.[271] Nephrocalcinosis does occur.[271]

In the past, progression of bone and soft tissue abnormalities was noted during maintenance hemodialysis.[179, 273] Progression of uremic osteopathy may be halted or reversed by beginning dialysis earlier in the course of renal failure[189] and by using shorter and more frequent dialysis treatments,[31] with more careful control of serum phosphate and calcium levels.[189] A decrease in vascular calcification has been noted after treatment with intestinal phosphate binders (aluminum hydroxide) and vitamin D.[376]

Treatment of uremic patients with $1,25(OH)_2D_3$ has shown encouraging results in both short-term[41, 43, 45] and long-term[159, 189, 343] treatment programs. Improvements in calcium absorption from the gut, reversal of negative calcium balance, and a return to normal levels of parathyroid hormone have been recorded.[45] Bone biopsies have shown

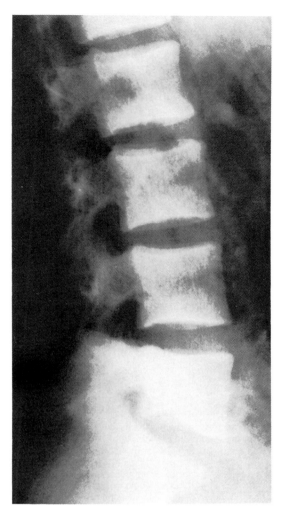

FIGURE 53–17. Areas of increased sclerosis subjacent to the cartilaginous plates (rugger-jersey spine) are demonstrated in a patient with chronic renal failure.

improvement, particularly in the changes of secondary hyperparathyroidism[45] and, to a lesser extent, in the osteomalacic abnormalities.

Although our knowledge of uremic bone disease has been expanded considerably, many questions remain unanswered.[319] The influence of uremic toxins, acidosis, and other factors accompanying the uremic state must be considered.[115] Of considerable interest are the studies by Russell and coworkers,[324, 326] who have shown defects in maturation of both the collagen and the mineral components of bone during experimental renal insufficiency.

Aluminum Toxicity

Aluminum, a "trace substance," is excreted primarily by the kidneys. Patients with chronic renal disease may develop aluminum toxicity, resulting in a low-turnover osteomalacia, termed dialysis osteomalacia[487] or aluminum osteomalacia. Rickets may develop in children.[501–504] This problem is important to recognize as it has been associated with significant morbidity and even death.[484]

Aluminum toxicity in uremia was first described as a complication of excess amounts of aluminum in the dialy-

sate,[486] due to either excess aluminum in the local water supply or aluminum sulfate added to the dialysate as a flocculating agent to remove particulate matter, or both factors.[487] The subsequent control of high aluminum concentration in dialysate water[487] has markedly reduced the prevalence of the disorder. Aluminum from oral phosphate binders[492] such as aluminum hydroxide, which lower serum phosphate levels by binding with phosphate in the intestine, now is implicated as the main source.[485, 493, 497] Aluminum "contamination" of parenteral fluids may contribute to rachitic and osteomalacic bone disease, particularly in premature infants receiving long-term parenteral nutrition and in patients receiving plasmapheresis therapy with albumin.[506]

Although the exact mechanism for the production of bone disease is unknown,[490] aluminum accumulation at the bone-osteoid junction (calcification front) appears to inhibit mineralization.[487, 502] Although biopsy specimens usually show marked increases in osteoid,[484, 487] some patients may show normal or reduced amounts of osteoid, referred to as "aplastic bone disease."[489] Because skeletal uptake of calcium is blocked, patients reveal a tendency to hypercalcemia and relative *hypo*parathyroidism.[487] Early symptoms and signs of aluminum toxicity include bone pain, muscle weakness, dementia, microcytic anemia, and hypercal-

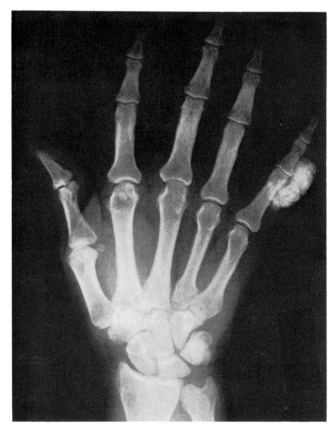

FIGURE 53–18. Tumoral calcinosis adjacent to the proximal interphalangeal joint of the little finger in a patient with chronic renal failure. Note the septated appearance of the calcium deposits. This patient had received large doses of vitamin D. Secondary hyperparathyroidism is reflected by the unsharpness of the phalangeal tufts and subperiosteal bone resorption on the radial aspects of the middle phalanges of the index and long fingers.

cemia.[484] Advanced complications may include pathologic fractures, seizures, encephalopathy, and death.[484, 485] Definitive diagnosis requires bone biopsy.[488] In addition to control of exogenous aluminum, treatment with deferoxamine (DFO), a potent chelating agent, may be useful, although results are not consistent and there are potential serious side effects.[491, 498]

Radiographs may be helpful in predicting aluminum toxicity without resorting to biopsy. Kriegshauser and associates found that aluminum toxicity was associated with (1) an increased frequency of fractures, (2) a *lack* of osteosclerosis, (3) a relative *decrease* in subperiosteal resorption (hyperparathyroidism) compared to patients without aluminum toxicity, and (4) a significant increase in osteonecrosis after transplantation.[484] They point out that fractures of the second, third, or fourth ribs, which almost always are pathologic, were seen almost exclusively in their patients with aluminum toxicity.[484]

Although the ribs, vertebral bodies, hips, and pelvis are the most common sites of fracture in uremia, Sundaram and colleagues[485] have described atypical fractures occurring in the long bones and dens in aluminum toxicity. These fractures were associated with vague, subacute symptoms, were nontraumatic and isolated, and showed no evidence of healing.[485] The authors suggest that this type of fracture presentation occurring in a uremic patient receiving dialysis should alert the physician to the possibility of aluminum-induced osteomalacia.[485]

Aluminum-associated bone disease also has been reported in azotemic, nondialyzed infants and children as a consequence of use of aluminum-containing phosphate binders.[501–505] Radiographs show osteopenia, rachitic changes at the physeal zones, and pathologic fractures. Findings of hyperparathyroidism, such as subperiosteal resorption, notably are *absent,* a feature suggestive of aluminum intoxication in a child with renal insufficiency.[502] Healing of the rachitic lesions after discontinuation of aluminum intake was distinctly unusual.[502] Calcification first appeared at the most recently formed osteoid, leaving a radiolucent area between newly calcified and previously calcified bone.[502] Calcification of epiphyseal secondary centers also began peripherally, resulting in a "bone in bone" appearance.[502]

Hereditary Vitamin D–Dependent Rickets

Hereditary vitamin D–dependent rickets, also termed pseudovitamin D–deficiency rickets, is a rare, autosomal recessive[507] disorder characterized by the clinical, radiographic, and biochemical features of vitamin D deficiency.[122, 335, 336, 410, 421] Vitamin D intake is normal, however, and no evidence exists of other disease states, such as intestinal malabsorption and liver or kidney disorders, that would account for derangement in vitamin D metabolism. Symptoms may be present as early as 3 months of age (in contrast to the later onset of nutritional rickets), with most patients being symptomatic by 1 year of age.[121] Rachitic bone changes may be severe and rapidly progressive, with pathologic fractures (Fig. 53–19). Although hypophosphatemia is present, the primary rachitogenic factor is hypocalcemia, which results from a decrease in intestinal calcium absorption, often apparent soon after birth; secondary hyperparathyroidism follows.[122] The effect of elevated para-

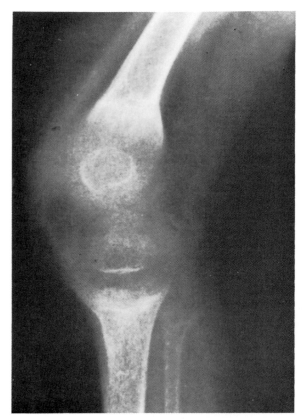

FIGURE 53–19. Vitamin D–dependent rickets. Typical rachitic changes are present at the growth plates with widening, demineralization, and disorganization of the metaphyseal bone. Observe the latitudinal widening (cupping) of the distal femoral and proximal tibial metaphyseal regions. The proximal tibial epiphysis has an unsharp bony margin. (Courtesy of Drs. Jequier and Nogrady, Montreal, Quebec, Canada.)

thyroid hormone levels on the kidney is responsible for the hyperphosphaturia, aminoaciduria, and hypophosphatemia.

Two types of hereditary vitamin D–dependent rickets have been recognized.[48, 410, 413, 414, 418, 419, 421] The type I disorder results from a deficiency in the production or response of the renal enzyme 1α-hydroxylase, which converts 25-OH-D to $1,25(OH)_2D$.[516] Serum levels of vitamin D and $25(OH)_2D$ are normal but serum levels of $1,25(OH)_2D$ are *low.* Affected patients show clinical improvement with large doses of vitamin D or 25-OH-D[120]; however, minute physiologic doses of $1,25(OH)_2D$ or 1α-OH-D promptly initiate healing, which supports the probability that the defect resides in deficient conversion of $25(OH)_2D$ to $1,25(OH)_2D$ by the kidney.[311] Uncommonly, presentation may occur in late infancy[418] or later in childhood,[416] suggesting heterogeneity in this disorder. In the type II disorder, levels of vitamin D and $25-OH_2-D$ are normal. Serum levels of $1,25(OH)_2D$ are moderately to extremely *elevated,*[508] however, indicating a problem with end-organ responsiveness to $1,25(OH)_2D$.[508] The type II disease, also called hereditary $1,25(OH)_2D$ resistant rickets,[420, 506] shows biochemical and clinical heterogeneity.[411, 417, 421] Common features include an elevation of parathyroid hormone and high levels of $1,25(OH)_2D$ during treatment. There is a variable clinical response to prolonged treatment with high doses of calciferol analogues.[411, 511, 514, 520] The rickets often is severe, and affected children may die of respiratory infection or generalized debility.[510, 521] Alopecia of early onset is present in approximately one half of the reported kindreds[417, 421] and does not improve with therapy.[514, 519] A delay may occur in the manifestation of full symptoms and signs[417] and in the dose of calciferol required for therapy.[417] Receptors for 1,25(OH)$_2$D have been found not only in the classic target organs of vitamin D (i.e., intestine, bone, and kidney) but also in calcium-transport organs (breast, placenta), endocrine glands (parathyroid, pituitary), ovary, skin, brain, and hematopoietic marrow myeloid progenitor cells.[509] Defective 1,25(OH)$_2$D receptors in cultured skin and bone fibroblasts, lymphocyte cell lines,[515] and the failure of 1,25(OH)$_2$D to induce the differentiation of marrow myeloid progenitor cells in vitro[509] in the type II disorder indicate that the condition results from a cellular defect at target organ sites.[411, 412, 415, 420, 506, 511–515, 517, 522, 523] Weisman and coworkers have made the prenatal diagnosis of the type II disorder by demonstrating the inability of 1,25(OH)$_2$D binding to amniotic fluid cells.[518] Of interest is the study by Scriver and associates,[338] who measured low levels of 1,25(OH)$_2$D in patients with hereditary vitamin D–dependent rickets who had been receiving sufficient amounts of vitamin D therapy to support normal serum levels of calcium and phosphorus and prevent rickets. The authors suggest that the low levels of 1,25(OH)$_2$D may meet the physiologic requirements of these patients.

Osteoporosis

Because vitamin D is a major determinant of intestinal calcium absorption and bone mineralization, attention has been directed to possible aberrations of vitamin D in senile osteoporosis. Available data are conflicting.[398, 469] Some studies have reported subnormal circulating 1,25(OH)$_2$D levels in osteoporotic persons.[466, 467] Presumably, suboptimal levels of circulating 1,25(OH)$_2$D could result in decreased intestinal calcium absorption, a finding noted in many but not all persons in the older age groups.[469] This would create a homeostatic need to maintain serum calcium levels at the expense of bone. However, the finding of low 1,25(OH)$_2$D levels in the serum in osteoporosis is not constant; normal levels of serum 1,25(OH)$_2$D in osteoporotic patients also have been recorded.[468, 469] Therefore, simple depressions of serum 1,25(OH)$_2$D levels alone do not seem to account for clinically significant osteoporosis.[469] It is likely that 1,25(OH)$_2$D interactions with estrogen, parathyroid hormone, and other, yet undefined factors all are contributory to senile osteoporosis.

Rickets and Osteomalacia Secondary to Phosphate Loss

A number of rachitic and osteomalacic syndromes have been identified, which, although differing in genetic and clinical features, share one or several renal tubular abnormalities. These disorders first were appreciated in the late 1920s[29] but were described in detail in the 1930s, notably by Albright and associates, DeToni, and Fanconi. "Rickets resistant to vitamin D therapy" was reported by Albright and associates in 1937.[7] Their patient most likely had X-linked hypophosphatemia.[122] The term vitamin D "resis-

tance" has persisted, although the designation of "refractory," in the sense of difficult to manage, might be more appropriate.[122, 272] DeToni in 1933 and Fanconi in 1936 described patients with multiple renal tubular dysfunctions, including urinary loss of various amino acids.[95] Multiple additional complex syndromes have been described subsequently, which share common renal tubular dysfunctions: renal phosphate loss with secondary hypophosphatemia, glycosuria, aminoaciduria, renal tubular acidosis, hypokalemia, and vasopressin-resistant polyuria. In recognition of Fanconi's studies, these diseases are collectively designated Fanconi syndromes. The most common is cystinosis[332, 457, 458]; tyrosinemia and the oculocerebrorenal syndrome (Lowe's syndrome)[2] are other, less common examples. Dent's historical review traces the medical recognition of these disorders.[95]

In addition to congenital diseases, acquired renal tubular disorders with similar clinical and biochemical features may be secondary to drug toxicity,[552] heavy metal poisoning, paraproteinemias, and tumors.

Dent[95] and later Mankin[231] have suggested a practical classification of the renal tubular disorders based on the site of involvement: the proximal renal tubule, the distal renal tubule, and combinations of proximal and distal tubular sites. Inorganic phosphate, glucose, and amino acids are absorbed in the proximal tubule; acidification of urine in exchange for a fixed base and concentration of urine occur in the distal tubule. A spectrum of dysfunction would include progressive proximal tubular abnormalities followed by combined proximal and distal tubular defects: loss of phosphate, as in X-linked hypophosphatemia; loss of inorganic phosphate and glucose; loss of phosphate, glucose, and amino acids; and combinations of above, with additional defects in urine acidification and concentration.

X-Linked Hypophosphatemia. X-linked hypophosphatemia (also known as familial vitamin D–resistant rickets) is the most common form of renal tubular rickets and osteomalacia.[231, 544] The classic syndrome is transmitted genetically as an X-linked dominant trait.[549, 550] As expected with X-linked transmission, men are affected to a greater degree than women.

Approximately one third of cases result from spontaneous mutation or the mothers show no evidence of disease.[536] The syndrome is characterized by lifelong hypophosphatemia that is secondary to renal tubular phosphate loss, decreased intestinal absorption of calcium, and normal serum levels of calcium. Early diagnosis is important as treatment can prevent many of the deformities.[535, 546] Rickets generally appears between 12 and 18 months of age.[121] Remission usually follows growth plate closure but recurrence of symptoms is common later in life.[272, 453] Patients typically are short, bowlegged, and stocky.[382, 532, 546] Short stature is primarily a result of decrease in growth of the legs[541, 543]; the trunk usually is normal.[541, 543] Systemic signs such as muscle weakness and hypotonia, which may accompany nutritional rickets, are absent. The development and severity of rickets may differ among patients with the classic syndrome. The degree of hypophosphatemia does not correlate with the severity of the skeletal abnormalities.[544] In addition, radiographs of affected patients may be normal. Reliance on radiographic abnormalities for the diagnosis will cause some patients with the disorder to be overlooked.[535] Variations of X-linked hypophosphatemia

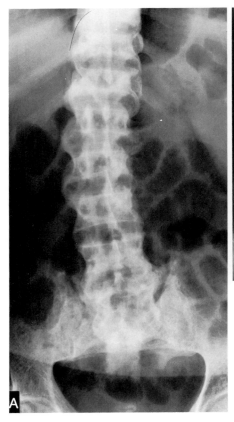

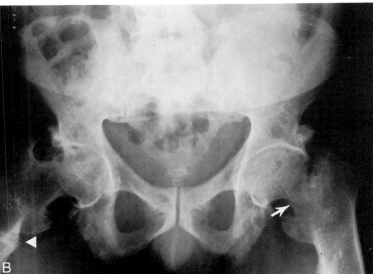

FIGURE 53–20. X-linked hypophosphatemia in an adult man.
A Multifocal areas of paravertebral ossification are similar to those in diffuse idiopathic skeletal hyperostosis or ankylosing spondylitis. Abnormalities of both sacroiliac joints result from ossification of the anterior sacroiliac ligaments.
B In the same patient, enthesopathic new bone is seen bilaterally at the supra-acetabular attachments of the rectus femoris muscles and at the adductor muscle attachments to the ischia. A Looser's zone is present in the right proximal femur (arrowhead). The patient had an intracapsular fracture of the left hip (arrow).

are reported,[547, 548, 551] particularly a late, adult-onset presentation without evidence of childhood rickets.[453, 454]

Radiographic features may allow for the specific diagnosis of this syndrome. In children, rachitic changes at the growth plates, in themselves nonspecific, may be only mild or moderate in degree. Osteopenia is not prominent. Bowing of long bones, particularly of the lower extremities,[537] may occur, but deformity frequently is minimal, and the condition may be overlooked.[280] With increasing age, the trabecular pattern becomes coarsened. Looser's zones are more prevalent[533] and can be complicated by complete fractures.[424] By adulthood, a generalized increase in bone density, especially in the axial skeleton, is characteristic.[280, 357, 422, 533] Enthesopathic calcification and ossification develop in the paravertebral ligaments, anulus fibrosus, and capsules of apophyseal and appendicular joints[533, 534] (Figs. 53–20 and 53–21). This ossification, paradoxic in a disease in which the basic problem is faulty mineralization of bone, increases with age but is not related to sex.[422] The spinal changes may resemble those of ankylosing spondylitis[280] or diffuse idiopathic skeletal hyperostosis.[422] In contrast to ankylosing spondylitis, however, the sacroiliac joints in X-linked hypophosphatemia show no bone erosions.

Narrowing of the spinal canal is common[423] and can lead to cord compression requiring surgical intervention.[538] Facet joint hypertrophy and laminar thickening are found in most patients. However, the most important cause of narrowing is ossification of the ligamentum flavum; this is most pronounced in the lower thoracic region.[538]

In the pelvis, multiple sites of calcification may involve the acetabulum, iliolumbar ligaments, and the sacroiliac ligaments, calcification of the last partially obscuring the sacroiliac joints (Fig. 53–20B). The appendicular skeleton shows multiple sites of new bone formation at various muscle and ligament attachments.[534] Osteoarthritis is common, particularly in the ankles, knees, feet, wrists, and sacroiliac joints.[533, 534] Separate small ossicles may develop around various joints, particularly those in the carpus[272, 280] (Fig. 53–21). The radiographic findings in the axial and appendicular skeleton are distinctive and may suggest the diagnosis prior to the clinical recognition of the disorder.

X-linked hypophosphatemia and the various Fanconi syndromes produce rickets and osteomalacia principally by renal tubular phosphate loss[336, 421]; relative deficiency of $1,25(OH)_2D$ also is a factor. The pathophysiologic mechanisms underlying the tubular loss of phosphate have been studied best in X-linked hypophosphatemia. Albright believed that the disorder was due primarily to decreased intestinal absorption of calcium. In this model, phosphaturia would be a result of secondary hyperparathyroidism evoked by the low serum calcium level. However, parathyroid hormone levels are normal,[12, 325, 361] and radiographic changes of secondary hyperparathyroidism are not present.[325] The most likely explanation for the phosphaturia has been provided by Glorieux and Scriver.[131] Their study of X-linked hypophosphatemia suggests two separate renal tubular mechanisms for phosphate resorption: a parathyroid hormone-sensitive component, which is responsible for about two thirds of the total net resorption, and an additional system, which is responsive to the serum calcium level. The parathyroid hormone-sensitive component is completely absent in male patients with X-linked hypophosphatemia and

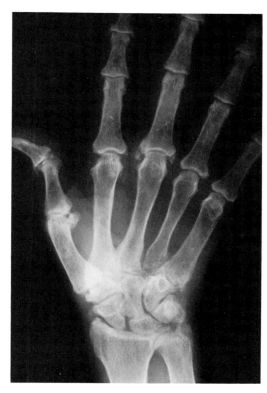

FIGURE 53–21. X-linked hypophosphatemia. Same patient as in Figure 53–20. Small ossicles are noted at the radial aspect of the wrist, and ossification of the triangular fibrocartilage complex is present. Capsular ossification is noted at multiple interphalangeal and metacarpophalangeal joints.

is partially absent in female patients. A similar defect in intestinal mucosal transport of inorganic phosphate in X-linked hypophosphatemic rickets also has been demonstrated.[345] Similarly, several studies by Popovtzer and associates indicate that renal tubular phosphate absorption results from two separate mechanisms, one of which is parathyroid hormone-dependent.[293–295]

Abnormalities in vitamin D metabolism have been demonstrated in both X-linked hypophosphatemia[153, 338] and the Fanconi syndromes.[38, 39, 553] In X-linked hypophosphatemia, serum $1,25(OH)_2D$ levels usually are normal or slightly below normal.[153, 425–428, 455] Expected levels of $1,25(OH)_2D$, however, should be higher for the degree of hypophosphatemia that is present, suggesting an inadequate response or regulation of the renal 1α-hydroxylase system with respect to its usual stimuli.[39, 153, 305] This postulation is supported by the observation that patients with X-linked hypophosphatemia who develop secondary hyperparathyroidism subsequent to oral phosphate therapy showed no concomitant increase in $1,25(OH)_2D$ formation.[305] In addition, both human[455] and Hyp mice[456] (the X-linked hypophosphatemic [Hyp] mouse serves as a model for the human genetic disease X-linked hypophosphatemia) fail to show increases in $1,25(OH)_2D$ with low phosphate diets. The relative importance of the $1,25(OH)_2D$ abnormality (or abnormalities) is uncertain but it may contribute to the pathogenesis of the bone disease.[103, 425]

Current therapy of X-linked hypophosphatemia combines oral phosphate supplementation with vitamin D,[428–432, 544, 545] resulting in improvement in growth,[540] limiting deformi-

ties,[429] and correcting both growth plate[539] and endosteal mineral defects.[428, 430–432] Nephrocalcinosis[540] (but not nephrolithiasis) may be a complication of this treatment, and renal failure has been reported.[541] Some have questioned whether any medical treatment has an effect on the clinical outcome.[541, 542] Scriver and associates have reported low serum levels of $1,25(OH)_2D$ in X-linked hypophosphatemia.[338] Patients studied were children who were receiving vitamin D therapy; these factors may explain the discrepancy with the normal levels measured by Haussler and colleagues.[153] It should be noted that inadequate therapeutic responses to both $1,25(OH)_2D$[42, 130, 325] and 1α-OH-D[305] have been observed in X-linked hypophosphatemia.

Brewer and coworkers[39] have found evidence for abnormal vitamin D metabolism in the Fanconi syndromes. Experimentally, a decrease in 25-OH-D-1α hydroxylase activity was noted after the induction of proximal tubular dysfunction (Fanconi syndrome) by maleic acid administration.[39] Clinically, they found significant depression of $1,25(OH)_2D$ formation in patients with Fanconi syndromes.[38]

Tumor-Associated Rickets and Osteomalacia

Hypophosphatemic vitamin D-refractory rickets and osteomalacia in association with various neoplasms have been recognized with increasing frequency since Prader and coworkers'[297] first description in 1959. In 1976, Linovitz and associates[214] reviewed 11 cases and added two new patients. Since then, additional reports have appeared.[15, 100, 313, 393, 407–409, 564]

The associated neoplasms have occurred in children and adults, are located in soft tissues or bone, and vary in size. The lesions typically are vascular and often show foci of new bone formation; the most frequent histologic diagnosis has been hemangiopericytoma. Although most of the neoplasms have been of mesenchymal origin, the syndrome has been reported in association with prostatic carcinoma[452] and with oat cell carcinoma of the lung.[408] Bone lesions have included nonossifying fibroma,[291] giant cell tumor,[100, 101] osteoblastoma,[393] and non-neoplastic diseases such as fibrous dysplasia[96] and neurofibromatosis.[563] Although the tumors usually are benign histologically, some may be malignant.[214] Patients frequently have generalized muscle weakness and proximal myopathy. Radiographic changes of rickets and osteomalacia may be advanced. Hypophosphatemia is the predominant biochemical feature and is secondary to failure of renal tubular reabsorption of phosphate. Serum calcium level is within normal limits. Serum alkaline phosphatase concentration usually is elevated. Parathyroid hormone levels generally are within normal limits, and a normal parathyroid response has been elicited in some patients with calcium infusions.

The cause of the decreased renal tubular absorption of phosphate remains unidentified. Circumstantial evidence suggests the presence of a tumor-elaborated humoral substance that affects renal phosphate absorption in the proximal tubule directly.[147] Injection of extract from a rickets-associated fibroangioma resulted in excessive phosphaturia in a puppy.[15] Altered vitamin D metabolism with selective decreases in $1,25(OH)_2D$ has been demonstrated.[100, 101, 407, 408, 452] Drezner and Feinglos reported on a patient with osteomalacia associated with a giant cell tumor of bone.[100, 101]

Measurement of serum 25-OH-D was within normal range, but 1,25(OH)$_2$D levels were depressed. Administration of 1,25(OH)$_2$D corrected the biochemical abnormalities and improved bone mineralization. After removal of the tumor, 1,25(OH)$_2$D therapy could be eliminated. Sweet and collaborators reported similar vitamin D abnormalities in a patient with a hemangiopericytoma of the nasal turbinates.[407]

Certainly, additional information is necessary before the pathogenesis of tumor-associated rickets and osteomalacia can be explained. Hypophosphatemia undoubtedly is the major contributor to the bone disease. The findings of low 1,25(OH)$_2$D levels might be considered in the context of the abnormal values of 1,25(OH)$_2$D also found in X-linked hypophosphatemia and the Fanconi syndromes (see previous discussion). The presence of normal serum calcium concentration and normal parathyroid hormone levels[147] and the absence of osteitis fibrosa cystica in the majority of patients would be a vote against a major role for 1,25(OH)$_2$D deficiency in the development of bone disease.

Fanconi syndromes with hypophosphatemic rickets and osteomalacia have been recognized as a complication of high dose ifosfamide, a chemotherapeutic agent used in the treatment of solid tumors, particularly in children.[554-562] This complication, which is seen in both children and adults, is a result of nephrotoxic metabolites of the drug and may be irreversible.[559] Renal toxicity is predominantly tubular, although glomerular abnormalities also may occur.[557] Hyperphosphaturia with resulting hypophosphatemia is the major cause of the rickets and osteomalacia. However, any part of the nephron may be damaged by ifosfamide and different combinations of clinical features may be present.[558] Urinary abnormalities also may include an excess loss of amino acids,[556] glycosuria,[558] and renal tubular acidosis.[556]

It is important for the radiologist to be aware of the association between various neoplasms and the development of rickets and osteomalacia. A careful search for these lesions should be made in patients with hypophosphatemic vitamin D–refractory states for which the more common causes have not been identified. In addition, any patient with a primary tumor who is being treated with ifosfamide may develop rickets and osteomalacia as a complication of drug nephrotoxicity rather than tumor elaboration of a humoral product.

Atypical Axial Osteomalacia

Atypical axial osteomalacia is a rare condition first described by Frame and associates in 1961.[118] Radiographic changes are characteristic[79, 118, 256]: skeletal involvement is axial, with sparing of appendicular sites (Figs. 53–22 and 53–23). A dense, coarse trabecular pattern involves primarily the cervical spine but also is present in the lumbar spine, pelvis, and ribs. Looser's zones have not been identified.[79, 118]

All reported patients have been men. Their general health is good, symptoms are minimal, and the biochemical findings are within normal limits. Biopsy of the involved areas demonstrates typical osteomalacia. Patients do not respond to vitamin D therapy.

Nelson and coworkers[256] reported four additional patients, two of whom had features of ankylosing spondylitis.

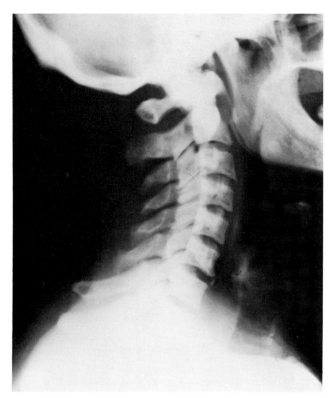

FIGURE 53–22. Atypical axial osteomalacia: A dense, coarse trabecular pattern involves the cervical spine. The appendicular skeleton was normal. (Courtesy of D. Resnick, M.D., San Diego, California.)

The relationship between these two syndromes is uncertain at present.

Hypophosphatasia

Hypophosphatasia is a rare disorder, transmitted genetically in an autosomal recessive pattern[309] and characterized by defective skeletal mineralization resembling that of rickets and osteomalacia, low serum alkaline phosphatase levels (only bone and liver isoenzymes),[254] and abnormal amounts of phosphoethanolamine in the urine and blood.[86] First described by Rathbun in 1948, it has been recorded in many parts of the world and involves both sexes.[86]

A wide spectrum of clinical severity is noted. Although most patients are diagnosed during infancy or childhood, in some patients the condition may not be recognized until adult life.[9, 24, 187] The most severely affected neonates usually die soon after birth. Generalized deficient or absent mineralization is noted radiologically. Fractures with deformity and shortening of the extremities may suggest a dwarfing syndrome. Hypercalcemia may be present in addition to the decreased serum alkaline phosphatase level and phosphoethanolamine levels in urine and blood. Multiple factors probably contribute to death, including a lack of bony support for the intracranial and thoracic structures.[254]

Patients surviving infancy display varying degrees of skeletal involvement. Radiographic changes at the growth plates may be identified soon after birth. These abnormalities are similar to those of rickets but characteristically

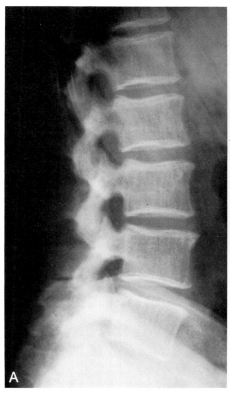

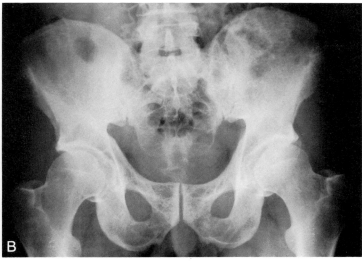

FIGURE 53–23. Atypical axial osteomalacia.

A The spine is osteopenic. The remaining vertically oriented trabeculations of the vertebral bodies show a coarse pattern. The appendicular skeleton was normal.

B In the same patient, a radiograph of the pelvis shows a coarsened trabecular pattern, particularly in the pubic bones. The proximal femora appear within normal limits.

demonstrate irregular, often prominent, lucent extensions into the metaphysis representing uncalcified bone matrix (Fig. 53–24). Generalized deossification with a coarse trabecular pattern, bowing deformities with or without healing fractures, and subperiosteal new bone accumulation may be present. Craniosynostosis involving all sutures is common,[86] and wormian (intersutural) bones may be identified. Spontaneous healing usually occurs[86]; there is no effective form of treatment.

Children with milder cases may demonstrate only delay in walking or early loss of deciduous teeth.

Uncommonly, the disease may be manifested first in adulthood, with fractures occurring after minor trauma.[9, 24, 187] Fracture healing is delayed, with only minimal peripheral callus developing.[9] Radiography in adults suggests osteomalacia with a coarse trabecular pattern, bowing deformities compatible with previous rickets, Looser's zones, and subperiosteal bone formation. A small skull may be present as a result of craniosynostosis. Calcification of ligamentous and tendinous attachments to bone and in paravertebral areas has been described. The findings of low serum alkaline phosphatase levels and phosphoethanolamine levels in blood and urine confirm the diagnosis; however, a few patients with this syndrome have been reported in whom no associated phosphoethanolamine accumulations were found.[9] The condition of a patient reported by Scriver and colleagues closely resembled hypophosphatasia, except that the alkaline phosphatase level was within normal range.[337] This syndrome was designated pseudohypophosphatasia.

Metaphyseal Chondrodysplasia (Type Schmid)

Metaphyseal chondrodysplasias encompass a variety of disorders that have in common generalized symmetric disturbance of endochondral bone formation, primarily at the metaphyses. The type described by Schmid is the most common and has radiologic features very similar to those of X-linked hypophosphatemic rickets (vitamin D-resistant rickets).[97, 360] Normal levels of serum phosphorus, alkaline phosphatase, and calcium differentiate these disorders from other rachitic syndromes.

The disease becomes manifested in childhood with short stature, bowing of long bones, and an accentuated lumbar lordosis with a waddling gait. General health is excellent, and the course is benign. The disease is transmitted in an autosomal dominant pattern, but spontaneous mutations occur.[97]

In the child, radiographs reveal widening of the growth plates, which, similarly to rickets, show most severe involvement in the more rapidly growing areas.[97] In contrast to usual rickets, the metaphysis is well mineralized and actually may show increased density. Fine, spurlike projections of organized bone may extend into the growth plate from the metaphysis.[97, 360] The long bones are bowed but show excellent mineralization. Growth recovery lines are infrequent.[97] The absence of Looser's zones or signs of secondary hyperparathyroidism is notable. The skull is normal. The lesions tend to heal spontaneously, particularly after periods of bedrest.[97] The patients do not improve with

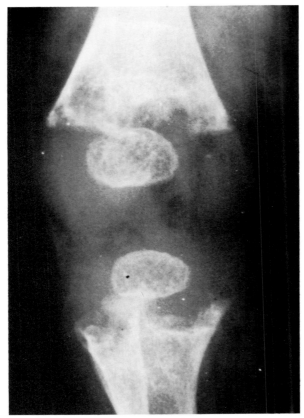

FIGURE 53–24. Hypophosphatasia. Deossification is present adjacent to the growth plates. Characteristic radiolucent areas extend from the growth plates into the metaphysis.

vitamin D therapy and in this sense are "resistant." In fact, confusion of this disorder with rachitic syndromes has resulted in vitamin D intoxication.[97]

Parathyroid Gland Abnormalities

The important role of parathyroid hormone as a major stimulus to $1,25(OH)_2D$ production has been considered in depth in earlier sections of this chapter (see Fig. 53–3). It might be anticipated that the clinical syndromes of hyperparathyroidism, hypoparathyroidism, and pseudohypoparathyroidism would be associated with abnormalities of vitamin D metabolism. This indeed is the case. Decreased levels of $1,25(OH)_2D$ are found in patients with hypoparathyroidism and pseudohypoparathyroidism (type I).[104, 153] Evidence suggests that conversion of 25-OH-D to $1,25(OH)_2D$ is impaired. Serum levels of 25-OH-D are normal. Low doses of $1,25(OH)_2D$ are effective in increasing intestinal calcium absorption and correcting hypocalcemia in patients with hypoparathyroidism[200] and pseudohypoparathyroidism.[200, 389] In contrast, pharmacologic doses of vitamin D and 25-OH-D are required to obtain similar responses.[200] These findings help to explain the refractory nature of hypoparathyroidism to large doses of vitamin D.[16] Patients with primary hyperparathyroidism demonstrate significant elevations of $1,25(OH)_2D$ levels.[153, 155]

Pseudohypoparathyroidism and Pseudopseudohypoparathyroidism. Early descriptions of these syndromes

were based on physical examination and routine laboratory data.[5, 6] The term pseudohypoparathyroidism was introduced by Albright and associates in 1942.[6] The three patients described presented a characteristic phenotype consisting of short stature, round face, short neck, and shortening of metacarpal bones, particularly the first, fifth, and fourth (Fig. 53–25). Low serum calcium and high serum phosphorus levels were consistent with hypoparathyroidism; however, administration of parathyroid hormone did not result in the normally expected increase in urinary phosphate levels. Albright and his collaborators correctly postulated an end-organ (kidney) unresponsiveness to parathyroid hormone.[6] They subsequently described patients with the characteristic phenotype of pseudohypoparathyroidism who had normal blood chemistry values and applied the term pseudopseudohypoparathyroidism to this condition.[5] The renal response to parathyroid hormone in this latter group of patients is normal.

Both pseudohypoparathyroidism (the classic syndrome is termed type I) and pseudopseudohypoparathyroidism have the same phenotype. The parathyroid glands are intrinsically normal. Parathyroid hormone levels are normal in pseudopseudohypoparathyroidism and elevated in pseudohypoparathyroidism, the latter a consequence of the ineffective hormone action at the kidney with secondary hyperphosphatemia and hypocalcemia. Patients have been reported who exhibit the phenotype described by Albright and colleagues but who have true hypoparathyroidism.[253] Parathyroid hormone levels are low, and they have a proper target-organ response to the administration of parathyroid hormone. These patients would be classified as having pseudopseudohypoparathyroidism. To clarify the distinctions between these disorders, it has been proposed[233, 253] that the condition with the phenotypic changes originally described by Albright be termed Albright's hereditary osteodystrophy (distinct from Albright's syndrome, which consists of fibrous dysplasia, precocious puberty, and café-au-lait spots). Hypoparathyroid states should be classified as either true hormone-deficient or hormone-resistant forms. Patients with Albright's hereditary osteodystrophy may exhibit target-organ (kidney and bone) unresponsiveness to parathyroid hormone (pseudohypoparathyroidism) or may exhibit a normal target-organ responsiveness (pseudopseudohypoparathyroidism with normal parathyroid hormone levels or pseudopseudohypoparathyroidism with true deficiency of parathyroid hormone). Biochemical research, beginning in the late 1960s, has uncovered specific biochemical abnormalities responsible for the syndrome and identified variations of the disorder. The genetic defect is indeed pleiotrophic.[102]

Albright's Hereditary Osteodystrophy: Pertinent Biochemistry. The actions of nonsteroidal hormones (i.e., parathyroid hormone, growth hormone, vasopressin) are mediated through cyclic adenosine monophosphate (cAMP). Initially the hormone interacts with a specific receptor site on the target cell surface membrane. Once this hormone-receptor reaction occurs, adenylate cyclase is activated, forming cAMP from ATP. The effect of the hormone then is mediated by cAMP (the "second messenger").[474, 475] In the late 1960s Chase and coworkers demonstrated that the biochemical defect in classic pseudohypoparathyroidism was an insufficient response of renal adenylate cyclase to parathyroid hormone stimulation, with

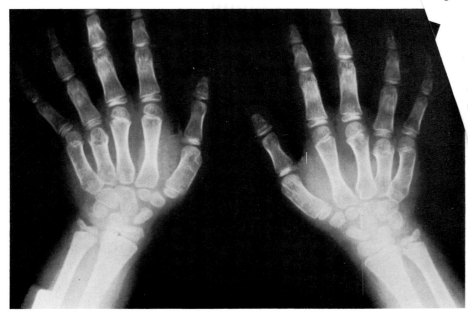

FIGURE 53–25. Pseudohypoparathyroidism (Albright's hereditary osteodystrophy) in a 9 year old boy, demonstrating shortening of all metacarpal bones, particularly the fourth.

inadequate formation of cAMP.[63] This defect also was presumed to be present in bone. This type of pseudohypoparathyroidism has been termed pseudohypoparathyroidism type I. Patients with pseudopseudohypoparathyroidism do not demonstrate the defect in cAMP production.[63]

At the renal level, cAMP is responsible for the parathyroid hormone-induced renal phosphaturic effect and (probably) also for the stimulation of the enzyme 1α-hydroxylase, which forms $1,25(OH)_2D$. Patients with pseudohypoparathyroidism demonstrate low levels of $1,25(OH)_2D$.[470] Hypocalcemia in these patients results from several factors, including the deficiency of $1,25(OH)_2D$ with subsequent decreased intestinal absorption of calcium, decreased skeletal responsiveness to parathyroid hormone (which requires an active form of vitamin D for adequate response), and hyperphosphatemia, which depresses serum calcium levels reciprocally.

Persons with pseudohypoparathyroidism also may demonstrate other hormonal dysfunctions, including deficient production of prolactin,[476] decreased thyrotropin with resultant hypothyroidism, and failure to respond to glucagon.[472, 473] The common denominator in these hormonal dysfunctions may be deficiency in a guanine nucleotide-binding protein (G unit). The G unit apparently couples the hormone-receptor reaction on the target cell surface with the adenylate cyclase system.[471] Because the G unit is common to all tissues, as opposed to hormone receptors, which are tissue-specific, a defective G unit could lead to resistance to multiple hormones that act by stimulating adenylate cyclase.[472]

Albright's Hereditary Osteodystrophy: Variant Forms. Although most patients with chemical pseudohypoparathyroidism demonstrate deficiency in both renal phosphaturic response and $1,25(OH)_2D$ production when stimulated by parathyroid hormone, a few patients maintain their ability to form $1,25(OH)_2D$. These patients demonstrate normal serum calcium levels and have what is termed normocalcemic pseudohypoparathyroidism[102] or pseudohyperparathyroidism.[478, 479] The phenotype of Albright's hereditary osteodystrophy may[479] or may not[477, 478] be present. Because parathyroid hormone levels are elevated and $1,25(OH)_2D$ is present, these patients may also show radiographic evidence of hyperparathyroidism.[481, 483] In children with this variation, the radiographic presentation suggests renal osteodystrophy.[482]

The term pseudohypoparathyroidism type II[44, 105] refers to the condition in which patients show normal parathyroid hormone activation of the renal adenylate cyclase system with production of cAMP but lack the expected phosphaturic response. These patients do not have the phenotype characteristic of Albright's hereditary osteodystrophy. Basal ganglion calcification, demonstrated by CT but not seen with routine radiography, has been reported in a patient with pseudohypoparathyroidism type II.[480]

When physiologic supplements of $1,25(OH)_2D$ or larger amounts of vitamin D are administered to patients with pseudohypoparathyroidism type I, normal bone response to parathyroid hormone and correction of hypocalcemia occur.[200, 389]

SUMMARY OF THE RADIOLOGIC APPROACH TO RICKETS AND OSTEOMALACIA (Fig. 53–26)

The general nonspecificity of the radiographic features of rickets and osteomalacia has been stressed. There are, however, specific radiographic findings that may identify or be suggestive of a particular cause. As with radiologic diagnoses in general, correlation with clinical history, physical findings, and laboratory data is essential. Of particular importance in this regard are the age at onset of disease, duration of symptoms, family history of similar problems, presence of renal or gastrointestinal disorders, and social and environmental conditions.

The following points may be useful in diagnosing specific syndromes:

Rickets / Radiographic
Osteomalacia / approach

1. Nonspecific changes
2. Renal Osteodystrophy (Uremic Osteopathy)
3. X-linked Hypophosphatemia
4. Axial Osteomalacia
5. Primary Biliary Cirrhosis
6. Hypophosphatasia
   Metaphyseal Chondrodysplasia

FIGURE 53–26. Radiographic approach to rickets and osteomalacia. See text for discussion.

1. Nonspecific radiographic changes of rickets and osteomalacia
   a. In patients less than 6 months of age: Consider biliary atresia, vitamin D-dependent rickets, hypophosphatasia, and rickets associated with prematurity.
   b. If resistance occurs to usual doses of vitamin D (in the absence of chronic glomerular renal disease): Consider a renal tubular disorder, tumor association, hypophosphatasia, or metaphyseal chondrodysplasia, type Schmid. Note: *Mild* changes of secondary hyperparathyroidism may be present.
2. Renal osteodystrophy (uremic osteopathy): Radiographic changes of secondary hyperparathyroidism usually are present and predominate over the pattern of deossification. Osteosclerotic foci, particularly in the spine adjacent to the cartilaginous endplates (rugger-jersey spine), are characteristic. Vascular calcification of the Mönckeberg type and, less commonly, large "tumoral" deposits of amorphous calcification may be identified, particularly around joints.
3. X-linked hypophosphatemia
   a. Children: Rachitic changes at the growth plates may be only mild to moderate. General osteoporosis is uncommon and the bones, although bowed, may be "strong" in appearance.
   b. Adults: Generalized increase in bone density may be present, particularly in the axial skeleton. Changes may suggest ankylosing spondylitis. Characteristic is paravertebral calcification, multiple small ossified dense areas near joints, and new bone formation at ligamentous and tendinous attachments in the extremities. Biochemical tests reveal hyperphosphaturia with low serum phosphate concentration.
4. Axial osteomalacia: Radiographic abnormalities are confined to the axial skeleton. Dense, coarse trabecular pattern is most marked in the cervical region. Lumbar spine, pelvis, and ribs also are involved. The skull is normal. This disorder affects adult men, symptoms are minimal, and biochemical values are within normal limits.
5. Primary biliary cirrhosis[262]: Mild to moderate generalized deossification. Hands show small, asymmetric, intracapsular marginal erosions involving predominantly distal interphalangeal joints but also found in proximal interphalangeal joint regions. Intramedullary defects also may be present. Symptoms are mild; the arthritis is nondeforming.
6. Hypophosphatasia: Varies in severity. Newborn infants may show advanced demineralization. Rachitic growth plates show characteristic multiple lucent extensions into the metaphyses. Wormian bones and craniosynostosis may be present.
7. Metaphyseal chondrodysplasia (type Schmid): Changes of rickets are more developed in the proximal portions of the femur. Multiple small bony projections extend from the proximal femoral metaphyses into the rachitic growth plates. Long bones maintain normal density. Skull is within normal limits. Spontaneous healing occurs.

ACKNOWLEDGMENTS: I extend my deep appreciation to Sandra Boltinghouse for her patience, care, and assistance during preparation of this chapter. Dr. Mark Haussler, Professor of Biochemistry, College of Medicine, University of Arizona, has provided considerable stimulation and advice for this chapter.

References

1. Aaron JE, Gallagher JC, Nordin BEC: Seasonal variation of histological osteomalacia in femoral-neck fractures. Lancet 2:84, 1974.
2. Abbassi V, Lowe C, Calcagno P: Oculo-cerebro-renal syndrome, a review. Am J Dis Child 115:145, 1968.
3. Aegerter E, Kirkpatrick J: Orthopedic Diseases. 4th Ed. Philadelphia, WB Saunders Co, 1975.
4. Ajdukiewicz AB, Agnew JE, Byers PD, et al: The relief of bone pain in primary biliary cirrhosis with calcium infusions. Gut 15:788, 1974.
5. Albright F, Forbes AP, Henneman PH: Pseudo-pseudohypoparathyroidism. Trans Assoc Am Physicians 65:337, 1952.
6. Albright F, Burnett CH, Smith PH, et al: Pseudohypoparathyroidism—an example of Seabright-Bantam syndrome (report of 3 cases). Endocrinology 30:922, 1942.
7. Albright F, Butler AM, Bloomberg E: Rickets resistant to vitamin D therapy. Am J Dis Child 54:529, 1937.
8. Amirhakimi GH: Rickets in a developing country—observations of general interest from southern Iran. Clin Pediatr 12:88, 1973.
9. Anderton JM: Orthopedic problems in adult hypophosphatasia. J Bone Joint Surg [Br] 61:82, 1979.
10. Anwar M: Nutritional hypovitaminosis-D and the genesis of osteomalacia in the elderly. J Am Geriatr Soc 26:309, 1978.
11. Arnaud SB, Arnaud CD, Bordier PJ, et al: The interrelationships between vitamin D and parathyroid hormone in disorders of mineral metabolism in man. *In* Vitamin D and Problems Related to Uremic Bone Disease. Proceedings of the Second Workshop on Vitamin D, Wiesbaden, Germany, October 1974, p 397. New York, Walter de Gruyter, 1975.
12. Arnaud C, Glorieux F, Scriver C: Serum parathyroid hormone in X-linked hypophosphatemia. Science 173:845, 1971.
13. Arnaud SB, Goldsmith RS, Lambert PW, et al: 25-Hydroxyvitamin D_3: Evidence of an enterohepatic circulation in man. Proc Exp Biol Med 149:570, 1975.
14. Arnaud SB, Stickler GB: Recent developments in vitamin D research. Clin Pediatr 13:444, 1974.
15. Aschinberg LC, Solomon LM, Zeis PM, et al: Vitamin D resistant rickets associated with epidermal nevus syndrome: Demonstration of a phosphaturic substance in the dermal lesions. J Pediatr 91:56, 1977.
16. Avioli LV: The therapeutic approach to hypoparathyroidism. Am J Med 57:34, 1974.
17. Avioli LV: Vitamin D metabolism in uremia. Kidney Int 8:1, 1975.
18. Avioli LV, Russell J: The pathogenesis of the bone lesion in experimental renal osteodystrophy. *In* Vitamin D and Problems Related to Uremic Bone Disease. Proceedings of the Second Workshop on Vitamin D, Wiesbaden, Germany, October 1974, p 119. New York, Walter de Gruyter, 1975.
19. Baker MR, McDonnell H, Peacock M, et al: Plasma 25-hydroxy vitamin D concentrations in patients with fractures of the femoral neck. Br Med J 1:589, 1979.
20. Baxter LA, DeLuca HF: Stimulation of 25-hydroxyvitamin D_3-1α-hydroxylase by phosphate depletion. J Biol Chem 251:3158, 1976.
21. Bayard F, Bec P, That HT, et al: Plasma 25-hydroxycholecalciferol in chronic renal failure. Eur J Clin Invest 3:447, 1973.
22. Bekemeier H, Pfennigsdorf, GF: Versuche zur erschöpfenden UV-Aktivierung des Provitamins D in Schwein eschwarte. Hoppe-Seylers Z Physiol Chem 314:120, 1959.
23. Belsey RE, DeLuca HF, Potts JT: Selective binding properties of vitamin D transport protein in chick plasma in vitro. Nature 247:208, 1974.
24. Bethune JE, Dent CE: Hypophosphatasia in the adult. Am J Med 28:615, 1960.

25. Bilezikian JP, Canfield RE, Jacobs TP, et al: Response of 1,25-dihydroxyvitamin D_3 to hypocalcemia in human subjects. N Engl J Med 299:437, 1978.

26. Bishop MC, Ledingham JGG, Oliver DO: Phosphate deficiency in haemodialysed patients. Proc Eur Dialysis Transplant Assoc 8:106, 1971.

27. Blomstrand R, Forsgren L: Intestinal absorption and esterification of vitamin D_3-1,2^3H in man. Acta Chem Scand 21:1662, 1967.

28. Bloom WL, Flinchum D: Osteomalacia with pseudofractures caused by ingestion of aluminum hydroxide. JAMA 174:1327, 1960.

29. Bloomberg MW: The treatment of persistent rickets. Am J Dis Child 34:624, 1927.

30. Blunt JW, DeLuca HF, Schnoes HK: 25-Hydroxycholecalciferol. A biologically active metabolite of vitamin D_3. Biochemistry 7:3317, 1968.

31. Bonomini V, Bortolotti GC: Serial bone biopsies in patients on maintenance hemodialysis. In Vitamin D and Problems Related to Uremic Bone Disease. Proceedings of the Second Workshop on Vitamin D, Wiesbaden, Germany, October 1974, p 531. New York, Walter de Gruyter, 1975.

32. Bonucci E, Maschio G, D'Angelo A, et al: Morphological aspects of bone tissue in chronic renal disease. A histological and electron microscopic study. In Vitamin D and Problems Related to Uremic Bone Disease. Proceedings of the Second Workshop on Vitamin D, Wiesbaden, Germany, October 1974, p 523. New York, Walter de Gruyter, 1975.

33. Bordier PJ, Chot ST, Eastwood JB, et al: Lack of histological evidence of vitamin D abnormality in the bones of anephric patients. Clin Sci 44:33, 1973.

34. Bouillon R, Reynaert J, Claes JH, et al: The effect of anticonvulsant therapy on serum levels of 25-hydroxy-vitamin D, calcium, and parathyroid hormone. J Clin Endocrinol Metab 41:1130, 1975.

35. Bouillon R, Van Baelen H, DeMoor P: The measurement of the vitamin D-binding protein in human serum. J Clin Endocrinol Metab 45:225, 1977.

36. Boyle IT, Gray RW, DeLuca HF: Regulation by calcium of in vivo synthesis of 1,25-dihydroxycholecalciferol and 21,25-dihydroxycalciferol. Proc Natl Acad Sci USA 68:2131, 1971.

37. Boyle IT, Miravet L, Gray RW, et al: The response of intestinal calcium transport to 25-hydroxy and 1,25 dihydroxy vitamin D in nephrectomized rats. Endocrinology 90:605, 1972.

38. Brewer ED, Tsai H, Morris RC Jr: Fanconi syndrome and its relationship to vitamin D. In Vitamin D: Biochemical, Chemical and Clinical Aspects Related to Calcium Metabolism. Proceedings of the Third Workshop on Vitamin D, Asilomar, Pacific Grove, California, January 1977. New York, Walter de Gruyter, 1977.

39. Brewer ED, Tsai HC, Szeto S, et al: Maleic acid induced impairment of conversion of 25-hydroxyvitamin D_3 (25-OH-D_3) to 1,25-dihydroxyvitamin for Fanconi's syndrome (FS). Clin Res 24:395A, 1976.

40. Bricker NS, Slatopolsky E, Reiss E, et al: Calcium, phosphorus, and bone in renal disease and transplantation. Arch Intern Med 123:543, 1969.

41. Brickman AS, Coburn JW, Norman AW: Action of 1,25 dihydroxycholecalciferol, a potent, kidney-produced metabolite of vitamin D_3 in uremic man. N Engl J Med 287:891, 1972.

42. Brickman AS, Coburn JW, Kurokawa K, et al: Actions of 1,25-dihydroxycholecalciferol in patients with hypophosphatemic, vitamin-D-resistant rickets. N Engl J Med 289:495, 1973.

43. Brickman AS, Coburn JW, Norman AW, et al: Short-term effects of 1,25 dihydroxycholecalciferol on disordered calcium metabolism of renal failure. Am J Med 57:28, 1974.

44. Brickman AS, Norman AW, Coburn JW: Vitamin D and pseudohypoparathyroidism. In Vitamin D: Biochemical, Chemical and Clinical Aspects Related to Calcium Metabolism. Proceedings of the Third Workshop on Vitamin D, Asilomar, Pacific Grove, California, January 1977. New York, Walter de Gruyter, 1977.

45. Brickman AS, Sherrard DJ, Jowsey J, et al: 1,25-dihydroxycholecalciferol. Effect on skeletal lesions and plasma parathyroid hormone levels in uremic osteodystrophy. Arch Intern Med 134:883, 1974.

46. Brighton CT: Structure and function of the growth plate. Clin Orthop 136:22, 1978.

47. Bronner F: Vitamin D deficiency and rickets. Am J Clin Nutr 29:1307, 1976.

48. Brooks MH, Bell NH, Love L, et al: Vitamin-D-dependent rickets type II: Resistance of target organs to 1,25 dihydroxyvitamin D. N Engl J Med 298:996, 1978.

49. Brumbaugh PF, Haussler MR: 1,25-dihydroxyvitamin D_3 receptor: competitive binding of vitamin D analogs. Life Sci 13:1737, 1973.

50. Brumbaugh PF, Haussler MR: Specific binding of 1,25-dihydroxycholecalciferol to nuclear components of chick intestine. J Biol Chem 250:1588, 1975.

51. Brumbaugh PF, Haussler DH, Bressler R, et al: Radioreceptor assay for 1,25-dihydroxyvitamin D_3. Science 183:1089, 1974.

52. Brumbaugh PF, Haussler DH, Bursac KM, et al: Filter assay of 1,25-dihydroxyvitamin D_3. Utilization of the hormone's target tissue chromatin receptor. Biochemistry 13:4091, 1974.

53. Brumbaugh PF, Hughes MR, Haussler MR: Cytoplasmic and nuclear binding components for 1,25-dihydroxyvitamin D_3 in chick parathyroid glands. Proc Natl Acad Sci 72:4871, 1975.

54. Buchan DJ, Mitchell DM: Hypertrophic osteoarthropathy in portal cirrhosis. Ann Intern Med 66:130, 1967.

55. Caffey J: Pediatric X-ray Diagnosis. 6th Ed. Vols 1, 2. Chicago, Year Book Medical Publishers, 1972.

56. Campbell JM, Hunt TK, Karam JH, et al: Jejunoileal bypass as a treatment for morbid obesity. Arch Intern Med 137:602, 1977.

57. Canas F, Brand JS, Neuman WF, et al: Some effects of vitamin D_3 on collagen synthesis in rachitic chick cortical bone. Am J Physiol 216:1092, 1969.

58. Caspary WF, Hesch RD, Matte R, et al: Intestinal calcium absorption in epileptics under anticonvulsant therapy. In Vitamin D and Problems Related to Uremic Bone Disease. Proceedings of the Second Workshop on Vitamin D, Wiesbaden, Germany, October 1974, p 737. New York, Walter de Gruyter, 1975.

59. Chan GM, Tsang RC, Chen IW, et al: The effect of $1,25(OH)_2$ vitamin D supplementation in premature infants. J Pediatr 93:91, 1978.

60. Chase LR, Aurbach GD: Renal adenyl cyclase; anatomically separate sites for parathyroid hormone and vasopressin. Science 159:545, 1968.

61. Chase LR, Aurbach GD: Cyclic AMP and the mechanism of action of parathyroid hormone. In RV Talmage, LF Belanger (Eds): Parathyroid Hormone and Thyrocalcitonin (Calcitonin). Amsterdam, Excerpta Medica Foundation, 1968, p 247.

62. Chase LR, Fedak SA, Aurbach GD: Activation of skeletal adenyl cyclase by parathyroid hormone in vitro. Endocrinology 84:761, 1969.

63. Chase LR, Melson GL, Aurbach GD: Pseudohypoparathyroidism: Defective excretion of 3',5'-AMP in response to parathyroid hormone. J Clin Invest 48:1832, 1969.

64. Chertow BS, Baylink DJ, Wergedal JE, et al: Decrease in serum immunoreactive parathyroid hormone in rats and in parathyroid hormone secretion in vitro by 1,25-dihydroxycholecalciferol. J Clin Invest 56:668, 1975.

65. Chesney RW, Hamstra AM, Mazess RB, et al: Reduction of serum-1,25-dihydroxyvitamin-D, in children receiving glucocorticoids. Lancet 2:1123, 1978.

66. Christiansen C, Kristensen M, Rodbro P: Latent osteomalacia in epileptic patients on anticonvulsants. Br Med J 3:738, 1972.

67. Christiansen C, Rodbro P: Anticonvulsant osteomalacia treated with different doses of vitamin D_3 and 25-OH-D_3. In Vitamin D and Problems Related to Uremic Bone Disease. Proceedings of the Second Workshop on Vitamin D, Wiesbaden, Germany, October 1974, p 743. New York, Walter de Gruyter, 1975.

68. Christiansen C, Rodbro P, Lund M: Incidence of anticonvulsant osteomalacia and effect of vitamin D: Controlled therapeutic trial. Br Med J 4:695, 1973.

69. Christiansen C, Rodbro P, Munck O: Actions of vitamin D_2 and D_3 and 25-OH-D_3 in anticonvulsant osteomalacia. Br Med J 2:363, 1975.

70. Christiansen C, Rodbro P, Nielsen CT: Iatrogenic osteomalacia in epileptic children. Acta Paediatr Scand 64:219, 1975.

71. Clark CG, Crooks J, Dawson AA, et al: Disordered calcium metabolism after Polya partial gastrectomy. Lancet 1:734, 1964.

72. Coburn JW, Brickman AS, Hartenblower DL: Clinical disorders of calcium metabolism in relation to vitamin D. In Vitamin D and Problems Related to Uremic Bone Disease. Proceedings of the Second Workshop on Vitamin D, Wiesbaden, Germany, October 1974, p 219. New York, Walter de Gruyter, 1975.

73. Coburn JW, Hartenblower DL, Brickman AS: Advances in vitamin D metabolism as they pertain to chronic renal disease. Am J Clin Nutr 29:1283, 1976.

74. Colston KW, Evans IMA, Galante L, et al: Regulation of vitamin D metabolism: Factors influencing the rate of formation of 1,25-dihydroxycholecalciferol by kidney homogenates. Biochem J 134:817, 1973.

75. Committee on Nutrition of the American Academy of Pediatrics: Infantile scurvy and nutritional rickets in the United States. Pediatrics 29:646, 1962.

76. Compston J, Creamer B: Plasma levels and intestinal absorption of 25-hydroxyvitamin D after small intestinal resection. In Vitamin D: Biochemical, Chemical, and Clinical Aspects Related to Calcium Metabolism. Proceedings of the Third Workshop on Vitamin D, Asilomar, Pacific Grove, California, January 1977. New York, Walter de Gruyter, 1977.

77. Compston JE, Ayers AB, Horton LWL, et al: Osteomalacia after small-intestinal resection. Lancet 1:9, 1978.

78. Compston JE, Thompson RPH: Intestinal absorption of 25-hydroxyvitamin D and osteomalacia in primary biliary cirrhosis. Lancet 1:721, 1977.

79. Condon JR, Nassim JR: Axial osteomalacia. Postgrad Med J 47:817, 1971.

80. Contiguglia SR, Alfrey A, Miller NL, et al: Nature of soft tissue calcification in uremia. Kidney Int 4:229, 1973.

81. Cooke WT, Asquith P, Ruck N, et al: Rickets, growth, and alkaline phosphatase in urban adolescents. Br Med J 2:293, 1974.

82. Cooke WT, Swan CH, Asquith P, et al: Serum alkaline phophatase and rickets in urban school children. Br Med J 1:324, 1974.

83. Cork DJ: The homeostatic control of the kidney 25-hydroxyvitamin D_3-1-hydroxylase. Master's Thesis, University of Arizona, 1974.

84. Corless D, Boucher BJ, Cohen RD, et al: Vitamin-D status in long-stay geriatric patients. Lancet 1:1404, 1975.

85. Crosley CJ, Chee C, Berman PH: Rickets associated with long-term anticonvulsant therapy in a pediatric outpatient population. Pediatrics 56:52, 1975.

86. Currarino G: Hypophosphatasia. In HJ Kaufmann (Ed): Progress in Pediatric Radiology. Vol 4. Intrinsic Diseases of Bones. New York, S Karger, 1973, p 464.

87. Daum F, Rosen JF, Roginsky M, et al: 25-hydroxycholecalciferol in the management of rickets associated with extrahepatic biliary atresia. J Pediatr 88:1041, 1976.

88. DeLuca HF: The kidney as an endocrine organ for the production of 1,25-dihydroxyvitamin D_3, a calcium mobilizing hormone. N Engl J Med 289:359, 1973.

89. DeLuca HF: Recent advances in our understanding of the vitamin D endocrine system. J Lab Clin Med 87:7, 1976.

90. DeLuca HF: Recent advances in our understanding of the metabolism of vitamin D and its regulation. Clin Endocrinol 5(Suppl):97S, 1976.

91. DeLuca HF: The kidney as an endocrine organ involved in the function of vitamin D. Am J Med 58:39, 1975.

92. DeLuca HF: Vitamin D—1973. Am J Med 57:1, 1974.

93. DeLuca HF: Vitamin D: The vitamin and the hormone. Fed Proc 33:2211, 1974.

94. Dent CE, Stamp TCB: Vitamin D, rickets and osteomalacia. In L Avioli, S Krane (Eds): Metabolic Bone Disease. New York, Academic Press, 1977, p 237.

95. Dent CE: Rickets (and osteomalacia), nutritional and metabolic (1919–1969). Proc R Soc Med 63:401, 1970.

96. Dent CE, Gertner JM: Hypophosphataemic osteomalacia in fibrous dysplasia. Q J Med 45:411, 1976.

97. Dent CE, Normand ECS: Metaphysial dysostosis, type Schmid. Arch Dis Child 39:444, 1964.

98. Dickstein SS, Frame B: Urinary tract calculi after intestinal shunt operations for treatment of obesity. Surg Gynecol Obstet 136:257, 1973.

99. Dodds GS, Cameron HC: Studies on experimental rickets in rats. IV. The relation of rickets to growth with special reference to the bones. Am J Pathol 19:169, 1943.

100. Drezner MK, Feinglos MN: Tumor induced 1-25 dihydroxycholecalciferol (1,25-DHCC) deficiency: A cause of oncogenic osteomalacia. Clin Res 25:31A, 1977.

101. Drezner MK, Feinglos MN: Tumor induced 1,25-dihydroxycholecalciferol (1,25-[OH]₂D₃) deficiency: A cause of oncogenic osteomalacia. In Vitamin D: Biochemical, Chemical and Clinical Aspects Related to Calcium Metabolism. Proceedings of the Third Workshop on Vitamin D, Asilomar, Pacific Grove, California, January 1977, New York, Walter de Gruyter, 1977, p 863.

102. Drezner MK, Haussler MR: Normocalcemic pseudohypoparathyroidism, association with normal vitamin D₃ metabolism. Am J Med 66:503, 1979.

103. Drezner MK, Haussler MR: Serum, 1,25-dihydroxyvitamin D in bone disease. N Engl J Med 300:434, 1979.

104. Drezner MK, Neelon FA, Haussler M, et al: 1,25-dihydroxycholecalciferol deficiency: The probable cause of hypocalcemia and metabolic bone disease in pseudohypoparathyroidism. J Clin Endocrinol Metab 42:621, 1976.

105. Drezner MK, Neelon FA, Lebovitz HE: Pseudohypoparathyroidism type II: A possible defect in the reception of the cyclic AMP signal. N Engl J Med 289:1056, 1973.

106. Dwyer JT, Dietz WH Jr, Hass G, et al: Risks of nutritional rickets among vegetarian children. Am J Dis Child 133:134, 1979.

107. Eastwood MA, Girdwood RH: Lignin: A bile-salt sequestrating agent. Lancet 2:1170, 1968.

108. Eastwood JB, Phillips ME, de Wardener HE, et al: Biochemical and histological effects of 1,25-dihydroxycholecalciferol (1,25-DHCC) in the osteomalacia of chronic renal failure. In Vitamin D and Problems Related to Uremic Bone Disease. Proceedings of the Second Workshop on Vitamin D, Wiesbaden, Germany, October 1974, p 595. New York, Walter de Gruyter, 1975.

109. Eddy RL: Metabolic bone disease after gastrectomy. Am J Med 50:442, 1971.

110. Eisman JA, DeLuca HF, Kream BE: A sensitive competitive binding assay for 1,25-dihydroxyvitamin D₃ (1,25-[OH]₂-D₃) applicable to human blood. Clin Res 24:457A, 1976.

111. Ellis G, Cooke WT: Serum concentrations of 25-hydroxy vitamin D in Europeans and Asians after oral vitamin D₃. Br Med J 1:685, 1978.

112. Erhard D: The new vegetarians. Part 2. Nutr Today 9:20, 1974.

113. Favus MJ, Walling MW, Kimberg DV: Effects of dietary calcium restriction and chronic thyroparathyroidectomy on the metabolism of ³H 25-hydroxyvitamin D₃ and the active transport of calcium by rat intestine. J Clin Invest 53:1139, 1974.

114. Favus MJ, Wezeman FH: Localization of ³H-1,25-dihydroxycholecalciferol in rat bone and cartilage. In Vitamin D: Biochemical, Chemical and Clinical Aspects Related to Calcium Metabolism. Proceedings of the Third Workshop on Vitamin D, Asilomar, Pacific Grove, California, January 1977, p 369. New York, Walter de Gruyter, 1977.

115. Feest TG, Ward MK, Ellis HA, et al: Renal bone disease—what is it and why does it happen? Clin Endocrinol 7(Suppl):19S, 1977.

116. Finberg, L: Human choice, vegetable deficiencies, and vegetarian rickets. Am J Dis Child 133:129, 1979.

117. Fleischman AR, Rosen JF, Nathenson G: 25-Hydroxycholecalciferol for early neonatal hypocalcemia. Am J Dis Child 132:973, 1978.

118. Frame B, Frost HM, Ormond RS, et al: Atypical osteomalacia involving the axial skeleton. Ann Intern Med 55:632, 1961.

119. Fraser DR, Kodicek E: Unique biosynthesis by kidney of a biologically active vitamin D metabolite. Nature 228:764, 1970.

120. Fraser D, Kooh SW, Kind HP, et al: Pathogenesis of hereditary vitamin-D-dependent rickets. An inborn error of vitamin D metabolism involving defective conversion of 25-hydroxyvitamin D to 1,25-dihydroxyvitamin D. N Engl J Med 289:817, 1973.

121. Fraser D, Kooh SW, Scriver CR: Vitamin D resistant rickets—pathophysiology of the various syndromes. In Vitamin D: Biochemical, Chemical and Clinical Aspects Related to Calcium Metabolism. Proceedings of the Third Workshop on Vitamin D, Asilomar, Pacific Grove, California, January 1977, p 771. New York, Walter de Gruyter, 1977.

122. Fraser D, Scriver CR: Familial forms of vitamin D-resistant rickets revisited. X-linked hypophosphatemia and autosomal recessive vitamin D dependency. Am J Clin Nutr 29:1315, 1976.

123. Frolik CA, DeLuca HF: 1,25-dihydroxycholecalciferol: The metabolite of vitamin D responsible for increased intestinal calcium transport. Arch Biochem Biophys 147:143, 1971.

124. Frymoyer JW: Fracture healing in rats treated with diphenylhydantoin (Dilantin). J Trauma 16:368, 1976.

125. Garabedian M, Holick MF, DeLuca HF, et al: Control of 25-hydroxycholecalciferol metabolism by parathyroid glands. Proc Natl Acad Sci 69:1673, 1972.

126. Garabedian M, Tanaka Y, Holick MR, et al: Response of intestinal calcium transport and bone calcium mobilization to 1,25-dihydroxyvitamin D₃ in thyroparathyroidectomized rats. Endocrinology 94:1022, 1974.

127. Gertner JM, Lilburn M, Domenech M: 25-hydroxycholecalciferol absorption in steatorrhoea and postgastrectomy osteomalacia. Br Med J 1:1310, 1977.

128. Glasgow JFT, Thomas PS: Rachitic respiratory distress in small preterm infants. Arch Dis Child 52:268, 1977.

129. Glisson F: De Rachitide Sive Morbo Puerili qui vulgo The Rickets Dicitur Tractatus. Adscitis in operis societatem Georgio Bate et Ahasuero Regemortero. London, G Du-Gardi, 1650.

130. Glorieux FH, Holick MF, Scriver CR, et al: X-linked hypophosphataemic rickets: Inadequate therapeutic response to 1,25-dihydroxycholecalciferol. Lancet 2:287, 1973.

131. Glorieux FH, Scriver CR: Loss of a parathyroid hormone-sensitive component of phosphate transport in X-linked hypophosphatemia. Science 175:997, 1972.

132. Goel KM, Logan RW, Arneil GC, et al: Florid and subclinical rickets among immigrant children in Glasgow. Lancet 1:1141, 1976.

133. Gray R, Boyle I, DeLuca HF: Vitamin D metabolism: The role of kidney tissue. Science 172:1232, 1971.

134. Gray RW, Caldas AE, Wilz DR, et al: Metabolism and excretion of ³H-1,25-(OH)₂-Vitamin D₃ in healthy adults. J Clin Endocrinol Metab 46:756, 1978.

135. Griscom NT, Craig JN, Neuhauser EBD: Systemic bone disease developing in small premature infants. Pediatrics 48:883, 1971.

136. Gutcher GR, Chesney RW: Iatrogenic rickets as a complication of a total parenteral nutrition program. Clin Pediatr 17:817, 1978.

137. Haddad JG, Chyu KJ: Competitive protein-binding radioassay for 25-hydroxycholecalciferol. J Clin Endocrinol Metab 33:992, 1971.

138. Haddad JG, Hahn TJ: Natural and synthetic sources of circulating 25-hydroxyvitamin D in man. Nature 244:515, 1973.

139. Hahn TJ: Corticosteroid-induced osteopenia. Arch Intern Med 138:882, 1978.

140. Hahn TJ, Avioli LV: Hepatic bioactivation of vitamin D and clinical implications. In Vitamin D: Biochemical, Chemical and Clinical Aspects Related to Calcium Metabolism. Proceedings of the Third Workshop on Vitamin D, Asilomar, Pacific Grove, California, January 1977, p 737. New York, Walter de Gruyter, 1977.

141. Hahn TJ, Birge SJ, Scharp CR, et al: Phenobarbital-induced alterations in vitamin D metabolism. J Clin Invest 51:741, 1972.

142. Hahn TJ, Hendin BA, Scharp CR, et al: Serum 25-hydroxycalciferol levels and bone mass in children on chronic anticonvulsant therapy. N Engl J Med 292:550, 1975.

143. Hahn TJ, Scharp CR, Avioli LV: Effect of phenobarbital administration on the subcellular distribution of vitamin D₃-³H in rat liver. Endocrinology 94:1489, 1974.

144. Hahn TJ, Squires AE, Halstead LR, et al: Reduced serum 25-hydroxyvitamin D concentration and disordered mineral metabolism in patients with cystic fibrosis. J Pediatr 94:38, 1979.

145. Harris HA: Rickets. In Bone Growth in Health and Disease. London, Oxford Medical Publications, Oxford University Press, 1933, p 87.

146. Harris WH, Heaney RP: Skeletal renewal and metabolic bone disease. N Engl J Med 280:193, 1969.

147. Harrison HE: Oncogenous rickets: Possible elaboration by a tumor of a humoral substance inhibiting tubular reabsorption of phosphate. Pediatrics 72:432, 1973.

148. Harrison HE, Harrison HC: Intestinal transport of phosphate: Action of vitamin D, and potassium. Am J Physiol 201:1007, 1961.

149. Harrison HE, Harrison HC: Rickets then and now. J Pediatr 87:1144, 1975.

150. Harrison HE, Harrison HC: The renal excretion of inorganic phosphate in relation to the action of vitamin D and parathyroid hormone. J Clin Invest 20:27, 1941.

151. Haussler MR: Personal communication, 1979.

152. Haussler MR: Vitamin D: Mode of action and biomedical applications. Nutr Rev 32:257, 1974.

153. Haussler MR, Baylink DJ, Hughes MR, et al: The assay of 1α 25-dihydroxyvitamin D₃: Physiologic and pathologic modulation of circulating hormone levels. Clin Endocrinol 5:151S, 1976.

154. Haussler MR, Boyce DW, Littledike ET, et al: A rapidly acting metabolite of vitamin D₃. Proc Natl Acad Sci 68:177, 1971.

155. Haussler MR, Bursac KM, Bone H, et al: Increased circulating 1α 25-dihydroxyvitamin D₃ in patients with primary hyperparathyroidism. Clin Res 23:A322, 1975.

156. Haussler M, Hughes M, Baylink D, et al: Influence of phosphate depletion on the biosynthesis and circulating level of 1α, 25-dihydroxyvitamin D. Adv Exp Med Biol 81:233, 1977.

157. Haussler MR, Myrtle JF, Norman AW: The association of a metabolite of vitamin D₃ with intestinal mucosa chromatin in vivo. J Biol Chem 243:4055, 1968.

158. Haussler MR, Rasmussen H: The metabolism of vitamin D$_3$ in the chick. J Biol Chem *247:*2328, 1972.

159. Henderson RG, Ledingham JGG, Oliver DO, et al: Effects of 1,25-dihydroxy-cholecalciferol on calcium absorption, muscle weakness, and bone disease in chronic renal failure. Lancet *1:*379, 1974.

160. Henry HL, Norman AW: Studies on the mechanism of action of calciferol. VII. Localization of 1,25-dihydroxyvitamin D$_3$ in chick parathyroid glands. Biochem Biophys Res *62:*781, 1975.

161. Henry HL, Midgett RJ, Norman AW: Regulation of 25-hydroxyvitamin D$_3$-1-hydroxylase in vivo. J Biol Chem *249:*7584, 1974.

162. Hepner GW, Roginsky M, Moo HF: Low serum 25-hydroxyvitamin D levels in patients with hepatic dysfunction. *In* Vitamin D and Problems Related to Uremic Bone Disease. Proceedings of the Second Workshop on Vitamin D, Wiesbaden, Germany, October 1974, p 325. New York, Walter de Gruyter, 1975.

163. Hess AF, Unger LJ: Prophylactic therapy for rickets in a Negro community. JAMA *69:*1583, 1917.

164. Hill LF, Mawer EB, Taylor ECM: Determination of plasma levels of 1,25-dihydroxycholecalciferol in man. *In* Vitamin D and Problems Related to Uremic Bone Disease. Proceedings of the Second Workshop on Vitamin D, Wiesbaden, Germany, October 1974, p 755. New York, Walter de Gruyter, 1975.

165. Hillman LS, Haddad JG: Perinatal vitamin D metabolism. J Pediatr *86:*928, 1975.

166. Hoff N, Haddad J, Teitelbaum S, et al: Serum concentration of 25-hydroxyvitamin D in rickets of extremely premature infants. J Pediatr *94:*460, 1979.

167. Hoffbrand BI: Chronic pancreatitis (?alcoholic) with osteomalacia. Proc R Soc Med *58:*697, 1965.

168. Franck WA, Hoffman GS, Davis JS, et al: Osteomalacia and weakness complicating jejunoileal bypass. J Rheumatol *6:*51, 1979.

169. Belsey RE, Clark MB, Bernat M, et al: The physiologic significance of plasma transport of vitamin D and metabolites. Am J Med *57:*50, 1974.

170. Holick MF, Frommer J, McNeil S, et al: Conversion of 7-dihydrocholesterol to vitamin D$_3$ in vivo: Isolation and identification of previtamin D$_3$ from skin. *In* Vitamin D: Biochemical, Chemical and Clinical Aspects Related to Calcium Metabolism. Proceedings of the Third Workshop on Vitamin D, Asilomar, Pacific Grove, California, 1977, p 135. New York, Walter de Gruyter, 1977.

171. Holick MF, Garabedian M, DeLuca HF: 1,25-dihydroxycholecalciferol: Metabolite of vitamin D$_3$ active on bone in anephric rats. Science *176:*1146, 1972.

172. Holick MR, Schnoes HF, DeLuca HF, et al: Isolation and identification of 1,25-dihydroxycholecalciferol. A metabolite of vitamin D active in intestine. Biochemistry *10:*2799, 1971.

173. Holmes AM, Enoch BA, Taylor JL, et al: Occult rickets and osteomalacia amongst the Asian immigrant population. Q J Med *42:*125, 1973.

174. Howarth AT: Biochemical indices of osteomalacia in pregnant Asian immigrants in Britain. J Clin Pathol *29:*981, 1976.

175. Howland J, Kramer B: Calcium and phosphorus in the serum in relation to rickets. Am J Dis Child *22:*105, 1921.

176. Park EA, Howland J: The dangers to life of severe involvement of the thorax in rickets. Bull Johns Hopkins Hosp *32:*101, 1921.

177. Hubbard VS, Farrell PM, diSant' Agnese PA: 25-Hydroxycholecalciferol levels in patients with cystic fibrosis. J Pediatr *94:*84, 1979.

178. Huffer WE, Kuzela D, Popovtzer MM, et al: Metabolic bone disease in chronic renal failure. II. Renal transplant patients. Am J Pathol *78:*385, 1975.

179. Huffer WE, Kuzela D, Popovtzer MM: Metabolic bone disease in chronic renal failure. I. Dialyzed uremics. Am J Pathol *78:*365, 1975.

180. Huldschinsky K: Heilung von Rachitis durch künstliche Hohensonne. Dstch Med Wochenschr *45:*712, 1919.

181. Hunt SP, O'Riordan JLH, Windo J, et al: Vitamin D status in different subgroups of British Asians. Br Med J *2:*1351, 1976.

182. Hunter R: Rickets, ruckets, rekets, or rackets? Lancet *1:*1176, 1972.

183. Hughes MR, Baylink DJ, Jones PG, et al: Radioligand receptor assay for 25-hydroxyvitamin D$_2$/D$_3$ and 1α, 25-dihydroxyvitamin D$_2$/D$_3$. J Clin Invest *58:*61, 1976.

184. Hughes MR, Brumbaugh PF, Haussler MR, et al: Regulation of serum 1α,25-dihydroxyvitamin D$_3$ by calcium and phosphate in the rat. Science *190:*578, 1975.

185. Ivey JL, Morey ER, Liu C-C, et al: Effects of vitamin D and its metabolites on bone. *In* Vitamin D: Biochemical, Chemical and Clinical Aspects Related to Calcium Metabolism. Proceedings of the Third Workshop on Vitamin D, Asilomar, Pacific Grove, California, January 1977, p 349. New York, Walter de Gruyter, 1977.

186. Jaffe HL: Metabolic, Degenerative and Inflammatory Diseases of Bones and Joints. Philadelphia, Lea & Febiger, 1972, p 381.

187. Jardon OM, Burney DW, Fink RL: Hypophosphatasia in an adult. J Bone Joint Surg [Am] *52:*1477, 1970.

188. Jaworski AFG: Pathophysiology, diagnosis, and treatment of osteomalacia. Orthop Clin North Am *3:*623, 1972.

189. Johnson WJ, Goldsmith RS, Jowsey J, et al: The influence of maintaining normal serum phosphate and calcium on renal osteodystrophy. *In* Vitamin D and Problems Related to Uremic Bone Disease. Proceedings of the Second Workshop on Vitamin D, Wiesbaden, Germany, October 1974, p 561. New York, Walter de Gruyter, 1975.

190. Jones CR, De Silva KL: Jejunal diverticulosis with malabsorption leading to osteomalacia and probable rickets. Gerontol Clin *12:*80, 1970.

191. Jowsey J, Massry SG, Coburn JW, et al: Microradiographic studies of bone in renal osteodystrophy. Arch Intern Med *124:*539, 1969.

192. Jubiz W, Haussler MR, McCain TA, Plasma 1,25-dihydroxyvitam in patients receiving anticonvulsant drugs. J Clin Endocrinol Meta*els* 1977. *7,*

193. Jubiz W, Haussler MR, Tolman KG, et al: Plasma 1,25-dihydroxyv' levels in patients receiving anticonvulsant drugs. J Clin Endocrino *44:*379, 1977.

194. Kanis JA, Adams ND, Earnshaw M, et al: Vitamin D, osteomalaci chronic renal failure. *In* Vitamin D: Biochemical, Chemical and Clinic pects Related to Calcium Metabolism. Proceedings of the Third Worksh Vitamin D, Asilomar, Pacific Grove, California, January 1977, p 671. York, Walter de Gruyter, 1977.

195. Klein RG, Arnaud SB, Gallagher JC, et al: Intestinal calcium absorption exogenous hypercortisonism. Role of 25-hydroxyvitamin D and corticostero dose. J Clin Invest *60:*253, 1977.

196. Koch H-U, Kraft D, Von Herrath D, et al: Influence of diphenylhydantoin an phenobarbital on intestinal calcium transport in the rat. Epilepsia *13:*829, 1972.

197. Kocian J, Sotornik I: Intestinal ^{47}Ca absorption in hepatic and renal diseases with respect to conversion of vitamin D. *In* Vitamin D and Problems Related to Uremic Bone Disease. Proceedings of the Second Workshop on Vitamin D, Wiesbaden, Germany, October 1974, p 391. New York, Walter de Gruyter, 1977.

198. Kodicek E: The metabolism of vitamin D. Proc Int Congress Biochem, 4th Vienna, Vol 11, pp 198–208. New York, Pergamon Press, 1960.

199. Kodicek E: The story of vitamin D from vitamin to hormone. Lancet *1:*325, 174.

200. Kooh SW, Fraser D, DeLuca HF, et al: Treatment of hypoparathyroidism and pseudohypoparathyroidism with metabolites of vitamin D: Evidence for impaired conversion of 25-hydroxyvitamin D to 1α,25-dihydroxyvitamin D. N Engl J Med *293:*840, 1975.

201. Kooh SW, Fraser D, Reilly BJ, et al: Rickets due to calcium deficiency. N Engl J Med *297:*1264, 1977.

202. Kooh SW, Fraser D, Toon R, et al: Response of protracted neonatal hypocalcaemia to 1α,25-dihydroxyvitamin D$_3$. Lancet *1:*1105, 1976.

203. Kruse R: Osteopathein bei antiepileptischer Langzeittherapie (Vorläufige Mitteilung). Monatsschr Kinderheilkd *116:*378, 1968.

204. Laditan AAO, Adeniyi A: Rickets in Nigerian children—response to vitamin D. J Trop Med Hyg *78:*206, 1975.

205. Lakdawala DR. Widdowson EM: Vitamin-D in human milk. Lancet *1:*167, 1977.

206. Larkins RG, Colston KW, Galante LS, et al: Regulation of vitamin D metabolism without parathyroid hormone. Lancet *2:*289, 1973.

207. Larkins RG, MacAuley SJ, MacIntyre I: Feedback control of vitamin D metabolism by a nuclear action of 1,25-dihydroxycholecalciferol on the kidney. Nature *252:*412, 1974.

208. LeMay M, Blunt JW: A factor determining the location of pseudofractures in osteomalacia. J Clin Invest *28:*521, 1949.

209. Lewin PK, Reid M, Reilly BJ, et al: Iatrogenic rickets in low-birth-weight infants. J Pediatr *78:*207, 1971.

210. Liakokos D, Papadopoulos Z, Vlachos P, et al: Serum alkaline phosphatase and urinary hydroxyproline values in children receiving phenobarbital with and without vitamin D. J Pediatr *87:*291, 1975.

211. Lifshitz F, Maclaren NK: Vitamin D-dependent rickets in institutionalized, mentally retarded children receiving long-term anticonvulsant therapy. I. A survey of 288 patients. J Pediatr *83:*612, 1973.

212. Lifshitz F, Maclaren NK: Vitamin D$_2$ (vit D) dihydrotachysterol (DHT) and 25-hydroxycholecalciferol (25-OHCC) treatment of vitamin D dependency rickets associated with anticonvulsants. Fed Proc *32:*918, 1973.

213. Lilienfeld-Toal HV, Mackes KG, Kodrat G, et al: Plasma 25-hydroxyvitamin D and urinary cyclic AMP in German patients with subtotal gastrectomy (Billroth II). Digest Dis *22:*633, 1977.

214. Linovitz RJ, Resnick D, Keissling P, et al: Tumor-induced osteomalacia and rickets: A surgically curable syndrome, report of two cases. J Bone Joint Surg [Am] *58:*419, 1976.

215. Livingston S, Berman W, Pauli LL: Anticonvulsant drugs and vitamin D metabolism. JAMA *224:*1634, 1973.

216. Llach F, Massry SG, Singer FR, et al: Skeletal resistance to endogenous parathyroid hormone in patients with early renal failure. A possible cause for secondary hyperparathyroidism. J Clin Endocrinol Metab *41:*339, 1975.

217. Long RG, Skinner RK, Wills MR, et al: Serum 25-hydroxyvitamin-D in untreated parenchymal and cholestatic liver disease. Lancet *2:*650, 1976.

218. Long RG, Skinner RK, Meinhard E, et al: Serum 25-hydroxyvitamin D values in liver disease and hepatic osteomalacia. Gut *17:*824, 1976.

219. Loomis WF: Rickets. Sci Am *223:*77, 1970.

220. Loomis WF: Skin-pigment regulation of vitamin-D biosynthesis in man. Science *157:*501, 1967.

221. Lorenc R, Tanaka Y, DeLuca HF, et al: Lack of effect of calcitonin on the regulation of vitamin D metabolism in the rat. Endocrinology *100:*468, 1977.

222. Lukert BP, Adams JS: Vitamin D metabolism in man: Effect of corticosteroids. Arch Intern Med *136:*1241, 1976.

223. Lumb GA, Mawer EB, Stanbury SW: The apparent vitamin D resistance of chronic renal failure, a study of the physiology of vitamin D in man. Am J Med *50:*421, 1971.

224. Lund J, DeLuca HF: Biologically active metabolite of vitamin D$_3$ from bone, liver, and blood serum. J Lipid Res *7:*739, 1966.

225. Lund B, Sorensen OH, Christensen AB: 25-hydroxycholeciferol and fractures of the proximal femur. Lancet *1:*300, 1975.

acLennan WJ, Hamilton JC: Vitamin D supplements and 25-hydroxyvitamin D concentrations in the elderly. Br Med J 2:859, 1977.

Mallette LE: Acetazolamide-accelerated anticonvulsant osteomalacia. Arch Intern Med 137:1013, 1977.

8. Malluche HH, Ritz E, Kutschera J, et al: Calcium metabolism and impaired mineralization in various stages of renal insufficiency. In Vitamin D and Problems Related to Uremic Bone Disease. Proceedings of the Second Workshop on Vitamin D, Wiesbaden, Germany, October 1974, p 513. New York, Walter de Gruyter, 1975.

229. Maltz HE, Fish MB, Holliday MA: Calcium deficiency rickets and the renal response to calcium infusion. Pediatrics 46:865, 1970.

230. Manicourt DH, Orloff S: Osteomalacia complicating a blind loop syndrome from congenital megaesophagus-megaduodenum. J Rheumatol 6:57, 1979.

231. Mankin HJ: Rickets, osteomalacia, and renal osteodystrophy—Part II. J Bone Joint Surg [Am] 56:352, 1974.

232. Mankin HJ: Rickets, osteomalacia, and renal osteodystrophy—Part I. J Bone Joint Surg [Am] 56:101, 1974.

233. Mann JB, Alterman S, Hills AG: Albright's hereditary osteodystrophy comprising pseudohypoparathyroidism and pseudo-pseudohypoparathyroidism. With a report of two cases representing the complete syndrome occurring in successive generations. Ann Intern Med 56:315, 1962.

234. Mariam TW, Sterky G: Severe rickets in infancy and childhood in Ethiopia. J Pediatr 82:876, 1973.

235. Marx WJ, O'Connell DJ: Arthritis of primary biliary cirrhosis. Arch Intern Med 139:213, 1979.

236. Massry SG: An evaluation of hypocalcemia pathogenesis. Dial Transplant 5:38, 1976.

237. Massry SG, Coburn JW, Lee DBN, et al: Skeletal resistance to parathyroid hormone in renal failure. Studies in 105 human subjects. Ann Intern Med 78:357, 1973.

238. Massry SG, Ritz E: The pathogenesis of secondary hyperparathyroidism of renal failure: Is there a controversy? Arch Intern Med 138:853, 1978.

239. Matheson R, Tolman KG, Herbst JJ, et al: Absorption and biotransformation of cholecalciferol in drug-induced osteomalacia. Clin Res 21:244, 1973.

240. McCollum EV, Simmonds N, Becker JE, et al: Studies on experimental rickets. XXI. An experimental demonstration of the existence of a vitamin which promotes calcium deposition. J Biol Chem 53:293, 1922.

241. Meema HE, Oreopoulos DG, Rabinovich S, et al: Periosteal new bone formation (periosteal neostosis) in renal osteodystrophy. Radiology 110:513, 1974.

242. Mellanby E: An experimental investigation on rickets. Lancet 1:407, 1919.

243. Mellanby E: Experimental Rickets. Privy Council. Medical Research Council Special Report Series No 93. London, His Majesty's Stationery Office, 1925, pp 4, 20, 38, 62.

244. Midgett RJ, Spielvogel AM, Coburn JW, et al: Studies on calciferol metabolism. VI. The renal production of the biologically active form of vitamin D, 1,25-dihydroxycholecalciferol; species, tissue and subcellular distribution. J Clin Endocrinol Metab 36:1153, 1973.

245. Milkman LA: Multiple spontaneous idiopathic symmetrical fracture. AJR 32:622, 1934.

246. Milkman LA: Pseudofractures (hunger osteopathy, late rickets, osteomalacia). AJR 24:29, 1930.

247. Moorhead JF, Wills MR, Ahmet KY, et al: Hypophosphataemic osteomalacia after cadaveric renal transplantation. Lancet 1:694, 1974.

248. Morgan DB, Paterson CR, Woods CG, et al: Search for osteomalacia in 1,228 patients after gastrectomy and other operations on the stomach. Lancet 2:1085, 1965.

249. Morii H, DeLuca HF: Relationship between vitamin D deficiency, thyrocalcitonin, and parathyroid hormone. Am J Physiol 213:358, 1967.

250. Morimoto T, Morii H, Okamoto T, et al: 25-hydroxycholecalciferol metabolism in hepatobiliary diseases. In Vitamin D: Biochemical, Chemical and Clinical Aspects Related to Calcium Metabolism. Proceedings of the Third Workshop on Vitamin D, Asilomar, Pacific Grove, California, January 1977, p 801. New York, Walter de Gruyter, 1977.

251. Morse JL: The frequency of rickets in infancy in Boston and vicinity. JAMA 34:724, 1900.

252. Mosekilde L, Christensen MS, Lund B, et al: The interrelationships between serum 25-hydroxycholecalciferol, serum parathyroid hormone and bone changes in anticonvulsant osteomalacia. Acta Endocrinol 84:559, 1977.

253. Moses AM, Rao KJ, Coulson R, et al: Parathyroid hormone deficiency with Albright's hereditary osteodystrophy. J Clin Endocrinol Metab 39:496, 1974.

254. Mulivor RA, Mennuti M, Zackai EH, et al: Prenatal diagnosis of hypophosphatasia: Genetic, biochemical, and clinical studies. Am J Hum Genet 30:271, 1978.

255. Neer RM: The evolutionary significance of vitamin D, skin pigment, and ultraviolet light. Am J Phys Anthropol 43:409, 1975.

256. Nelson AM, Riggs BL, Jowsey JO: Atypical axial osteomalacia, report of four cases with two having features of ankylosing spondylitis. Arthritis Rheum 21:715, 1978.

257. Neville PF, DeLuca HF: The synthesis of (1,2-³H) vitamin D₃ and the tissue localization of a 0.25-μg (10 IU) dose per rat. J Biochem 5:2201, 1966.

258. Norfray J, Calenoff L, DelGreco F, et al: Renal osteodystrophy in patients on hemodialysis as reflected in the bony pelvis. AJR 125:352, 1975.

259. Norman AW: 1,25-dihydroxyvitamin D₃: A kidney-produced steroid hormone essential to calcium homeostasis. Am J Med 57:21, 1974.

260. Norman AW, Haussler MR, Adams TH, et al: Basic studies on the mechanism of action of vitamin D. Am J Clin Nutr 22:396, 1969.

261. Norman AW, Henry H: The role of the kidney and vitamin D metabolism in health and disease. Clin Orthop 98:258, 1974.

262. O'Connell DJ, Marx WJ: Hand changes in primary biliary cirrhosis. Radiology 129:31, 1978.

263. Oettinger CW, Merrill R, Blanton T, et al: Reduced calcium absorption after nephrectomy in uremic patients. N Engl J Med 291:458, 1974.

264. Offermann G, Kruse R: Prophylactic vitamin D supplementation in chronic anticonvulsant therapy. In Vitamin D: Biochemical, Chemical and Clinical Aspects Related to Calcium Metabolism. Proceedings of the Third Workshop on Vitamin D, Asilomar, Pacific Grove, California, January 1977, p 805. New York, Walter de Gruyter, 1977.

265. Oldham SB, Fischer JA, Shen LH, et al: Isolation and properties of a calcium-binding protein from porcine parathyroid glands. Biochemistry 13:4790, 1974.

266. Oldham SB, Smith R, Hartenbower D, et al: The effects of 1,25-dihydroxyvitamin D₃ (1,25-[OH]₂-D₃) on serum calcium (SCa), immunoreactive parathyroid hormone (IPTH) and the intestinal and parathyroid calcium binding proteins (ICaBP and PCaBP) in the dog (Abstr). Clin Res 24:118A, 1976.

267. Omdahl JL, DeLuca HF: Regulation of vitamin D metabolism and function. Physiol Rev 53:327, 1973.

268. Page CM, Hulme B, Papapoulos SE, et al: Avascular necrosis of bone after renal transplantation: Role of parathyroid hormone and vitamin D. Br Med J 3:664, 1978.

269. Park E, Howland J: The dangers to life of severe involvement of the thorax in rickets. Bull Johns Hopkins Hosp 31:101, 1921.

270. Parfitt AM: Renal osteodystrophy. Orthop Clin North Am 3:681, 1972.

271. Parfitt AM: Soft-tissue calcification in uremia. Arch Intern Med 124:544, 1969.

272. Parfitt AM, Chir B: Hypophosphatemic vitamin D refractory rickets and osteomalacia. Orthop Clin North Am 3:653, 1972.

273. Parfitt AM, Massry SG, Winfield AC, et al: Disordered calcium and phosphorus metabolism during maintenance hemodialysis. Am J Med 51:319, 1971.

274. Parfitt AM, Miller MJ, Frame B, et al: Metabolic bone disease after intestinal bypass for treatment of obesity. Ann Intern Med 89:193, 1978.

275. Park EA: Observations on the pathology of rickets with particular reference to the changes at the cartilage-shaft junctions of the growing bones. Bull NY Acad Med 15:495, 1939.

276. Park EA: The Blackader lecture on some aspects of rickets. Can Med Assoc J 26:3, 1932.

277. Park EA: The influence of severe illness on rickets. Arch Dis Child 29:369, 1954.

278. Parsons LG: The bone changes occurring in renal and coeliac infantilism, and their relationship to rickets. Part I. Renal rickets. Arch Dis Child 2:1, 1927.

279. Parsons LG: The bone changes occurring in renal and coeliac infantilism and their relationship to rickets. Part II. Coeliac rickets. Arch Dis Child 2:198, 1927.

280. Patton JT: Skeletal Changes in Hypophosphataemic Osteomalacia. Symposium Ossium. London, E&S Livingstone Ltd, 1970, p 299.

281. Pavlovitch H, Garabedian M, Balsan S: Calcium-mobilizing effect of large doses of 25-hydroxycholecalciferol in anephric rats. J Clin Invest 52:2656, 1973.

282. Peacock M: Renal bone disease. Practitioner 220:913, 1978.

283. Petith MM, Wilson HD, Schedl HP: Vitamin D dependence of in vivo calcium transport and mucosal calcium binding protein in rat large intestine. Gastroenterology 76:99, 1979.

284. Pettifor JM, Ross FP, Solomon L: Seasonal variation in serum 25-hydroxycholecalciferol concentrations in elderly South African patients with fractures of femoral neck. Br Med J 1:826, 1978.

285. Piel CF, Roof BS, Avioli LV: Metabolism of tritiated 25-hydroxycholecalciferol in chronically uremic children before and after successful renal homotransplantation. J Clin Endocrinol Metab 37:944, 1973.

286. Pierides AM, Ellis HA, Kerr DNS: Phosphate-deficiency osteomalacia during regular haemodialysis. Lancet 2:746, 1976.

287. Pierides AM, Ellis HA, Ward M, et al: Barbiturate and anticonvulsant treatment in relation to osteomalacia with haemodialysis and renal transplantation. Br Med J 1:190, 1976.

288. Pietrek J, Preece MA, Windo J, et al: Prevention of vitamin-D deficiency in Asians. Lancet 1:1145, 1976.

289. Pitt MJ, Haussler MR: Vitamin D: Biochemistry and clinical applications. Skel Radiol 1:191, 1977.

290. Pitt MJ, Haussler MR, Davis JR: Current concepts of vitamin D metabolism: Correlation with clinical syndromes. Crit Rev Radiol Sci 10:129, 1977.

291. Pollack JA, Schiller AL, Crawford JD: Rickets and myopathy cured by removal of a nonossifying fibroma of bone. Pediatrics 52:363, 1973.

292. Ponchon G, Kennan AL, DeLuca HF: "Activation" of vitamin D by the liver. J Clin Invest 48:2032, 1969.

293. Popovtzer MM, Robinette JB: The effect of 25-OH-Vit D₃ on renal handling of phosphorus. Evidence for two reabsorptive mechanisms for phosphorus (Abstr). Clin Res 22:477A, 1974.

294. Popovtzer MM, Robinette JB, DeLuca HF, et al: The acute effect of 25-hydroxycholecalciferol on renal handling of phosphorus. Evidence for a parathyroid hormone-dependent mechanism. J Clin Invest 53:913, 1974.

295. Popovtzer MM, Robinette JB, McDonald KM, et al: Effect of Ca⁺⁺ on renal handling of PO₄⁻: Evidence for two reabsorptive mechanisms. Am J Physiol 229:901, 1975.

296. Potter DE: Renal osteodystrophy in children. Dial Transplant 5:53, 1976.

297. Prader A, Illig R, Uehlinger RE, et al: Rachitis infolge Knochen-tumors. Helv Paediatr Acta 14:554, 1959.

298. Preece MA, O'Riordan JLH, Lawson DEM, et al: A competitive protein-binding assay for 25-hydroxycholecalciferol and 25-hydroxyergocalciferol in serum. Clin Chim Acta 54:235, 1974.
299. Preece MA, Tomlinson S, Ribot CA, et al: Studies of vitamin D deficiency in man. Q J Med 44:575, 1975.
300. Preece MA, Valman HB: Vitamin D status after resection of ileum in childhood. Arch Dis Child 50:283, 1975.
301. Puschett JB, Moranz J, Kurnick WS: Evidence for a direct action of cholecalciferol and 25-hydroxycholecalciferol on the renal transport of phosphate, sodium, and calcium. J Clin Invest 51:373, 1972.
302. Pylupchuk G, Oreopoulos DG, Wilson DR, et al: Calcium metabolism in adult outpatients with epilepsy receiving long-term anticonvulsant therapy. Can Med Assoc J 118:635, 1978.
303. Rab SM, Baseer A: Occult osteomalacia amongst healthy and pregnant women in Pakistan. Lancet 2:1211, 1976.
304. Rang M: The Growth Plate and Its Disorders. Baltimore, Williams & Wilkins Co, 1969.
305. Rasmussen H, Anast C, Parks J, et al: 1-(OH)D₃ in treatment of hypophosphatemic rickets. Clin Res 24:486A, 1976.
306. Rasmussen H, Bordier P, Kurokawa K, et al: Hormonal control of skeletal and mineral homeostasis. Am J Med 56:751, 1974.
307. Rasmussen H, DeLuca HF, Arnaud C, et al: The relationship between vitamin D and parathyroid hormone. J Clin Invest 42:1940, 1963.
308. Rasmussen H, Wong M, Bikle D, et al: Hormonal control of the renal conversion of 25-hydroxycholcalciferol to 1,25-dihydroxycholecalciferol. J Clin Invest 51:2502, 1972.
309. Rathbun JC, MacDonald JW, Robinson HMC, et al: Hypophosphatasia: A genetic study. Arch Dis Child 36:540, 1961.
310. Ravid M, Robson M: Proximal myopathy caused by iatrogenic phosphate depletion. JAMA 236:1380, 1976.
311. Reade TM, Scriver CR, Glorieux FH, et al: Response to crystalline 1α-hydroxyvitamin D₃ in vitamin D dependency. Pediatr Res 9:593, 1975.
312. Reinhold JG: Rickets in Asian immigrants. Lancet 2:1132, 1976.
313. Renton P, Shaw DG: Hypophosphatemic osteomalacia secondary to vascular tumors of bone and soft tissue. Skel Radiol 1:21, 1976.
314. Resnick D, Niwayama G: Subchondral resorption of bone in renal osteodystrophy. Radiology 118:315, 1976.
315. Reynolds WA, Karo JJ: Radiologic diagnosis of metabolic bone disease. Orthop Clin North Am 3:521, 1972.
316. Richards IDG, Sweet EM, Arneil GC: Infantile rickets persists in Glasgow. Lancet 1:803, 1968.
317. Rikkers H, Kletziens RF, DeLuca HF: Vitamin D binding globulin in the rat: Specificity for the vitamins D. Proc Soc Exp Biol Med 130:1321, 1969.
318. Ritchie WGM, Winney RJ, Davison AM, et al: Periosteal new bone formation developing during haemodialysis for chronic renal failure. Br J Radiol 48:656, 1975.
319. Ritz E, Mehls O, Malluche H, et al: Unanswered problems in uremic bone disease. In Vitamin D and Problems Related to Uremic Bone Disease. Proceedings of the Second Workshop on Vitamin D, Wiesbaden, Germany, October 1974, p 497. New York, Walter de Gruyter, 1975.
320. Rodbro P, Christiansen C: Anticonvulsant osteomalacia treated with different doses of vitamin D₂. In Vitamin D and Problems Related to Uremic Bone Disease. Proceedings of the Second Workshop on Vitamin D, Wiesbaden, Germany, October 1974, p 749. New York, Walter de Gruyter, 1975.
321. Rojanasathit S, Haddad JG: Ontogeny and effect of vitamin D deprivation on rat serum 25-hydroxyvitamin D binding protein. Endocrinology 100:642, 1977.
322. Rose E, Espinoza LR, Osterland K: Intestinal bypass arthritis: Association with circulating immune complexes and HLA B27. J Rheumatol 4:129, 1977.
323. Rowe JC, Wood DH, Rowe DW, et al: Nutritional hypophosphatemic rickets in a premature infant fed breast milk. N Engl J Med 300:293, 1979.
324. Russell JE, Avioli LV: Effect of experimental chronic renal insufficiency on bone mineral and collagen maturation. J Clin Invest 51:3072, 1972.
325. Russell RGG, Smith R, Preston C, et al: The effect of 1,25-dihydroxycholecalciferol on renal tubular reabsorption of phosphate, intestinal absorption of calcium, and bone histology in hypophosphataemic renal tubular rickets. Clin Sci Mol Med 48:177, 1975.
326. Russell J, Termine JD, Avioli LV: Abnormal bone mineral maturation in the chronic uremic state. J Clin Invest 52:2848, 1973.
327. Salimpour R: Rickets in Tehran—study of 200 cases. Arch Dis Child 50:63, 1975.
328. Schachter D, Finkelstein JD, Kowarski S: Metabolism of vitamin D. I. Preparation of radioactive vitamin D and its intestinal absorption in the rat. J Clin Invest 43:787, 1964.
329. Schaefer K, Kraft D, VonHerrath D, et al: Intestinal absorption of vitamin D₃ in epileptic patients and phenobarbital-treated rats. Epilepsia 13:509, 1972.
330. Schull MW, Reed RB, Valadian I, et al: Velocities of growth in vegetarian preschool children. Pediatrics 60:410, 1977.
331. Schmorl G: Die pathologische Anatomie de rachitischen Knochenerkrankung mit besonderer Berucksichtigung iher Histologie und Pathogenese. Ergebn inn Med Kinder 4:403, 1909.
332. Schulman JD, Schneider JA: Cystinosis and the Fanconi syndrome. Pediatr Clin North Am 23:779, 1976.
333. Schuster W: Radiological follow-up examination of the mineral salt content in the various vitamin-D resistant forms of rachitis of renal origin. Pediatr Radiol 2:191, 1974.
334. Scott J, Elias E, Moult PJA, et al: Rickets in adult cystic fibrosis with myopathy, pancreatic insufficiency and proximal renal tubular dysfunction. Am J Med 63:488, 1977.
335. Scriver CR: Familial hypophosphatemia: The dilemma of treatment. N Engl J Med 289:531, 1973.
336. Scriver CR: Rickets and the pathogenesis of impaired tubular transport of phosphate and other solutes. Am J Med 57:43, 1974.
337. Scriver CR, Cameron D: Pseudohypophosphatasia. N Engl J Med 281:604, 1969.
338. Scriver CR, Reade TM, DeLuca HF, et al: Serum 1,25-dihydroxyvitamin D levels in normal subjects and in patients with hereditary rickets or bone disease. N Engl J Med 299:976, 1978.
339. Shagrin JW, Frame B, Duncan H: Polyarthritis in obese patients with intestinal bypass. Ann Intern Med 75:377, 1971.
340. Shany S, Hirsh J, Berlyne GM: 25-Hydroxycholecalciferol levels in the bedouins in the Negev. Am J Clin Nutr 29:1104, 1976.
341. Shapiro R: Radiologic aspects of renal osteodystrophy. Radiol Clin North Am 10:557, 1972.
342. Shaw JCL: Evidence for defective skeletal mineralization in low birthweight infants: The absorption of calcium and fat. Pediatrics 57:16, 1976.
343. Sherk HH, Cruz M, Stambaugh J: Vitamin D prophylaxis and the lowered incidence of fractures in anticonvulsant rickets and osteomalacia. Clin Orthop 129:251, 1977.
344. Sherrard DJ: Bone disease in uremia. Dial Transplant 5:12, 72, 1975–76.
345. Short EM, Binder HJ, Rosenberg LE: Familial hypophosphatemic rickets: Defective transport of inorganic phosphate by intestinal mucosa. Science 179:700, 1973.
346. Silverberg DS, Bettcher KB, Dossetor JB, et al: Effect of 1,25-dihydroxycholecalciferol in renal osteodystrophy. Can Med Assoc J 112:190, 1975.
347. Sitrin M, Meredith S, Rosenberg IH: Vitamin D deficiency and bone disease in gastrointestinal disorders. Arch Intern Med 138:886, 1978.
348. Skinner RK, Long RG, Sherlock S, et al: 25-Hydroxylation of vitamin D in primary biliary cirrhosis. Lancet 1:720, 1977.
349. Slatopolsky E, Rutherford WE, Hruska K, et al: How important is phosphate in the pathogenesis of renal osteodystrophy? Arch Intern Med 138:848, 1978.
350. Smith R: The pathophysiology and management of rickets. Orthop Clin North Am 3:601, 1972.
351. Somerville PJ, Kaye M: Resistance to parathyroid hormone in renal failure. Role of vitamin D metabolites. Kidney Int 14:245, 1978.
352. Sorensen OH, Lund B, Hilden M, et al: 25-hydroxylation in chronic alcoholic liver disease. In Vitamin D and Problems Related to Uremic Bone Disease. Proceedings of the Second Workshop on Vitamin D, Wiesbaden, Germany, October 1974, p 843. New York, Walter de Gruyter, 1975.
353. Sotaniemi EA, Hakkarainen HK, Puranen JA, et al: Radiologic bone changes and hypocalcemia with anticonvulsant therapy in epilepsy. Ann Intern Med 77:389, 1972.
354. Stamp TCB, Exton-Smith AN, Richens A: Classical rickets and osteomalacia in Britain. Lancet 2:308, 1976.
355. Stamp TCB, Round JM: Seasonal changes in human plasma levels of 25-hydroxyvitamin D. Nature 247:563, 1974.
356. Stanbury SW, Lumb GA, Mawer EB: Osteodystrophy developing spontaneously in the course of chronic renal failure. Arch Intern Med 124:274, 1969.
357. Steinbach HL, Kolb FO, Crane JT: Unusual roentgen manifestations of osteomalacia. AJR 82:875, 1959.
358. Steinbach HL, Kolb FO, Gilfillan R: A mechanism of the production of pseudofractures in osteomalacia (Milkman's syndrome). Radiology 62:388, 1954.
359. Steinbach HL, Noetzli M: Roentgen appearance of the skeleton in osteomalacia and rickets. AJR 91:955, 1964.
360. Sutcliffe J, Stanley P: Metaphyseal chondrodysplasia. In HJ Kaufmann (Ed): Progress in Pediatric Radiology. Vol 4. Intrinsic Diseases of Bones. New York, S Karger, 1973, p 250.
361. Talwalkar YB, Musgrave JE, Buist NRM, et al: Vitamin D-resistant rickets and parathyroid adenomas. Am J Dis Child 128:704, 1974.
362. Tanaka A, Castillo L, DeLuca HF: Control of renal vitamin D hydroxylases in birds by sex hormones. Proc Natl Acad Sci 73:2701, 1976.
363. Tanaka Y, DeLuca HF: Role of 1,25-dihydroxyvitamin D₃ in maintaining serum phosphorus and curing rickets. Proc Nat Acad Sci 71:1040, 1974.
364. Tanaka Y, DeLuca HF: The control of 25 hydroxyvitamin D metabolism by inorganic phosphorus. Arch Biochem Biophys 154:566, 1973.
365. Taylor CM: The measurement of 24,25-dihydroxycholecalciferol in human serum. Vitamin D: Biochemical, Chemical, and Clinical Aspects Related to Calcium Metabolism. Proceedings of the Third Workshop on Vitamin D, Asilomar, Pacific Grove, California, January 1977, p 541. New York, Walter de Gruyter, 1977.
366. Taylor AN, Wasserman RH: Immunofluorescent localization of vitamin D-dependent calcium-binding protein. J Histochem Cytochem 18:107, 1969.
367. Taylor AN, Wasserman RH: Vitamin D-induced calcium-binding protein: Comparative aspects in kidney and intestine. Am J Physiol 223:110, 1972.
368. Teitelbaum SL, Halverson JD, Bates M, et al: Abnormalities of circulating 25-OH vitamin D after jejunal-ileal bypass for obesity. Evidence of an adaptive response. Ann Intern Med 86:289, 1977.
369. Thomas PS, Obst D, Glasgow JFT: The "mandibular mantle"—a sign of rickets in very low birth weight infants. Br J Radiol 51:93, 1978.
370. Thompson GR, Lewis B, Neale G, et al: Mechanisms of vitamin D deficiency in patients with lesions of the gastrointestinal tract. N Engl J Med 272:486, 1965.

371. Tolman KG, Jubiz W, Sannella JJ, et al: Osteomalacia associated with anticonvulsant drug therapy in mentally retarded children. Pediatrics 56:45, 1975.
372. Tryfus H: Hepatic rickets. Ann Pediatr 192:81, 1959.
373. Tucker G, Gagnon RE, Haussler MR: Vitamin D₃-hydroxylase tissue occurrence and apparent lack of regulation. Arch Biochem Biophys 155:47, 1973.
374. Tulloch AL: Rickets in the premature. Med J Aust 1:137, 1974.
375. Velentzas C, Oreopoulos DG, From G, et al: Vitamin D levels in thyrotoxicosis. Lancet 1:370, 1977.
376. Verberckmoes R, Bouillon R, Krempien B: Disappearance of vascular calcifications during treatment of renal osteodystrophy—two patients treated with high doses of vitamin D and aluminum hydroxide. Ann Intern Med 82:529, 1975.
377. Villareale ME, Chiroff RT, Bergstron WH, et al: Bone changes induced by diphenylhydantoin in chicks on a controlled vitamin D intake. J Bone Joint Surg [Am] 60:911, 1978.
378. Villareale M, Gould LV, Wasserman RH, et al: Diphenylhydantoin: Effects on calcium metabolism in the chick. Science 183:671, 1974.
379. Wagonfeld JB, Bolt M, Boyer JL, et al: Comparison of vitamin D and 25-hydroxy-vitamin D in the therapy of primary biliary cirrhosis. Lancet 2:391, 1976.
380. Walker ARP: Does a low intake of calcium cause or promote the development of rickets? Am J Clin Nutr 3:114, 1955.
381. Walker ARP: The human requirement of calcium: Should low intakes be supplemented? Am J Clin Nutr 25:518, 1972.
382. Walton J: Familial hypophosphatemic rickets; a delineation of its subdivisions and pathogenesis. Clin Pediatr 15:1007, 1976.
383. Wasserman RH, Taylor AN: Evidence for a vitamin D₃-induced calcium-binding protein in New World primates. Proc Soc Exp Biol Med 136:25, 1971.
384. Wasserman RH, Taylor AN: Intestinal absorption of phosphate in the chick: Effect of vitamin D₃ and other parameters. J Nutr 103:586, 1973.
385. Wasserman RH, Taylor AN: Vitamin D₃-induced calcium-binding protein in chick intestinal mucosa. Science 152:791, 1966.
386. Weber JC, Pons V, Kodicek E: The localization of 1,25-dihydroxycholecalciferol in bone cell nuclei of rachitic chicks. Biochem J 125:147, 1971.
387. Weick, MT: A history of rickets in the United States. Am J Clin Nutr 20:1234, 1967.
388. Winnacker JL, Yeager H, Saunders JA, et al: Rickets in children receiving anticonvulsant drugs. Am J Dis Child 131:286, 1977.
389. Werder EA, Kind HP, Egert F, et al: Effective long-term treatment of pseudohypoparathyroidism with oral 1-hydroxy- and 1,25-dihydroxycholecalciferol. J Pediatr 89:266, 1976.
390. Whelton MJ, Kehayoglou AK, Agnew JE, et al: Calcium absorption in parenchymatous and biliary liver disease. Gut 12:978, 1971.
391. Wong RG, Norman AW, Reddy CR, et al: Biologic effects of 1,25-dihydroxycholecalciferol (a highly active vitamin D metabolite) in acutely uremic rats. J Clin Invest 51:1287, 1972.
392. Wright JA: Trinuride in the treatment of major epilepsy. Epilepsia 6:67, 1965.
393. Yoshikawa S, Nakamura T, Takagi M, et al: Benign osteoblastoma as a cause of osteomalacia, a report of two cases. J Bone Joint Surg [Br] 59:279, 1977.
394. Yu JS, Walker-Smith JA, Burnard ED: Rickets: A common complication of neonatal hepatitis. Med J Aust 1:790, 1971.
395. Zanzi I, Schoen M, Roginsky MS, et al: Skeletal mass and serum levels of 25-hydroxyvitamin D in postgastrectomy patients. In Vitamin D: Biochemical, Chemical and Clinical Aspects Related to Calcium Metabolism. Proceedings of the Third Workshop on Vitamin D, Asilomar, Pacific Grove, California, January 1977, p 859. New York, Walter de Gruyter, 1977.
396. Zerwekh JE: Vitamin D-dependent intestinal calcium absorption. Gastroenterology 76:404, 1979.
397. Zerwekh JE, Haussler MR, Lindell TJ: Rapid enhancement of chick intestinal DNA-dependent RNA polymerase II activity by 1α,25-dihydroxyvitamin D₃, in vivo. Proc Natl Acad Sci 71:2337, 1974.
398. Avioli LV, Haddad JG: Editorial retrospective: The vitamin D family revisited. N Engl J Med 311:47, 1984.
399. Koide Y, Kugai N, Kimura S, et al: Increased 1,25-dihydroxycholecalciferol as a cause of abnormal calcium metabolism in sarcoidosis. J Clin Endocrinol Metab 52:494, 1981.
400. Barbour GL, Coburn JW, Slatopolsky E, et al: Hypercalcemia in an anephric patient with sarcoidosis: Evidence for extrarenal generation of 1,25-dihydroxyvitamin D. N Engl J Med 305:440, 1981.
401. Bell NH, Stern PH, Pantzer E, et al: Evidence that increased circulating 1α,25-dihydroxyvitamin D is the probable cause for abnormal calcium metabolism in sarcoidosis. J Clin Invest 64:218, 1979.
402. Sandler LM, Winearls CG, Fraher LJ, et al: Studies of the hypercalcaemia of sarcoidosis: Effect of steroids and exogenous vitamin D₃ on the circulating concentrations of 1,25-dihydroxyvitamin D₃. Q J Med 53:165, 1984.
403. Turner RT, Howard GA, Puzas JE, et al: Calvarial cells synthesize 1α,25-dihydroxyvitamin D₃ from 25-hydroxyvitamin D₃. Biochemistry 22:1073, 1983.
404. Mason RS, Frankel T, Chan YL, et al: Vitamin D conversion by sarcoid lymph node homogenate. Ann Intern Med 100:59, 1984.
405. Davies M, Hayes ME, Mawer EB, et al: Abnormal vitamin D metabolism in Hodgkin's lymphoma. Lancet 1:1186, 1985.
406. Rosenthal N, Insogna KL, Godsall JW, et al: Elevations in circulating 1,25-dihydroxyvitamin D in three patients with lymphoma-associated hypercalcemia. J Clin Endocrinol Metab 60:29, 1985.
407. Sweet RA, Males JL, Hamstra AJ, et al: Vitamin D metabolite levels in oncogenic osteomalacia. Ann Intern Med 93:279, 1980.
408. Taylor HC, Fallon MD, Velasco ME: Oncogenic osteomalacia and inappropriate antidiuretic hormone secretion due to oat-cell carcinoma. Ann Intern Med 101:786, 1984.
409. Turner ML, Dalinka MK: Osteomalacia: Uncommon causes. AJR 133:539, 1979.
410. Silver J, Landau H, Bab I, Shvil Y, et al: Vitamin D-dependent rickets types I and II: Diagnosis and response to therapy. Isr J Med Sci 21:53, 1985.
411. Gamblin GT, Liberman UA, Eil C, et al: Vitamin D-dependent rickets type II. Defective induction of 25-hydroxyvitamin D₃-24-hydroxylase by 1,25-dihydroxyvitamin D₃ in cultured skin fibroblasts. J Clin Invest 75:954, 1985.
412. Eil C, Liberman UA, Rosen JF, et al: A cellular defect in hereditary vitamin-D-dependent rickets type II: Defective nuclear uptake of 1,25-dihydroxyvitamin D in cultured skin fibroblasts. N Engl J Med 304:1588, 1981.
413. Harrison HE, Finberg L: Rickets: Primary hypophosphatemic and vitamin D-dependent varieties. J Pediatr 99:84, 1981.
414. Delvin EE, Glorieux FH, Marie PJ, et al: Vitamin D dependency: Replacement therapy with calcitriol. J Pediatr 99:26, 1981.
415. Feldman D, Chen T, Cone C, et al: Vitamin D resistant rickets with alopecia: Cultured skin fibroblasts exhibit defective cytoplasmic receptors and unresponsiveness to 1,25(OH)₂D₃. J Clin Endocrinol 55:1020, 1982.
416. Cowen J, Harris F: Late presentation of vitamin D-dependent rickets. Arch Dis Child 55:964, 1980.
417. Tsuchiya Y, Matsuo N, Cho H, et al: An unusual form of vitamin D-dependent rickets in a child: Alopecia and marked end-organ hyposensitivity to biologically active vitamin D. J Clin Endocrinol Metab 51:685, 1980.
418. Alpan G, Mogle P, Patz D, et al: Respiratory failure and multiple fractures in vitamin D-dependent rickets. Acta Paediatr Scand 74:300, 1985.
419. Bell NH: Vitamin D-dependent rickets Type II. Calcif Tissue Int 31:89, 1980.
420. Chen TL, Hirst MA, Cone CM, et al: 1,25-dihydroxyvitamin D resistance, rickets, and alopecia: Analysis of receptors and bioresponse in cultured fibroblasts from patients and parents. J Clin Endocrinol Metab 59:383, 1984.
421. Marx SJ, Liberman UA, Eil C, et al: Hereditary resistance to 1,25-dihydroxyvitamin D. Recent Prog Horm Res 40:589, 1984.
422. Polisson RP, Martinez S, Khoury M, et al: Calcification of entheses associated with X-linked hypophosphatemic osteomalacia. N Engl J Med 313:1, 1985.
423. Cartwright DW, Masel JP, Latham SC: The lumbar spinal canal in hypophosphataemic vitamin D-resistant rickets. Aust NZ J Med 11:154, 1981.
424. Milgram JW, Compere CL: Hypophosphatemic vitamin D refractory osteomalacia with bilateral femoral pseudofractures. Clin Orthop 160:78, 1981.
425. Lyles KW, Clark AG, Drezner MK: Serum 1,25-dihydroxyvitamin D levels in subjects with X-linked hypophosphatemic rickets and osteomalacia. Calcif Tissue Int 34:125, 1982.
426. Meyer RA, Gray RW, Roos BA, et al: Increased plasma 1,25-dihydroxyvitamin D after low calcium challenge in X-linked hypophosphatemic mice. Endocrinology 111:174, 1982.
427. Mason RS, Rohl PG, Lissner D, et al: Vitamin D metabolism in hypophosphatemic rickets. Am J Dis Child 136:909, 1982.
428. Glorieux FH, Marie PJ, Pettifor JM, et al: Bone response to phosphate salts, ergocalciferol, and calcitriol in hypophosphatemic vitamin D-resistant rickets. N Engl J Med 303:1023, 1980.
429. Evans GA, Arulanantham K, Gage JR: Primary hypophosphatemic rickets. J Bone Joint Surg [Am] 62:1130, 1980.
430. Chesney RW, Mazess RB, Rose P, et al: Long-term influence of calcitriol (1,25-dihydroxyvitamin D) and supplemental phosphate in X-linked hypophosphatemic rickets. Pediatrics 71:559, 1983.
431. Price HV, Woodhead JS: Hypophosphataemic vitamin-D resistant rickets may need phosphate supplements. Br Med J 284:1442, 1982.
432. Marie PJ, Travers R, Glorieux FH: Bone response to phosphate and vitamin D metabolites in the hypophosphatemic male mouse. Calcif Tissue Int 34:158, 1982.
433. Elidrissy ATH, Sedrani SH, Lawson DEM: Vitamin D deficiency in mothers of rachitic infants. Calcif Tissue Int 36:266, 1984.
434. Greer FR, Hollis BW, Cripps DJ, et al: Effects of maternal ultraviolet B irradiation on vitamin D content of human milk. J Pediatr 105:431, 1984.
435. Niesen KC, Lilienfeld-Toal HV, Burmeister W: Vitamin D,25-hydroxyvitamin D and 1,25-dihydroxy-vitamin D in cow's milk, infant formulas and breast milk during different stages of lactation. Int J Vitam Nutr Res 54:141, 1984.
436. Fetter WPF, Mettau JW, Degenhart HJ, et al: Plasma 1,25-dihydroxyvitamin D concentrations in preterm infants. Acta Paediatr Scand 74:549, 1985.
437. Hillman LS, Hoff N, Salmons S, et al: Mineral homeostasis in very premature infants: Serial evaluation of serum 25-hydroxyvitamin D, serum minerals, and bone mineralization. J Pediatr 106:970, 1985.
438. Hillman LS, Hollis B, Salmons S, et al: Absorption, dosage, and effect on mineral homeostasis of 25-hydroxycholecalciferol in premature infants: Comparison with 400 and 800 IU vitamin D₂ supplementation. J Pediatr 106:981, 1985.
439. Hillman LS, Salmons S, Dokoh S: Serum 1,25-dihydroxyvitamin D concentrations in premature infants: Preliminary results. Calcif Tissue Int 37:223, 1985.
440. Hellebostad M, Markestad T, Halvorsen KS: Vitamin D deficiency rickets and vitamin B₁₂ deficiency in vegetarian children. Acta Paediatr Scand 74:191, 1985.
441. Lamberg-Allardt C: Vitamin D intake, sunlight exposure and 25-hydroxyvitamin D levels in the elderly during one year. Ann Nutr Metab 28:144, 1984.
442. McKenna MJ, Freaney R, Meade A, et al: Prevention of hypovitaminosis D in the elderly. Calcif Tissue Int 37:112, 1985.

443. Le Vay D: On the derivation of the name "rickets." Proc R Soc Med 68:46, 1975.
444. Weinstein RS, Bryce GF, Sappington LJ, et al: Decreased serum ionized calcium and normal vitamin D metabolite levels with anticonvulsant drug treatment. J Clin Endocrinol Metab 58:1003, 1984.
445. Hahn TJ, Halstead LR: Sequential changes in mineral metabolism and serum vitamin D metabolite concentrations produced by phenobarbital administration in the rat. Calcif Tissue Int 35:376, 1983.
446. Adams JS, Sharma OP, Gacad MA, et al: Metabolism of 25-hydroxyvitamin D₃ by cultured pulmonary alveolar macrophages in sarcoidosis. J Clin Invest 72:1856, 1983.
447. McCrea ES, Rao K, Diaconis JN: Roentgenographic changes during long-term diphenylhydantoin therapy. South Med J 73:312, 1980.
448. Davie MWJ, Lawson DEM, Emberson C, et al: Vitamin D from skin: Contribution to vitamin D status compared with oral vitamin D in normal and anticonvulsant-treated subjects. Clin Sci 63:461, 1982.
449. Hoikka V, Savolainen K, Alhava EM, et al: Anticonvulsant osteomalacia in epileptic outpatients. Ann Clin Res 14:129, 1982.
450. Blayney DW, Jaffe ES, Fisher RI, et al: The human T-cell leukemia/lymphoma virus, lymphoma, lytic bone lesions, and hypercalcemia. Ann Intern Med 98:144, 1983.
451. Mundy GR, Luben RA, Raisz LG, et al: Bone-resorbing activity in supernatants from lymphoid cell lines. N Engl J Med 290:867, 1974.
452. Lyles KW, Berry WR, Haussler M, et al: Hypophosphatemic osteomalacia: Association with prostatic carcinoma. Ann Intern Med 93:275, 1980.
453. Frymoyer JW, Hodgkin W: Adult-onset vitamin D-resistant hypophosphatemic osteomalacia. J Bone Joint Surg [Am] 59:101, 1977.
454. Dent CE, Stamp TCB: Hypophosphataemic osteomalacia presenting in adults. Q J Med, 40:303, 1971.
455. Insogna K, Stewart A, Gertner J: Impaired response to acute phosphorus (P) deprivation in sex-linked hypophosphatemic rickets (Abstr). Calcif Tissue Int 33:315, 1981.
456. Meyer RA, Gray RW, Meyer MH: Abnormal vitamin D metabolism in the X-linked hypophosphatemic mouse. Endocrinology 107:1577, 1979.
457. Zurbrugg RP, Lavanchy P, Blumberg A, et al: Long-term treatment of infantile nephropathic cystinosis with cysteamine. N Engl J Med 313:1460, 1985.
458. Schneider JA: Therapy of cystinosis. N Engl J Med 313:1473, 1985.
459. Hillman LS, Salmons S, Dokoh S: Serum 1,25-dihydroxyvitamin D concentrations in premature infants: Preliminary results. Calcif Tissue Int 37:223, 1985.
460. Haussler MR: Personal communication, 1986.
461. Perry HM, Weinstein RS, Teitelbaum SL, et al: Pseudofractures in the absence of osteomalacia. Skel Radiol 8:17, 1982.
462. Clements MR, Chalmers TM, Fraser DR: Enterohepatic circulation of vitamin D: A reappraisal of the hypothesis. Lancet 1:1376, 1984.
463. Editorial: Hepatic osteomalacia and vitamin D. Lancet 1:943, 1982.
464. Wills MR, Savory J: Vitamin D metabolism and chronic liver disease. Ann Clin Lab Sci 14:189, 1984.
465. Bengoa JM, Sitrin MD, Meredith S, et al: Intestinal calcium absorption and vitamin D status in chronic cholestatic liver disease. Hepatology 4:261, 1984.
466. Riggs BL, Hamstra A, DeLuca HF: Assessment of 25-hydroxyvitamin D 1α-hydroxylase reserve in postmenopausal osteoporosis by administration of parathyroid extract. J Clin Endocrinol Metab 53:833, 1981.
467. Sorensen OH, Lumholtz B, Lund B, et al: Acute effects of parathyroid hormone on vitamin D metabolism in patients with the bone loss of aging. J Clin Endocrinol Metab 54:1258, 1982.
468. Slovik DM, Adams JS, Neer RM, et al: Deficient production of 1,25-dihydroxyvitamin D in elderly osteoporotic patients. N Engl J Med 305:372, 1981.
469. Haussler MR, Donaldson CA, Allegretto EA, et al: New actions of 1,25-dihydroxyvitamin D₃: Possible clues to the pathogenesis of postmenopausal osteoporosis. In C Christiansen, CD Arnaud, BEC Nordin, et al (Eds): Osteoporosis Copenhagen, Aalborg Stift Sbogtrykkeri, 1984, p 725.
470. Sinha TK, DeLuca HF, Bell NH: Evidence for a defect in the formation of 1α,25-dihydroxyvitamin D in pseudohypoparathyroidism. Metabolism 26:731, 1977.
471. Spiegel AM, Levine MA, Marx SJ, et al: Pseudohypoparathyroidism: The molecular basis for hormone resistance—a retrospective. N Engl J Med 307:679, 1982.
472. Levine MA, Downs RW, Moses AM, et al: Resistance to multiple hormones in patients with pseudohypoparathyroidism. Am J Med 74:545, 1983.
473. Marx SJ, Aurbach GD: Heterogeneous hormonal disorder in pseudohypoparathyroidism. N Engl J Med 296:169, 1977.
474. Grodsky GM: General Characteristics of Hormones, Harper's Review of Biochemistry. Los Altos, CA, Lange Medical Publications, 1983.
475. Morel F, Chabardes D, Imbert-Teboul M, et al: Multiple hormonal control of adenylate cyclase in distal segments of the rat kidney. Kidney Int 21(Suppl 11):S-55, 1982.
476. Carlson HE, Brickman AS, Bottazzo GF: Prolactin deficiency in pseudohypoparathyroidism. N Engl J Med 296:140, 1977.
477. Kidd GS, Schaaf M, Adler RA, et al: Skeletal responsiveness in pseudohypoparathyroidism: A spectrum of clinical disease. Am J Med 68:772, 1980.
478. Singleton EB, Teng CT: Pseudohypoparathyroidism with bone changes simulating hyperparathyroidism. Radiology 78:388, 1962.
479. Kolb FO, Steinbach HL: Pseudohypoparathyroidism with secondary hyperparathyroidism and osteitis fibrosa. J Clin Endocrinol Metab 22:59, 1962.
480. Windeck R, Menken U, Benker G, et al: Basal ganglia calcification in pseudohypoparathyroidism type II. Clin Endocrinol 15:57, 1981.
481. Wilson JD, Hadden DR: Pseudohypoparathyroidism presenting with rickets. J Clin Endocrinol Metab 51:1184, 1980.
482. Hall FM, Segall-Blank M, Genant HK, et al: Pseudohypoparathyroidism presenting as renal osteodystrophy. Skel Radiol 6:43, 1981.
483. Burnstein MI, Kottamasu SR, Petitifor JM, et al: Metabolic bone disease in pseudohypoparathyroidism: Radiologic features. Radiology 155:351, 1985.
484. Kriegshauser JS, Swee RG, McCarthy JT, et al: Aluminum toxicity in patients undergoing dialysis: Radiographic findings and prediction of bone biopsy results. Radiology 164:399, 1987.
485. Sundaram M, Dessner D, Ballal S: Solitary, spontaneous cervical and large bone fracture in aluminum osteodystrophy. Skel Radiol 20:91, 1991.
486. Ward MK, Feest TG, Ellis HA, et al: Osteomalacic dialysis osteodystrophy: Evidence for a water-borne aetiological agent, probably aluminum. Lancet 4:841, 1978.
487. Smith GD, Winney RJ, McLean A, et al: Aluminum-related osteomalacia: Response to reverse osmosis water treatment. Kidney Int 32:96, 1987.
488. Mousson C, Charhon SA, Ammar M, et al: Aluminium bone deposits in normal renal function patients after long-term treatment by plasma exchange. Int J Artif Organs 12:664, 1989.
489. Andress DL, Maloney NA, Coburn JW, et al: Osteomalacia and aplastic bone disease in aluminum-related osteodystrophy. J Clin Endocrinol Metab 65:11, 1987.
490. Boyce BF, Byars J, McWilliams S, et al: Histological and electron microprobe studies of mineralisation in aluminium-related osteomalacia. J Clin Pathol 45:502, 1992.
491. Rapoport J, Chaimovitz C, Abulfil A, et al: Aluminum-related osteomalacia: Clinical and histological improvement following treatment with desferrioxamine (DFO). Isr J Med Sci 23:1242, 1987.
492. Heaf JG, Podenphant J, Joffe P, et al: The effect of oral aluminium salts on the bone of non-dialysed uremic patients. Scand J Urol Nephrol 21:229, 1987.
493. Quarles LD, Drezner MK: Aluminum accumulation in patients with chronic renal disease. N Engl J Med 325:208, 1991.
494. Neumann L, Jensen BG: Osteomalacia from Al and Mg antacids. Report of a case of bilateral hip fracture. Acta Orthop Scand 60:361, 1989.
495. Spencer H, Kramer L: Antacid-induced calcium loss. Arch Intern Med 143:657, 1983.
496. Insogna KL, Bordley DR, Caro JF, et al: Osteomalacia and weakness from excessive antacid ingestion. JAMA 244:2544, 1980.
497. Turner MW, Ardila M, Hutchinson T, et al: Sporadic aluminum osteomalacia: identification of patients at risk. Am J Kidney Dis 11:51, 1988.
498. Colussi G, Rombola G, DeFerrari ME, et al: Vitamin D treatment: A hidden risk factor for aluminum bone toxicity? Nephron 47:78, 1987.
499. McKenna MJ, Kleerekoper M, Ellis BI, et al: Atypical insufficiency fractures confused with Looser zones of osteomalacia. Bone 8:71, 1987.
500. Pitt MJ: Rickets and osteomalacia are still around. Radiol Clin North Am 29:97, 1991.
501. Andreoli SP, Bergstein JM, Sherrard DJ: Aluminum intoxication from aluminum-containing phosphate binders in children with azotemia not undergoing dialysis. N Engl J Med 310:1079, 1984.
502. Andreoli SP, Smith JA, Bergstein JM: Aluminum bone disease in children: Radiographic features from diagnosis to resolution. Radiology 156:663, 1985.
503. Vukicevic S: Letter to the Editor. Bone 13:119, 1992.
504. Foldes J, Balena R, Ho A, et al: Hypophosphatemic rickets with hypocalciuria following long-term treatment with aluminum-containing antacid. Bone 12:67, 1991.
505. Klein GL: The aluminum content of parenteral solutions: current status. Nutr Rev 49:74, 1991.
506. Ritchie HH, Hughes MR, Thompson ET, et al: An ochre mutation in the vitamin D receptor gene causes hereditary 1,25-dihydroxyvitamin D₃-resistant rickets in three families. Proc Natl Acad Sci USA 86:9783, 1989.
507. De Braekeleer M, Larochelle J: Population genetics of vitamin D-dependent rickets in northeastern Quebec. Ann Hum Genet 55:283, 1991.
508. Sone T, Marx SJ, Liberman UA: A unique point mutation in the human vitamin D receptor chromosomal gene confers hereditary resistance to 1,25-dihydroxyvitamin D₃. Mol Endocrinol 4:623, 1990.
509. Nagler A, Merchave S, Fabian I, et al: Myeloid progenitors from the bone marrow of patients with vitamin D resistant rickets (type II) fail to respond to 1,25(OH)₂D₃. Br J Haematol 67:267, 1987.
510. Feldman D, Malloy PJ: Hereditary 1,25-dihydroxyvitamin D resistant rickets: Molecular basis and implications for the role of 1,25(OH)₂D₃ in normal physiology. Mol Cell Endocrinol 72:C57, 1990.
511. Balsan S, Garabedian M, Liberman UA, et al: Rickets and alopecia with resistance to 1,25-dihydroxyvitamin D: Two different clinical courses with two different cellular defects. J Clin Endocrinol Metab 57:803, 1983.
512. Liberman UA, Eil C, Holst P, et al: Hereditary resistance to 1,25-dihydroxyvitamin D: Defective function of receptors for 1,25-dihydroxyvitamin D in cells cultured from bone. J Clin Endocrinol Metab 57:958, 1983.
513. Castells S, Greig F, Fusi MA, et al: Severely deficient binding of 1,25-dihydroxyvitamin D to its receptors in a patient responsive to high doses of this hormone. J Clin Endocrinol Metab 63:252, 1986.
514. Takeda E, Kuroda Y, Saijo T, et al: 1α-hydroxyvitamin D₃ treatment of three patients with 1,25-dihydroxyvitamin D–receptor-defect rickets and alopecia. Pediatrics 80:97, 1987.
515. Koeffler HP, Bishop JE, Reichel H, et al: Lymphocyte cell lines from vitamin D-dependent rickets type II show functional defects in the 1,25-dihydroxyvitamin D₃ receptor. Mol Cell Endocrinol 70:1, 1990.

516. Mandla S, Jones G, Tenenhouse H: Normal 24-hydroxylation of vitamin D metabolites in patients with vitamin D-dependency rickets type I. Structural implications for the vitamin D hydroxylases. J Clin Endocrinol Metab 74:814, 1992.
517. Malloy PJ, Hochberg Z, Pike JW, et al: Abnormal binding of vitamin D receptors to deoxyribonucleic acid in a kindred with vitamin D-dependent rickets, type II. J Clin Endocrinol Metab 68:263, 1989.
518. Weisman Y, Jaccard N, Legum C, et al: Prenatal diagnosis of vitamin D-dependent rickets, type II: Response to 1,25-dihydroxyvitamin D in amniotic fluid cells and fetal tissues. J Clin Endocrinol Metab 71:937, 1990.
519. Manandhar DS, Sarkawi S, Hunt MCJ: Rickets with alopecia—remission following a course of 1-α-hydroxy vitamin D₃ therapy. Eur J Pediatr 148:761, 1989.
520. Takeda E, Kokota I, Kawakami I, et al: Two siblings with vitamin-D–dependent rickets type II: No recurrence of rickets for 14 years after cessation of therapy. Eur J Pediatr 149:54, 1989.
521. Walka MM, Daumling S, Hadorn HB, et al: Vitamin D dependent rickets type II with myelofibrosis and immune dysfunction. Eur J Pediatr 150:665, 1991.
522. Malloy PJ, Hochberg Z, Tiosano D, et al: The molecular basis of hereditary 1,25-dihydroxyvitamin D₃ resistant rickets in seven related families. J Clin Invest 86:2071, 1990.
523. Marx SJ, Barsony J: Tissue-selective 1,25-dihydroxyvitamin D₃ resistance: Novel applications of calciferols. J Bone Mineral Res 3:481, 1988.
524. Cooke RJ: Rickets in a very low birth weight infant. J Pediatr Gastroenterol Nutr 9:397, 1989.
525. Lyon AJ, McIntosh N, Wheeler K, et al: Radiological rickets in extremely low birthweight infants. Pediatr Radiol 17:56, 1987.
526. Metabolic bone disease of prematurity. Lancet, p. 200, 1987.
527. Airede AI: Rickets of prematurity: A case report. East Afr Med J 68:1006, 1991.
528. Johnson CB: Neonatal rickets: Metabolic bone disease of prematurity. Neonatal Network 9:13, 1991.
529. Salle BL, Glorieux FH, Delvin EE: Perinatal vitamin D metabolism. Biol Neonate 54:181, 1988.
530. Salle BL, Senterre J, Glorieux FH, et al: Vitamin D metabolism in preterm infants. Biol Neonate 52:119, 1987.
531. Koo WWK, Sherman R, Succop P, et al: Fractures and rickets in very low birth weight infants: Conservative management and outcome. J Pediatr Orthop 9:326, 1989.
532. Fettis B, Walker C, Jackson A, et al: The orthopaedic management of hypophosphataemic rickets. J Pediatr Orthop 11:367, 1991.
533. Hardy DC, Murphy WA, Siegel BA, et al: X-linked hypophosphatemia in adults: Prevalence of skeletal radiographic and scintigraphic features. Radiology 171:402, 1989.
534. Burnstein MI, Lawson JP, Kottamasu SR, et al: The enthesopathic changes of hypophosphatemic osteomalacia in adults: Radiologic findings. AJR 153:785, 1989.
535. Econs MJ, Feussner JR, Samsa GP, et al: X-linked hypophosphatemic rickets with ''rickets.'' Skel Radiol 20:109, 1991.
536. Stamp TCB: Rickets. In CBD Brook (Ed): Clinical Pediatric Endocrinology. Oxford, Blackwell Scientific, 1981, p 547.
537. McAlister WH, Kim GS, Whyte MP: Tibial bowing exacerbated by partial premature epiphyseal closure in sex-linked hypophosphatemic rickets. Radiology 162:461, 1987.
538. Adams JE, Davies M: Intra-spinal new bone formation and spinal cord compression in familial hypophosphataemic vitamin D resistant osteomalacia. Q J Med 61:1117, 1986.
539. Block JE, Piel CF, Selvidge R, et al: Familial hypophosphatemic rickets: Bone mass measurements in children following therapy with calcitriol and supplemental phosphate. Calcif Tiss Int 44:86, 1989.
540. Verge CF, Lam A, Simpson JM, et al: Effects of therapy in X-linked hypophosphatemic rickets. N Engl J Med 325:1843, 1991.
541. Stickler GB, Morgenstern BZ: Hypophosphataemic rickets: Final height and clinical symptoms in adults. Lancet 2:902, 1989.
542. Chan JCM, Chinchilli VM: Growth velocity data and hypophosphatemic rickets. Am J Dis Child 142:14, 1988.
543. Steendijk R, Hauspie RC: The pattern of growth and growth retardation of patients with hypophosphataemic vitamin D–resistant rickets: A longitudinal study. Eur J Pediatr 151:422, 1992.
544. Hanna JD, Niimi K, Chan JCM: X-linked hypophosphatemia. Genetic and clinical correlates. Am J Dis Child 145:865, 1991.
545. Balsan S, Tieder M: Linear growth in patients with hypophosphatemic vitamin D-resistant rickets: Influence of treatment regimen and parental height. J Pediatr 116:365, 1990.
546. Lubani MM, Khuffash FA, Reavey PC, et al: Familial hypophosphataemic rickets: Experience with 24 children from Kuwait. Ann Trop Paediatr 10:377, 1990.
547. Tieder M, Modai D, Shaked U, et al: ''Idiopathic'' hypercalciuria and hereditary hypophosphatemic rickets. Two phenotypical expressions of a common genetic defect. N Engl J Med 316:125, 1987.
548. Tieder M, Arie R, Bab I, et al: A new kindred with hereditary hypophosphatemic rickets with hypercalciuria: Implications for correct diagnosis and treatment. Nephron 62:176, 1992.
549. Thakker RV, Farmery MR, Sakati NA, et al: Genetic linkage studies of X-linked hypophosphataemic rickets in a Saudi Arabian family. Clin Endocrinol 37:338, 1992.
550. Thakker RV, Read AP, Davies KE, et al: Bridging markers defining the map position of X linked hypophosphataemic rickets. J Med Genet 23:756, 1987.
551. Kainer G, Chan JCM: Ask the expert. Pediatr Nephrol 3:372, 1989.
552. Labib M, Marks V: Hypophosphataemic osteomalacia and alcoholism: A possible link. Alcohol Alcoholism 23:111, 1988.
553. Tieder M, Arie R, Modai D, et al: Elevated serum 1,25-dihydroxyvitamin D concentrations in siblings with primary Fanconi's syndrome. N Engl J Med 319:845, 1988.
554. Heney D, Lewis IJ, Bailey CC: Acute ifosfamide-induced tubular toxicity. Lancet 2:103, 1989.
555. Hilgard P, Burkert H: Sodium-2-mercaptoethanesulfonate (MESNA) and ifosfamide nephrotoxicity. Eur J Cancer Clin Oncol 20:1451, 1984.
556. Mewbury-Ecob RA, Noble VW, Barbor PRH: Ifosfamide-induced Fanconi syndrome. Lancet 1:1328, 1989.
557. Skinner R, Pearson ADJ, Price L, et al: Hypophosphataemic rickets after ifosfamide treatment in children. Br Med J 298:1560, 1989.
558. Skinner R, Pearson ADJ, Price L, et al: Nephrotoxicity of ifosfamide in children. Lancet 2:159, 1989.
559. Smeitink J, Verreussel M, Schroder C, et al: Nephrotoxicity associated with ifosfamide in children. Eur J Pediatr 148:164, 1988.
560. Skinner R, Pearson ADJ, Price L, et al: Hypophosphataemic rickets after ifosfamide treatment in children. Br Med J 298:1560, 1989.
561. Burk CD, Restaino I, Kaplan BS, et al: Ifosfamide-induced renal tubular dysfunction and rickets in children with Wilms tumor. J Pediatr 117:331, 1990.
562. Silberzweig JE, Haller JO, Miller S: Ifosfamide: A new cause of rickets. AJR 158:823, 1992.
563. Lambert J, Lips P: Adult hypophosphataemic osteomalacia with Fanconi syndrome presenting in a patient with neurofibromatosis. Neth J Med 35:309, 1989.
564. Skovby F, Svejgaard, Moller J: Hypophosphatemic rickets in linear sebaceous nevus sequence. J Pediatr 11:855, 1987.
565. Quarles LD, Murphy G, Econs MJ, et al: Uremic tumoral calcinosis; preliminary observations suggesting an association with aberrant vitamin D homeostasis. Am J Kidney Dis 18:706, 1991.
566. Mankin HJ: Rickets, osteomalacia, and renal osteodystrophy. Orthop Clin North Am 21:81, 1990.
567. Rafter GW: Elmer McCollum and the disappearance of rickets. Perspect Biol Med 30:527, 1987.
568. DeLuca HF, Krisinger J, Darwish H: The vitamin D system: 1990. Kidney Int 38:S2, 1990.
569. Norman AW: Intestinal calcium absorption: A vitamin D–hormone-mediated adaptive response. Am J Clin Nutr 51:290, 1990.
570. Holick MF, Smith E, Pincus S: Skin as the site of vitamin D synthesis and target tissue for 1,25-dihydroxyvitamin D₃. Arch Dermatol 123:1677a, 1987.
571. Carpenter TO: Mineral regulation of vitamin D metabolism. Bone Mineral 5:259, 1989.
572. Reichel H, Koeffler HP, Norman AW: The role of the vitamin D endocrine system in health and disease. N Engl J Med 320:980, 1989.
573. Jiang Y, Wang Y, Zhao J, et al: Bone remodeling in hypervitaminosis D3: Radiologic-microangiography-pathologic correlations. Invest Radiol 26:213, 1991.

54

Paget's Disease

Donald Resnick, M.D., and Gen Niwayama, M.D.

Paget's disease (osteitis deformans) is a condition of unknown cause affecting approximately 3 per cent of the population over the age of 40 years.[1] Initially described by Paget in 1877,[2] the disease varies considerably in severity: Commonly it is a process localized to one or several regions of the skeleton without significant clinical findings; occasionally it is widespread and severe, producing extensive osseous abnormality and deformity. Paget's disease demonstrates certain geographic and racial characteristics: It appears to be particularly common in inhabitants of Australia, Great Britain, and certain areas of continental Europe; it is not uncommon in the United States; and it is extremely rare among the Chinese.[158, 163] It also is rare in most areas of Africa.[263, 277] Reports of cases affecting several members of a family in various generations and identical twins suggest a genetic basis,[3–7] although this has not been documented clearly in most patients.[8]

The disease is characterized by excessive and abnormal remodeling of bone. Its active phase is associated with aggressive bone resorption and formation, whereas its quiescent phase is associated with a diminished rate of bone turnover. The combination of osseous resorption and apposition produces a diagnostic pathologic and radiographic appearance in which irregular bony fragments with a thickened and disorganized trabecular (mosaic) pattern are visualized as coarsened and enlarged osseous trabeculae on radiographs.

This chapter summarizes the clinical, pathologic, and radiologic features of Paget's disease of bone. Its classification in this book under the heading of metabolic diseases in no way suggests that all of the questions regarding the etiologic basis of the disorder have been answered.

HISTORICAL ASPECTS

Sir James Paget was a superb observer and diagnostician who spoke and wrote of disease with words rich in content and description.[157] On November 14, 1876, he presented to the Medical and Chirurgical Society of London a series of five cases that illustrated a slowly progressive disorder leading to enlargement and deformity of bones. The following year, a detailed report of one of these patients, whom Paget had observed for approximately 20 years, as well as a brief summary of several other persons with the same disorder, was published in the Medico-Chirurgical Transactions.[2] Although other descriptions of the disease preceded his, Paget's account is a lesson in accurate and lucid medical writing, and, in recognition of his work, the disorder simply is called Paget's disease. Paget's words have been quoted in numerous subsequent reports, including the excellent monograph by Hamdy[158]; they also are used in this chapter to emphasize the accuracy of Paget's initial descriptions and to dramatize the clinical manifestations as only Sir James Paget could have done.

It is often said or implied that, in our profession, a man cannot be both practical and scientific; science and practice seem to some people to be incompatible. Each man, they say, must devote himself to the one or the other. The like of this has long been said, and it is sheer nonsense.[159]

SIR JAMES PAGET (1894)

CLINICAL FEATURES

It begins in middle age or later, is very slow in progress, . . . and may give no other trouble than those which are due to changes of shape, size and direction of the diseased bones.

SIR JAMES PAGET (1877)

Paget's disease is common, particularly in middle-aged and elderly persons.[158, 160–162] Schmorl[1] detected 138 cases of this disorder in a study of cadavers of persons over the age of 40 years, a frequency of 3 per cent. Collins[9] reported a frequency of 3.7 per cent in an investigation of 650 unselected necropsies. In this latter study, the disease was exceptional in persons below the age of 40 years, uncommon between the ages of 40 and 55 years, common (3 to 4 per cent) after the age of 55 years, and frequent (10 per cent) in very old people. Other investigators confirm that the disease is present in approximately 10 to 11 per cent of patients over the age of 80 years.[10] Rarely, Paget's disease is documented in patients under 40 years old. Barry[11] noted that 3.7 per cent of 2320 patients with Paget's disease were younger than 40 years, whereas others have reported the frequency of involvement in young adults to be slightly higher.[12, 13] The classic features of Paget's disease are present even in younger patients, allowing accurate diagnosis.[14] Paget's disease is more common in men than in women,[15] although the difference in frequency between the two sexes may not be great.[16] The age of onset of the disease may be slightly lower in men than in women.[244]

Clinical findings in patients with Paget's disease are extremely variable. In many patients, the disorder is diagnosed first as an incidental finding on radiographs obtained for unrelated purposes; it has been suggested that approximately one fifth of persons with pagetic skeletal involvement detectable on radiographs are entirely asymptomatic.[15] Conversely, on occasion the disease is manifested initially with severe symptoms and signs, which may include skeletal, neuromuscular, and cardiovascular complications. In the presence of widespread skeletal involvement, patients appear apathetic, somnolent, and without energy.[158]

In patients with symptoms, clinical findings vary with the distribution of the disease. Although Paget's disease has predilection for the axial skeleton and may be widespread at the time of initial diagnosis, it may affect just one bone and remain limited in its distribution throughout the course of the disease. At other times, the disorder which was first localized to one or two sites may progress to involve much of the skeleton. Local pain and tenderness frequently are present at an affected skeletal site. Pain often is worse at night and unrelated to exercise. Increasing size of a bone may produce clinical findings, such as enlarging head size (the patient may note that his or her hat size constantly is changing) or progressing prominence of the shins. Skeletal deformities include kyphosis and bowing of the long bones of the extremities. Osseous involvement may lead to pathologic fracture, with resulting pain and angulation, or to stiffness and reduced mobility of joints.[245]

Neuromuscular complications are not infrequent.[17] Neurologic deficits, such as muscle weakness, paralysis, and rectal and vesical incontinence, resulting from impingement on the spinal cord, can be apparent in patients with compression fractures of the vertebral bodies.[18] Similar deficits may accompany platybasia owing to involvement of the base of the skull. Compression of cranial nerves in their foramina is not common, although deafness may be apparent. In fact, some investigators suggest that Beethoven's deafness resulted from Paget's disease.[164] Impingement on the auditory nerves usually is the result of pagetic involvement of the temporal bone and labyrinth,[19–21] although structural abnormality of the ossicles of the middle ears also has been observed.[22]

Congestive heart failure has been noted in patients with Paget's disease. Initially, investigators stressed that this complication was due to the presence of arteriovenous shunts in the involved bone, but these observations have not been confirmed.[23] It now seems probable that high output congestive failure is related to hyperemia and increased blood flow in pagetic bone.[24]

Reports have indicated that Paget's disease may be associated with arterial calcification,[16, 25] cardiac valvular calcification,[26] Hashimoto's thyroiditis,[27] and pseudoxanthoma elasticum.[24, 27]

Laboratory analysis in Paget's disease generally reveals elevation of alkaline phosphatase and hydroxyproline levels in the serum and of hydroxyproline levels in the urine.[28–30] The raised serum levels of alkaline phosphatase may be related to an increased rate of bone formation,[31] whereas the elevated urinary levels of hydroxyproline may indicate an increased rate of bone resorption.[32] Urinary hydroxylysine (and hydroxylysine glycoside) excretion also increases in patients with Paget's disease.[165, 264] These chemical abnormalities vary with the distribution and activity of disease; in patients with limited skeletal involvement or inactive disease, aberrations in laboratory values may be absent or not pronounced. Generally, serum alkaline phosphatase is thought to be a less sensitive parameter of pagetic activity than urinary hydroxyproline,[158] although the former may rise sharply in the presence of neoplastic degeneration.[31] Usually serum levels of calcium and phosphorus are normal in patients with Paget's disease, although in affected persons who have developed fractures or are immobilized, hypercalcemia may be found. Serum acid phosphatase values also are normal in this disease, whereas uric acid levels in the serum commonly are elevated. Increased serum levels of procollagen extension fragments reflect increased synthesis of type I collagen (bone matrix) and type III collagen (marrow fibrosis); increased serum levels of γ-carboxyglutamic acid-protein presumably reflect primarily synthesis of bone matrix but indicate bone resorption as well.[264]

As summarized by Hamdy,[158] assessment of both the serum alkaline phosphatase levels and the urinary hydroxyproline levels at frequent intervals is useful in gauging the activity of Paget's disease, especially in cases of monostotic involvement or involvement confined to only a few bones. As urinary hydroxyproline levels are reflective of osteoclastic activity, an increase in excretion of hydroxyproline suggests an osteolytic phase of the disease. In the mixed osteolytic-osteosclerotic phase, osteoclastic activity decreases, accompanied by stationary or decreasing levels of urinary hydroxyproline, and osteoblastic activity increases in association with an elevation in serum levels of alkaline phosphatase. In the inactive sclerotic stage of Paget's disease, serum alkaline phosphatase levels decrease. Too rigid an application of these laboratory parameters is not recommended, owing to fluctuation in serum and urinary values of the enzymes and to enzymatic changes associated with immobilization. Furthermore, in recent years, additional biochemical markers of bone metabolism have been used to assess the activity of Paget's disease. The intermolecular collagen crosslinking compounds pyridinoline and deoxypyridinoline appear to be more specific and less cumbersome to measure than urinary hydroxyproline.[327, 328] Assays for these compounds in the urine correlate well with rates of bone resorption. Scintigraphy also may be valuable in assessing activity of Paget's disease.[256]

ETIOLOGY

With regard to the nature of the process . . . only 3 things could produce so great an increase in the size of a bone, namely, new growth (tumor), hypertrophy, and chronic inflammation. The first of these may be at once set aside as out of the question, nor is the second much more probable than the first. . . . Of the three causes, chronic inflammation alone remains.

SIR JAMES PAGET (1877), QUOTING MR. BUTLIN

The precise cause of Paget's disease is unknown. An inflammatory cause has been suggested by some investigators, including Paget,[2] a view that has gained some support from the clinical improvement that may be observed in patients treated with anti-inflammatory agents.[33] Other proposed etiologic conditions have included a generalized disorder of connective tissue, a vascular or infectious disease, and an autoimmune disorder.[24] The role of parathyroid hormone in Paget's disease also has been emphasized, and elevated parathormone levels in the serum of patients with this disease have been observed.[166] Such levels may reflect active bone apposition, which decreases serum calcium and stimulates parathormone secretion. Although reports of coexistent Paget's disease and hyperparathyroidism have appeared,[131] there is no firm evidence linking the two disorders. In fact, Paget's disease has been recognized in a patient with idiopathic hypoparathyroidism.[132]

Reports of familial aggregation of cases[133–134] have led some investigators to argue that an autosomal dominant pattern of inheritance is present,[135] a concept strengthened by the observation that Paget's disease may be linked to an HLA haplotype.[136] The prevalence of the disease among identical twins is less than expected, however, and the role of heredity in Paget's disease has been questioned.[158]

A neoplastic cause was suggested by Rasmussen and Bordier,[137] in which the primary event was the activation of an abnormally large number of osteoprogenitor cells.

It is a viral cause of the disease that has gained support by observations in a number of more recently published articles. Active pagetic bone is characterized by the presence of giant osteoclasts containing large numbers of nuclei. Intranuclear inclusion bodies have been identified in these cells,[138, 156, 168] which are not observed in osteoblasts or osteocytes of pagetic bone or in osseous tissue derived from patients with a variety of other skeletal disorders, even those characterized by osteoclastic proliferation.[158] Ultra-

structural characteristics of the pagetic osteoclasts suggested that the inclusions were viral in nature (Fig. 54–1). Similar cellular characteristics are observed in disorders produced by certain viruses, specifically subacute sclerosing panencephalitis related to a paramyxovirus of the measles group.[168, 267] Additional morphologic evidence for a viral cause is cited: The dense fibrillar material associated with some of the inclusions is similar to that found in the nuclei of virus-infected cells; filament bundles and spindle-shaped structures enclosed in double membranes observed in the cytoplasm of some osteoclasts are considered an indirect cellular response to viral attack; and the very presence of enormous osteoclasts in pagetic bone is compatible with abnormalities noted with in vitro measles virus infection.[167] The identification of similar intranuclear inclusions within giant cell tumors in patients with Paget's disease[171, 172] is further evidence supporting a viral cause of the disorder (although identical inclusions have been described within giant cell tumors in patients who do not have evidence of Paget's disease[246, 247]), and certain immunocytologic data have reinforced this viral hypothesis.[169, 170, 173, 174] Furthermore, significant and sustained viral antibody titers against the measles virus have been detected in a few patients with Paget's disease; the minimum degree of inflammation and the absence of considerable inflammatory cells in bone and peripheral blood in Paget's disease are compatible with a response to a chronic infection; viral infections may require several years for clinical expression, consistent with the advanced age of most patients with Paget's disease; geographic and familial clustering is typical of an infectious process; and viruses may affect a single organ system selectively, such as the skeletal tissue of patients with Paget's disease.[158] Further support for a viral cause of Paget's disease are the identification of similar intranuclear virus-like microcylindric structures within the osteoclasts in bone affected by familial chronic hyperphosphatasemia, which may be a juvenile form of Paget's disease[265]; and the documentation of a higher frequency of HLA-DR2 in the serum of Ashkenazi Jews with Paget's disease, an antigen that may predispose the bone cells to viral infection.[266] No virus has been cultured from pagetic tissue, however, and no evidence has been found for measles virus, respiratory syncytial virus, canine distemper virus, or related paramyxoviruses in RNA extracted from such tissue.[329] Therefore, the basic nature of the disease is not much clearer than it was at the time of Paget's original description over a century ago.[139]

PATHOPHYSIOLOGY

Paget's disease is a remarkable disorder of bone that evolves through various stages or phases of activity, followed by an inactive or quiescent stage. Its initial characteristic is an intense wave of osteoclastic activity with resorption of normal bone by giant multinucleated cells.[10, 175] Subsequently, excessive and disorganized new bone formation owing to a vigorous osteoblastic response leads to the appearance of osseous tissue that is abnormal architecturally, consisting of primitive or woven bone with increased vascularity and a pronounced connective tissue reaction.[158, 175] Thus, it is a combination of osteoclastic and osteoblastic activity that accounts for marked elevation of the rate of osseous turnover, with succeeding waves of bone

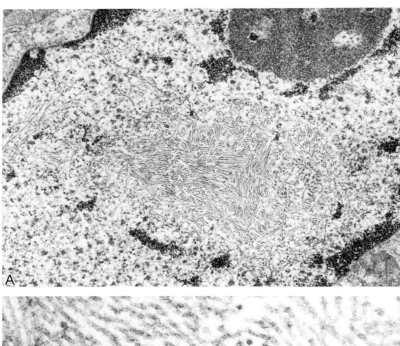

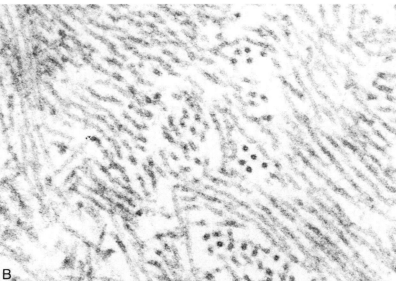

FIGURE 54–1. Viral cause of Paget's disease.

A Nucleus of an osteoclast from a patient with Paget's disease shows a typical example of a nuclear filamentous inclusion. Note the variable orientation of the filaments without obvious attachment to the nucleolus (32,000×).

B A higher magnification photomicrograph illustrates the tubular structure of the microfilaments, cut both in cross section and in parallel to the long axis of the tubules (180,000×).

(From Singer FR, Mills BG: Clin Orthop *178*:245, 1983.)

destruction and bone formation. The coarse-fibered pagetic bone reveals distinct avidity for both calcium and phosphorus[158]; this phenomenon is well documented in isotopic studies in which injected radioactive ions reveal rapid intraosseous incorporation.[176] An increase in regional blood flow, manifested clinically as a rise in skin temperature, is related to hypervascularity of the pagetic bone[177] and cutaneous vasodilation.[178] The osseous tissue contains an increased number of patent capillaries and dilated arterioles; the venous sinuses also are larger than normal.[158] With a decrease in peripheral resistance, the heart rate is increased, and the cardiac output may be elevated.[158] High output cardiac failure is associated with extensive skeletal involvement.

After a variable period of time, osteoclastic activity may decrease, although continued deposition of abnormal bone occurs. Some of the immature woven bone may be replaced by normal-appearing lamellar bone. Microscopic evaluation reveals distortion of the normal trabecular appearance with a mosaic pattern of irregular cement lines joining areas of lamellar bone (Fig. 54–2). As the pagetic bone shows no tendency to form haversian systems or to center on blood vessels, the bones are ivory-hard, difficult to cut, and heavier than normal.[158] Eventually, osteoblastic activity also declines, and the condition becomes quiescent or inactive. In this stage, sclerotic bone is observed, and evidence of continued resorption and increased cellular activity is minimal or absent.[24]

Although the aforementioned changes emphasize a regular sequence of events characterized by an initial increase in osteoclastic activity, followed by increased osteoblastic and decreased osteoclastic activity and, finally, a decrease in osteoblastic activity, this response is not invariable. Furthermore, as Paget's disease commonly is accompanied by widespread involvement of the skeleton, each lesion demonstrates its own pathophysiology with a unique rate of progression. At any one time, multiple stages or phases of the disease process can be identified in different skeletal regions. As indicated previously, a variety of laboratory parameters as well as certain imaging techniques, such as

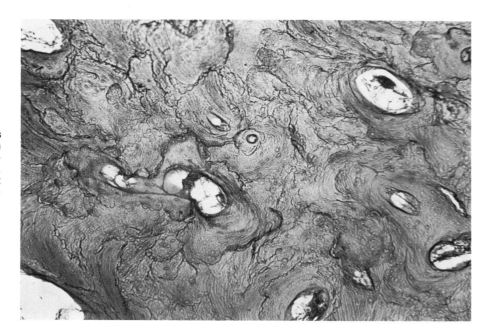

FIGURE 54–2. Histologic abnormalities of Paget's disease: Mosaic pattern. In this photomicrograph (80×) from a femur that is involved by Paget's disease, the typical mosaic pattern of cement lines joining areas of lamellar bone can be seen.

scintigraphy, will allow an overall assessment of the progress of Paget's disease as well as provide information about individual osseous lesions. In addition, the radiographic examination will document in its own fashion the nature and the distribution of the process.

RADIOGRAPHIC-PATHOLOGIC CORRELATION

General Stages of the Disease
(Table 54–1)

The pathologic stages already described have their radiographic counterparts. An initial phase of intense osteoclastic activity with resorption of bone trabeculae may be detected on radiographs as an "osteolytic" form of the disease (Fig. 54–3).[34, 35] This imaging appearance particularly is common in the skull, at which site it is termed osteoporosis circumscripta.[36–38] Osteolysis in the cranial vault is observed most frequently in the frontal or occipital regions and may progress to involve the entire skull. The advancing radiolucent lesion may be sharply delineated from the adjacent normal bone. When a segment of the cranium that is involved with osteoporosis circumscripta is inspected by removing the pericranium and dura, the bone appears dark and red.[16] On cross section, the enlarging diploic bone is found to encroach on the outer and inner tables of the skull. This bone is porous, accounting for its increased radiolucency. Diploic trabeculae are thin and sparse and exhibit increased osteoclastic activity. As elsewhere in the skeleton, this osteolytic phase may be followed by bone sclerosis and condensation.

The osteolytic phase of Paget's disease may be apparent elsewhere in the skeleton, particularly in the long bones, although occasionally other sites may be involved, including the pelvis, the spine, and the small bones of the hands and feet.[34, 39, 179, 252, 321, 330] In tubular bones, osteolysis begins almost invariably in the subchondral regions of the epiphysis and extends subsequently into the metaphysis and diaph-

ysis; occasionally, the disease may appear at both ends of an involved bone, but only exceptionally is Paget's disease apparent in the diaphysis without involvement of the epiphysis. When present, this latter feature typically occurs in the tibia,[180, 257] although other bones, particularly the radius, also may show initial diaphyseal involvement (Fig. 54–3E). As the disease progresses, osteolysis may advance into the diaphysis as a V- or wedge-shaped radiolucent area, clearly demarcated from the adjacent bone. This appearance has

TABLE 54–1. Stages of Paget's Disease

Stage	Most Common Sites	Appearance
Active		
Osteolytic	Cranial vault	Osteoporosis circumscripta
	Long tubular bones	Subchondral location; advancing wedge of radiolucency
Osteolytic or osteosclerotic, or both	Cranial vault	Osteoporosis circumscripta; focal radiodense areas
	Pelvis	Patchy radiolucency and radiodensity
	Long tubular bones	Diaphyseal radiolucency; epiphyseal and metaphyseal radiodensity
Inactive		
Osteosclerotic	Cranial vault	"Cotton-wool" appearance; thickened cranial vault; basilar invagination
	Spine	"Picture frame" vertebral body; ivory vertebral body
	Pelvis	Thickening of pelvic ring; focal or diffuse radiodensity
	Long tubular bones	Epiphyseal predilection; coarse trabeculae; widened and deformed bone

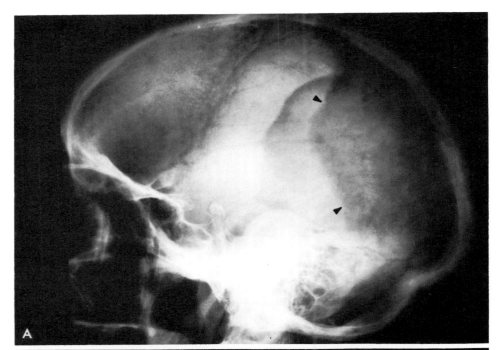

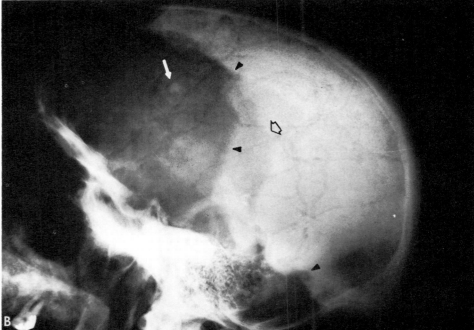

FIGURE 54–3. General stages of Paget's disease: Osteolytic stage.

A, B Cranial vault. Two examples of osteoporosis circumscripta. The osteolytic bone usually commences in the frontal or occipital areas of the skull. Its advancing edge (arrowheads) is well demarcated from adjacent normal bone. Focal radiodense areas (arrow) within the areas of osteolysis are apparent. In some locations, involvement of a portion of the cranial vault has created beveled margins (open arrow).

Illustration continued on opposite page

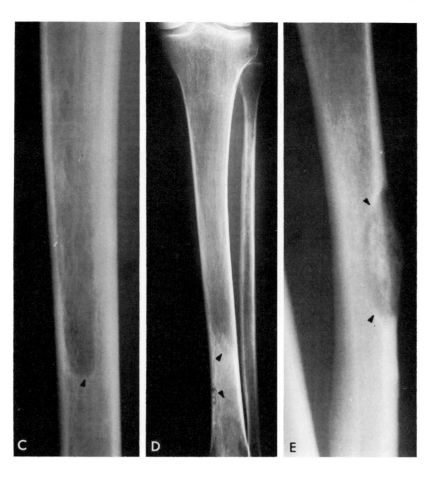

FIGURE 54–3 *Continued*
C–E Tubular bones. **C** An advancing wedge-shaped radiolucent edge (arrowhead) is observed in the femur. **D** Osteolytic edges (arrowheads) are advancing from either end of the tibia separated by a small zone of normal bone. **E** An unusual example of biopsy-proved Paget's disease appears as an osteolytic cortical lesion (arrowheads) in the midshaft of the radius.

been likened to a blade of grass or flame. Within the area of radiolucency, remaining trabeculae may appear thickened, although frequently they are obliterated and a hazy "ground glass" or "washed-out" pattern is observed. The involved bone commonly is enlarged or widened, and pathologic fractures may be evident.

Radiographic evidence of increased density or sclerosis of bone may be seen in the active or inactive stages of the disease (Figs. 54–4 and 54–5). Coarsened trabeculae produce focal or widespread areas of radiodensity, which may be superimposed on lytic foci. In the cranium, bone sclerosis may produce circular radiodense lesions in one area, whereas osteoporosis circumscripta is noted elsewhere. Similarly, in the long bones, as the flame-shaped advancing edge of osteolysis proceeds toward the shaft, focal radiodensity may become evident in the epiphysis and metaphysis. Cortical thickening, enlargement of bone, and coarsened trabeculae are prominent. On histologic examination, the sclerotic areas contain closely meshed trabeculae with a typical mosaic pattern. Eventually, radiographic evidence of osteolysis may be absent, and the imaging picture is entirely that of osteosclerosis. The radiographic appearance of Paget's disease may be influenced by the administration of various therapeutic drugs, such as diphosphonates, mithramycin, and calcitonin[154, 155] (see later discussion). Arrest of the lytic front and remineralization of cortical and trabecular bone can be observed. Radionuclide studies, particularly those with gallium, also may document improvement during therapy.[152]

General Distribution of the Disease (Fig. 54–6)

The most frequent seats of the osteitis have been . . . the tibiae, femora, clavicles, spine, and vault of the skull.
                                                    SIR JAMES PAGET (1889)

As noted previously, Paget's disease predominates in the axial skeleton. Particularly characteristic is involvement of the pelvis (30 to 75 per cent); sacrum (30 to 60 per cent); spine (30 to 75 per cent), especially the lumbar segment; and skull (25 to 65 per cent).[1, 9, 158, 181] Additionally, the proximal portions of the long bones, particularly the femur (25 to 35 per cent), commonly are affected. Abnormalities of the axial skeleton or proximal part of the femur are present in approximately 75 to 80 per cent of cases.[9, 13] Furthermore, the shoulder girdle is altered not infrequently, and at this site abnormalities of the proximal portion of the humerus, scapula (particularly the acromion and coracoid process), and clavicle can be seen.[248] In some patients, widespread skeletal involvement is evident in both the axial and the appendicular skeleton; in fact, no bone is exempt, although changes in the ribs, fibula,[268] and small bones in the hand and foot are infrequent. In other patients, the disease is initially or totally monostotic, a pattern that is evident in 10 to 35 per cent of cases. Monostotic Paget's disease is not infrequent in the axial skeleton, even though any portion of the skeleton may represent the sole site of involvement.[269, 270, 330] Although Paget's disease confined to one bone or a portion of one bone may be more difficult to diagnose, the characteristic radiographic findings generally

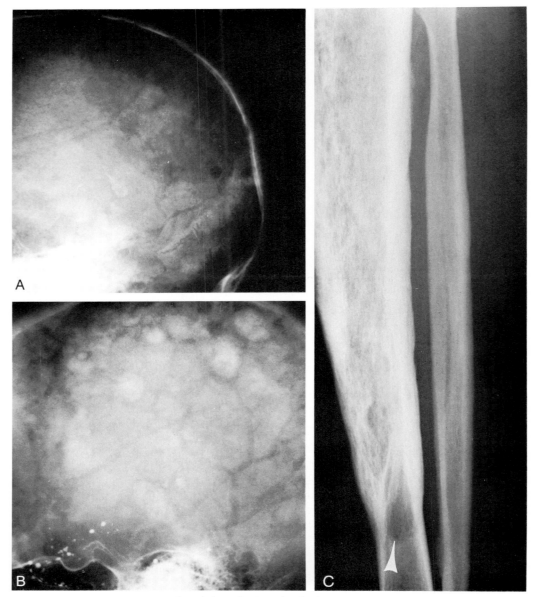

FIGURE 54–4. General stages of Paget's disease: Osteolytic and osteosclerotic stage.

A, B These two examples of cranial involvement show both osteolysis and osteosclerosis. Radiodense foci in **A** are occurring in an area of osteoporosis circumscripta. In **B,** more extensive osteosclerosis, producing the "cotton-wool" appearance, is seen.

C In the tibia, new bone formation in the epiphysis, metaphysis, and diaphysis is combined with an osteolytic focus (arrowhead) distally.

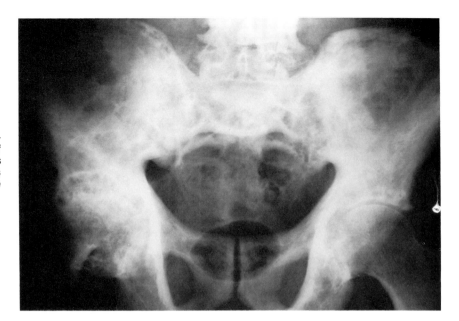

FIGURE 54–5. General stages of Paget's disease: Osteosclerotic stage. In this example of long-standing disease, diffuse osteosclerosis throughout the pelvis, including the sacrum, is evident. Note degenerative joint disease in the right hip.

are observed, allowing accurate differentiation from other conditions.

The specific characteristics of osseous distribution in Paget's disease (axial involvement, a preference for the lower extremities, and a tendency for right-sided altera-

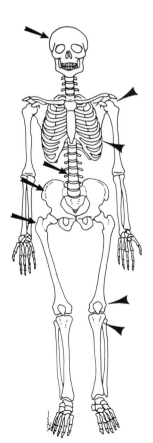

FIGURE 54–6. General distribution of Paget's disease. Very common (arrows) and common (arrowheads) sites are indicated.

tions) are interesting. The central distribution corresponds to that of hematopoietic red marrow, so that the locations of Paget's disease and skeletal metastases are similar; however, the relative frequency of tibial involvement and infrequency of rib involvement are features of Paget's disease not shared by osseous metastases.[158] The spinal distribution of Paget's disease, with preferential involvement of the upper and lower cervical, low thoracic, and third and fourth lumbar vertebrae, is similar to that of spondylosis deformans, suggesting the importance of bone stress in site selection.[181]

Involvement of Specific Sites

The skull became gradually larger, so that nearly every year, for many years, his hat and the helmet that he wore as a member of a Yeomanry Corps needed to be enlarged.

The length of the spine thus seemed lessened, and from a height of six feet one inch, he sank to about five feet nine inches. . . .

The left tibia had become larger, and had a well-marked anterior curve, as if lengthened while its ends were held in place by their attachments to the unchanged fibula.

SIR JAMES PAGET (1877)

Cranium (Fig. 54–7). Pagetic alterations of the skull vary from typical osteoporosis circumscripta to widespread sclerosis. Focal radiodense areas may be observed, termed the "cotton-wool" appearance. These islands obscure the differentiation of outer and inner tables from the diploë. Cranial thickening occasionally is extensive, particularly in frontal regions, and both bony sclerosis and thickening may be distributed asymmetrically. Bone apposition on the inner margins of the cranial vault may be irregular, producing areas of brain compression that may be responsible for altered mentality and dementia.[40] Similar irregularities on the outer surface of the skull, although they are less frequent, may be associated with striking corrugation or a wavy appearance.[41] As opposed to exuberant facial changes

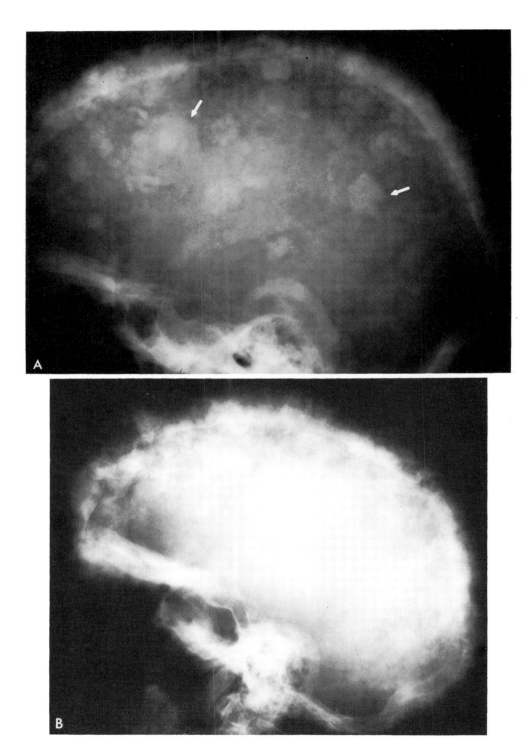

FIGURE 54–7. Radiographic abnormalities in Paget's disease: Skull.

A "Cotton-wool" appearance. Observe focal radiodense regions (arrows) simulating osteoblastic skeletal metastasis. The cranial vault is thickened.

B More extensive involvement includes increased sclerosis, thickening of the cranial vault, particularly anteriorly, alterations of the base of the skull, and platybasia.

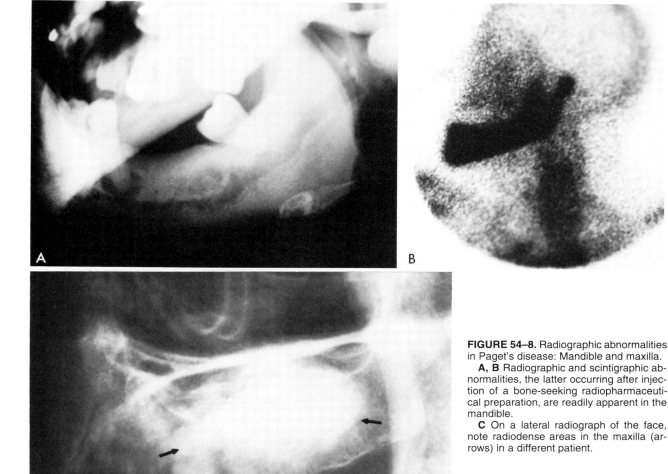

FIGURE 54–8. Radiographic abnormalities in Paget's disease: Mandible and maxilla.

A, B Radiographic and scintigraphic abnormalities, the latter occurring after injection of a bone-seeking radiopharmaceutical preparation, are readily apparent in the mandible.

C On a lateral radiograph of the face, note radiodense areas in the maxilla (arrows) in a different patient.

that may be seen in fibrous dysplasia, extensive alterations of the facial bones in Paget's disease are infrequent, although maxillary and mandibular changes may be observed,[271] including radiodense lesions termed cementomas, which can displace teeth and result in malocclusion (Fig. 54–8).[142, 145] As opposed to the situation in nonpagetic hypercementosis, the cementomas in Paget's disease obscure the lamina dura.[182, 183]

Basilar invagination is seen in about one third of patients with Paget's disease of the skull. This complication is more frequent in women than in men and increases in frequency with progressive severity of the disease. Basilar invagination is characterized by upward protrusion of the foramen magnum and surrounding bone owing to the effect of gravity and muscle pull. It may be associated with neurologic symptoms and signs caused by compression of the contents of the upper cervical canal and posterior fossa. Additional clinical findings relate to impingement on other cranial nerves by the enlarging pagetic bone. These findings include sensory abnormalities, impaired motor function, deafness, atrophy of the optic nerve, and obstruction of the lacrimal duct. Stretching or occlusion of the vertebral or basilar arteries is possible. Internal hydrocephalus results from obstruction of the flow of the cerebrospinal fluid.

Syringomyelia of the cervical cord may be an associated feature.[272]

The diagnosis of basilar invagination, basilar impression, and platybasia is accomplished with plain film radiography through the use of a number of lines (Chamberlain's, McGregor's, and other lines) that are described elsewhere in this textbook. Other techniques, including conventional tomography, CT scanning, and MR imaging, also can be helpful diagnostically in this situation.[184, 272]

Vertebral Column (Figs. 54–9 to 54–11). Paget's disease frequently involves the vertebral column, particularly the lumbar spine and the sacrum.[42] Thoracic and cervical involvement[43–47] and monostotic disease of the spine[48, 49, 269, 273–275] can be observed. Five mechanisms have been emphasized in the pathogenesis of neurologic complications of such involvement: collapse of affected vertebral bodies; increased vascularity of pagetic bone, which "steals" blood from the spinal cord; mechanical interference with the spinal cord blood supply; narrowing of the spinal canal owing to new bone formation or soft tissue and ligament ossification; and stenosis of neural foramina resulting from involvement of vertebral posterior elements.[158, 185, 197, 258, 259, 276, 278, 281] Additional reported causes of neurologic compromise in pagetic spines have included epidural hematoma[279]

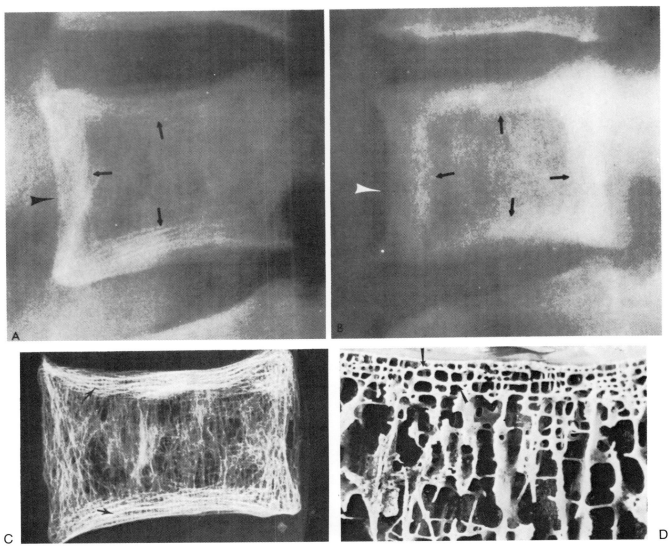

FIGURE 54–9. Radiographic abnormalities in Paget's disease: Spine.

A, B "Picture-frame" vertebral bodies. Condensation of bone can be seen along the peripheral margins of the vertebral bodies (arrows) on lateral radiographs of the spine in two patients with Paget's disease. Observe straightening or convexity of the anterior surface of the bone (arrowheads), and involvement of the pedicles.

C, D In a cadaver, a sectional radiograph and photograph reveal the increased thickness of the marginal trabeculae in the vertebral body. Observe the linear, horizontal direction of the trabeculae (arrows).

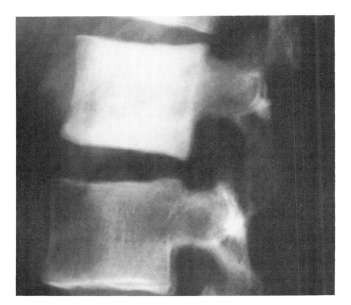

FIGURE 54–10. Radiographic abnormalities in Paget's disease: Spine. In this case, observe a relatively homogeneous pattern of osteosclerosis of the vertebral body. The pedicles also are affected. The resulting ivory vertebra resembles that of skeletal metastasis and lymphoma. (Courtesy of R. Kerr, M.D., Los Angeles, California.)

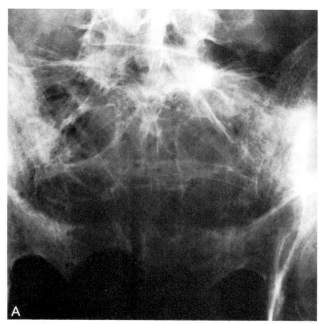 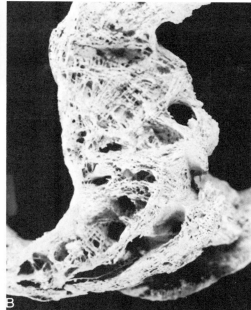

FIGURE 54–11. Radiographic abnormalities in Paget's disease: Sacrum.
  A Although the sacrum reveals few trabeculae and the entire bone is osteopenic, the remaining trabecular pattern is coarsened, diagnostic of Paget's disease.
  B A photograph of a sagittal section through the lower lumbar spine and sacrum shows coarsened trabeculae throughout, although cystic lesions are present in the sacrum.

and osteoarthritis,[280] although a meaningful association of these conditions with Paget's disease is not proved. Extramedullary hematopoiesis represents another potential cause of spinal cord compression in such spines.[326] Clinical manifestations of Paget's disease of the vertebral column also depend on the level of involvement. In the lumbar spine, Paget's disease can lead to compression of the cauda equina[17, 50, 140] and encroachment on the foramina.[17] In the thoracic spine, cord compression, most frequent in the upper thoracic region because of the relatively small size of the vertebral canal, and intervertebral foraminal impingement may be seen.[51, 52] With cervical involvement, Paget's disease can lead to cord compression and even spastic quadriplegia.[43, 44, 46] Pagetic abnormalities of the vertebral body at any level can lead to collapse, a complication that may induce acute compression of the spinal cord.[48]

Gross pathologic and radiographic aberrations of the spine in Paget's disease are characteristic. The vertebral bodies and posterior elements may be altered, the changes being more apparent in the vertebral bodies. Enlarged, coarsened trabeculae are observed, and condensation of bone may be especially prominent along the contours of the vertebral body. In this situation, the highlighted contour of the involved vertebra resembles a picture frame, an appearance that is diagnostic of this condition. Although thickening of vertical trabeculae of the vertebra may be reminiscent of changes in osteoporosis or hemangioma, the accompanying radiodensity of the periphery of the vertebral bodies permits an accurate diagnosis of Paget's disease. In some patients, uniform increase in osseous density is seen, producing an ivory vertebra (Fig. 54–10), and differentiation of Paget's disease from other causes of ivory vertebrae, such as metastasis and lymphoma, may be difficult.[141] In this situation, if the vertebra is enlarged, the diagnosis of

Paget's disease usually is assured. It must be stressed, however, that such enlargement may not be apparent. Occasionally Paget's disease of one vertebra may extend into an adjacent osteophytic outgrowth.

Alterations in shape of involved vertebral bodies in Paget's disease are common, reflecting the structural weakness of the altered bone. Biconcave deformities termed fish vertebrae are identical to those occurring in metabolic disorders such as osteoporosis, osteomalacia, and hyperparathyroidism. These deformities are due to compression of "softened" vertebrae by the adjacent intervertebral disc. Secondary degenerative alterations in the intervertebral discs may lead to disc space narrowing and osseous bridging of the vertebral bodies. Resulting ankylosis of adjacent vertebral bodies resembles that accompanying congenital fusions.[282] Complicating accurate diagnosis is the rarely reported occurrence of Paget's disease in congenitally fused vertebral bodies.[283] Infrequently, complete collapse of the vertebral bodies is observed in Paget's disease, and an adjacent soft tissue mass can be seen.[179] More commonly, loss of vertebral height is a manifestation of gradual remodeling of bone rather than acute compression.

Pagetic changes in the posterior elements may occur in conjunction with vertebral body abnormalities[186] or as an isolated spinal manifestation of the disease. With pediculate involvement, increased radiodensity may simulate osteoblastic metastasis. An increase in the interpediculate distance is more suggestive of Paget's disease than of metastasis.[187] Sacral alterations usually are associated with involvement of additional areas of the pelvis. Osteolytic features commonly predominate in the sacrum and, in such instances, missed diagnosis is not infrequent.

Pelvis (Fig. 54–12). Manifestations of Paget's disease in the pelvis usually include both bone resorption and bone

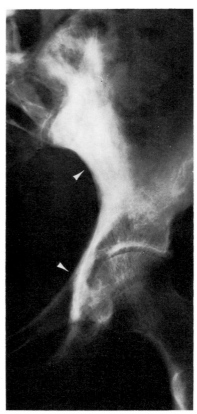

FIGURE 54–12. Radiographic abnormalities in Paget's disease: Pelvis. Trabecular thickening and sclerosis are apparent in the ilium and along the iliopubic line (arrowheads). Note the involvement of the subchondral bone of the ilium about the sacroiliac joint and acetabulum.

formation. Initial trabecular thickening may be evident along the inner contour of the pelvis, termed the pelvic ring. The iliopubic and ilioischial lines may be prominent, with little other osseous abnormality of the pelvis. Thickening in these areas must be distinguished from irregularity of the iliopubic contour, which is frequent in normal elderly persons, and from calcification of Cooper's ligament. The periphery of the iliac bone may appear radiodense, with a relatively lucent central portion. Iliac sclerosis adjacent to the sacroiliac joint can simulate osteitis condensans ilii.[53] Furthermore, when sclerosis of both the ilium and the sacrum is apparent about the articulation, the joint margins frequently are indistinct, mimicking the findings of sacroiliitis (see discussion later in this chapter). Involvement of the pubis and ischium frequently is associated with enlarged osseous contours. Para-acetabular alterations can lead to acetabular protrusion.

Diffuse abnormalities of the pelvis are not infrequent in Paget's disease. These changes are commonly asymmetric in distribution, and, in fact, widespread alterations of the pelvis on one side may occur in the absence of changes on the contralateral side. This unilaterality rarely is encountered with widespread osteoblastic metastasis, providing one clue to differentiation of these two conditions.

Additional Sites (Figs. 54–13 to 54–15). Paget's disease can affect any part of the skeleton. Involvement of the tubular bones of the extremities is most common in the femur, the tibia, and the humerus.[284] As noted previously, the involvement is characterized by epiphyseal predilection, an advancing wedge of radiolucency, periosteal apposition of new bone leading to widening of the osseous surface, and deformity and fracture. Cortical thickening with encroachment on the medullary canal is evident. In rare instances, the involved bone reveals narrowing or contraction.[253] Diaphyseal changes without epiphyseal abnormality are extremely unusual but may be observed, particularly in the tibia.[180, 188] In the tibia, pagetic involvement may begin in the middiaphysis, although a far more characteristic site of initial involvement in cases of "diaphyseal" Paget's disease is the anterior tibial tubercle.[285] Patients with this latter, unique mode of involvement tend to be younger than those with more classic Paget's disease, may have monostotic disease and normal serum levels of alkaline phosphatase, and have radiographic evidence of purely osteolytic or purely osteosclerotic abnormalities, or a combination of the two.[285] Other bone protuberances, such as the femoral trochanters or humeral tuberosities, may show initial involvement in Paget's disease,[286] but this is less common than localization in the tibial tuberosity. The radius appears to be the second most common site of diaphyseal Paget's disease, after the tibia.

Peculiarities in the distribution of stress in the lower extremity lead to typical patterns of deformity; most characteristically, exaggerated lateral curvature of the femur and anterior curvature of the tibia become apparent. Lateral bowing of the humerus also is seen. The fibula frequently is spared.

Paget's disease of the bones of the feet and hands is less common. In the foot, changes show predilection for the calcaneus, although other tarsal and metatarsal bones may be altered.[54] When present, Paget's disease in the hands reveals typical radiographic findings.[55, 56] In this location, involvement of a single hand or even a single bone is typical.[189]

Rib involvement is not common in Paget's disease. This involvement may be localized to one or two ribs or distributed throughout the thorax. The major differential diagnostic consideration at this site is the Paget's disease–like appearance in the posterior portion of one or more ribs that accompanies bone ankylosis of the adjacent costovertebral joints. Scapular and clavicular changes are not infrequent, and even the patella may be affected, leading to patellofemoral compartmental changes.[148, 287] Pagetic involvement of heterotopic ossification about the patella has been described.[190]

Rare manifestations of Paget's disease include its development at a site of bone grafting when pagetic bone is used inadvertently in the graft and extension of the disease across joints after arthrodesis.[288]

OTHER DIAGNOSTIC METHODS

Scintigraphy

Bone scintigraphy has been employed in the evaluation of patients with Paget's disease (Figs. 54–16 and 54–17).[57–60] As would be expected, areas of skeletal disease are depicted as sites of increased uptake of bone-seeking radiotracers and, in appropriate locations, of marrow replacement.[61, 289, 290] The immediate accumulation of radionuclide reflects

Text continued on page 1942

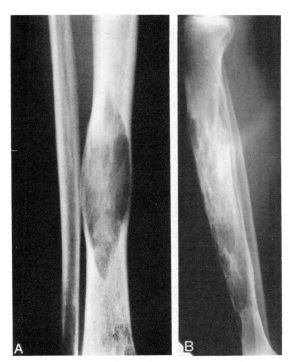

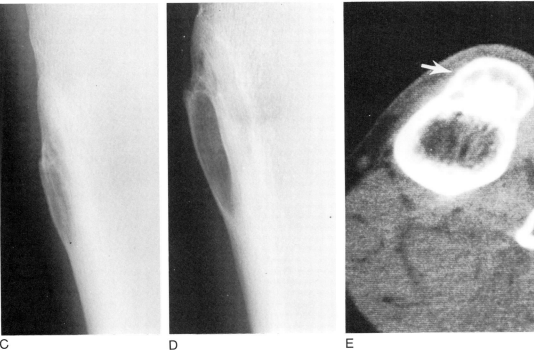

FIGURE 54–13. Radiographic abnormalities in Paget's disease: Tibia.

A Diaphyseal involvement, as in this case, is unusual, but, when seen, typically is located in the tibia. (Courtesy of T. Yochum, D.C., Denver, Colorado.)

B In a second patient, observe classic findings of Paget's disease confined to the diaphysis of the tibia.

C–E In a 50 year old male radiologist with increased local skin temperature and knee pain, radiographs obtained 1 year apart and CT scan reveal a progressing osteolytic focus of Paget's disease. On the transaxial CT image at the level of the tibial tuberosity, observe the intracortical location of the lesion (arrow). (Courtesy of H. Rodriguez, M.D., Santa Barbara, California.)

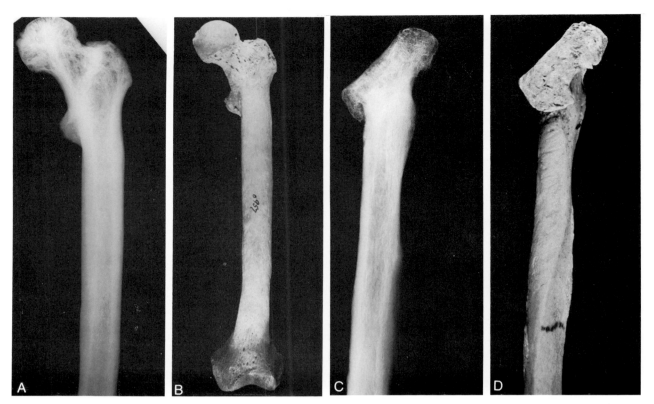

FIGURE 54–14. Radiographic abnormalities in Paget's disease: Long tubular bones.
   A, B Femur. Note the enlarged bone with abnormal shape and coarse trabeculae.
   C, D Radius. The bone is large and the radial head is deformed and angulated, presumably as a result of a previous fracture.

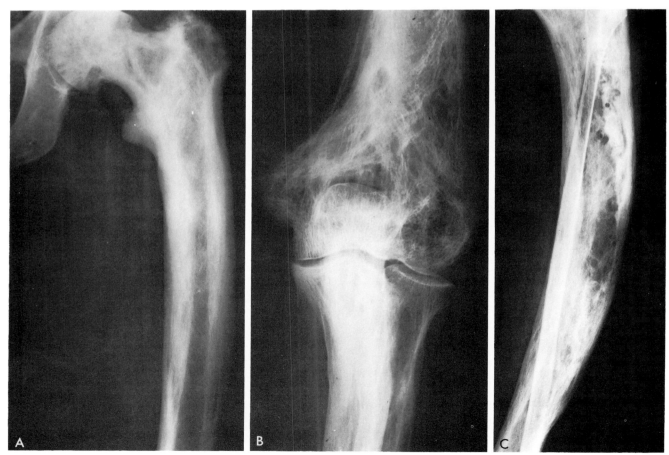

FIGURE 54–15 *See legend on opposite page*

1938

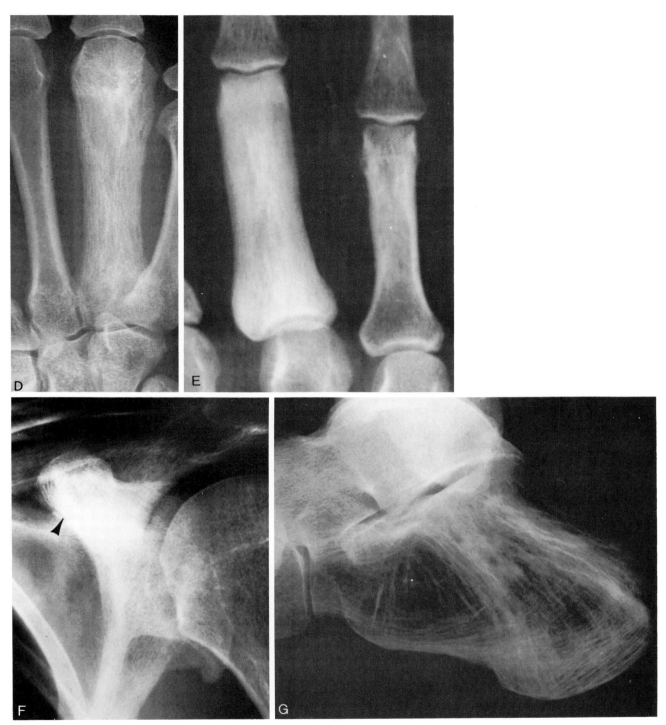

FIGURE 54–15. Radiographic abnormalities in Paget's disease: Additional sites.

A Femur. Alterations extend from the femoral head to the middiaphyseal region. The cortex is thickened and there is cortical encroachment on the medullary canal. Observe the coarse trabecular pattern.

B Humerus, radius, and ulna. Coarsely trabeculated bone is associated with radiolucent regions of varying size. The osseous outlines are enlarged.

C Tibia. On a lateral radiograph, typical Paget's disease of the tibia is associated with exaggerated anterior curvature. Note the lack of fibular involvement.

D, E Hand. The characteristic findings of Paget's disease are observed throughout an entire metacarpal **(D)** and proximal phalanx **(E).**

F Scapula. Observe the prominent coracoid process (arrowhead) and enlargement of the glenoid cavity and acromion.

G Calcaneus. The entire bone is affected. A pathologic fracture was present but not well seen in this radiograph.

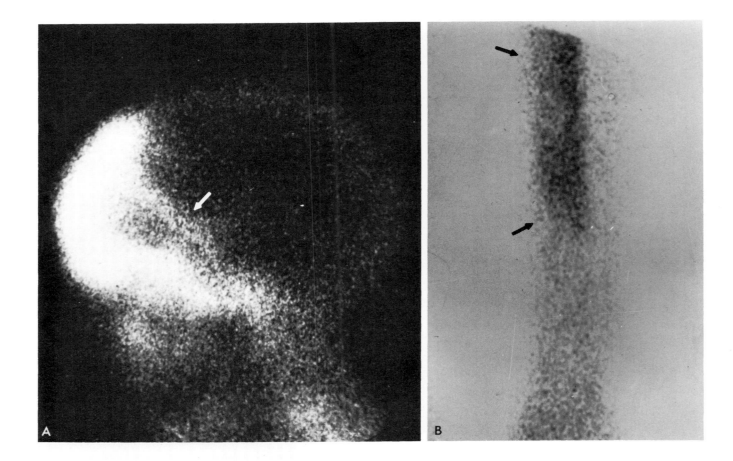

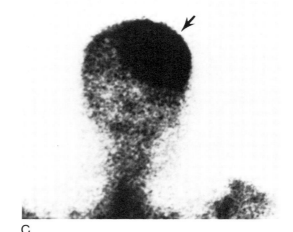

FIGURE 54–16. Scintigraphic abnormalities in Paget's disease: Bone-seeking agents (technetium polyphosphate).

A, B Osteolytic phase. On a lateral view of the skull **(A)** the area of increased uptake in the frontal region corresponded to the site of osteoporosis circumscripta. Note the "hot" curvilinear region (arrow) reflecting the location of the advancing edge of osteolysis. On a frontal view of the tibia **(B),** accumulation of radioisotope (arrows) corresponded to sites of lytic changes of Paget's disease.

C One additional example is shown of intense radionuclide activity (arrow) in the cranial vault of a person with osteoporosis circumscripta.

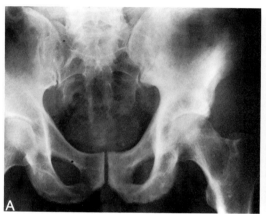
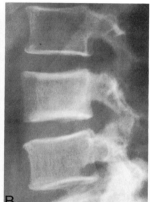
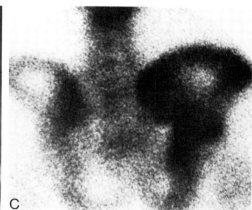
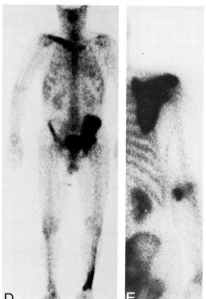

FIGURE 54–17. Scintigraphic abnormalities in Paget's disease: Bone-seeking agents (technetium polyphosphate). Osteosclerotic phase.

A–C Radiographs reveal typical changes of Paget's disease affecting the left hemipelvis and third lumbar vertebra. Increased radionuclide activity is evident in these sites.

D In a different patient, observe the accentuated uptake of radionuclide in the left hemipelvis, distal portion of the left tibia, and right clavicle. The scintigraphic pattern is virtually diagnostic of Paget's disease.

E In a third patient, intense scintigraphic activity is evident in the scapula.

(**E,** Courtesy of V. Vint, M.D., San Diego, California.)

an increased blood supply to bone, which may explain false-positive brain scintiscans in patients with calvarial Paget's disease.[62] Scintigraphic abnormalities may precede radiographic changes, underscoring the greater sensitivity of radionuclide versus radiographic examination. In addition, scintigraphy can document the extent of the initial lytic phase of Paget's disease.[63, 191, 249] In this phase, increased radionuclide activity may be particularly prominent at the advancing edge of bone lysis,[192] corresponding to sites of prominent vascularity, osteoclastosis, and new bone formation. Serial bone scintigraphs may provide objective evidence of the effect of various therapeutic agents (see later discussion).[64, 65] Thermography also has been utilized in this situation,[66] as has gallium scanning.[152] Indium-labeled leukocyte imaging may show regions of decreased uptake of the radiopharmaceutical owing to marrow replacement in sites of Paget's disease.[291]

As is generally recognized, bone scanning monitors physiologic parameters more accurately than radiography. It therefore is not surprising that scintigraphic abnormalities may be observed prior to radiographic changes in Paget's disease, although, in the quiescent or inactive stage of the disease, pagetic lesions may be detected radiographically but not scintigraphically. It is the active phase of Paget's disease that is well evaluated by radionuclide examination. The concentration of the bone-seeking radiopharmaceutical agent in a pagetic lesion correlates with the grade of radiologic deformation and the frequency of pain; the total skeletal uptake correlates with the severity of the biochemical aberrations,[193] particularly the serum level of alkaline phosphatase and the urinary level of hydroxyproline.[158]

Computed Tomography

CT scanning generally is not required in the evaluation of uncomplicated Paget's disease. When used, this technique will reveal the coarsened trabecular pattern that is typical of the disorder,[194] whether it be in the skull, spine, pelvis, or tubular bones (Fig. 54–18). On the other hand, CT is useful in the further delineation of a number of complications of Paget's disease, including articular abnormalities, especially in the hip,[195] neoplastic degeneration (Fig. 54–19), and vertebral involvement with neurologic compromise.[196, 259]

Magnetic Resonance Imaging

MR imaging is not required for the diagnosis of Paget's disease of bone, which is better accomplished with routine radiography. Furthermore, owing to the variability in the MR appearance of Paget's disease, diagnostic difficulty may arise when the MR findings are interpreted in the absence of routine radiographs.

MR imaging alterations are most characteristic in those patients who have long-standing inactive phases of Paget's disease (Fig. 54–20). In this situation, the morphologic features observed during the MR imaging examination are identical to those evident with routine radiography and include cortical thickening, coarse trabeculation, enlargement of the bone, reduction in the size of the medullary cavity, and, in tubular bones, bowing. Typically but not invariably, the cortex remains devoid of signal on all imaging sequences. Thickened trabeculae in the medullary cavity also

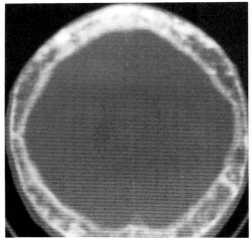

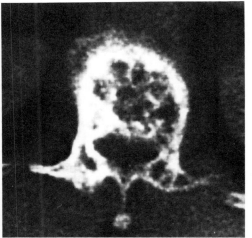

A   B   C

FIGURE 54–18. CT abnormalities in Paget's disease: Uncomplicated disease. The transaxial images of the cranial vault **(A)**, vertebra **(B)**, and pelvis **(C)** show a coarsened trabecular pattern and enlarged osseous contour, typical of Paget's disease. In the skull, the diploic space is widened throughout; in the pelvis, unilateral abnormalities are seen on the left side; and in the spine, alterations involve both the vertebral body and the posterior elements.

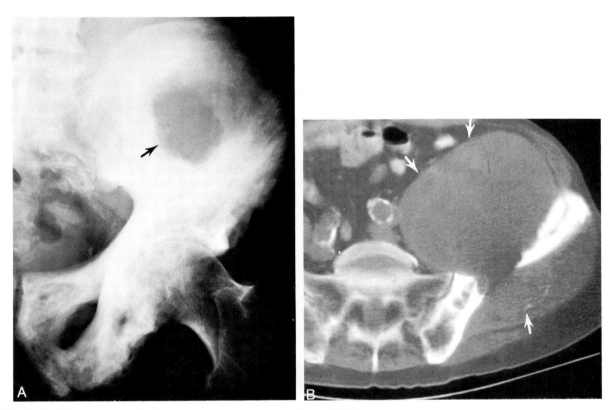

FIGURE 54–19. CT abnormalities in Paget's disease: Sarcomatous degeneration.
  A The plain film demonstrates pagetic involvement of the left hemipelvis and sacrum, and a large osteolytic lesion in the ilium (arrow).
  B A transaxial CT image at the level of the lesion shows osseous destruction and a large soft tissue mass (arrows). The final diagnosis was osteosarcoma in Paget's disease.
  (Courtesy of P. Kaplan, M.D., Charlottesville, Virginia.)

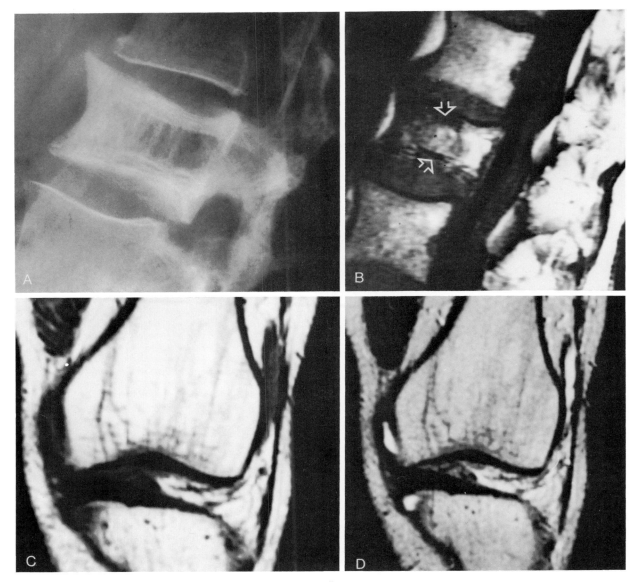

FIGURE 54–20. MR imaging abnormalities in Paget's disease: Inactive disease.

A, B Spine. A routine radiograph **(A)** shows classic pagetic abnormalities with a "picture frame" appearance. The vertebral body is mildly compressed, and osteophytes are seen. Note involvement of the posterior osseous elements. On a sagittal T1-weighted (TR/TE, 600/20) spin echo MR image **(B),** coarse trabeculation appears as regions of low signal intensity (arrows).

C, D Femur. On proton density weighted (TR/TE, 2000/12) **(C)** and T2-weighted (TR/TE, 2000/70) **(D)** coronal MR images, note the linear regions of low signal intensity, corresponding to sites of trabecular thickening. The normal signal intensity of the medullary fat is preserved. A joint effusion is present.

(C, D, Courtesy of T. Pope, M.D., Winston-Salem, North Carolina.)

Illustration continued on opposite page

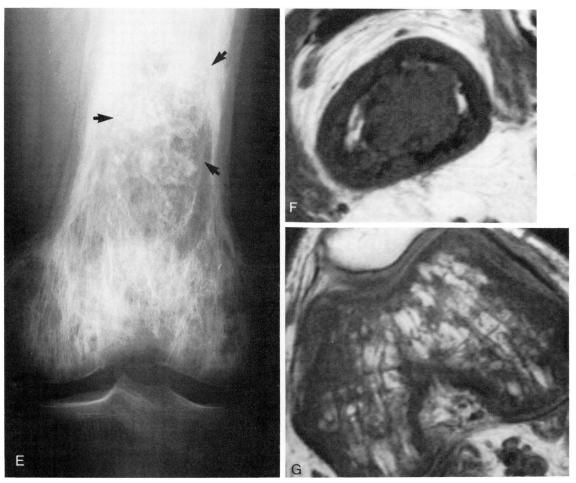

FIGURE 54–20 *Continued*

E–G In this patient, a frontal radiograph **(E)** shows typical features of Paget's disease of the femur as well as an osteolytic region (arrows) containing calcification. A transaxial T-weighted (TR)TE, 690/15) spin echo MR image through the osteolytic region **(F)** reveals a lesion of low signal intensity in the marrow, which histologically proved to be an enchondroma. A transaxial T1-weighted (TR/TE, 690/15) spin echo MR image through the distal femur **(G)** shows thickened trabeculae of Paget's disease with intertrabecular islands of fat.

(**E–G,** Courtesy of M. Recht, M.D., Cleveland, Ohio.)

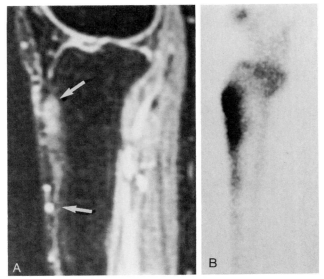

FIGURE 54–21. MR imaging abnormalities in Paget's disease: Active disease. In an elderly woman with Paget's disease of the tibial tuberosity, STIR imaging (TR/TE, 2800/20; inversion time, 150 ms) in the sagittal plane **(A)** shows high signal intensity (between arrows) in the anterior portion of the tibia. With bone scintigraphy **(B)**, increased radionuclide accumulation is evident. (Courtesy of W. Glenn, M.D., Los Angeles, California.)

reveal a signal void. In the tubular bones of the extremities, the trabeculae reveal a criss-crossing appearance and are separated by normal-appearing fatty bone marrow with its typical signal characteristics.[292–294] Indeed, Kaufman and coworkers[294] emphasized the persistence of signal from normal fat as a potential way of differentiating osteosclerotic Paget's disease alone from that associated with fracture or tumor in symptomatic patients. Obliteration of areas of normal fatty marrow would be expected in the presence of edematous or neoplastic tissue. In some instances of long-standing, uncomplicated Paget's disease, the signal intensity of the bone marrow in involved regions is similar to that of fat but even more intense and more homogeneous.[293] Cystlike areas, representing fat-filled marrow spaces, are surrounded by thickened and somewhat distorted trabeculae, resulting in a characteristic MR appearance.[293]

The active stage of Paget's disease leads to variability in the MR findings, making diagnostic difficulty more likely (Fig. 54–21). In this stage, the hematopoietic marrow is replaced by fibrous connective tissue with numerous, large vascular channels. These histologic characteristics resemble those of granulation tissue and account for the MR features that may resemble findings in tumor or infection.[293] With spin echo imaging, the signal intensity of the involved bone marrow may be decreased on the T1-weighted sequences and increased on the T2-weighted sequences.[322] These signal characteristics differ from those of fibrosis alone, which would be expected to be of low signal intensity on both types of sequences.[295, 296] Although prominent trabeculae that are not destroyed about such regions of marrow may allow a correct MR diagnosis of Paget's disease alone, elimination of the possibility of secondary tumor or fracture may be impossible in some cases.

In common with CT, MR imaging in patients with Paget's disease may be employed to evaluate effectively some

of the neurologic complications of the disease. Basilar impression and spinal stenosis, two of the causes of such complications, are studied well with both CT scanning and MR imaging, although the latter method provides superior visualization of the brain, spinal cord, and cauda equina. Also, in common with CT, MR imaging provides useful information about the extent and neurovascular compromise of pagetic sarcomas.[296, 297]

COMPLICATIONS OF PAGET'S DISEASE
(Table 54–2)

Numerous complications can be observed in patients with Paget's disease. Reference has been made earlier in this chapter to deformities of the long bones, spine, and skull, some of which can lead to neurologic deficits; articular problems in Paget's disease are discussed later. Additional complications are fractures and neoplasms.

Fractures

. . . as he was riding and suddenly raised his arm the bone broke near the shoulder . . . and I amputated the arm at the shoulder joint.

SIR JAMES PAGET (1877)

Partial or complete insufficiency (stress) and acute true fractures can complicate Paget's disease (Fig. 54–22).[198, 199] Cortical stress fractures are prominent in the lower extremity, particularly in the femur and the tibia. They appear as single or multiple horizontal radiolucent areas with predilection for the convex aspect of the bone (lateral aspect of the femoral neck and shaft; anterior aspect of the tibia). Although the appearance of these linear radiolucent areas that partially traverse the bone simulates that of Looser's zones, which are apparent in osteomalacia, the involvement of convex surfaces rather than concave surfaces is distinctive. In Paget's disease, the horizontal clefts are filled with cartilaginous callus that does not fully mineralize, explaining their relative radiolucency.[39] These stress fractures appear most frequently in patients with long-standing (inactive) disease. In some instances, healing of these fractures may be observed on their periosteal and endosteal surfaces,[67] isolating a permanent cortical radiolucent area. In other patients, the partial fracture remains unchanged indefinitely, suggesting inactivity of adjacent pagetic bone,[68] or it may progress, extending across the entire bone.[147] Patho-

TABLE 54–2. Musculoskeletal Complications of Paget's Disease

Neurologic abnormalities
Osseous deformities
Fractures
Neoplasms
Soft tissue masses
Osteomyelitis
Extramedullary hematopoiesis
Crystal deposition
Monosodium urate
Calcium pyrophosphate dihydrate*
Calcific periarthritis
Degenerative joint disease
Rheumatoid arthritis and its variants*

*Questionable association.

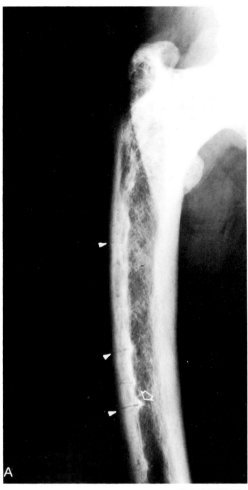

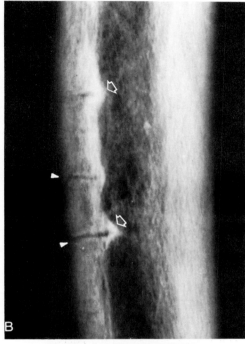

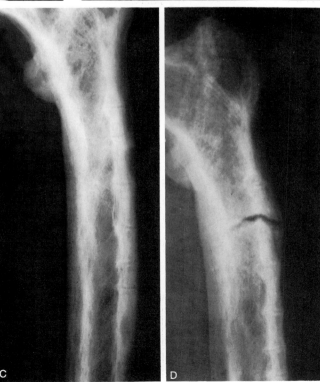

FIGURE 54–22. Complications of Paget's disease: Insufficiency (stress) fractures.

A, B Radiographs of the proximal portion of the femur outline multiple linear radiolucent areas (arrowheads) on the outer aspect of the thickened femoral cortex. Some of the fractures traverse the entire cortex, whereas others do not. Endosteal callus is evident (open arrows).

(**A, B,** Courtesy of C. Wackenheim, M.D., and Y. Dirheimer, M.D., Strasbourg, France.)

C, D Observe the progression of the stress fractures of the proximal portion of the femur in this patient with Paget's disease. On the later film, a large fracture line extends partially across the bone.

(**C, D,** Courtesy of G. Greenway, M.D., Dallas, Texas.)

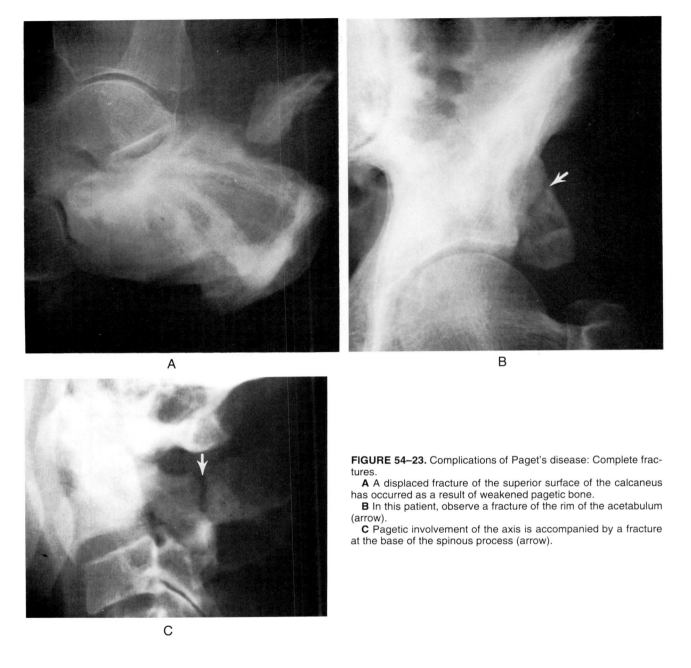

A

B

C

FIGURE 54–23. Complications of Paget's disease: Complete fractures.
  A A displaced fracture of the superior surface of the calcaneus has occurred as a result of weakened pagetic bone.
  B In this patient, observe a fracture of the rim of the acetabulum (arrow).
  C Pagetic involvement of the axis is accompanied by a fracture at the base of the spinous process (arrow).

logic fractures in Paget's disease are the most common orthopedic complication of the disorder, may be its presenting manifestation, and are more frequent in women than in men.[158] They typically are seen in the femur, humerus, tibia, spine, and pelvis; multiple fractures in a single bone or in several bones are described.[200, 323] With regard to frequency, the commonest site of fracture is the femur. In the femur, such complete fractures most commonly are subtrochanteric in location,[69] followed in frequency by the upper third of the femoral shaft and the femoral neck.[158] Complete fractures also may be seen after biopsy[252] or significant or minor trauma[70] (Fig. 54–23). These may occur in tubular bones[146, 147] or in the vertebral column, and the fractures generally heal when the injured part is immobilized,[298] although the rate of healing may be slow. The frequency of nonunion of femoral fractures may be quite high, and the developing callus may be involved in the pagetic process.[147]

Refracture at the same site as a previous fracture has been described. Furthermore, as the risk of sarcoma is substantial in cases of pathologic fractures in Paget's disease, a biopsy is recommended whenever such a fracture develops.[158]

Neoplasms

In three out of the five well-marked cases that I have seen or read of cancer appeared late in life . . . suggesting careful inquiry.

SIR JAMES PAGET (1877)

Neoplastic involvement in Paget's disease includes sarcomatous degeneration, giant cell tumor, and superimposition of another tumorous condition, such as metastatic disease, plasma cell myeloma, and lymphoma.

Sarcomatous transformation in this disease first was rec-

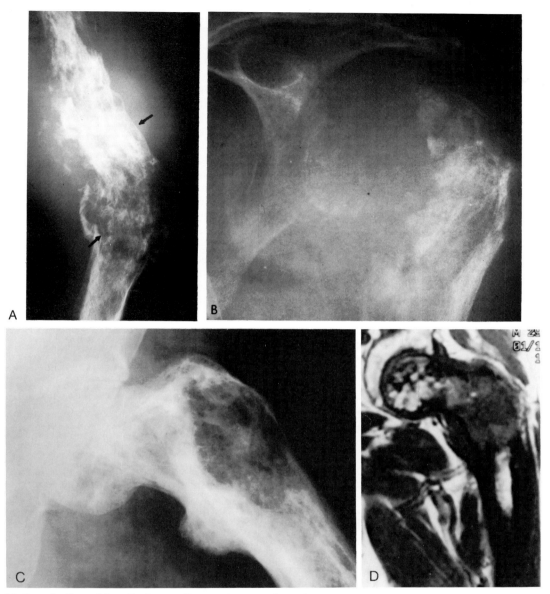

FIGURE 54–24. Complications of Paget's disease: Sarcomatous transformation.

 A Osteosarcoma. A large tumor is involving the midshaft of a humerus, which is affected by Paget's disease. Radiographic findings of neoplasm include a soft tissue mass, areas of bone lysis and sclerosis (arrows), and pathologic fractures.

 B Osteosarcoma. An extensive lesion has replaced the entire humeral head. Changes of Paget's disease can be visualized in the metaphysis and diaphysis of the humerus.

 C, D Osteosarcoma. The initial radiograph **(C)** in this 80 year old man shows pagetic involvement of the left femur, with an osteolytic lesion of the greater trochanter. A coronal T1-weighted (TR/TE, 400/11) spin echo MR image **(D)** reveals inhomogeneous signal intensity in the left femoral head. Note the region of low signal intensity in the intertrochanteric region, which, on analysis of a biopsy specimen, was found to be an osteosarcoma.

 (C, D, Courtesy of T. Armbuster, M.D., Fort Wayne, Indiana.)

ognized by Paget in some of his original five patients.[2] Its reported frequency has varied: In patients with widespread skeletal involvement, sarcomatous degeneration may occur in as many as 5 to 10 per cent of cases; with less extensive skeletal disease, this complication may be apparent in fewer than 1 per cent of persons.[16, 71] Currently it generally is believed that approximately 1 per cent of patients with Paget's disease develop malignant changes,[158, 201, 202] although higher figures, on the order of 5 per cent, still are suggested.[203] The tumor is apparent in areas of pagetic involvement (Fig. 54–24). Although generally a single fo-

cus of neoplasm is seen, in some instances multiple foci are observed, which may represent independent multicentric origin of the tumor.[204, 299] In certain cases, multiple sites of neoplasm indicate metastases from a single lesion.

Patients with sarcomatous degeneration in Paget's disease usually are between 55 and 80 years of age. Men are affected slightly more frequently than women and at a younger age.[158] Clinical findings include pain and swelling. The bones most commonly affected are the femur, the pelvis, and the humerus[72]; however, any bone may be involved, including the skull and vertebral column.[73–75, 143, 149]

Except for the higher frequency of neoplastic changes in the humerus and lower frequency in the skull and vertebrae, the distribution of sarcomas in Paget's disease is similar to that of the disorder itself.[158] Sarcomas arising in the skull almost invariably are associated with Paget's disease.[158, 205] Pagetic sarcomas may occur close to sites of previous, healed fractures.[299] Although sarcomas in Paget's disease vary widely in their cellularity and cytologic details, they appear to arise from the substratum of fibrous tissue in the pagetic bone.[76] Predominance of certain cells most commonly leads to a diagnosis of osteosarcoma (50 to 60 per cent)[206–208] or fibrosarcoma (20 to 25 per cent), although additional diagnoses such as chondrosarcoma (10 per cent) and sarcoma of myeloid and mesenchymal[209] elements may be entertained. No matter which cell type predominates, the prognosis for the patient is ominous, particularly in those persons with multicentric tumors.

Osteolysis rather than osteosclerosis is the major radiographic characteristic of the sarcoma,[71] although extensive osteosclerosis is seen in some cases.[324] In addition to bone destruction, findings include a soft tissue mass, cortical disruption, bony spiculation, and a persistent fracture without evidence of healing.[77] Periostitis is infrequent.[299]

Giant cell tumors are another type of neoplasm associated with Paget's disease, although this association is not well known or frequent.[78, 300] Giant cell tumors in this disease are almost always confined to the skull or the facial bones, although on rare occasions other skeletal sites are involved, particularly the pelvis[79–85, 150, 210] but also the clavicle,[203, 211] the spine,[212] and the tubular bones.[203, 301] The tumors invariably affect regions of the skeleton involved in the pagetic process, although the pagetic involvement may be inconspicuous radiographically and demonstrated only on histologic analysis. Patients with this neoplasm generally are elderly and have polyostotic (or, rarely, monostotic) Paget's disease. The histologic pattern of the tumor more frequently is benign than malignant. A lytic lesion, expansile in nature, with a soft tissue mass is observed. MR imaging analysis will reveal an osseous component with the variable signal characteristics of pagetic bone (see previous discussion) and a soft tissue component that is prominent with intermediate signal intensity on T1-weighted spin echo images and foci of increased signal intensity on T2-weighted spin echo images.[300] The prognosis usually is good. Dramatic reduction in tumor bulk may occur with the use of steroids alone.[300] The occurrence of a giant cell tumor in the facial bones should suggest the presence of underlying Paget's disease. Similarly, the occurrence of multiple giant cell tumors should suggest underlying Paget's disease, although, rarely, such multiple tumors can occur in the absence of pagetic skeletal involvement.[151] In some cases of giant cell tumor complicating Paget's disease, familial and geographic clustering is evident.[150] In other cases of Paget's disease, giant cell reparative granulomas and other benign processes and tumors are described.[254, 307]

Plasma cell myeloma may complicate Paget's disease, although the association may be fortuitous.[86–89, 213, 214, 302] Patients are elderly, and the two disorders usually involve different bones. Hodgkin's disease, other lymphomas, and leukemias occasionally are evident in patients with Paget's disease.[158, 215]

Metastatic disease and Paget's disease also may coexist,[90, 91, 216–218, 255, 303–306] and it is interesting to speculate that increased local blood flow in the latter disorder may make the bone more susceptible to metastasis.[92] Typical sites of the primary tumor are the breast, lung, kidney, prostate, and colon. A lytic lesion within sclerotic bone is detected in patients with metastatic foci superimposed on Paget's disease (Fig. 54–25). A soft tissue mass may be apparent. Of interest, metastasis to uninvolved skeletal sites in patients with Paget's disease is recorded.[207]

The diagnosis of neoplasm complicating Paget's disease usually is not difficult. Clinically, increased pain and a soft tissue mass are observed. Laboratory analysis may reveal further elevation of serum levels of alkaline phosphatase, although the finding is not invariable. Changes in concentrations of serum calcium or phosphorus or the erythrocyte sedimentation rate generally are not evident in the situation of sarcomatous degeneration in Paget's disease. On radiographs, soft tissue swelling and a lytic lesion may be seen, and in some tumors the presenting sign may be a pathologic fracture. It is rare to note bone formation in tumors occurring in Paget's disease even when the predominant cell type suggests osteosarcoma; therefore, any enlarging lytic lesion within pagetic bone should be evaluated carefully. These lytic neoplasms must be differentiated from the osteolytic phase of Paget's disease. In addition, cystic lesions, representing fat-filled marrow spaces, can be apparent in Paget's disease, simulating tumor[93] (Fig. 54–26). These radiolucent cysts may represent liquefactive degeneration and necrosis of proliferating fibrous tissue.[35] One additional mechanism producing lysis in Paget's disease is localized osteoporosis associated with an immobilized fracture.[94]

An enlarging soft tissue mass in patients with Paget's disease also must be regarded with suspicion, as such a mass may be the first indication of a superimposed neoplasm. Periosteal bone proliferation in uncomplicated Paget's disease can produce a radiodense soft tissue lesion that may contain new bone, however[95, 219, 308, 309] (Fig. 54–27). This may occur about involved long bones, especially the femur, or even in the spine, where a paraspinal mass can produce extradural compression of contrast material during myelography.[96]

Radionuclide abnormalities have been recorded in patients with Paget's disease with malignant degeneration. A decrease in accumulation of bone-seeking radiopharmaceutical agents, which may lead even to a "cold" area of absent uptake, and an increase in accumulation of gallium are regarded as characteristic of a neoplastic focus.[207, 220] The decrease in uptake probably is related to tumor necrosis. A decrease in gallium accumulation has been suggested as a radionuclide feature indicative of tumor response to therapy.[220]

Miscellaneous Complications

Lately her sight had become much impaired and still more lately she has been becoming deaf.

SIR JAMES PAGET (1882)

Neurologic dysfunction in Paget's disease may relate to changes at the base of the skull or the spine. Compression of the spinal cord can be due to expansion of bone, liga-

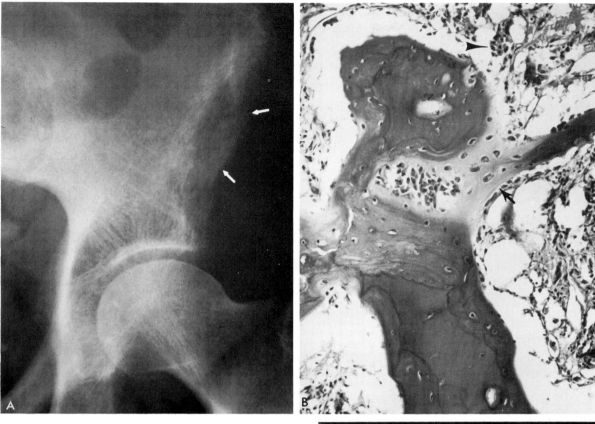

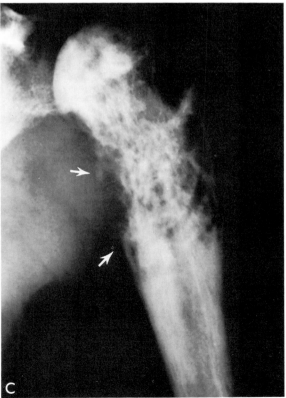

FIGURE 54–25. Complications of Paget's disease: Skeletal metastasis.

A The changes of Paget's disease are subtle but include a slightly coarsened trabecular pattern in the acetabular region and thickening of the iliopubic line. A lytic area (arrows) represents a metastatic focus from a poorly differentiated adenocarcinoma.

B On a photomicrograph (200×) of the involved bone, observe osteoblastic proliferation (arrow) and poorly differentiated adenocarcinoma cells (arrowhead).

C In a different patient, osteolysis and cortical destruction (arrows) in the medial aspect of a pagetic humerus were the result of metastatic adenocarcinoma, although the appearance is identical to that of sarcomatous degeneration.

(**C,** Courtesy of L. Cooperstein, M.D., Pittsburgh, Pennsylvania.)

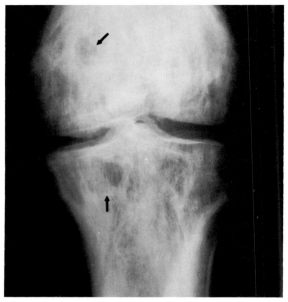

FIGURE 54–26. Paget's disease: Pseudoneoplastic cystic lesions. Osteolytic lesions of varying size (arrows) in Paget's disease represent degeneration and necrosis of proliferating fibrous tissue. They should not be mistaken for neoplasm.

ments, or soft tissue from the pagetic process, collapse with hemorrhage, deformity, vascular compromise, or neoplastic degeneration.[17, 44, 46, 50–52, 97–103] Cauda equina compression in this disease also has been attributed to ossification of extradural fat.[104] Additionally, the sciatic nerve may be compressed in external rotation between an enlarged ischium and lesser trochanter of the femur or in internal rotation between the ilium and piriformis muscle.[17]

Additional complications of Paget's disease include osteomyelitis and extramedullary hematopoiesis.[105]

ARTICULAR ABNORMALITIES

The bones of both hands and feet were healthy unless for some nodular enlargement of the phalanges such as one sees due to gout.

SIR JAMES PAGET (1882)

A variety of rheumatic manifestations have been described in association with Paget's disease.[162]

Crystal Deposition

Franck and collaborators[106] detected hyperuricemia in 40 per cent of 55 patients with symptomatic Paget's disease. This chemical abnormality was more common in men than in women and appeared to be related to overproduction of urate. Serum levels of uric acid correlated with total urinary hydroxyproline excretion, serum alkaline phosphatase level, and activity of bone involvement, suggesting that hyperuricemia was attributable to turnover of nucleic acids in the active cells of pagetic bone. Patients may demonstrate typical clinical and radiographic features of gout.[310]

Coexistence of calcium pyrophosphate dihydrate (CPPD) crystal deposition and Paget's disease also has been noted (Fig. 54–28). McCarty observed Paget's disease in 3.4 per cent of 238 patients with CPPD crystal deposition disease.[107] The reported frequency of CPPD crystal deposition in patients with Paget's disease has varied from 4 to 43 per cent.[106, 108, 109] In two of these three reports, the frequency of crystal deposition in patients with Paget's disease did not differ significantly from that in controls; in the third study, a high frequency in Paget's disease may have been related to the small number of patients with this disorder who had had an adequate radiographic examination. A well-documented association of CPPD crystal deposition disease and Paget's disease has yet to be defined.

Soft tissue calcification and ossification have been observed in patients with Paget's disease,[325] particularly those receiving large doses of vitamin D or those with associated scleroderma or calcinosis circumscripta.[110–113] Franck and coworkers reported periarticular calcification in 36 per cent of 55 patients with Paget's disease; 44 per cent of involved sites demonstrated an acute inflammatory response. This is the first report that provides strong evidence of an association between Paget's disease and calcific periarthritis presumably related to calcium hydroxyapatite (HA) crystal deposition.

Vascular calcification, especially that in arteries, attracted the attention of early observers of Paget's disease and appears to be common; the calcium is deposited in the media of the arteries, and the lumen usually is preserved.[158]

Rheumatoid Arthritis and Related Disorders

Rheumatoid arthritis and psoriatic arthritis have been detected in patients with Paget's disease, in whom maximum articular symptoms and signs occurred adjacent to pagetic bone.[106] A definite association between Paget's disease and these two arthritides has not been delineated. Reports of patients with both Paget's disease and ankylosing spondylitis are more frequent.[106, 114, 115] Some of these patients may have had pagetic involvement of periarticular regions of sacrum and ilium obscuring the sacroiliac joint, simulating ankylosing spondylitis, although other patients had typical radiographic changes of sacroiliitis and spondylitis (Figs. 54–29 and 54–30).[144] Our pathologic examination of sacroiliac joints in pagetic patients with articular obscuration has revealed degenerative changes without evidence of moderate or severe inflammatory disease, an observation confirmed by other investigators.[106] Irregularity of subchondral bone, particularly in the ilium, and ossification of the interosseous ligament are encountered. On microscopy, cartilaginous fusion of the joint space is evident. Although it can be argued that clinical findings, such as limitation of chest expansion and spinal flexion, and radiographic findings, such as obliteration of the sacroiliac joints, in patients with Paget's disease support the simultaneous occurrence of ankylosing spondylitis, these abnormalities may be related to Paget's disease itself. The absence of HLA-B27 antigen in some of these persons[106] further underscores the fact that a definite association between Paget's disease and ankylosing spondylitis has not been proved.[162]

A relationship between Paget's disease and diffuse idiopathic skeletal hyperostosis has been suggested[153] but not proved.[162]

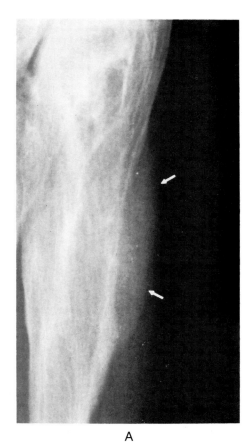

A

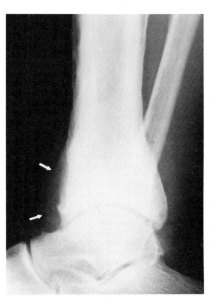

B

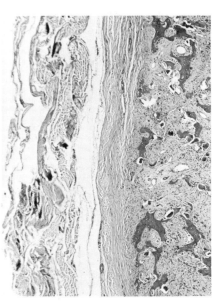

C

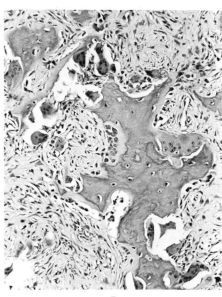

D

FIGURE 54–27. Paget's disease: Soft tissue extension.

A In this radiograph of the distal portion of the fibula, Paget's disease is evident. In addition, a soft tissue mass can be seen on the lateral aspect of the bone (arrows). This represents periosteal bone proliferation in the disease and should not be interpreted as neoplastic degeneration. (Courtesy of M. J. Palayew, M.D., Montreal, Quebec, Canada.)

B–D In a 60 year old man with a 4 month history of pain in the leg, a radiograph reveals Paget's disease and a fusiform soft tissue mass (arrows) extending from the anterior aspect of the distal end of the tibia. Photomicrographs (7×, 29×) prepared from biopsy material of the mass show subperiosteal bony elements with irregular borders in a vascular fibromyxoid connective tissue background. The spicules are bordered by osteoblasts and osteoclasts. No malignant cells are present. (From Resnik CS, et al: Skel Radiol *9*:145, 1982.)

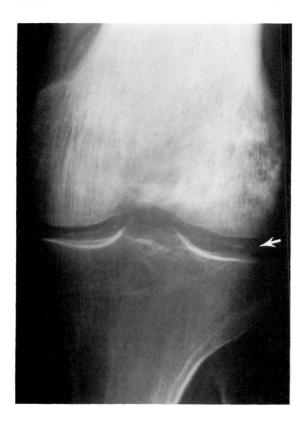

FIGURE 54–28. Paget's disease and CPPD crystal deposition. A frontal radiograph of the knee demonstrates pagetic involvement of the distal femur and chondrocalcinosis of the meniscus (arrow).

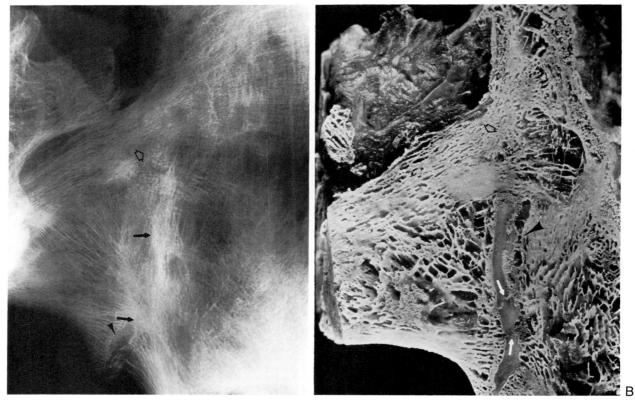

A   B

FIGURE 54–29. Paget's disease: Sacroiliac joint abnormalities. Cadaver with Paget's disease and apparent bony ankylosis of the sacroiliac joint. On the radiograph of the intact specimen **(A)** much of the sacroiliac joint appears ankylosed (arrows). The inferior aspect of the joint is open (arrowhead), and ligamentous ossification may be seen (open arrow). Observe the thickened pagetic bone in both sacrum and ilium. A coronal section **(B)** of the anterior aspect of the joint reveals the coarsened trabeculae of sacrum and ilium, ligamentous ossification (open arrow), and irregularity of subchondral bone, particularly in the ilium (arrowhead). One or two focal areas reveal trabeculae that are traversing the joint (arrows). Elsewhere fibrocartilaginous ankylosis of the joint is apparent.

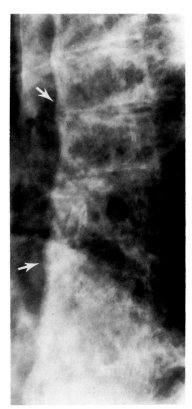

FIGURE 54–30. Paget's disease: Spinal ankylosis. A lateral radiograph of the thoracolumbar spine demonstrates Paget's disease in multiple vertebrae and flowing ossification along the anterior aspect of the spine (arrows), which resembles the findings of diffuse idiopathic skeletal hyperostosis (DISH).

Degenerative Joint Disease

Clinical and radiographic features of degenerative joint disease may be apparent in patients with Paget's disease. This complication is reported most frequently in the hip and the knee, although similar abnormalities are seen rarely in other articulations.[260]

Observation of hip joint abnormalities associated with Paget's disease was made by Collins in 1931[116] and subsequently by numerous other investigators,[117-123] although Guyer and Dewbury[124] were unable to document an increased frequency of articular abnormalities of the hip in patients with Paget's disease. Hip complaints are not unusual in pagetic patients, although these findings are not always attributable to articular pathology.[125]

In some reports, the frequency of joint space narrowing in the hip in patients with Paget's disease has varied from 50 to 96 per cent. Some of this variation relates to selection of patients and radiographic techniques. The pattern of narrowing of the articular space in this disease depends on whether the acetabulum or the femur is involved, although this pattern generally can be differentiated from primary degenerative joint disease.[126] In the last-mentioned disease, the most frequent area of joint space loss is at the superior aspect of the articulation (80 to 85 per cent); in 10 to 20 per cent of patients with primary degenerative joint disease, the medial joint space may be narrowed, but it is unusual to observe symmetric (axial) joint space diminution in this disease. With acetabular involvement in Paget's disease,

either medial or axial joint space narrowing can be seen (Fig. 54–31); with Paget's disease of both the acetabulum and the femoral head, axial joint space loss is particularly frequent, although medial joint space diminution also can be observed (Figs. 54–32 and 54–33); and with isolated femoral head involvement in Paget's disease (which is not a common distribution of the disease), superior joint space loss can occur. These patterns of joint space abnormality are only guidelines, although they do underscore the fact that degenerative joint disease of the hip in Paget's disease frequently differs in appearance from primary degenerative joint disease. Acetabular protrusion may complicate Paget's disease of the acetabulum (Fig. 54–34). Osteophyte formation usually is a mild feature of the disease.

Hip abnormalities accompanying Paget's disease may require surgical intervention. Prosthetic replacement of the femoral head is not always successful because of acetabular pagetic involvement. Although difficulties might be anticipated in performing total hip arthroplasties in patients with Paget's disease because of the presence of sclerotic bone, deformities such as acetabular protrusion and coxa vara, and increased vascularity,[221] Stauffer and Sim[123] experienced no particular technical problems in performing this operation in these persons, although postoperative persistence of pain and induction of heterotopic bone formation may be encountered. Results of more recent reviews of total hip (or knee) arthroplasties in pagetic patients with osteoarthritis of the hip (or knee) have indicated generally successful outcomes.[311-313] In one report, however, rapidly developing osteolysis occurred about the proximal portion of the femoral component of a total hip arthroplasty in a patient with Paget's disease.[331]

With pagetic involvement of the distal femur or proximal tibia, joint space narrowing may be observed in the knee[106] (Fig. 54–35). The glenohumeral joint, too, occasionally is abnormal in Paget's disease (Fig. 54–36). Accompanying symptoms and signs are pain, tenderness, and limitation of motion.

The pathogenesis of arthritic changes associated with Paget's disease is not clear. Goldman and coworkers[121] described pathologic changes about involved hips, which supported the concept that the basis of the joint disease is related, at least in part, to disturbance of endochondral ossification. Hypervascularity and rapid bone turnover in pagetic subchondral bone may lead to accelerated endochondral bone formation, which occurs at the expense of the articular cartilage. The cartilaginous surface can be eroded from beneath.[261] Superimposed on this interference with dynamics at the chondro-osseous junction are mechanical abnormalities about the articulation. Enlargement of the femoral head or decreased size of the acetabulum combined with adjacent bone deformity (femoral bowing, coxa vara, protrusio acetabuli) leads to abnormal stress across the articulation, producing cartilaginous and osseous degeneration.

Other Rheumatic Syndromes

Although certain reports have indicated the coexistence of Paget's disease and specific rheumatic syndromes such as Dupuytren's contracture, Peyronie's disease, and pigmented villonodular synovitis,[162, 222] the relationships between the disorders appear insignificant.

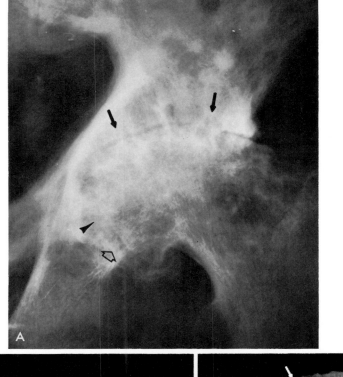

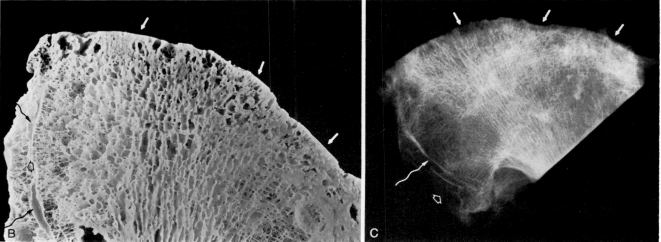

FIGURE 54–31. Paget's disease with secondary degenerative joint disease: Acetabular involvement alone.

A The radiograph demonstrates Paget's disease isolated to the acetabulum with loss of both superior and axial joint space (arrows). The medial joint space is narrowed only slightly (arrowhead). A medial femoral osteophyte is evident (open arrow).

B A photograph of a macerated coronal section of the removed femoral head confirms the widespread distribution of subchondral sclerotic bone (straight arrows) and the presence of a medial femoral osteophyte (open arrow). Some cartilaginous layers have been left behind as the osteophyte has grown (wavy arrows). Paget's disease has not involved the femoral head.

C A radiograph of the macerated section outlines considerable irregularity of subchondral bone over a long segment of the femoral head (straight arrows) with bony eburnation and cyst formation. The osteophyte (open arrow) and original zone of calcified cartilage (wavy arrow) are identified.

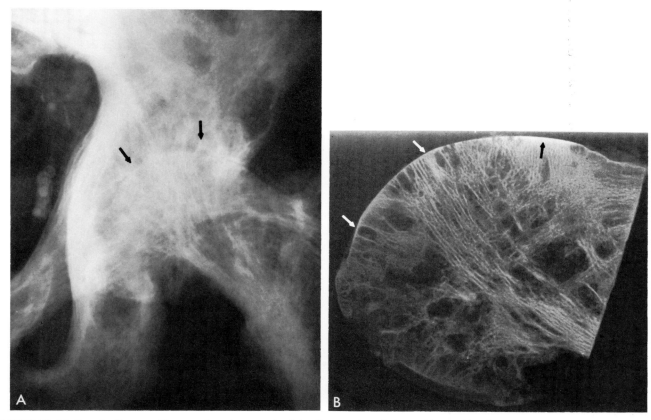

FIGURE 54–32. Paget's disease with secondary degenerative joint disease: Acetabular and femoral involvement.

A The radiograph reveals widespread joint space loss in the superior and axial aspects of the articulation (arrows). Paget's disease is clearly evident in both femur and acetabulum. Osteophytes are not prominent.

B The radiograph of a coronal section of the removed femoral head indicates the coarsened trabeculae of Paget's disease. Note the widespread loss of articular cartilage (arrows), the presence of multiple cystic lesions, and the absence of prominent osteophytes.

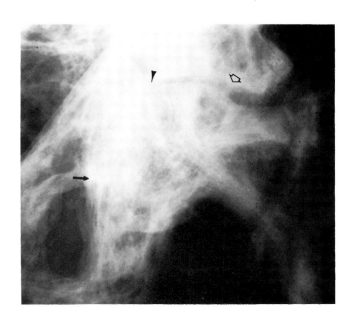

FIGURE 54–33. Paget's disease with secondary degenerative joint disease: Acetabular and femoral involvement. The radiograph reveals severe medial loss of joint space (arrow), with less narrowing of the axial joint space (arrowhead), and relative preservation of the superior joint space (open arrow). Widespread Paget's disease is apparent.

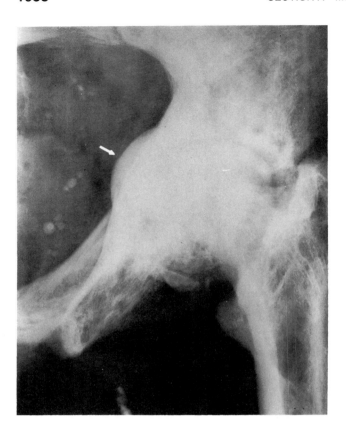

FIGURE 54–34. Paget's disease with acetabular protrusion: Acetabular and femoral involvement. In association with severe Paget's disease of acetabulum and femur, protrusion deformity is apparent (arrow).

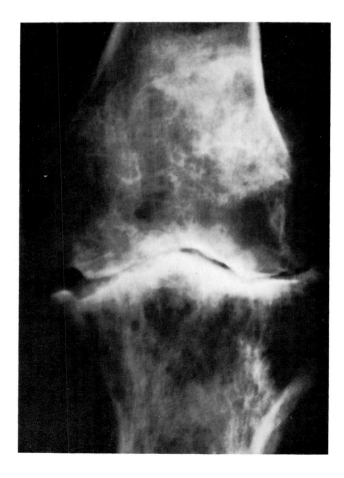

FIGURE 54–35. Paget's disease with secondary degenerative joint disease: Femoral and tibial involvement. Observe considerable loss of articular space in the medial femorotibial and lateral femorotibial compartments. Bone sclerosis is extensive in the subchondral regions, but osteophytes are not prominent.

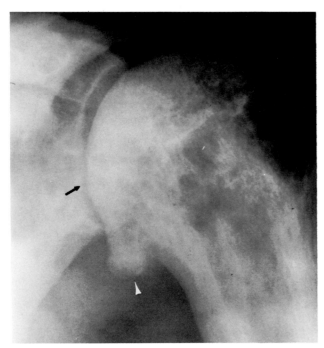

FIGURE 54–36. Paget's disease with secondary degenerative joint disease: Glenohumeral joint involvement. The changes of Paget's disease are readily apparent in the scapula and humerus. Observe glenohumeral joint space narrowing (arrow) and a large humeral osteophyte (arrowhead).

IMAGING ASPECTS OF THERAPY

Since the 1950s, effective therapeutic agents have been used in Paget's disease. One such agent is calcitonin, a potent inhibitor of bone resorption, which can lead to relief of pain within weeks of its administration to patients with Paget's disease and to a reduction in serum alkaline phosphatase levels and urinary hydroxyproline excretion. Radiographic improvement in the appearance of the pagetic bone during calcitonin treatment has been reported by numerous investigators, a finding that is evident in both cortical and trabecular bone, especially during the osteolytic phases of the disease.[223–225, 250, 314, 315] After cessation of the therapy, a period of rapid bone resorption, even greater than that typical of untreated Paget's disease, has been observed[223]; this rapid resorption responds well to re-treatment with calcitonin. Side effects of calcitonin therapy include flushing, nausea, and vomiting, and they occur in about 30 per cent of patients.

A second agent used in the therapy of Paget's disease is disodium etidronate (EHDP), a diphosphonate.[316, 319] Diphosphonates inhibit bone resorption and mineralization by binding to the hydroxyapatite crystals and inhibiting their growth and dissolution.[158] In a majority of patients with this disorder their administration results in a decrease in skeletal pain, a reduction in serum alkaline phosphatase and urinary hydroxyproline levels,[233, 234] and, on evaluation of material derived from bone biopsies, a conversion of pagetic bone to a more normal tissue.[226–228] Radiographic improvement, however, has not been a consistent feature,[316] although it has been apparent in some instances (Fig. 54–37). Several reports have indicated an increased frequency of fractures in patients with Paget's disease treated with EHDP,[229–231] a complication that may relate to drug dosage[231] and to the occurrence of osteomalacia.[175, 232, 262, 317] Other diphosphonates, such as dichloromethylene diphosphonate (Cl$_2$MDP) and 3-amino-1-hydroxypropylidene-1,1-biphosphonate (APD), have been suggested as therapeutic alternatives to EHDP.[235, 316, 318] Such agents delivered intravenously can lead to remissions of 2 years or longer in patients with mild or moderate involvement with Paget's disease.[327]

Mithramycin is an antibiotic with cytotoxic activity that has been used successfully in the treatment of Paget's disease, leading to a decrease in bone pain and an improvement in laboratory parameters of disease activity.[175] Radiographic and scintigraphic assessment of the skeletal disease during therapy also indicates a return to a more normal situation,[236] although radiographic change is less frequent and dramatic after the use of mithramycin than after calcitonin.[225] Owing to its significant toxicity, mithramycin administration is best reserved for cases of Paget's disease resistant to other forms of treatment.[175, 332]

Any of the aforementioned therapeutic agents,[251] but especially calcitonin,[238] can be accompanied by an improvement in the radiographic abnormalities of Paget's disease. The changes generally are subtle, however, and the radio-

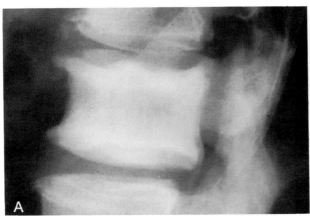
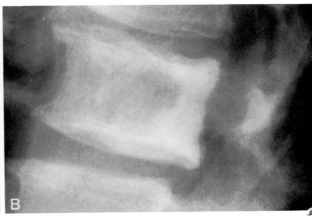

FIGURE 54–37. Treatment of Paget's disease: Disodium etidronate (EHDP)—radiographic improvement. Radiographs obtained 1 year after initial presentation of the disease **(A)** and 4 years 6 months after discontinuity of treatment with EHDP **(B)** reveal improvement in the abnormalities of the second lumbar vertebra on the later examination. (From Nicholas JJ, et al: Arthritis Rheum 32:776, 1989.)

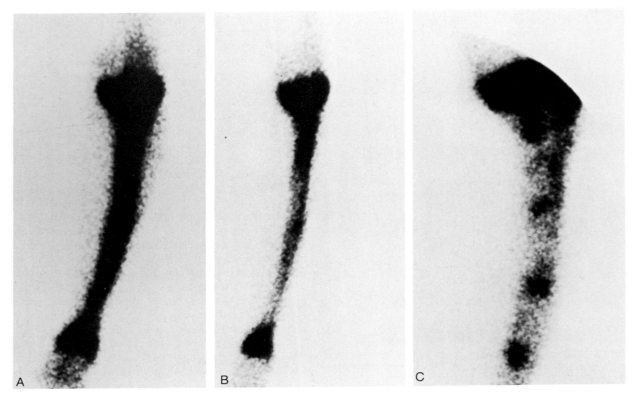

FIGURE 54–38. Treatment of Paget's disease: Thyrocalcitonin—scintigraphic improvement. Bone scans obtained 1 year apart show, initially, intense accumulation of the radionuclide in the tibia with partial resolution over a 2 year period during treatment with thyrocalcitonin. The residual activity on the last scan corresponded in position to sites of insufficiency fractures.

logic assessment is limited further by the influence of such factors as patient position and alterations in radiation exposure on the radiographic image and the variability in progress of untreated Paget's disease. When present, radiographic features of improvement depend on the stage of the disease at the time of treatment and include a conversion of osteolytic lesions to osteosclerotic ones (which also may be seen in uncontrolled Paget's disease), consolidation of the layered new bone, reappearance of a cortex of uniform density, restoration of corticomedullary differentiation, widening of the medullary canal, thinning of the cortex, a reduction in the external volume of the bone, and a return to normal osseous shape.[158]

Scintigraphy, in comparison to radiography, possesses advantages in monitoring the response of pagetic bone to any of these therapeutic agents. The uptake of a bone-seeking radiopharmaceutical preparation is influenced by such factors as the vascularity, bone metabolism, exchangeable bone pool, amount of osteoid, and microscopic architecture.[239] A distinct decrease in radionuclide accumulation in diseased areas is characteristic of the pagetic response to treatment (Fig. 54–38).[64, 65, 239–243] Quantitative measurement of such accumulation has been stressed in some investigations of Paget's disease as a technique superior to qualitative analysis. In general, there is good correlation of scintigraphic and biochemical parameters of disease activity. A remission of Paget's disease is associated with residual activity on the bone scan, presumably indicative of permanent changes in the macro- and microarchitecture of the bone.[239] Recurrence of the disorder typically is accompanied scintigraphically by a rise in activity in one or more bones in a diffuse or circumscribed pattern, or by spread of disease into an adjacent normal bone.[237, 239] Such radionuclide deterioration is not constant in cases of disease recurrence; when present, however, it may precede biochemical indicators of recurrent disease.

DIFFERENTIAL DIAGNOSIS

There are, I think, only two other diseases, namely rachitis and osteomalacia, from which it can be necessary to discriminate the osteitis deformans, and the differences between them are very wide.

SIR JAMES PAGET (1877)

General Features

Although the initial lytic phase of Paget's disease may present some difficulties for the inexperienced observer, its radiographic features are diagnostic. Epiphyseal involvement, sharply demarcated bone lysis, and an advancing wedge of radiolucency allow accurate diagnosis. Widespread sclerosis, which can be apparent in Paget's disease of long duration, also has specific characteristics, such as bony enlargement and a coarsened trabecular pattern, which can be distinguished from findings associated with other diseases. Diffuse increased skeletal radiodensity may be observed in bony metastasis (particularly from prostatic carcinoma) (Fig. 54–39), myelofibrosis (Fig. 54–40), fluorosis, mastocytosis (urticaria pigmentosa), renal osteodystrophy, fibrous dysplasia, and tuberous sclerosis. Additional findings in these other disorders ensure their recognition.

FIGURE 54–39. Skeletal metastasis from carcinoma of the prostate. Patchy osteosclerosis is observed in the pelvis, spine, sacrum, and proximal femora. A coarsened trabecular pattern, which is evident in Paget's disease, is not seen in skeletal metastases.

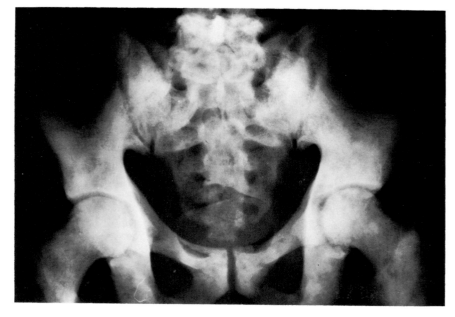

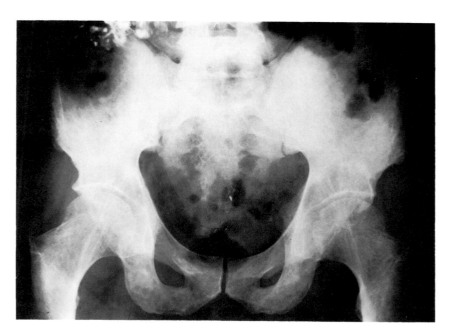

FIGURE 54–40. Myelofibrosis. Lucent and sclerotic areas can be found in the pelvis and proximal femora. The cortices are not thickened, nor is a prominent trabecular pattern in evidence.

For example, hepatosplenomegaly (myelofibrosis, mastocytosis), ligamentous ossification (fluorosis), focal radiodensity (mastocytosis and tuberous sclerosis), characteristic bowing deformities and ''ground glass'' appearance (fibrous dysplasia), and subperiosteal and subchondral bone resorption (renal osteodystrophy) are abnormalities associated with these other diseases.

Axial osteomalacia[127] is a rare disorder, confined to the axial skeleton, associated with a coarsened trabecular pattern on radiographic examination and with abundant osteoid seams on histologic examination. The radiographic findings may simulate those of Paget's disease, although ''spongy''-appearing trabeculae in the cervical spine are especially characteristic in axial osteomalacia.

Fibrogenesis imperfecta ossium[128] is another rare disease observed in elderly patients, associated with coarse trabeculation, spontaneous fractures, and deformity. Pathologically, the condition is characterized by a generalized deficiency in collagen fiber formation. When examined with a polarizing microscope, this collagen lacks normal birefringency, being optically inactive. This feature ensures correct identification of the disease.

Familial idiopathic hyperphosphatasia (osteitis deformans in children, ''juvenile'' Paget's disease, hyperostosis corticalis)[129] is a rare disorder of bone occurring in children, associated with progressive skeletal deformities, coarsely trabeculated and widened bone, and elevation of serum levels of alkaline phosphatase and of urinary levels of hydroxyproline. Additional features include premature loss of teeth and dwarfism. Although some characteristics of this disorder resemble those of Paget's disease, familial idiopathic hyperphosphatasia occurs in younger patients, and epiphyses may not be involved.

Familial expansile osteolysis is a rare, autosomal dominant bone dysplasia, which is characterized by radiographic features that resemble those of Paget's disease.[320] The clinical onset is in the second through fourth decades of life.

Progressive osteoclastic resorption is accompanied by medullary expansion of bone, with a tendency to pain, pathologic fracture, and skeletal deformity.[320] Loss of dentition and an early onset of deafness are associated clinical features. The serum levels of alkaline phosphatase and the urinary levels of hydroxyproline may be elevated.

Calvarial Hyperostosis

Paget's disease of the skull can be confused with other disorders associated with calvarial hyperostosis. These include hyperostosis frontalis interna, fibrous dysplasia, anemias, and skeletal metastasis. Hyperostosis frontalis interna predominates in women and produces thickening of the inner table of the frontal squama.[130] The cause and significance of this condition are not known. Slowly progressive changes may be apparent. Fibrous dysplasia may cause gross enlargement of the skull, although facial involvement is particularly characteristic (Fig. 54–41). Certain anemias, such as sickle cell anemia and thalassemia, produce thickening of the cranial vault and a radiating trabecular pattern (hair-on-end appearance). The base of the skull generally is spared. Osteoblastic metastasis can simulate the ''cotton-wool'' radiodense lesions of Paget's disease.

Vertebral Sclerosis

Condensation of the periphery of a vertebral body, the picture frame vertebra, is diagnostic of Paget's disease. It differs from the accentuated vertical trabeculae of hemangiomas and the rugger-jersey spine of renal osteodystrophy. Some patients with Paget's disease reveal diffuse sclerosis of an entire vertebral body, the ivory vertebra, which can simulate skeletal metastasis and lymphoma (Fig. 54–42). Others reveal a vertebral pattern similar to that of a hemangioma, although the relatively common involvement of the

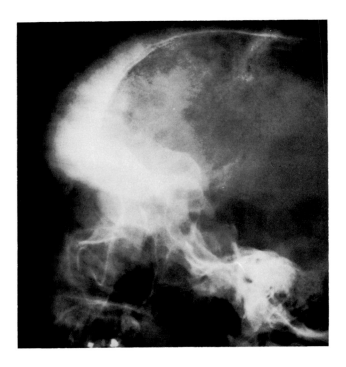

FIGURE 54–41. Fibrous dysplasia. Characteristic hyperostosis and calvarial thickening can be seen in the frontal regions. The facial bones also are affected.

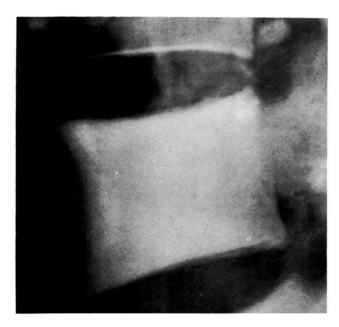

FIGURE 54–42. Skeletal metastasis from carcinoma of the prostate: Ivory vertebral body. Note the homogeneous increase in skeletal density of the involved vertebral body. The disc spaces are preserved.

posterior spinal elements in Paget's disease usually is not seen in hemangiomas.

Pelvic Abnormalities

Although pelvic sclerosis in Paget's disease can mimic the findings of osteoblastic metastasis, asymmetric or unilateral distribution, accentuated trabecular pattern, and enlargement of the involved bone are typical of Paget's disease. In elderly patients, thickening of the iliopubic line and Cooper's ligament calcification should not be interpreted as early radiographic signs of Paget's disease (Fig. 54–43).

SUMMARY

Paget's disease is a common disorder of middle-aged and elderly patients, characterized by excessive and abnormal remodeling of bone. Its radiographic features are virtually diagnostic, including an initial osteolytic phase, most common in the skull and tubular bones, and a subsequent osteosclerotic phase, particularly in the axial skeleton. An enlarged bone with increased radiodensity and accentuated trabecular pattern is typical. Involvement of specific sites leads to characteristic radiographic signs, including the cotton-wool cranial vault and the picture frame vertebral body.

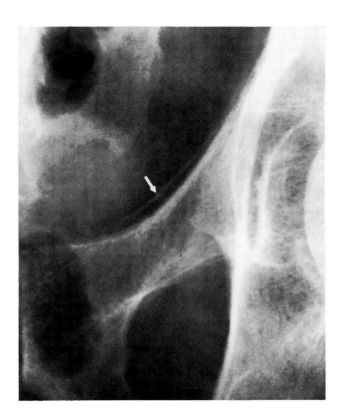

FIGURE 54–43. Cooper's ligament calcification. A curvilinear radiodense area (arrow) adjacent to the pubic bone represents calcification of Cooper's ligament. The appearance is not reminiscent of Paget's disease.

Complications associated with Paget's disease are insufficiency fractures, neurologic symptoms and signs, skeletal deformities, neoplasms, and articular alterations. The most important articular abnormality associated with this disorder is degenerative joint disease, particularly of the hip and knee. Additionally, crystal deposition and rheumatoid variant disorders have been reported in this condition.

References

1. Schmorl G: Ueber Ostitis deformans Paget. Virchows Arch (Pathol Anat) 283:694, 1932.
2. Paget J: On a form of chronic inflammation of bones (osteitis deformans). Med Chir Tr 60:37, 1877.
3. Jones JV, Reed MF: Paget's disease. Family with six cases. Br Med J 4:90, 1967.
4. Gutman AB, Kasabach H: Paget's disease (osteitis deformans). Analysis of 116 cases. Am J Med Sci 191:361, 1936.
5. Rast H, Weber FP: Paget's bone disease in three sisters. Br Med J 1:918, 1937.
6. Aschner BM, Hurst LA, Roizin L: A genetic study of Paget's disease (osteitis deformans) in monozygotic twin brothers. Acta Genet Med Gemellol 1:67, 1952.
7. Montagu MFA: Paget's disease (osteitis deformans) and heredity. Am J Hum Genet 1:94, 1949.
8. Nagant de Deuxchaisnes C, Krane SM: Paget's disease of bone: Clinical and metabolic observations. Medicine 43:233, 1964.
9. Collins DH: Paget's disease of bone. Incidence and subclinical forms. Lancet 271:51, 1956.
10. Harris ED Jr, Krane SM: Paget's disease of bone. Bull Rheum Dis 18:506, 1968.
11. Barry HC: Paget's Disease of Bone. Edinburgh, E&S Livingstone, 1969, p 16.
12. Kasabach HH, Gutman AB: Osteoporosis circumscripta of the skull and Paget's disease; 15 new cases and a review of the literature. AJR 37:577, 1937.
13. Dickson DD, Camp JD, Ghormley RK: Osteitis deformans: Paget's disease of the bone. Radiology 44:449, 1945.
14. Greenspan A, Normon A, Sterling AP: Precocious onset of Paget's disease—a report of three cases and review of the literature. J Can Assoc Radiol 28:69, 1977.
15. Edeiken J, DePalma AF, Hodes PJ: Paget's disease: Osteitis deformans. Clin Orthop 146:141, 1966.
16. Jaffe HL: Metabolic, Degenerative and Inflammatory Diseases of Bones and Joints. Philadelphia, Lea & Febiger, 1972, p 240.
17. Hartman JT, Down JDF: Paget's disease of the spine with cord or nerve root compression. J Bone Joint Surg [Am] 48:1079, 1966.
18. Lake M: Studies of Paget's disease (osteitis deformans). J Bone Joint Surg [Br] 33:323, 1951.
19. Nager GT: Paget's disease of the temporal bone. Ann Otol Rhinol Laryngol 84(Suppl 22):1, 1975.
20. Davies DG: Paget's disease of the temporal bone. Acta Otolaryngol 242(Suppl):1, 1968.
21. Lindsay JR, Lehman RH: Histopathology of the temporal bone in advanced Paget's disease. Laryngoscope 79:213, 1969.
22. Waltner JG: Stapedectomy in Paget's disease. Arch Otolaryngol 82:355, 1965.
23. Howarth S: Cardiac output in osteitis deformans. Clin Sci 12:271, 1953.
24. Potts JT Jr, Deftos LJ: Parathyroid hormone, calcitonin, vitamin D, bone and bone mineral metabolism. In PK Bondy, LE Rosenberg (Eds): Duncan's Diseases of Metabolism. 7th Ed. Vol II. Endocrinology. Philadelphia, W.B. Saunders Co, 1974, p 1381.
25. O'Reilly TJ, Race J: Osteitis deformans. Q J Med 1:471, 1932.
26. Harrison CV, Lennox B: Heart block in osteitis deformans. Br Heart J 10:167, 1948.
27. Luxton RW: Paget's disease of bone associated with Hashimoto's struma lymphomatosa. Lancet 1:441, 1957.
28. Bodansky A, Jaffe HL: Phosphatase studies. III. Serum phosphatase in diseases of bone: Interpretation and significance. Arch Intern Med 54:88, 1934.
29. Jaffe HL, Bodansky A: Diagnostic significance of serum alkaline and acid phosphatase values in relation to bone disease. Bull NY Acad Med 19:831, 1943.
30. Woodard HQ, Twombly GH, Coley BL: A study of the serum phosphatase in bone disease. J Clin Invest 15:193, 1936.
31. Woodard HQ: Long term studies of the blood chemistries in Paget's disease of bone. Cancer 12:1226, 1959.
32. Dull TA, Henneman PH: Urinary hydroxyproline as an index of collagen turnover in bone. N Engl J Med 268:132, 1963.
33. Henneman PH, Dull TA, Avioli LV, et al: Effects of aspirin and corticosteroids on Paget's disease of bone. Trans Stud Coll Physicians Phila 31:10, 1963.
34. Jacobs P: Osteolytic Paget's disease. Clin Radiol 25:137, 1974.
35. Anderson JT, Dehner LP: Osteolytic form of Paget's disease. Differential diagnosis and pathogenesis. J Bone Joint Surg [Am] 58:994, 1976.
36. Kasabach HH, Dyke CG: Osteoporosis circumscripta of the skull as a form of osteitis deformans. AJR 28:192, 1932.
37. Kasabach HH, Gutman AB: Osteoporosis circumscripta of the skull and Paget's disease. Fifteen new cases and a review of the literature. AJR 37:577, 1937.
38. Collins DH, Winn JM: Focal Paget's disease of the skull (osteoporosis circumscripta). J Pathol Bacteriol 69:1, 1955.
39. Milgram JW: Radiographical and pathological assessment of the activity of Paget's disease of bone. Clin Orthop 127:43, 1977.
40. Grunthal E: Über den Hirnbefund bei Pagetscher Krankheit des Schädels. Zugleich ein Beitrag zur Kenntnis der Entstehung systematischer Kleinhirnatrophien. Ztschr Neurol Psychiat 136:656, 1931.
41. Chakravorty NK, Das SK, Kataria MS: Corrugation of the skull in Paget's disease of bone. Postgrad Med J 53:40, 1977.
42. Steinbach HL: Some roentgen features of Paget's disease. AJR 86:950, 1961.
43. Brown HP, LaRocca H, Wickstrom JK: Paget's disease of the atlas and axis. J Bone Joint Surg [Am] 53:1441, 1971.
44. Feldman F, Seaman WB: The neurologic complications of Paget's disease in the cervical spine. AJR 105:375, 1969.
45. Janetos GP: Paget's disease in the cervical spine. AJR 97:655, 1966.
46. Ramamurthi B, Visvanathan GS: Paget's disease of the axis causing quadriplegia. J Neurosurg 14:580, 1957.
47. Whalley N: Paget's disease of atlas and axis. J Neurol Neurosurg Psychiatry 9:84, 1946.
48. Schreiber MH, Richardson GA: Paget's disease confined to one lumbar vertebra. AJR 90:1271, 1963.
49. Lewis RJ, Jacobs B, Marchisello PJ, et al. Monostotic Paget's disease of the spine. Clin Orthop 127:208, 1977.
50. Klenerman L: Cauda equina and spinal cord compression in Paget's disease. J Bone Joint Surg [Am] 48:365, 1966.
51. Turner JWA: The spinal complications of Paget's disease (osteitis deformans). Brain 63:321, 1940.
52. Robinson RG: Paraplegia due to Paget's disease (osteitis deformans). Br Med J 2:542, 1953.
53. Burgener FA, Perry PE: Pitfalls in the radiographic diagnosis of Paget's disease of the pelvis. Skel Radiol 2:231, 1978.
54. Claustre J, Blotman F, Simon L: Les atteintes du pied au cours de la maladie osseuse de Paget. Rev Rhum Mal Osteoartic 43:45, 1976.
55. Haverbush TJ, Wilde AH, Phalen GS: The hand in Paget's disease of bone. Report of two cases. J Bone Joint Surg [Am] 54:173, 1972.
56. Wilner D, Sherman RS: Roentgen diagnosis of Paget's disease (osteitis deformans). Med Radiogr Photogr 42:35, 1966.
57. Lentle BC, Russell AS, Heslip PG, et al: The scintigraphic findings in Paget's disease of bone. Clin Radiol 27:129, 1976.
58. Lentle BC, Russell AS, Percy JS, et al: Bone scintiscanning updated. Ann Intern Med 84:297, 1976.
59. Khairi MRA, Wellman HN, Robb JA, et al: Paget's disease of bone (osteitis deformans): Symptomatic lesions and bone scan. Ann Intern Med 79:348, 1973.
60. Miller SW, Castronovo FP, Pendergrass HP, et al: Technetium-99m labeled diphosphonate bone scanning in Paget's disease. AJR 121:177, 1974.
61. Fletcher JW, Butler RL, Henry RE, et al: Bone marrow scanning in Paget's disease. J Nucl Med 14:928, 1973.
62. Andrews JT: Osteoporosis circumscripta cranii: Its importance in brain scintiscanning. Australas Radiol 20:273, 1976.
63. Rausch JM, Resnick D, Goergen TG, et al: Bone scanning in osteolytic Paget's disease: Case report. J Nucl Med 18:699, 1977.
64. Waxman AD, Ducker S, McKee D, et al: Evaluation of ^{99m}Tc diphosphonate kinetics and bone scans in patients with Paget's disease before and after calcitonin treatment. Radiology 125:761, 1977.
65. Lavender JP, Evans IMA, Arnot R, et al: A comparison of radiography and radioisotope scanning in the detection of Paget's disease and in the assessment of response to human calcitonin. Br J Radiol 50:243, 1977.
66. Camus JP, Tricoire J, Mariel L, et al: La maladie de Paget. Poussées évolutives traitées par la calcitonine. Étude thermographique. Nouv Presse Med 2:2517, 1973.
67. Allen ML, John RL: Osteitis deformans (Paget's disease) fissure fractures—their etiology and clinical significance. AJR 38:109, 1937.
68. Looser E: Osteitis deformans und Unfall. Arch Klin Chir 180:379, 1934.
69. Grundy M: Fractures of the femur in Paget's disease of bone, their etiology and treatment. J Bone Joint Surg [Br] 52:252, 1970.
70. Nicholas JA, Killoran P: Fracture of the femur in patients with Paget's disease. Results of treatment in twenty-three cases. J Bone Joint Surg [Am] 47:450, 1965.
71. Price CHG, Goldie W: Paget's sarcoma of bone. J Bone Joint Surg [Br] 51:205, 1969.
72. Ross FGM, Middlemiss JH, Fitton JM: Sarcoma in Paget's disease (Abstr). J Bone Joint Surg [Br] 55:880, 1973.
73. Shannon FT, Hopkins JS: Paget's sarcoma of the vertebral column with neurological complications. Acta Orthop Scand 48:385, 1977.
74. Campbell E, Whitfield RD: Osteogenic sarcoma of vertebrae secondary to Paget's disease. NY State J Med 43:931, 1943.
75. Poretta CA, Dahlin DC, Janes JM: Sarcoma in Paget's disease of bone. J Bone Joint Surg [Am] 39:1314, 1957.
76. Von Albertini A: Über Sarkombildung auf dem Boden der Ostitis deformans Paget (Kasuistischer Beitrag). Virchows Arch (Pathol Anat) 268:259, 1928.
77. McKenna RJ, Schwinn CP, Soong KY, et al: Osteogenic sarcoma arising in Paget's disease. Cancer 17:42, 1964.
78. Bonakdarpour A, Harwick R, Pickering J: Case report 34. Skel Radiol 2:52, 1977.
79. Hutter RV, Foote FW, Frazell EL, et al: Giant cell tumors complicating Paget's disease of bone. Cancer 16:1044, 1963.

80. Shklar G, Meyer I: A giant-cell tumor of the maxilla in an area of osteitis deformans (Paget's disease of bone). Oral Surg *11:*835, 1958.

81. Hilton G: Osteoclastoma associated with generalized bone disease. Br J Radiol *23:*437, 1950.

82. Goldstein BH, Laskin DM: Giant cell tumor of the maxilla complicating Paget's disease of bone. J Oral Surg *32:*209, 1974.

83. Brook RI: Giant cell tumor in patients with Paget's disease. J Oral Surg *30:*230, 1970.

84. Miller AS, Cuttino CL, Elzay RP, et al: Giant cell tumor of the jaws associated with Paget's disease of bone. Arch Otolaryngol *100:*233, 1974.

85. Barry HC: Sarcoma in Paget's disease of bone in Australia. J Bone Joint Surg [Am] *43:*1122, 1961.

86. Price CHG: Myeloma occurring with Paget's disease of bone. Skel Radiol *1:*15, 1976.

87. Gross RJ, Yelin G: Multiple myeloma complicating Paget's disease. AJR *65:*585, 1951.

88. Verdier JM, Commandre F, Rivollier P, et al: Triple association pelvispondylite, Paget et myélome. Rev Rhum Mal Osteoartic *41:*353, 1974.

89. Scurr JA: Myeloma occurring in Paget's disease. Proc R Soc Med *65:*725, 1972.

90. Burgener FA, Perry PE: Solitary renal cell carcinoma metastasis in Paget's disease simulating sarcomatous degeneration. AJR *128:*853, 1977.

91. Agha FP, Norman A, Hirschl S, et al: Paget's disease. Coexistence with metastatic carcinoma. NY State J Med *76:*734, 1976.

92. Jacobson HG, Siegelman SS: Some miscellaneous solitary bone lesions. Semin Roentgenol *1:*314, 1966.

93. Jaffe HL: Paget's disease of bone. Arch Pathol *15:*83, 1933.

94. Reifenstein EC Jr, Albright F: Paget's disease: Its pathologic physiology and the importance of this in the complications arising from fracture and immobilization. N Engl J Med *231:*343, 1944.

95. Bowerman JW, Altman J, Hughes JL, et al: Pseudo-malignant lesions in Paget's disease of bone. AJR *124:*57, 1975.

96. Latimer FR, Webster JE, Gurdjian ES: Osteitis deformans with spinal cord compression. J Neurosurg *10:*583, 1953.

97. Sadar ES, Walton RJ, Grossman HH: Neurological dysfunction in Paget's disease of the vertebral column. J Neurosurg *37:*661, 1972.

98. Colclough JA: Compression of the spinal cord by osteitis deformans: Report of a case. Surgery *25:*760, 1949.

99. Direkze M, Milnes JN: Spinal cord compression in Paget's disease. Br J Surg *57:*239, 1970.

100. Hunt JH: Paget's disease with spinal compression improving after laminectomy. Proc R Soc Med *28:*1519, 1935.

101. Miller JD: Spinal compression due to Paget's disease of bone. Scott Med J *12:*441, 1967.

102. Schwarz GA, Reback S: Compression of the spinal cord in osteitis deformans (Paget's disease) of the vertebrae. AJR *42:*345, 1939.

103. Siegelman SS, Levine SA, Walpin L: Paget's disease with spinal cord compression. Clin Radiol *19:*421, 1968.

104. Clarke PRR, Williams HI: Ossification in extradural fat in Paget's disease of the spine. Br J Surg *62:*571, 1975.

105. Kadir S, Kalisher L, Schiller AL: Extramedullary hematopoiesis in Paget's disease of bone. AJR *129:*493, 1977.

106. Franck WA, Bress NM, Singer FR, et al: Rheumatic manifestations of Paget's disease of bone. Am J Med *56:*592, 1974.

107. McCarty DJ Jr: Pseudogout: Articular chondrocalcinosis. *In* JL Hollander, DJ McCarty Jr (Eds): Arthritis and Allied Conditions. 8th Ed. Philadelphia, Lea & Febiger, 1972, p 1140.

108. Radi I, Epiney J, Reiner M: Chondrocalcinose et maladie osseuse de Paget. Rev Rhum Mal Osteoartic *37:*385, 1970.

109. Boussina I, Gerster JC, Epiney J, et al: A study of the incidence of articular chondrocalcinosis in Paget's disease of bone. Scand J Rheumatol *5:*33, 1976.

110. Wells HG, Holley SW: Metastatic calcification in osteitis deformans (Paget's disease of bone). Arch Pathol *34:*435, 1942.

111. Seligman B, Nathanson L: "Metastatic" calcification in soft tissues of legs in osteitis deformans; case report. Ann Intern Med *23:*82, 1945.

112. Davidson JC: Case of calcinosis circumscripta with Paget's disease of bone. Cent Afr J Med *7:*240, 1961.

113. Commandre FA, Berato J, Bonnefond O, et al: Association d'une sclerodermie type Thibierge-Weissenbach et d'une maladie de Paget. Rhumatologie *19:*179, 1967.

114. Layani F, Francon J, Wattebled R: A propos de l'association cinq fois constatée, de spondylarthrite ankylosante et de maladie de Paget. Sem Hôp Paris *37:*1037, 1961.

115. Bitar E: Maladie osseuse pagetoide avec ossification des ligaments prevertébraux chez un homme jeune. Rev Med Moyen Orient *18:*477, 1961.

116. Collins DH (Ed): The Pathology of Articular and Spinal Diseases. London, Edward Arnold, 1949, p 108.

117. Machtey I, Rodnan GP, Benedek TG: Paget's disease of the hip joint. Am J Med Sci *251:*524, 1966.

118. Graham J, Harris WH: Paget's disease involving the hip joint. J Bone Joint Surg [Br] *53:*650, 1971.

119. Roper BA: Paget's disease involving the hip joint. A classification. Clin Orthop *80:*33, 1971.

120. Detenbeck LC, Sim FH, Johnson EW Jr: Symptomatic Paget disease of the hip. JAMA *224:*213, 1973.

121. Goldman AB, Bullough P, Kammermans S, et al: Osteitis deformans of the hip joint. AJR *128:*601, 1977.

122. Roper BA: Paget's disease of the hip with osteoarthrosis: Results of intertrochanteric osteotomy. J Bone Joint Surg [Br] *53:*660, 1971.

123. Stauffer RN, Sim FH: Total hip arthroplasty in Paget's disease of the hip. J Bone Joint Surg [Am] *58:*476, 1976.

124. Guyer PB, Dewbury KC: The hip joint in Paget's disease (Paget's "coxopathy"). Br J Radiol *51:*574, 1978.

125. Chambers GM, Pearson JR: Femoral osteotomy in Paget's disease affecting the hip joint. Br J Clin Pract *24:*107, 1970.

126. Resnick D: Patterns of migration of the femoral head in osteoarthritis of the hip: Roentgenographic-pathologic correlation and comparison with rheumatoid arthritis. AJR *124:*62, 1975.

127. Frame B, Frost HM, Ormond RS, et al: Atypical osteomalacia involving the axial skeleton. Ann Intern Med *55:*632, 1961.

128. Baker SL, Dent CE, Friedman M, et al: Fibrogenesis imperfecta ossium. J Bone Joint Surg [Br] *48:*804, 1966.

129. Eyring EJ, Eisenberg E: Congenital hyperphosphatasia. A clinical, pathological, and biochemical study of two cases. J Bone Joint Surg [Am] *50:*1099, 1968.

130. Salmi A, Voutilainen A, Holsti LR, et al: Hyperostosis cranii in a normal population. Am J Roentgenol *87:*1032, 1962.

131. Bhate DV, Supan WAP, Sparagana M, et al: Case report 94. Skel Radiol *4:*115, 1979.

132. Genuth SM, Klein L: Hypoparathyroidism and Paget's disease: The effect of parathyroid hormone administration. J Clin Endocrinol Metab *35:*693, 1972.

133. Jones JV, Reed MF: Paget's disease. A family with six cases. Br Med J *4:*90, 1967.

134. Melick RA, Martin TJ: Paget's disease in identical twins. Aust NZ J Med *5:*564, 1974.

135. McKusick VA: Heritable Disorders of Connective Tissue. 4th Ed. St Louis, CV Mosby Co, 1972.

136. Fotino M, Haymovits A, Falk CT: Evidence for linkage between HLA and Paget's disease. Transplant Proc *9:*1867, 1977.

137. Rasmussen H, Bordier P: The cellular basis of metabolic bone disease. N Engl J Med *289:*25, 1973.

138. Mills BG, Singer FR: Nuclear inclusions in Paget's disease of bone. Science *194:*201, 1976.

139. Medical Staff Conference, University of California: Paget disease of bone. West J Med *129:*210, 1978.

140. Walpin LA, Singer FR: Paget's disease. Reversal of severe paraparesis using calcitonin. Spine *4:*213, 1979.

141. Harris DJ, Hons Ch B, Fornasier VL: An ivory vertebra. Monostotic Paget's disease of bone. Clin Orthop *136:*173, 1978.

142. Smith NHH: Monostotic Paget's disease of the mandible presenting with progressive resorption of the teeth. Oral Surg *46:*246, 1978.

143. Henin D, Weiss AM, Dairow A, et al: Sarcome ostéogéne cranien sur maladie de Paget. Ann Med Intern *130:*169, 1970.

144. Fried K: Das Uberwachsen von Knorpel- und Bindegewebestrukturen der Wirbelsäule in der deformierenden Osteodystrophie. Radiologe *18:*362, 1978.

145. Stafne EC, Austin LT: A study of dental roentgenograms in cases of Paget's disease (osteitis deformans), osteitis fibrosa cystica and osteoma. J Am Dent Assoc *25:*1202, 1938.

146. Ogilvie-Harris DJ, Hons ChB, Fornasier VL: Pathologic fractures of the hand in Paget's disease. Clin Orthop *143:*168, 1979.

147. Dove J: Complete fractures of the femur in Paget's disease of bone. J Bone Joint Surg [Br] *62:*12, 1980.

148. Weinert CR, Wiss DA: Paget's disease of the patella. Clin Orthop *142:*139, 1979.

149. Huang TL, Cohen NJ, Sahgal S, et al: Osteosarcoma complicating Paget's disease of the spine with neurological complications. Clin Orthop *141:*260, 1979.

150. Jacobs TP, Michelsen J, Polay JS, et al: Giant cell tumor in Paget's disease of bone. Familial and geographic clustering. Cancer *44:*742, 1979.

151. Feldman F: Case report 115. Skel Radiol *5:*119, 1980.

152. Waxman AD, McKee D, Siemsen JK, et al: Gallium scanning in Paget's disease of bone: Effect of calcitonin. AJR *134:*303, 1980.

153. Mazières B, Jung-Rozenfarb M, Arlet J: Rapports de la maladie de Paget avec l'hyperostose vértébrale ankylosante et l'hyperostose frontale interne. Sem Hôp Paris *54:*521, 1978.

154. Murphy WA, Whyte MP, Haddad JG Jr: Healing of lytic Paget bone disease with diphosphonate therapy. Radiology *134:*635, 1980.

155. Murphy WA, Whyte MP, Haddad JG Jr: Paget bone disease: Radiologic documentation of healing with human calcitonin therapy. Radiology *136:*1, 1980.

156. Rebel A, Baslé M, Pouplard A, et al: Viral antigens in osteoclasts from Paget's disease of bone. Lancet *2:*344, 1980.

157. Shenoy BV, Scheithauer BW: Sir James Paget, F.R.S. Mayo Clin Proc *58:*51, 1983.

158. Hamdy RC: Paget's Disease of Bone. Assessment and Management. New York, Praeger Publishers, 1981.

159. Paget S: Memoirs and Letters of Sir James Paget. Fifth impression. London, Longmans, Green and Company, 1901 (cited in Shenoy and Scheithauer[157]).

160. Woodhouse NJY: Paget's disease. Clin Rheum Dis *7:*647, 1981.

161. Dalinka MK, Aronchick JM, Haddad JG Jr: Paget's disease. Orthop Clin North Am *14:*3, 1983.

162. Altman RD, Collins B: Musculoskeletal manifestations of Paget's disease of bone. Arthritis Rheum *23:*1121, 1980.

163. Detheridge FM, Guyer PB, Barker DJP: European distribution of Paget's disease of bone. Br Med J 285:1005, 1982.

164. Naiken VS: Did Beethoven have Paget's disease of bone? Ann Intern Med 74:995, 1971.

165. Askenasi R, Debacker M, Devos A: The origin of urinary hydroxylysyl glycosides in Paget's disease of bone and in primary hyperparathyroidism. Calcif Tissue Res 22:35, 1976.

166. Chapuy MC, Zucchelli Ph, Meunier RJ: Parathyroid function in Paget's disease of bone. Rev Rhum Mal Osteoartic 50:336, 1983.

167. Rebel A, Basle M, Pouplard A, et al: Toward a viral etiology for Paget's disease of bone. Metab Bone Dis Rel Res 4–5:235, 1981.

168. Raine CS, Powers JM, Kinuko-S: Acute multiple scleroses. Confirmation of "paramyxovirus like" intranuclear inclusions. Arch Neurol 30:39, 1974.

169. Mills BG, Singer FR, Weiner LP, et al: Evidence for both respiratory syncytial virus and measles virus antigens in the osteoclasts of patients with Paget's disease of bone. Clin Orthop 183:303, 1984.

170. Singer FR, Mills BG: Evidence for a viral etiology of Paget's disease of bone. Clin Orthop 178:245, 1983.

171. Mirra JM, Bauer H, Grant TT: Giant cell tumor with viral-like intranuclear inclusions associated with Paget's disease. Clin Orthop 158:243, 1981.

172. Mirra JM, Gold RH: Case report 186. Skel Radiol 8:67, 1982.

173. Basle MF, Rebel A, Renier JC, et al: Bone tissue in Paget's disease treated by ethane-1, hydroxy-1, 1 diphosphonate (EHDP). Structure, ultrastructure, and immunocytology. Clin Orthop 184:281, 1984.

174. Rebel A, Basle M: Maladie osseuse de Paget et virus. Ann Pathol 1:21, 1981.

175. Frame B, Marel GM: Paget disease: A review of current knowledge. Radiology 141:21, 1981.

176. Lauffenberger T, Olah AJ, Dambacher MA, et al: Bone remodeling and calcium metabolism; a correlated histomorphometric, calcium kinetic and biochemical study in patients with osteoporosis and Paget's disease. Metabolism 26:589, 1977.

177. Wootton R, Tellez M, Green JR, et al: Skeletal blood flow in Paget's disease of bone. Metab Bone Dis Rel Res 4–5:263, 1981.

178. Wootton R, Reeve J, Veall N: The clinical measurement of skeletal blood flow. Clin Sci Molec Med 50:261, 1976.

179. Rosenthal DI, Raymond K: Case report 148. Skel Radiol 6:205, 1981.

180. Schubert F, Siddle KJ, Harper JS: Diaphyseal Paget's disease: An unusual finding in the tibia. Clin Radiol 35:71, 1984.

181. Guyer PB, Chamberlain AT, Ackery DM, et al: The anatomic distribution of osteitis deformans. Clin Orthop 156:141, 1981.

182. Lucas RB: The jaws and teeth in Paget's disease of bone. J Clin Pathol 8:195, 1955.

183. Rao VM, Karasick D: Hypercementosis—an important clue to Paget disease of the maxilla. Skel Radiol 9:126, 1982.

184. Bewermeyer H, Dreesbach HA, Hunermann B, et al: MR imaging of familial basilar impression. J Comput Assist Tomogr 8:953, 1984.

185. Herzberg L, Bayliss E: Spinal cord syndrome due to non-compressive Paget's disease of bone: A spinal artery steal phenomenon reversible with calcitonin. Lancet 2:13, 1980.

186. Godefroy D, Chevrot A, Ranoux C, et al: L'arc posterieur de la vertébre d'ivoire pagetique. A propos de six cas biopsies. J Radiol 61:611, 1980.

187. Maldague B, Malghem J: Aspects radiologiques de la maladie de Paget. J Belge Rheum Med Phys 29:293, 1974.

188. Schlesinger A, Naimark A, Lee VW: Diaphyseal presentation of Paget's disease in long bones. Radiology 147:83, 1983.

189. Friedman AC, Orcutt J, Madewell JE: Paget disease of the hand: Radiographic spectrum. AJR 138:691, 1982.

190. Hadjipavlou A, Lander P, Boudreau R, et al: Pagetoid changes in a heterotopic center of ossification. A case report. J Bone Joint Surg [Am] 63:1339, 1981.

191. Kattapuram SV, Gadziala NA, Kirkham SE: Case report 191. Skel Radiol 8:81, 1982.

192. Dionne D, Taillefer R, Leblond R, et al: Osteoporosis circumscripta cranii. A cause for "doughnut" sign on cerebral and bone scans. Clin Nucl Med 8:377, 1983.

193. Vellenga CJLR, Pauwels EKL, Bijvoet OLM, et al: Untreated Paget's disease of bone studied by scintigraphy. Radiology 153:799, 1984.

194. Newmark H III: Paget's disease of a vertebral body seen on computerized tomography. Comput Radiol 6:7, 1982.

195. Heller M, Dihlmann W: Computertomographie der Paget-koxopathie. ROFO 138:427, 1983.

196. Weisz GM: Lumbar spinal canal stenosis in Paget's disease. Spine 8:192, 1983.

197. Ravichandran G: Spinal cord function in Paget's disease of spine. Paraplegia 19:7, 1981.

198. Barry HC: Orthopedic aspects of Paget's disease of bone. Arthritis Rheum 23:1128, 1980.

199. Stevens J: Orthopaedic aspects of Paget's disease. Metab Bone Dis Rel Res 4–5:271, 1981.

200. Louyot P, Pourel J, Delagoutte JP, et al: Quelques aspects inhabituels de fracture d'os pagetique. Rev Rhum Mal Osteoartic 42:653, 1975.

201. Wick MR, McLeod RA, Siegal GP, et al: Sarcomas of bone complicating osteitis deformans (Paget's disease). Fifty years' experience. Am J Surg Pathol 5:47, 1981.

202. Greditzer HG III, McLeod RA, Unni KK, et al: Bone sarcomas in Paget disease. Radiology 146:327, 1983.

203. Schajowicz F, Araujo ES, Berenstein M: Sarcoma complicating Paget's disease of bone. A clinicopathological study of 62 cases. J Bone Joint Surg [Br] 65:299, 1983.

204. Choquette D, Haraoui B, Altman RD, et al: Simultaneous multifocal sarcomatous degeneration in Paget's disease of bone. A hypothesis. Clin Orthop 179:308, 1983.

205. Miller C, Rao VM: Sarcomatous degeneration of Paget's disease in the skull. Skel Radiol 10:102, 1983.

206. Huvos AG, Butler A, Bretsky SS: Osteogenic sarcoma associated with Paget's disease of bone. A clinicopathologic study of 65 patients. Cancer 52:1489, 1983.

207. Smith J, Botet JF, Yeh SDJ: Bone sarcomas in Paget's disease: A study of 85 patients. Radiology 152:583, 1984.

208. Yochum TR: Paget's sarcoma of bone. Radiologe 24:428, 1984.

209. Griffin JF, Colclough A, Twentyman O, et al: Chordoid sarcoma complicating Paget's disease of bone: A case report and review of the literature. Br J Radiol 57:836, 1984.

210. Francis R, Lewis E: CT demonstration of giant cell tumor complicating Paget disease. J Comput Assist Tomogr 7:917, 1983.

211. Nusbacher N, Sclafani SJ, Birla SR: Case report 155. Skel Radiol 6:233, 1981.

212. Song IS, Chan KF, Tey PH, et al: Case report 159. Skel Radiol 6:299, 1981.

213. Wong DF, Bobeehko PE, Becker EJ, et al: Coexistent multiple myeloma and Paget's disease of bone. J Can Assoc Radiol 32:251, 1981.

214. Dine G, Cheriot J, Hopfner C, et al: Association d'une maladie de Paget et d'une maladie de Kahler. Presse Med 12:361, 1983.

215. Molle D, Bard H, Kuntz D, et al: Osteolyse revelatrice d'un lymphome developpe sur un os pagetique. Rev Rhum Mal Osteoartic 50:217, 1983.

216. Kalinowski DT, Goodwin CA: Case report 179. Skel Radiol 7:229, 1981.

217. Taillandier J, de Lara AC, Manigand G: Metastase osseuse d'un adenocarcinome similant, au cours d'une maladie de Paget, une dégénérescence sarcomateuse. Sem Hop Paris 60:2019, 1984.

218. Powell N: Metastatic carcinoma in association with Paget's disease of bone. Br J Radiol 56:582, 1983.

219. Resnik CS, Walter RD, Haghighi P, et al: Case report 218. Skel Radiol 9:145, 1982.

220. Yeh SDJ, Rosen G, Benua RS: Gallium scans in Paget's sarcoma. Clin Nucl Med 7:546, 1982.

221. Merkow RL, Pellicci PM, Hely DP, et al: Total hip replacement for Paget's disease of the hip. J Bone Joint Surg [Am] 66:752, 1984.

222. Mirra JH, Finerman G, Lindholm S: Diffuse pigmented villonodular synovitis in association with Paget's disease of bone. Report of a case. Clin Orthop 149:305, 1980.

223. Doyle FH, Banks LM, Pennock JM: Radiologic observations on bone resorption in Paget's disease. Arthritis Rheum 23:1205, 1980.

224. Hamilton CR Jr: Effects of synthetic salmon calcitonin in patients with Paget's disease of bone. Am J Med 56:315, 1974.

225. Mallette LE: An unusual morphologic evolution of Paget's disease of bone. Arthritis Rheum 24:1544, 1981.

226. Russell RG, Smith R, Preston C, et al: Diphosphonates in Paget's disease. Lancet 1:894, 1974.

227. Hosking D, Bijvoet OL: Combined diphosphonate and calcitonin therapy for Paget's disease of bone. Calcif Tissue Res (Suppl) 21:321, 1976.

228. Smith R, Russell RG, Bishop M: Diphosphonates and Paget's disease of bone. Lancet 1:945, 1971.

229. Canfield R, Rosner W, Skinner J, et al: Diphosphonate therapy of Paget's disease of bone. Clin Endocrinol Metab 44:96, 1977.

230. Finerman GAM, Gonick HC, Smith RK, et al: Diphosphonate treatment of Paget's disease. Clin Orthop 120:115, 1976.

231. Johnston CC Jr, Altman RD, Canfield RE, et al: Review of fracture experience during treatment of Paget's disease of bone with etidronate disodium (EHDP). Clin Orthop 172:186, 1983.

232. Boyce BF, Smith L, Fogelman I, et al: Focal osteomalacia due to low-dose diphosphonate therapy in Paget's disease. Lancet 1:821, 1984.

233. Johnston CC Jr, Khairi MRA, Meunier RJ: Use of etidronate (EHDP) in Paget's disease of bone. Arthritis Rheum 23:1172, 1980.

234. Siris ES, Canfield RE, Jacobs TP, et al: Long-term therapy of Paget's disease of bone with EHDP. Arthritis Rheum 23:1177, 1980.

235. Douglas DL, Duckworth T, Kanis JA, et al: Biochemical and clinical responses to dichloromethylene disphosphonate (Cl$_2$MDP) in Paget's disease of bone. Arthritis Rheum 23:1185, 1980.

236. Ryan WG, Schwartz TB: Mithramycin treatment of Paget's disease of bone: Exploration of combined mithramycin-EHDP therapy. Arthritis Rheum 23:1155, 1980.

237. Vellenga CJLR, Pauwels EKJ, Bijvoet OLM, et al: Scintigraphic aspects of the recurrence of treated Paget's disease of bone. J Nucl Med 22:510, 1981.

238. Doyle FH, Pennock J, Greenberg PB, et al: Radiological evidence of a dose-related response to long-term treatment of Paget's disease with human calcitonin. Br J Radiol 47:9, 1974.

239. Vellenga CJLR, Pauwels EKJ, Bijvoet OLM, et al: Bone scintigraphy in Paget's disease treated with combined calcitonin and diphosphonate (EHDP). Metab Bone Dis Rel Res 4:103, 1982.

240. Lentle BC, Russell AS, Heslip PG, et al: The scintigraphic findings in Paget's disease of bone. Clin Radiol 27:129, 1976.

241. Khairi MRA, Wellman HN, Robb JA, et al: Paget's disease of bone; symptomatic lesions and bone scan. Ann Intern Med 79:348, 1973.

242. Wellman HN, Schauwecker D, Robb JA, et al: Skeletal scintimaging and

radiography in the diagnosis and management of Paget's disease. Clin Orthop *127:*55, 1977.

243. Lee JY: Bone scintigraphy in evaluation of Didronel therapy for Paget's disease. Clin Nucl Med *6:*356, 1981.

244. Ziegler R, Holz G, Rotzler B, et al: Paget's disease of bone in West Germany. Prevalence and distribution. Clin Orthop *194:*199, 1985.

245. Winfield J, Stamp TCB: Bone and joint symptoms in Paget's disease. Ann Rheum Dis *43:*769, 1984.

246. Schajowicz F, Ubios AM, Araujo ES, et al: Virus-like intranuclear inclusions in giant cell tumor of bone. Clin Orthop *201:*247, 1985.

247. Fornasier VL, Flores L, Hastings D, et al: Virus-like filamentous intranuclear inclusions in a giant-cell tumor, not associated with Paget's disease of bone. A case report. J Bone Joint Surg [Am] *67:*333, 1985.

248. Heuck F, Buck J: Seltene Lokalisationen der Osteodystrophia deformans Paget am Skelett. Radiologe *24:*422, 1984.

249. Vellenga CJLR, Pauwels EKJ, Bijvoet OLM: Some characteristics of local scintigraphic and radiologic patterns of Paget's disease of bone (Osteitis deformans). Diagn Imaging Clin Med *54:*273, 1985.

250. Whyte MP, Daniels EH, Murphy WA: Osteolytic Paget's bone disease in a young man. Rapid healing with human calcitonin therapy. Am J Med *78:*326, 1985.

251. Vellenga CJLR, Mulder JD, Bijvoet OLM: Radiological demonstration of healing in Paget's disease of bone treated with ADP. Br J Radiol *58:*831, 1985.

252. Eisman JA, Martin TJ: Osteolytic Paget's disease. Recognition and risks of biopsy. J Bone Joint Surg [Am] *68:*112, 1986.

253. Lander PH, Hadjipavlou AG: Paget disease with contraction of long bones. Radiology *159:*471, 1986.

254. Case records of the Massachusetts General Hospital. N Engl J Med *314:*105, 1986.

255. Roberts JA: Paget's disease and metastatic carcinoma. A case report. J Bone Joint Surg [Br] *68:*22, 1986.

256. Lander PH, Hadjipavlou AG: A dynamic classification of Paget's disease. J Bone Joint Surg [Br] *68:*431, 1986.

257. Levine RB, Rao VM, Karasick D, et al: Paget's disease: Unusual radiographic manifestations. CRC Crit Rev Diagn Imag *25:*209, 1986.

258. Weisz GM: Lumbar canal stenosis in Paget's disease. The staging of the clinical syndrome, its diagnosis, and treatment. Clin Orthop *206:*223, 1986.

259. Zlatkin MB, Lander PH, Hadjipavlou AG, et al: Paget's disease of the spine: CT with clinical correlation. Radiology *160:*155, 1986.

260. Lakhanpal S, O'Duffy JD: Paget's disease and osteoarthritis. Arthritis Rheum *29:*1414, 1986.

261. Hadjipavlou A, Lander P, Srolovitz H: Pagetic arthritis. Pathophysiology and management. Clin Orthop *208:*15, 1986.

262. Mautalen C, Gonzalez D, Blumenfeld EL, et al: Spontaneous fractures of uninvolved bones in patients with Paget's disease during unduly prolonged treatment with disodium etidronate (EHDP). Clin Orthop *207:*150, 1986.

263. Dahniya MH: Paget's disease of bone in Africa. Br J Radiol *60:*113, 1987.

264. Krane SM, Simon LS: Metabolic consequences of bone turnover in Paget's disease of bone. Clin Orthop *217:*26, 1987.

265. Mirra J: Pathogenesis of Paget's disease based on viral etiology. Clin Orthop *217:*162, 1987.

266. Foldes J, Shamir S, Brautbar C, et al: HLA-D antigens and Paget's disease of bone. Clin Orthop *217:*301, 1987.

267. Baslé MF, Rebel A, Fournier JG, et al: On the trail of paramyxoviruses in Paget's disease of bone. Clin Orthop *217:*9, 1987.

268. Clarke AM, Douglas DL: Paget's disease of the fibula. J Orthop Rheumatol *4:*109, 1991.

269. Groh JA: Mono-osteitic Paget's disease as a clinical entity. Roentgenologic observations in nine cases. AJR *50:*230, 1943.

270. Resnick D: Paget's disease of bone: Current status and a look back to 1943 and earlier. AJR *150:*249, 1988.

271. Som PM, Hermann G, Sacher M, et al: Paget disease of the calvaria and facial bones with an osteosarcoma of the maxilla: CT and MR findings. J Comput Assist Tomogr *11:*887, 1987.

272. Pryce AP, Wiener SN: Syringomyelia associated with Paget disease of the skull. AJR *155:*881, 1990.

273. Rosen MA, Wesolowski DP, Herkowitz HN: Osteolytic monostotic Paget's disease of the axis. A case report. Spine *13:*125, 1988.

274. Rosen MA, Matasar KW, Irwin BR: Osteolytic monostotic Paget's disease of the fifth lumbar vertebra. A case report. Clin Orthop *262:*119, 1991.

275. Dinneen SF, Buckley TF: Spinal nerve root compression due to monostotic Paget's disease of a lumbar vertebra. Spine *12:*948, 1987.

276. Hadjipavlou A, Lander P: Paget disease of the spine. J Bone Joint Surg [Am] *73:*1376, 1991.

277. Guyer PB, Chamberlain AT: Paget's disease of bone in South Africa. Clin Radiol *39:*51, 1988.

278. Nicholson DA, Roberts T, Sanville PR: Spinal cord compression in Paget's disease due to extradural pagetic ossification. Br J Radiol *64:*864, 1991.

279. Richter RL, Semble EL, Turner RA, et al: An unusual manifestation of Paget's disease of bone: Spinal epidural hematoma presenting as acute cauda equina syndrome. J Rheumatol *17:*975, 1990.

280. Altman RD, Brown M, Gargano F: Low back pain in Paget's disease of bone. Clin Orthop *217:*152, 1987.

281. Hadjipavlou A, Shaffer N, Lander P, et al: Pagetic spinal stenosis with extradural pagetoid ossification. Spine *13:*128, 1988.

282. Meloux J, Bussière JL, Épifanie JL, et al: Maladie de Paget et blocs vertébraux. A propos de 9 observations. Rev Rhum Mal Osteoartic *55:*271, 1988.

283. Geil GE, Staple TW: Case report 530. Skel Radiol *18:*140, 1989.

284. Mitchell ML, Ackerman LV, Tsutsumi A: Case report 438. Skel Radiol *16:*498, 1987.

285. Moser RP Jr, Vinh TN, Ros PR, et al: Paget's disease of the anterior tibial tubercle. Radiology *164:*211, 1987.

286. Hermann G, Abdelwahab IF, Klein MJ, et al: Case report 644. Skel Radiol *19:*613, 1990.

287. Stuhl MA, Moser RP Jr, Vinh TN, et al: Paget's disease of the patella. Skel Radiol *19:*407, 1990.

288. O'Driscoll SW, Hastings DE: Extension of monostotic Paget disease from the femur to the tibia after arthrodesis of the knee. A case report. J Bone Joint Surg [Am] *71:*129, 1989.

289. Brixen K, Hansen HH, Mosekilde L, et al: SPECT bone scintigraphy in assessment of cranial Paget's disease. Acta Radiol *31:*549, 1990.

290. Rudberg U, Ahlbäck S-O, Udén R: Bone marrow scintigraphy in Paget's disease of bone. Acta Radiol *31:*141, 1990.

291. Iles SE: Extensive Paget's disease demonstrated on In-III WBC Scanning. Clin Nucl Med *15:*652, 1990.

292. Neuerburg J, Bohndorf K, Krasny R: M. Paget des skeletts: MR-charakteristika bei 1,5 T. ROFO *149:*609, 1988.

293. Roberts MC, Kressel HY, Fallon MD, et al: Paget disease: MR imaging findings. Radiology *173:*341, 1989.

294. Kaufmann GA, Sundaram M, McDonald DJ: Magnetic resonance imaging in symptomatic Paget's disease. Skel Radiol *20:*413, 1991.

295. Tjon-A-Tham RTO, Bloem JL, Falke THM, et al: Magnetic resonance imaging in Paget disease of the skull. AJNR *6:*879, 1985.

296. Kelly JK, Denier JE, Wilner HI, et al: MR imaging of lytic changes in Paget disease of the calvarium. J Comput Assist Tomogr *13:*27, 1989.

297. Som PM, Hermann G, Sacher M, et al: Paget disease of the calvaria and facial bones with an osteosarcoma of the maxilla: CT and MR findings. J Comput Assist Tomogr *11:*887, 1987.

298. Eyres KS, O'Doherty D, McCutchan D, et al: Paget's disease of bone: The outcome after fracture. J Orthop Rheumatol *4:*63, 1991.

299. Moore TE, King AR, Kathol MH, et al: Sarcoma in Paget disease of bone: Clinical, radiologic, and pathologic features in 22 cases. AJR *156:*1199, 1991.

300. Potter HG, Schneider R, Ghelman B, et al: Multiple giant cell tumors and Paget disease of bone: Radiographic and clinical correlations. Radiology *180:*261, 1991.

301. Pazzaglia UE, Barbieri D, Ceciliani L: An epiphyseal giant cell tumor associated with early Paget's disease. A case report. Clin Orthop *234:*217, 1988.

302. Dowling K, Hutto RL, Dowling EA: Sternal mass in a patient with Paget's disease. Invest Radiol *26:*615, 1991.

303. Roblot P, Alcalay M, Payen J, et al: Metastases of a lingual epidermoid carcinoma in a femur affected by Paget disease. J Bone Joint Surg [Am] *69:*1440, 1987.

304. Schajowicz F, Velan O, Araujo ES, et al: Metastases of carcinoma in the pagetic bone. A report of two cases. Clin Orthop *228:*290, 1988.

305. Crouzet J, Beraneck L: Maladie de Paget et métastase d'épithéliomas sur le même os. Rev Rhum Mal Osteoartic *57:*517, 1990.

306. Fenton P, Resnick D: Metastases to bone affected by Paget's disease. A report of three cases. Int Orthop (SICOT) *15:*397, 1991.

307. Hillmann JS, Mesgarzadeh M, Tang C-K, et al: Case report 481. Skel Radiol *17:*356, 1988.

308. Monson DK, Finn HA, Dawson PJ, et al: Pseudosarcoma in Paget disease of bone. J Bone Joint Surg [Am] *71:*453, 1989.

309. Khraishi M, Howard B, Fam AG: Paget's pseudosarcoma. Arthritis Rheum *34:*241, 1991.

310. Lluberas-Acosta G, Hansell JR, Schumacher HR Jr: Paget's disease of bone in patients with gout. Arch Intern Med *146:*2389, 1986.

311. Gabel GT, Rand JA, Sim FH: Total knee arthroplasty for osteoarthrosis in patients who have Paget disease of bone at the knee. J Bone Joint Surg [Am] *73:*739, 1991.

312. McDonald DJ, Sim FH: Total hip arthroplasty in Paget's disease. J Bone Joint Surg [Am] *69:*766, 1987.

313. Ludkowski P, Willis-MacDonald J: Total arthroplasty in Paget's disease of the hip. A clinical review and review of the literature. Clin Orthop *255:*160, 1991.

314. De Deuxchaisnes CN, Devogelaer JP, Huaux JP: New modes of administration of Salmon calcitonin in Paget's disease. Clin Orthop *217:*56, 1987.

315. Maldague B, Malghem J: Dynamic radiologic patterns of Paget's disease of bone. Clin Orthop *217:*126, 1987.

316. Dodd GW, Ibbertson HK, Fraser TRC, et al: Radiological assessment of Paget's disease of bone after treatment with the biphosphonates EHDP and APD. Br J Radiol *60:*849, 1987.

317. Bitaudeau Ph, Tabaraud F, Papapietro PM, et al: Deux complications osseuses de l'éthane, hydroxy, diphosphonate dans le traitement de la maladie de Paget: L'ostéolyse et l'ostéomalacie. Sem Hôp Paris *63:*337, 1987.

318. Harinck HIJ, Bijvoet OLM, Blanksma HJ, et al: Efficacious management with aminobisphosphonate (APD) in Paget's disease of bone. Clin Orthop *217:*79, 1987.

319. Nicholas JJ, Helfrich DJ, Cooperstein L, et al: Clinical and radiographic improvement of bone of the second lumbar vertebra in Paget's disease following therapy with etidronate disodium: A case report. Arthritis Rheum *32:*776, 1989.

320. Osterberg PH, Wallace RGH, Adams DA, et al: Familial expansile osteolysis. A new dysplasia. J Bone Joint Surg [Br] *70:*255, 1988.
321. Korber J, McCarthy S, Marsden W: Case report 782. Skel Radiol *22:*222, 1993.
322. Steinbach LS, Johnston JO: Case report 777. Skel Radiol *22:*203, 1993.
323. Kumar A, Poon PY, Aggarwal S: Value of CT in diagnosing nonneoplastic osteolysis in Paget disease. J Comput Assist Tomogr *17:*144, 1993.
324. Breton CL, Méziou M, Laredo JD, et al: Sarcoma complicating Paget's disease of the spine. A study of 8 cases. Rev Rhum Mal Osteoartic [Engl Ed] *60:*17, 1993.
325. Kuo JS, Fallon MD, Gannon FH, et al: The articular manifestations of Paget's disease of bone. A case report. Clin Orthop *285:*250, 1992.
326. Ducloux JM, Maugars Y, Moreau A, et al: Extramedullary hematopoiesis. An unusual cause for Pagetic spinal cord compression. Rev Rhum Mal Osteoartic [Engl Ed] *60:*24, 1993.
327. Matfin G, McPherson F: Paget's disease of bone: recent advances. J Orthop Rheumatol *6:*127, 1993.
328. Eyre D: New biomarkers of bone resorption. J Clin Endocrinol Metab *74:*470, 1992.
329. Ralston SH, DiGiovine FS, Gallacher SJ, et al: Failure to detect paramyxovirus sequences in Paget's disease of bone using the polymerase chain reaction. J Bone Min Res *6:*1243, 1991.
330. Rodriguez-Peralto JL, Ro JY, McCabe KM, et al: Case report 806. Skeletal Radiol *23:*55, 1994.
331. Marr DS, Rosenthal DI, Cohen GL, et al: Rapid postoperative osteolysis in Paget disease. A case report. J Bone Joint Surg [Am] *76:*274, 1994.
332. Bone HG, Kleerekoper M: Paget's disease of bone. J Clin Endocrinol Metab *7:*1179, 1992.

Endocrine Diseases

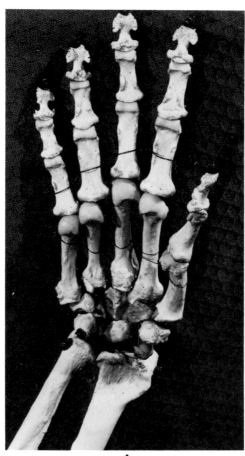

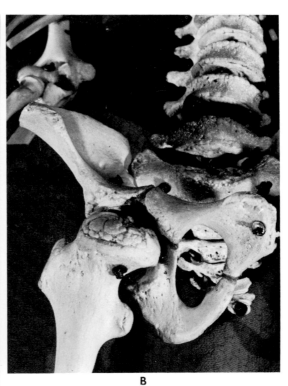

B

A

A Acromegaly: The "arrowhead" appearance of the terminal tufts and broad caliber of all of the phalanges are characteristic of this disease.

B Hypothyroidism: Observe the multiple epiphyseal centers with delayed physeal closure in the femur and flattened vertebrae in a 37 year old hypothyroid woman.

(From Ortner DJ, Putschar WGJ: Identification of Pathological Conditions in Human Skeletal Remains. Washington, DC, Smithsonian Institution Press, 1981.)

Pituitary Disorders

Donald Resnick, M.D.

ACROMEGALY AND GIGANTISM

Growth hormone (somatotropin) hypersecretion can be associated with acidophilic or chromophobic adenomas of the anterior lobe of the pituitary gland. Less frequently, such hypersecretion is associated with diffuse hyperplasia of the acidophil cells or no histologic abnormality at all. Malignant change is rare. In the immature skeleton, in which the growth plates still are open, growth hormone hypersecretion leads to excessive proportional growth of bone (e.g., in both length and width). This results from direct hormonal stimulation of endochondral bone formation at the physeal growth plates. The resulting syndrome is termed hyperpituitary gigantism and is characterized by extreme height. In the mature skeleton, in which the growth plates have closed and endochondral bone formation has ceased, growth hormone hypersecretion may reactivate endochondral bone formation at various existing cartilage-bone junctions (such as the costochondral junctions) and induce periosteal bone formation, leading to widening of osseous structures. This overgrowth of bone in association with enlargement of soft tissue is prominent particularly in the acral parts (hands, feet, lower jaw) of the skeleton, leading to use of the term acromegaly for this condition.[1] Patients with acromegaly demonstrate distinctive symptoms and signs, which relate to morphologic, biochemical, and metabolic effects of growth hormone excess[2-4] (Table 55–1).

General Clinical Features

Typically the onset of symptoms and signs of acromegaly is in the third or fourth decade of life; however, older and younger patients are affected, and the occurrence of acromegaly (as distinct from gigantism) is recorded in children. Although the physical appearance of a patient with hyperpituitary gigantism essentially is that of a tall, normally proportioned person, the characteristics of acromegaly may include dramatic features.[2] Facial characteristics are a large mandible, producing a "lantern jaw" appearance, poor dental occlusion with separation of the teeth, coarsening of facial features related to overgrowth of bone and soft tissue, prominence of the forehead produced by calvarial thickening, and enlargement of the frontal sinuses, deepening of the voice, and prominence of the tongue. The hands appear broad and spadelike, and the fingers are separated and blunted. The entire frame enlarges as a result of overgrowth of osseous tissue. Hypersecretion of growth hormone also affects other organ systems, producing thickening and coarsening of the skin and enlargement of the kidneys, liver, pancreas, spleen, thyroid gland, and heart. Associated endocrine alterations may be observed, including diabetes mellitus (12 to 25 per cent), persistent lactation (4 per cent), increased secretion of cortisol by the adrenal cortex, and increased frequency of parathyroid and pancreatic islet cell adenomas (Table 55–2).

TABLE 55–1. Actions of Growth Hormone*

Morphologic Effects

1. Increased growth of bone and cartilage
   a. In immature skeleton with open physes, proportional increase in length and width of bone
   b. In mature skeleton, increase in width of bone due to periosteal overgrowth
2. Increased growth of muscle and connective tissue
3. Increased mass of viscera, including liver, kidneys, intestines, adrenals, pancreas, lungs, heart

Biochemical Effects

1. Protein synthesis (bone, cartilage, muscle, liver, other viscera)
   a. Increased transport of amino acids into cells
   b. Increased protein synthesis, perhaps due to alterations in translational mechanisms
   c. Increased total RNA synthesis
   d. Increased DNA synthesis and cell number
2. Fat metabolism (biphasic effects)
   a. Acutely, increased lipogenesis in fat cells
   b. Chronically, increased lipolysis with elevation in plasma free fatty acids
   c. Increased fatty acid oxidation
   d. Accentuation of ketogenesis in diabetic patients

3. Carbohydrate metabolism (biphasic effects)
   a. Acutely, increased glucose uptake and utilization by fat cells
   b. Acutely, decrease in serum glucose
   c. Chronically, decreased glucose utilization by fat cells and muscle
   d. Increased gluconeogenesis
   e. Chronically, normal or increased serum glucose
   f. Chronically, insulin resistance
4. Connective tissue metabolism
   a. Stimulation of chondroitin sulfate synthesis
   b. Stimulation of collagen synthesis
   c. Increased urinary hydroxyproline
5. Changes in calcium, phosphorus, and bone metabolism
   a. Increased intestinal absorption of calcium
   b. Hypercalciuria
   c. Increased renal tubular reabsorption of phosphorus with increased serum inorganic phosphate
   d. Increased serum alkaline phosphatase

Changes in Metabolic Balance

1. Positive nitrogen balance; decreased urea excretion
2. Positive phosphorus balance
3. Decreased excretion and positive balances of sodium and potassium
4. Positive calcium balance

*From Ney RL: The anterior pituitary gland. *In* PK Bundy, LE Rosenberg (Eds): Duncan's Diseases of Metabolism. 7th Ed. Vol II. Endocrinology. Philadelphia, WB Saunders Co, 1974, p 966.

The clinical manifestations of acromegaly may stabilize after the disease has progressed to a certain degree. This fact, in addition to the insidious nature of the disease, may lead to considerable delay before the acromegalic patient

TABLE 55–2. Signs and Symptoms of Acromegaly*

	Per Cent
Enlargement of acral parts	100
Enlargement of sella turcica on radiograph	93
Disturbances of menstrual cycle	87
Headaches	87
Complete amenorrhea	73
Increased basal metabolic rate	70
Visual disturbances	62
Excessive perspiration	60
Hypertrichosis	53
Cutaneous pigmentation	46
Drowsiness and lethargy	42
Gain in weight	39
Diminished libido	38
Fibromata mollusca of skin	27
Enlarged thyroid gland	25
Glycosuria	25
Rhinorrhea	15
Clinical diabetes mellitus	12
Uncinate attacks	7
Persistent lactation	4
Failure of breasts to develop	4
Papilledema	3

*From Ney RL: The anterior pituitary gland. *In* PK Bondy, LE Rosenberg (Eds): Duncan's Diseases of Metabolism. 7th Ed. Vol II. Endocrinology. Philadelphia, WB Saunders Co, 1974, p 1000.

seeks medical attention. Headaches and visual disturbances, which are findings related to the pressure exerted by an enlarging pituitary gland, eventually may lead the patient to a physician. Degeneration of an enlarged anterior lobe of the pituitary gland, perhaps related to hemorrhage, can produce symptoms and signs of hypopituitarism, such as loss of libido in men and cessation of menstruation in women.

Rheumatic complaints are common in patients with acromegaly. The initial clinical descriptions of these complaints were those of Marie in 1886[1] and Middleton in 1894.[5] The fundamental morphologic abnormality leading to articular symptoms and signs appears to be overstimulation of cartilaginous tissue, manifested as increased chondrocyte activity in the basal and middle layers of cartilage, with excess ground substance, leading to thickened, friable matrix.[6, 7] Rheumatic manifestations generally begin after 20 years of age and are equally frequent in men and women.[8] These clinical findings may be observed at either early or late stages of the disease,[81, 83] and they may persist even after the hyperpituitarism has been treated successfully. Five types of rheumatic complaints may be encountered[8, 70, 80] (Table 55–3).

Backache. Approximately 50 per cent of acromegalic patients have backache, particularly of the lower spine.[6] This symptom, which usually is insidious in onset, may be associated with local tenderness and a normal or increased range of spinal and hip motion. Painful kyphosis of the thoracic spine may be observed. It has been suggested that backache relates to irregularity of cartilaginous endplates, degenerative changes, osteophytosis, and ligamentous ossi-

TABLE 55–3. Rheumatic Complaints in Acromegaly

Backache
Limb arthropathy
Compression neuropathy
Neuromuscular symptoms
Raynaud's phenomenon

fication, whereas normal or increased range of motion can be attributed to increased thickness of the intervertebral discs.[8]

Limb Arthropathy. Arthropathy is most common in the large joints, such as the knees, shoulders, and hips. Coarse crepitus throughout the full range of joint motion may be seen, perhaps related to increased cartilage thickness. The finding of crepitus in a joint with little or no pain is suggestive of the diagnosis of acromegaly. Symptoms and signs, which frequently are mild, include soft tissue swelling and minimal pain and tenderness. Synovial effusions are uncommon, and when they are detected, analysis reveals non-inflammatory fluid with low polymorphonuclear leukocyte counts. Rarely, crystal-induced synovitis attributable to calcium pyrophosphate dihydrate (CPPD) crystal deposition may be seen.[9, 10, 82] In later stages of the articular disease, secondary degenerative changes, particularly in the hip and knee, may produce pain, limitation of motion, deformity, and angulation.

Compression Neuropathy. Compression neuropathies are due to connective tissue and bony overgrowth. The carpal tunnel syndrome is particularly characteristic, occurring in 30 per cent of patients, frequently with a bilateral distribution. Spinal cord compression with long tract signs has been noted in some patients with acromegaly.[11] This may relate to narrowing of the spinal canal from soft tissue overgrowth and hypertrophy of the vertebrae.[67, 84, 87] Control of pituitary function and surgical removal of enlarged tissue may produce clinical relief from this problem.[12]

Neuromuscular Symptoms. Fatigue and lethargy are two common clinical findings in acromegaly. Muscle wasting generally is not a prominent feature. A specific myopathy has been described in acromegaly,[13] consisting of mild proximal muscle weakness associated with an elevated serum level of creatine kinase and a decreased mean action potential duration on electromyography. Nonspecific muscle fiber hypertrophy is observed on histologic study.

Neurologic changes also are encountered. Increased connective tissue formation may occur between nerve fibers.[14] Lewis,[15] observing peripheral neuropathy in two patients with pituitary gigantism, has suggested that endoneural fibroblasts may be affected by growth hormone, resulting in connective tissue enlargement and subsequent neuropathy.

Raynaud's Phenomenon. Raynaud's phenomenon is a relatively uncommon manifestation of the disease, more marked in the hands than in the feet.

Pathologic Features of Skeletal Involvement

Characteristic pathologic aberrations accompany acromegaly[3, 6–8, 12, 16, 17] (Table 55–4).

Stimulation of Endochondral Ossification. In patients whose growth plates are not yet closed, excessive growth hormone results in exaggerated longitudinal growth of the skeleton. In the young, true gigantism may result, whereas in persons in whom the cartilaginous growth plates are near fusion, some increase in longitudinal growth is observed, but gigantism is relatively mild. After closure of the growth plates, excessive secretion of growth hormone can result in reactivation of endochondral bone formation at certain chondro-osseous junctions. One such site is the costochondral area of the rib[3, 16, 18] (Fig. 55–1). Thickening of the costal cartilages results from deposition of new cartilage on

TABLE 55–4. Radiographic-Pathologic Correlation in Acromegaly

Stimulation of endochondral bone formation	Enlargement of costochondral junctions Thickening of intervertebral discs
Stimulation of periosteal bone formation	Mandibular enlargement Thickening of the cranial vault Prominence of the supraorbital ridges and facial structures Cortical thickening of tubular bones Enlargement of phalangeal tufts Increase in sagittal and transverse diameters of vertebral bodies
Stimulation of subligamentous bone formation	Calcaneal enthesophytes Excrescences on patella, tuberosities, trochanters
Stimulation of bone resorption	Overtubulation of phalanges, metacarpals, metatarsals Intracortical striations Medullary widening Vertebral scalloping
Proliferation of articular cartilage	Widening of articular spaces
Cartilaginous degeneration and regeneration	Narrowing of articular spaces Periarticular calcifications and ossifications Osteophytosis
Connective tissue hyperplasia	Increased thickness of skin (e.g., heel-pad)
Pituitary neoplasm	Sella turcica abnormalities

preexisting cartilage, and enlargement of the costochondral junctions, termed the acromegalic rosary,[85] relates to stimulation of endochondral ossification.

Stimulation of Periosteal Bone Formation. In acromegaly, subperiosteal bone formation is observed at specific sites. In the skull, this form of bony proliferation is apparent on the alveolar margins of the maxilla and mandible, with resultant deepening of the alveolar sockets and separation of the teeth. Subperiosteal new bone formation and articular cartilage stimulation produce distinctive changes along the mental eminence of the mandible and mandibular rami, with enlargement and forward protrusion of the entire mandible.[71] Bony deposition also is characteristic in the supraorbital ridges, facial bones, and calvarial vault.

The long and short tubular bones likewise are modified. Subperiosteal and subligamentous bone formation may result in thickening and irregularity of the cortices of the bony shafts, prominence of various tuberosities, and osteophytosis. These alterations account for the enlargement of the phalanges, metacarpals, and metatarsals. Proliferation of the phalangeal tufts particularly is characteristic.

In the vertebral column, there is an increase of both the transverse and sagittal diameters of the vertebral bodies owing to prominent subperiosteal bone deposition (Fig. 55–2). This produces an altered vertebral shape, in which the vertebral bodies appear short in height and elongated in sagittal and transverse planes. These vertebral abnormalities are associated with an increase in size of the intervertebral disc, which is produced by marginal subperichondrial formation of cartilage. Reactivation of endochondral bone formation occurs at the chondro-osseous junction between the intervertebral disc and the vertebral body. Osteophytes of

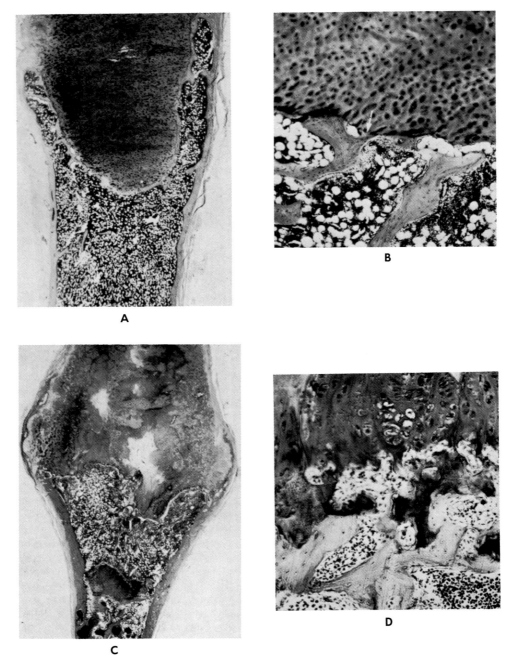

FIGURE 55–1. Acromegaly: Endochondral ossification of costochondral junction.

A, B In the normal situation, photomicrographs (7×, 35×) outline a smooth, tongue-like projection of cartilage into the shaft of the rib. The costal cartilage is in an inactive stage and bony trabeculae of the rib abut on (close off) the costal cartilage (arrow).

C, D In acromegaly, photomicrographs (7×, 35×) reveal reactivation of endochondral ossification, indicated by the irregular chondro-osseous junctions, and the proliferation and columnar arrangement of the cartilage cells, with formation of bony trabeculae.

(From Jaffe HL: Metabolic, Degenerative, and Inflammatory Diseases of Bones and Joints. Philadelphia, Lea & Febiger, 1972.)

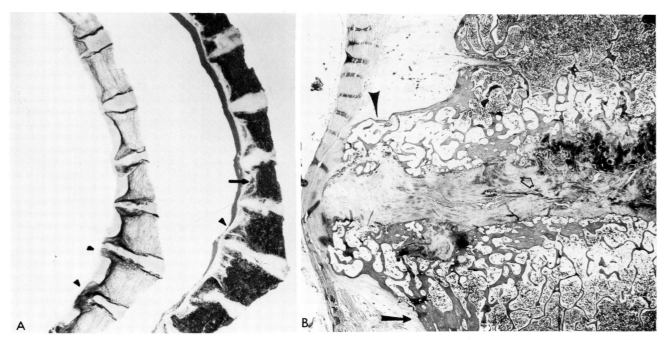

FIGURE 55–2. Acromegaly: Periosteal and endochondral ossification of spine. A radiograph and gross pathologic photograph **(A)** and a photomicrograph (18×) **(B)** of a sagittal section of a thoracic spine outline osteophytosis (arrowheads), periosteal proliferation on the anterior surface of the vertebrae (solid arrows), and disruption of the chondro-osseous junction with cartilage within the bone marrow of the vertebra (open arrow). Increased anteroposterior diameter of the vertebral bodies results from periosteal bone formation. (From Bluestone R, et al: Ann Rheum Dis *30*:243, 1971.)

the vertebral column may be a prominent feature, perhaps related to excessive spinal mobility, with laxity of paraspinal ligaments and thickening of intervertebral discs.

Bone Formation and Bone Resorption. It appears that subperiosteal and endosteal bone proliferation in acromegaly occurs simultaneously with increased bone resorption.[19] Kinetic studies using various agents demonstrate an increased miscible calcium pool. Radiologic and pathologic evidence that cortical bone formation and resorption are occurring simultaneously is seen in the finding of overtubulation of the phalanges and metatarsals, with normal or increased cortical thickness,[12, 20, 86] and periosteal apposition of bone on the anterolateral aspect of the vertebral bodies, with concomitant increased concavity along their posterior margins. In most sites, bony apposition exceeds bony resorption; occasionally however, the opposite may be true, in which case decreased bone thickness is observed, a finding that has been described in relation to the cranial vault.[12, 21] In the hand, increased bone formation and resorption in acromegaly (or cerebral gigantism) can be detected by careful analysis of total bone width, medullary cavity width, and cortical thickness.[22, 23] This analysis reveals increased bone formation at one cortical surface (enlargement of total bone width due to periosteal bone apposition), which may be associated with increased bone resorption at another surface (increased width of the medullary cavity). In acromegaly, there is poor documentation of reduction in total bone mass, although bone mass may be reduced in one bone but be normal or increased in another.

Articular Cartilage Alterations. Increased growth hormone secretion can lead to proliferation of articular carti-

lage[3, 6, 72] (Figs. 55–3 to 55–6). Increased chondrocytic activity is distributed irregularly in the deeper layers of the cartilage; cellular proliferation begins in the radial zone and spreads to adjacent areas. The cartilaginous coat eventually thickens. These cartilaginous changes presumably reflect the effect of excess circulating growth hormone on chondrocyte metabolism, although in vitro studies suggest that the effects of growth hormone on cartilage are mediated in vivo by the release of somatomedin, produced in the liver in response to growth hormone stimulation.[24] Ulceration and fissuring of superficial cartilage may progress to involve deeper layers, producing sharply demarcated ulcers with undermined edges. A continuous cycle apparently occurs, with progressive cartilaginous fragmentation and denudation, disordered joint mechanics, and tissue repair with remodeling (Fig. 55–7). Bluestone[7] emphasized that briskness of the reparative process is the most characteristic manifestation of acromegalic arthropathy. The regeneration process is associated with fibrocartilaginous plugs within cartilage and articular margins and capsule that become hypertrophied, calcified, and ossified. Widespread osteophytic outgrowths are seen in association with subchondral cyst formation. The eventual features of the exuberant regenerative process of acromegaly are an enlarged joint with thickened ulcerative cartilage, hypertrophied periarticular tissue, calcinosis, osteophytosis, and periosteal bone formation at insertion sites of tendons, ligaments, and capsule.

The synovial membrane may show a mild, nonspecific, villous synovitis with a fatty tissue core and increased vascularity[17] (Fig. 55–8). In association with structural joint damage, synovial inflammatory changes have been seen.[72]

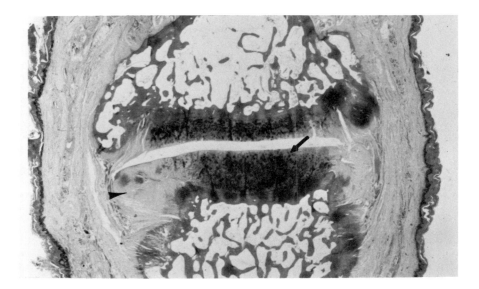

FIGURE 55–3. Acromegaly: Articular cartilage abnormalities—distal interphalangeal joint. Histologic examination (6×) of a coronal section through the joint outlines hypertrophied articular cartilage (arrow), marginal fibrocartilage (arrowhead), and calcification and ossification of the capsular insertions. (From Bluestone R, et al: Ann Rheum Dis *30*:243, 1971.)

Thickened subcutaneous tissue reveals noninflammatory connective tissue hyperplasia that is replaced, in part, by subcutaneous fat.[12] Skin hypertrophy also is apparent.

Radiologic Features of Skeletal Involvement

Radiologic changes of the skeleton in patients with acromegaly are well known.[17, 25–33]

Changes in Skin Thickness (Fig. 55–9). Collagen tissue demonstrates a marked response to excessive amounts of growth hormone. Manifestations of this response are an increase in the periportal connective tissues, an increase in the connective tissue of the bronchi, alterations in the connective tissues of the renal and pancreatic parenchyma, and thickening of the skin.[34–36] Numerous articles have reported the potential use of radiographic measurements of skin thickness in the diagnosis of acromegaly. In 1964, Meema and coworkers,[37] using radiographs of the soft tissues in the forearm, reported an increased thickness of this tissue in patients with acromegaly. In the same year, Steinbach and Russell[38] emphasized the diagnostic significance of a thickened heel-pad in acromegaly, stating that a measurement greater than 21 mm was suggestive of the diagnosis if other causes of skin thickening, such as injury, infection, myxedema, or peripheral edema, were excluded. This measurement was obtained by calculating the shortest distance between the calcaneus and plantar surface of the skin. Three years later, Puckette and Seymour[39] reported fallibility in the measurement of heel-pad thickness because of a wide variation of values in normal persons. In 1968, Jackson[40] found increased heel-pad thickness in obese persons. Sheppard and Meema[28] responded to this criticism of skin thickness measurements as a diagnostic aid by again emphasizing the role of this measurement in patients with acromegaly.

The controversy over the reliability of measurements of heel-pad thickness in diagnosing acromegaly has continued, leading some investigators to use more sophisticated calculations. Gonticas and colleagues[41] proposed that relating the heel-pad thickness to body weight was a more accurate method of separating normal and abnormal values. Kho and associates[42] were able to achieve good separation of the values of heel-pad thickness in acromegalic and normal patients by applying a statistical method of discriminant analysis to heel-pad thickness and body weight. These authors noted that the thickness of the heel-pad in acromegaly probably is related to the severity of disease, increases in patients whose disease is of long duration, and is correlated with serum levels of growth hormone.

Despite some inconsistencies in the value of heel-pad thickness measurements because of its variation with body weight and even race,[65] values greater than 23 mm in men and 21.5 mm in women are suggestive of acromegaly, and values greater than 25 mm in men and 23 mm in women are even more diagnostic of this disease if local causes of skin thickening are excluded.

Abnormalities of the Skull (Fig. 55–10). Radiographic manifestations of the skull in patients with acromegaly include sella turcica alterations (such as enlargement, rarefaction, and destruction of the dorsum of the sella and osteopenia of the anterior and posterior clinoid processes), prominence and enlargement of the frontal and maxillary sinuses,[73] excessive pneumatization of the mastoids, prominence of the occipital protuberance (particularly in men), thickening or, less commonly, thinning of the cranial vault, prominence of the supraorbital ridges and zygomatic arches, enlargement and elongation of the mandible, widening of the mandibular angle, and anterior tilting, separation, and hypercementosis of the teeth.[25, 29, 69]

Abnormalities of the Hand and Wrist (Fig. 55–11). Initial reports of the radiographic findings of acromegaly stressed characteristic findings in the hand.[25, 29] Abnormalities included soft tissue thickening of the fingers, thickening and squaring of the phalanges and metacarpals, tubulation or overconstriction of the shafts of the phalanges, abnormally wide articular spaces, bony excrescences at sites of tendon and ligament attachment to bone, and prominence of the ungual tufts. Bony enlargement could be observed about the wrist as well.

In 1966, Kleinberg and coworkers[27] introduced the sesamoid index in the early diagnosis of acromegaly. The index consisted of measurement of the size of the medial sesamoid at the first metacarpophalangeal joint. On a nonmagnified radiograph of the hand exposed at a 36 inch focus-

Text continued on page 1984

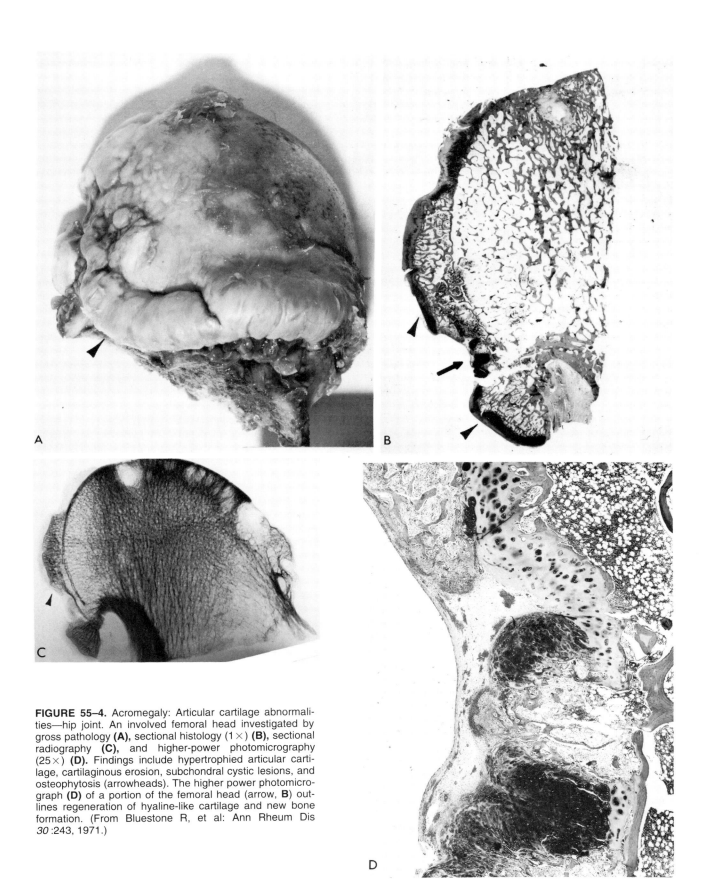

FIGURE 55–4. Acromegaly: Articular cartilage abnormalities—hip joint. An involved femoral head investigated by gross pathology **(A)**, sectional histology (1×) **(B)**, sectional radiography **(C)**, and higher-power photomicrography (25×) **(D)**. Findings include hypertrophied articular cartilage, cartilaginous erosion, subchondral cystic lesions, and osteophytosis (arrowheads). The higher power photomicrograph **(D)** of a portion of the femoral head (arrow, **B**) outlines regeneration of hyaline-like cartilage and new bone formation. (From Bluestone R, et al: Ann Rheum Dis *30*:243, 1971.)

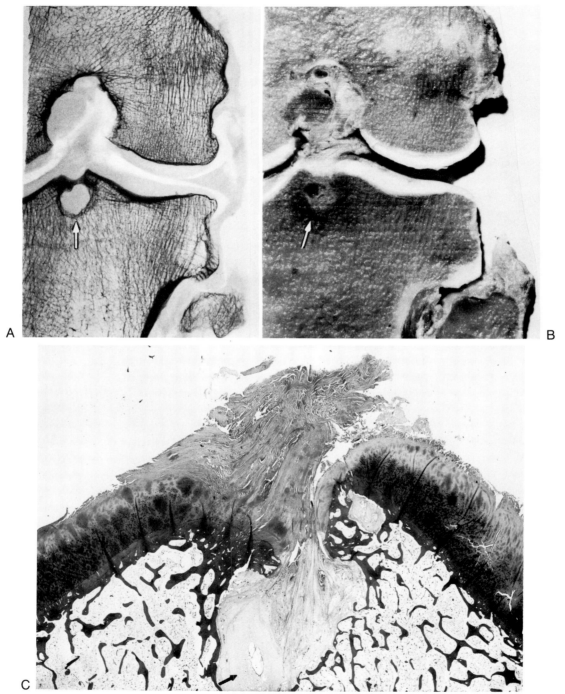

FIGURE 55–5. Acromegaly: Articular cartilage abnormalities—knee. Femoral and tibial involvement. Radiograph **(A)**, gross photograph **(B)**, and photomicrograph (6×) **(C)** of a coronal section through the knee demonstrate thickened articular cartilage and a tibial cyst (arrows). Histologic section shows midzone basophilic proliferation and intercondylar cyst formation.

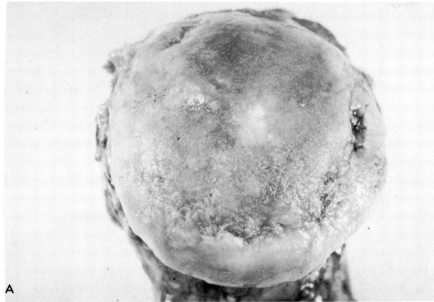

FIGURE 55–6. Acromegaly: Articular cartilage abnormalities—glenohumeral joint.

A A photograph of the articular surface of an involved humeral head outlines area of cartilaginous hypertrophy intermingled with areas of cartilaginous loss. Marginal osteophytes are present. (Courtesy of R. Bluestone, M.D., Los Angeles, California.)

B In this photomicrograph from a different humeral specimen, note the irregular surface of the articular cartilage. The chondral surface is thickened with proliferation of chondrocytes (16×).

C In the same specimen as in **B**, the cancellous bone is markedly thickened with an apparent increase in the number of osteocytes (16×).

(**B, C,** Courtesy of P. Haghighi, M.D., San Diego, California.)

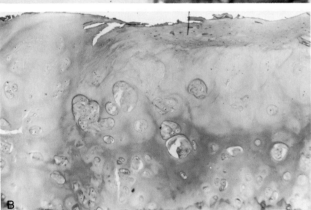

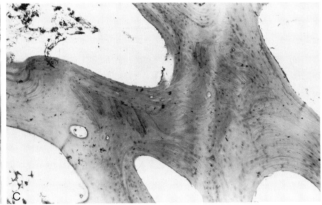

FIGURE 55–7. Acromegalic arthropathy: Summary of pathophysiology. Excess circulating growth hormone stimulates chondrocyte proliferation. Hypertrophy of both hyaline cartilage and fibrocartilage occurs. Fissuring, ulceration, and denudation of the hyaline cartilage lead to degeneration of the articular surface. Calcification and ossification of fibrocartilage are associated with formation of osteophytes and calcinosis. Brisk fibrocartilaginous regeneration is characteristic, producing thickened cartilage, enlarged bones, and hypertrophy of periarticular soft tissues.

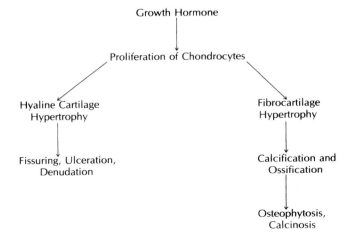

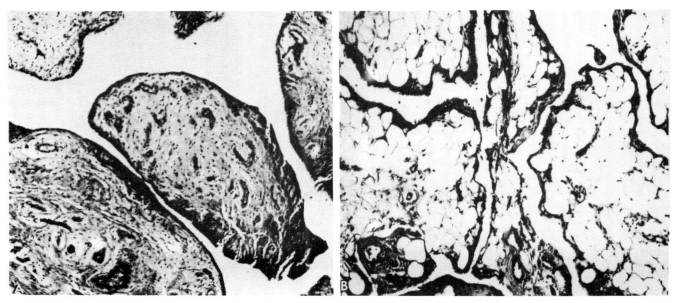

FIGURE 55–8. Acromegalic arthropathy: Synovial membrane abnormalities.
A Nonspecific villous synovitis is associated with increased vascularity (40×).
B Cores of fatty tissue also are apparent (40×).
(From Detenbeck LC, et al: Clin Orthop *91*:119, 1973.)

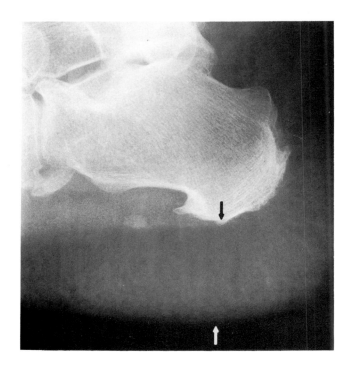

FIGURE 55–9. Acromegaly: Radiographic features—increase in skin thickness. Observe prominence of the soft tissues of the heel with associated hyperostosis and enthesophytosis of the calcaneus. One technique of measurement of these soft tissues evaluates the shortest distance between the calcaneus and plantar skin surface (between arrows).

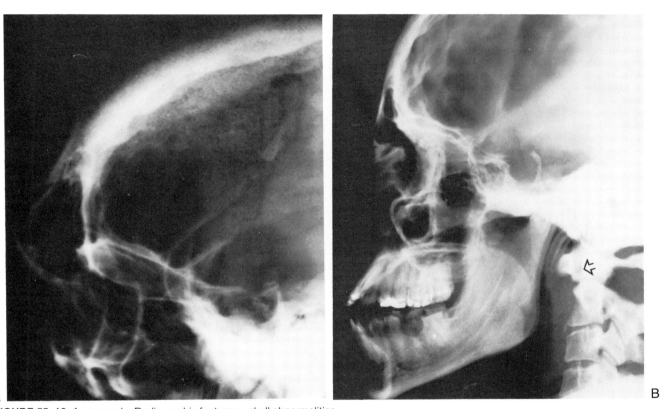

FIGURE 55–10. Acromegaly: Radiographic features—skull abnormalities.

A Findings include increased thickness of the cranial vault, prominent sinuses and supraorbital ridges, and enlarged sella turcica.

B In a different patient, findings include prominence of the mandible, widening of the anterior median atlantoaxial joint (arrow), and enlargement of the sella turcica.

(Courtesy of K. Kortman, M.D., San Diego, California.)

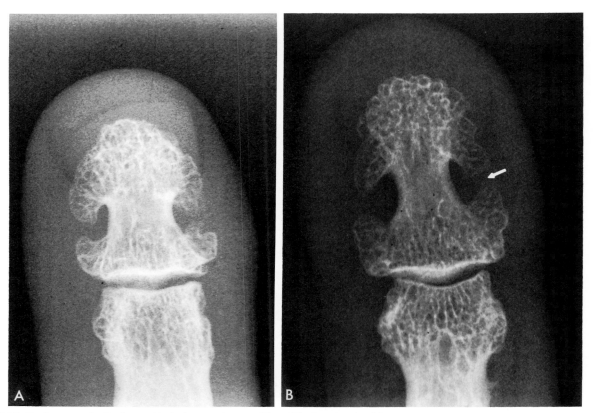

FIGURE 55–11. Acromegaly: Radiographic features—abnormalities of the hand and wrist.
A, B Terminal phalanges: Two examples demonstrate typical findings, including soft tissue prominence and enlargement of the tuft and base of the terminal phalanges. Note the formation of pseudoforamina (arrow).

Illustration continued on opposite page

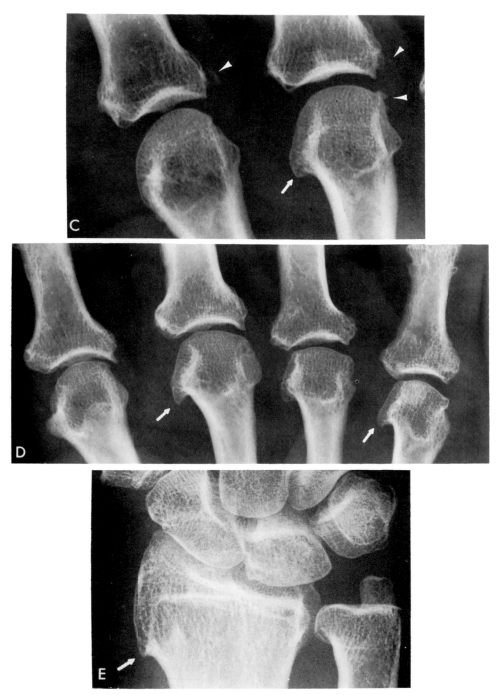

FIGURE 55-11 *Continued*
  C, D Metacarpophalangeal joints. Observe widening of some articular spaces and narrowing of others, beaklike osteophytes on the medial aspect of the metacarpal heads (arrows), and periarticular calcific deposits (arrowheads).
  E Wrist. Note enlargement of the distal end of the radius and ulna as well as the ulnar styloid. A beaklike outgrowth on the lateral aspect of the radius can be seen (arrow).

film distance, the greatest diameter of this bone was multiplied by the greatest diameter of the same sesamoid image that was perpendicular to the first measurement. In controls, the sesamoid index was 20 (range, 12 to 29); in patients with acromegaly, the sesamoid index in men was 40 (range, 30 to 63) and in women it was 33 (range, 31 to 35). These investigators noted a direct correlation between age and sesamoid index in acromegalic patients.

The reliability of the sesamoid index in diagnosing acromegaly subsequently was challenged by Anton[43] and Duncan[44]; both investigators noted variations in this measurement in normal men and women. Anton reported that a sesamoid index of greater than 40 in men and greater than 32 in women was suggestive of acromegaly, whereas Duncan observed that a sesamoid index below 30 militates against but does not exclude the diagnosis of acromegaly.

Anton[43] calculated other measurements of the hand in patients with acromegaly and normal controls, including a determination of tufting, joint space thickness, and hand length. Highly significant sex differences were found. Anton observed that a tuft breadth of the third digit of 12 mm or more in men and of 10 mm or more in women was virtually diagnostic of acromegaly. Additionally, this investigator stressed the usefulness of joint space thickening of the second metacarpophalangeal joint in evaluating women with acromegaly and the unreliability of hand length measurements in detecting patients with gigantism.

Lin and Lee[45] also investigated the value of certain measurements of the hand in the early diagnosis of acromegaly (Fig. 55–12). These authors calculated soft tissue width of the fingers, width of the phalanges, width of the metacarpophalangeal joints, sesamoid index, and interstyloid distance. Each of the measurements demonstrated significant differences between the acromegalic and control groups, and most measurements revealed significant variations between the sexes. Although no single measurement was specific for acromegaly, the concomitant findings of increased soft tissue thickness of the fingers and widening of the metacarpophalangeal joints with exostoses and marginal spurs were sufficient to establish the diagnosis of acromegaly. In addition, increased width of the phalanges, a large sesamoid index, and an increased interstyloid distance were helpful signs in borderline cases.

Abnormalities of the Foot (Fig. 55–13). Radiographic changes in the foot resemble those in the hand. Thickening of the soft tissues of the toes, enlargement of the sesamoid bones[74] and articular spaces (particularly at the metatarsophalangeal joints), and prominence of the metatarsal heads are seen. The terminal tufts become prominent, and bone outgrowths arise from the terminal phalangeal base, extending distally. Proliferation at sites of tendon and ligament attachments such as the calcaneus, thickening of the metatarsal shafts, and constriction of the shafts of the proximal phalanges may be observed. With regard to the metatarsal shafts, resorption of the cortex in the plantar aspects of these bones leads to a V- or keel-shaped deformity that is seen best with CT in the coronal plane.[86]

Abnormalities of the Vertebral Column (Fig. 55–14). Elongation and widening of the vertebral bodies are noted in some patients with acromegaly. These findings are more frequent in the thoracic and lumbar spinal regions and less common in the cervical region.[67] Anterior and lateral osteophytes of the thoracic and lumbar vertebrae may be exten-

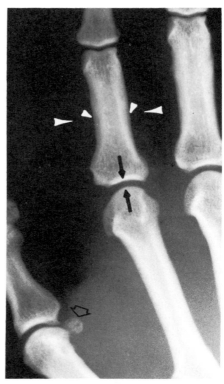

FIGURE 55–12. Acromegaly: Radiographic features—hand measurements. The width of the soft tissues about the proximal phalanx of the second finger (between large arrowheads) and the width of the phalanx (between small arrowheads) are calculated. The soft tissue index represents the ratio of the bone measurement over the soft tissue measurement. The width of the second metacarpophalangeal joint (between arrows) also is indicated. The sesamoid index is the product of the height and length of the sesamoid bone of the first digit (open arrow). The interstyloid distance between the radial and ulnar styloid processes is not indicated on this radiograph. (This is a radiograph from a normal person.)

sive, resembling the findings of spondylosis deformans and diffuse idiopathic skeletal hyperostosis. Posterior deposition of bone is less frequent. Ossification of the anterior portion of the disc may be observed in association with osteophyte formation. Increased height of the intervertebral disc space, particularly in the lumbar region, hypertrophic changes about apophyseal joints, increased thoracic kyphosis, and increased lumbar lordosis are additional manifestations of acromegaly.

Exaggeration of the normal concavity on the posterior aspect of the vertebral bodies is a recognized abnormality in this disease. This finding, related to excessive resorption of bone, frequently is associated with apposition of bone on the anterior margin of the vertebrae, although the findings of apposition and resorption may occur at different levels. Dorsal vertebrae more commonly demonstrate apposition, whereas the lumbar vertebral bodies more frequently demonstrate resorption.[25, 31]

The cause of scalloping of the posterior margins of the vertebral bodies in acromegaly is not clear. Steinbach and associates[29] theorized that the changes could be secondary to pressure erosion from enlarged soft tissue or could be related to resorption and modeling as a direct result of elevated levels of growth hormone. Although it is reasonable to attribute scalloping to the well-documented hyperpla-

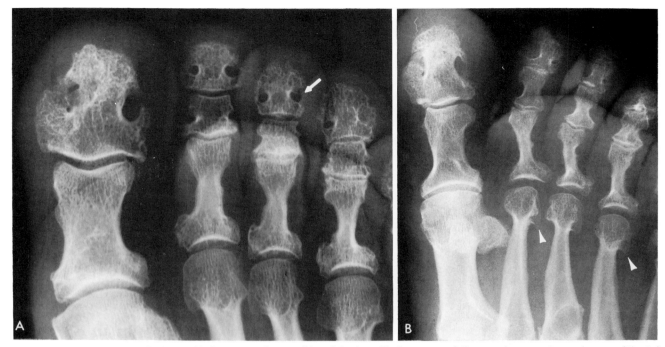

FIGURE 55–13. Acromegaly: Radiographic features—abnormalities of the foot. Findings are soft tissue enlargement, prominence of the tufts and bases of the terminal phalanges, pseudoforamina (arrow), widening of some of the metatarsophalangeal joints, and beaklike outgrowths of the metatarsal heads (arrowheads). A cystic lesion is seen in the proximal aspect of the third metatarsal in **B.**

sia of soft tissue that occurs in acromegaly, this theory does not explain adequately the predilection of the changes for the lumbar region and the absence of more widespread canal enlargement.[31] It also should be recognized that scalloping of vertebral bodies is not diagnostic of this condition, being found in a variety of disease processes.[46]

Cauda equina compression may be apparent in patients with acromegaly.[33] Back pain can simulate the findings of a herniated intervertebral disc. The changes may be due to soft tissue and bony overgrowth superimposed on a narrow lumbar spinal canal. Myelography can reveal characteristic changes, including extradural defects related to bony and soft tissue hypertrophy.[84] Similar changes can be detected with CT scanning[67] and MR imaging.

Abnormalities of the Thoracic Cage. The thorax may appear enlarged owing to elongation of the ribs. Elevation of the lower portion of the sternum and an increased angulation of the sternal angle have been observed,[29] which may be attributable to disproportionate enlargement of the lower and middle ribs. Prominence of the costochondral junction[21] is due to reactivation of endochondral ossification at this site. Rarely, resorption of portions of the ribs is seen.

Abnormalities of the Pelvis (Fig. 55–15). In addition to articular alterations at the sacroiliac joints and hips, enlargement and beaking of the symphysis pubis can be recognized in some patients with acromegaly.

Abnormalities of the Long Bones. The simultaneous occurrence of osseous proliferation and resorption is evident in the tubular bones of the extremities. In some of these bones, resorption is predominant, producing a narrow diaphysis with apparent flaring of the metaphysis and epiphysis.[14, 20, 29, 47]

Miscellaneous Osseous Abnormalities. Bone proliferation occurs at sites of tendon and ligament attachment to

bone (Fig. 55–16). Particularly characteristic are excrescences on the undersurface of the calcaneus, the anterior margin of the patella, the trochanters of the femur, the tuberosities of the humerus, and the undersurface of the distal end of the clavicle.

Localized and generalized osteoporosis has been described in acromegaly.[14, 20, 25, 48] More accurately, bone resorption accompanies bone proliferation in this disease. Widening of the medullary canal and intracortical "tunneling" are seen. In rare instances, resorptive abnormalities may indicate coincidental hyperparathyroidism.[49] Aloia and coworkers[66] have postulated that in untreated acromegaly, an increase in cortical bone is accompanied by a reduced trabecular bone mass. These authors further speculate that during treatment of acromegaly, cortical apposition decreases, increasing the patient's risk of fractures, a risk that may be further accentuated by the hypogonadism that may arise secondary to pituitary irradiation or surgery.

Articular Abnormalities. Radiologic abnormalities of the peripheral joints in acromegaly are seen most frequently in the knees, hips, and shoulders, although they may be apparent at more distant sites, including the elbows, ankles, hands, wrists, and feet. These abnormalities can be divided into two types: cartilage hypertrophy and cartilaginous and osseous degeneration.[6, 7, 17, 25, 26, 29]

Cartilage Hypertrophy (Fig. 55–17). Gross thickening of the cartilage is associated with radiographically evident widening of the articular space. This finding may be combined with soft tissue prominence due to soft tissue and synovial hypertrophy. Initially, the subchondral bone appears morphologically normal, although enlargement of the osseous surface may be seen. Widening of the joint space may be apparent in any joint, although it is observed most frequently in the metacarpophalangeal, metatarsophalan-

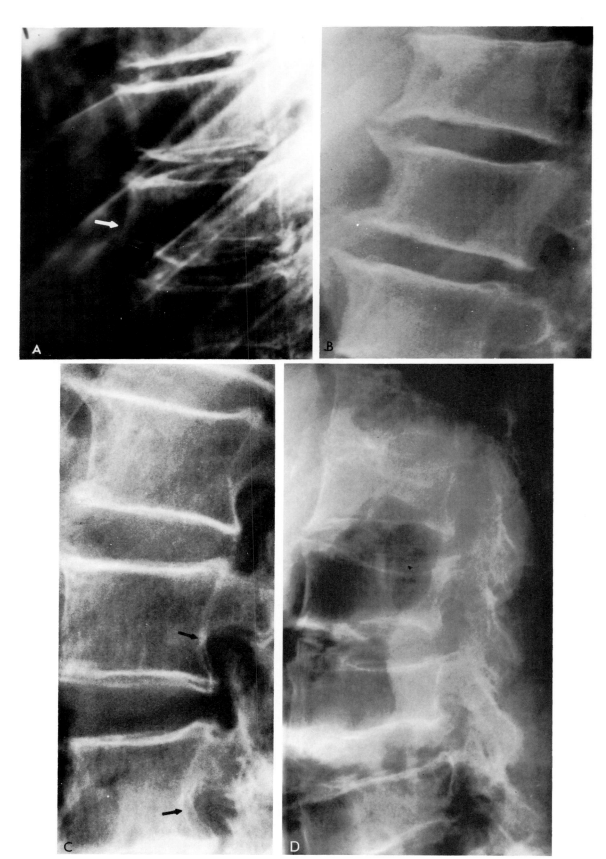

FIGURE 55–14. Acromegaly: Radiographic features—abnormalities of the spine.

A In the thoracic spine, note bone formation on the anterior aspect of the vertebrae (arrow) producing an increase in the anteroposterior diameter of the vertebral bodies.

B In the lumbar spine, similar bone production can be seen.

C In a second patient, observe exaggerated concavity on the posterior aspect of multiple lumbar vertebral bodies (arrows).

D In a third patient, findings include osteopenia, increased anteroposterior dimensions of the vertebral bodies, decreased height of the vertebral bodies, and mild osteophytosis.

(Courtesy of C. Chen, M.D., Kaohsiung, Taiwan.)

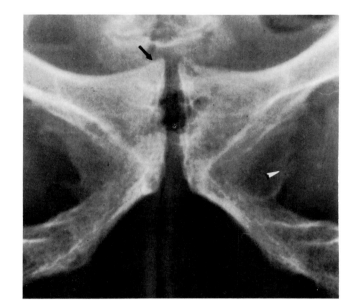

FIGURE 55–15. Acromegaly: Radiographic features—abnormalities of the pubis. Findings include "beaking" of the superior aspect of the symphysis (arrow) and hyperostosis at sites of ligament attachment to bone (arrowhead).

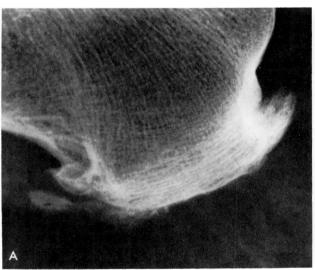

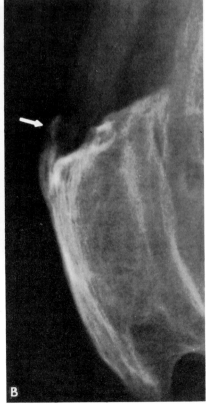

FIGURE 55–16. Acromegaly: Radiographic features—bone proliferation at sites of tendon and ligament attachment to bone.

   A Note proliferation along the posterior and inferior aspects of the calcaneus.

   B Lateral radiograph of the knee reveals hyperostosis on the anterior surface of the patella with ossification at the site of attachment of the quadriceps mechanism (arrow).

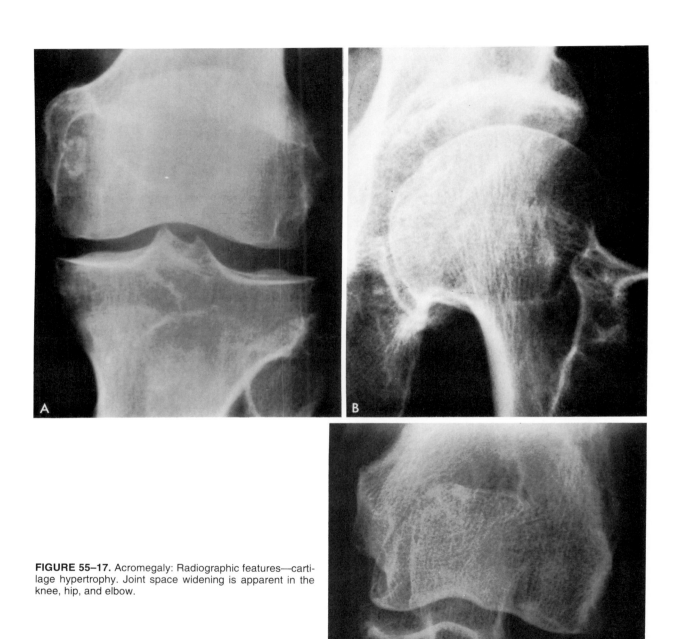

FIGURE 55–17. Acromegaly: Radiographic features—cartilage hypertrophy. Joint space widening is apparent in the knee, hip, and elbow.

geal, and interphalangeal joints. Large joints also reveal this finding, and enlargement of the median atlantoaxial articulation has been reported in acromegaly (Fig. 55–10).[32] At this latter location, as well as in other sites, softening and thickening of the capsular and ligamentous structures produce joint laxity, which contributes to the prominence of the joint cavity. Thickening of the intervertebral discs is another manifestation of joint space widening in acromegaly.

Cartilaginous and Osseous Degeneration (Fig. 55–18). In later stages of the disease, cartilage fibrillation and erosion lead to secondary degenerative alterations. Initially, osteophytes are seen, and the combination of osteophyte formation and a normal or widened joint space is suggestive of acromegaly. With continued cartilage and bone degen-

eration, limitation of joint motion becomes apparent. Articular space narrowing, cyst formation, sclerosis, and progressive osteophytosis are seen. The eventual appearance resembles that of primary degenerative disease, and the differentiation of the radiographic features of these two disorders becomes increasingly difficult as the joint manifestations progress. Involvement of articular sites such as the glenohumeral joint and elbow, which are not affected commonly in degenerative joint disease, the presence of prominent osteophytes and bony excrescences, and the documentation of typical findings of acromegaly elsewhere in the skeleton usually allow accurate diagnosis of this disease. Beaklike osteophytes on the inferior aspect of the humeral head, lateral aspect of the acetabulum, medial portion of the femoral head, superior margin of the symphysis

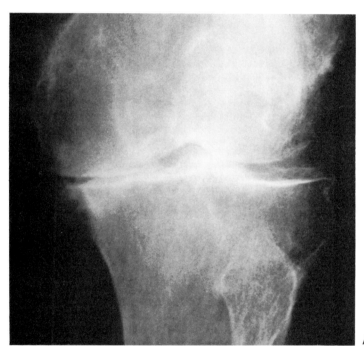

FIGURE 55–18. Acromegaly: Radiographic features—cartilaginous and osseous degeneration.

A In the knee, narrowing of both the medial and the lateral femorotibial compartments is seen with sclerosis and osteophytosis.

B Glenohumeral joint involvement is characterized by mild narrowing of the articular space, beaklike osteophytes of the inferior aspect of the humeral head (arrow), sclerosis, and bony fragmentation (arrowhead).

C At the metacarpophalangeal joints, articular space narrowing is evident.

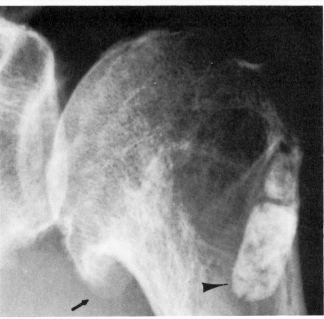

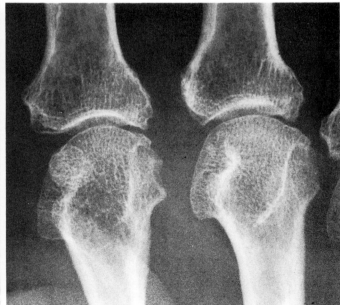

A

B

C

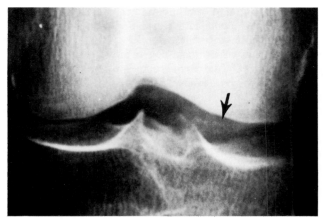

FIGURE 55–19. Acromegaly: Radiographic features—calcium pyrophosphate dihydrate crystal deposition. Observe chondrocalcinosis (arrow) and an enlarged articular space.

pubis, and radial or tibial aspect of the metacarpals or metatarsals, respectively, are characteristic of acromegaly. Small collections of calcification or ossification within or around the articular space have been described in patients with acromegaly,[6, 7] and chondrocalcinosis due to calcium pyrophosphate dihydrate (CPPD) crystal deposition, particularly in the knee, occasionally is encountered in these persons (Fig. 55–19). In rare instances, severe collapse of the osseous structure, especially in the knee, hip, and shoulder, is apparent.[17, 26] An association of acromegaly and ischemic necrosis of bone, noted in some reports,[75] is not proved and may be related, in part, to misinterpretation of the cause of such collapse.

Differential Diagnosis

The combination of radiographic findings in acromegaly is sufficiently characteristic that accurate diagnosis is not difficult, particularly in advanced cases, although individual radiographic signs, such as increased soft tissue width, tuftal prominence, and vertebral scalloping, which are apparent in this disease, may be noted in other disorders. The early radiographic diagnosis of acromegaly relies on a variety of measurements, especially in the hands and feet, which discriminate patients with this disease from normal persons (Table 55–5).

General Radiographic Features. The general radiographic features of acromegaly are differentiated easily from those of most skeletal disorders. An acromegaly-like

TABLE 55–5. Bone and Soft Tissue Measurements Suggestive of Acromegaly

Heel-pad thickness	>23 mm (men)
	>21.5 mm (women)
Sesamoid index (first MCP joint)	>40 (men)
	>32 (women)
Tuftal width (third finger)	≥12 mm (men)
	≥10 mm (women)
Joint space thickness (second MCP joint)	>2.5 mm (men and women)
Phalangeal soft tissue thickness (proximal midphalanges)	≥27 mm (men)
	≥26 mm (women)

syndrome has been associated with pachydermoperiostosis.[50] The characteristic features of this familial syndrome are digital clubbing, coarsening of facial features, furrowing and oiliness of the skin, and periosteal new bone formation. In the "forme fruste" of this condition, skin thickening, coarsening of facial features, and furrowing of the scalp (cutis verticis gyrata) simulate the appearance of acromegaly. Although laboratory analysis reveals normal serum levels of growth hormone in pachydermoperiostosis, radiographic findings are similar to those of acromegaly, with enlarged sinuses, prominent supraorbital ridges, and thickening of the phalanges (Fig. 55–20). The sella turcica is not enlarged, and severe prominence of the phalangeal tufts and enlargement of articular space are not observed. Thickening of the heel-pad in pachydermoperiostosis occasionally is apparent.

Enlargement of the Phalangeal Tufts. Widening and prominence of the tufts of the distal phalanges of the hand (and foot) are well-recognized signs of acromegaly. In judging the significance of these signs, however, it is necessary to take into account the patient's sex and occupation.[51] Phalangeal tufts are more prominent in men than in women and in persons who perform heavy manual labor than in those who have more sedentary occupations (Fig. 55–21). Furthermore, irregular excrescences on the tuft occasionally are apparent in elderly persons.

Thickening of Soft Tissues. Although soft tissue thickening at certain sites, such as the phalanges and heel, can

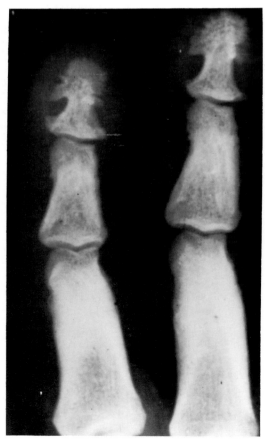

FIGURE 55–20. Pachydermoperiostosis. Findings include soft tissue prominence, thickening of all of the phalanges, and enlargement of phalangeal tufts.

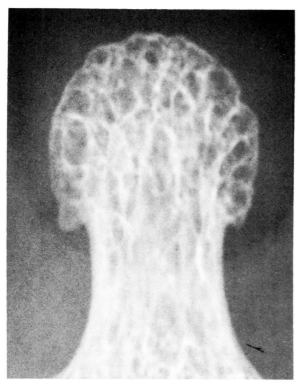

FIGURE 55–21. Prominent phalangeal tuft in a normal person. Tuftal enlargement can be a normal finding.

be reliable indicators of acromegaly, similar thickening can be seen in other diseases, related to edema, hemorrhage, exudation, or fatty tissue infiltration. Long-term phenytoin therapy has been accompanied by thickening of the heel-pad.[76]

Scalloped Vertebrae. Exaggerated concavity of the posterior surface of the vertebral bodies is recognized in acromegaly. It also is seen in a variety of other disease processes[46] (Table 55–6). The mechanism for accentuated concavity of vertebral bodies in some of these diseases may relate to increased intraspinal pressure; this may explain the occurrence of scalloped vertebrae in association with intraspinal neoplasms and cysts and in syringomyelia. It has

TABLE 55–6. Some Causes of Scalloped Vertebral Bodies*

1. Increased intraspinal pressure
   a. Intradural neoplasms
   b. Intraspinal cysts
   c. Syringomyelia and hydromyelia
   d. Communicating hydrocephalus

2. Dural "ectasia"
   a. Marfan's syndrome
   b. Ehlers-Danlos syndrome
   c. Neurofibromatosis

3. Bone resorption
   a. Acromegaly

4. Congenital disorders
   a. Achondroplasia
   b. Morquio's disease
   c. Hurler's syndrome

5. Physiologic scalloping

*From Mitchell GE, et al: Radiology 89:67, 1967.

been suggested that scalloped vertebrae also may be caused by dural ectasia, in which weakness of the dura predisposes the vertebral bodies to deformity. Thus, abnormality of vertebral body contour may be apparent in Marfan's syndrome, neurofibromatosis, and Ehlers-Danlos syndrome (Fig. 55–22). Scalloped vertebrae also are recognized in additional skeletal disorders, such as achondroplasia, Hurler's syndrome, and Morquio's disease.

Articular Abnormalities. The initial phase of acromegalic joint disease is manifested as increased articular space and enlargement of the osseous surfaces. These radiographic findings are differentiated easily from those accompanying other disease processes. The later stages of acromegalic joint disease include findings such as joint space narrowing, cyst formation, sclerosis, and osteophytosis, which are similar to the abnormalities of primary degenerative joint disease. Differentiation between these two disorders may be difficult. In some patients with acromegaly, involvement of weight-bearing joints such as the hip and knee simulates the distribution of primary degenerative joint disease, although in other patients, non–weight-bearing joints such as the glenohumeral joint and elbow are involved, a distribution that is unusual in primary degenerative joint disease. Furthermore, prominent osteophytes and beaklike excrescences of articular bony surfaces are characteristic in acromegaly. In fact, these outgrowths may be apparent before joint space loss becomes evident.

The distribution of degenerative alterations in acromegaly may be similar to that in alkaptonuria and CPPD crystal deposition disease. In the former disorder, vertebral osteo-

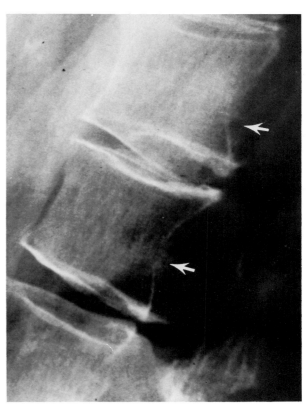

FIGURE 55–22. Vertebral scalloping in Ehlers-Danlos syndrome. A lateral radiograph of the spine delineates prominent scalloping of the posterior surface of multiple vertebral bodies (arrows). (Courtesy of M. Dalinka, M.D., Philadelphia, Pennsylvania.)

porosis, discal calcification, and widespread loss of disc height ensure proper diagnosis; in the latter disorder, the presence of articular and periarticular calcification and more severe and progressive joint destruction are important diagnostic clues, although both acromegaly and CPPD crystal deposition disease may occur in the same person.

Summary

The osseous manifestations of acromegaly are the result of the effects of elevated serum growth hormone on the adult skeleton. Reactivation of endochondral bone formation and stimulation of periosteal bone formation in association with connective tissue proliferation are apparent, leading to characteristic radiographic findings, including increased soft tissue thickness and bony overgrowth. Joint abnormalities result from chondrocyte proliferation in articular cartilage. The excessively stimulated cartilage is vulnerable to fissuring, fragmentation, and ulceration, which are followed by a brisk reparative response. These histologic alterations have their radiographic counterparts. Initial joint space widening is followed by joint space narrowing, bone sclerosis, cyst formation, and osteophytosis. The latter radiographic abnormalities simulate those of primary degenerative joint disease.

HYPOPITUITARISM

Damage to the anterior lobe of the pituitary gland during the period of skeletal growth leads to abnormality of osseous development. The cause of damage is variable and includes neoplasms (adenomas, craniopharyngioma, pituitary carcinoma, metastasis), infection (pyogenic, tuberculous, fungal), granulomas (histiocytosis, sarcoidosis), injury, and vascular insult (Table 55–7). In approximately 10 per cent of cases, hypopituitarism is familial, probably related to transmission of a recessive gene or, less commonly, a dominant one. The effect on the skeleton is a delay in appearance and growth of ossification centers and a similar delay in their fusion and disappearance (Fig. 55–23). On histologic examination, the growth plate is observed to remain open and its metaphyseal side is "closed off" as osseous tissue abuts on the cartilaginous tissue[3] (Fig. 55–24). Eventually the growth plate may disappear, although osseous fusion occurs at an advanced age.

Clinically, growth failure usually is recognized when the child is 1 to 3 years of age and, if the condition is untreated, continued slow growth at the rate of 50 to 60 per cent of normal occurs throughout childhood. Findings include immature body proportions and facial features, abnormal distribution of fat, and delay in eruption of secondary teeth. Mental development generally parallels the chronological age.

Radiographic abnormalities are reported in association with hypopituitarism,[51–53, 64] but articular manifestations rarely are noted, although nonspecific and diffuse myalgia and arthralgia have been identified in a man with hypothalamic hypopituitarism, presumably related to adrenal gland insufficiency.[77] In patients with hypopituitarism, treatment with human growth hormone results in an increase in skeletal maturation paralleling the increase in chronological age[54–56, 68] and an increase in cortical thickness. The growth plates may widen.[57] In rare instances, slipping of the femo-

TABLE 55–7. Causes of Hypopituitarism*

Primary Involvement of the Pituitary
Neoplasms
  1. Chromophobe, acidophilic, and mixed adenomas
  2. Craniopharyngioma
  3. Pituitary carcinoma
  4. Metastatic carcinoma
Granulomas
  1. Histiocytosis
  2. Sarcoidosis
Infection
  1. Mycotic, monilial
  2. Tuberculous
  3. Luetic
  4. Pyogenic
Hemochromatosis
Aneurysm of internal carotid artery
Infarction
  1. Postpartum necrosis
  2. Cerebrovascular disease (in diabetes mellitus)
Idiopathic

Primary Involvement of the Hypothalamus
Neoplasms
  1. Meningioma, ependymoma, pinealoma
  2. Craniopharyngioma
  3. Metastatic carcinoma

Therapeutic Ablation
Surgery
Stalk section
Radioisotope implants (yttrium-99)
Cryohypophysectomy
Heavy particle irradiation (protons, neutrons)

*From Ney RL: The anterior pituitary gland. In PK Bondy, LE Rosenberg (Eds): Duncan's Diseases of Metabolism. 7th Ed. Vol II. Endocrinology. Philadelphia, WB Saunders Co, 1974, p 989.

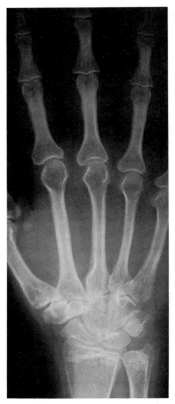

FIGURE 55–23. Hypopituitarism: Delayed skeletal maturation. In this 23 year old woman, a marked reduction in the rate of skeletal maturation is confirmed by the absence of closure of the physes of the distal portions of the radius and ulna. Osteopenia is evident.

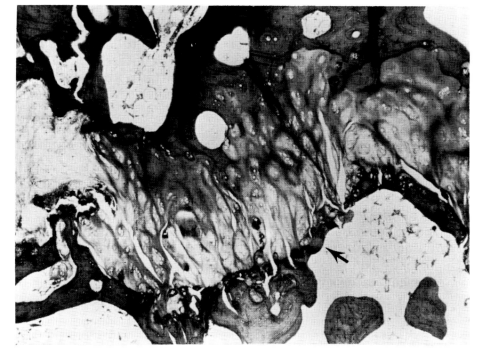

FIGURE 55–24. Hypopituitarism: Cessation of endochondral ossification. A photomicrograph (35×) of an open growth plate in a 38 year old man with hypopituitarism demonstrates that metaphyseal bone (arrow) abuts on the cartilaginous plate, and endochondral ossification is lacking despite the columnar arrangement of the cartilage cells. (From Jaffe HL: Metabolic, Degenerative, and Inflammatory Diseases of Bones and Joints. Philadelphia, Lea & Febiger, 1972.)

ral capital epiphysis may occur before or during growth hormone therapy[58–61, 78] in patients with pituitary dysfunction. The exact mechanism for epiphyseal displacement in these persons is not known, although Harris has demonstrated a reduction in shearing stress in the tibial growth plate in rats given growth hormone or estrogen.[62] Femoral

capital epiphyseal necrosis has been reported during human growth hormone therapy.[63] Of interest in this regard, depressed levels of secretion of growth hormone have been implicated in the pathogenesis of Legg-Calvé-Perthes disease in some investigations.[79]

The differential diagnosis of pituitary dwarfism includes psychosocial dwarfism, hypothyroidism, gonadal dysgenesis (Turner's syndrome), malnutrition, diabetes mellitus, occult systemic inflammatory diseases, chronic renal disease, and a variety of skeletal disorders, including achondroplasia, forms of rickets, pseudohypoparathyroidism, and neurofibromatosis (Table 55–8). Most of these conditions are differentiated easily from pituitary dwarfism, which is important as the latter disease probably accounts for fewer than 10 per cent of cases of short stature in children.

TABLE 55–8. Some Causes of Short Stature

Endocrine Disorders
 Hypopituitarism
 Hypothyroidism
 Diabetes mellitus
 Hypercortisolism
 Congenital adrenal hyperplasia
 Deficient somatomedin production (Laron dwarfism)

Chronic Disorders of Major Organ Systems
 Chronic renal disease
 Congenital heart disease
 Juvenile chronic arthritis
 Sickle cell anemia
 Malabsorption syndromes

Skeletal Disorders
 Achondroplasia
 Osteochondrodysplasias
 Pseudohypoparathyroidism and pseudopseudohypoparathyroidism
 Rickets

Chromosomal Aberrations
 Gonadal dysgenesis
 Trisomy conditions

Miscellaneous Disorders
 Malnutrition
 Familial short stature
 Inborn errors of metabolism
 Intrauterine infections
 Systemic inflammatory diseases
 Renal tubular disorders
 Psychosocial dwarfism
 Neurologic disorders

References

1. Marie P: Sur deux cas d'acromegalie; hypertrophie singulière noncongenitale des extremites superieures, inferieures et cephalique. Rev Med 6:297, 1886.
2. Ney RL: The anterior pituitary gland. *In* PK Bondy, LE Rosenberg (Eds): Duncan's Diseases of Metabolism. 7th Ed. Vol II. Endocrinology. Philadelphia, WB Saunders Co, 1974, p 961.
3. Jaffe HL: Metabolic, Degenerative and Inflammatory Diseases of Bones and Joints. Philadelphia, Lea & Febiger, 1972, p 332.
4. Davis JC, Hipkin LJ: Clinical Endocrine Pathology. Oxford, England, Blackwell Scientific Publications, 1977, p 11.
5. Middleton GS: A marked case of acromegaly with joint affections. Glasgow Med J 41:401, 1894.
6. Bluestone R, Bywaters EGL, Hartog M, et al: Acromegalic arthropathy. Ann Rheum Dis 30:243, 1971.
7. Bluestone R: Rheumatological complications of some endocrinopathies. Clin Rheum Dis 1:95, 1975.
8. Holt PJL: Endocrine disorders and metabolic bone disease. *In* JT Scott (Ed): Copeman's Textbook of the Rheumatic Diseases. 5th Ed. Edinburgh, Churchill Livingstone, 1978, p 707.
9. Silcox DC, McCarty DJ: Measurement of inorganic pyrophosphate in biological fluids. Elevated levels in some patients with osteoarthritis, pseudogout, acromegaly and uremia. J Clin Invest 52:1863, 1973.
10. Lamotte M, Segrestaa JM, Krassinine G: Arthrite microcristalline calique (pseudogoutte) chez un acromegale. Sem Hôp Paris 42:2420, 1966.
11. Horenstein S, Hambrook G, Eyerman E: Spinal cord compression by vertebral acromegaly. Trans Am Neurol Assoc 96:254, 1971.

12. Longson D, Isherwood I: Personal communication (1975).
13. Mastaglia FL, Barwick DD, Hall R: Myopathy in acromegaly. Lancet 2:907, 1970.
14. Kellgren JH, Ball J, Tutton GK: Articular and other limb changes in acromegaly; a clinical and pathological study of 25 cases. Q J Med 21:405, 1952.
15. Lewis PD: Neuromuscular involvement in pituitary gigantism. Br Med J 2:499, 1972.
16. Waine H, Bennett GA, Bauer W: Joint disease associated with acromegaly. Am J Med Sci 209:671, 1945.
17. Detenbeck LC, Tressler HA, O'Duffy JD, et al: Peripheral joint manifestations of acromegaly. Clin Orthop 91:119, 1973.
18. Erdheim J: Über Wirbelsäulenveranderungen bei Akromegalie. Virchows Arch (Pathol Anat) 281:197, 1931.
19. Doyle FH: Radiologic assessment of endocrine effects on bone. Radiol Clin North Am 5:289, 1967.
20. Curshmann H: Über regressive Knochenveranderungen bei Akromegalie. ROFO 9:83, 1905–1906.
21. Finlay JM, MacDonald RI: Acromegaly. Can Med Assoc J 71:345, 1954.
22. Garn SM, Poznanski AK, Nagy JM: Bone measurement in the differential diagnosis of osteopenia and osteoporosis. Radiology 100:509, 1971.
23. Memma HE: Recognition of cortical bone resorption in metabolic bone disease in vivo. Skel Radiol 2:11, 1977.
24. Sledge CB: Growth hormone and articular cartilage. Fed Proc 32:1503, 1973.
25. Lang EK, Bessler WT: The roentgenologic features of acromegaly. AJR 86:321, 1961.
26. Good AE: Acromegalic arthropathy. A case report. Arthritis Rheum 7:65, 1964.
27. Kleinberg DL, Young IS, Kupperman HS: The sesamoid index. An aid in the diagnosis of acromegaly. Ann Intern Med 64:1075, 1966.
28. Sheppard RH, Meema HE: Skin thickness in endocrine disease. A roentgenographic study. Ann Intern Med 66:531, 1967.
29. Steinbach HL, Feldman R, Goldberg MB: Acromegaly. Radiology 72:535, 1959.
30. Bluestone R, Bywaters EGL, Hartog M, et al: Acromegalic arthropathy. Arthritis Rheum 14:371, 1971.
31. Stuber JL, Palacios E: Vertebral scalloping in acromegaly. AJR 112:397, 1971.
32. Lin SR, Lee KF: Widening of the median atlanto-axial joint in acromegaly. J Can Assoc Rad 24:36, 1973.
33. Gelman MI: Cauda equina compression in acromegaly. Radiology 112:357, 1974.
34. Cushing H, Davidoff LM: Pathological findings in four autopsied cases of acromegaly with discussion of their significance. Monograph No 22. New York, Rockefeller Institute for Medical Research, 1927.
35. Gershberg H, Heinemann HO, Stumpf HH: Renal function studies and autopsy report in a patient with gigantism and acromegaly. J Clin Endocrinol 17:377, 1957.
36. Hejtmancik MR, Bradfield JY Jr, Herrmann GR: Acromegaly and heart: Clinical and pathologic study. Ann Intern Med 34:1445, 1951.
37. Meema HE, Sheppard RH, Rapoport A: Roentgenographic visualization and measurement of skin thickness and its diagnostic application in acromegaly. Radiology 82:411, 1964.
38. Steinbach HL, Russell W: Measurement of the heel pad as an aid to diagnosis of acromegaly. Radiology 82:418, 1964.
39. Puckette SE Jr, Seymour EQ: Fallibility of the heel pad thickness in the diagnosis of acromegaly. Radiology 88:982, 1967.
40. Jackson DM: Heel-pad thickness in obese persons. Radiology 90:129, 1968.
41. Gonticas SK, Ikkos DG, Stergiou LH: Evaluation of the diagnostic value of heel-pad thickness in acromegaly. Radiology 92:304, 1969.
42. Kho KM, Wright AD, Doyle FH: Heel pad thickness in acromegaly. Br J Radiology 43:119, 1970.
43. Anton HC: Hand measurements in acromegaly. Clin Radiol 23:445, 1972.
44. Duncan TR: Validity of the sesamoid index in the diagnosis of acromegaly. Radiology 115:617, 1975.
45. Lin SR, Lee KF: Relative value of some radiographic measurements of the hand in the diagnosis of acromegaly. Invest Radiol 6:426, 1971.
46. Mitchell GE, Lourie H, Berne AS: The various causes of scalloped vertebrae with notes on their pathogenesis. Radiology 89:67, 1967.
47. Von Bonin G: Study of a case of dyspituitarism. Q J Med 6:125, 1913.
48. Reinhardt WO, Li CH: Experimental production of arthritis in rats by hypophyseal growth hormone. Science 117:295, 1953.
49. Hartog M: Acromegaly and hyperparathyroidism. Proc R Soc Med 60:477, 1967.
50. Harbison JB, Nice CM Jr: Familial pachydermoperiostosis presenting as an acromegaly-like syndrome. AJR 112:532, 1971.
51. Poznanski AK: The Hand in Radiologic Diagnosis. Philadelphia, WB Saunders Co, 1974, p 510.
52. Hernandez R, Poznanski AK, Kelch RP, et al: Hand radiographic measurement in growth hormone deficiency before and after treatment. AJR 129:487, 1977.
53. Hernandez RJ, Poznanski AK, Hopwood NJ, et al: Incidence of growth lines in psychosocial dwarfs and idiopathic hypopituitarism. AJR 131:477, 1978.
54. Prader A, Zachmann M, Poley JR, et al: Long term treatment with human growth hormone (Raben) in small doses. Evaluation of 18 hypopituitary patients. Helv Paediatr Acta 22:423, 1967.
55. Tanner JM, Whitehouse RH: Growth response of 26 children with short stature given human growth hormone. Br Med J 2:69, 1967.
56. Soyka LF, Bode HH, Crawford JD, et al: Effectiveness of long term human growth hormone therapy for short stature in children with growth hormone deficiency. J Clin Endocrinol Metab 30:1, 1970.
57. Greenspan FS, Li CH, Simpson ME, et al: Bioassay of hypophyseal growth hormone: The tibia test. Endocrinology 45:455, 1949.
58. Semple JC, Goldschmidt RG: Epiphyseal maturation and slipping femoral epiphysis in a hypopituitary dwarf. Orthopedics (Oxford) 2:31, 1969.
59. Fidler MW, Brook CGD: Slipped upper femoral epiphysis following treatment with human growth hormone. J. Bone Joint Surg [Am] 56:1719, 1974.
60. Rennie W, Mitchell N: Slipped femoral capital epiphysis occurring during growth hormone therapy. J Bone Joint Surg [Br] 56:703, 1974.
61. Heatley FW, Greenwood RH, Boase DL: Slipping of the upper femoral epiphysis in patients with intracranial tumors causing hypopituitarism and chiasmal compression. J Bone Joint Surg [Br] 58:169, 1976.
62. Harris WR: The endocrine basis for slipping of the upper femoral epiphysis. An experimental study. J Bone Joint Surg [Br] 52:5, 1950.
63. Bjerkreim I, Trygstad O: Necrosis of the femoral capital epiphysis occurring during human growth hormone therapy. Acta Orthop Scand 47:189, 1976.
64. Hernandez RJ, Poznanski AW, Hopwood NJ: Size and skeletal maturation of the hand in children with hypothyroidism and hypopituitarism. AJR 133:405, 1979.
65. Bohrer SP, Ude AC: Heel pad thickness in Nigerians. Skel Radiol 3:108, 1978.
66. Aloia JF, Petrak Z, Ellis K, et al: Body composition and skeletal metabolism following pituitary irradiation in acromegaly. Am J Med 61:59, 1976.
67. Efird TA, Genant HK, Wilson CB: Pituitary gigantism with cervical spinal stenosis. AJR 134:171, 1980.
68. Shore RM, Mazess RB, Bargman GJ: Bone mineral status in growth hormone deficiency. J Pediatr 96:393, 1980.
69. Shapiro R, Schorr S: A consideration of the systemic factors that influence frontal sinus pneumatization. Invest Radiol 15:191, 1980.
70. Holt PJL: Locomotor abnormalities in acromegaly. Clin Rheum Dis 7:689, 1981.
71. Petrovic A, Stutzmann J: Hormone somatotrope: Modalities d'action sur la croissance des diverses variétés de cartilage. Pathol Biol 28:43, 1980.
72. Johanson NA, Vigorita VJ, Goldman AB, et al: Acromegalic arthropathy of the hip. Clin Orthop 173:130, 1983.
73. Copya P, Uriel C, Gilsanz A, et al: Los senos frontales en la acromegalia. Med Esp 81:161, 1982.
74. Sabet D, Stark AR: Sesamoid index of the foot in acromegaly. J Am Podiatry Assoc 71:625, 1981.
75. Chaouat D, Lambrozo J, Baffet A, et al: Osteonecrose aseptique bilaterale de la tête femorale au cours d'une acromegalie. Rev Rhum Mal Osteoartic 51:215, 1984.
76. Kattan KR: Thickening of the heel-pad associated with long-term Dilantin therapy. AJR 124:52, 1975.
77. Yunus M, Masi AT, Allen JP: Hypothalamic hypopituitarism presenting with rheumatologic symptoms. Arthritis Rheum 24:632, 1981.
78. McAfee PC, Cady RB: Endocrinologic and metabolic factors in atypical presentations of slipped capital femoral epiphysis. Clin Orthop 180:188, 1983.
79. Tanaka H, Tamura K, Takano K, et al: Serum somatomedin A in Perthes' disease. Acta Orthop Scand 55:135, 1984.
80. Lacks S, Jacobs RP: Acromegalic arthropathy: A reversible rheumatic disease. J Rheumatol 13:634, 1986.
81. Layton MW, Fudman EJ, Barkan A, et al: Acromegalic arthropathy. Characteristics and response to therapy. Arthritis Rheum 31:1022, 1988.
82. Dupond JL, de Wazières B, Morin G: Acromégalie et chondrocalcinose articulaire chez une femme de 26 ans. Rev Rhum Mal Osteoartic 59:83, 1992.
83. Melo-Gomes J, Viana-Queiroz M: Acromegalic arthropathy: A reversible rheumatic disease. J Rheumatol 14:393, 1987.
84. Parikh M, Iyer K, Elias AN, et al: Spinal stenosis in acromegaly. Spine 12:627, 1987.
85. Ibbertson HK, Manning PJ, Holdaway IM, et al: The acromegalic rosary. Lancet 337:154, 1991.
86. Doppman JL, Sharon M, Gorden P: Metatarsal pencilling in acromegaly: A proposed mechanism based on CT findings. J Comput Assist Tomogr 12:708, 1988.
87. Mikawa Y, Watanabe R, Nishishita Y: Cervical myelopathy in acromegaly. Report of a case. Spine 17:1542, 1992.

56

Thyroid Disorders

Donald Resnick, M.D.

Thyroxine and triiodothyronine are active thyroid hormones that increase the turnover of protein, carbohydrate, fat, and mineral. They circulate in the blood, largely bound to serum proteins, although small quantities are in an active free form. Excessive thyroid hormone produces catabolism of protein and loss of connective tissue; deficiency of thyroid hormone has a dramatic effect on the body, causing defects in bone growth and development.[1] Various factors produce abnormality in thyroid function, including alteration in autoimmune mechanisms, which may lead to Hashimoto's thyroiditis and other diseases.[2] Thyroid disorders, in addition, may be associated with other articular and autoimmune diseases, including systemic lupus erythematosus and rheumatoid arthritis.[2-4] In this regard, thyroid fibrosis and thyroiditis have been detected in 12 per cent of patients with rheumatoid arthritis, and both rheumatoid arthritis and systemic lupus erythematosus may occur with increased frequency in patients with Hashimoto's thyroiditis. Furthermore, antithyroid drugs, such as thiouracil and thionamide, can induce a lupus erythematosus–like syndrome,[5, 6] and hyperuricemia may be apparent in persons with hypothyroidism.[7]

This chapter summarizes skeletal and articular manifestations of thyroid disorders.

HYPERTHYROIDISM

General Characteristics

Thyrotoxicosis is a general term indicating biochemical and physiologic abnormalities that result from excessive quantities of the thyroid hormones; the term hyperthyroidism is used to describe this syndrome when it is the result of overproduction of these hormones by the thyroid gland itself rather than of abnormalities that have not originated in this gland.[8] Of the many forms of thyrotoxicosis, toxic diffuse goiter (Graves' disease or Basedow's disease) and toxic nodular goiter produced by single or multiple adenomas are most common. Other causes of thyrotoxicosis include toxic adenoma, trophoblastic diseases (hydatidiform mole, choriocarcinoma, metastatic embryonal carcinoma of the testes), iodine-induced hyperthyroidism, thyrotoxicosis factitia, subacute or chronic thyroiditis, and ectopic thyroid tissue.[8] Clinical manifestations of thyrotoxicosis that generally allow accurate diagnosis include symptoms such as fatigue, weakness, nervousness, hypersensitivity to heat, hyperhidrosis, weight loss, tachycardia, palpitation, eye complaints, and diarrhea; physical signs may include enlargement of the neck, rapid heart beat, tremor, thyroid bruit, and abnormalities of the eye (Tables 56–1 and 56–2).

Bone Resorption

In patients with hyperthyroidism, whether endogenous or exogenous[9] in origin, elevation of serum calcium concentration is apparent, although hypercalcemia generally is not severe or sustained.[10-12] Additional laboratory findings are elevated levels of serum phosphorus and alkaline phosphatase and hypercalciuria.[12] These features underscore the presence of excessive bone turnover with a negative calcium balance, although the mechanism by which this occurs is not known.[1, 11] Despite evidence that suggests an increased frequency of hyperparathyroidism in patients with hyperthyroidism,[13, 14] calcium mobilization by thyroid hor-

TABLE 56–1. Prevalence of Symptoms and Signs in Thyrotoxicosis*

Symptoms	Per Cent of Patients	Signs	Per Cent of Patients
Nervousness	99	Goiter	97–100
Hyperhidrosis	91	Tachycardia	97–100
Hypersensitivity to heat	89	Skin changes	97
Palpitation	89	Tremor	97
Fatigue	88	Thyroid bruit	77
Weight loss	85	Eye signs	71
Weight gain	2	Thyroid heart disease	15
No weight change	13		
Tachycardia	82	Atrial fibrillation	10
Dyspnea	75	Splenomegaly	10
Weakness	70	Gynecomastia	10
Hyperorexia	65	Liver palms	8
Anorexia	9		
Eye complaints	54		
Swelling of legs	35		
Increased frequency of bowel movement	33		
Diarrhea	23		

*From Robbins J, et al: The thyroid and iodine metabolism. *In* PK Bondy, LE Rosenberg (Eds): Metabolic Control and Disease. 8th Ed. Philadelphia, WB Saunders Co, 1980, p 1375. (After Williams.)

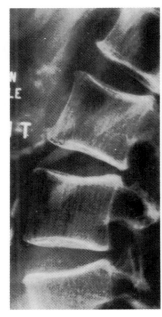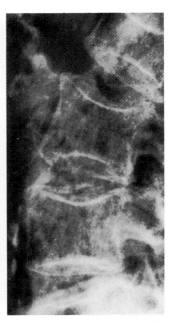

FIGURE 56–1. Hyperthyroidism: Spinal abnormalities. Radiographs obtained 5 months apart reveal the rapid course of vertebral osteoporosis that may accompany thyrotoxicosis. On the later film (right), increased radiolucency of the vertebral bodies and biconcave deformities are apparent. (From Meunier PJ, et al: Orthop Clin North Am 3:745, 1972.)

mone apparently does not depend on the presence of the parathyroid glands and, in fact, hyperthyroidism with its hypercalcemia decreases secretion of both thyrocalcitonin and parathyroid hormone.[12, 15]

The laboratory evidence of elevation of cellular activity and bony resorption in hyperthyroidism[16] may have its counterpart in radiographic changes. The reported frequency of radiographically detectable bone disease in patients with hyperthyroidism has varied from 3.5 to 50 per cent,[17–21] some of the variation resulting from different criteria used by various investigators. The changes are more common in men than in women, and, in women, predominate after the menopause. Symptomatic hyperthyroid bone disease also is more common in older persons in whom the process of bone loss already has been initiated, and in whom the classic features of Graves' disease are less obvious, so that the disease may escape detection for a longer period of time. Most persons with bone abnormalities have had hyperthyroidism for longer than 5 years,[22] although osseous changes may be apparent in less than 1 year.[18] Hyperthyroid bone disease does not appear to be linked to the severity of the thyroid dysfunction but is more frequent in patients with exophthalmos.[18]

The findings of Meunier and associates[18] may be summarized as follows: bone abnormalities in hyperthyroidism

TABLE 56–2. Musculoskeletal Abnormalities of Hyperthyroidism

Hyperthyroid osteopathy
Accelerated skeletal maturation
Myopathy

may be associated with pain, fracture, and deformity. Discomfort is due to dorsalgia and lumbar pain and may be accentuated with the onset of vertebral collapse. Deformities include reduction in height and exaggerated dorsal kyphosis. Spontaneous fractures in hyperthyroidism are frequent and, in addition to vertebral body collapse, may be seen in the femoral neck, other long bones, and even the metacarpals.[18, 22] Clinical as well as radiographic findings may appear quickly, progress rapidly, and stabilize or improve with appropriate treatment of thyrotoxicosis.

The radiographic features of bone loss in hyperthyroidism simulate those associated with other varieties of osteoporosis, although hyperthyroid osteopathy may lead to bone loss not only in the vertebral column but also in the pelvis, cranium, hands, and feet.[18, 23, 24] In the spine, osteoporosis, vertebral compression, and kyphosis (or kyphoscoliosis) are seen (Fig. 56–1). Osteoporosis produces typical rarefaction of the midportion of the vertebral body and fish vertebrae with exaggerated biconcave deformity of the vertebral body. These changes are more pronounced in the thoracic and lumbar vertebrae but may be observed in the cervical region as well.

In the skull, focal rarefaction of bone, particularly in the frontal region, may produce a radiographic picture reminiscent of that in multiple myeloma[18] (Fig. 56–2). Increased radiolucency and cystic lesions[25] also may be apparent in long bones, clavicles, and ribs.[26] Rarely, a pathologic fracture is seen.[27]

Osteoporosis also is observed in the hands and feet of patients with hyperthyroidism[18, 26, 28] (Fig. 56–3). Findings include a lattice-like appearance in the phalanges, and "flaky" cortices due to radiolucent longitudinal striations within the cortical bone. Using magnification techniques in examining the second metacarpal, Meema and Schatz[28] ob-

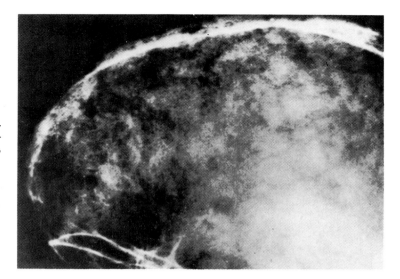

FIGURE 56–2. Hyperthyroidism: Cranial abnormalities. Severe patchy radiolucency of the skull in a patient with hyperthyroidism simulates multiple myeloma. (From Meunier PJ, et al: Orthop Clin North Am *3*:745, 1972.)

served cortical striations in over 50 per cent of patients with moderate to severe hyperthyroidism. These striations correlated well with the mineralization of the distal radius and poorly with metacarpal thickness. Fraser and associates,[29] using radiodensitometry techniques, noted osseous rarefaction of the third metacarpal in untreated women with hyperthyroidism but not in controls.

Rarely, bone loss in hyperthyroidism may be associated with an osteomalacic pattern[18, 30] in which radiolucent areas or Looser's zones may be observed in the femoral neck or elsewhere.

Descriptions of the histology of bone in patients with hyperthyroidism emphasize bone resorption[18, 31, 32] (Fig. 56–4). Initial reports stressed perforations of compact bone and the presence of fibrosis within Howship's lacunae.[32, 33] Meunier and associates[18] confirmed the presence of hyperosteoclastosis in cortical bone, resulting in longitudinal

splitting or striations, and stressed that the cancellous bone was relatively spared, differing from the findings of hyperparathyroidism, in which osteoclasia is equally prominent in cortical and cancellous bone. Osteoblastic foci also are seen in hyperthyroidism. Hypervascularity is apparent both on gross inspection (stripping the periosteum from an involved bone reveals a hyperemic cortex) and on histologic examination (engorged blood vessels are observed).[31] Rarefaction of cancellous bone with thin trabeculae has been confirmed.[32] Reports of morphologic changes of osteomalacia in hyperthyroidism have described osteoid seams.[32] As noted by Meunier and coworkers,[18] these osteoid seams represent overproduction of preosseous tissue by osteoblasts rather than arrested calcification of this tissue.[34–36]

Quantitative histologic study of bone in thyrotoxicosis confirms a significant increase in cortical porosity, a reduction in absolute bone volume of spongy bone without in-

FIGURE 56–3. Hyperthyroidism: Abnormalities of the hands and feet.

A, B Before the onset of the disease, a radiograph of the finger essentially is normal **(A)**. Five years after the onset of hyperthyroidism, increased radiolucency of the phalanges is associated with intracortical striations **(B)**.

C Similar abnormalities in the foot can be seen. Observe a stress fracture of the proximal phalanx of the fifth toe.

(From Chevrot A, et al: J Radiol Electrol Med Nucl *59*:167, 1978.)

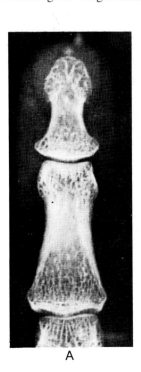

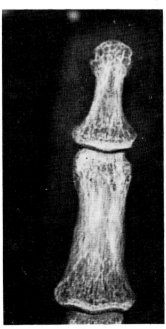

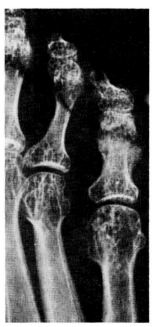

A B C

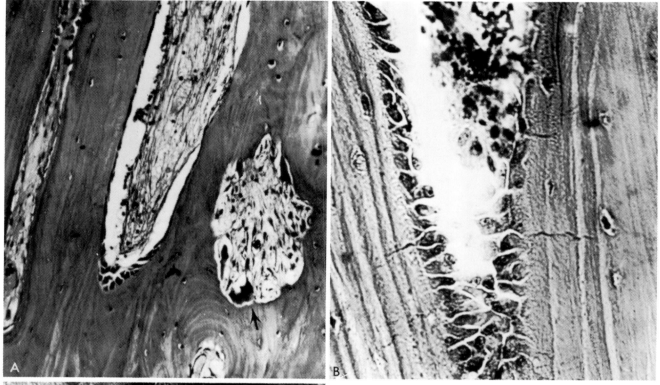

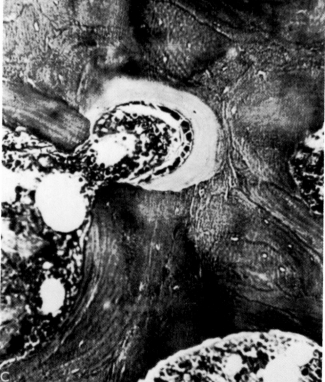

FIGURE 56–4. Hyperthyroidism: Pathologic abnormalities.
A The cortex is perforated with osteoclastic foci (arrow).
B Elsewhere, an osteoblastic focus is observed within the cortex.
C A thick osteoid seam is apparent in the spongy bone.
(From Meunier PJ, et al: Orthop Clin North Am *3*:745, 1972.)

creased osteoid volume, an extension of trabecular osteoclastic resorption sites, and the absence of periosteocytic enlargement.[18]

In summary, the qualitative and quantitative histologic findings in hyperthyroid osteopathy suggest the presence of both hyperosteoclastosis and hyperosteoblastosis, which are more prominent in cortical bone than in trabecular bone.[18] Both bone resorption and bone formation are increased, but in the presence of reduced skeletal mass, bone resorption is the more dominant abnormality. Osteopenia, deformity, and even pathologic fracture are the observed radiologic alterations. Although appropriate therapy with the establishment of a euthyroid state is accompanied by some degree of recovery in bone mineral content, the latter may remain depressed compared with that of normal persons.

Additional Musculoskeletal Abnormalities

Occasionally patients with hyperthyroidism may reveal prominent calcification of costal cartilage as well as of other structures, including the tracheal rings.[18, 38, 39] A minor radiographic sign in hyperthyroidism is the visualization of Plummer's nails (onycholysis), characterized by separation of tissue from the undersurface of the nail with accumulation of dirt.[40]

Hyperthyroidism in children is associated with different osseous manifestations than in adults. Acceleration of skeletal maturation can be seen, which may reach severe proportions.[41] Riggs and coworkers[42] described one child 5 weeks old whose skeletal maturation was that of a 2½ year old child. Similar observations have been noted by others.[43–45] Premature craniosynostosis can be evident.[46]

Myopathy is frequent in hyperthyroidism, especially in men, and its symptoms and signs may simulate arthritis. Weakness, cramps, and muscular tenderness are observed,[47] particularly in the proximal muscles of the extremities, although peripheral musculature also may be affected. Muscle wasting out of proportion to the generalized loss of tissue associated with the disease sometimes is observed.[48] Although the findings may resemble those of polymyositis, biopsy documents the absence of significant muscle inflammation and the presence of atrophy and infiltration with fat cells and lymphocytes. With effective treatment of hyperthyroidism, the symptoms and signs may decrease in intensity or even disappear.[49]

Neurologic manifestations of hyperthyroidism include peripheral neuropathy, corticospinal tract disease, chorea, seizures, and psychiatric disorders.[50, 51]

When hyperthyroidism is seen in association with other disorders, the clinical and radiologic findings of these concomitant diseases may be observed. Scleroderma-like skin thickening in the extremities occasionally is seen in hyperthyroidism, and a patient with both hyperthyroidism and scleroderma has been described in whom typical soft tissue and osseous radiographic manifestations of scleroderma were depicted.[52] In addition, reports have appeared of patients with rheumatoid arthritis who developed toxic adenomas[53, 54] and patients with thyrotoxicosis who developed rheumatoid arthritis.[55] An association between hyperthyroidism and systemic lupus erythematosus also has been suggested.[56] Hyperthyroidism occurs in approximately 3 to 5 per cent of patients with myasthenia gravis, and about 1 per cent of patients with Graves' disease develop myasthe-

nia gravis.[8] Unlike thyrotoxic myopathy, the association of myasthenia gravis and Graves' disease has a distinct female sex preponderance.[8]

Finally, the possibility of secretion of a thyroid-stimulating substance by tumors in nonendocrine organs has been noted.[57, 58]

THYROID ACROPACHY

General Characteristics

Thyroid acropachy is an unusual manifestation of thyroid disease that may be seen in approximately 0.5 to 1 per cent of patients with thyrotoxicosis.[59] This condition usually is observed after treatment of hyperthyroidism, at which time the patient may be euthyroid or hypothyroid, although it has been described in the hyperthyroid state as well.[41, 60] It can occur at any age, even in teenagers.[61] Men and women are affected equally. Thyroid acropachy usually occurs several years after the onset of hyperthyroidism, although it may be one of the initial findings of the disease.[60]

Clinical findings in thyroid acropachy include exophthalmos, which may be severe and progressive, painless symmetric or asymmetric soft tissue swelling of the fingers and toes, which may be erythematous and fluctuant, pretibial myxedema, and clubbing of the fingers (Table 56–3).

Radiographic and Pathologic Findings

Radiographic abnormalities are virtually diagnostic[41, 59–68] (Figs. 56–5 and 56–6). Periosteal bone formation is seen in the diaphyses of the metacarpals, metatarsals, and proximal and middle phalanges, although this change may be visualized occasionally at other sites, including the long bones. Periostitis is asymmetric in distribution and more prominent on the radial aspect of the bone, and it tends to be dense and solid in appearance, with a feathery contour. Soft tissue swelling in the hands and feet, phalangeal tufts, and anterior tibial region is observed. Soft tissue deformity rarely may require surgical intervention.[68] The osseous abnormalities generally are not progressive[66, 68]; correcting the thyroid function has little or no effect on the acropachy. Increased radionuclide activity in areas of bony alteration has been observed.[69, 70]

A limited number of reports of histologic alterations in this condition note soft tissue infiltration with myxedematous tissue and periosteal nodular fibrosis with new bone formation.[71]

The cause of thyroid acropachy is not known. Initial theories emphasized the role of vascular changes[72] and pituitary dysfunction.[73] More recently, long-acting thyroid stimulator (LATS) and human thyroid stimulator (HTS) also have been implicated.[74]

TABLE 56–3. Clinical and Radiographic Features of Thyroid Acropachy

Exophthalmos
Soft tissue swelling
Pretibial myxedema
Clubbing
Periostitis

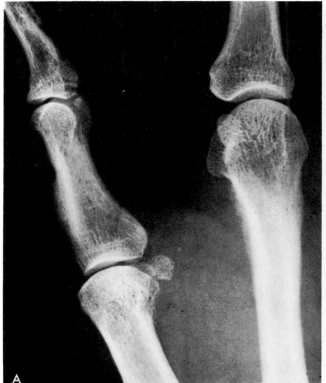

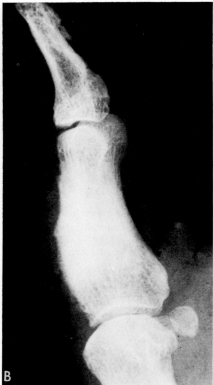

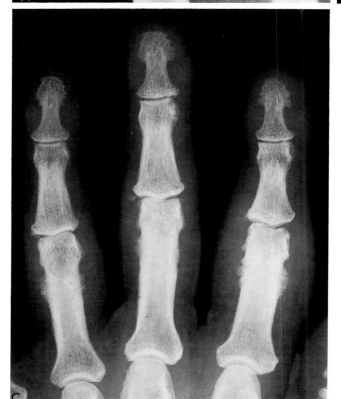

FIGURE 56–5. Thyroid acropachy.

A Observe thick shaggy periostitis, asymmetric in distribution, which has predilection for the radial aspect of the proximal phalanx of the first digit and the second metacarpal.

B In another hand, more extensive deposition of periosteal bone on the radial aspect of the proximal phalanx has produced irregular enlargement of the bone.

(**A, B,** Courtesy of V. Schiappacasse, M.D., Santiago, Chile.)

C In a different patient, observe soft tissue swelling, clubbing, and spiculated or feathery periostitis in the proximal phalanges. Less extensive changes in middle phalanges and terminal tufts are seen.

(**C,** Courtesy of L. Santini, M.D., Danville, Pennsylvania.)

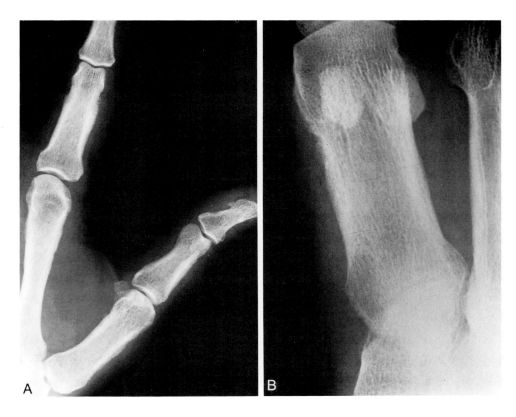

FIGURE 56–6. Thyroid acropachy. This 51 year old woman had intermittent painless swelling and soft tissue thickening in the hands and feet of several months' duration. Her past medical history included hyperthyroidism, which had been treated with radioactive iodine. Evaluation documented a euthyroid state despite the presence of proptosis and pretibial myxedema. Observe shaggy periosteal new bone formation in the diaphyses of the phalanges and metacarpal bones of the hand, predominating along the radial aspect of the digits, and along the medial and lateral aspects of the first metatarsal bone. (Courtesy of G. Greenway, M.D., Dallas, Texas.)

Differential Diagnosis

Thyroid acropachy must be differentiated from other disorders associated with periosteal bone formation (Table 56–4) (Fig. 56–7). Hypertrophic osteoarthropathy, which commonly is associated with thoracic neoplasm, is characterized by bony proliferation and soft tissue swelling of the hands and tufts, but the distribution of osseous abnormality differs from that of thyroid acropachy. In hypertrophic osteoarthropathy, periosteal bone formation is observed most commonly in the tibia, fibula, radius, and ulna. Changes limited to the hands and feet are unusual in this condition. Furthermore, the feathery pattern of bony proliferation that is seen in thyroid acropachy is not typical of hypertrophic osteoarthropathy.

Pachydermoperiostosis is associated with typical facies, soft tissue prominence of the hands, and periostitis.[75, 76] Periosteal bone formation generally is apparent in a symmetric pattern in the tibia, fibula, radius, and ulna, although the hands also may be affected. Periostitis in this disorder is not limited to the diaphysis but may be exuberant at the metaphyseal and epiphyseal areas.

Hypervitaminosis A and venous stasis may produce periosteal bone proliferation, but clinical and radiographic features allow accurate diagnosis of these conditions. Fluorosis is associated with more extensive abnormality of the axial skeleton and long bones. Leukemic acropachy is particularly prominent in the terminal phalanges.[77] Periosteal bone formation in acromegaly and vasculitides such as periarteritis nodosa is readily distinguished from changes of thyroid acropachy. Infectious and traumatic disorders reveal alterations in addition to periostitis.

HYPOTHYROIDISM

General Characteristics

Hypothyroidism and myxedema are terms describing a clinical state of thyroxine and triiodothyronine deficiency. The deficiency may be divided into a primary form, in which the thyroid gland itself is involved, and a secondary form, characterized by a deficiency in thyroid stimulating hormone. Hypothyroidism may have many causes, including atrophy; thyroid gland destruction after radioactive iodine therapy or surgery; thyroiditis, which may be acute or chronic (Hashimoto's disease); infiltrative disorders such as lymphoma, cystinosis, amyloidosis, and metastasis; deficiency in iodine or iodine metabolism; use of certain medications; and a variety of pituitary disorders.

In infants, thyroid deficiency results in cretinism, and in children it produces juvenile myxedema, with mental retardation and developmental abnormalities. Symptoms and signs include lethargy, constipation, enlarged tongue, abdominal distention, hypotonia, dry hair and skin, and delayed dentition. In adults, the disease is more frequent in women than in men and can be associated with dry, coarse skin and hair, fatigue, lethargy, edema, hoarseness, consti-

TABLE 56–4. Conditions Associated with Periostitis of Multiple Bones

Hypertrophic osteoarthropathy	Fluorosis
Pachydermoperiostosis	Leukemia
Thyroid acropachy	Vascular insufficiency
Hypervitaminosis A	Infection
Venous stasis	Trauma

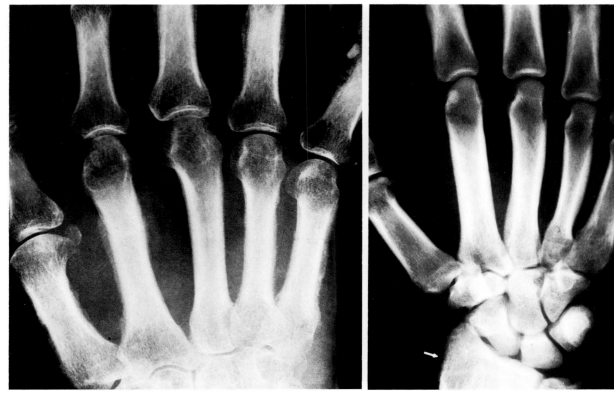

FIGURE 56–7. Differential diagnosis of periosteal new bone formation in the hand.
A Hypertrophic osteoarthropathy. In this condition, typical findings are linear or irregular bone proliferation on the distal diaphyseal and metaphyseal portions of the metacarpals and phalanges.
B Pachydermoperiostosis. Note thickening and sclerosis of the metacarpal bones and phalanges and irregular new bone formation of the metaphysis and epiphysis of the radius (arrow).

pation, paresthesias, and bradycardia as well as other symptoms and signs (Tables 56–5 and 56–6).

In adult-onset hypothyroidism, bone abnormalities are mild. Altered kinetics in bone indicate a consistent reduc-

tion in the exchangeable pool of calcium and its rate of turnover and a decrease in the rates of bone formation and resorption.[8, 78] These changes may result in a decreased excretion of calcium and phosphorus in urine and stool and a decrease in calcium deposition within osseous tissue.[1, 79] Occasionally, the bone may appear more compact, with increased radiodensity.[31] The serum calcium and phosphorus levels generally are normal, although calcium infusion may induce an exaggerated response with elevation of calcium levels.[1, 80] Articular and muscular alterations also may be seen in adult patients with hypothyroidism.

In cretinism and juvenile myxedema, skeletal manifesta-

TABLE 56–5. Symptoms and Signs of Hypothyroidism*

	Percentage of Cases
Dry coarse skin and hair	70–97
Fatigue, lethargy, mental or physical slowness	70–91
Edema, puffy hand, face, or eyes	67–95
Pallor	50–59
Cold intolerance	58–95
Decreased sweating	68–89
Hoarseness	48–74
Constipation	36–61
Weight gain	48–76
Loss or thinning of hair	32–57
Paresthesias	56
Enlarged tongue	19
Bradycardia	14
Menstrual disturbance	16–30
Decreased hearing	6

*From Robbins J, et al: The thyroid and iodine metabolism. *In* PK Bondy, LE Rosenberg (Eds): Metabolic Control and Disease. 8th Ed. WB Saunders Co, Philadelphia, 1980, p 1390.

TABLE 56–6. Reported Musculoskeletal Abnormalities of Hypothyroidism

Retarded skeletal maturation
Accessory sutural bones
Epiphyseal dysgenesis
Epiphyseal deformity with secondary degenerative joint disease
Gibbus deformity
Dystrophic calcification
Carpal tunnel syndrome
Synovial effusion; tenosynovitis
Myopathy
Neuropathy
Soft tissue edema
Osteoporosis
Slipped capital femoral epiphysis
Ligamentous laxity
CPPD crystal deposition
Erosive arthritis

tions are more marked. Delayed bony maturation is most characteristic,[81] and in the infant, absence of the distal femoral and proximal tibial epiphyses is an important radiographic clue. In older children, abnormal epiphyseal maturation leads to distinctive radiographic findings, with fragmented irregular epiphyseal contours, termed epiphyseal dysgenesis. Delayed dental development is a concomitant feature of the disease. Retardation in growth in these persons may simulate that associated with growth hormone deficiency.

Altered Development of Bone

A fundamental radiographic feature of hypothyroidism of infants, children, and young adults is retardation of skeletal maturation (Fig. 56–8). Although this finding may be seen in other disorders, skeletal retardation usually is more severe in hypothyroidism than in these other conditions, and the diagnosis of hypothyroidism is suspect if a child has normal maturation.[41] Even in patients with precocious puberty, skeletal development, as determined by bone age, remains retarded.[82, 83] The radiographic confirmation of delayed skeletal maturation relies on a delay in appearance and growth of epiphyseal ossification centers and is most facilitated in the infant by examination of the knees (or

feet). Evaluation of the bones of the hand is less helpful, as in normal situations the carpal bones are not ossified at birth. This abnormality of epiphyseal development is accompanied by alterations in development of synchondroses (e.g., between segments of sternum and sacrum) and sutures; physeal growth plates and sutures may persist well beyond the age at which they normally should have disappeared.[84, 85]

On histologic examination, the persisting physeal growth plate reveals little evidence of cartilage cellular proliferation.[31] The plate is "closed off" by osseous tissue of the metaphysis, which is apposed to the cartilage growth zone. This mechanical impediment accounts for the fact that despite persistence of the physeal growth plate, longitudinal growth of the skeleton is diminished.

In the skull, growth retardation is particularly striking at the base of the cranium. Decreased growth of the sphenooccipital synchondrosis produces brachycephaly. Enlargement of the sella turcica is observed,[86–92] which has been related, in part, to rebound hypertrophy of the pituitary gland and which may be reversible with adequate early treatment of the hypothyroid state (Fig. 56–9). Additional cranial findings in hypothyroidism include prominent sutures with accessory (wormian) bones (which also can be seen in osteogenesis imperfecta, cleidocranial dysostosis,

FIGURE 56–8. Hypothyroidism: Delayed ossification of epiphyses.

A In a 3 year old child with hypothyroidism, the capital femoral epiphysis has not yet ossified.

B On a photomicrograph (35×) of a growth zone that has not developed normally in a child with hypothyroidism, the cartilage of the growth plate has lined up in columns, but cores of calcified cartilage matrix are not extending into the shaft, as would be expected at a site of active endochondral bone formation. On the shaft side of the growth plate, osseous tissue is apposed to cartilage (arrow), impeding proper osseous development.

(**B,** From Jaffe HL: Metabolic, Degenerative and Inflammatory Diseases of Bones and Joints. Philadelphia, Lea & Febiger, 1972.)

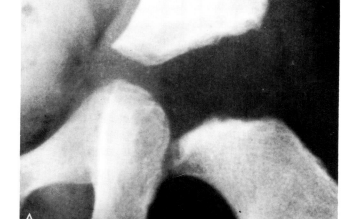

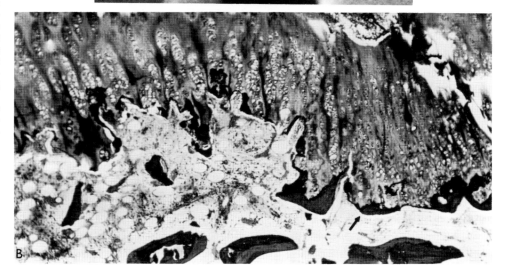

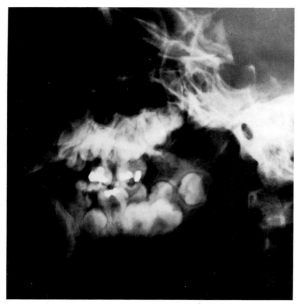

FIGURE 56–9. Hypothyroidism: Cranial and facial abnormalities. In a 21 year old man with cretinism, findings include an enlarged sella turcica, prominent lower jaw, and delayed dental development. (Courtesy of S. Hilton, M.D., San Diego, California.)

and other conditions), underdevelopment of the paranasal sinuses and mastoid air cells, and a prognathous lower jaw (Fig. 56–10).

In addition to delay in the appearance of epiphyseal centers, the pattern of ossification within these centers may be altered in hypothyroidism. In affected epiphyses, ossification proceeds from multiple centers rather than from a single site, and the resulting irregular appearance is termed epiphyseal dysgenesis[93–97] (Fig. 56–11). Epiphyseal dysgenesis is particularly frequent in the femoral and humeral heads and tarsal navicular bone, although it may be observed in almost any other epiphysis as well. The fragmented epiphysis can simulate the appearance of other dis-

eases, particularly osteonecrosis. With involvement of the femoral head, this leads to a mistaken diagnosis of Legg-Calvé-Perthes disease. It is important to realize that although osteonecrosis and osteochondritis dissecans rarely have been described in patients with hypothyroidism,[93, 98] epiphyseal dysgenesis is not due to vascular insufficiency. It relates to an aberration of the ossification pattern in the involved epiphysis,[31, 99] in which islands of endochondral ossification are observed. When the patient is treated, coalescence of the fragments may lead to disappearance of epiphyseal dysgenesis within a year or two. With delayed or inadequate therapy, epiphyseal abnormalities may result in secondary articular degeneration, intra-articular osseous and cartilaginous bodies, and angular deformities. In the hip, coxa plana, coxa magna, and coxa vara have been described.

Epiphyseal dysgenesis is an important radiographic sign of hypothyroidism but must be differentiated from other conditions, including osteonecrosis and epiphyseal dysplasias, as well as from the irregularity of the growing epiphysis that may be encountered in normal children (Fig. 56–12).

Increased radiopacity of epiphyses as well as metaphyses also has been noted in patients with hypothyroidism (Fig. 56–13).[41] Unfused apophyses may be seen.[96] An additional helpful diagnostic sign of hypothyroidism is the rapid improvement in ossification that results during therapy, although delayed growth spurts may lead to mechanical deformity, including epiphyseal slipping, especially of the femoral head (see later discussion).

Abnormality of the vertebral column also is common in hypothyroidism.[93, 96, 100, 101] Spinal findings are particularly prominent at the thoracolumbar junction, at which site short and bullet-shaped twelfth thoracic and first lumbar vertebral bodies may be visualized (Fig. 56–14). A gibbus deformity may result, although this deformity may improve with thyroid treatment.[101] Although more widespread spinal changes may be apparent, including osteoporosis and delayed development and fusion of the apophyses, with irregularity of vertebral body contour, the findings at the thoracolumbar

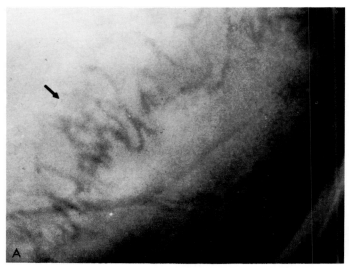
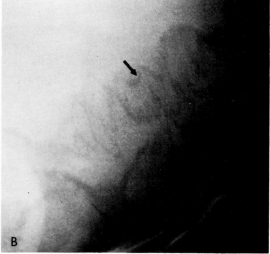

FIGURE 56–10. Hypothyroidism: Prominent sutures with accessory (wormian) bones. Examples of intrasutural bones (arrows), which are characteristic of hypothyroidism.

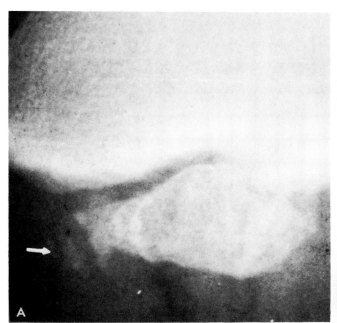

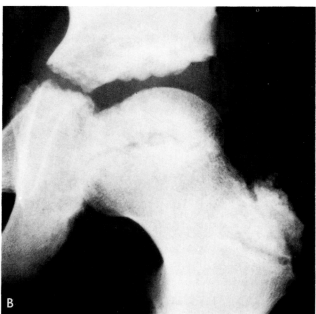

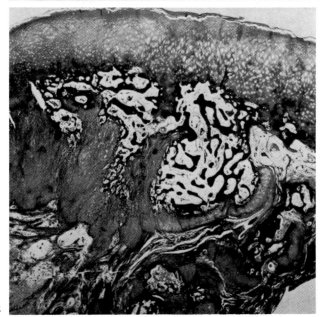

FIGURE 56–11. Hypothyroidism: Epiphyseal dysgenesis.

A Note fragmentation of the distal femoral epiphysis (arrow).

B Irregularity of the apophysis of the greater trochanter and acetabular margin is associated with flattening and deformity of the proximal capital femoral epiphysis.

C A photomicrograph (8×) of part of a femoral head in a 39 year old patient with hypothyroidism reveals irregular islands of endochondral ossification surrounded by degenerative cartilage in the interior of the head below the articular cartilage.

(**C,** From Jaffe HL: Metabolic, Degenerative and Inflammatory Diseases of Bones and Joints. Philadelphia, Lea & Febiger, 1972.)

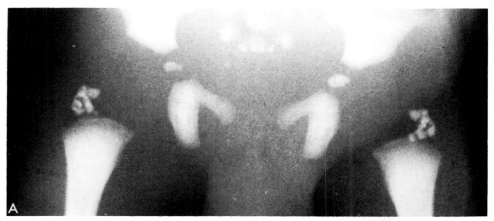

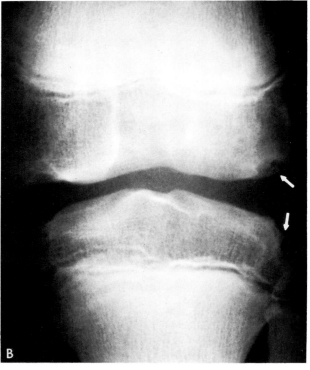

FIGURE 56–12. Differential diagnosis of "fragmented" epiphyses.
  A Chondrodysplasia punctata. Irregular calcification of the epiphyses can be seen.
  B Normal development. Small, separate islands of ossification can appear in the normal developing epiphysis (arrows).

FIGURE 56–13. Hypothyroidism: Metaphyseal abnormalities. Same patient as in Figure 56–9. Findings include delayed skeletal maturation, linear sclerosis in the metaphyses of the proximal femora, and irregularity in ossification of apophyses. (Courtesy of S. Hilton, M.D., San Diego, California.)

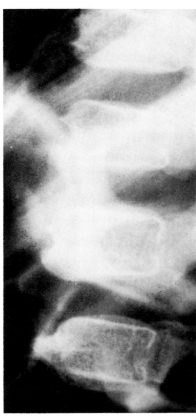

FIGURE 56–14. Hypothyroidism: Spinal abnormalities. Note bullet-shaped vertebrae and beaklike anterior surfaces of the vertebral bodies.

area are most characteristic. Predilection for this segment may be due to inordinate stress at the thoracolumbar level and a relative insensitivity to pain.[102] Additional vertebral alterations that have been noted in hypothyroidism are relatively widened intervertebral disc spaces and increased distance between the anterior arch of the atlas and the odontoid process of the axis.[102] Thoracic cage deformities may be apparent.[103] Also, a distinctive osseous projection in the mid-portion of the metaphyses of the distal phalanges has been described.[104]

Abnormal Calcification

In hypothyroidism, abnormal calcium metabolism and excretion are present.[79, 80, 105] Retention of calcium with increased bone sclerosis may be seen in association with soft tissue calcific deposits.[106] Increased bony eburnation in the periorbital region is termed the ''lunette'' sign.[96] Hypersensitivity to vitamin D[107] secondary to delayed breakdown of steroids may lead to increased absorption of calcium from the intestinal tract, hypercalcemia, nephrocalcinosis, and dystrophic calcification in various organs and soft tissues.[96, 108, 109] Parotid calcification and premature atherosclerosis are two examples of abnormal calcific deposition in hypothyroidism.

Additional Rheumatologic Manifestations

Rheumatic syndromes may be observed in patients with hypothyroidism. An entrapment neuropathy, including the carpal tunnel syndrome caused by median nerve compression at the wrist (or, rarely, median plantar nerve compression in the foot), is seen in approximately 7 per cent of patients with hypothyroidism.[50, 110–113] The carpal tunnel syndrome, which is produced by nerve impingement by the myxedematous tissue and accompanying tenosynovitis, may be persistent, showing little response to hydrocortisone injections, although it can improve rapidly after thyroid replacement.[114] Descriptions have appeared of accompanying noninflammatory synovial thickening and effusion, especially in the metacarpophalangeal and metatarsophalangeal joints, wrists, and knees.[113] Analysis of synovial fluid in these patients reveals low total cell counts, normal protein concentrations, and high viscosity. Hyperuricemia and elevation of erythrocyte sedimentation rate can be detected.[7, 115] A symmetric peripheral sensory neuropathy rarely has been described.[116]

Muscular cramps and stiffness are common in hypothyroidism, with predilection for the calves, thighs, and shoulders. Symptoms and signs, which include pain and tenderness that increase after exercise, are similar to those accompanying polymyalgia rheumatica[109, 112, 117] or, more rarely, dermatomyositis[118] and fibrositis.[119] Prominent soft tissues are due to myxomatous infiltration of soft tissues, and tendon reflexes characteristically are slow, with delayed relaxation.[120] Hypothyroid myopathy, with proximal muscular pain, weakness, and hypotonia, may be associated with abnormal serum levels of muscle enzymes and histologic changes in muscle, including focal necrosis and regeneration, variable muscle fiber size, and mucinous deposits.[121-123] A rare pattern of muscle involvement in hypothyroidism, termed Hoffman's or Kocher-Debré-Sémélaigne syndrome, is characterized by a massive increase in muscle mass, decrease in muscle strength, slowness in muscular activity, and low serum levels of thyroxine.[124]

Articular findings are less prominent than those related to neuropathy and myopathy. Abnormalities due to abnormal epiphyseal development already have been noted. Thickening of periarticular soft tissues and effusions are encountered rarely,[113] although tenosynovitis may be observed in the hands, wrists, and feet.[125] Furthermore, synovial cyst formation and calcium pyrophosphate dihydrate (CPPD) crystal deposition in association with hypothyroidism (a questionable association[126]) may produce characteristic radiographic and arthrographic findings.[125] Joint space narrowing, ligament laxity, and intra-articular osseous bodies can be visualized. In these instances, needle biopsy of synovium reveals only mild inflammation with cellular infiltration. In general, these articular manifestations decrease with proper therapy.[110]

Juxta-articular osteoporosis has been noted in patients with hypothyroidism.[110, 125] Collapse of osseous surfaces, similar to that observed in osteonecrosis and hyperparathyroidism, may be secondary to weakening of subchondral bone. These findings have been described in the tibial plateau[127] with intra-articular cartilaginous and osseous debris.[110] Osteolytic lesions of the epiphyses have been noted.[128]

The occurrence of a destructive arthropathy involving the hands or feet, or both, in middle-aged and elderly women with primary hypothyroidism has been noted.[127, 129] This arthropathy may appear in the absence of myopathy, neuropathy, and CPPD crystal deposition.[129] Bilateral involve-

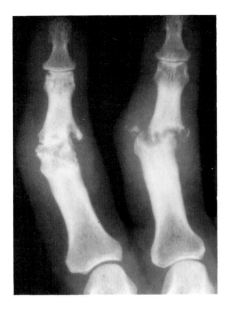

FIGURE 56–15. Hypothyroidism: Articular destruction. This 60 year old woman developed painful deformity of her fingers with swelling of the proximal interphalangeal joints. Other clinical and laboratory manifestations confirmed the diagnosis of primary hypothyroidism occurring as a consequence of previous autoimmune thyroiditis. The radiograph of the second and third digits reveals findings similar to those of inflammatory (erosive) osteoarthritis with soft tissue swelling, osteophytosis, bone erosions, and subluxation of the proximal interphalangeal joints. Other digits on both hands were affected similarly. (Courtesy of J. C. Gerstner, M.D., Lausanne, Switzerland.)

FIGURE 56–16. Hypothyroidism: Slipped capital femoral epiphyses. In a 13 year old girl, bilateral hip pain developed over a 1 year period. A frontal radiograph of the pelvis **(A)** and frog-leg views of both hips **(B, C)** show bilateral slipped capital femoral epiphyses. Evaluation revealed decreased bone age and, subsequently, the diagnosis of hypothyroidism was verified. (Courtesy of G. Greenway, M.D., Dallas, Texas.)

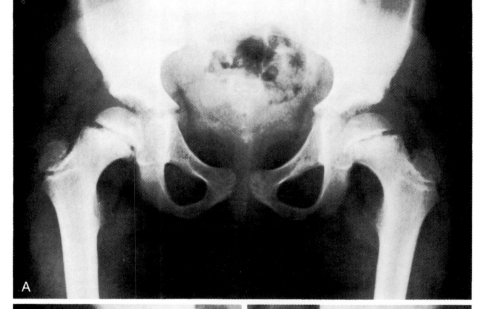
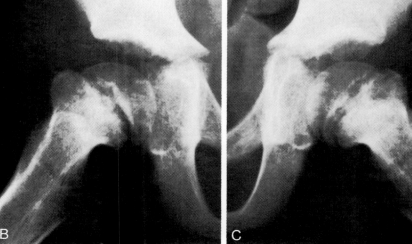

ment of the hands, with predilection for the proximal inter-phalangeal joints, appears typical. Resulting radiographic abnormalities appear identical to those of severe inflammatory (erosive) osteoarthritis (Fig. 56–15). Histologic findings include fibrinous synovial hyperplasia, fibroblastic pannus, and shards of articular cartilage in the synovial membrane.

Finally, it should be emphasized that various connective tissue diseases have been described in patients with Hashimoto's thyroiditis, including rheumatoid arthritis, seronegative polyarthritis, systemic lupus erythematosus, Sjögren's syndrome, and scleroderma.[2, 3, 130] This may relate to an autoimmune reaction, which is common to both Hashimoto's disease and collagen vascular disorders.

Slipped Capital Femoral Epiphysis

Slipped capital femoral epiphyses may occur in patients with hypothyroidism who may or may not have been started on treatment.[131–135] Although usually seen in prepubescent subjects, the complication occasionally is apparent in the more sexually mature man or woman.[136] A bilateral or unilateral distribution is evident.[137] Typical radiographic features are encountered. The cause of this complication in treated or untreated hypothyroidism is not known. Hypotheses include abnormalities in the chondrocytes and extracellular matrix owing to the hypothyroid state, changes related to the introduction of thyroid hormone during treatment, and a relative surge of growth hormone secretion related to regranulation of the pituitary acidophilic cells during therapy for hypothyroidism.[131, 138–140] Whatever the cause, slipped capital femoral epiphyses are an important manifestation of hypothyroidism and, in fact, may be the presenting feature of the disease[137] (Fig. 56–16).

SUMMARY

Distinctive osseous, articular, and soft tissue alterations may accompany hyperthyroid and hypothyroid states. These alterations underscore the importance of thyroid hormone in regulating normal growth, development, and maturation of tissue. Radiographs may provide an important clue to the proper diagnosis when clinical findings are not specific and may serve as a useful parameter for assessing the adequacy of therapy.

References

1. Robbins J, Rall JE, Gorden P: The thyroid and iodine metabolism. *In* PK Bondy, LE Rosenberg (Eds): Metabolic Control and Disease. 8th Ed. Philadelphia, WB Saunders Co, 1980, p 1375.
2. Becker KL, Ferguson RH, McConahey WM: The connective tissue diseases and symptoms associated with Hashimoto's thyroiditis. N Engl J Med 268:277, 1963.
3. Mulhern LM, Masi AT, Shulman LE: Hashimoto's disease. A search for associated disorders in 170 clinically detected cases. Lancet 2:508, 1966.
4. Gardner D: Pathology of the rheumatic diseases. *In* WSC Copeman (Ed): Textbook of Rheumatic Diseases. 4th Ed. Edinburgh, E&S Livingstone, 1969.
5. Amrhein JA, Kenny RM, Ross D: Granulocytopenia, lupus-like syndrome and other complications of propylthiouracil therapy. J Pediatr 76:54, 1970.
6. Librik L, Sussman L, Bejar R, et al: Thyrotoxicosis and collagen-like diseases in three sisters of American Indian extraction. J Pediatr 76:64, 1970.
7. Leeper RD, Benua RA, Brener JL, et al: Hyperuricemia in myxedema. J Clin Endocrinol Metab 20:1457, 1960.
8. Ingbar SH, Woeber KA: The thyroid gland. *In* RH Williams (Ed): Textbook of Endocrinology. 6th Ed. Philadelphia, WB Saunders Co, 1981, p 117.
9. Fallon MD, Perry HM III, Bergfeld M, et al: Exogenous hyperthyroidism with osteoporosis. Arch Intern Med 143:442, 1983.
10. Baxter JD, Bondy PK: Hypercalcemia of thyrotoxicosis. Ann Intern Med 65:429, 1966.
11. Parfitt AM, Dent CE: Hyperthyroidism and hypercalcaemia. Q J Med 39:171, 1970.
12. Epstein RH: Bone and mineral metabolism in hyperthyroidism. Ann Intern Med 68:490, 1968.
13. Man EB, Gildea EF, Peters JP: Serum lipoids and proteins in hyperthyroidism. J. Clin Invest 19:43, 1940.
14. Richards AJ: Hypercalcaemia in thyrotoxicosis with and without hyperparathyroidism. Postgrad Med J 46:440, 1970.
15. Auwerx J, Bouillon R: Mineral and bone metabolism in thyroid disease: A review. Q J Med 60:737, 1986.
16. Bianchi GS, Meunier P, Courpron P, et al: Le retentissement osseux des hyperthyroïdies. Rev Rhum Mal Osteoartic 39:19, 1972.
17. Williams RH, Morgan HJ: Thyrotoxic osteoporosis. Int Clinic 2:48, 1940.
18. Meunier PJ, S-Bianchi GG, Edouard CM, et al: Bony manifestations of thyrotoxicosis. Orthop Clin North Am 3:745, 1972.
19. Beaumont GE, Dodds EC, Robertson JD: Calcium and phosphorus metabolism in thyrotoxicosis. J Endocrinol 2:237, 1940.
20. Golden R, Abbott H: The relation of the thyroid, the adrenals and the islands of Langerhans to malacic diseases of bone. AJR 30:641, 1933.
21. Nielsen H: The bone system in hyperthyroidism. A clinical and experimental study. Acta Med Scand (Suppl)266:783, 1952.
22. Ryckewaert A, Bordier P, Miravet L, et al: L'osteose thyroïdienne. Sem Hôp Paris 44:222, 1968.
23. Fraser SA, Smith DA, Anderson JB, et al: Osteoporosis and fractures following thyrotoxicosis. Lancet 1:981, 1971.
24. Chevrot A, Pallardy G, Ledoux-Lebard G: Manifestations squelettiques de l'hyperthyroïdie. J Radiol Electrol Med Nucl 59:167, 1978.
25. Leroux JL, Mery C, Amor B, et al: Osteite fibrokystique hyperthyroïdienne. Rev Rhum Mal Osteoartic 48:257, 1981.
26. Doyle FH: Radiologic assessment of endocrine effects on bone. Radiol Clin North Am 5:289, 1967.
27. Chmell S: Pathological fracture in hyperthyroidism. Orthopedics 4:1019, 1981.
28. Meema HE, Schatz DL: Simple radiologic demonstration of cortical bone loss in thyrotoxicosis. Radiology 97:9, 1970.
29. Fraser S, Smith DA, Wilson GM: Effet des troubles thyroïdiens sur le metabolisme et la densité osseuse actualités endocrinologiques 11° serie. Paris, Expansion Scientifique Française, 1967, p 3.
30. Legrand R, Linquette M, Gerard A, et al: Osteose hyperthyroïdienne et syndrome de Looser-Milkman. Guerison après iode 131. Lille Med 4:236, 1959.
31. Jaffe HL: Metabolic, Degenerative and Inflammatory Diseases of Bones and Joints. Philadelphia, Lea & Febiger, 1972, p 346.
32. Follis RH Jr: Skeletal changes associated with hyperthyroidism. Bull Johns Hopkins Hosp 92:405, 1953.
33. von Recklinghausen FC: Die fibrose oder deformierende Ostitis, die Osteomalacie und die osteoplastische Karzinose in ihren gegenseitigen Beziehungen. *In* Festschrift fur Rudolf Virchow, Berlin, G Reimer, 1891, p 1.
34. Bianchi GS, Meunier P, Courpron P, et al: Le retentissement osseux des hyperthyroïdies. Rev Rhum Mal Osteoartic 7:19, 1972.
35. Bordier P, Miravet L, Matrajt H, et al: Bone changes in adult patients with abnormal thyroid function (with special reference to 45-Ca kinetics and quantitative histology). Proc R Soc Med 60:1132, 1967.
36. Melsen F, Mosekilde L: Dynamic studies of trabecular bone formation and osteoid maturation in normal and certain pathological conditions. Metab Bone Dis Rel Res 1:45, 1978.
37. Toh SH, Claunch BC, Brown PH: Effect of hyperthyroidism and its treatment on bone mineral content. Arch Intern Med 145:883, 1985.
38. Creyx M, Levy J, Daurios J: Deux cas d'osteose thyroïdienne. Sem Hôp Paris 24:2819, 1948.
39. Senaj MO Jr, Lee FA, Gilsanz V: Early costochondral calcification in adolescent hyperthyroidism. Radiology 156:375, 1985.
40. Lentino W, Poppel MH: The roentgen manifestations of Plummer's nails (onycholysis) in hyperthyroidism. AJR 84:941, 1960.
41. Poznanski AK: The Hand in Radiologic Diagnosis. Philadelphia, WB Saunders Co, 1974, p 502.
42. Riggs W Jr, Wilroy RS Jr, Etteldorf JN: Neonatal hyperthyroidism with accelerated skeletal maturation, craniosynostosis, and brachydactyly. Radiology 105:621, 1972.
43. Bonakdarpour A, Kirkpatric JA, Renzi A, et al: Skeletal changes in neonatal thyrotoxicosis. Radiology 102:149, 1972.
44. Robinson DC, Hall R, Munro DS: Graves' disease, an unusual complication: Raised intracranial pressure due to premature fusion of skull sutures. Arch Dis Child 44:252, 1969.
45. Schlesinger B, Fisher OD: Accelerated skeletal development from thyrotoxicosis and thyroid overdosage in childhood. Lancet 2:289, 1951.
46. Johnsonbaugh RE, Bryan RN, Hierlwimmer UR, et al: Premature craniosynostosis: A common complication of juvenile thyrotoxicosis. J Pediatr 93:188, 1978.
47. Segal AM, Sheeler LR, Wilke WS: Myalgia as the primary manifestation of spontaneously resolving hyperthyroidism. J Rheumatol 9:459, 1982.
48. Wohlgethan JR: Frozen shoulder in hyperthyroidism. Arthritis Rheum 30:936, 1987.
49. Ramsay ID: Muscle dysfunction in hyperthyroidism. Lancet 2:931, 1966.
50. Swanson JW, Kelly JJ Jr, McConahey WM: Neurological aspects of thyroid dysfunction. Mayo Clin Proc 56:504, 1981.

51. Beard L, Kumar A, Estep HL: Bilateral carpal tunnel syndrome caused by Graves' disease. Arch Intern Med 145:345, 1985.

52. Shoaleh-var M, Momtaz AH, Jamshidi C: Scleroderma and hyperthyroidism. Report of a case. JAMA 235:752, 1976.

53. Rampon S, Bussière JL, Prin PH, et al: Polyarthrite rhumatoïde et hyperthyroïdie. A propos de l'association rhumatoïde et adénome toxique. Rev Rhum Mal Osteoartic 40:503, 1973.

54. Gibberd FB: A survey of 406 cases of rheumatoid arthritis. Acta Rheumatol Scand 11:62, 1965.

55. Bach F: Rheumatoid arthritis following thyrotoxicosis. Proc R Soc Med 43:314, 1950.

56. Pousset G, Tourniaire J, Perrot H, et al: Hyperthyroide et lupus érythémateux aigu disséminé; à propos de deux observations. Lyon Med 226:141, 1971.

57. Lipsett MB, Odell WD, Rosenberg LE, et al: Humoral syndromes associated with nonendocrine tumors. Ann Intern Med 61:733, 1964.

58. Curry JT, Zallen RD: Ossifying fibroma of the maxilla occurring with hyperthyroidism. Oral Surg 35:28, 1973.

59. Gimlette TMD: Thyroid acropachy. Lancet 1:22, 1960.

60. Nixon DW, Samols E: Acral changes associated with thyroid diseases. JAMA 212:1175, 1970.

61. Thomas J, Collipp PJ, Sharma RK: Thyroid acropachy. Am J Dis Child 125:745, 1973.

62. Scanlon GT, Clemett AR: Thyroid acropachy. Radiology 83:1039, 1964.

63. Torres-Reyes E, Staple TW: Roentgenographic appearance of thyroid acropachy. Clin Radiol 21:95, 1970.

64. Moule B, Grant MC, Boyle IT, et al: Thyroid acropachy. Clin Radiol 21:329, 1970.

65. Verney GI: Thyroid acropachy. Br J Radiol 35:644, 1962.

66. Kinsella RA Jr, Back DK: Thyroid acropachy. Med Clin North Am 52:393, 1968.

67. Wietersen FK, Balow RM: The radiologic aspects of thyroid disease. Radiol Clin North Am 5:255, 1967.

68. McCarty J, Twersky J, Lion M: Thyroid acropachy. J Can Assoc Radiol 26:199, 1975.

69. Seigel RS, Thrall JH, Sisson JC: 99mTc-pyrophosphate scan and radiographic correlation in thyroid acropachy: Case report. J Nucl Med 17:791, 1976.

70. Bieler E, Albrecht HJ: Das szintigraphische Bild der Osteoarthropathie hypertrophiante. Nucl Med (Stuttg) 10:196, 1971.

71. King LR, Braunstein H, Chambers D, et al: A case study of peculiar soft tissue and bony changes in association with thyroid disease. J Clin Endocrinol Metab 19:1323, 1959.

72. Thomas HM: Secondary sub-periosteal new bone formation. Arch Intern Med 51:571, 1933.

73. Greene R: Thyroid acropachy. Proc R Soc Med 44:159, 1951.

74. Lynch PJ, Maize JC, Sisson JC: Pretibial myxedema and nonthyrotoxic thyroid disease. Arch Dermatol 107:107, 1973.

75. Shawarby K, Ibrahim MS: Pachydermoperiostosis. Br Med J 1:763, 1962.

76. Lazarus JH, Galloway JK: Pachydermoperiostosis. AJR 118:308, 1973.

77. Glatt W, Weinstein A: Acropachy in lymphatic leukemia. Radiology 92:125, 1969.

78. Enksen EF, Mosekilde L, Melsen F: Kinetics of trabecular bone resorption and formation in hypothyroidism: Evidence for a positive balance per remodeling cycle. Bone 7:101, 1986.

79. Krane SM, Brownell GL, Stanbury JB, et al: The effect of thyroid disease on calcium metabolism in man. J Clin Invest 35:874, 1956.

80. Lowe CE, Bird ED, Thomas WC: Hypercalcemia in myxedema. J Clin Endocrinol 22:261, 1962.

81. Hernandez RJ, Poznanski AW, Hopwood NJ: Size and skeletal maturation of the hand in children with hypothyroidism and hypopituitarism. AJR 133:405, 1979.

82. Van Wyk JJ, Grumbach MM: Syndrome of precocious menstruation and galactorrhea in juvenile hypothyroidism: An example of hormonal overlap in pituitary feedback. J Pediatr 57:416, 1960.

83. Pabst HF, Pueschel S, Hillman DA: Etiologic interrelationship in Down's syndrome, hypothyroidism and precocious sexual development. Pediatrics 40:590, 1967.

84. Langhans T: Anatomische Beitrage zur Kenntniss der Cretinen (Knochen, Geschlechtsdrüsen, Muskeln und Muskelspindeln nebst Bemerkungen über die physiologische Bedeutung der Letzteren). Arch Pathol Anat 149:155, 1897.

85. Benda CE: Mongolism and Cretinism. 2nd Ed. New York, Grune & Stratton, 1949.

86. Bower BF: Pituitary enlargement secondary to untreated primary hypogonadism. Ann Intern Med 69:107, 1968.

87. Boyce R, Beadles CF: Enlargement of the hypophysis cerebri in myxoedema: With remarks upon hypertrophy of the hypophysis associated with changes in the thyroid body. J Pathol Bacteriol 1:223, 1892.

88. Barnes ND, Hayles AB, Ryan RJ: Sexual maturation in juvenile hypothyroidism. Mayo Clin Proc 48:849, 1973.

89. Comas AP: Hypothyroidism and precocious sexual development: Another case. Pediatrics 52:149, 1973.

90. Lawrence AM, Wilber JF, Hagen TC: The pituitary and primary hypothyroidism. Enlargement and unusual growth hormone secretory responses. Arch Intern Med 132:327, 1973.

91. McCarten KM, Kuhns LR: The area and volume of the sella turcica in childhood primary hypothyroidism. Radiology 119:645, 1976.

92. Swischuk LE, Sarwar M: The sella in childhood hypothyroidism. Pediatr Radiol 6:1, 1977.

93. Wilkins L: Epiphysial dysgenesis associated with hypothyroidism. Am J Dis Child 61:13, 1941.

94. Reilly WA, Smyth FS: Cretinoid epiphyseal dysgenesis. J Pediatr 11:786, 1937.

95. Albright F: Changes simulating Legg-Perthes disease (osteochondritis deformans juvenilis) due to juvenile myxoedema. J Bone Joint Surg 20:764, 1938.

96. Borg SA, Fitzer PM, Young LW: Roentgenologic aspects of adult cretinism. Two case reports and review of the literature. AJR 123:820, 1975.

97. Parker BR: Hypothyroidism with epiphyseal dysgenesis. Pediatric case of the day. AJR 136:1030, 1981.

98. Rubinstein HM, Brooks MH: Aseptic necrosis of bone in myxedema. Ann Intern Med 87:580, 1977.

99. Looser E: Über die Ossifikationsstorungen die Kretinismus. Verh Dtsch Ges Pathol 24:352, 1929.

100. Andersen HJ: Changes of the spine in children with myxoedema. Acta Paediatr 44(Suppl 103):102, 1955.

101. Evans PR: Deformity of vertebral bodies in cretinism. J Pediatr 41:706, 1952.

102. Moosa A, Dubowitz V: Slow nerve conduction velocity in cretins. Arch Dis Child 46:852, 1971.

103. Lintermans JP, Seyhnaeve V: Hypothyroidism and vertebral anomalies. A new syndrome? Am J Roentgenol 109:294, 1970.

104. Hernandez RJ, Poznanski AK: Distinctive appearance of the distal phalanges in children with primary hypothyroidism. Radiology 132:83, 1979.

105. Aub JC, Bauer W, Heath C, et al: Studies of calcium and phosphorus metabolism. III. The effects of the thyroid hormone and thyroid disease. J Clin Invest 7:97, 1929.

106. Bateson EM, Chandler S: Nephrocalcinosis in cretinism. Br J Radiol 38:581, 1965.

107. Fanconi G, de Chastonay E: Die D-Hypervitaminose im Säuglingsalter. Helv Paediatr Acta 5:5, 1950.

108. Tumay SB, Bilger M, Hatemi N: Skeletal changes and nephrocalcinosis in a case of athyreosis. Arch Dis Child 37:543, 1962.

109. Burke JW, Williamson BRJ, Hurst RW: "Idiopathic" cerebellar calcification: Association with hypothyroidism? Radiology 167:533, 1988.

110. Bland JH, Frymoyer JW: Rheumatic syndromes of myxedema. N Engl J Med 282:1171, 1970.

111. Golding DN: The musculoskeletal features of hypothyroidism. Postgrad Med J 47:611, 1971.

112. Golding DN: Hypothyroidism presenting with musculoskeletal symptoms. Ann Rheum Dis 29:10, 1970.

113. Frymoyer JW, Bland J: Carpal tunnel syndrome in patients with myxedematous arthropathy. J Bone Joint Surg [Am] 55:78, 1973.

114. Fincham RW, Cape CA: Neuropathy in myxedema. A study of sensory nerve conduction in the upper extremities. Arch Neurol 19:464, 1968.

115. Lillington GA, Gastineau CF, Underdahl LO: Clinics on endocrine and metabolic diseases. I. The sedimentation rate in primary myxedema. Proc Mayo Clin 34:605, 1959.

116. Nickel SN, Frame B, Bebin J, et al: Myxedema neuropathy and myopathy. A clinical and pathological study. Neurology 11:125, 1961.

117. Wilson J, Walton JN: Some muscular manifestations of hypothyroidism. J Neurol Neurosurg Psychiatry 22:320, 1959.

118. Newman AJ, Lee C: Hypothyroidism simulating dermatomyositis. J Pediatr 97:772, 1980.

119. Wilke WS, Sheeler LR, Makarowski WS: Hypothyroidism with presenting symptoms of fibrositis. J Rheumatol 8:626, 1981.

120. Spiro AJ, Hirano A, Beilin RL, et al: Cretinism with muscular hypertrophy (Kocher-Debré-Sémélaigne syndrome). Arch Neurol 23:340, 1970.

121. Layey F: Quadriceps test for the myasthenia of thyroidism. JAMA 87:754, 1926.

122. Salick AI, Colachis SC, Pearson CM: Myxedema myopathy: Clinical, electrodiagnostic and pathologic findings in an advanced case. Arch Phys Med Rehabil 49:230, 1968.

123. Fessel WJ: Myopathy of hypothyroidism. Ann Rheum Dis 27:590, 1968.

124. Klein I, Parker M, Shebert R, et al: Hypothyroidism presenting as muscle stiffness and pseudohypertrophy: Hoffman's syndrome. Am J Med 70:891, 1981.

125. Dorwart BB, Schumacher HR: Joint effusions, chondrocalcinosis and other rheumatic manifestations in hypothyroidism. A clinicopathologic study. Am J Med 59:780, 1975.

126. Ellman MH: Hypothyroidism and calcium pyrophosphate dihydrate deposition disease. Ann Rheum Dis 42:112, 1982.

127. Neeck G, Riedel W, Schmidt KL: Neuropathy, myopathy and destructive arthropathy in primary hypothyroidism. J Rheumatol 17:1697, 1990.

128. Weissbein AS, Darby JP, Lawson JD: An unusual bone lesion in an adult with myxoedema. Report of a case and review of the literature. Arch Intern Med 104:643, 1959.

129. Gerster JC, Valceschini P: Destructive arthropathy of fingers in primary hypothyroidism without chondrocalcinosis. Report of 3 cases. J Rheumatol 19:637, 1992.

130. LeRiche NGH, Bell DA: Hashimoto's thyroiditis and polyarthritis: a possible subset of seronegative polyarthritis. Ann Rheum Dis 43:594, 1984.

131. Zubrow AB, Lane JM, Parks JS: Slipped capital femoral epiphysis occurring during treatment for hypothyroidism. J Bone Joint Surg [Am] 60:256, 1978.

132. Moorefield WG, Urbaniak JR, Ogden WS, et al: Acquired hypothyroidism and

slipped capital femoral epiphysis. Report of three cases. J Bone Joint Surg [Am] *58:*705, 1976.

133. Crawford AH, MacEwen GD, Fonte D: Slipped capital femoral epiphysis co-existent with hypothyroidism. Clin Orthop *122:*135, 1977.

134. Benjamin B, Miller PR: Hypothyroidism as a cause of disease of the hip. Am J Dis Child *55:*1189, 1938.

135. Epps CH Jr, Martin ED: Slipped capital femoral epiphysis in a sexually mature myxedematous female. JAMA *183:*287, 1963.

136. Hennessy MJ, Jones KL: Slipped capital femoral epiphysis in a hypothyroid adult male. Clin Orthop *165:*204, 1982.

137. Puri R, Smith CS, Malhotra D. Slipped upper femoral epiphysis and primary juvenile hypothyroidism. J Bone Joint Surg [Br] *67:*14, 1985.

138. Wilkins JN, Mayer SE, Vanderlaan WP: The effects of hypothyroidism and 2,4-dinitrophenol on growth hormone synthesis. Endocrinology *95:*1259, 1974.

139. Dearden LC: Enhanced mineralization of the tibial epiphyseal plate in the rat following propylthiouracil treatment: A histochemical, light and electron microscopic study. Anat Rec *178:*671, 1974.

140. Heyerman W, Weiner D: Slipped epiphysis associated with hypothyroidism. J Pediatr Orthop *4:*569, 1984.

57

Parathyroid Disorders and Renal Osteodystrophy

Donald Resnick, M.D., and Gen Niwayama, M.D.

Parathyroid hormone influences many tissues in the human body. It is essential for the proper transport of calcium and other ions in bone, intestine, and kidney. Parathyroid hormone has dramatic effects on osseous tissue.[1] Its initial effect is to promote release of calcium into the blood from bone whereas a second action is to stimulate extensive bone remodeling. Alterations of parathyroid function cause breakdown in calcium homeostasis, leading to characteristic pathologic and radiographic abnormalities. A voluminous amount of literature is available for the interested reader who wishes to know all the bodily changes associated with parathyroid diseases. This chapter, which discusses hyperparathyroidism, renal osteodystrophy, hypoparathyroidism, pseudohypoparathyroidism, and pseudopseudohypoparathyroidism, summarizes skeletal manifestations in these diseases.

HYPERPARATHYROIDISM

Background and General Features

Hyperparathyroidism is a general term indicating an increased level of parathyroid hormone in the blood. The condition generally is divided into three types: primary, secondary, and tertiary.

Primary hyperparathyroidism is characterized by increased parathyroid hormone secretion occurring as a result of abnormality in one or more of the parathyroid glands. Autonomous hyperfunction of these glands results from a variety of causes, including diffuse hyperplasia (10 to 40 per cent of cases), single (50 to 80 per cent) or multiple (10 per cent) adenomas, and, rarely, carcinoma.[1, 2, 264] The fundamental biochemical parameter of the disease is persistent hypercalcemia, reflecting the importance of parathyroid hormone in the control of serum calcium levels, although some patients with primary hyperparathyroidism demonstrate intermittent hypercalcemia or normal total serum calcium concentrations.[264–267]

Secondary hyperparathyroidism is associated with abnormalities in function of the parathyroid glands induced by a sustained hypocalcemic stimulus, usually resulting from chronic renal failure or, occasionally, from malabsorption states, including pancreatic insufficiency, nontropical sprue, and gluten enteropathy.[268–271] Pathologic examination generally reveals hyperplasia of all four parathyroid glands, plasma calcium levels are normal or low, and serum inorganic phosphate levels are high (chronic renal disease) or low (intestinal malabsorption).[264] Renal abnormality is associated with additional soft tissue and skeletal changes, and the entire complex is termed *renal osteodystrophy.*

Tertiary hyperparathyroidism occurs in patients with chronic renal failure or malabsorption and long-standing secondary hyperparathyroidism who develop relatively autonomous parathyroid function and hypercalcemia; although the glands normally regress after reversal of the initial abnormality, some instances of tertiary hyperparathyroidism require surgical removal of autonomously hyperfunctioning parathyroid tissue.[264]

It is the elevation of serum levels of parathyroid hormone that provides the most important clue in establishing the diagnosis of hyperparathyroidism, and, in fact, the diagnosis is tenuous in the absence of this laboratory aberration. Diagnostic difficulty arises in those few persons with normocalcemic hyperparathyroidism or as a result of the unreliability of serum calcium measurements in routine clinical laboratories and the disregard of age-dependent changes in the normal values of serum calcium.[264] Furthermore, hypercalcemia is a known complication of other disease states (Table 57–1), such as neoplasms; 10 to 20 per cent of patients with malignancy reveal elevation in serum calcium levels. The majority of these patients have direct involvement of the skeleton by a malignant lesion, although a significant number of persons with malignancies demonstrate hypercalcemia in the absence of skeletal metastasis.[272] Resection of the malignant tumor may result in a correction of the hypercalcemia, suggesting that the tumors are synthesizing and secreting a humoral substance, such as prostaglandin E, vitamin D metabolites, osteoclast-activating factor, parathyrotrophic factor, or parathyroid hormone, that is capable of influencing the serum calcium concentration.[273] The syndrome consisting of hypercalcemia of malignancy in the absence of demonstrable skeletal metastasis or primary hyperparathyroidism is termed *pseudohyperparathyroidism.*[274, 275] Histologic examination of the bone in this syndrome has revealed an increase in both osteoclastic resorption and fibrous connective tissue in the marrow; similar examination of the parathyroid glands has indicated a normal size and secondary evidence of hyperplasia.[274] Serum biochemical parameters are consistent with a status of suppressed parathyroid function and support the concept of a humoral substance, distinct from parathyroid hormone, that is elaborated by the tumors.[274]

In addition to hypercalcemia, laboratory abnormalities in

TABLE 57–1. Differential Diagnosis of Hypercalcemia

Artifactual Disorders
  Hyperproteinemia
    Venous stasis during blood collection
    Hyperalbuminemia (e.g., hyperalimentation)
    Hypergammaglobulinemia (e.g., myeloma, sarcoidosis)
Malignancy
  Solid tumors (primarily breast cancer)
  Hematologic disorders
    Myeloma
    Lymphoma
    Leukemia
Endocrinologic Disorders
  Primary hyperparathyroidism
  Multiple endocrine adenomatoses, types I and II
  Ectopic hyperparathyroidism (malignancy, predominantly lung cancer)
  Secondary hyperparathyroidism (e.g., renal failure)
  Hyperthyroidism
  Hypoadrenalism (usually following acute steroid withdrawal)
Drugs
  Vitamin A intoxication
  Vitamin D intoxication
  Thiazides
  Calcium
    Milk-alkali syndrome (ingestion of absorbable antacid calcium-containing preparations—e.g., calcium carbonate)
    Dialysis (with dialysate calcium concentration >7.0 mg/dl)
Granulomatous Disorders
  Sarcoidosis
  Tuberculosis
  Histoplasmosis
  Berylliosis
  Rheumatoid arthritis (primarily during immobilization)
Pediatric Disorders
  Infantile hypercalcemia
  Hypophosphatasia
Immobilization
  Paget's disease
  Growth
Miscellaneous Disorders
  Pheochromocytoma
  Idiopathic periostitis
  Post renal transplant surgery
  Benign familial hypercalcemia
  Diuretic phase of acute renal failure

(From Aviolo LV, Raisz LG: Bone metabolism and disease. *In* PK Bondy, LE Rosenberg [Eds]: Metabolic Control and Disease. 8th Ed. Philadelphia, WB Saunders, 1980, p 1734.)

hyperparathyroidism include hypophosphatemia, hyperphosphatasia, hypercalciuria, and, less constantly, a tendency toward hyperchloremic acidosis, hydroxyprolinuria, hyperglycemia, hyperuricemia, and hypomagnesemia.[264]

The variability of the symptoms and signs of primary hyperparathyroidism relates to the many organ systems that can be involved in the disease. In general, clinical findings most commonly are attributable to renal, skeletal, and gastrointestinal changes. The patient's initial complaints frequently are due to the presence of urinary tract calculi and nephrolithiasis, peptic ulcer disease, or pancreatitis. Symptomatic bone disease may be observed in 10 to 25 per cent of patients[1, 3] and may consist of tenderness and aching of the peripheral joints and the vertebral column, which eventually may progress to severe pain, swelling, and deformity. Alterations in the central nervous system, skin, and cardiovascular system also may contribute to the initial clinical picture, producing personality disturbance, coma, muscular weakness, fatigue, dry skin, itching, hypertension, and congestive heart failure. Increased awareness of these various manifestations of the disease has led to earlier diagnosis before devastating and irreparable effects on the skeleton and kidney have occurred. In fact, many patients with primary hyperparathyroidism are being diagnosed accurately before radiographic evidence of bone disease is encountered. In such cases, however, the use of advanced imaging techniques, such as photon absorptiometry, CT, and total body neutron activation analysis, will allow detection of osteopenia[366] (see Chapter 52).

Fundamental Characteristics of Bone Involvement

Although initial descriptions considered the bone alterations in hyperparathyroidism to be due to osteomalacia, von Recklinghausen[4] in 1891 stressed differences in the skeletal abnormalities of hyperparathyroidism and osteomalacia. Subsequently the distinctive hyperparathyroid osseous changes were termed Recklinghausen's disease of bone or generalized osteitis fibrosa cystica. In 1926, Mandl[5] emphasized that the primary abnormality leading to skeletal alteration was hyperfunctioning of the parathyroid glands.

In experimental or clinical situations, hyperparathyroidism is accompanied by an increase in the ratio of osteoclasts to osteoblasts. Accordingly, speculation developed that the osteoclasts are the primary target of parathyroid hormone in bone. In fact, the observed increase in the number of osteoclasts in hyperparathyroid bone raised the possibility that an actual conversion of osteoblasts to osteoclasts is mediated by parathyroid hormone, a theory that is incompatible with recent evidence suggesting an extraskeletal origin for the osteoclasts. It now appears certain that this hormone influences all three types of bone cells—osteoclasts, osteoblasts, and osteocytes.[276] Mobilization of calcium from the bone has been attributed to the process of osteocytic osteolysis,[8] as evidenced by an apparent increase in the extracellular space of bone lacunae. Extensive bone remodeling may be due to alterations of both osteoblasts and osteoclasts[9]; evidence of an effect of parathyroid hormone on the former cells includes the known inhibition of collagen formation, a primary function of osteoblasts, by the hormone. As bone remodeling requires the resorption of older osteons and their subsequent replacement with new bone, excessive remodeling in hyperparathyroidism necessitates altered behavior of both the osteoclasts, which are responsible for degradation of the bone, and the osteoblasts, which are responsible for the synthesis of new collagen and the remineralization of replacement osteons.[276] The stimulation of bone formation by parathyroid hormone is consistent with the occurrence of osteosclerosis in some cases of hyperparathyroidism.

Histologic examination of osseous tissue in hyperparathyroidism demonstrates great variation in the pathologic findings. Abnormalities include those of osteitis fibrosa cystica, with replacement of marrow elements by highly vascular fibrous tissue, as well as the changes of osteoporosis and osteomalacia. It has been suggested that the latter abnormality may be related to the persistent hypophosphatemia that can be seen in hyperparathyroidism.[1]

In hyperparathyroidism, initial bone changes may be so slight as to be imperceptible on radiographic or gross pathologic examination, although microscopic evaluation reveals exaggerated osteoclastic activity on the surface of trabecu-

lae within the cancellous bone and on the walls of the haversian canals within the cortical bone.[10] At these sites of osseous resorption, substitutive fibrosis is apparent. Subsequently, more severe skeletal involvement may lead to the characteristic pathologic findings of osteitis fibrosa cystica, in which osteofibrosis is associated with localized cysts or brown tumors, rarefied and thinned cortices, distorted and blurred cancellous trabeculae, infractions, fractures, and deformities. These pathologic aberrations have specific radiographic counterparts that have been well described.[11–20]

Bone Resorption

Resorption of osseous tissue is evident on histologic and radiologic examination in patients with primary (or secondary) hyperparathyroidism. In a radiographic search for evidence of abnormal bone resorption in hyperparathyroidism, the physician must have knowledge of the typical target areas of the disease. As will be noted in the following pages, such sites are scattered throughout the skeleton, which might appear to indicate that a skeletal survey consisting of a great number of radiographs is required. This generally is not the case. The sensitivity of bone resorption in the hands in the early stages of the disease has been documented repeatedly, indicating that high quality radiography (with macroradiography or digitized radiography) of this region is adequate in detecting and monitoring the course of skeletal changes in primary and secondary hyperparathyroidism.[277, 404]

It is convenient to categorize bone resorption as subperiosteal, intracortical, endosteal, subchondral, trabecular, and subligamentous and subtendinous. Localized lesions or brown tumors also may be seen.

Subperiosteal Bone Resorption (Figs. 57–1 and 57–2). Subperiosteal resorption of cortical bone virtually is diagnostic of hyperparathyroid bone disease. It was described initially by Camp and Ochsner[21] in 1931 in patients with primary hyperparathyroidism and identified subsequently by Albright and coworkers[22] in 1937 in patients with chronic renal disease. Although this change may be visualized in various skeletal locations, it is most frequent along the radial aspect of the phalanges of the hand, particularly in the middle phalanges of the index and middle fingers. The ulnar aspect is affected less significantly.[235] Early findings at this site may be subtle and are detected more readily using fine-grain (industrial) film and optical or radiographic magnification. A lacelike appearance of the phalangeal bone may progress to a spiculated contour and, eventually, to complete resorption of the entire cortex. Pugh[15] and others[23, 24] have noted additional sites of subperiosteal resorption. These include the phalangeal tufts; medial aspect of the proximal ends of the tibia, humerus, and femur; superior and inferior margins of the ribs; and lamina dura. Some investigations have shown that the earliest changes of subperiosteal bone resorption occur not on the radial aspect of the phalanges but in the phalangeal tufts, where a loss of the cortical line is an important indicator of disease.[236] Complicating the analysis of alterations at these sites is the normal irregular contour of the tufts, which must not be misinterpreted as evidence of hyperparathyroidism.[277] Once the observer is comfortable in his or her ability to differentiate abnormal from normal, attention to the tuftal regions of the terminal phalanges in the hands allows an early radiographic diagnosis of the disease as well as provides a sensitive means to evaluate the effects of treatment on the course of the disorder.[278] Furthermore, a distinctive pattern of acro-osteolysis in the terminal phalanges of the hands (and, less commonly, the feet), consisting of bandlike radiolucent areas that may separate the tuft and the base of the phalanx completely, is observed in primary and secondary hyperparathyroidism and is reminiscent of that occurring in certain familial forms of acro-osteolysis (see Chapter 94). The precise cause of this finding in hyperparathyroidism is not clear. With osseous healing, soft tissue clubbing[421] or phalangeal brachydactyly,[422] or both, may be evident.

Subperiosteal resorption of bone also may be apparent at the *margins* of certain joints, accounting for one "articular" manifestation of hyperparathyroidism (Table 57–2) (Fig. 57–3). Although this may be noted about the acromioclavicular, sternoclavicular, and sacroiliac joints and symphysis pubis, periarticular subperiosteal resorption may be especially prominent in the hand, wrist, and foot.[25, 26, 279, 420] The erosions that are created can simulate the appearance of rheumatoid arthritis,[279, 280] although they may be located slightly farther from the joint margin and almost always are associated with typical subperiosteal resorption of the adjacent phalangeal shafts. Furthermore, in the authors' experience, they predominate on the ulnar aspect of the metacarpal heads (compared with a radial predilection in rheumatoid arthritis), involve the distal interphalangeal joints with relative sparing of the proximal interphalangeal joints (compared with the opposite situation in rheumatoid arthritis), are associated with a normal-appearing joint space (whereas early joint space narrowing is typical of rheumatoid arthritis), and are characterized by a shaggy, irregular osseous contour with bony "whiskering" (in comparison to rheumatoid arthritis, in which bone proliferation is mild or absent).

It should be stressed that although other forms of bone resorption are frequent in hyperparathyroidism, subperiosteal resorption is the most useful diagnostic sign, and changes in the phalanges are among the initial bony manifestations of the disease. In very rare instances of hyperparathyroidism, however, another form of bone resorption may predominate or distant skeletal sites can be altered without presence of typical abnormalities of the hand.[363]

Furthermore, other disorders occasionally can be associated with subperiosteal resorption of bone, particularly as a localized phenomenon. Thus, loss of lamina dura may accompany dental sepsis, fibrous dysplasia, Paget's disease, Cushing's syndrome, hyperphosphatasemia, and osteomalacia; in addition, cortical erosion in the phalanges may be apparent adjacent to various soft tissue processes.

Intracortical Bone Resorption (Fig. 57–4). Osteoclastic resorption of bone within cortical haversian canals can produce radiographically detectable intracortical linear striations. These are best observed in the cortex of the second metacarpal.[23] The findings are not specific, being seen in other disorders with rapid bone turnover, such as acromegaly and hyperthyroidism. In all of these disorders, multiple intracortical lucent areas may be visualized, whereas in normal situations, two or fewer striae are observed in the metacarpal cortex. In hyperparathyroidism, intracortical resorption of bone almost always is associated with subperiosteal resorption. This association, coupled with analysis of serial radiographs in patients with this disease, has led to speculation that extensive intracortical bone resorption in juxtaperiosteal locations can lead to disruption of subperiosteal bone from within.[281] Certainly, a similar mechanism of superficial intracortical bone loss produces pseudoperiostitis.

Endosteal Bone Resorption (Fig. 57–5). Osteoclastic resorption occurs along the endosteal surface of bone, particularly in the hands. Radiographic features include localized pocket-like or scalloped defects along the inner margin of the cortex, which are reminiscent of abnormalities occurring in multiple myeloma, and more generalized thinning of the cortex, which can simulate the appearance of osteoporosis. Endosteal bone resorption rarely is an isolated or predominant feature of hyperparathyroidism, being overshadowed by adjacent intracortical and subperiosteal resorption.

Subchondral Bone Resorption (Figs. 57–6 to 57–10). Subchondral resorption of bone is a common manifestation of hyperparathyroidism, accounting for a second "articular" finding in this disease.[26–33] This type of resorption can be seen at multiple sites but is most frequent in the joints of the axial skeleton, such as the sacroiliac, sternoclavicular, and acromioclavicular joints, symphysis pubis, and discovertebral junctions, although it also is observed in large

Text continued on page 2021

TABLE 57–2. Articular Manifestations of Hyperparathyroidism

Mechanism	Characteristic Sites	Characteristic Appearance
Subperiosteal bone resorption	Hands, wrists, feet	Marginal erosions with adjacent bone resorption and proliferation
Subchondral bone resorption	Sacroiliac, sternoclavicular, and acromioclavicular joints; symphysis pubis; discovertebral junction; large and small joints of the appendicular skeleton	Subchondral erosions, weakening, and collapse
Subligamentous and subtendinous bone resorption	Trochanters, ischial tuberosities, humeral tuberosities, calcanei, distal clavicles	Osseous erosion with reactive bone formation
CPPD crystal deposition	Knees, wrists, and symphysis pubis	Chondrocalcinosis; pyrophosphate arthropathy (rare)
Urate crystal deposition	Various sites	Soft tissue swelling, osseous erosions
Tendon and ligament laxity	Sacroiliac and acromioclavicular joints; spine	Joint instability, soft tissue swelling, osseous erosion, dislocation, and subluxation
Tendon avulsion and rupture	Quadriceps, patellar, triceps, flexor and extensor finger tendons	Subluxation and dislocation

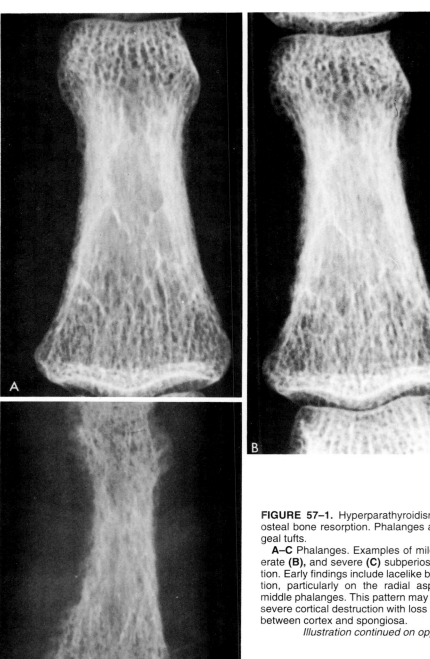

FIGURE 57–1. Hyperparathyroidism: Subperiosteal bone resorption. Phalanges and phalangeal tufts.

A–C Phalanges. Examples of mild **(A)**, moderate **(B)**, and severe **(C)** subperiosteal resorption. Early findings include lacelike bone resorption, particularly on the radial aspect of the middle phalanges. This pattern may progress to severe cortical destruction with loss of definition between cortex and spongiosa.

Illustration continued on opposite page

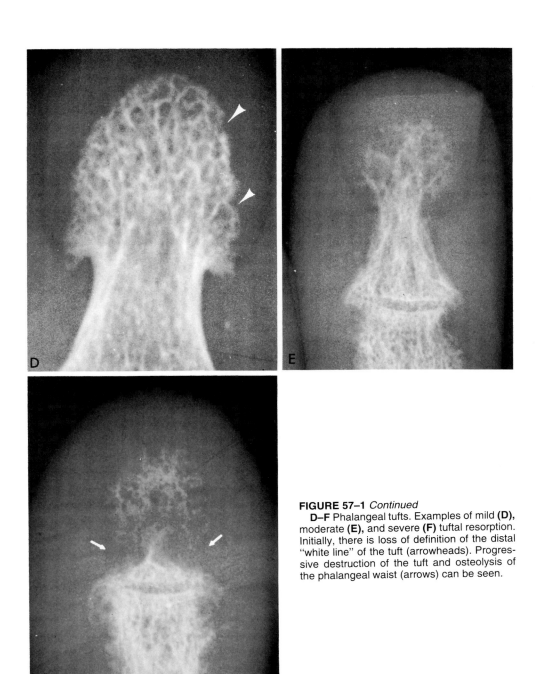

FIGURE 57–1 *Continued*
   D–F Phalangeal tufts. Examples of mild **(D)**, moderate **(E)**, and severe **(F)** tuftal resorption. Initially, there is loss of definition of the distal "white line" of the tuft (arrowheads). Progressive destruction of the tuft and osteolysis of the phalangeal waist (arrows) can be seen.

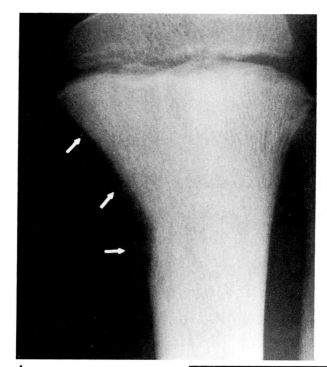

A

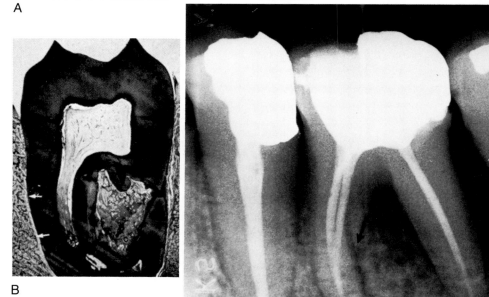

B

C

FIGURE 57–2. Hyperparathyroidism: Subperiosteal bone resorption. Other sites.

A Proximal portion of the tibia. Subperiosteal resorption is particularly prominent on the medial aspect of this bone (arrows).

B, C Lamina dura. Note resorption and fibro-osseous transformation of the lamina dura on a photomicrograph (5×) and radiograph (arrows).

(**B,** Courtesy of Jaffe HL: Metabolic, Degenerative and Inflammatory Diseases of Bones and Joints. Philadelphia, Lea & Febiger, 1972.)

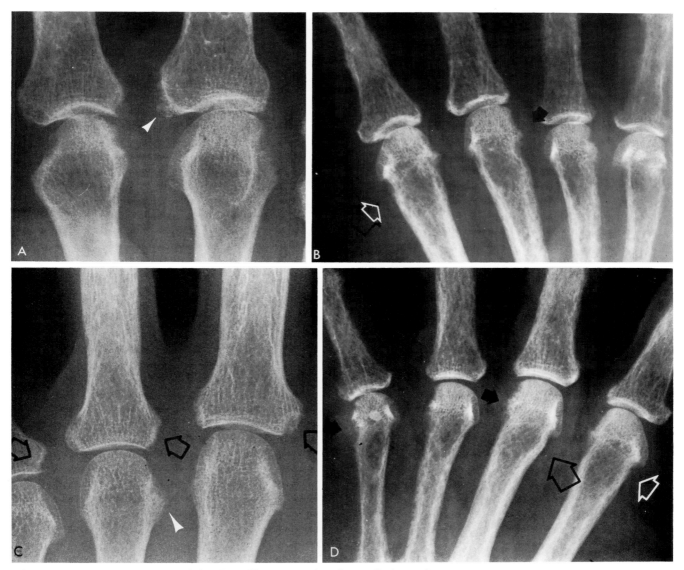

FIGURE 57–3. Hyperparathyroidism: Subperiosteal bone resorption—juxta-articular erosions.

A–D Metacarpophalangeal joint abnormalities. Erosions occur on the radial (open arrows) and ulnar (solid arrows) aspects of the metacarpal heads and proximal phalanges. Note their hooklike quality. Although in some places the erosions are intra-articular, they extend outside the joint. Observe the shaggy irregular osseous contour (arrowheads). The articular spaces are relatively normal. Subperiosteal bone resorption also is evident.

(**A–D,** From Resnick D: Radiology *110*:263, 1974.)

Illustration continued on following page

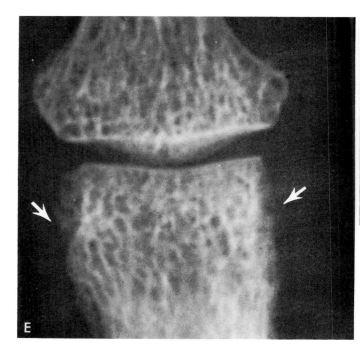

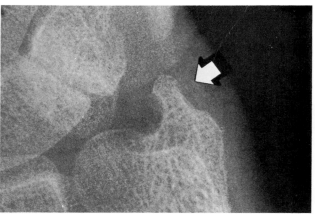

FIGURE 57–3 *Continued*

E Interphalangeal joint abnormalities. At the distal interphalangeal joints, subperiosteal resorption at the corners of the joints (arrows) is continuous with intra-articular erosion, producing a squared appearance of the phalangeal bone.

F Distal ulnar abnormalities. Pointing of the ulnar styloid has resulted from adjacent osseous erosions on either side (arrow).

(**F**, From Resnick D: Radiology *110*:263, 1974.)

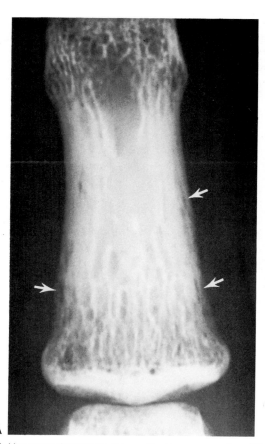

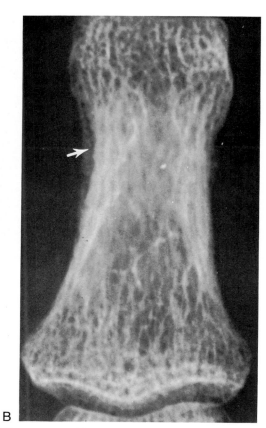

FIGURE 57–4. Hyperparathyroidism: Intracortical bone resorption. Slightly exaggerated linear radiolucency of the phalangeal cortices can be observed (arrows) in two different patients.

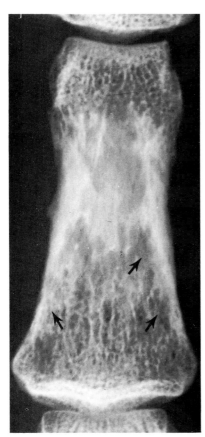

FIGURE 57–5. Hyperparathyroidism: Endosteal bone resorption. Observe scalloped erosions on the endosteal margin of the cortex (arrows).

and small joints of the appendicular skeleton. The fundamental pathologic aberration is osteoclastic resorption of trabeculae beneath the cartilaginous surface with fibrous replacement and new bone formation. Weakening and collapse of the osseous surface are accompanied by depression of the overlying cartilage. Juxta-articular bony surfaces may demonstrate concomitant subperiosteal resorption. An associated "osteogenic" synovitis has been described,[27, 28, 30] perhaps related to synovial irritation produced by collapse of subchondral bone at sites of mechanical stress, intra-articular cartilaginous and osseous debris, surface irregularity, and secondary cartilaginous and bony degeneration. With healing, intraosseous callus and fibrocartilage may become apparent.

The role of subchondral microfracture and collapse in the production of joint abnormalities is not clear, although these alterations do predominate in tight articulations, such as the sacroiliac, sternoclavicular, acromioclavicular, and temporomandibular joints[34, 35] and the symphysis pubis, which are subject to excessive shearing forces. More frequent involvement of joints in patients on maintenance dialysis might be expected, as this form of therapy apparently may result in a new type of osteodystrophy caused by a severe depression of bone formation and reduction in bone mass.[36] Radiographic surveys of patients undergoing renal dialysis (or after kidney transplantation) have revealed progressive skeletal alterations, including changes in trabecular

pattern, reduction in cortical thickness, subarticular sclerosis, and pathologic fractures[37] as well as exaggerated subchondral resorption about the sacroiliac joints.[38–40]

Subchondral resorption in hyperparathyroidism perhaps is most distinctive at the sacroiliac joints and, at this location, radiographic findings may mimic those of ankylosing spondylitis. The ilium is involved more severely than the sacrum. Overlying cartilage fibrillation and erosion may be accompanied by focal intra-articular fibrous adhesions. On radiographs, osseous erosion and reactive new bone formation produce a poorly defined and sclerotic articular margin and "pseudo-widening" of the joint space. CT confirms the presence of these joint manifestations (Fig. 57–11).[282] Although this constellation of findings is similar to that observed with true sacroiliitis, the absence of joint space narrowing and severe surface irregularity in hyperparathyroidism may allow accurate diagnosis. As in ankylosing spondylitis, the classic sacroiliac joint changes in hyperparathyroidism usually are bilateral and symmetric and can be associated with alterations in the symphysis pubis. At this latter site, symmetric subchondral resorption on both sides of the pubic disc can be accompanied by splitting and cleft formation within the central cartilage and adjacent subperiosteal resorption of bone.

Subchondral resorption also is common at the acromioclavicular and sternoclavicular joints.[16, 28, 41] The changes usually are symmetric. They are equally severe on the sternum and clavicle at the sternoclavicular joint and more severe on the clavicle than on the acromion at the acromioclavicular joint. Although resorption of the distal end of the clavicle is not a specific sign of hyperparathyroidism, it is helpful in diagnosis. At both sternoclavicular and acromioclavicular joints, subperiosteal resorption also may be encountered.

Subchondral resorption also is evident at the discovertebral junctions.[28] Changes in the vertebral bodies beneath the cartilaginous endplates produce areas of structural weakening, allowing displacement of disc material or formation of cartilaginous (Schmorl's) nodes. Although such displacements can be widespread in the spine of hyperparathyroid patients, they have received little attention. Eugenidis and coworkers[42] described a patient with tertiary hyperparathyroidism who demonstrated multiple cartilaginous nodes and mild surrounding sclerosis on conventional tomograms of the lumbar spine. Four years later, a typical rugger-jersey spine was evident, with bandlike sclerosis of the superior and inferior margins of the vertebral bodies. This sequence of events suggests that scrutiny of serial spinal radiographs in other patients with renal osteodystrophy and subchondral vertebral sclerosis may disclose additional examples of initial intraosseous disc displacement. Although the increased bone density at the margins of the vertebral bodies that is characteristic of the rugger-jersey spine may reflect generalized osteitis fibrosa cystica in its healing stage, subchondral condensation of bone may be an additional factor. This has been suggested by Jaffe[43] in cases of primary hyperparathyroidism, in which he described a layer of newly formed trabeculae of condensed bone surrounded by osteoclasts and fibrous tissue. Aitken and colleagues[44] verified these histologic findings in the spine of an additional patient with primary hyperparathyroidism and noted similar changes in the subchondral zones of the sternum and the

Text continued on page 2026

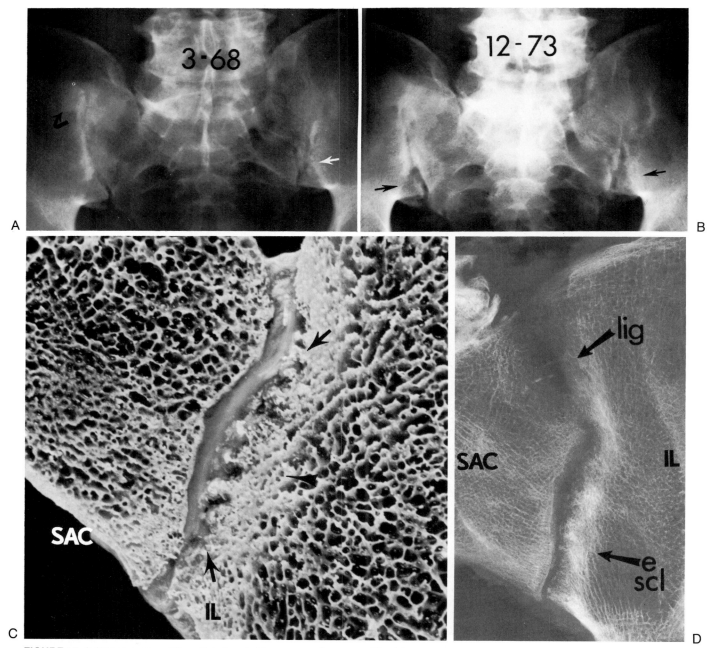

FIGURE 57–6. Hyperparathyroidism: Subchondral bone resorption—sacroiliac joint.

A, B Progressive subchondral resorption of bone (straight arrows) about both sacroiliac joints over a 5 year period in a 73 year old man with renal osteodystrophy. Observe the irregular osseous surface on the ilium and adjacent reactive sclerosis. A para-articular osteophyte also is apparent (curved arrow).

C, D Photograph and radiograph of a coronal section of the involved sacroiliac joint. The sacrum (SAC) and ilium (IL) are indicated. Observe subchondral erosion (arrows, e), predominantly on the ilium, and reactive sclerosis (arrowhead, scl). Mild ligamentous (lig) ossification is apparent.

(**C, D** From Resnick D, Niwayama G: Radiology *118*:315, 1976.)

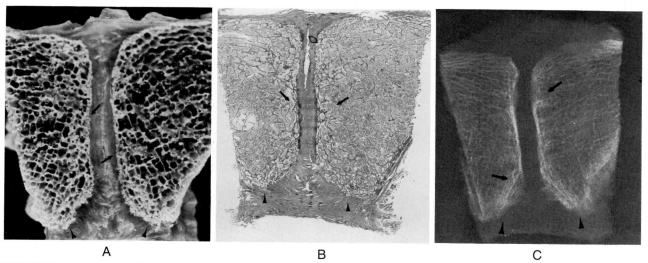

FIGURE 57–7. Hyperparathyroidism: Subchondral bone resorption—symphysis pubis.

A, B Gross photograph of a macerated coronal section through the symphysis pubis **(A)** and a corresponding photomicrograph (2×) **(B)** demonstrate erosion and sclerosis of subchondral bone (arrows). Subperiosteal resorption and sclerosis also are apparent (arrowheads). Note cartilaginous cleft formation (open arrow).

C A radiograph of the section reveals subchondral (arrows) and subperiosteal (arrowheads) erosion and sclerosis, which are continuous in some places.

(From Resnick D, Niwayama G: Radiology *118*:315, 1976.)

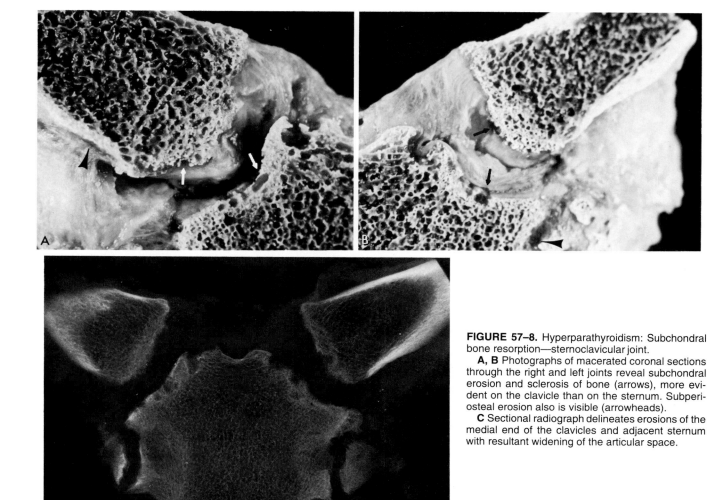

FIGURE 57–8. Hyperparathyroidism: Subchondral bone resorption—sternoclavicular joint.

A, B Photographs of macerated coronal sections through the right and left joints reveal subchondral erosion and sclerosis of bone (arrows), more evident on the clavicle than on the sternum. Subperiosteal erosion also is visible (arrowheads).

C Sectional radiograph delineates erosions of the medial end of the clavicles and adjacent sternum with resultant widening of the articular space.

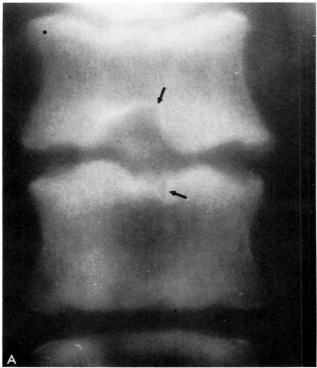

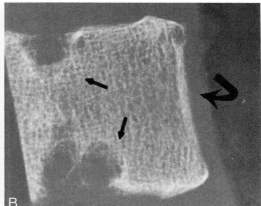

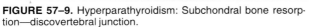

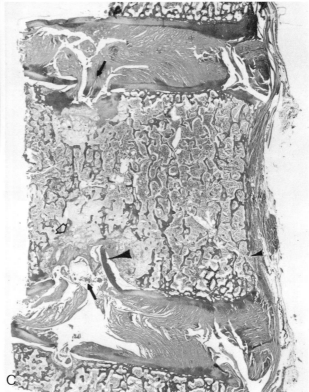

FIGURE 57–9. Hyperparathyroidism: Subchondral bone resorption—discovertebral junction.

A Frontal tomography in a patient with renal osteodystrophy reveals extensive subchondral resorption of bone at the discovertebral junction. Note cartilaginous (Schmorl's) nodes (arrows) producing irregular depressions in the osseous surface, reactive sclerosis, and narrowing of the disc space.

(**A,** Courtesy of J. Mink, M.D., Los Angeles, California.)

B Radiograph of a macerated sagittal section of such a spine reveals irregular subchondral erosion of bone with intraosseous discal displacement or cartilaginous node formation (straight arrows) and minimal subperiosteal bone irregularity on the anterior portion of the vertebral body (curved arrow).

C A photomicrograph (4×) of the section outlines prolapse of portions of the nucleus pulposus through gaps in the cartilaginous endplates (straight arrows). Displacement of the endplates into the vertebral bodies also has occurred (large arrowhead). The subchondral bone demonstrates features of osteitis fibrosa cystica with extensive resorption and fibrous replacement (open arrow). Subperiosteal resorption of bone along the anterior aspect of the vertebral body has occurred (small arrowhead).

(**B, C** From Resnick D, Niwayama G: Radiology *118*:315, 1976.)

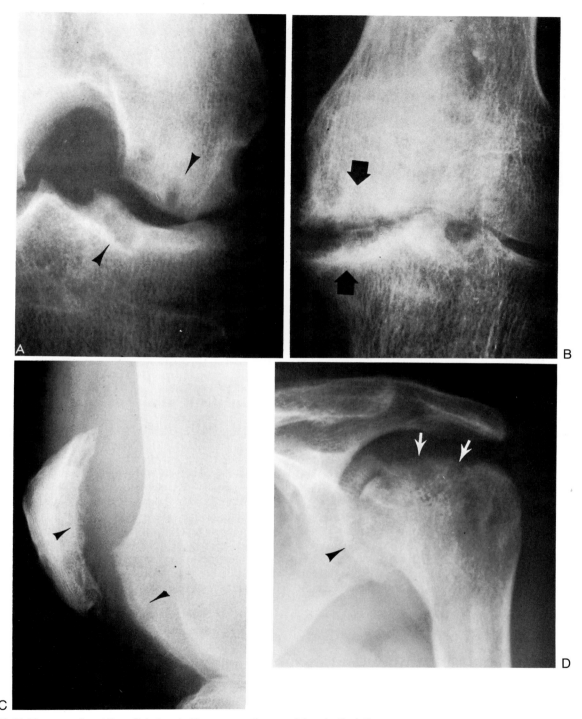

FIGURE 57–10. Hyperparathyroidism: Subchondral bone resorption—peripheral articulations.

A, B Femorotibial joints. These findings begin as subchondral radiolucent areas with adjacent sclerosis (arrowheads) and progress with irregularity and depression of the articular surface simulating infection (arrows).

(**B,** From Resnick D, Niwayama G: Radiology *118*:315, 1976.)

C Patellofemoral joint. Observe considerable erosion with deformity of the posterior surface of the patella and resorption on the anterior surface of the femur (arrowheads). An effusion is present.

(**C,** Courtesy of R. Shapiro, M.D., and K. Weisner, M.D., Sacramento, California.)

D Glenohumeral joint. Prominent subchondral resorption is seen in the humeral head (arrows) and glenoid cavity (arrowhead). Additional findings include subchondral resorption about the acromioclavicular joint and subperiosteal resorption in the medial aspect of the proximal humerus.

(**D,** Courtesy of G. Greenway, M.D., Dallas, Texas.)

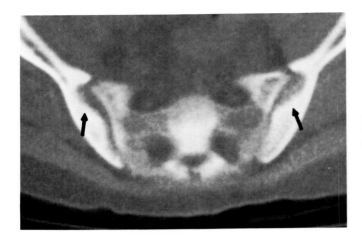

FIGURE 57–11. Hyperparathyroidism: Subchondral bone resorption—sacroiliac joints. A transaxial CT scan reveals bilateral and symmetric abnormalities (arrows).

pubis. These investigators suggested that physical stress produced a local stimulus in each of these locations that resulted in osteosclerosis. This evidence may indicate that both trabecular compression (subchondral condensation) and increased bone formation during the healing phase of osteitis fibrosa cystica may contribute to increased radiodensity in some patients with the rugger-jersey spine.

Subchondral bone resorption in hyperparathyroidism is not confined to the axial skeleton. Subchondral bone collapse in the peripheral skeleton has been described.[26–28, 259, 283–285, 288, 290] This finding is particularly frequent in the knee but also may be observed in other large and small appendicular joints. It often is difficult to ascertain the exact contribution of subchondral resorption to the radiographic appearance of peripheral joint abnormalities in hyperparathyroidism, particularly those about the hand, wrist, and patellofemoral areas, as subperiosteal resorption, "osteogenic" synovitis, and crystal-induced arthritis also may occur in this disease. Furthermore, many of the descriptions of joint manifestations in hyperparathyroidism have been provided through analyses of groups of patients with chronic renal disease undergoing dialysis. In this situation, numerous and complex skeletal alterations, related to renal osteodystrophy and dialysis bone disease, complicate the identification of a specific pathogenesis for the articular abnormalities, and it is likely that several distinct mechanisms are contributory. Although secondary hyperparathyroidism usually is evident in these patients,[288] suggesting that subchondral and subperiosteal bone resorption plays a definite role in the production of intra- and periarticular "erosive" alterations, the importance of other factors, such as calcium pyrophosphate dihydrate (CPPD), urate, calcium hydroxyapatite, and oxalate crystal deposition and amyloidosis, must be considered (see later discussion).

Subphyseal Bone Resorption (see Fig. 57–29). In children with primary or secondary hyperparathyroidism, irregular radiolucent areas may appear in the metaphysis adjacent to the growth plate. This finding is seen in tubular bones, especially those in the hand and foot, and is reminiscent of the abnormalities accompanying rickets.[121–123] The absence of similar changes at other skeletal sites, the occurrence of these findings in patients with primary hyperparathyroidism, and the absence of histologic evidence of osteomalacia suggest that such metaphyseal alterations are a manifestation of hyperparathyroidism itself. Physical stress may be an aggravating factor in some cases. Sequential radiographic examinations have revealed progressive metaphyseal sclerosis in some children, which may persist even after the adjacent physis has fused.[423]

Trabecular Bone Resorption (Fig. 57–12). Trabecular resorption within medullary bone occurs throughout the skeleton in hyperparathyroidism, particularly in the advanced stages of the disease. Bone assumes a granular appearance, with loss of distinct trabecular detail. Such resorption within the cranium is especially striking. The diploë is replaced by connective tissue containing newly formed trabeculae, and definition between the diploic portion of the skull and the inner and outer tables is lost. On radiographs, an osteopenic (decreased radiodensity) and speckled appearance is termed the "salt and pepper" skull. Focal areas of osseous thickening in the cranial vault may be observed on radiographs as well-defined or poorly defined radiopaque areas.

Similar histologic and radiologic findings in the spongy trabeculae may be seen throughout the skeleton, with involvement of the tubular bones, pelvis, and facial bones, including the mandible. Osseous deformities may resemble the changes of osteomalacia.

Subligamentous and Subtendinous Bone Resorption (Fig. 57–13). Osseous resorption occurs at sites of tendon and ligament attachment to bone. This is particularly frequent at the femoral trochanters, ischial and humeral tuberosities, elbow, inferior surface of the calcaneus, and inferior aspect of the distal end of the clavicle.[45, 277, 286, 287]

Brown Tumors (Fig. 57–14). Brown tumors or osteoclastomas were described initially as characteristic of primary hyperparathyroidism, although, more recently, they have been noted with increasing frequency in secondary hyperparathyroidism as well.[46–50, 289] Brown tumors represent localized accumulations of fibrous tissue and giant cells, which can replace bone and even may produce osseous expansion.[237] They subsequently may undergo necrosis and liquefaction, producing cysts.[51] Brown tumors appear as single or multiple well-defined lesions of the axial or appendicular skeleton, frequently eccentric or cortical in location. Common sites of involvement are the facial bones, pelvis, ribs, and femora. Other manifestations of hyperparathyroidism generally are apparent, although occasionally a

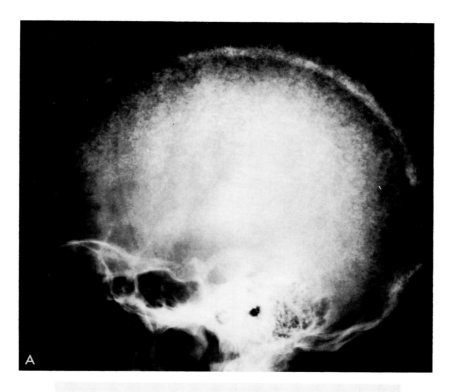

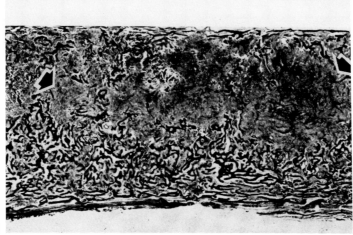

FIGURE 57–12. Hyperparathyroidism: Trabecular bone resorption—cranial vault.

A The lateral radiograph outlines the characteristic mottling of the vault. Alternating areas of lucency and sclerosis produce the "salt and pepper" appearance.

B Photomicrograph (6×) illustrates the histologic changes in the skull. Connective tissue containing new bone has replaced trabeculae within the diploë (arrows). The tables have been obliterated.

(**B,** From Jaffe HL: Metabolic, Degenerative and Inflammatory Diseases of Bones and Joint. Philadelphia, Lea & Febiger, 1972.)

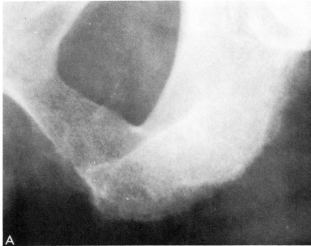

FIGURE 57–13. Hyperparathyroidism: Subligamentous and subtendinous bone resorption.

A Ischial tuberosity. Erosion of bone has produced a poorly defined, irregular osseous surface.

B, C Inferior calcaneal surface. In two patients, mild **(B)** and severe **(C)** subligamentous (subaponeurotic) erosion of bone can be detected (arrowheads). The osseous surface is irregular, and proliferation can be seen in **C**, creating a poorly defined enthesophyte.

D Inferior aspect of the distal end of the clavicle. Resorption of the clavicular surface beneath the coracoclavicular ligament (arrowhead) is characteristic of this disorder. A similar change may be observed in rheumatoid arthritis and ankylosing spondylitis.

E Ulnar olecranon process. Note the poorly defined osseous surface (arrowheads) and an enthesophyte.

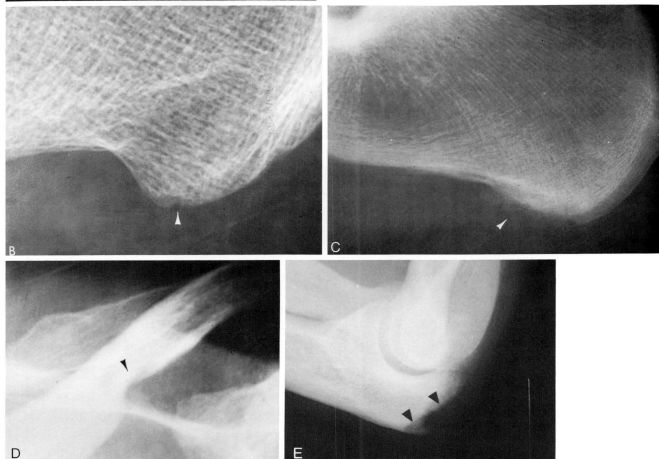

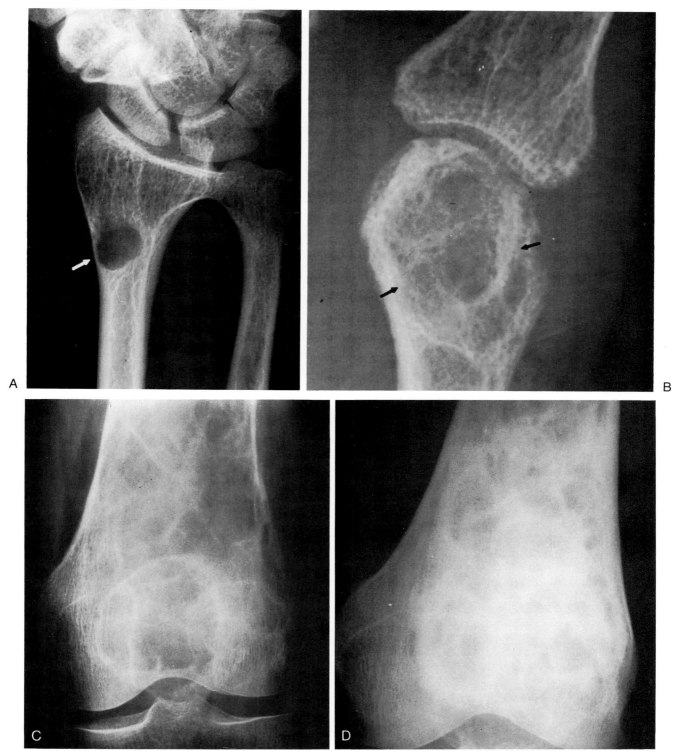

FIGURE 57–14. Hyperparathyroidism: Brown tumors.

A, B Examples of brown tumors (arrows) in the distal portion of the radius and metacarpal head. They can be single or multiple, well demarcated or poorly defined, and eccentric or central in location.

C, D Brown tumor of the distal portion of the femur before **(C)** and after **(D)** removal of parathyroid adenoma. Increased radiodensity of the lesion after surgery is evident.

brown tumor is the presenting finding in the disease. Rarely, brown tumors of the vertebral column may cause spinal cord compression or acute paraplegia.[246, 247] With removal of the parathyroid adenoma, brown tumors may demonstrate healing with increased radiodensity. Persistence of the fibro-osseous lesions after such surgery may indicate that they are not the brown tumors of hyperparathyroidism but are related to some other cause.[291] In this regard, the simultaneous occurrence of hyperparathyroidism and fibrous dysplasia or ameloblastoma has been recorded.[292–294, 405]

It should be emphasized that although advanced cases of hyperparathyroidism with severe bone resorption were not infrequent in the past (Fig. 57–15), more sophisticated diagnostic techniques coupled with an increased awareness of the condition have led to earlier diagnosis, at a time when the degree of bone resorption is somewhat limited. Fine-detail and magnification radiography are two such techniques.[253] Genant and coworkers[14] have emphasized that fine-detail skeletal radiography in primary hyperparathyroidism will not only detect mild disease but also reveal intracortical, endosteal, and trabecular resorption without the classic features of osteitis fibrosa cystica that were apparent in earlier cases of fulminant hyperparathyroidism. A prominent radiographic feature of the disease may be generalized osteopenia, perhaps resulting from osteocytic osteolysis rather than osteoclastosis. On radiographs, osteopenia frequently is a subjective finding that is difficult to interpret and is identifiable only after 25 to 50 per cent of mineral is lost.[14, 52, 53] This difficulty can be overcome by using quantitative bone mineral analysis,[54, 55] which will indicate not only the degree and rate of bone loss in the disease but also a partial recovery of this loss that may ensue after successful parathyroidectomy.[295]

Bone Sclerosis

Increased amounts of trabecular bone can occur in patients with hyperparathyroidism and create abnormal radiodensity on skeletal radiographs.[11] This is observed far more frequently in patients with renal osteodystrophy and secondary hyperparathyroidism,[56–61] although it may be apparent in primary hyperparathyroidism as well.[12, 44, 58–64, 364, 507] In some of these latter cases, sclerosis may be due to impairment of renal function secondary to parathyroid gland malfunctioning. In patients with secondary hyperparathyroidism and bone sclerosis, diffuse increase in bone density may be seen. In patients with primary hyperparathyroidism, bone sclerosis may be localized or patchy, apparent in the metaphyseal regions of the long bones, the skull, or the vertebral endplates (Fig. 57–16). Diffuse bone sclerosis rarely is noted in primary hyperparathyroidism.[12, 65, 66, 364] Deposition of bone in the subchondral areas of the vertebral bodies results in the appearance of radiodense bands across the superior and inferior margins (rugger-jersey spine). This manifestation, too, is much more frequent in secondary hyperparathyroidism than in primary hyperparathyroidism.

The mechanism of bone sclerosis in hyperparathyroidism is not defined clearly. Administration of small doses of parathyroid hormone to rats has led to metaphyseal sclerosis.[67, 68] Furthermore, as it is known that parathyroid hormone can increase bone-forming surfaces and stimulate

osteoblastic activity,[7] it is possible that bone formation may be more dramatic than bone resorption in some patients with hyperparathyroidism, leading to osseous eburnation. Alternatively, some investigators attribute bone sclerosis in association with hyperparathyroidism to the effect of thyrocalcitonin.[12] Secretion of this latter substance inhibits bone resorption,[69] producing hypocalcemia and, in experimental situations, osteosclerosis.[70–72] The role of thyrocalcitonin in humans is less clear, although syndromes of thyrocalcitonin excess leading to hypocalcemia and bone sclerosis have been suggested.[70, 73] Whatever the mechanism of osteosclerosis in hyperparathyroidism, increased radiodensity of bones may become a prominent radiographic feature, particularly in the axial skeleton, associated with close-meshed thickened spongy trabeculae on gross pathologic and histologic examination.[10]

Chondrocalcinosis (Calcium Pyrophosphate Dihydrate Crystal Deposition)

The association of primary hyperparathyroidism and CPPD crystal deposition is well known. CPPD crystal deposition also may occur in chronic renal disease, although its frequency is much lower than that in primary hyperparathyroidism. Radiographic evidence of such crystal deposition has been reported in 18 to 40 per cent of patients with hyperparathyroidism,[74–76] usually related to the presence of cartilage calcification (chondrocalcinosis), although deposits in other intra-articular structures also may be observed. Persistence of chondrocalcinosis and pseudogout attacks[25] after parathyroidectomy has been reported. Pritchard and Jessop[77] were unable to relate the presence of chondrocalcinosis to hypercalcemia in hyperparathyroid patients, although patients with cartilage calcification had higher serum levels of alkaline phosphatase and more severe radiologic bone disease. Although patients with hyperparathyroidism and CPPD crystal deposition may develop structural joint damage (pyrophosphate arthropathy) (Fig. 57–17), this complication is much more frequent in patients with idiopathic or sporadic CPPD crystal deposition disease. A patient has been described with hyperparathyroidism, CPPD crystal deposition manifested as chondrocalcinosis and synovial calcification, and carpal tunnel syndrome.[78]

Additional Rheumatic Manifestations

In addition to subchondral osseous resorption leading to collapse and fragmentation of bone, subperiosteal osseous resorption leading to periarticular (and possibly intra-articular) erosions, subligamentous and subtendinous osseous resorption with erosion at ligamentous and tendinous attachments to bone, and CPPD crystal deposition that may lead to the pseudogout syndrome, other rheumatic manifestations of hyperparathyroidism may be encountered (Fig. 57–18).

Parathyroid hormone may affect ligaments and tendons themselves, either by direct effect on collagen[79] or by influencing its enzymatic degradation.[80, 81] The resultant capsular and ligamentous laxity, as well as rupture, may contribute to joint instability, traumatic synovitis, and cartilaginous and osseous destruction (Figs. 57–19 and 57–20). The acromioclavicular and sacroiliac joints[82] may be particularly

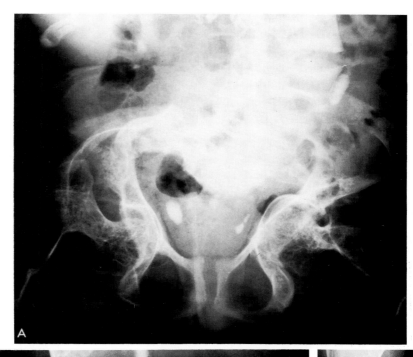

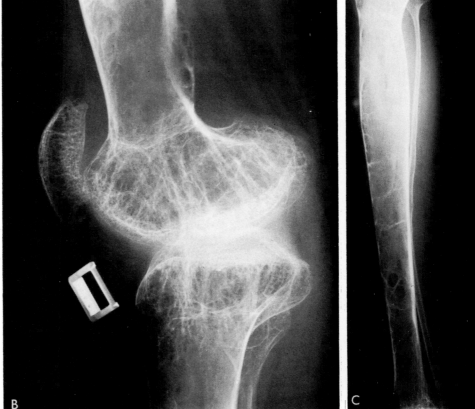

FIGURE 57–15. Hyperparathyroidism: Advanced case. This 18 year old Mexican girl had had clinical symptoms and signs since the age of 8 years. Progressive deformities and shortening were observed. The patient also was found to have renal and ureteral lithiasis. A parathyroid adenoma was removed. Severe alterations are characterized by fibroosseous transformation producing osteopenia, cortical thinning, medullary expansion, and deformity.

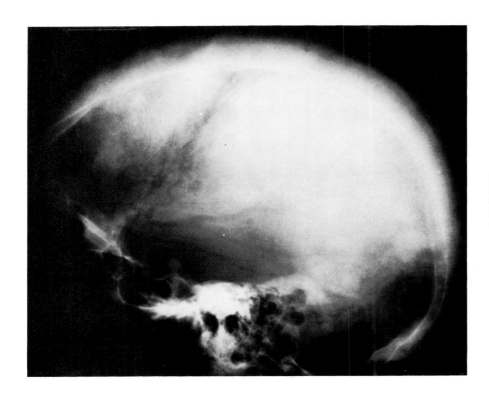

FIGURE 57–16. Hyperparathyroidism: Bone sclerosis—cranial vault. Patchy osteosclerosis of the skull is associated with thickening of the cranial vault and loss of delineation between tables and diploë.

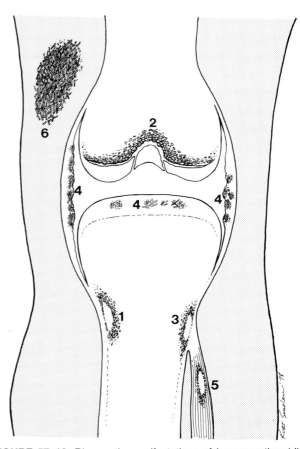

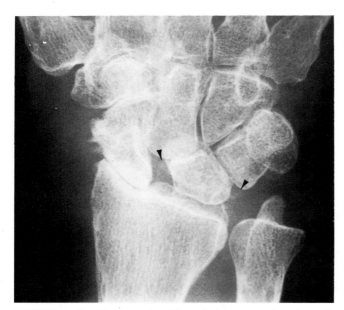

FIGURE 57–17. Hyperparathyroidism: Calcium pyrophosphate dihydrate (CPPD) crystal deposition disease. In a patient with primary hyperparathyroidism and CPPD crystal deposition documented by joint aspiration, observe intra-articular calcification (arrowheads) and structural joint damage (pyrophosphate arthropathy) characterized by joint space narrowing, sclerosis, and osteophytosis.

FIGURE 57–18. Rheumatic manifestations of hyperparathyroidism (and renal osteodystrophy). Findings may relate to subperiosteal resorption at the margins of the joint (1), subchondral resorption leading to cartilage and bone disintegration and fragmentation (2), subligamentous and subtendinous resorption (3), intra-articular crystal deposition (CPPD, monosodium urate) in cartilage, synovium, and capsule (4), tendinous and ligamentous injury and rupture (5), and periarticular crystal deposition (monosodium urate, calcium hydroxyapatite) in soft tissues (6).

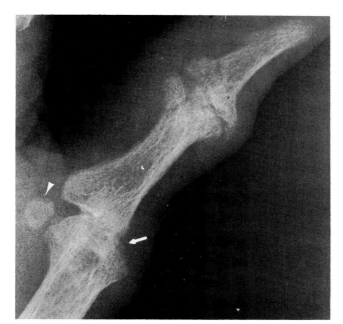

FIGURE 57–19. Hyperparathyroidism: Ligamentous laxity. A minor degree of subluxation (arrow) at the first metacarpophalangeal joint is apparent in a patient with other typical osseous abnormalities. Observe erosion and poor definition of the sesamoid bone (arrowhead). (From Resnick D: Radiology *110*:263, 1974.)

vulnerable because of their dependence on soft tissues for support. Bywaters[83] alluded to this action of parathyroid hormone when he described possible dislocations of the spine related to softening of the tendinous and ligamentous attachments in patients with hyperparathyroidism. McKusick[84] noted a patient with both hyperparathyroidism and Ehlers-Danlos syndrome in whom joint laxity decreased after parathyroidectomy. Furthermore, the occurrence of spontaneous tendon avulsion in patients with hyperparathyroidism has been attributed to the direct effect of parathyroid hormone on connective tissue.[85] Similar reports of tendinous ruptures have been seen in patients on chronic hemodialysis with secondary hyperparathyroidism,[86–90] suggesting an alternative theory that chronic acidosis in these patients may lead to degeneration of tendons with a change in their tensile characteristics. Tendon rupture in either primary or secondary hyperparathyroidism can involve one or multiple sites, including the quadriceps, patellar, and triceps tendons, as well as the flexor and extensor tendons of the fingers[260, 365, 418, 419] (Fig. 57–21).

Even in the absence of demonstrable rupture of tendons, patients with hyperparathyroidism may reveal pain and tenderness at sites of tendon insertion, such as those related to the thigh adductors, gluteal muscles, and quadriceps mechanism, which when combined with weakness from neuropathy and myopathy can lead to abnormalities of gait.[91] Clinically, these symptoms and signs can resemble the enthesopathy of ankylosing spondylitis. On rare occasions, this similarity may be accentuated by the occurrence of paravertebral calcification and ankylosis of sacroiliac joints in patients with primary hyperparathyroidism.[92] In these latter cases it is not clear whether there is a distinct syndrome or the chance occurrence of two diseases.

Monosodium urate crystals and clinical gout have been described in patients with hyperparathyroidism[93, 94]; in these

patients, gouty arthritis may become manifest only after parathyroidectomy.[248] In addition, an association between rheumatoid arthritis or rheumatoid arthritis–like syndromes and hyperparathyroidism has been suggested.[79, 85, 95]

Hyperparathyroidism in Infants and Children

Primary hyperparathyroidism may be evident in infants and children. Congenital primary hyperparathyroidism is a rare disorder occurring in infants, demonstrating autosomal recessive inheritance.[96, 97, 296] Symptoms and signs include hypotonicity, respiratory distress, fever, dehydration, constipation, anorexia, lethargy, vomiting, dysphagia, craniotabes, and hepatosplenomegaly.[296, 367] Hypercalcemia generally, but not universally, is present and may require serial blood sampling for detection. Elevated levels of blood urea nitrogen, reflecting the presence of dehydration and nephrocalcinosis, and anemia, due to fibrosis of the bone marrow or concurrent infections, have been observed. Radiographs may reveal severe bone disease with subperiosteal resorption, periosteal bone formation, trabecular reduction,

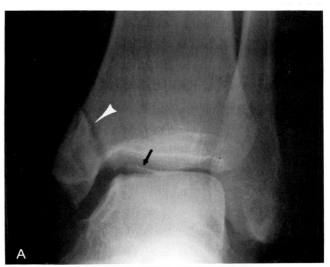

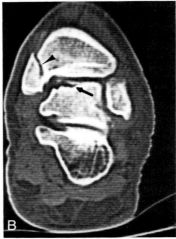

FIGURE 57–20. Hyperparathyroidism: Joint instability. In this 58 year old man with primary hyperparathyroidism, ankle pain, swelling, and "giving way" occurred in the absence of trauma.

A Findings include an osteochondral fracture of the talar dome (arrow) and an oblique fracture of the medial malleolus (arrowhead).

B A direct coronal CT scan illustrates the same findings as in **A**.

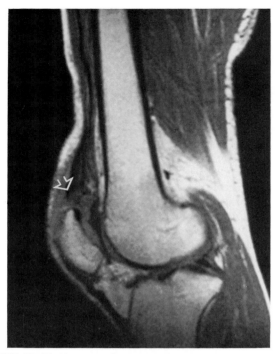

FIGURE 57–21. Hyperparathyroidism: Tendon rupture. In this patient with renal osteodystrophy and secondary hyperparathyroidism, spontaneous bilateral ruptures of the quadriceps mechanism occurred. A sagittal T1-weighted (TR/TE, 700/30) spin echo MR image reveals interruption of the quadriceps tendon (arrow). Note the low position of the patella, buckling of the patellar tendon, and prepatellar soft tissue edema. (Courtesy of R. Stiles, M.D., Atlanta, Georgia.)

extensive erosions of tubular bones, and pathologic fractures. Subperiosteal resorption of bone involves both metaphyses and diaphyses. Rib fractures with callus formation resemble pulmonary infiltrates, and periodontal osteopenia accentuates the density of the teeth.[296] The degree of periostitis may be so severe as to simulate the findings of syphilis. Unless parathyroidectomy is performed, the infants usually die.

A second disorder, transient hyperparathyroidism of the neonate, occurs secondary to hypoparathyroidism in the mother.[98, 250] The radiographic changes are similar to congenital primary hyperparathyroidism, although they resolve rapidly. Similarly, histologic abnormalities resemble those of congenital primary hyperparathyroidism, and these too may improve with time.[250] Because of its self-limited na-

ture, the disorder usually is benign, although fractures and hypercalcemia may occur.

In older children, skeletal involvement in hyperparathyroidism is characterized by osteopenia, genu valgum, fractures, cystic lesions of bone, and clubbing of the fingers. Renal involvement and rickets-like changes with metaphyseal irregularity may be observed. A possible association of primary hyperparathyroidism and slipping of the capital femoral epiphysis has been noted,[99] a complication that is much more frequent in renal osteodystrophy.

Familial Hypercalcemia

Specific and distinct syndromes of familial hypercalcemia have been identified including several types of disorders accompanied by tumors of multiple endocrine glands and familial hypocalciuric hypercalcemia (Table 57–3).

Familial multiple endocrine neoplasia (MEN), type I, which also is referred to as multiple endocrine adenomatosis (MEA) and Wermer's syndrome, is an autosomal dominant disease (due to changes in chromosome 11[407]) associated with primary hyperparathyroidism (95 per cent of cases) and, less frequently, excessive secretion of gastrin (20 to 40 per cent of cases), insulin (2 to 10 per cent of cases), other pancreatic islet peptides (rare), and anterior pituitary peptides (rare).[276, 368, 369, 372] The hyperparathyroidism usually is attributable to diffuse hyperplasia of chief cells or to multiple adenomas; pancreatic islet cell hyperplasia or islet cell tumors are present in 50 to 85 per cent of cases.[406] Nonsecretory neoplastic masses, including lipomas, pituitary chromophobe adenomas (30 to 65 per cent of cases), carcinoid tumors, and adrenal and thyroid adenomas, also occur but rarely metastasize. MEN syndrome, type I, generally becomes manifest clinically in the third, fourth, or fifth decade of life. Clinical manifestations are variable but include those related to renal calculi. Hypercalcemia usually is not severe, and the frequency of bone pain and tenderness and pathologic fractures is low.[406] Indeed, the prevalence of osseous changes of hyperparathyroidism does not differ from that in primary hyperparathyroidism.

Familial MEN type IIA, also called Sipple's syndrome, is inherited as an autosomal dominant trait with very high penetrance for medullary thyroid carcinoma in adults.[276, 370] Abnormalities of other endocrine glands, particularly primary parathyroid hyperplasia and pheochromocytoma, occur in approximately one third of cases, but malignant change related to these other endocrine aberrations is rare. A variant of this type of familial MEN, type IIB or III,

TABLE 57–3. Major Features in Syndromes of Familial Hypercalcemia

	Multiple Endocrine Neoplasia, Type I	Multiple Endocrine Neoplasia, Type II*	Hypocalciuric Hypercalcemia
Inheritance	Autosomal dominant	Autosomal dominant	Autosomal dominant
Penetrance of hypercalcemia, first decade	Low	Low	High
Associated endocrinopathy	Islet cell; anterior pituitary	Medullary thyroid cancer; pheochromocytoma	None
Unique biochemical features	Hypergastrinemia	Hypercalcitoninemia	Relative hypocalciuria
Subtotal parathyroidectomy	Useful	Useful	Usually no benefit

*Multiple endocrine neoplasia, type IIB, rarely has hypercalcemia or hyperparathyroidism. (From Aurbach GD, Marx SJ, Spiegel AM: Parathyroid hormone, calcitonin, and the calciferols. *In* RH Williams [Ed]: Textbook of Endocrinology. 7th Ed. Philadelphia, WB Saunders Co, 1985, p 1176.)

characterized by overgrowth of neural elements and the development of mucosal neuromas, thickened corneal nerves, and intestinal ganglioneuromatosis, has been identified.[276, 361] Additional abnormalities, including joint laxity, slender body habitus, pes cavus, talipes equinovarus, abnormal spinal curvature, muscle weakness, and pectus excavatum or carinatum, resemble findings in Marfan's syndrome. It is a serious disorder with a high mortality rate, owing mainly to metastasis from the medullary thyroid carcinoma. This complication can lead to the patient's death as a teenager, although some persons survive for decades. Early diagnosis, provided by the nonendocrine manifestations of the disease, is important.

One additional pattern of MEN is the combination of pheochromocytoma and pancreatic islet cell tumor.[362]

The MEN syndromes are uncommon but important disorders. Their oncogenic trigger is not yet known,[392] although multiple theories regarding the pathogenesis of these syndromes exist.[406]

Familial hypocalciuric hypercalcemia, also called familial benign hypercalcemia, is a rare disorder of unknown cause characterized by autosomal dominant inheritance with high penetration for expression of hypercalcemia at all ages.[276] It was first described by Foley and collaborators in 1972[355] and was studied more extensively by Marx and colleagues in 1981.[356] The syndrome is associated with lifelong hypercalcemia, low urinary calcium excretion, the absence of prominent symptoms and signs, and the failure of subtotal parathyroidectomy to decrease plasma calcium levels.[357] Muscle weakness and fatigability are typical, although nephrolithiasis or peptic ulcer disease is seen in approximately 10 per cent of cases. Superficially, familial hypocalciuric hypercalcemia resembles asymptomatic primary hyperparathyroidism; in the former condition, however, there is no significant reduction of bone mass in the axial or appendicular skeleton, and the prevalence of fractures is not increased.[357, 371] With regard to the size and the histologic composition of the parathyroid glands in this disease, conflicting data have been reported[358]; normal findings or minor aberrations in size and a decrease in parenchymal tissue are recorded in some studies. Data further indicate that basal levels of serum parathyroid hormone are normal or slightly increased, and the levels are not suppressed in a normal fashion during standard calcium infusions.[358, 359] It has been suggested that the hypercalcemia in familial hypocalciuric hypercalcemia is due primarily to excessive renal conservation of calcium and that this element prevents the development of parathyroid hyperplasia.[358] Of interest in this regard, neonates born of parents who are members of kindreds with the disease may have severe hyperparathyroidism.[360]

Differential Diagnosis

In most patients with hyperparathyroidism, the radiographic findings are pathognomonic, whereas in others, they are highly suggestive of the disease process. Some of the individual radiographic findings may lack specificity, but the combination of abnormalities is much easier to interpret.

Subperiosteal bone resorption is the most helpful diagnostic clue on the radiographs. Widespread subperiosteal resorption is confined to hyperparathyroid bone disease; focal areas of subperiosteal bone resorption may be seen adjacent to a variety of soft tissue processes, including tumor, infection, and even articular disorders, such as xanthomatosis and gout, but the resulting contour defects in the bone, particularly in the latter disorders, generally are much better defined than the defects in hyperparathyroidism. Intracortical bone resorption may be noted in disease states characterized by rapid bone turnover, such as hyperthyroidism and acromegaly, whereas endosteal bone resorption can be produced by osteoporosis or marrow-containing disorders, such as multiple myeloma. Some degree of subchondral bone resorption may accompany osteoporosis, but extensive resorption and collapse of articular surfaces are not common features of this condition. The severely depressed and fragmented subchondral bone surface that may accompany hyperparathyroidism may simulate the findings of septic arthritis, osteonecrosis, or crystal-induced arthropathy. In addition, the presence of these changes in certain joints necessitates inclusion of other differential diagnostic possibilities: In the interphalangeal joints of the hand, the findings may resemble inflammatory osteoarthritis, psoriasis, or even rheumatoid arthritis; in the sacroiliac articulations and symphysis pubis, the differential diagnosis includes ankylosing spondylitis and its variants; in the acromioclavicular and sternoclavicular joints, hyperparathyroid subchondral bone resorption may simulate the changes of rheumatoid arthritis or ankylosing spondylitis; in the patellofemoral joints, the appearance almost is identical to that in Wilson's disease and CPPD crystal deposition disease; and at the discovertebral junction, hyperparathyroidism with subchondral resorption resembles infection, neuropathic osteoarthropathy, or degenerative disc disease. Subligamentous bone resorption in hyperparathyroidism may produce a radiographic appearance that simulates the changes that can be seen in ankylosing spondylitis and related disorders. Localized areas of osseous resorption (brown tumors) in hyperparathyroidism resemble a variety of neoplastic or neoplastic-like diseases, particularly giant cell tumor and fibrous dysplasia.

Bone sclerosis is a radiographic finding of hyperparathyroidism that also can be confused with changes in other diseases. The rugger-jersey spine is a relatively specific finding of the disease, although a somewhat similar vertebral sclerosis may occur in Paget's disease (leading to the "picture frame" vertebral body), osteopetrosis, osteomesopyknosis,[424] and osteoporosis (particularly that associated with excess endogenous or exogenous steroid hormones).[297] Diffuse bone sclerosis, which is more frequent in secondary hyperparathyroidism, also is seen in many other diseases, such as myelofibrosis, fluorosis, mastocytosis (urticaria pigmentosa), anemia (particularly sickle cell anemia), neoplasm (especially metastasis), irradiation, hypoparathyroidism, sarcoidosis, and Paget's disease. Specific differences in the appearance and distribution of the increased bone density as well as associated radiographic findings allow differential diagnosis of these conditions.

CPPD crystal deposition in primary and (less commonly) secondary hyperparathyroidism is identical to that occurring in idiopathic CPPD crystal deposition disease and hemochromatosis. Any patient with chondrocalcinosis should be evaluated for the presence of hyperparathyroidism. In most patients with chondrocalcinosis and hyperparathyroidism, typical radiographic findings of the latter disease are identified readily. Monosodium urate crystal deposition in hyperparathyroidism leads to secondary gout, which resembles primary gout. Involvement of unusual articular sites is more common in secondary gout, however.

In infants and children, periostitis and extensive bone resorption in hyperparathyroidism may simulate the findings of syphilis or leukemia, whereas metaphyseal destruction in the long bones in hyperparathyroidism produces a radiographic picture identical to that of rickets.

RENAL OSTEODYSTROPHY

Background and General Features

In the presence of chronic renal insufficiency, the parathyroid glands undergo hyperplasia of the chief cells, the effect generally being attributable to phosphate retention and consequent lowering of serum calcium level. In childhood or adolescence, the underlying renal disorder frequently is related to structural abnormalities of the urinary tract or, rarely, to chronic inflammatory disease of the kidney. In adults, the underlying renal abnormality may be one of many possible causative conditions including inflammatory disorders, congenital disorders, or obstructive uropathy. Secondary hyperparathyroidism, which is observed as a complication of chronic renal disease, also is seen in other conditions, such as malabsorption states, osteomalacia, and pseudohypoparathyroidism. It is but one of the skeletal changes that occur in patients with chronic renal disease. As normal function of the kidney is fundamental to the proper metabolism of vitamin D, renal diseases can lead to rickets and osteomalacia. Additional changes also are observed in patients with chronic renal disorders. The reader should refer to Chapters 20 and 53 for a discussion of the biochemical aspects of bone changes in patients with chronic renal disease.

Renal osteodystrophy is a term applied to the bone disease that is apparent in patients with chronic renal failure. The term was introduced by Liu and Chu in 1943.[100] Renal osteodystrophy is characterized by radiologic findings that allow precise diagnosis in many persons; it also is associated with characteristic histologic findings. These latter findings can be detected on trocar bone biopsy specimens of the iliac crest, and serial biopsies of this bone may provide important information regarding the progress of the disease.[101]

Osseous abnormalities of renal osteodystrophy have been well outlined.[17–20, 28, 30, 36, 38, 102–108, 396, 408, 409] The pathologic and radiologic findings can be divided into hyperparathyroidism, rickets and osteomalacia, osteoporosis, soft tissue and vascular calcification, and miscellaneous alterations.

Hyperparathyroidism

The abnormalities associated with hyperparathyroidism may become manifest in renal osteodystrophy, including subperiosteal, intracortical, endosteal, trabecular, subchondral, and subligamentous and subtendinous bone resorption, brown tumors, bone sclerosis, and chondrocalcinosis (Fig. 57–22). The frequency of some of these findings is different in renal osteodystrophy with secondary hyperparathyroidism in comparison to primary hyperparathyroidism (Table 57–4). It should be noted, however, that modern techniques

TABLE 57–4. Primary Versus Secondary Hyperparathyroidism

Findings	Primary Hyperparathyroidism	Secondary Hyperparathyroidism*
Brown tumors	Common	Less common
Osteosclerosis	Rare	Common
Chondrocalcinosis	Not infrequent	Rare
Periostitis	Rare	Not infrequent

*Additional findings of renal osteodystrophy are observed in association with secondary hyperparathyroidism, including rickets, osteomalacia, and soft tissue and vascular calcification.

allow the diagnosis of primary hyperparathyroidism to be made at an early stage, when bone abnormalities are not extensive; therefore, many of the osseous changes originally believed to be more frequent in primary than in secondary hyperparathyroidism currently are found to be more typical of the latter.[366]

The frequency of brown tumors in association with renal osteodystrophy and secondary hyperparathryoidism is reported to be lower than the frequency in primary hyperparathyroidism.[19, 46–49, 109–112, 508] In two large series of patients with secondary hyperparathyroidism, the cited prevalence of brown tumors has been 1.5 and 1.7 per cent,[50, 113] although with the introduction of more effective modes of therapy, such as dialysis, the frequency of brown tumors in secondary hyperparathyroidism is expected to change.[289] Brown tumors in renal osteodystrophy generally are single, although Brown and coworkers described a patient with multiple tumors[46] (Fig. 57–23). Rarely, one or more brown tumors are the presenting feature of the disease.[410] As in primary hyperparathyroidism, sites of brown tumors are subject to fracture, and brown tumors may cause pain because of expansion of the cortex.[408] Decrease in size or disappearance of these lesions with or without bone sclerosis has been described after adequate treatment in patients with either primary or secondary hyperparathyroidism.[13, 238]

Osteosclerosis is a well-known feature of renal osteodystrophy (Fig. 57–24). It predominates in the axial skeleton with involvement of the pelvis, ribs, and superior and inferior portions of the vertebral bodies (rugger-jersey spine), although the appendicular skeleton (Fig. 57–25) also may be involved, particularly the metaphyseal regions of long bones. Less commonly, epiphyseal sclerosis resembling ischemic necrosis is seen (Fig. 57–26).[298, 299] Involvement of facial bones may produce a form of leontiasis ossea.[408] It is popular to ascribe osteosclerosis in renal osteodystrophy to hyperparathyroidism, as increased bony radiodensity also is seen in primary hyperparathyroidism (see previous discussion), although other theories for increased bone density have been suggested. Increased bone density probably results from redistribution of mineral rather than from an increase in total skeletal calcium. In patients with osteosclerosis, iliac crest biopsies reveal trabecular thickening and significant fibrosis.[114, 115] It has been suggested that the severe degree of fibrosis and sclerosis in some patients with renal osteodystrophy may compromise marrow function, with hematologic decompensation.[108] Radiologists generally have believed that radiographic monitoring of the distribution and extent of bone sclerosis, especially that of the

Text continued on page 2042

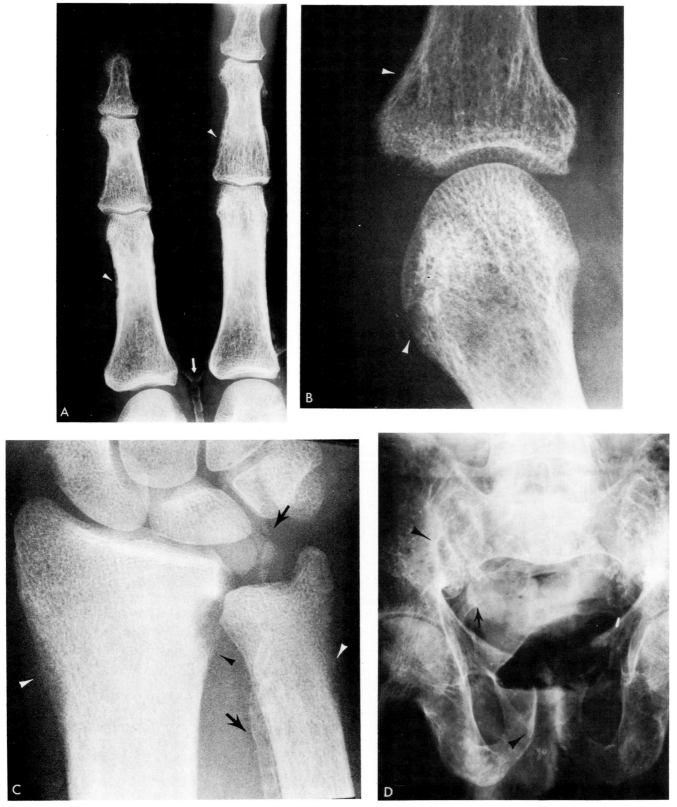

FIGURE 57–22. Renal osteodystrophy: Hyperparathyroidism with bone resorption. **A–D,** In four patients with renal osteodystrophy manifested as vascular and soft tissue calcification (arrows), observe the osseous findings of hyperparathyroidism, including subperiosteal resorption (small arrowheads) and subchondral resorption (large arrowheads).

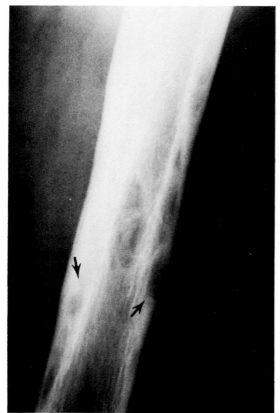

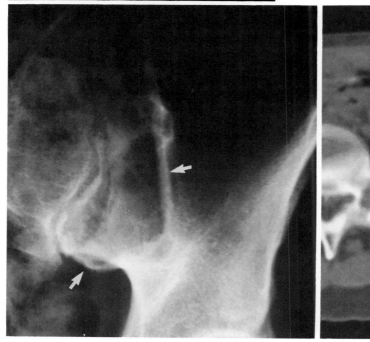

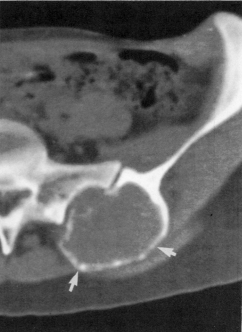

FIGURE 57–23. Renal osteodystrophy: Hyperparathyroidism with brown tumors.

A Multiple cortical radiolucent areas (arrows) represent brown tumors in a patient with chronic renal disease.

B,C In a second patient, a brown tumor has produced an expansile lesion (arrows) adjacent to the left sacroiliac joint.

(**B, C,** Courtesy of A. Newberg, M.D., Boston, Massachusetts.)

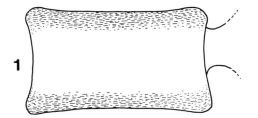

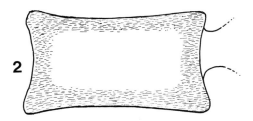

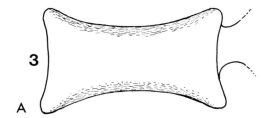

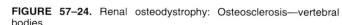

FIGURE 57–24. Renal osteodystrophy: Osteosclerosis—vertebral bodies.

A Vertebral osteosclerosis in renal osteodystrophy is characterized by bandlike sclerosis on the superior and inferior surfaces of the vertebral body (1), an appearance that is termed the rugger-jersey spine. In Paget's disease (2), sclerosis around the entire vertebral body resembles a picture frame. In osteoporosis (3), particularly that associated with steroid excess, biconcave vertebral bodies (fish vertebrae) may be associated with condensation of bone.

B, C Two examples of rugger-jersey spine. In one **(B),** condensation of bone in the superior and inferior margins of the vertebral bodies (arrows) is not associated with osseous collapse. In the other **(C),** similar condensation is associated with biconcave and collapsed vertebral bodies, producing angular kyphosis.

Illustration continued on following page

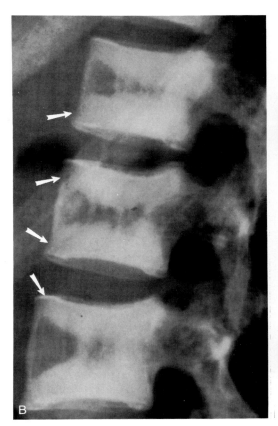

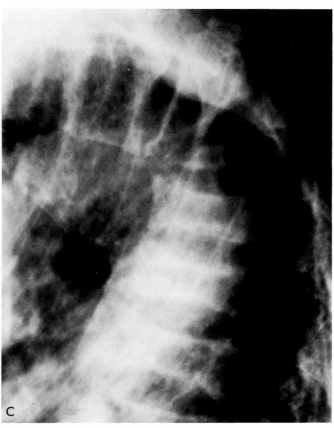

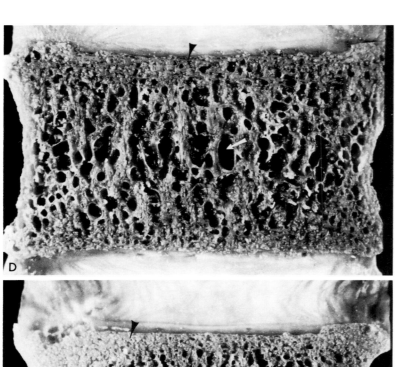

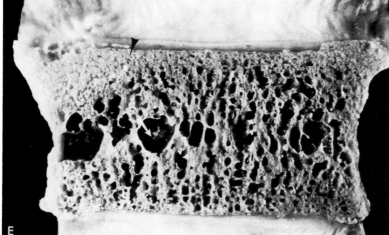

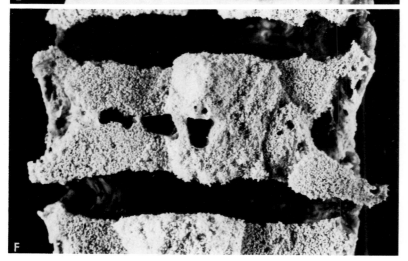

FIGURE 57–24 *Continued*

D–F Photographs of macerated coronal sections of the vertebral bodies reveal progressive findings of osteosclerosis in renal osteodystrophy. Initially **(D, E)** central trabecular resorption (arrows) is associated with mild marginal sclerosis (arrowheads). The process of sclerosis and collapse may become extreme **(F).**

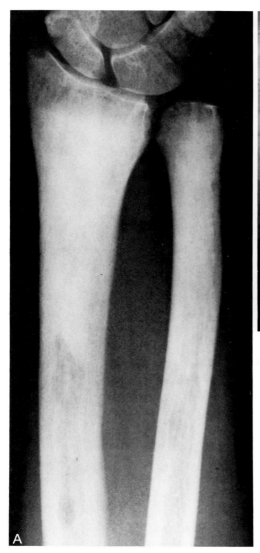

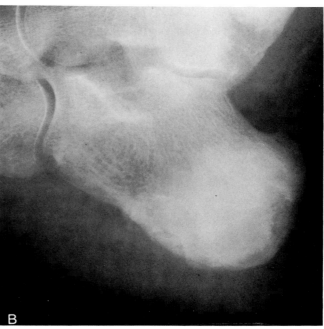

FIGURE 57–25. Renal osteodystrophy: Osteosclerosis—appendicular skeleton. Findings include osteosclerosis of the diaphyses and metaphyses of the radius and ulna and of the posterior surface of the calcaneus. The last-mentioned location is a stressed region in a patient who is bedridden. (Courtesy of L. Cooperstein, M.D., Pittsburgh, Pennsylvania.)

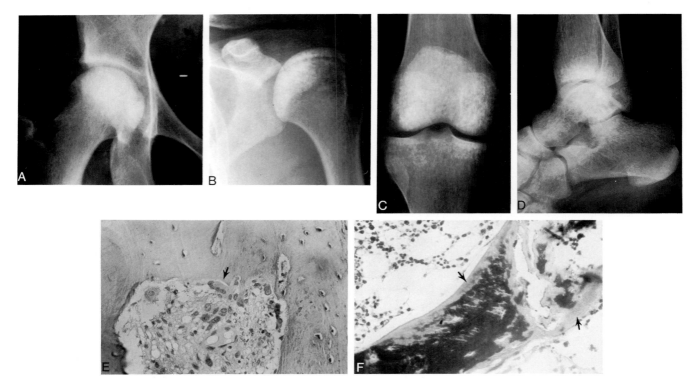

FIGURE 57–26. Renal osteodystrophy: Osteosclerosis—appendicular skeleton. This 25 year old woman with renal failure underwent renal transplantation with subsequent rejection of the donor kidney and has since been on chronic hemodialysis. After removal of diffusely hyperplastic parathyroid glands, some parathyroid tissue was transplanted into the left deltoid muscle. Subsequently, serum calcium levels fluctuated between normal and hypocalcemic values. The patient had not received corticosteroid medication.

A–D Multiple small, punctuate, mottled radiodense lesions, resembling the findings of ischemic necrosis, are evident in the epiphyseal regions of the tubular bones and throughout the tarsus.

E, F A biopsy of the iliac crest revealed changes of hyperparathyroidism, including increased osteoclastic activity and peritrabecular fibrosis (arrows). Similar changes were evident on examination of tissue derived from the medial malleolus.

(From Garver P, et al: AJR *136*:1239, 1981. Copyright 1981, American Roentgen Ray Society.)

vertebrae, is an inaccurate means of studying the progression or remission of renal osteodystrophy.[408]

Chondrocalcinosis due to CPPD crystal deposition is much more frequent in primary hyperparathyroidism than in renal osteodystrophy. The authors have observed carti-lage calcification in the fibrocartilage of the wrist, knee, and symphysis pubis with renal osteodystrophy, but widespread chondrocalcinosis and pyrophosphate arthropathy are unusual manifestations of this disorder (Fig. 57–27).[483]

Periosteal neostosis is a term applied to periosteal bone

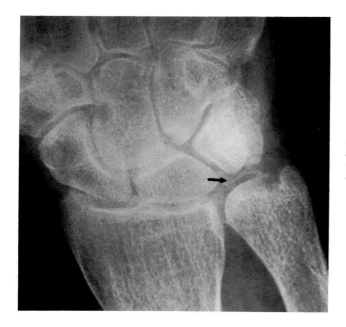

FIGURE 57–27. Renal osteodystrophy: CPPD crystal deposition. Typical chondrocalcinosis (arrow) in the triangular fibrocartilage of the wrist is apparent in a patient with renal osteodystrophy. The bones appear diffusely abnormal.

formation in patients with renal osteodystrophy[116–118] (Fig. 57–28). Its frequency is estimated to be 8 to 25 per cent in such patients,[300] and periostitis is more frequent in those with severe skeletal abnormalities.[373] Periosteal neostosis is observed most commonly in the metatarsals, femur, and pelvis, particularly the pubic rami, although it may be visualized elsewhere, including the humerus, radius, ulna, tibia, metacarpals, and phalanges. A symmetric distribution generally is apparent.[411] Monostotic involvement is infrequent. Frequently, a zone of radiolucency is seen between the periosteal and parent bone, although fusion of the two areas eventually may occur. Periosteal neostosis generally has been considered to be a manifestation of hyperparathyroidism for three reasons[116]: Iliac bone biopsies in patients with periostitis demonstrate predominantly osteitis fibrosa cystica and osteosclerosis; new bone formation is more common in patients with severe hyperparathyroid bone disease; and the woven type of periosteal bone predominates, which is typical of bone disease in hyperparathyroidsm. Periostitis, however, is not a feature of primary hyperparathyroidism. Furthermore, its presence in patients on hemodialysis who do not have findings of hyperparathyroidism has led some investigators to consider periosteal neostosis to be a manifestation of aluminum intoxication with osteomalacia.[380]

Rickets and Osteomalacia

The cause of the osteomalacia seen in chronic renal disease prior to dialysis treatment is not clear; osteomalacia occurring in association with dialysis is discussed later in this chapter. As the kidney is essential in the further hydroxylation of 25-hydroxycholecalciferol to 1,25-dihydroxycholecalciferol, which is an active metabolite of vitamin D, absence of this metabolite in patients with chronic renal disease theoretically could lead to abnormality of bone. Furthermore, patients with renal failure have malabsorption of calcium from the gut, which also can contribute to bone disease. Therefore, osseous change in association with renal disease is easy to explain, although it is much more difficult to pinpoint the exact cause of osteomalacia. Osteomalacia also may relate to vitamin D deficiency as well as resistance, the deficiency occurring as a result of anorexia and inadequate diet, increased requirement of hyperparathyroid bone, and abnormality of the hepatic enzyme system.[119–120] Osteomalacia accompanying renal osteodystrophy has been associated with specific types of kidney disorders, especially chronic pyelonephritis and obstructive uropathy, acidosis, hypocalcemia, and normophosphatemia; its association with the length and severity of uremia is inconsistent.[301] Rachitic abnormalities of bone are common in children with chronic renal disease (Fig. 57–29).[409] These same abnormalities may be noted in children with primary hyperparathyroidism[64, 121–123] (subphyseal bone resorption may be the cause) so that it is difficult to be certain that rickets-like changes occurring in renal osteodystrophy are related to osteomalacia.[124, 302] In fact, histologic evidence of osteomalacia or rickets in patients with chronic renal failure is an infrequent finding; its frequency may increase in children.[303]

The radiographic features of osteomalacia in chronic renal disease are not prominent or easily separated from those related to other forms of bone disease in renal osteo-

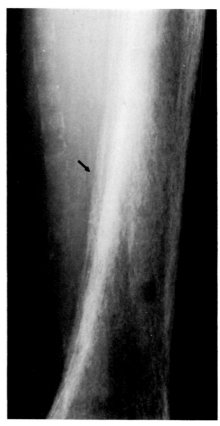

FIGURE 57–28. Renal osteodystrophy: Periosteal neostosis. Frontal radiograph of the femur in a patient with renal osteodystrophy outlines laminated periosteal new bone formation (arrow). Vascular calcification and bony abnormalities are present.

dystrophy; in fact, it generally is believed that renal osteomalacia can be diagnosed confidently only by biopsy.[301] When present, such features include osteopenia (decrease in radiodensity of bone), which also is a sign of osteitis fibrosa cystica itself, and Looser's zones[125, 304] (Fig. 57–30). The latter abnormalities are narrow radiolucent bands, frequently symmetric and oriented perpendicular to the osseous surface. Looser's zones are most common in the pubic rami, ilii, ribs, femoral necks, scapulae, and long bones. They are not common in renal osteodystrophy, having been observed in 1 per cent of patients with chronic renal disease.[40] Radiographic features consistent with rickets include osteopenia, irregularity and widening of the growth plate, and poor definition of the epiphysis (Fig. 57–31).

Slipped epiphyses have been described in chronic renal disease in children.[126–131, 254, 305] Mehls and coworkers[128] observed this finding in approximately 10 per cent of children with this disorder. The capital femoral epiphysis is the most common site of involvement by far, although similar changes may be seen at other skeletal locations, including the proximal end of the humerus; the distal portion of the radius, ulna, or femur; and rarely the small bones of the hands and feet.[414] Bilateral involvement is frequent. Goldman and coworkers[131] have indicated three radiographic signs that may precede slipping of the capital femoral epiphysis in renal osteodystrophy: bilateral subperiosteal erosion on the medial aspect of the femoral neck; increase

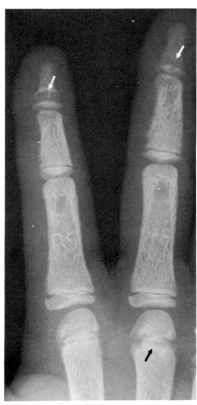

FIGURE 57–29. Renal osteodystrophy: Rickets-like abnormalities. In a child with chronic renal disease, irregularities and widening of the physes (arrows), especially in the metacarpal bones and distal phalanges, are associated with subperiosteal resorption of bone. The physeal alterations could potentially relate to hyperparathyroidism rather than rickets. (Courtesy of C. Resnik, M.D., Baltimore, Maryland.)

in width of the cartilaginous growth plate; and bilateral coxa vara. These imaging signs should alert the physician that a slipped epiphysis may follow, an important warning, as such slips initially may be asymptomatic and a high index of suspicion is required so that diagnosis is established before the onset of irreversible damage. Particular attention should be paid to male adolescents who have been uremic for longer than 2 years or who are beginning hemodialysis or undergoing renal transplantation close to the onset of puberty.[126, 131, 132] Histologically, iliac bone biopsy in patients with epiphysiolysis reveals severe osteitis fibrosa cystica, and metaphyseal regions may contain disorganized trabeculae and woven bone.[133] This histologic evidence may indicate that epiphyseal slipping in chronic renal disease is related to hyperparathyroidism itself, and a similar complication has been seen in patients with primary hyperparathyroidism.[99, 374]

Predilection of this complication for the capital femoral epiphysis is noteworthy, although the cause of this localization is not entirely understood. Subperiosteal resorption on the medial aspect of the femoral neck can result in weakening and collapse, a decrease in the neck-shaft angle, and a change in alignment of the growth plate from horizontal to vertical.[131] This alteration in alignment accentuates shearing forces across the plate, which, coupled with a metaphysis already compromised by the disease process, leads to epiphysiolysis. A similar change in alignment may

explain the occurrence of ischemic necrosis of the femoral head in uremic children who have not received steroid medication or undergone transplantation.[309, 340]

Osteoporosis

A diminution of bone volume occurs in renal osteodystrophy,[134] which, although it is not entirely accurate, may be characterized as osteoporosis. On radiographs, decreased bone density or osteopenia is evident, although the diminished radiodensity is due not only to osteoporosis but also to osteitis fibrosa cystica and osteomalacia. Histologic measurements of iliac bone volume (cancellous bone) have revealed osteopenia in zero to 25 per cent of patients with renal osteodystrophy.[114, 135]

It should be expected that osteoporosis will produce diminution of cortical bone as well. In fact, thinning of cortices is recognized in renal osteodystrophy, although it results not only from osteoporosis but also from endosteal and subperiosteal resorption of hyperparathyroidism.[239]

Fractures

Pathologic fractures (Fig. 57–32) are a recognized complication of renal osteodystrophy and also may occur in primary hyperparathyroidism. Potential causes of such fractures include hyperparathyroidism itself, osteomalacia, osteoporosis, and aluminum intoxication. In the spine, vertebral compression in association with a rugger-jersey appearance commonly is encountered. Fractures in regions of brown tumors also are characteristic. Insufficiency fractures, which in some instances represent Looser's zones of osteomalacia, are seen in patients with renal osteodystrophy. The medial aspect of the femoral neck is an important and common site of such insufficiency fractures.[412] Bilateral involvement at this site is reported in 50 per cent of patients, and the compressive or tensile side of the femoral neck may be affected.[412] Complete fractures of the femoral neck, in a unilateral or bilateral distribution, may be an early manifestation of renal osteodystrophy (or primary hyperparathyroidism).[510] The fracture line typically is vertically oriented near the base of the femoral neck.[413] Other long or short tubular bones and the ribs represent additional sites of fracture in renal osteodystrophy.[511]

Soft Tissue and Vascular Calcification

Although calcification may be observed in the soft tissues and vessels of patients with primary hyperparathyroidism, it is much more frequent in patients with renal osteodystrophy and, in the latter persons, such soft tissue calcification can lead to symptoms and signs that simulate the findings of articular disease. Soft tissue calcification in patients with chronic renal failure occurs when multiplication of the respective concentrations (in mg/dl) of plasma calcium and plasma phosphorus produces a value greater than 70.[136, 137]

Soft tissue deposits can occur in multiple sites, including corneal and conjunctival tissue, viscera, vasculature, and subcutaneous and periarticular tissue (Fig. 57–33).[512] Accumulated evidence has suggested that the chemical nature of the deposited crystal varies according to the anatomic site that is involved[138, 139]: In subcutaneous tissues, vessels, and periarticular regions, hydroxyapatite material (Ca:Mg:P ra-

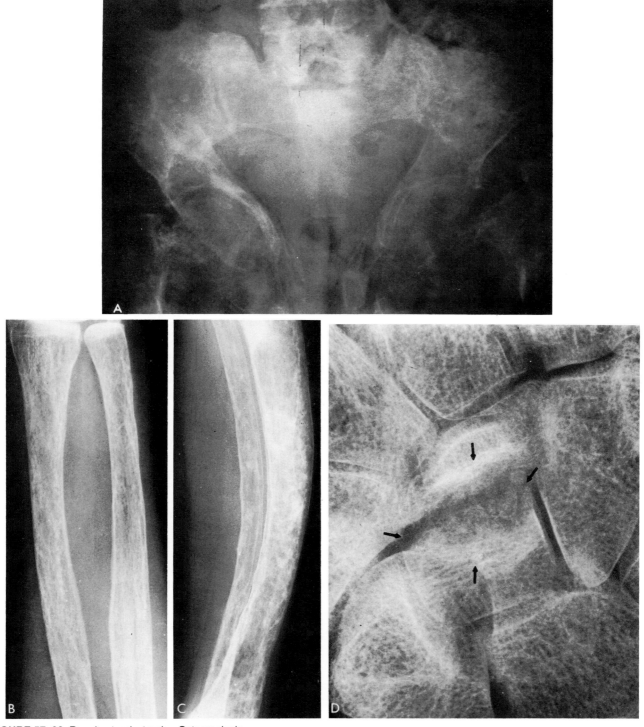

FIGURE 57–30. Renal osteodystrophy: Osteomalacia.
   A–C Observe the bony deformities of the pelvis and tubular bones. Acetabular protrusion, coxa vara, and bowing of the radius, ulna, tibia, and fibula are seen. Trabecular detail virtually is absent.
   D Pseudofracture of the capitate. A spontaneously occurring complete fracture (arrows) has resulted in separation of bony fragments and reactive sclerosis.

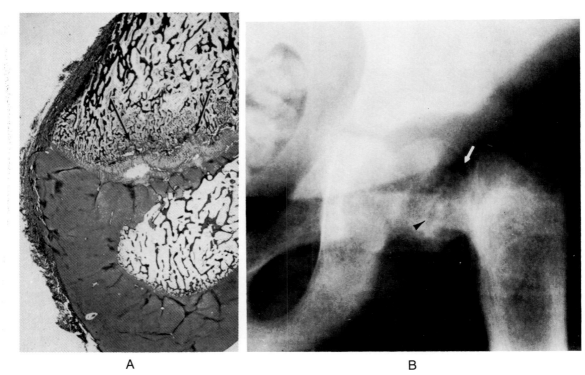

A   B

FIGURE 57–31. Renal osteodystrophy: Rickets.

  A Photomicrograph (4×) of the distal end of the femur in a 3 year old child with chronic renal disease and secondary hyperparathyroidism. The changes of rickets include widening of the proliferating cartilage zone at the cartilaginous growth plate (arrows) with scarring of the intertrabecular marrow and destruction of spongy trabeculae.

  B Note metaphyseal irregularity and resorption (arrow), with surrounding sclerosis, and severe coxa vara. The growth plate (arrowhead) is oriented in a vertical position, which may predispose to epiphyseal slipping.

  (**A,** From Jaffe HL: Metabolic, Degenerative and Inflammatory Diseases of Bones and Joints. Philadelphia, Lea & Febiger, 1972.)

tio of 30:1:18) is observed; in viscera such as the heart, lung, and muscle, magnesium whitlockite-like material (Ca:Mg:P ratio of 4.9:1:4.6) is found. Visceral calcific deposits produce little tissue reaction, whereas the nonvisceral deposits in the soft tissues provoke a fibrotic reaction with encapsulation of the material. This latter response is similar to that observed in idiopathic hydroxyapatite rheumatism, which is discussed in a previous chapter.

  Numerous descriptions have been published of the soft tissue calcifications of chronic renal disease and their response to therapy.[140–142] These deposits are very frequent on histologic examination, particularly in the heart, lungs, stomach, and kidneys,[143] and are less common on radiographic examination.[144] When located in periarticular regions, they may evoke an acute aseptic inflammatory response of soft tissues, including tendon sheaths, which may respond to phenylbutazone.[140, 145, 146] The deposits may occur in patients with chronic uremia who have not been treated, although they appear to be more frequent and extensive in uremic patients who have undergone hemodialysis[140, 142–146] or renal transplantation[147, 148] (see discussion later in this chapter). In one patient with kidney failure and progressive soft tissue calcification, parathyroidectomy was followed by acute apatite-induced periarthritis.[306] Periarticular deposits may reach considerable size and produce striking patchy or tumoral radiodense areas, particularly in the hips, knees, shoulders, and wrists. Bilateral symmetric deposits about multiple joints are not uncommon and, in some

instances, may be associated with radiodense lesions in the joint capsule. Ligamentous calcification (e.g., coracoclavicular and coracoacromial ligaments) also is seen.[417] Osseous erosions beneath periarticular calcific collections[307] and in association with intra-articular hydroxyapatite crystal deposition[308] have been described. In the latter situation, cloud-like calcification in the joint is identical to that seen in idiopathic hydroxyapatite crystal deposition disease (Fig. 57–34).

  Vascular collections involve not only the heart and great vessels but also the peripheral arteries, especially the dorsalis pedis artery of the foot. Calcifications in this location usually appear as linear or circular radiodense areas between the first and second metatarsal bones.[149] Arterial calcification can lead to vascular obstruction with gangrene[137] or heart failure and death.[50] Ischemic skin ulcerations of the fingers, toes, legs, ankles, and thighs, which can be observed in advanced renal failure, may be associated with arterial calcification.[249]

  Meema and Oreopoulos[375] have described in great detail the patterns of vascular calcification in patients with end-stage renal disease, many of whom were receiving hemodialysis or peritoneal dialysis. In addition to linear, pipe stem-like arterial calcifications, small nodular calcifications were noted, often external to the linear deposits. These investigators divided calcifications in the media of the arteries into two types: a benign, slowly progressive type with little or no narrowing of the arterial lumen; and a rapidly progressive type in which massive and often nodular calcification led to displacement of the elastica interna toward the lumen, causing luminal narrowing.

Miscellaneous Abnormalities

Patients with chronic renal insufficiency have hyperuricemia and may develop secondary gouty arthritis (Fig. 57–35). The frequency of acute attacks of gout in these persons is not high, perhaps related to the poor tissue inflammatory response generated in uremic patients. Radiographic features resemble those of primary gout, with asymmetric soft tissue swelling and eccentric osseous erosions, although in secondary gout, atypical articular sites may be affected. Oxalosis of bone may develop as a rare secondary manifestation of chronic renal failure,[150, 151] although similar deposits in the kidney and heart of patients with chronic renal disease are not uncommon,[150, 152, 261, 415] and a familial or primary form of the disease also has been described (see Chapter 48).[153, 258] A possible association of oxalate deposition and dialysis is discussed subsequently.

Musculoskeletal Abnormalities Occurring After Hemodialysis

Although many of the musculoskeletal manifestations in patients treated with hemodialysis, peritoneal dialysis, or

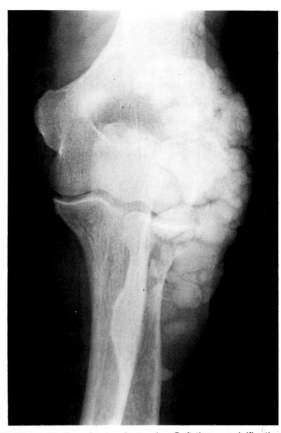

FIGURE 57–33. Renal osteodystrophy: Soft tissue calcification. Extensive "tumoral" calcification is apparent in the periarticular regions of the elbow.

renal transplantation are due to renal osteodystrophy, some of these manifestations are modified during treatment, and additional manifestations may be encountered that relate to the specific mode of therapy (Table 57–5).

In the vast majority of patients with chronic renal failure who are placed on maintenance hemodialysis, many of the bone changes of renal osteodystrophy resolve provided that the hemodialysis is of adequate quality and duration (Fig. 57–36). It should be emphasized, however, that a general statement regarding the osseous response to hemodialysis is difficult owing to the complex histologic aberrations in renal osteodystrophy. With regard to the effect of hemodialysis on hyperparathyroid bone disease, the concentration of calcium in the dialysis fluid is important, as low concentrations may not be sufficient to suppress hyperplastic parathyroid glands, and subsequent parathyroidectomy is required.[50] With higher levels of calcium in the dialysate (7.0 to 8.0 mg/dl), the changes of hyperparathyroidism rarely progress and usually decrease in severity,[154] although other factors also are important, including the intake and plasma level of phosphorus. The effect of hemodialysis on the osteomalacia of chronic renal disease largely is unknown, although some authors suggest osteomalacia may not develop or, when present before dialysis, may not progress during hemodialysis,[40, 155] whereas others support the view that osteomalacia may worsen after hemodialysis.[156, 381] In poorly managed patients on dialysis, increasing osteopenia may be observed in association with spontaneous fractures

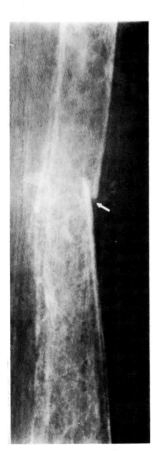

FIGURE 57–32. Renal osteodystrophy: Osteoporosis. On a lateral view of the femur, severe osteoporosis has resulted in medullary widening, cortical diminution, and a pathologic fracture (arrow) of the diaphysis. The cortices, although thinned, appear relatively distinct.

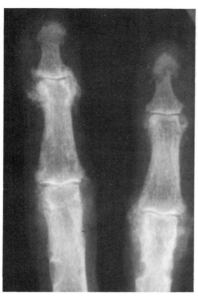

FIGURE 57–34. Renal osteodystrophy: Periarticular and intra-articular calcification. Findings include radiodense foci within and about multiple interphalangeal joints. Acro-osteolysis and subperiosteal bone resorption are additional features. (Courtesy of T. Broderick, M.D., Orange, California.)

TABLE 57–5. Musculoskeletal Abnormalities Following Dialysis and Renal Transplantation

Hyperparathyroidism
Osteomalacia and rickets
Osteosclerosis
Fractures
Soft tissue and vascular calcification
Osteomyelitis and septic arthritis
Osteonecrosis
Crystal deposition
Destructive spondyloarthropathy
Amyloidosis
Carpal tunnel syndrome
Digital clubbing
Aluminum toxicity
Dialysis cysts
Olecranon bursitis

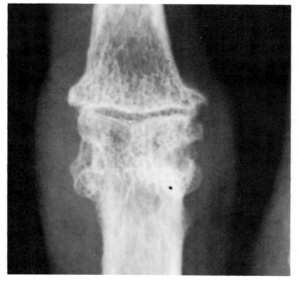

A

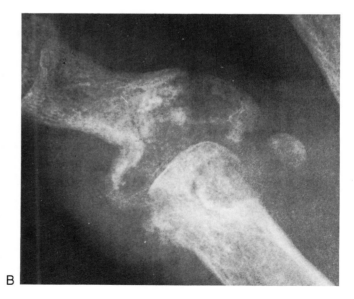

B

FIGURE 57–35. Renal osteodystrophy: Secondary gout.
  A Observe considerable osseous proliferation and soft tissue swelling about the proximal interphalangeal joint in a patient with chronic renal disease and documented gout.
  B In a different patient with chronic renal disease, monosodium urate crystals were recovered from this destroyed first metacarpophalangeal joint.
  (**B,** Courtesy of D. Alarcón-Segovia, M.D., Mexico City, Mexico.)

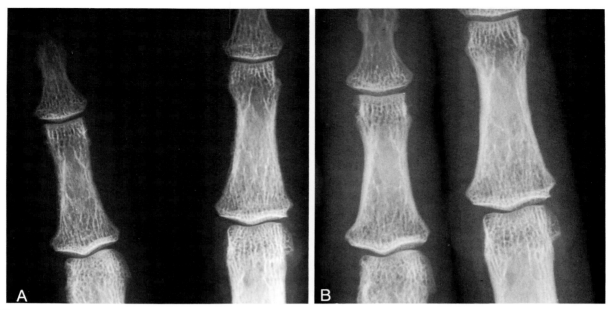

FIGURE 57–36. Renal osteodystrophy: Resolution of skeletal abnormalities during hemodialysis. In this 38 year old man on maintenance hemodialysis, radiographs obtained 4 years apart reveal significant improvement in the osseous abnormalities.

(Fig. 57–37).[157] These fractures are most frequent in the ribs, although they are seen at other skeletal sites, including the femoral necks, vertebrae, pubic rami, tibiae, and metatarsals. The fractures may be symmetric, and it is not uncommon to see multiple bilateral rib fractures in this clinical setting.

Aluminum Intoxication. It now is generally believed that the primary cause of the progression of skeletal abnormalities in patients (adults or children) on chronic regular hemodialysis is osteomalacia due to aluminum intoxication (Fig. 57–37).[301, 310–313, 376–378, 425, 427, 429, 431] Clinical characteristics of this syndrome include bone pain, myopathy, fracture, and dialysis encephalopathy accompanied by dementia, speech disorder, seizures, and dyspraxia.[314–320, 379] Fractures of the ribs and proximal portion of the femora are characteristic,[427, 428, 488] although the spine and other tubular bones may be affected.[430, 432] (Fig. 57–37). High aluminum levels in tissues, including the brain and bone[324] as well as various articular structures (synovial membrane, cartilage, joint fluid),[322] support the speculation that aluminum toxicity is involved in this syndrome.[316] The source of the aluminum can be related to the contents of phosphate binding gels or the ambient water or dialysate; elevation of serum levels of this metal and a higher frequency of this syndrome are evident when the dialysate or ambient water contains high concentrations of aluminum. Aluminum-induced changes, however, are documented in patients with chronic renal disease who have not undergone dialysis, and, in such cases, considerable evidence exists that aluminum is absorbed from the orally administered aluminum-containing phosphate-binding medications that are prescribed for patients with renal failure.[426] Reversal of the findings may follow the removal of sources of aluminum contamination[316, 321, 323]; clinical improvement precedes radiographic improvement, the latter characterized by healing of fractures and osteosclerosis, especially in the metaphyseal regions.[321] Other factors, not completely understood, probably contribute to dialysis encephalopathy and osteopathy. A more complete discussion of aluminum intoxication is contained in Chapter 76.

It is obvious that the issues concerning the effects of hemodialysis on the bone aberrations of renal osteodystrophy are complex. Furthermore, no uniformly reliable clinical, biochemical, or radiologic findings are found that are predictive of the specific type of histologic abnormality that is present (i.e., hyperparathyroidism, osteomalacia, osteoporosis). Symptoms and signs bear no relation to the type and severity of the histologic changes; serum concentrations of alkaline phosphatase and parathyroid hormone are of some use in detecting hyperparathyroidism but are of little value in assessing osteomalacia; and radiographic signs are not sufficiently sensitive for diagnostic purposes.[381] Ultimately, bone biopsy may be required in the evaluation of dialysis osteopathy.

Soft Tissue and Vascular Calcification. Soft tissue and vascular calcification is frequent in patients undergoing hemodialysis (Fig. 57–38).[145, 146, 148] In an autopsy study of 56 dialyzed patients, Kuzela and associates[143] observed foci of soft tissue calcification in more than one internal viscus in approximately 80 per cent of patients. Calcification was classified as severe in 35 per cent of these dialysis patients. Metastatic calcification has been reported to progress during maintenance hemodialysis therapy[158] and to worsen with increasing duration of dialysis.[159] Other investigators have found no relationship between the presence and severity of soft tissue calcification and the duration of dialysis, patient's age, degree of parathyroid gland hyperplasia, radiographic evidence of soft tissue calcification, serum calcium and phosphorus levels, serum calcium and phosphorus products, or type and severity of metabolic bone disease.[143] Reversal of periarticular and, less commonly, vascular calcification may be seen during dialysis.[136, 160, 240] Progression

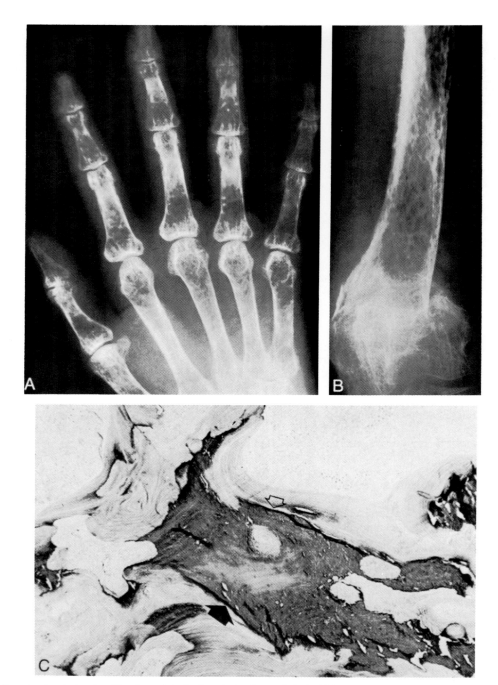

FIGURE 57–37. Renal osteodystrophy: Aluminum intoxication during hemodialysis. This 52 year old man with end-stage renal disease was maintained on hemodialysis for 18 years. He developed gradually progressive and severe skeletal pain in both the upper and lower extremities. Pain was unresponsive to administration of oral vitamin D compounds and calcium and to total parathyroidectomy. The patient had been ingesting oral aluminum hydroxide gels. The serum calcium, phosphorus, and alkaline phosphatase levels remained within normal limits.

　A A radiograph of the hand reveals marked osteopenia with indistinctness of the cortical margins and trabeculae.

　B The radiograph of the lower femur shows osteopenia, cortical tunneling, and a supracondylar fracture with insignificant callus formation 1 year after the injury.

　C A biopsy specimen of the iliac crest with histologic analysis shows large quantities of excessive lamellar osteoid, the absence of active hyperparathyroidism, and the presence of aluminum deposition at the interface between the mineralized bone and excessive osteoid (arrows).

　(From Llewellyn CH, et al: Skel Radiol *12*:223, 1984.)

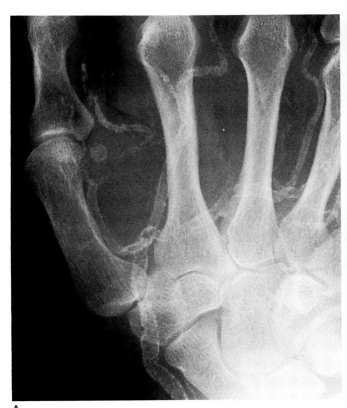

A

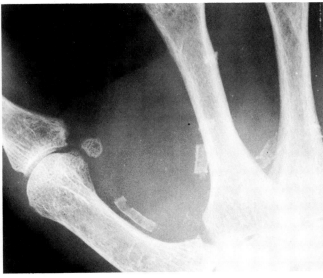

B

FIGURE 57–38. Vascular calcification: Effect of hemodialysis. Observe the extreme vascular calcification that was present prior to the onset of dialysis **(A)** and its marked improvement after dialysis **(B)**.

of such calcification, however, is a more typical finding and, in the case of vascular calcification, may lead to narrowing of the lumen of the artery.[375]

Musculoskeletal Infection. Septicemia, osteomyelitis, and septic arthritis are well-recognized complications of hemodialysis (as well as renal transplantation).[161, 393] External or internal arteriovenous fistulae provide an ideal site of entry for infectious organisms.[257] This fact, combined with impaired host resistance related to the presence of a chronic debilitating illness and the use of immunosuppressive agents and adrenal steroids, increases the risk of infection in these persons. Osteomyelitis and septic arthritis may occur at any site,[162] and any type of organism may be implicated, including Staphylococcus, Streptococcus, Pseudomonas, Mycobacterium, and fungi.[161] Typical radiologic signs of infection will become apparent, although radionuclide examination usually will allow earlier diagnosis of infection in these patients. In interpreting the bone scan, the physician must be aware of the radionuclide patterns related to hyperparathyroidism or renal osteodystrophy itself.[163, 164, 251, 252, 262, 263, 325] These patterns may be characterized by a diffuse increase in skeletal radionuclide uptake, although bone scintigraphy in uremic patients is complicated by delayed or absent renal radiotracer excretion, which itself may lead to increased skeletal uptake and elevated soft tissue levels of activity.[252] Despite this complication, bone scintigraphy may be useful in monitoring patients with renal osteodystrophy, as total skeletal activity appears dependent on the severity of the osseous changes, particularly those of hyperparathyroidism and osteomalacia.

Osteonecrosis. Ischemic necrosis of bone may complicate the administration of steroids in patients with chronic renal disease undergoing dialysis. (This same complication is well recognized as occurring after renal transplantation and is discussed later in this chapter.) Bailey and coworkers, however, reported 23 dialysis patients with osteonecrosis of the femoral heads in whom recent corticosteroid therapy had not been used.[165] Although the radiographic manifestations of osseous collapse and fragmentation in these persons may have been due to subchondral resorption of bone, additional reports of osteonecrosis in dialysis patients who were not receiving corticosteroids have appeared.[433, 434] Affected sites have included the femoral and humeral heads and the talus.

Destructive Spondyloarthropathy. A peculiar pattern of spondyloarthropathy has been identified in patients with chronic renal disease who have been undergoing hemodialysis.[326, 327, 394, 397–399, 435–445, 489] Middle-aged or elderly men or women who have been hemodialyzed for a period of years are affected. The estimated frequency of destructive spondyloarthropathy in patients undergoing hemodialysis has varied from five per cent to 23 per cent. Evidence of secondary hyperparathyroidism commonly is lacking. Mild to moderate back or neck pain is seen. Single or multiple spinal levels, especially in the cervical or lumbar segment, reveal rapidly progressive radiographic abnormalities characterized by loss of intervertebral disc space, erosion of subchondral bone in the neighboring vertebral bodies, and new bone formation (Fig. 57–39). The findings resemble infection, neuropathic osteoarthropathy, severe intervertebral (osteo)chondrosis, or calcium pyrophosphate dihydrate crystal deposition disease.

Histologic analysis has indicated consistently the absence of infection, although the precise cause of the spinal abnor-

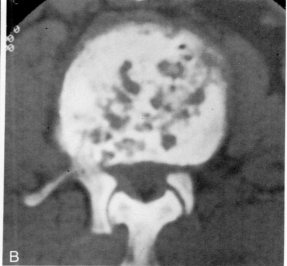

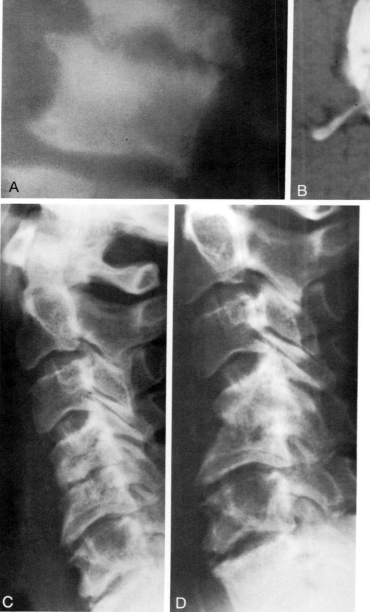

FIGURE 57–39. Renal osteodystrophy: Spondyloarthropathy during hemodialysis.

A, B In this patient with chronic renal disease who was maintained on hemodialysis, clinical and radiographic abnormalities in the lumbar spine progressed over an 11 year period. Serum parahormone levels were slightly elevated. A lateral conventional tomogram of the spine **(A)** delineates loss of height of the intervertebral disc, erosion of the subchondral bone of two adjacent vertebral bodies, extreme bone sclerosis, and subluxation. The findings resemble those of infection, CPPD crystal deposition disease, cartilaginous node formation, or neuropathic osteoarthropathy. A transaxial CT scan **(B)** shows multiple radiolucent foci within a sclerotic vertebral body. Histologic analysis of material derived from a biopsy of the spinal lesion indicated cartilage debris and osseous reaction with no evidence of infection or crystal accumulation. A search for amyloidosis was not undertaken.

C, D In a different patient with chronic renal failure who was receiving hemodialysis, radiographs obtained 7 months apart show progressive destruction of the C4-C5 intervertebral disc and both adjacent vertebral bodies. An osteolytic lesion in C6 also is evident.

(A, B, Courtesy of P. Kaplan, M.D., Charlottesville, Virginia.)

malities has been debated. Initial reports emphasized the importance of hydroxyapatite or oxalate crystal deposition in the pathogenesis of the spondyloarthropathy of hemodialysis.[436] Such crystal accumulation appears to be a secondary phenomenon, however. Some investigators have suggested that severe hyperparathyroidism, possibly resulting in subchondral bone resorption, is a causative factor, citing the occurrence of spinal changes in those patients who have undergone hemodialysis for years, in those with elevated levels of immunoreactive parathyroid hormone, and in those whose bone biopsies show histologic evidence of severe hyperparathyroidism.[439, 442] The documentation of similar vertebral abnormalities in patients with chronic renal failure who have not received hemodialysis therapy indirectly supports the etiologic importance of secondary hyperparathyroidism in this condition.[446] Dynamic radiography, accomplished with flexion and extension views of the affected cervical spine, has revealed evidence of ligament laxity, implicating a possible role of spinal instability in the causation of this destructive spondyloarthropathy.[440] Although each of these factors may contribute to the development or progression of the vertebral alterations, accumulating data underscore the importance of amyloid deposition in regions of spinal destruction.[382, 400, 435, 437, 438, 444, 445] Amyloid masses, composed of beta-2-microglobulins, have been documented repeatedly not only in the vertebral column but also in other skeletal and extraskeletal sites in patients undergoing chronic hemodialysis (see later discussion).

Of further interest has been the documentation of unusual forms of destructive spondyloarthropathy accompanying chronic dialysis, as well as the investigation of such spondyloarthropathy with newer imaging methods, such as MR imaging. Although the typical features of spinal involvement in chronic hemodialysis include erosion of adjacent vertebral bodies, disc space loss, and subchondral bone sclerosis at one or several levels in the cervical or lumbar segment, more localized areas of bone destruction may become evident. Osteolytic lesions within a vertebral body may be accompanied by pathologic fracture, simulating the

appearance of an aggressive bone tumor.[445] Similar "amyloidomas" have been encountered in other skeletal sites in patients with chronic renal disease receiving hemodialysis therapy (see later discussion). Furthermore, long segments of the cervical spine may be involved, and the appearance of multiple subluxations in some patients resembles that seen in rheumatoid arthritis.[443]

Extensive alterations of the occipitoatlantoaxial region may accompany long-term hemodialysis (Fig. 57–40). Cystic lesions in the atlas or axis, including the odontoid process, have been encountered.[447, 448] Synovial hypertrophy in the anterior and posterior median atlantoaxial joints produces soft tissue masses that surround the dens.[449, 450] The odontoid process may be eroded or it may fracture, and atlantoaxial subluxation is an accompanying feature. The resulting radiographic features resemble those of rheumatoid arthritis. Although affected patients may be asymptomatic,[448] such changes can produce local and referred pain.[450] The cause of occipitoatlantoaxial destruction in hemodialyzed patients with chronic renal failure again appears to be accumulation of amyloid masses composed of beta-2-microglobulins.

MR imaging has been used to study the spondyloarthropathy that accompanies long-term hemodialysis.[438, 441, 444, 448–452] In an analysis of three patients with cervical spine involvement using MR imaging, Rafto and coworkers[441] indicated that the observed findings differed from those of infective spondylitis, being characterized by low signal intensity in the involved intervertebral discs on T1-weighted spin echo MR images that persisted on T2-weighted spin echo images and the absence of paraspinal masses. Naidich and collaborators,[438] however, described one patient with similar cervical alterations who revealed increased signal intensity in the affected disc and adjacent portions of the vertebral bodies on T2-weighted spin echo MR images. Naito and coworkers,[444] in common with Rafto's group,[441] emphasized the persistence of low signal intensity in affected regions of the cervical and lumbar segments of the spine in T2-weighted (as well as T2*-weighted) MR im-

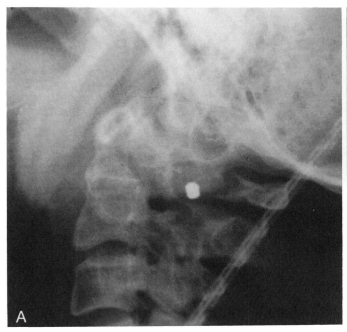

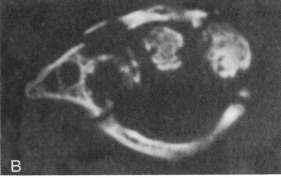

FIGURE 57–40. Renal osteodystrophy: Spondyloarthropathy during hemodialysis. In this patient on long-term hemodialysis, findings include bone destruction of the atlas, odontoid erosions, a pathologic fracture at the base of the dens, fractures of the ring of the atlas, and posterior atlantoaxial subluxation. (Courtesy of S. Moreland, M.D., San Diego, California.)

FIGURE 57–41. Renal osteodystrophy: Carpal tunnel syndrome and amyloid deposition during hemodialysis.

A In this 56 year old man who had been maintained on hemodialysis for 5 years owing to renal failure secondary to chronic glomerulonephritis, wrist pain of several months' duration was accompanied by soft tissue swelling and findings of a carpal tunnel syndrome. A radiograph of the wrist that had been obtained 2 years previously was normal. Observe soft tissue swelling and cystic lesions in the scaphoid, lunate, capitate, and ulna. During a carpal tunnel release, a biopsy of the synovium and distal portion of the ulna revealed tissue that demonstrated chronic synovitis with amyloid deposition in both the synovium and the bone.

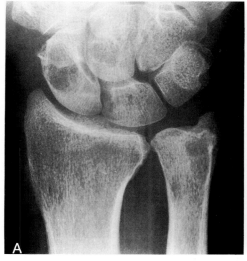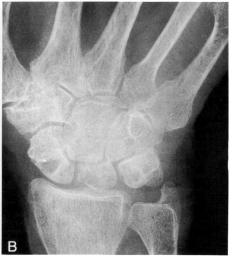

B In a 73 year old woman with chronic renal failure who had been undergoing hemodialysis for several years, a carpal tunnel syndrome developed in both wrists requiring bilateral operative releases. A radiograph of the wrist prior to surgery shows cystic lesions in the scaphoid, lunate, and triquetrum. Histologic analysis of the synovium and material in the lunate showed synovial thickening and amyloid deposition. Similar radiographic and pathologic findings were present on the opposite side.

(Courtesy of G. Greenway, M.D., Dallas, Texas.)

ages. Inconsistent results employing MR imaging also have been encountered in the analysis of occipitoatlantoaxial destruction accompanying hemodialysis. Persistent low signal intensity about the odontoid process on both T1-weighted and T2-weighted spin echo MR images has been observed by Rousselin and associates[449]; however Stäbler and collaborators,[452] using both spin echo and gradient echo MR images, reported cases in which regions of high signal intensity in and about the odontoid process were observed on the gradient echo images. The effectiveness of MR imaging in delineating the spinal cord and its relationship to displaced vertebral bodies and any paraspinal masses has been established repeatedly in patients with dialysis spondyloarthropathy. It is the specificity of the MR findings, particularly with regard to those of infective spondylitis, that is in question.

Carpal Tunnel Syndrome. The carpal tunnel syndrome, with pain, dysesthesias, weakness, and sensory changes in the hands of uremic patients receiving hemodialysis, is well recognized and usually is attributed to alterations in vascular hemodynamics at the access site, resulting in edema, venous distention, and secondary compression of the median nerve within the carpal canal.[241, 328–330, 383, 453] Men and women both are affected, findings are unilateral or bilateral, and the rate of occurrence of the abnormalities is related directly to the length of dialysis.[328] Histologic features indicate amyloid deposition in the synovium and adjacent tendons.[331, 384, 385, 395, 401, 402, 454, 509] Amyloid accumulation also occurs in accompanying small cystic lesions in the carpal bones (Fig. 57–41). As such lesions occasionally are observed elsewhere in the hands of patients undergoing chronic hemodialysis and are termed dialysis cysts, it is interesting to speculate that secondary amyloidosis is the cause of these cysts.

Amyloid Deposition. The association of amyloid deposition with hemodialysis now is well established. Although multiple skeletal sites may be affected, the accumulation of beta-2-microglobulin in patients undergoing hemodialysis

appears to have first been emphasized in the wrist and as an accompaniment of the carpal tunnel syndrome. As summarized by Ullian and associates,[454] beta-2-microglobulin is a protein consisting of 100 amino acid residues and one disulfide bridge. Its daily production normally is 150 to 200 mg. Virtually all of the beta-2-microglobulin that is unassociated with cells is filtered freely by the normal glomerulus, reabsorbed by the epithelium in the proximal tubules of the kidney, and catabolized to amino acids. Serum concentrations of beta-2-microglobulin in patients with normal renal function range from 1 to 2 mg/liter; concentrations in patients undergoing chronic hemodialysis are 40 to 50 times higher.

Beta-2-microglobulin–associated amyloidosis accompanying chronic hemodialysis appears to affect predominantly the musculoskeletal system. Accumulating data related to its importance in the pathogenesis of destructive spondyloarthropathy and carpal tunnel syndrome have been cited earlier in this chapter, but its effects are far more widespread. Periarticular soft tissue masses, cystic lesions in long and short tubular bones and in flat and irregular bones, pathologic fractures, joint subluxations and dislocations, digital contractures, and other abnormalities may be observed in one or more sites in the axial and appendicular skeleton. Amyloid deposition may lead to arthralgias and arthropathies, especially in the shoulders but also in the hips, wrists, and other joints; amyloidomas in periarticular bone may produce radiolucent lesions of variable size that may fracture, particularly in the femoral necks and vertebrae but in additional sites as well; amyloid accumulation in soft tissues may produce neurovascular compromise, most evident about the wrist; and masses of amyloid may extend from affected vertebral bodies and intervertebral discs into the spinal canal, leading to significant neurologic compromise. Although other factors (including hyperparathyroidism, deposition of calcium oxalate, hydroxyapatite, and pyrophosphate dihydrate crystals, and accumulation of iron[455] and aluminum[456]) may be contributory, especially

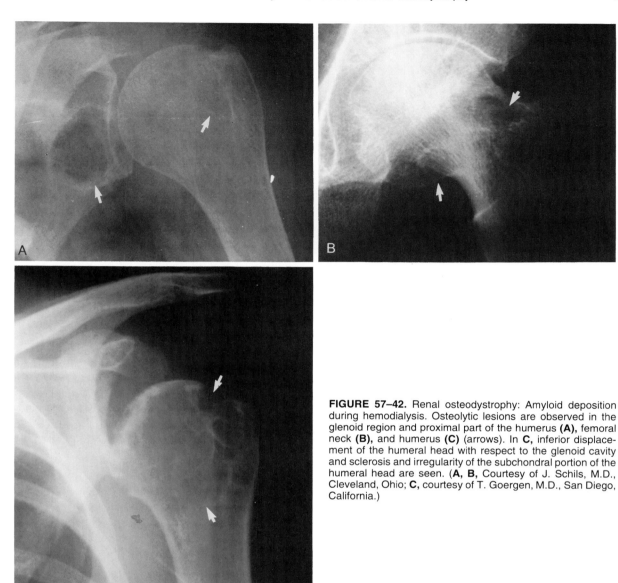

FIGURE 57–42. Renal osteodystrophy: Amyloid deposition during hemodialysis. Osteolytic lesions are observed in the glenoid region and proximal part of the humerus **(A),** femoral neck **(B),** and humerus **(C)** (arrows). In **C,** inferior displacement of the humeral head with respect to the glenoid cavity and sclerosis and irregularity of the subchondral portion of the humeral head are seen. **(A, B,** Courtesy of J. Schils, M.D., Cleveland, Ohio; **C,** courtesy of T. Goergen, M.D., San Diego, California.)

with regard to the arthropathy of hemodialysis, gross pathologic and histologic evidence of amyloid infiltration in bones, joints, and soft tissues of patients with chronic renal disease undergoing hemodialysis is undeniable.[457]

Amyloid deposition in soft tissue, joint capsule, and synovium may lead to prominent periarticular masses about the shoulders, knees, hips, wrists, and other sites.[458] Such deposition can be verified on histologic examination of the synovial membrane[459] as well as by microscopic evaluation of the synovial fluid.[460] Amyloid accumulation also can be documented in capsular and ligamentous tissue.[461] Osteolytic lesions are identified in the femoral neck,[461, 463–466] acetabulum,[461, 463, 464] carpal bones,[461, 462, 464, 465] humerus,[461, 462, 464–466] radius,[461] patella,[462] talus,[464] clavicle,[466] pubic bones,[466] glenoid cavity,[466] and many other sites (Fig. 57–42). They frequently are multiple, may be bilateral, and can increase in size and number.[462] The lesions are well defined,

with geographic bone destruction, and may be septated with a sclerotic margin. They affect both central and marginal regions of periarticular bone and, when large, may lead to collapse of the articular surface. Pathologic fractures of these cystic lesions are well documented,[436, 467–471] especially in the femoral neck (Fig. 57–43). Histologic examination confirms that amyloid accumulation is a common, although not invariable, finding in regions of bone destruction. Other alterations associated with amyloidosis in hemodialyzed patients include spontaneous tendon rupture, trigger finger, and flexor tendon contracture.[470]

The articular manifestations of dialysis-associated amyloidosis also are varied. An oligoarticular distribution is typical. A preference for involvement of large joints has been noted in some reports,[472] although widespread and severe alterations in small joints, even those of the hand, have been observed.[473, 474] It should be noted, however, that

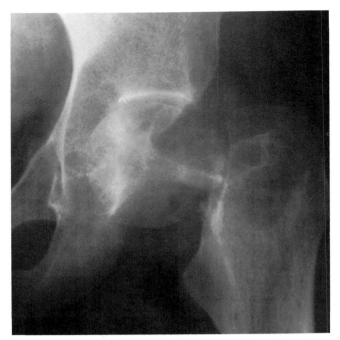

FIGURE 57–43. Renal osteodystrophy: Amyloid deposition during hemodialysis leading to pathologic fracture. Note the displaced fracture of the femoral neck with osteolytic destruction of the femoral head and neck. Additional destructive lesions of the acetabulum and pubic ramus are present. (Courtesy of A. Newberg, M.D., Boston, Massachusetts.)

mechanisms other than amyloid deposition may be operative in some patients with dialysis-related arthropathy, and it is difficult to define the importance of hyperparathyroidism itself and of aluminum, iron, and crystalline accumulation in this regard. That beta-2-microglobulin amyloid can infiltrate a variety of articular structures in the clinical setting of long-term hemodialysis is clear, however. Indeed, the type and severity of clinical manifestations related to joint involvement may be dependent on the distribution and extent of intra-articular amyloid deposition. Asymptomatic patients may have such deposition in the synovial membrane, but it is mainly in a superficial location and is less extensive; more prominent amyloid accumulation in the synovial membrane can explain the frequency of joint effusions owing to disturbances in the turnover of synovial fluid, and massive accumulation of amyloid in deeper intra-articular and periarticular structures may account for soft tissue prominence that is detected on physical examination.[472] The occurrence of articular destruction in dialysis-related arthropathy, even if related solely to amyloidosis, can be the result of several different mechanisms. Osseous involvement in subchondral locations may produce weakening, fracture, and collapse of joint surfaces; synovial collections of amyloid may invade marginal regions of intra-articular bone directly; and amyloid accumulation in cartilage also may be a causative factor in joint destruction. As deposition of amyloid in articular cartilage is a well-documented occurrence in asymptomatic, elderly persons,[475] the clinical significance of beta-2-microglobulin accumulation in such cartilage in patients receiving long-term hemodialysis could be questioned. Solé and coworkers,[472] however, have presented histologic evidence that this accumulation of amyloid may not be innocuous. These inves-

tigators noted the prominence of amyloid deposition in capsulosynovial insertions in dialysis-related arthropathy, contrasting this pattern of deposition with the localized chondral collections that characterize benign senile amyloidosis. Furthermore, Solé and colleagues[472] have speculated that beta-2-microglobulin amyloid may spread from these insertional sites along the superficial layers of cartilage, leading initially to surface fibrillation and irregularities and subsequently to deep fissures.

MR imaging has been used to investigate dialysis-related arthropathy.[476–478] This method is effective in the demonstration of the full extent of intra-articular involvement and reveals generally that subchondral intraosseous collections of amyloid communicate with the articular surface.[476, 478] The reported signal characteristics of dialysis-related arthropathy have not been uniform, however. Kokubu and associates[476] showed regions of low signal intensity corresponding to sites of amyloid accumulation. Claudon and investigators[477] described a more variable MR appearance; the reported findings included regions of low signal intensity on both T1- and T2-weighted spin echo MR images, of high signal intensity on both T1- and T2-weighted images, and of low signal intensity on T1-weighted images with high signal intensity on T2-weighted images (Fig. 57–44). Of these patterns, the first and third were most frequent and were consistent with either fibrous tissue (persistent low signal intensity on both T1- and T2-weighted images) or fluid (low signal intensity on T1-weighted images and high signal intensity on T2-weighted images) within the intraosseous lesions. The second pattern (high signal intensity on both T1- and T2-weighted spin echo images), combined with the results of short tau inversion recovery (STIR) imaging, in which persistent low signal intensity was seen, suggested the presence of a fatty component. As histologic evidence of amyloid deposition was lacking in this report, the precise cause of the various MR patterns was not clear. Cobby and associates,[478] using MR imaging to investigate four patients with histologically proved (three patients) or radiographically suspected (one patient) dialysis-related amyloid arthropathy, found that the signal characteristics of the amyloid deposition were intermediate between those of fibrocartilage or muscle on all spin echo MR sequences, distinguishing the deposition from cellular lesions or those containing large amounts of water, such as inflammatory masses, acute or chronic synovitis, and brown tumors of hyperparathyroidism (Fig. 57–45). These investigators also used a fat-suppression technique (Dixon sequence) in two patients, which enhanced the visualization of amyloid deposits in one patient.

Although inconsistencies in results and variations in interpretation are evident, it is certain, on the basis of a review of available literature, that amyloid accumulation in osseous and articular structures is a prominent feature of hemodialysis in patients with chronic renal disease; that the prevalence and extent of such accumulation increase with the duration of hemodialysis; that periarticular soft tissue prominence, intraosseous and subchondral bone destruction, pathologic fracture, and the carpal tunnel syndrome are characteristic clinical and radiographic features of amyloid accumulation; that the variety of amyloid in this clinical setting is a beta-2-microglobulin; and that such amyloid deposition must be considered one important factor, in addition to hyperparathyroidism, aluminum intoxication, and

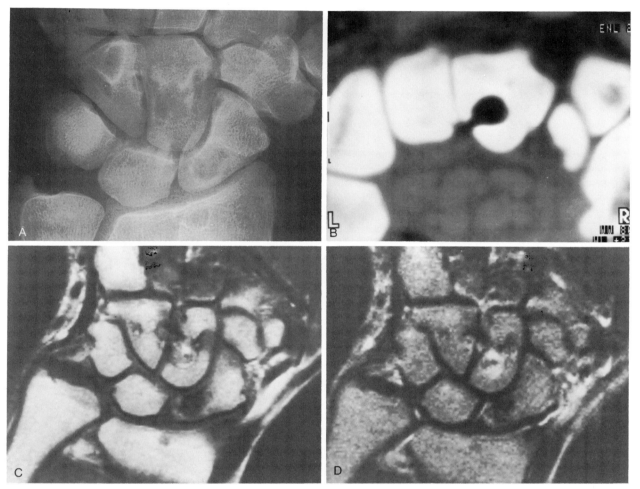

FIGURE 57–44. Renal osteodystrophy: Dialysis arthropathy with MR imaging abnormalities. This 45 year old man had a 10 year history of hemodialysis and had been treated with a renal allograft 5 years previously.

    A The conventional radiograph shows radiolucent lesions in the radius, scaphoid, capitate, and hamate. The articular spaces are normal.

    B CT reveals that the radiolucent lesion of the capitate communicates with the surface of the bone. The lesion had low attenuation values (−110 HU).

    C, D Coronal T1-weighted (TR/TE, 500/26) **(C)** and T2-weighted (TR/TE, 2000/150) **(D)** spin echo MR images are shown. In **C,** heterogeneous but high signal intensity is noted in the capitate lesion; in **D,** areas of high signal intensity persist. The scaphoid lesion is of low signal intensity in both images.

    (From Claudon M, et al: J Comput Assist Tomogr *14*:968, 1990.)

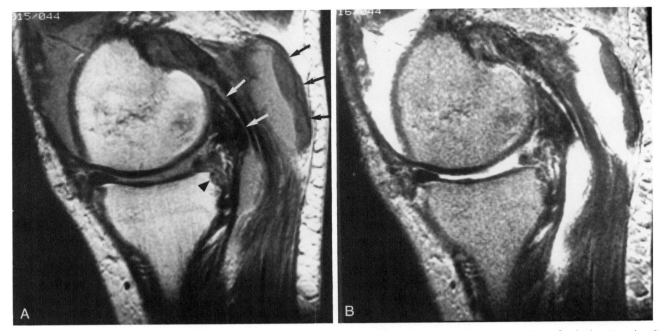

FIGURE 57–45. Renal osteodystrophy: Dialysis arthropathy related to amyloidosis with MR imaging abnormalities. Sagittal proton density (TR/TE, 2500/25) **(A)** and T2-weighted (TR/TE, 2500/80) **(B)** MR images are illustrated in a patient with biopsy-confirmed amyloidosis. The abnormal tissue (arrows) is of intermediate signal intensity in both images. A large popliteal cyst is present, and intra-articular and intrabursal fluid is of high signal intensity in **B.** Note the presence of a bone erosion of the tibia (arrowhead), filled with tissue demonstrating persistent low signal intensity. A tear of the posterior horn of the medial meniscus is evident.

(From Cobby MJ, et al: AJR *157*:1023, 1991. Copyright 1991, American Roentgen Ray Society.)

crystalline and iron accumulation, in the pathogenesis of the musculoskeletal manifestations of hemodialysis.[479–488]

Additional Manifestations. Several additional musculoskeletal manifestations of hemodialysis are worthy of note. Olecranon bursitis, called dialysis elbow, may be seen in patients on long-term hemodialysis as a consequence of the sustained pressure on the elbow related to the position of the arm during treatment.[166] Digital clubbing confined to one or more fingers may be induced by anoxia distal to the fistulae,[242] and aneurysms with or without calcification may appear at the site of shunt. Hemodialysis-induced alkalosis and hypomagnesemia and aluminum-induced encephalopathy are associated with tetany and convulsions, producing multiple fractures owing to direct trauma or forceful muscle contractions.[167, 332] Hemarthrosis also has been reported in hemodialyzed patients, perhaps related to heparin administration or abnormal platelet function.[333] Tendinous and ligamentous laxity may be observed, resulting in atlantoaxial subluxation, articular hypermobility, elongation of the patellar tendon, and reducible deformities of peripheral joints.[490]

Musculoskeletal Abnormalities Occurring After Peritoneal Dialysis

Bone disease and soft tissue calcification also have been observed in uremic patients undergoing peritoneal dialysis (Fig. 57–46). Some investigators suggest that the frequency and severity of the osseous and soft tissue changes are less in this therapeutic technique than in hemodialysis, but others have not found this to be true.[334] Indeed, examples of rapidly progressive calcific periarthritis[491] and soft tissue calcific deposits leading to tendon failure in the hand and

wrist[492] have been reported in patients receiving chronic peritoneal dialysis on an ambulatory basis. Calcium hydroxyapatite crystal deposition generally is the cause of tumoral deposits of calcification in this situation. Rarely, as has been described in hemodialysis,[493] subjacent bone erosion accompanying such tumor-like calcific collections may occur in patients undergoing peritoneal dialysis. Also, in both forms of dialysis therapy, CPPD crystal deposition may occur.[334]

Deposition of beta-2-microglobulin amyloid has been documented in patients with chronic renal disease receiving long-term peritoneal dialysis.[494] Although there are theoretical reasons why this form of dialysis might lead less frequently to such deposition (the peritoneum has been shown to be permeable to beta-2-microglobulin[495]), the known occurrence of arthralgias, destructive arthropathy and spondyloarthropathy, intraosseous lytic lesions, and carpal tunnel syndrome in association with chronic peritoneal dialysis appears to underscore the importance of amyloidosis as a complication of this form of therapy as well.[494, 496, 497]

Musculoskeletal Abnormalities Occurring After Renal Transplantation

Abnormalities of bone and soft tissue may be encountered after renal transplantation[113, 147, 148, 168, 403] (Fig. 57–47). After transplantation, normal renal function is restored; the nature and progress of bone disease depends on the state of the bones at the time of transplantation. Clinical findings resembling primary hyperparathyroidism (hypercalcemia, hypophosphatemia, low renal phosphorus threshold) may be apparent in those patients who had radiographically evident hyperparathyroidism prior to transplantation.[169–171] It

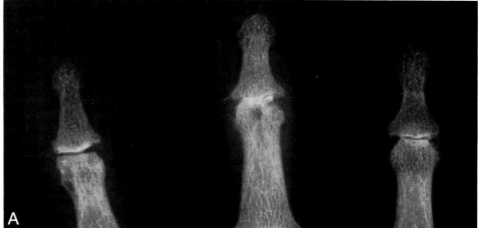
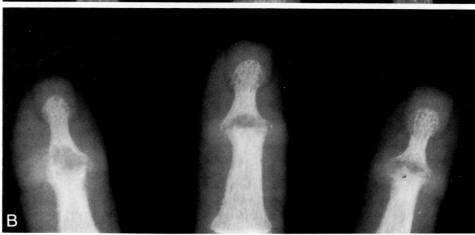

FIGURE 57–46. Renal osteodystrophy: Erosive arthritis during peritoneal dialysis. A 64 year old woman developed end-stage renal disease secondary to nephropathy as a result of analgesic abuse. She was maintained on peritoneal dialysis. Increasing pain and swelling of multiple interphalangeal joints in the hand appeared during a 5 year period. Radiographs obtained 2 years apart demonstrate progressive bone erosions about the distal interphalangeal joints as well as increasing subperiosteal resorption. The opposite side was affected similarly. The precise nature of the findings is unclear. (Courtesy of G. Greenway, M.D., Dallas, Texas.)

also has been suggested that skeletal resistance to parathyroid hormone, which is noted in uremia, is overcome, permitting the development of hypercalcemia and phosphaturia and a state of primary hyperparathyroidism. In most patients, this state is self-limited, although a few persons develop persistent hypercalcemia.[172] Other factors contributing to hypercalcemia after renal transplantation are phosphate depletion from antacids given in conjunction with steroid medication, injudicious vitamin D therapy in the pretransplant period, and mobilization of soft tissue calcium deposits.[36] Histologic[173] and radiologic features of hyperparathyroidism may be noted in patients after renal transplantation; in some patients, these features remain unchanged in the posttransplantation period, whereas in others, they may disappear or become exaggerated. After renal transplantation, osteopenia may remain unchanged or worsen; a few patients reveal an increase in bone mineral levels. The histologic features of osteomalacia may disappear after surgery,[174] and periarticular calcifications may resolve.[498]

The occurrence of osteonecrosis after renal transplantation is well known.[113, 148, 175–192, 243, 244, 255, 335–342, 386, 499] Osteonecrosis generally becomes evident from 4 to 36 months after the surgery.[342] It generally is assumed that osteonecrosis in the posttransplant period is due to steroid medications, although patients (including children) with severe secondary hyperparathyroidism being treated with chronic hemodialysis who have not received steroids or undergone renal transplantation may develop osteonecrosis.[165, 309, 340] The reported frequency of osteonecrosis after renal transplantation has varied from 1.4 to 40 per cent, although the occurrence of clinically occult ischemic bone necrosis, detected only by MR imaging, in patients with renal transplantation[500] makes analysis of the prevalence of osteonecrosis in these patients difficult when routine diagnostic tests alone are used. Some investigators suggest that the frequency of this complication depends on the exact schedule or dosage of steroid administration.[188, 335] Furthermore, patients with threatened rejection episodes or patients who have undergone a second renal transplant operation appear more prone to develop osteonecrosis. Additional factors in the production of osteonecrosis after renal transplantation may include structural osseous weakening due to osteopenia, the direct effect of parathyroid hormone in producing capillary leakage and permeability, hypophosphatemia, and an immune response to the donor kidney. Studies have failed to relate the frequency of posttransplantation osteonecrosis to patient sex, type of renal disease, or origin of the graft. Similarly, although renal osteodystrophy itself might be inducive of this complication, no association between duration of uremia or histologic evidence of severe bone involvement and ischemic necrosis has been defined clearly.[339] The precise mechanism by which corticosteroids induce osteonecrosis is not clear. Suggested mechanisms

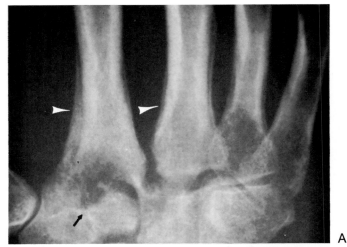

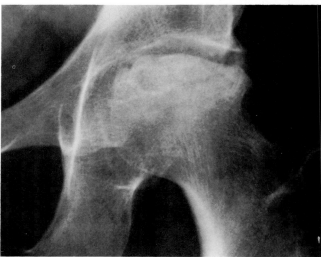

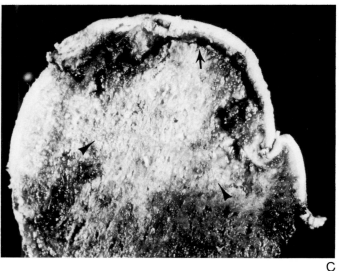

FIGURE 57–47. Renal osteodystrophy: Complications of renal transplantation.

A Osteomyelitis and septic arthritis. Note destruction at the common carpometacarpal joint (arrow) and metacarpal periostitis (arrowheads).

B, C Osteonecrosis. The radiographic features **(B)** are characteristic, including patchy radiolucency and sclerosis and collapse of the femoral head. In a coronal section of such a necrotic femoral head **(C)** observe the subchondral fracture (arrow) separating a portion of subchondral bone and overlying cartilage, as well as widespread bone necrosis (arrowheads).

A

B

C

are fatty infiltration of the liver, hyperlipidemia, and systemic fat embolization; osteoporosis and decreased pain sensation complicated by microfractures; defects in coagulation and vasculitis; fatty infiltration of marrow with compression of blood vessels; and infection.

The most common site of osteonecrosis after renal transplantation is the femoral head; additional sites are the distal end of the femur, humeral head, talus, humeral condyles, cuboid, and carpal bones. In fact, no bone is exempt, and multiple osseous surfaces may be altered in a single patient commonly in a bilateral distribution. In general, convex articular surfaces are affected. Clinical manifestations of osteonecrosis in these persons include joint pain and synovitis.

Radiographic and pathologic manifestations of osteonecrosis are characteristic. An early sign is a linear subchondral radiolucent shadow, which represents a fracture beneath the cartilaginous surface. Focal areas of sclerosis are observed about this lucent area, and bony eburnation soon increases to involve a large segment of bone, reflecting an attempt at healing. Displacement of the subchondral bone and overlying cartilage is noted. Later, fragmentation, collapse, sclerosis, and cyst formation are seen, although the articular space generally remains intact. This latter appear-

ance denotes the presence of relatively normal cartilage, which retains its integrity by nourishment from intrusion of the adjacent synovial fluid. Cartilage loss eventually may occur, heralding the onset of secondary degenerative joint disease related to incongruity of apposing articular surfaces. In some hips, concentric joint space narrowing differs from the pattern of primary degenerative joint disease and may be due to chondrolysis. With the onset of fragmentation and loss of cartilage, a low grade synovitis may ensue,[161] with synovial effusions. This may account for a ''nonspecific'' synovitis complicating renal transplantation that has been observed by some investigators.[184, 245] In non–weight-bearing joints, such as the glenohumeral joint, patchy sclerosis and lucency may appear without significant subchondral collapse of bone. Epiphyseal bone sclerosis, however, may occur in patients with renal osteodystrophy in the absence of osteonecrosis[501] (see Fig. 57–26).

With regard to the early diagnosis of osteonecrosis, the limitations of plain film radiography and conventional tomography are well known. Although CT reveals characteristic alterations in the trabecular pattern, particularly in the femoral head, these too are not evident in the preliminary stages of the process. Bone scintigraphy represents a more sensitive diagnostic technique and can be especially helpful in documenting changes on the less involved side, as in the femoral head, when radiographs are normal. MR imaging, however, has emerged as the most sensitive means to diagnose ischemic necrosis of bone (see Chapter 80).

Spontaneous fractures are not infrequent after renal transplantation.[336, 337] This complication is more common in older patients and occurs within 1 month or as long as 5 years after the surgery. Multiple fractures, particularly in the axial skeleton, are typical. The ribs, pubic rami, and vertebrae are favored fracture locations, although short and long tubular bones also may be affected.[511] Fracture healing generally is normal.

The precise cause of these fractures, which have been observed in 5 to 25 per cent of patients, is not known. A continuous reduction in bone mass in the posttransplantation period probably is significant in their development.[343, 344]

As in the case of hemodialysis, bone and joint infection may be noted after renal transplantation.[113, 148, 345, 346, 387, 393] The predisposing factors include decreased host resistance due to the presence of a chronic debilitating disease and the administration of steroids and immunosuppressive agents.

Tendinitis and spontaneous tendon ruptures have been identified in some patients who have had renal transplants.[502, 503] Such complications also occur in association with hyperparathyroidism, renal osteodystrophy, and dialysis, so the precise role of renal transplantation in this regard is difficult to determine. Corticosteroid therapy certainly may be a contributory factor. Typical sites of involvement are the Achilles, quadriceps, and rotator cuff tendons. Tendon disruption may occur within a year or two after the transplantation.

An increased rate of malignant change can be evident in patients with renal transplants.[256] Possible explanations for this increased risk of neoplasm are the presence of an underlying autoimmune renal disease and the transplantation of a kidney from a cancer patient. In one report, a patient developed a malignant fibrous histiocytoma of bone after renal transplantation; he had been receiving immunosuppressive therapy, which may have contributed to the development of the malignancy.[256]

Differential Diagnosis

In renal osteodystrophy, the radiographic features of hyperparathyroidism must be distinguished from those accompanying primary hyperparathyroidism. In secondary hyperparathyroidism, diagnostic features include an increased frequency of vascular and soft tissue calcification, more common and widespread bone sclerosis, and a decreased frequency of chondrocalcinosis. In addition, the radiographic abnormalities of renal osteodystrophy may be confused with those of other disorders. Diffuse osteosclerosis in this condition may be particularly prominent and, although usually accompanied by other radiographic changes of renal osteodystrophy, must be differentiated from the increased radiodensity associated with various other endocrine, metabolic, and neoplastic diseases. Periosteal neostosis in renal osteodystrophy produces diffuse periosteal bone formation, a finding that also can occur with hypertrophic osteoarthropathy, neoplasm, and infection.

Osteomalacia in chronic renal disease produces decreased radiodensity of bone, a finding that lacks specificity. Occasionally, Looser's zones appear identical to those accompanying other types of osteomalacia. Rachitic changes of renal osteodystrophy almost are identical to those accompanying rickets related to dietary deficiencies and chronic renal tubular disorders. The presence of slipped epiphyses and genu valgum deformities are features that may be more common in the rickets of renal osteodystrophy.

Periarticular calcification is found not only in renal osteodystrophy but also in various collagen vascular diseases, hypervitaminosis D, milk-alkali syndrome, idiopathic tumoral calcinosis, and idiopathic calcium hydroxyapatite crystal deposition disease. The periarticular, soft tissue, and vascular calcifications of renal osteodystrophy usually are accompanied by other radiographic changes of the disorder.

Radiographic findings in patients with renal disease who have undergone dialysis or transplantation include bone and joint infections and osteonecrosis. Osteomyelitis and septic arthritis in this clinical setting produce findings that are identical to those associated with infection in nondialyzed or nontransplant patients. Osteonecrosis after renal transplantation most commonly involves the femoral head. Osteonecrosis at this site also is observed in association with alcoholism, chronic liver disease, pancreatitis, endogenous or exogenous steroid excess, trauma, caisson disease, sickle cell anemia, Gaucher's disease, irradiation, and vasculitis. In all of these cases, the basic radiographic features of osteonecrosis are identical, although manifestations of the underlying process may be identified.

HYPOPARATHYROIDISM

Background and General Features

Hypoparathyroidism is characterized by hypocalcemia and its neuromuscular symptoms and signs. The disease may result from a deficiency in parathyroid hormone production or an end-organ resistance to the action of the hormone. Deficiency of parathyroid hormone most commonly occurs as a result of excision or trauma to the parathyroid glands during thyroid surgery, although it also can occur as idiopathic hypoparathyroidism in which the parathyroid glands usually are absent or atrophied. End-organ unresponsiveness to parathyroid hormone is seen in pseudohypoparathyroidism and pseudopseudohypoparathyroidism, which are discussed in the next section. Rare forms of hypoparathyroidism are seen after radiation damage to the gland and as a response of an infant to hyperparathyroidism in the mother owing to transplacental transport of calcium with suppression of fetal parathyroid activity.

Postsurgical hypoparathyroidism occurs in fewer than 13 per cent of thyroidectomies,[347] may be unrecognized for years, and becomes evident clinically during pregnancy and lactation. Immediately evident hypoparathyroidism, documented with laboratory tests, after such surgery commonly is a transient phenomenon. Mechanisms for postoperative hypoparathyroidism may include vascular abnormalities, suppression of parathyroid function in thyrotoxicosis, increased secretion of thyrocalcitonin, or, rarely, inadvertent removal of most of the parathyroid tissue at the time of surgery.

Idiopathic hypoparathyroidism usually occurs in childhood, girls being more commonly affected than boys.[3] The disease is rare in blacks.[193] A familial occurrence is noted occasionally, particularly in association with pernicious anemia and hypoadrenalism.[194] The disorder may be characterized by the presence of circulating antibodies to the parathyroid, adrenal, and thyroid glands, supporting the concept that idiopathic hypoparathyroidism may be a part of a generalized autoimmune disease.[195, 196] Multisystem involvement with deficiency of other endocrine glands can lead to an array of features, including abnormalities of skin, hair, and nails, epilepsy, cataracts, mental deficiency, tetany, and ectopic calcification. Despite the diversity of these findings, symptoms and signs may be insidious in onset so that the diagnosis may not be established until adulthood. In fact the diagnosis of hypoparathyroidism may be uncovered when an affected mother gives birth to a child with hyperparathyroidism.[1] Confirmation of the clinical diagnosis in these cases can be obtained from appropriate laboratory and radiologic examinations. Histologic studies reveal parathyroid atrophy with fatty replacement.

General radiographic abnormalities of this condition have been described,[197, 198] which include thickening of the cranial vault and facial bones[199]; increased intracranial pressure with sutural diastasis[200]; calcification of the basal ganglia and rarely the choroid plexus and the cerebellum[198, 201]; ventricular dilation[202]; dental abnormalities such as hypoplasia of enamel and dentin, delay or failure of eruption, blunting of the roots, and thickening of the lamina dura[198, 199, 201]; and gastrointestinal hypersecretion and spasm.[198]

Skeletal Abnormalities (Table 57–6)

Osteosclerosis, which may be generalized or localized, is the most common skeletal abnormality of hypoparathyroidism. In fact, the original patient with this syndrome was investigated primarily because of increased osseous density.[203] Bronsky and associates[201] reported generalized increased radiodensity of bone in 9 per cent of patients and localized increased radiodensity in 23 per cent of patients. A similar frequency of osteosclerosis was reported by Steinberg and Waldron.[197] Typically radiographic findings of hypoparathyroidism (and pseudohypoparathyroidism) include increased radiodensity of the skeleton, calvarial thickening, and hypoplastic dentition (Fig. 57–48). Also noteworthy are peculiar bandlike areas of increased radiodensity in the metaphyses of long bones associated with increased density of the iliac crest and marginal sclerosis of the vertebral bodies. Occasional reports indicate diminished bone radiodensity, particularly in pseudohypoparathyroidism,[201] apparently related to increased bone resorption.[204] Growth recovery lines also have been reported.[388]

Subcutaneous calcification may be seen,[197] especially about the hips and shoulders. The deposits generally are asymptomatic, although painful calcific periarthritis is reported in this condition, perhaps due to depression of serum

TABLE 57–6. Radiographic Features of the Skeleton in Hypoparathyroidism

Osteosclerosis
Calvarial thickening
Hypoplastic dentition
Subcutaneous calcification
Basal ganglion calcification
Premature physeal fusion
Spinal ossification

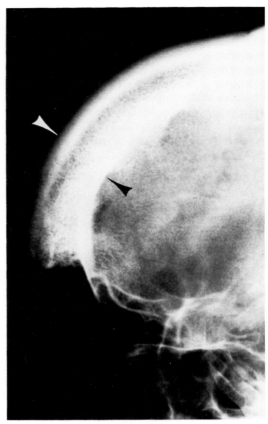

FIGURE 57–48. Hypoparathyroidism: Calvarial thickening. In a lateral radiograph of the anterior aspect of the skull, observe thickening of the cranial vault (arrowheads) with narrowing of the diploic space.

calcium levels.[348] Additionally, deformity and narrowing of the hip joint with sclerosis of the femoral head and acetabulum and premature fusion of the physes have been described.[201, 205]

In rare situations, distinctive abnormalities of the spine resembling those of ankylosing spondylitis or diffuse idiopathic skeletal hyperostosis have been reported in patients with hypoparathyroidism.[206–211] These patients reveal pain, stiffness, and limitation of spinal motion, especially on rotation. On physical examination, spinal and pelvic tenderness are not observed. Radiographic evaluation outlines calcification of the anterior longitudinal ligament and posterior paraspinal ligaments with spinal osteophytes (Fig. 57–49). In some cases, these spinal changes are associated with bony proliferation about the pelvis, hip, and long bones and soft tissue and tendon calcification.[389, 504, 505] The sacroiliac joints generally are spared, although periarticular ossification has been recorded in this location. These changes resemble or are identical to those of diffuse idiopathic skeletal hyperostosis, and a causative relationship between idiopathic hypoparathyroidism and diffuse idiopathic skeletal hyperostosis has been suggested.[504] The erythrocyte sedimentation rate is within normal limits in both conditions.

Differential Diagnosis

Widespread osteosclerosis, particularly of the axial skeleton, that may be identified in hypoparathyroidism also is

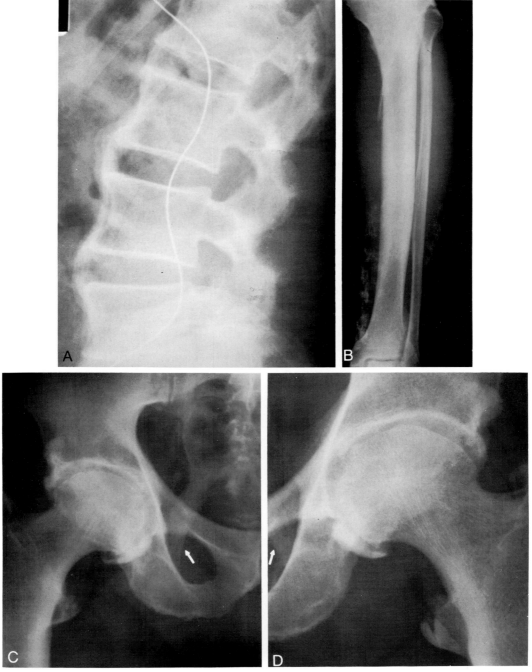

FIGURE 57–49. Hypoparathyroidism: Enthesopathy and soft tissue calcification. This 63 year old obese man had cataracts, a deep voice, first degree heart block, and cutaneous plaques. Serologic evaluation revealed decreased calcium and parathyroid hormone levels and increased phosphorus levels.

A Changes resemble those of diffuse idiopathic skeletal hyperostosis, including flowing anterior vertebral ossification.

B Soft tissue calcification in the calf and bone excrescences arising from the proximal portion of the tibia are evident.

C, D Radiographs of both hips reveal acetabular outgrowths, bone proliferation in the femoral trochanters, and sacrotuberous ligament ossification (arrows).

(Courtesy of P. Cockshott, M.D., Hamilton, Ontario, Canada.)

seen in certain other disorders, including osteoblastic metastasis, myelofibrosis, Paget's disease, fluorosis, renal osteodystrophy, sickle cell anemia, and mastocytosis. In these other diseases, other radiographic features usually are apparent, allowing accurate diagnosis. In hypoparathyroidism (and pseudohypoparathyroidism), additional findings such as calvarial thickening and hypoplastic dentition are helpful clues, although other causes of generalized sclerosis, such as Paget's disease, sickle cell anemia, and even metastasis, may produce increased thickness and sclerosis of the cranial vault. Hypoplastic dentition also is seen in a variety of congenital syndromes, including cleidocranial dysostosis and pyknodysostosis, and a number of other endocrine disorders, such as hypopituitarism and hypothyroidism. Sclerosis of the metaphyseal region of the long bones, which is seen in some patients with hypoparathyroidism, is not specific. A similar finding may be noted in systemic illnesses in infancy and childhood, leading to growth recovery lines, leukemia during treatment, heavy metal poisoning, hypothyroidism, healing scurvy, and hypervitaminoses, although additional radiographic and clinical features usually allow easy differentiation among these disorders.[212]

Basal ganglion calcification is particularly characteristic of hypoparathyroidism and pseudohypoparathyroidism. It also is seen without known cause in infectious disorders such as toxoplasmosis and cytomegalic inclusion disease, in Fahr's syndrome (ferrocalcinosis), after radiation therapy and exposure to toxic substances such as carbon monoxide, and rarely in certain other diseases.[213, 214] Also, subcutaneous calcification, seen in hypoparathyroidism and pseudohypoparathyroidism, is not a specific finding, being observed in collagen vascular disease, hypervitaminosis D, milk-alkali syndrome, and renal osteodystrophy.[215]

The "pseudospondylitic" manifestations of hypoparathyroidism are of particular interest. Descriptions of these manifestations bear a striking resemblance to those of diffuse idiopathic skeletal hyperostosis, including the tendency toward spinal and extraspinal ligament ossification, osteophytosis, and bony excrescences at sites of tendon and ligament attachment to bone. Similar spinal alterations may be seen in fluorosis and ankylosing spondylitis, although, as opposed to the latter disorder, thin vertical syndesmophytes, erosion, and intra-articular ankylosis of the sacroiliac joints are not characteristic of hypoparathyroidism.

PSEUDOHYPOPARATHYROIDISM AND PSEUDOPSEUDOHYPOPARATHYROIDISM

Background and General Features

Pseudohypoparathyroidism (PHP) is a heritable disorder that was first described in 1942 by Albright and coworkers.[216] The disease shares many features with idiopathic hypoparathyroidism, including hypocalcemia, hyperphosphatemia, and basal ganglion and soft tissue calcification. PHP differs from idiopathic hypoparathyroidism in several respects; it involves an end-organ resistance to the action of parathyroid hormone, and it is associated with a characteristic somatotype, which includes short stature, obesity, round face, and brachydactyly. Additional clinical findings of this disease are abnormal dentition, mental retardation, strabismus, dermatoglyphic abnormalities, and impaired taste and olfaction.[1, 217–219] Typical radiographic features of

PHP are short metacarpals, metatarsals, and phalanges, exostoses, cone epiphyses, and wide bones.[220] In some cases, changes of secondary hyperparathyroidism are seen (see later discussion).

PHP is more frequent in women than in men and appears to be transmitted as an X-linked dominant trait.[221] Cases of apparent male-to-male transmission have been reported but not fully documented. PHP usually is diagnosed in the second decade of life, although significant delays in diagnosis may occur.[353] Affected persons reveal increased levels of serum phosphorus, decreased levels of serum calcium, and diminished phosphaturia. Abnormalities of the glucose tolerance test and the simultaneous occurrence of hypothyroidism have been noted in patients with PHP.[1, 3, 222] In addition, because of similarities in somatotypic findings, some investigators suggest that PHP may be related to other hereditary syndromes, such as multiple epiphyseal dysplasia, basal cell nevus syndrome, and Turner's syndrome.[1, 223, 224]

It is probable that PHP results from an inability of end organs to respond to parathyroid hormone rather than from deficient secretion of the hormone or the presence of a biologically ineffective hormone.[203] On histologic examination, the parathyroid glands appear normal or hyperplastic.[3] Excessive secretion of parathyroid hormone has been demonstrated in patients with PHP.[1] In fact, reports have indicated an apparently rare variation of PHP characterized by renal unresponsiveness to parathyroid hormone but with a normal osseous response to the hormone. The condition, termed pseudohypohyperparathyroidism, is associated with histologic findings similar to those of renal osteodystrophy.[349–351] Abnormal somatic features may or may not be present. Radiographic abnormalities are those of hyperparathyroidism, including subperiosteal bone resorption, brown tumors, osteosclerosis, periosteal neostosis, and slipped capital femoral epiphyses.[390]

Pseudopseudohypoparathyroidism (PPHP) is the normocalcemic form of PHP. Patients with PPHP possess the same somatic abnormalities as those with PHP. The two diseases, PHP and PPHP, may occur in the same family, suggesting a close association of these disorders. Furthermore, mothers with PPHP may have children with PHP manifested as persistent hypocalcemia or hypocalcemia during stress.[218, 221] Both conditions have been grouped together under the term Albright's hereditary osteodystrophy.[225] In PHP, there is a deficient response of kidney 3′,5′-cyclic adenosine monophosphate (3′,5′-cAMP) to parathyroid hormone,[226] a finding that suggests a deficiency in membrane receptors or specific enzyme systems in the kidney in patients with this disease, perhaps explaining the end-organ refractoriness to parathyroid hormone[1]; a study of one patient with PPHP has revealed a normal rate of excretion of cAMP in urine in response to parathyroid hormones[227] (see also Chapter 53). Unresponsiveness to other hormones, perhaps related to deficient activity of the guanine nucleotide regulatory protein (G unit) of adenylate cyclase, is reported to be common in PHP.[352] Thus, abnormalities in thyroid function, in the hepatic response to glucagon, in prolactin secretion, and in gonadal function may be observed. Patients with PHP frequently come to medical attention with tetany and occasionally with convulsions in late childhood or adolescence. Additionally, they reveal hyperexcitability, cramping of the extremities, and stridor.

TABLE 57–7. Radiographic Features of the Skeleton in PHP and PPHP*

Soft tissue calcification and ossification
Basal ganglion calcification
Premature physeal fusion
Metacarpal and metatarsal shortening
Calvarial thickening
Exostoses
Abnormalities of bone density
Bowing deformities

*PHP, pseudohypoparathyroidism; PPHP, pseudopseudohypoparathyroidism.

Skeletal Abnormalities (Table 57–7)

Skeletal abnormalities are an integral part of PHP and PPHP.[207, 220] Steinbach and coworkers[228] outlined the evolution of these abnormalities in a detailed study of one patient with PHP. At 9 months of age, this patient revealed no characteristic skeletal lesions. Subsequently, radiographic findings included shortening of all the metacarpals, with premature fusion of the growth plates, broad and short phalanges with pseudoepiphyses, and soft tissue calcification. The calcification was characterized as plaquelike in appearance, asymmetrically distributed, and located beneath the skin surface (Fig. 57–50). In some areas, soft tissue ossification was seen, an interesting observation in view of a report emphasizing the association of PHP and myositis (fibrodysplasia) ossificans progressiva.[229] Ossification usually is limited and periarticular in distribution, nontender, unassociated with swelling, and without overlying erythema.[230]

In most reports of PHP and PPHP, metacarpal shortening frequently is observed in the first, fourth, and fifth digits;

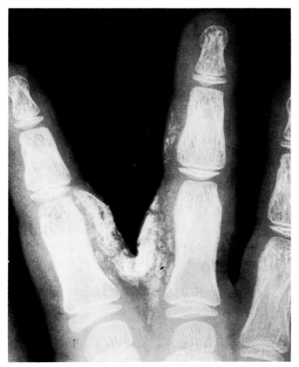

FIGURE 57–50. Pseudohypoparathyroidism: Soft tissue calcification. Plaquelike calcification of the subcutaneous tissue of the second and third digits is observed.

metatarsal shortening shows predilection for the first and fourth digits[231] (Fig. 57–51). It is rare to observe metatarsal shortening as an isolated skeletal abnormality. The first metacarpal bone may reveal excessive width and curvature, and the phalanges are short and wide, with cone-shaped epiphyses. Additional findings have included basal ganglion calcification, calvarial thickening, bowing of the extremities, and exostoses (Fig. 57–52). The exostoses frequently are located centrally and project at right angles to the bone, differing from the appearance of multiple hereditary exostoses, in which outgrowths usually are directed away from joints. Bone density may be increased, normal, or decreased in PHP and PPHP. The carpal angle may be reduced,[232] and spinal stenosis may occur.[354] Causes of such stenosis include vertebral anomalies and ectopic calcifications.[506] Ossification of the posterior longitudinal ligament in the cervical spine also has been noted.[391]

The shortening of the metacarpals may lead to a positive metacarpal sign (Fig. 57–53). Normally, a line drawn tangential to the heads of the fourth and fifth metacarpals does not intersect the third metacarpal or just contacts its distal aspect; in PHP and PPHP, such a line may intersect the third metacarpal, indicating disproportionate shortening of the fourth and fifth metacarpals. This sign is not specific, being positive in other congenital conditions, such as the basal cell nevus syndrome, multiple epiphyseal dysplasia, and Beckwith-Wiedemann syndrome, as well as in acquired conditions, such as juvenile chronic arthritis, sickle cell anemia with infarction, trauma, and neonatal hyperthyroidism.[220] In addition, this sign sometimes is unreliable in diagnosing PHP and PPHP because the third metacarpal also may be short in these conditions.

Radiographic findings of hyperparathyroidism may be seen in some patients with PHP and PPHP.[195, 228, 233, 350, 351, 390] In these patients, typical subperiosteal resorption is identified in the phalanges in association with cortical erosion of the distal portions of the radius and ulna. As indicated previously, brown tumors, periosteal neostosis, osteosclerosis, and even slipped capital femoral epiphyses also may be apparent.[390]

Differential Diagnosis

Radiographic abnormalities of the hand in PHP and PPHP almost are identical (except for a relatively higher rate of occurrence of short distal phalanges in PHP and relatively shorter metacarpals in PPHP).[220] Additionally, these hand abnormalities resemble findings in acrodysostosis (except for the much smaller size of the bones seen in this latter condition), Turner's syndrome (the changes in Turner's syndrome may be less severe than PHP and PPHP, and drumstick phalanges and thin bones may be apparent in Turner's syndrome) (Fig. 57–54), and brachydactyly E and D.[220, 234] Some radiographic features of PHP and PPHP resemble findings of myositis (fibrodysplasia) ossificans progressiva (Fig. 57–55)[229] and multiple hereditary exostoses (Fig. 57–56).

SUMMARY

It is readily apparent that parathyroid hormone excess or deficiency has a profound effect on the human skeleton. Elevated levels of parathyroid hormone occurring in pri-

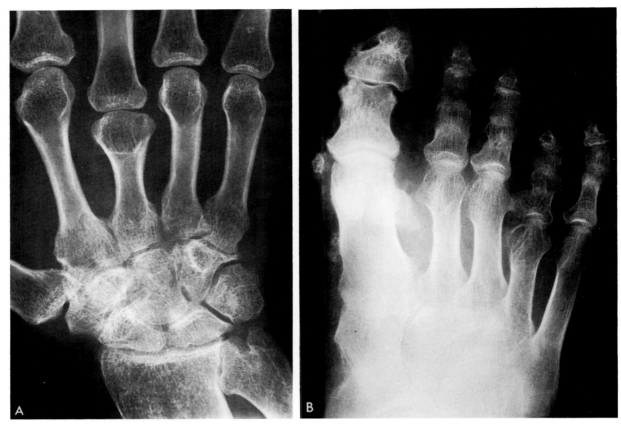

FIGURE 57–51. Pseudohypoparathyroidism: Metacarpal and metatarsal shortening.

A Shortening of all of the metacarpal bones is evident, although the most severe abnormality is present in the third digit. Note irregularity of the distal end of the ulna and carpal bones, with joint space narrowing and sclerosis.

B Shortening of all of the metatarsal bones, particularly the fourth, is associated with soft tissue ossification on the medial aspect of the first digit.

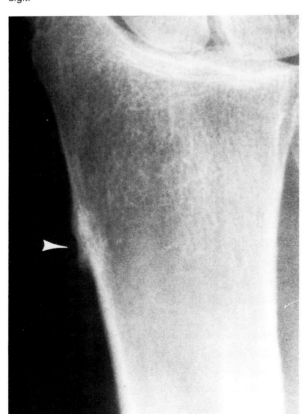

FIGURE 57–52. Pseudohypoparathyroidism: Exostosis. Observe a small, broad-based excrescence on the distal portion of the radius (arrowhead).

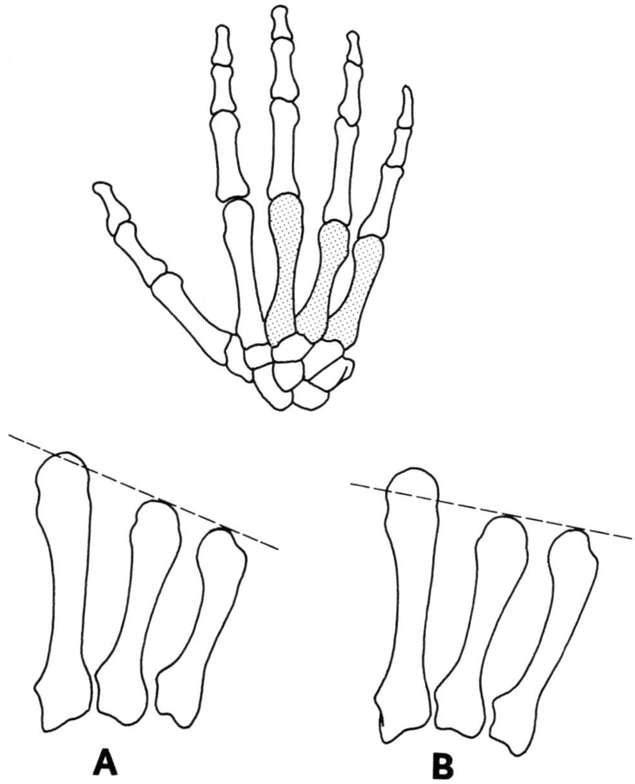

FIGURE 57–53. Pseudohypoparathyroidism and pseudopseudohypoparathyroidism: Positive metacarpal sign. Normally, a line drawn tangential to the heads of the fourth and fifth metacarpal bones will not intersect the end of the third metacarpal bone or will just contact its articular surface **(A).** A positive metacarpal sign is present when such a line intersects the third metacarpal bone **(B).**

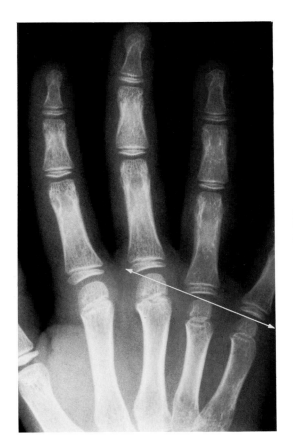

FIGURE 57–54. Turner's syndrome. A positive metacarpal sign (arrow) is related to mild shortening of the fourth metacarpal bone. Subtle cystic changes are present in the phalanges, including the tufts.

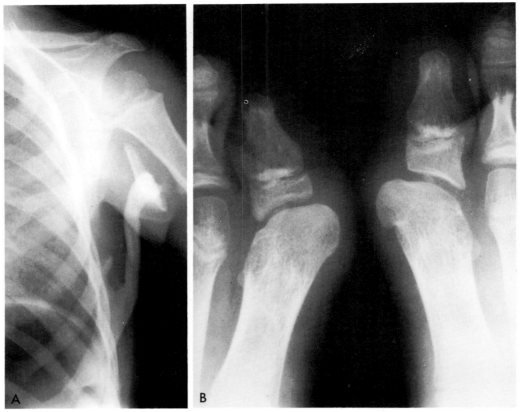

FIGURE 57–55. Myositis (fibrodysplasia) ossificans progressiva. Distinctive abnormalities include soft tissue ossification about the chest and axilla and deformities of the great toes, with overgrowth of the medial aspect of the first metatarsal bones and hypoplasia of the proximal phalanges.

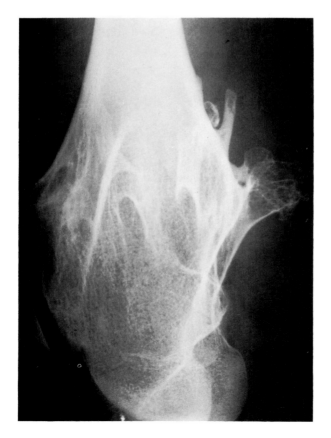

FIGURE 57–56. Multiple hereditary exostoses. On a lateral radiograph of the distal end of the femur, the bizarre exostoses arising from the posterior aspect of the bone are seen to be associated with metaphyseal widening. These outgrowths point away from the joint.

mary and secondary hyperparathyroidism produce considerable osseous erosion involving subperiosteal, intracortical, endosteal, trabecular, subchondral, subphyseal, and subtendinous and subligamentous foci. In renal osteodystrophy, the changes of secondary hyperparathyroidism are combined with additional radiographic and histologic features, including osteomalacia, osteoporosis, and soft tissue and vascular calcification, findings that may become exaggerated or arrested after hemodialysis and renal transplantation. A peculiar variety of amyloidosis occurs in dialyzed patients, whereas osteonecrosis is an important complication of renal transplantation. Depressed levels of parathyroid hormone may be associated with osteosclerosis, subcutaneous and basal ganglion calcification, and spinal abnormalities simulating diffuse idiopathic skeletal hyperostosis or ankylosing spondylitis. PHP and PPHP may be associated with abnormalities in skeletal maturation and development, peculiar exostoses, and soft tissue calcification and ossification.

References

1. Potts JT, Deftos LJ: Parathyroid hormone, calcitonin, vitamin D, bone, and bone mineral metabolism. In PK Bondy, LE Rosenberg (Eds): Duncan's Diseases of Metabolism. Vol II. Endocrinology. 7th Ed. Philadelphia, WB Saunders Co, 1974, p 1225.
2. Castleman B, Mallory TB: Pathology of the parathyroid glands in hyperparathyroidism. Am J Pathol 11:1, 1935.
3. Aurbach GD, Potts JT Jr: The parathyroids. Adv Metab Dis 1:45, 1964.
4. von Recklinghausen FC: Die Fibrose oder deformierende Ostitis, die Osteomalacie und die osteoplastische Karcinose in ihren gegenseitigen Beziehungen. In Festchrift fur Rudolf Virchow. Berlin, Reimer, 1891, p 1.
5. Mandl F: Klinisches und experimentelles zue Frage der lokalisierten und generalisierten Ostitis fibrosa. Arch Klin Chir 143:1, 1926.
6. Krane SM, Brownell GL, Stanbury JB, et al: The effect of thyroid disease on calcium metabolism in man. J Clin Invest 35:874, 1956.
7. Jowsey J: Quantitative microradiography—a new approach in the evaluation of metabolic bone disease. Am J Med 40:485, 1966.
8. Belanger LF: The parathyroid glands, ultrastructure, secretion, and function. In PJ Gaillard et al (Eds): Osteolysis. An Outlook on its Mechanisms and Causation. Chicago, University of Chicago Press, 1965.
9. Talmage RV: A study of the effect of parathyroid hormone on bone remodeling and on calcium homeostasis. Clin Orthop 54:163, 1967.
10. Jaffe HL: Metabolic, Degenerative, and Inflammatory Diseases of Bones and Joints. Philadelphia, Lea & Febiger, 1972, p 301.
11. Gleason DC, Potchen EJ: The diagnosis of hyperparathyroidism. Radiol Clin North Am 5:277, 1967.
12. Genant HK, Baron JM, Strauss FH II, et al: Osteosclerosis in primary hyperparathyroidism. Am J Med 59:104, 1975.
13. Steinbach HL, Gordan GS, Eisenberg E, et al: Primary hyperparathyroidism: A correlation of roentgen, clinical and pathologic features. AJR 86:329, 1961.
14. Genant HK, Heck LL, Lanzl LH, et al: Primary hyperparathyroidism. A comprehensive study of clinical, biochemical, and radiographic manifestations. Radiology 109:513, 1973.
15. Pugh DG: Subperiosteal resorption of bone. A roentgenologic manifestation of primary hyperparathyroidism and renal osteodystrophy. AJR 66:577, 1951.
16. Teng CT, Nathan MH: Primary hyperparathyroidism. AJR 83:716, 1960.
17. Debnam JW, Bates ML, Kopelman RC, et al: Radiological/pathological correlations in uremic bone disease. Radiology 125:653, 1977.
18. Jensen PS, Kliger AS: Early radiographic manifestations of secondary hyperparathyroidism associated with chronic renal disease. Radiology 125:645, 1977.
19. Johnson C, Graham CB, Kings F, et al: Roentgenographic manifestations of chronic renal disease treated by periodic hemodialysis. AJR 101:915, 1967.
20. Weller M, Edeiken J, Hodes PJ: Renal osteodystrophy. AJR 104:354, 1931.
21. Camp JD, Ochsner HC: The osseous changes in hyperparathyroidism associated with parathyroid tumor: A roentgenologic study. Radiology 17:63, 1931.
22. Albright F, Drake TG, Sulkowitch HW: Renal osteitis fibrosa cystica. Report of a case with discussion of metabolic aspects. Bull Johns Hopkins Hosp 60:377, 1937.
23. Meema HE, Meema S: Microradioscopic and morphometric findings in the hand bones with densitometric findings in the proximal radius in thyrotoxicosis and in renal osteodystrophy. Invest Radiol 7:88, 1972.
24. Berry HM Jr: The lore and lure o' the lamina dura. Radiology 109:525, 1973.
25. Zvaifler NJ, Reefe WE, Black RL: Articular manifestations in primary hyperparathyroidism. Arthritis Rheum 5:237, 1962.
26. Resnick D: Erosive arthritis of the hand and wrist in hyperparathyroidism. Radiology 110:263, 1974.
27. Bywaters EGL, Dixon ASJ, Scott JT: Joint lesions of hyperparathyroidism. Ann Rheum Dis 22:171, 1963.
28. Resnick D, Niwayama G: Subchondral resorption of bone in renal osteodystrophy. Radiology 118:315, 1976.
29. Cetina JA, Alarcon-Segovia D: Manifestaciones articulares del hiperparatiroidismo primario. Rev Invest Clin 25:143, 1973.
30. Resnick D, Dwosh IL, Niwayama G: Sacro-iliac joint in renal osteodystrophy: Roentgenographic-pathologic correlation. J Rheumatol 2:287, 1975.
31. Dihlmann W, Muller G: Iliosakralveränderungen als Frühsymptom des Hyperparathyreoidismus. Beitrag zur Differentialdiagnose der Spondylose ankylopoetica. ROFO 111:558, 1969.
32. Dihlmann W, Muller G: Sacroiliacalbefunde beim Hyperparathyreoidism (Röntgenologie, Histomorphologie). Radiologe 13:160, 1973.
33. Dihlmann W, Muller G: Pseudo-Bechterew-Befunde beim Hyperparathyreoidismus bzw, bei der renalen Osteopathie. Z Rheumaforsch 31:401, 1972.
34. Dick R, Jones DN: Temporomandibular joint changes in patients undergoing chronic haemodialysis. Clin Radiol 24:72, 1974.
35. Sellers A, Winfield AC, Massry SG: Resorption of condyloid process of the mandible. An unusual manifestation of renal osteodystrophy. Arch Intern Med 131:727, 1973.
36. Parfitt AM: Renal osteodystrophy. Orthop Clin North Am 3:681, 1972.
37. Simpson W, Kerr DNS, Hill AVL, et al: Skeletal changes in patients on regular hemodialysis. Radiology 107:313, 1973.
38. Shapiro R: The biochemical basis of the skeletal changes in chronic uremia. AJR 111:750, 1971.
39. Ritz E, Krempien B, Mehls O, et al: Skeletal abnormalities in chronic renal insufficiency before and during maintenance hemodialysis. Kidney Int 4:116, 1973.
40. Ritz E, Krempien B, Riedasch G, et al: Dialysis bone disease. Proc Eur Dial Transplant Assoc 8:131, 1971.
41. Teplick JG, Eftekhari F, Haskin ME: Erosion of the sternal ends of the clavicles. A new sign of primary and secondary hyperparathyroidism. Radiology 113:323, 1974.
42. Eugenidis N, Olah AJ, Haas HG: Osteosclerosis in hyperparathyroidism. Radiology 105:265, 1972.
43. Jaffe HL: Hyperparathyroidism (Recklinghausen's disease of bone). Arch Pathol 16:63, 1933.
44. Aitken RE, Kerr JL, Lloyd HM: Primary hyperparathyroidism with osteosclerosis and calcification in articular cartilage. Am J Med 37:813, 1964.
45. Schwartz EE, Lantieri R, Teplick JG: Erosion of the inferior aspect of the clavicle in secondary hyperparathyroidism. AJR 129:291, 1977.
46. Brown TW, Genant HK, Hattner RS, et al: Multiple brown tumors in a patient with chronic renal failure and secondary hyperparathyroidism. AJR 128:131, 1977.
47. Fordham CC, Williams TF: Brown tumors and secondary hyperparathyroidism. N Engl J Med 269:129, 1963.
48. Friedman WH, Pervez N, Schwartz AE: Brown tumor of the maxilla in secondary hyperparathyroidism. Arch Otolaryngol 100:157, 1974.
49. Idelson BA, Rudikoff J, Smith GW: Renal osteodystrophy. Unusual roentgenologic manifestations. JAMA 230:870, 1974.
50. Katz AI, Hampers CL, Merrill JP: Secondary hyperparathyroidism and renal osteodystrophy in chronic renal failure. Analysis of 195 patients with observations on the effects of chronic dialysis kidney transplantation and subtotal parathyroidectomy. Medicine 48:333, 1969.
51. Jaffe HL, Bodansky A, Blair JE: Influence of age and of duration of treatment on production and repair of bone lesions in experimental hyperparathyroidism. J Exp Med 55:139, 1932.
52. Feist JH: The biologic basis of radiologic findings in bone disease: Recognition and interpretation of abnormal bone architecture. Radiol Clin North Am 8:183, 1970.
53. Rose GA: Radiological diagnosis of osteoporosis, osteomalacia and hyperparathyroidism. Clin Radiol 15:75, 1961.
54. Evens RG, Pak YC, Ashburn W, et al: Clinical investigations in metabolic bone disease. Invest Radiol 4:364, 1969.
55. Goldsmith NF, Johnson JO, Ury H, et al: Bone mineral estimation in normal and osteoporotic women, a comparability trial of four methods and seven bone sites. J Bone Joint Surg [Am] 53:83, 1971.
56. Crawford T, Dent CE, Lucas P, et al: Osteosclerosis associated with chronic renal failure. Lancet 2:981, 1954.
57. Berner A: Les osteodystrophies d'origine renale (étude systematique du squelette dans 138 cas de maladies renale). Helv Med Acta 11:961, 1944.
58. Davis JG: Osseous radiographic findings of chronic renal insufficiency. Radiology 60:406, 1953.
59. Doyle FH: Ulnar bone mineral concentration in metabolic bone diseases. Br J Radiol 34:698, 1961.
60. Doyle FH: Some quantitative radiological observations in primary and secondary hyperparathyroidism. Br J Radiol 39:161, 1966.
61. Garner A, Ball J: Quantitative observations on mineralized and unmineralized bone in chronic renal azotaemia and intestinal malabsorption syndrome. J Pathol Bacteriol 91:545, 1966.
62. Adam A, Ritchie D: Hyperparathyroidism with increased bone density in the areas of growth. J Bone Joint Surg [Br] 36:257, 1954.
63. Dresser R: Osteitis fibrosa cystica associated with parathyroid overactivity. AJR 30:596, 1933.
64. Lloyd HM, Aitken RE, Ferrier TM: Primary hyperparathyroidism resembling rickets of late onset. Br Med J 2:853, 1965.

65. Templeton AW, Jaconette JR, Ormond RS: Localized osteosclerosis in hyperparathyroidism. Radiology 78:955, 1962.
66. Connor TB, Freijanes J, Stoner RE, et al: Generalized osteosclerosis in primary hyperparathyroidism. Trans Am Clin Climatol Assoc 85:185, 1973.
67. Seyle H: Mechanism of parathyroid hormone action. Arch Pathol 34:625, 1942.
68. Kalu DN, Doyle FH, Pennock J, et al: Parathyroid hormone and experimental osteosclerosis. Lancet 1:1363, 1970.
69. Copp DH: Endocrine regulation of calcium metabolism. Annu Rev Physiol 32:61, 1970.
70. Bell NH: On the possible clinical significance of thyrocalcitonin and of osteosclerosis. J Chron Dis 20:829, 1967.
71. Foster GV, Doyle FH, Bordier P, et al: Effect of thyrocalcitonin on bone. Lancet 2:1428, 1966.
72. Krook L, Lutwak L, McEntee K, et al: Nutritional hypercalcitoninism in bulls. Cornell Vet 61:625, 1971.
73. Mazzuoli GF, Coen G, Baschieri L: Thyrocalcitonin-excess syndrome. Lancet 2:1192, 1966.
74. Dodds WJ, Steinbach HL: Primary hyperparathyroidism and articular cartilage calcification. AJR 104:884, 1968.
75. Ryckewaert A, Solnica J, Lanham C, et al: Manifestations articulaires de l'hyperparathyroidie. Presse Med 74:2599, 1966.
76. Glass JS, Grahame R: Chondrocalcinosis after parathyroidectomy. Ann Rheum Dis 35:521, 1976.
77. Pritchard MH, Jessop JD: Chondrocalcinosis in primary hyperparathyroidism. Influence of age, metabolic bone disease and parathyroidectomy. Ann Rheum Dis 36:146, 1977.
78. Weinstein JD, Dick HM, Grantham SA: Pseudogout, hyperparathyroidism and carpal-tunnel syndrome. A case report. J Bone Joint Surg [Am] 50:1669, 1968.
79. Lipson RL, Williams LE: The ''connective tissue disorder'' of hyperparathyroidism. Arthritis Rheum 11:198, 1968.
80. Avioli LV, Prockop DJ: Collagen degradation and the response to parathyroid extract in the intact Rhesus monkey. J Clin Invest 46:217, 1967.
81. Kaufman EJ, Glimcher MJ, Mechanic GL, et al: Collagenolytic activity during active bone resorption in tissue culture. Proc Soc Exp Biol Med 120:632, 1965.
82. Colachis SC Jr, Worden RE, Bechtol CO, et al: Movement of the sacro-iliac joint in the adult male: A preliminary report. Arch Phys Med Rehabil 44:490, 1963.
83. Bywaters EGL: Discussion of simulation of rheumatic disorders by metabolic bone disease. Ann Rheum Dis 18:64, 1959.
84. McKusick VA: Heritable Disorders of Connective Tissue. St Louis, CV Mosby, 1966, p 218.
85. Preston FS, Adicoff A: Hyperparathyroidism with avulsion of three major tendons. N Engl J Med 266:968, 1962.
86. Murphy KJ, McPhee I: Tears of major tendons in chronic acidosis with elastosis. J Bone Joint Surg [Am] 47:1253, 1965.
87. Lotem M, Robson MD, Rosenfeld JB: Spontaneous rupture of the quadriceps tendon in patients on chronic haemodialysis. Ann Rheum Dis 33:428, 1974.
88. Cirincione RJ, Baker BE: Tendon ruptures with secondary hyperparathyroidism. A case report. J Bone Joint Surg [Am] 57:852, 1975.
89. Persch WF, Birkner H: Bilaterale traumatische Ruptur der Patellarsehne bei renaler Osteopathie. Akt Traumatol 6:51, 1976.
90. Morein G, Goldschmidt Z, Pauker M, et al: Spontaneous tendon ruptures in patients treated by chronic hemodialysis. Clin Orthop 124:209, 1977.
91. Patten BM, Bilezikian JP, Mallette LE, et al: Neuromuscular disease in primary hyperparathyroidism. Ann Intern Med 80:182, 1974.
92. Bunch TW, Hunder GG: Ankylosing spondylitis and primary hyperparathyroidism. JAMA 225:1108, 1973.
93. Mintz DH, Canary JJ, Carreon G, et al: Hyperuricemia in hyperparathyroidism. N Engl J Med 112:112, 1961.
94. Scott JT, Dixon AS, Bywaters EGL: Association of hyperuricemia and gout with hyperparathyroidism. Br Med J 1:1070, 1964.
95. Oppel VA: Pathogenesis and treatment of polyarthritis ankylotica. Vestnik Khir 9:7, 1927.
96. Grantmyre EB: Roentgenographic features of ''primary'' hyperparathyroidism in infancy. J Can Assoc Radiol 24:257, 1973.
97. Randall C, Lauchlan SC: Parathyroid hyperplasia in an infant. Am J Dis Child 105:364, 1963.
98. Bronsky D, Kiamko RT, Moncada R, et al: Intrauterine hyperparathyroidism secondary to maternal hypoparathyroidism. Pediatrics 42:606, 1968.
99. Chiroff RT, Sears KA, Slaughter WH III: Slipped capital femoral epiphyses and parathyroid adenoma. Case report. J Bone Joint Surg [Am] 56:1063, 1974.
100. Liu SH, Chu HI: Studies of calcium and phosphorus metabolism with special reference to pathogenesis and effects of dihydrotachysterol (A.T.10) and iron. Medicine 22:103, 1943.
101. Bordier PJ, Matrajt H, Miravet L, et al: Mesure histologique de la masse et de la resorption des travées osseuses. Pathol Biol 12:1238, 1964.
102. Ferran J-L, Luciani J-C, Meunier P, et al: Osteodystrophie rénale de l'enfant. J Radiol Electrol Med Nucl 58:173, 1977.
103. Gonick HC, Drinkard JP, Hertoghe J, et al: A calcium kinetic approach to the problem of renal osteodystrophy. Clin Orthop 100:315, 1974.
104. Griffiths HJ, Zimmerman RE, Bailey G, et al: The use of photon absorptiometry in the diagnosis of renal osteodystrophy. Radiology 109:277, 1973.
105. Agus ZS, Goldberg M: Pathogenesis of uremic osteodystrophy. Radiol Clin North Am 10:545, 1972.
106. Norfray J, Calenoff L, DelGreco F, et al: Renal osteodystrophy in patients on hemodialysis as reflected in the bony pelvis. AJR 125:352, 1975.
107. Greenfield GB: Roentgen appearance of bone and soft tissue changes in chronic renal disease. AJR 116:749, 1972.
108. Weinberg SG, Lubin A, Wiener SN, et al: Myelofibrosis and renal osteodystrophy. Am J Med 63:755, 1977.
109. Rao P, Solomon M, Avramides A, et al: Brown tumors associated with secondary hyperparathyroidism of chronic renal failure. J Oral Surg 36:154, 1978.
110. Lindenfelser R, Dihlmann W, Mann H, et al: Resorptives Riesenzellgranulom und sekundarer Hyperparathyreoidismus. ROFO 121:584, 1974.
111. Meema HE, Rabinovich S, Meema S, et al: Improved radiological diagnosis of azotemic osteodystrophy. Radiology 102:1, 1972.
112. Potter DE, Wilson CJ, Ozonoff MB: Hyperparathyroid bone disease in children undergoing long-term hemodialysis: Treatment with Vitamin D. J Pediatr 85:60, 1974.
113. Griffiths HJ, Ennis JT, Bailey G: Skeletal changes following renal transplantation. Radiology 113:621, 1974.
114. Ellis HA, Peart KM: Azotaemic renal osteodystrophy: A quantitative study on iliac bone. J Clin Pathol 26:83, 1973.
115. Garner A, Ball J: Quantitative observations on mineralized and unmineralized bone in chronic renal azotaemia and intestinal malabsorption syndrome. J Pathol Bacteriol 91:545, 1966.
116. Meema HE, Oreopoulos DG, Rabinovich S, et al: Periosteal new bone formation (periosteal neostosis) in renal osteodystrophy. Relationship to osteosclerosis, osteitis fibrosa, and osteoid excess. Radiology 110:513, 1974.
117. Ritchie WGM, Winney RJ, Davison AM, et al: Periosteal new bone formation developing during haemodialysis for chronic renal failure. Br J Radiol 48:656, 1975.
118. Heath DA, Martin DJ: Periosteal new bone formation in hyperparathyroidism associated with renal failure. Br J Radiol 43:517, 1970.
119. Woodhouse NJY, Doyle FH, Joplin GF: Vitamin-D deficiency and primary hyperparathyroidism. Lancet 2:283, 1971.
120. Fine A, Sumner D: Alteration of hepatic acetylation in uraemia. Proc Eur Dial Transplant Assoc 11:433, 1974.
121. Philips RN: Primary diffuse parathyroid hyperplasia in an infant of four months. Pediatrics 2:428, 1948.
122. Rajasuriya K, Peiris OA, Ratnaike VT, et al: Parathyroid adenomas in childhood. Am J Dis Child 107:442, 1964.
123. Lomnitz E, Sepulveda L, Stevenson C, et al: Primary hyperparathyroidism simulating rickets. J Clin Endocrinol Metab 26:309, 1966.
124. Mehls O, Ritz E, Krempien B, et al: Roentgenological signs in the skeleton of uremic children. Pediatr Radiol 1:183, 1973.
125. Looser E: Uber pathologische formen von infraktionen und callusbildungen bei rachitis und osteomalakie und andered knochenkrankungen. Zentrabl Chir 47:1470, 1920.
126. Brailsford JF: Slipping of the epiphysis of the head of the femur. Its relation to renal rickets. Lancet 1:16, 1933.
127. Shea D, Mankin HJ: Slipped capital femoral epiphysis in renal rickets. Report of three cases. J Bone Joint Surg [Am] 48:349, 1966.
128. Mehls O, Ritz E, Krempien B, et al: Slipped epiphyses in renal osteodystrophy. Arch Dis Child 50:545, 1975.
129. Kirkwood JR, Ozonoff MB, Steinbach HL: Epiphyseal displacement after metaphyseal fracture in renal osteodystrophy. AJR 115:547, 1972.
130. Floman Y, Yosipovitch Z, Licht A, et al: Bilateral slipped upper femoral epiphysis: A rare manifestation of renal osteodystrophy. Isr J Med Sci 11:15, 1975.
131. Goldman AB, Lane JM, Salvati E: Slipped capital femoral epiphyses complicating renal osteodystrophy: A report of three cases. Radiology 126:333, 1978.
132. Crutchlow WP, David DS, Whitsell J: Multiple skeletal complications in a case of chronic renal failure treated by kidney homotransplantation. Am J Med 50:390, 1971.
133. Krempien B, Mehls O, Ritz E: Morphological studies on pathogenesis of epiphyseal slipping in uremic children. Virchows Arch Pathol Anat Histol 362:129, 1974.
134. Avioli LV: Vitamin D, the kidney and calcium homeostasis. Kidney Int 2:241, 1972.
135. Ingham JP, Stewart JH, Posen S: Quantitative skeletal histology in untreated end-stage renal failure. Br Med J 2:745, 1973.
136. Parfitt AM: Soft-tissue calcification in uraemia. Arch Intern Med 124:544, 1969.
137. Massry SG, Coburn JW, Popovtzer MM, et al: Secondary hyperparathyroidism in chronic renal failure. Arch Intern Med 124:431, 1969.
138. Contiguglia SR, Alfrey AC, Miller NL, et al: Nature of soft tissue calcification in uremia. Kidney Int 4:229, 1973.
139. Legeros RZ, Contiguglia SR, Alfrey AC: Pathological calcifications associated with uremia. Two types of calcium phosphate deposits. Calcif Tissue Res 13:173, 1973.
140. Mirahmadi KS, Coburn JW, Bluestone R: Calcific periarthritis and hemodialysis. JAMA 223:548, 1973.
141. Hilbish TF, Bartter FC: Roentgen findings in abnormal deposition of calcium in tissues. AJR 87:1128, 1962.
142. Han SY, Witten DM: Diffuse calcification of the breast in chronic renal failure. AJR 129:341, 1977.
143. Kuzela DC, Huffer WE, Conger JD, et al: Soft tissue calcification in chronic dialysis patients. Am J Pathol 86:403, 1977.
144. Barber ND, Nakamoto S, McCormack LJ, et al: Pathologic anatomy of 13 patients after prolonged periodic hemodialysis. Trans Am Soc Artif Intern Organs 9:21, 1963.

145. Caner JE, Decker JL: Recurrent acute (gouty?) arthritis in chronic renal failure treated with periodic hemodialysis. Am J Med 36:571, 1964.
146. Moskowitz RW, Vertes V, Schwartz A, et al: Crystal induced inflammation associated with chronic renal failure treated with periodic hemodialysis. Am J Med 47:450, 1969.
147. Peterson R: Small vessel calcification and its relationship to secondary hyperparathyroidism in the renal homotransplant patient. Radiology 126:627, 1978.
148. Irby R, Edwards WM, Gatter R: Articular complications of homotransplantation and chronic renal hemodialysis. J Rheumatol 2:91, 1975.
149. Tatler GLV, Baillod RA, Varghese Z, et al: Evolution of bone disease over 10 years in 135 patients with terminal renal failure. Br Med J 4:315, 1973.
150. Salyer WR, Keren D: Oxalosis as a complication of chronic renal failure. Kidney Int 4:61, 1973.
151. Milgram JW, Salyer WR: Secondary oxalosis of bone in chronic renal failure. J Bone Joint Surg [Am] 56:387, 1974.
152. Bennett B, Rosenblum C: Identification of calcium oxalate crystals in the myocardium in patients with uremia. Lab Invest 10:947, 1961.
153. Stauffer M: Oxalosis. Report of a case with review of the literature and a discussion of the pathogenesis. N Engl J Med 263:386, 1960.
154. Fournier AE, Johnson WJ, Taves DR, et al: Etiology of hyperparathyroidism and bone disease during chronic renal hemodialysis. I. Association of bone disease with potential etiologic factors. J Clin Invest 50:592, 1971.
155. Bordier PJ, Chot ST, Eastwood JB, et al: Lack of histological evidence of vitamin D abnormality in the bones of anephric patients. Clin Sci 44:33, 1973.
156. DeVerber GA, Oreopoulos DG, Rabinovich S, et al: Changing pattern of renal osteodystrophy with chronic hemodialysis. Trans Am Soc Artif Intern Organs 16:479, 1970.
157. Simpson W, Kerr DNS, Hill AVL, et al: Skeletal changes in patients on regular hemodialysis. Radiology 107:313, 1971.
158. Pafitt AM, Massry SG, Winfield AC, et al: Disordered calcium and phosphorus metabolism during maintenance hemodialysis: Correlation of clinical, roentgenographic and biochemical changes. Am J Med 51:391, 1971.
159. Cadnapaphornchai P, Kuruvila KC, Holmes J, et al: Analysis of 5 year experience of home dialysis as a treatment modality for patients with end-stage renal failure. Am J Med 57:789, 1974.
160. Verberckmoes R, Bouillon R, Krempien B: Disappearance of vascular calcification during treatment of renal osteodystrophy. Two patients treated with high doses of vitamin D and aluminum hydroxide. Ann Intern Med 82:529, 1975.
161. Massry SG, Bluestone R, Klinenberg JR, et al: Abnormalities of the musculoskeletal system in hemodialysis patients. Semin Arthritis Rheum 4:321, 1975.
162. Leonard A, Comty CM, Shapiro FL, et al: Osteomyelitis in hemodialysis patients. Ann Intern Med 78:651, 1973.
163. Sy WM, Mittal AK: Bone scan in chronic dialysis patients with evidence of secondary hyperparathyroidism and renal osteodystrophy. Br J Radiol 48:878, 1975.
164. Wiegmann T, Rosenthall L, Kaye M: Technetium-99m-pyrophosphate bone scans in hyperparathyroidism. J Nucl Med 18:231, 1977.
165. Bailey GL, Griffiths HJL, Mocelin AJ, et al: Avascular necrosis of the femoral head in patients on chronic hemodialysis. Trans Am Soc Artif Intern Organs 18:401, 1972.
166. Cangiano JL, Ramirez-González RE, Ramirez-Muxó O: Bone disease and soft tissue calcification in chronic peritoneal dialysis. Am J Med Sci 264:301, 1972.
167. Sakai S, David D, Shoji H, et al: Bone injuries due to tetany of convulsions during hemodialysis. Clin Orthop 118:118, 1976.
168. Resnick D: Abnormalities of bone and soft tissue following renal transplantation. Semin Roentgenol 13:329, 1978.
169. Alfrey AC, Jenkins D, Groth CG, et al: Resolution of hyperparathyroidism, renal osteodystrophy and metastatic calcification after renal homotransplantation. N Engl J Med 279:1349, 1968.
170. David DS, Sakal S, Brennan BL, et al: Hypercalcemia after renal transplantation. N Engl J Med 289:398, 1973.
171. Ogg C: Parathyroidectomy in the treatment of secondary renal hyperparathyroidism. Kidney Int 4:168, 1973.
172. Hampers CL, Katz AI, Wilson RE, et al: Calcium metabolism and osteodystrophy after renal transplantation. Arch Intern Med 124:282, 1969.
173. Kleerekoper M, Ibels LS, Ingham JP, et al: Hyperparathyroidism after renal transplantation. Br Med J 3:680, 1975.
174. Pierides AM, Ellis HA, Peart KM, et al: Assessment of renal osteodystrophy following renal transplantation. Proc Eur Dial Transplant Assoc 11:481, 1974.
175. Harris RR, Niemann KMW, Diethelm AG: Skeletal complications after renal transplantation. South Med J 67:1016, 1974.
176. Murray WR: Hip problems associated with organ transplants. Clin Orthop 90:57, 1973.
177. Moreau JF, Pomarede D, Arfi S, et al: Aspects radiographiques des osteonecroses aseptiques de la transplantation renale. J Radiol Electrol Med Nucl 56:97, 1975.
178. Arfi S, Moreau JF, Heuclin C, et al: L'osteonecrose aseptique de la transplantation renale. A propos de 29 cas. Rev Rhum Mal Osteoartic 42:162, 1975.
179. Aichroth P, Branfoot AC, Huskisson EC, et al: Destructive joint changes following kidney transplantation. Report of a case. J Bone Joint Surg [Br] 53:488, 1971.
180. Creuss RL, Blennerhassett J, Macdonald FR, et al: Aseptic necrosis following renal transplantation. J Bone Joint Surg [Am] 50:1577, 1968.
181. Lecestre P, Dabos N, Benoit J, et al: L'osteonecrose aseptique chez le transplante renal. Rev Chir Orthop 63:373, 1977.
182. Habermann ET, Cristofaro RL: Avascular necrosis of bone as a complication of renal transplantation. Semin Arthritis Rheum 6:189, 1976.
183. Levine E, Erken EH, Price HI, et al: Osteonecrosis following renal transplantation. AJR 128:985, 1977.
184. Bravo JF, Herman JH, Smyth CJ: Musculoskeletal disorders after renal homotransplantation: A clinic and laboratory analysis of 60 cases. Ann Intern Med 66:87, 1967.
185. Irby R, Hume DM: Joint changes observed following renal transplants. Clin Orthop 57:101, 1968.
186. Hall MC, Elmore SM, Bright RW, et al: Skeletal complications in a series of human renal allografts. JAMA 208:1825, 1969.
187. Eremein J, Swaney WE, Marshall VC, et al: Avascular necrosis in cadaveric renal allografts. Aust NZ J Surg 39:41, 1969.
188. Harrington KD, Murray WR, Kountz SL, et al: Avascular necrosis of bone after renal transplantation. J Bone Joint Surg [Am] 53:203, 1971.
189. Evarts CM, Phalen CS: Osseous avascular necrosis associated with renal transplantation. Clin Orthop 78:330, 1971.
190. Rombouts JJ, Troch R, Vincent A, et al: Bone necrosis after renal transplantation. Acta Orthop Belg 38:588, 1972.
191. Francon F, Diaz R: Aseptic osteonecrosis after preventive and curative treatment with immunodepressive agents. Phenomena of rejection after renal transplantation. Brux Med 53:581, 1973.
192. Boerbooms AM, Van der Korst JK: Corticosteroids and femoral head necrosis. Neth J Med 16:267, 1973.
193. Dimich A, Bedrossian PB, Wallach S: Hypoparathyroidism. Arch Intern Med 120:449, 1967.
194. Hung W, Migeon CJ, Parrott RH: Possible autoimmune basis for Addison's disease in three siblings, one with idiopathic hypoparathyroidism, pernicious anemia and superficial moniliasis. N Engl J Med 269:658, 1963.
195. Kolb FO, Steinbach HL: Pseudohypoparathyroidism with secondary hyperparathyroidism and osteitis fibrosa. J Clin Endocrinol 22:59, 1962.
196. Blizzard RM, Chee D, Davis W: The incidence of parathyroid and other antibodies in the sera of patients with idiopathic hypoparathyroidism. Clin Exp Immunol 1:119, 1966.
197. Steinberg H, Waldron BR: Idiopathic hypoparathyroidism: Analysis of 52 cases, including report of new case. Medicine 31:133, 1952.
198. Taybi H, Keele D: Hypoparathyroidism: A review of the literature and report of two cases in sisters, one with steatorrhea and intestinal pseudo-obstruction. AJR 88:432, 1962.
199. Goldman R, Reynolds JL, Cummings HR, et al: Familial hypoparathyroidism: Report of a case. JAMA 150:1104, 1952.
200. Strom L, Winberg J: Idiopathic hypoparathyroidism. Acta Paediatr 43:574, 1954.
201. Bronsky D, Kushner DS, Dubin A, et al: Idiopathic hypoparathyroidism and pseudohypoparathyroidism: Case reports and review of the literature. Medicine 37:317, 1958.
202. Winer NJ: Hypoparathyroidism of probable encephalopathic origin. J Clin Endocrinol 5:86, 1945.
203. Albright F, Reifenstein EC: The Parathyroid Glands and Metabolic Bone Disease. Baltimore, Williams & Wilkins, 1948, p 40.
204. Jowsey J: Bone in parathyroid disorders in man. In RV Talmage, LF Belanger (Eds): Parathyroid Hormone and Thyrocalcitonin (Calcitonin) Amsterdam, Excerpta Medica, 1968, p 137.
205. Achenbach W, Bohm A: Skelettveränderungen bei parathyreogenen Tetanien. ROFO 79:95, 1953.
206. Jimenea CM, Frame B, Chaykin LB, et al: Spondylitis of hypoparathyroidism. Clin Orthop 74:84, 1971.
207. Cusmano JV, Baker DH, Finby N: Pseudohypoparathyroidism. Radiology 67:845, 1956.
208. Chaykin LB, Frame B, Sigler JW: Spondylitis: A clue to hypoparathyroidism. Ann Intern Med 70:995, 1970.
209. Salvesen HA, Boe J: Idiopathic hypoparathyroidism. Acta Endocrinol 14:214, 1953.
210. Gibberd FB: Idiopathic hypoparathyroidism with unusual bone changes and spastic paraplegia. Acta Endocrinol 48:23, 1965.
211. Ott VR, Stěpán J: Spondylitis ankylopoietica bei postoperativer Hypoparathyreose und Hypothyreose. Z Rheumaforsch 26:20, 1967.
212. Follis RH Jr, Park EA: Some observations on bone growth, with particular respect to zones and transverse lines of increased density in the metaphysis. AJR 68:709, 1952.
213. Bennett JC, Maffly RH, Steinbach HL: The significance of bilateral basal ganglia calcification. Radiology 72:368, 1959.
214. Harwood-Nash DCF, Reilly BJ: Calcification of the basal ganglia following radiation therapy. AJR 108:392, 1970.
215. Gayler BW, Brogdon BG: Soft tissue calcifications in the extremities in systemic disease. Am J Med Sci 249:590, 1965.
216. Albright F, Burnett CH, Smith PH, et al: Pseudohypoparathyroidism—an example of "Seabright-Bantam Syndrome." Report of 3 cases. Endocrinology 30:922, 1942.
217. Ritchie GM: Dental manifestations of pseudohypoparathyroidism. Arch Dis Child 40:565, 1965.
218. Henkin RI: Impairment of olfaction and of the tastes of sour and bitter in pseudohypoparathyroidism. J Clin Endocrinol Metab 28:624, 1968.
219. Forbes AP: Fingerprints and palm prints (dermatoglyphics) and palmar-flexion creases in gonadal dysgenesis, pseudohypoparathyroidism and Klinefelter's syndrome. N Engl J Med 270:1268, 1964.

220. Poznanski AK, Werder EA, Giedion A, et al: The pattern of shortening of the bones of the hand in PHP and PPHP—a comparison with brachydactyly E, Turner syndrome, and acrodysostosis. Radiology 123:707, 1977.

221. Gershberg H, Weseley AC: Pseudohypoparathyroidism in pregnancy. Is pseudo-pseudohypoparathyroidism a mild form of pseudohyperparathyroidism? J Pediatr 56:383, 1960.

222. Winnacker JL, Becker KL, Moore CF: Pseudohypoparathyroidism and selective deficiency of thyrotropin. An interesting association. Metabolism 16:644, 1967.

223. Van der Werff JJ: Syndrome of brachymetacarpal dwarfism: With and without gonadal dysgenesis. Lancet 1:69, 1959.

224. Block JB, Clendenning WE: Parathyroid hormone hyporesponsiveness in patients with basal-cell nevi and bone defects. N Engl J Med 268:1157, 1963.

225. Vignon E, Robert JM, Pansu D, et al: Osteodystrophie hereditaire de type 2 d'Albright (pseudo-pseudohypoparathyroidisme) chez deux soeurs (enquête génétique). Lyon Med 225:1083, 1971.

226. Chase LR, Melson GL, Aurbach GD: Metabolic abnormality in pseudohypoparathyroidism. Defective renal excretion of 3',5'-AMP in response to parathyroid hormone. J Clin Invest 47:18a, 1968.

227. Chase LR, Aurbach GD: Activation of skeletal adenyl cyclase by parathyroid hormone in vitro. Third International Congress of Endocrinology. Excerpta Medical Foundation International Congress Series 157:87, 1968.

228. Steinbach HL, Rudhe U, Jonsson M, et al: Evolution of skeletal lesions in pseudohypoparathyroidism. Radiology 85:670, 1965.

229. Malter IJ, McAlister WH: Pseudohypoparathyroidism and myositis ossificans progressiva in the same patient. J Can Assoc Radiol 23:27, 1972.

230. Mann J, Alterman S, Hills AG: Albright's hereditary osteodystrophy comprising pseudohypoparathyroidism and pseudopseudohypoparathyroidism. Ann Intern Med 56:315, 1962.

231. Elrick H, Albright F, Bartter FC, et al: Further studies on pseudo-hypoparathyroidism. Report of four new cases. Acta Endocrinol 5:199, 1950.

232. Steinbach HL, Young DA: The roentgen appearance of pseudohypoparathyroidism (PH) and pseudo-pseudohypoparathyroidism (PPH). Differentiation from other syndromes associated with short metacarpals, metatarsals and phalanges. AJR 97:49, 1966.

233. Bell NH, Gerard ES, Bartter FC: Pseudohypoparathyroidism with osteitis fibrosa cystica and impaired absorption of calcium. J Clin Endocrinol Metab 23:759, 1963.

234. Ablow RC, Hsia YE, Brandt IK: Acrodysostosis coinciding with pseudohypoparathyroidism and pseudo-pseudohypoparathyroidism. AJR 128:95, 1977.

235. Meema HE, Meema S, Oreopoulos DG: Periosteal resorption of finger phalanges: Radial versus ulnar surfaces. J Can Assoc Radiol 29:175, 1978.

236. Sundaram M, Joyce PF, Shields JB, et al: Terminal phalangeal tufts: Earliest site of renal osteodystrophy findings in hemodialysis patients. AJR 133:25, 1979.

237. Doppman JL, Marx S, Spiegel A, et al: Differential diagnosis of Brown tumor vs cystic osteitis by arteriography and computed tomography. Radiology 131:339, 1979.

238. Brown WT, Lyons KP, Winer RL: Changing manifestations of brown tumors on bone scan in renal osteodystrophy. J Nucl Med 19:1146, 1978.

239. Anton HC: Thinning of the clavicular cortex in adults under the age of 45 in osteomalacia and hyperparathyroidism. Clin Radiol 30:307, 1979.

240. Pfeiffer J, Bundschu HD: Reversible Muskelverkalkungen bei akutem Nierenversagen. Klin Wochenschr 56:1125, 1978.

241. Kenzora JE: Dialysis carpal tunnel syndrome. Orthopedics 1:195, 1978.

242. Leb DE, Sharma JK: Clubbing secondary to an arteriovenous fistula used for hemodialysis. JAMA 240:142, 1978.

243. Potter DE, Genant HK, Salvatierra O Jr: Avascular necrosis of bone after renal transplantation. Am J Dis Child 132:1125, 1978.

244. Uittenbogaart CH, Isaacson AS, Stanley P, et al: Aseptic necrosis after renal transplantation in children. Am J Dis Child 132:765, 1978.

245. Macfarlane JD, Filo RS, Brandt KD: Joint effusions after kidney transplantation. Arthritis Rheum 22:164, 1979.

246. Sundarim M, Scholz C: Primary hyperparathyroidism presenting with acute paraplegia. AJR 128:674, 1977.

247. Shaw MT, Davies M: Primary hyperparathyroidism presenting as spinal cord compression. Br Med J 4:230, 1968.

248. Kiss ZS, Neale FC, Posen S, et al: Acute arthritis and hyperuricemia following parathyroidectomy. Arch Intern Med 119:279, 1967.

249. Coburn JW, Gipstein RM, Mirahmadi KS, et al: Calciphylaxis in patients with renal disease. A unique syndrome manifested by soft tissue calcification and necrosis and linked to secondary hyperparathyroidism. Clin Res 21:281, 1973.

250. Stuart C, Aceto T Jr, Kuhn JP, et al: Intrauterine hyperparathyroidism. Postmortem findings in two cases. Am J Dis Child 133:67, 1979.

251. Krishnamurthy GT, Brickman AS, Blahd WH: Technetium-99m-Sn-pyrophosphate pharmaco-kinetics and bone image changes in parathyroid disease. J Nucl Med 18:236, 1977.

252. deGraaf P, Schict IM, Pauwels EKJ, et al: Bone scintigraphy in renal osteodystrophy. J Nucl Med 19:1289, 1978.

253. Carr D, Davidson JK, McMillan M, et al: Renal osteodystrophy: An underdiagnosed condition. Clin Radiol 31:55, 1980.

254. Nixon JR, Douglas JF: Bilateral slipping of the upper femoral epiphysis in end-stage renal failure. A report of two cases. J Bone Joint Surg [Br] 62:18, 1980.

255. Stern PJ, Watts HG: Osteonecrosis after renal transplantation in children. J Bone Joint Surg [Am] 61:851, 1979.

256. Barenfanger J, Mazur JM, Mody N, et al: Malignant fibrous histiocytoma of bone in a renal-transplant patient. Case report. J Bone Joint Surg [Am] 62:297, 1980.

257. Onorato IM, Axelrod JL, Lorch JA, et al: Fungal infections of dialysis fistulae. Ann Intern Med 91:50, 1979.

258. Fong PL, Jackson B, Tucker WG, et al: Progressive osteosclerosis associated with renal failure due to primary oxalosis. A case report. Australas Radiol 23:259, 1979.

259. Bonavita JA, Dalinka MK: Shoulder erosions in renal osteodystrophy. Skel Radiol 5:105, 1980.

260. Kricun R, Kricun ME, Arangio GA, et al: Patellar tendon rupture with underlying systemic disease. AJR 135:803, 1980.

261. Fayemi AO, Ali M: Sarcoid-like granulomas in secondary oxalosis: A case report. Mt Sinai J Med 47:255, 1980.

262. Fogelman I, Carr D: A comparison of bone scanning and radiology in the evaluation of patients with metabolic bone disease. Clin Radiol 31:321, 1950.

263. Fogelman I, Bessent RG, Beastall G, et al: Estimation of skeletal involvement in primary hyperparathyroidism. Use of 24-hour whole body retention of technetium-99m diphosphonate. Ann Intern Med 92:65, 1980.

264. Avioli LV, Raisz LG: Bone metabolism and disease. In PK Bondy, LE Resenberg (Eds): Metabolic Control and Disease. 8th Ed. Philadelphia, WB Saunders Co, 1980, p 1709.

265. Wills MR, Pak CYC, Hammond WG, et al: Normocalcemic primary hyperparathyroidism. Am J Med 47:384, 1969.

266. DeGroote JW: Acute intermittent hyperparathyroidism with hemorrhage into a parathyroid adenoma. JAMA 208:2160, 1969.

267. Frame B, Foroozanfar F, Patton RB: Normocalcemic primary hyperparathyroidism with osteitis fibrosa. Ann Intern Med 73:253, 1970.

268. Burkholder PK, DuBoff EA, Filmanowicz EV: Nontropical sprue with secondary hyperparathyroidism. Am J Dig Dis 10:75, 1965.

269. Davies DR, Dent CE, Wilcox A: Hyperparathyroidism and steatorrhea. Br J Med 2:1133, 1956.

270. Plough IC, Kyle LH: Pancreatic insufficiency and hyperparathyroidism. Ann Intern Med 47:590, 1957.

271. Ehrlich GW, Genant HK, Kolb FO: Secondary hyperparathyroidism and brown tumors in a patient with gluten enteropathy. AJR 141:381, 1983.

272. Singer FR, Sharp CF Jr, Rude RK: Pathogenesis of hypercalcemia in malignancy. Miner Electrolyte Metab 2:161, 1979.

273. Plimpton CH, Gelhorn A: Hypercalcemia in malignant disease without evidence of bone destruction. Am J Med 21:750, 1956.

274. Sharp CF Jr, Rude RK, Terry R, et al: Abnormal bone and parathyroid histology in carcinoma patients with pseudohyperparathyroidism. Cancer 49:1449, 1982.

275. Fry L: Pseudohyperparathyroidism with carcinoma of the bronchus. Br Med J 1:301, 1962.

276. Aurbach GD, Marx SJ, Spiegel AM: Parathyroid hormone, calcitonin, and the calciferols. In RH Williams (Ed): Textbook of Endocrinology. 6th Ed. Philadelphia, WB Saunders Co, 1981, p 922.

277. Resnick D, Deftos LJ, Parthemore JG: Renal osteodystrophy: Magnification radiography of target sites of absorption. AJR 136:711, 1981.

278. Sundaram M, Phillipp SR, Wolverson MK, et al: Ungual tufts in the follow-up of patients on maintenance dialysis. Skel Radiol 5:247, 1980.

279. Hamilton S, Knickerbocker WJ: Peri-articular erosions in the hands and wrists in haemodialysis patients. Clin Radiol 33:19, 1982.

280. Sundaram M, Wolverson MK, Heiberg E, Grider RD: Erosive azotemic osteodystrophy. AJR 136:363, 1981.

281. Meema HE, Oreopoulos DG: The mode of progression of subperiosteal resorption in the hyperparathyroidism of chronic renal failure. Skel Radiol 10:157, 1983.

282. Hooge WA, Li D: CT of sacroiliac joints in secondary hyperparathyroidism. J Can Assoc Radiol 31:42, 1981.

283. Kricun ME, Resnick D: Patellofemoral abnormalities in renal osteodystrophy. Radiology 143:667, 1982.

284. Ang JGP, Weinstein AS: Case report 279. Skel Radiol 12:63, 1984.

285. Griffin CN Jr: Severe erosive arthritis of large joints in chronic renal failure. Skel Radiol 12:29, 1984.

286. Kricun ME, Resnick D: Elbow abnormalities in renal osteodystrophy. AJR 140:577, 1983.

287. Meneghello A, Bertoli M: Tendon disease and adjacent bone erosion in dialysis patients. Br J Radiol 56:915, 1983.

288. Rubin LA, Fam AG, Rubenstein J, et al: Erosive azotemic osteoarthropathy. Arthritis Rheum 27:1086, 1984.

289. Kattan KR, Campana HA: Case report 232. Skel Radiol 10:47, 1983.

290. Nussbaum AJ, Doppman JL: Shoulder arthropathy in primary hyperparathyroidism. Skel Radiol 9:98, 1982.

291. Rosen IB, Palmer JA: Fibroosseous tumors of the facial skeleton in association with primary hyperparathyroidism: An endocrine syndrome or coincidence? Am J Surg 142:494, 1981.

292. Benedict PH: Endocrine features in Albright's syndrome (fibrous dysplasia of bone). Metabolism 11:30, 1962.

293. Benedict PH: Sexual precocity and polyostotic fibrosis dysplasia. Am J Dis Child 111:426, 1966.

294. Firat D, Stutzman L: Fibrous dysplasia of bone. Am J Med 44:421, 1968.

295. Leppla DC, Snyder W, Pak CYC: Sequential changes in bone density before and after parathyroidectomy in primary hyperparathyroidism. Invest Radiol 17:604, 1982.

296. Eftekhari F, Yousefzakeh DK: Primary infantile hyperparathyroidism: clinical, laboratory, and radiographic features in 21 cases. Skel Radiol 8:201, 1982.

297. Resnick D: The "rugger jersey" vertebral body. Arthritis Rheum 24:1191, 1981.
298. Garver P, Resnick D, Niwayama G, et al: Epiphyseal sclerosis in renal osteodystrophy simulating osteonecrosis. AJR 136:1239, 1981.
299. Lewis VL, Keats TE: Bone end sclerosis in renal osteodystrophy simulating osteonecrosis. Skel Radiol 8:275, 1982.
300. Tamarozzi R, Bedani PL, Scutellari PN, et al: Periosteal new bone in uraemic osteodystrophy. Skel Radiol 11:50, 1984.
301. Palma FJM, Ellis HA, Cook DB, et al: Osteomalacia in patients with chronic renal failure before dialysis or transplantation. Q J Med 52:332, 1983.
302. Hsu AC, Kooh SW, Fraser D, et al: Renal osteodystrophy in children with chronic renal failure: An unexpectedly common and incapacitating complication. Pediatrics 70:742, 1982.
303. Hodson EM, Evans RA, Dunstan CR, et al: Quantitative bone histology in children with chronic renal failure. Kidney Int 21:833, 1982.
304. Griffin CN Jr: Symmetrical iliac pseudofractures: A complication of chronic renal failure. A case review with a review of the literature. Skel Radiol 8:295, 1982.
305. McAfee PC, Cady RB: Endocrinologic and metabolic factors in atypical presentations of slipped capital femoral epiphysis. Report of four cases and review of the literature. Clin Orthop 180:188, 1983.
306. Schreiber S, Dupont P: Apatite-induced acute bursitides triggered by parathyroidectomy. Clin Rheum 2:419, 1983.
307. Meneghello A, Bertoli M, Romagnoli GF: Unusual complication of soft tissue calcifications in chronic renal disease: The articular erosions. Skel Radiol 5:251, 1980.
308. Schumacher HR, Miller JL, Ludivico C, et al: Erosive arthritis associated with apatite crystal deposition. Arthritis Rheum 24:31, 1981.
309. Mehls O, Ritz E, Oppermann HC, et al: Femoral head necrosis in uremic children without steroid treatment or transplantation. J Pediatr 99:926, 1981.
310. Ward MK, Feest TG, Ellis HA, et al: Osteomalacic dialysis osteodystrophy: Evidence for a water-borne aetiological agent, probably aluminum. Lancet 1:841, 1978.
311. Pierides AM, Edwards WG Jr, Callum UX Jr, et al: Hemodialysis encephalopathy with osteomalacic fractures and muscle weakness. Kidney Int 18:115, 1980.
312. Cochran M, Platts MM, Moorhead PJ, et al: Spontaneous hypercalcaemia in maintenance dialysis patients: An association with atypical osteomalacia and fractures. Miner Electrolyte Metab 5:280, 1981.
313. Maloney NA, Ott SM, Alfrey AC, et al: Histological quantitation of aluminum in iliac bone from patients with renal failure. J Lab Clin Med 99:206, 1982.
314. Alfrey AC: Dialysis encephalopathy syndrome. Ann Rev Med 29:93, 1978.
315. Lederman RJ, Henry CE: Progressive dialysis encephalopathy. Ann Neurol 4:199, 1978.
316. Prior JC, Cameron EC, Knickerbocker WJ, et al: Dialysis encephalopathy and osteomalacic bone disease. A case-controlled study. Am J Med 72:33, 1982.
317. Alfrey AC, LeGendre GR, Kaehny WD: The dialysis encephalopathy syndrome: Possible aluminum intoxication. N Engl J Med 294:184, 1976.
318. Flendrig JA, Kruis H, Das H: Aluminum and dialysis dementia. Lancet 1:1235, 1976.
319. Rozas VV, Port FK, Rutt WM: Progressive dialysis encephalopathy from dialysate aluminum. Arch Intern Med 138:1375, 1978.
320. McDermott JR, Smith AI, Ward MK, et al: Brain-aluminum concentration in dialysis encephalopathy. Lancet 1:901, 1978.
321. Barmeir E, Dubowitz B, Hudson GA, et al: Radiography of healing dialysis osteodystrophy. Acta Radiol (Diagn) 25:107, 1984.
322. Netter P, Kessler M, Burnel D, et al: Aluminum in the joint tissues of chronic renal failure patients treated with regular hemodialysis and aluminum compounds. J Rheumatol 11:66, 1984.
323. Bertholf RL, Roman JM, Brown S, et al: Aluminum hydroxide-induced osteomalacia, encephalopathy and hyperaluminemia in CAPD. Treatment with desferrioxamine. Peritoneal Dial Bull, Jan-Mar 1984, p 30.
324. Xipell JM, Ham KN, Brown DJ, et al: Case report 294. Skel Radiol 12:298, 1984.
325. de Graaf P, te Velde J, Pauwels EKJ, et al: Increased bone radiotracer uptake in renal osteodystrophy. Clinical evidence of hyperparathyroidism as the major cause. Eur J Nucl Med 7:152, 1982.
326. Kuntz D, Naveau B, Bardin T, et al: Destructive spondylarthropathy in hemodialyzed patients. A new syndrome. Arthritis Rheum 27:369, 1984.
327. Meneghello A, Bertolli M: Neuropathic arthropathy (Charcot's joint) in dialysis patients. ROFO 141:180, 1984.
328. Halter SK, DeLisa JA, Stolov WC, et al: Carpal tunnel syndrome in chronic renal dialysis patients. Arch Phys Med Rehabil 62:197, 1981.
329. Kumar S, Trivedi HL, Smith EKM: Carpal tunnel syndrome: Complication of arteriovenous fistula in hemodialysis patients. Can Med Assoc J 113:1070, 1975.
330. Emery JP, Geffray E, Lemant P: Le syndrome du canal carpien chez l'insuffisant rénal chronique traité par hémodialyse. Sem Hop Paris 59:1161, 1983.
331. Allieu Y, Asencio G, Mailhe D, et al: Syndrome du canal carpien chez l'hémodialysé chronique. Approche étio-pathogénique. A propos de 31 cas opérés. Rev Chir Orthop 69:28, 1983.
332. Mathews RE, Cocke TB, D'Ambrosia RD: Scapular fractures secondary to seizures in patients with osteodystrophy. Report of two cases and review of the literature. J Bone Joint Surg [Am] 65:850, 1983.
333. Marino C, Kazdin H: Spontaneous hemarthrosis in a patient treated with hemodialysis for chronic renal failure. Arthritis Rheum 25:1387, 1982.
334. Chalmers A, Reynolds WJ, Oreopoulos DG, et al: The arthropathy of maintenance intermittent peritoneal dialysis. Can Med Assoc J 123:635, 1980.
335. Elmstedt E: Incidence of skeletal complications in renal graft recipients. Effect of changes in pharmacotherapy. Acta Orthop Scand 53:853, 1982.
336. Elmstedt E, Svahn T: Skeletal complications following renal transplantation. Acta Orthop Scand 52:279, 1981.
337. Andresen J, Nielsen HE: Osteonecrosis and spontaneous fractures following renal transplantation. A longitudinal study of radiological bone changes and metacarpal bone mass. Acta Orthop Scand 52:397, 1981.
338. Charhon S, Baverey E, Malik MC, et al: L'ostéonecrose de la transplantation rénale. Etude clinique; apport de la biopsie osseuse transiliaque. Lyon Med 247:339, 1982.
339. Elmstedt E: Avascular bone necrosis in the renal transplant patient: A discriminant analysis of 144 cases. Clin Orthop 158:149, 1981.
340. Oppermann H-C, Mehls O, Willich E, et al: Osteonekrosen bei Kindern mit chronischen Nierenerkrankungen vor und nach Nierentransplantation. Radiologe 21:175, 1981.
341. Bouteiller G, Dehais-Goffinet F, That HT, et al: Apport de l'histopathologie osseuse à la pathogénie de l'ostéonecrose des transplantes rénaux. Rev Rhum Mal Osteoartic 47:323, 1980.
342. Andressen J, Nielsen HE: Osteonecrosis in renal transplant recipients. Early radiological detection and course. Acta Orthop Scand 52:475, 1981.
343. Elmstedt E: Spontaneous fractures in the renal graft recipient: A discriminant analysis of 144 cases. Clin Orthop 162:195, 1982.
344. Andresen J, Nielsen HE: Interrelationship between metacarpal bone mass and bone mineral content in renal transplant recipients. Acta Radiol (Diagn) 23:513, 1982.
345. Rao KV, O'Brien TJ, Andersen C: Septic arthritis due to Nocardia asteroides after successful kidney transplantation. Arthritis Rheum 24:99, 1981.
346. Leff RD, Smith EJ, Aldo-Benson MA, et al: Cryptococcal arthritis after renal transplantation. South Med J 74:1290, 1981.
347. Michie W, Stowers JM, Frazer SC, et al: Thyroidectomy and the parathyroids. Br J Surg 52:503, 1965.
348. Walton K, Swinson DR: Acute calcific periarthritis associated with transient hypocalcaemia secondary to hypoparathyroidism. Case report. Br J Rheumatol 22:179, 1983.
349. Nusynowitz ML, Frame B, Kolb FO: The spectrum of the hypoparathyroid states: A classification based on physiologic principles. Medicine 55:105, 1976.
350. Singleton EB, Teng CT: Pseudohypoparathyroidism with bone changes simulating hyperparathyroidism. Radiology 78:388, 1962.
351. Hall FM, Segall-Blank M, Genant HK, et al: Pseudohypoparathyroidism presenting as renal osteodystrophy. Skel Radiol 6:43, 1981.
352. Levine MA, Downs RW Jr, Moses AM, et al: Resistance to multiple hormones in patients with pseudohypoparathyroidism. Association with deficient activity of guanine nucleotide regulatory protein. Am J Med 74:545, 1983.
353. Frederiksen PK, Jacobsen JG: Pseudohypoparathyroidism. A 25-year delay in diagnosis. Acta Med Scand 207:341, 1980.
354. Halloran SL, Flannery DB, Kodroff MB, et al: Cheirolumbar dysostosis: A phenotype of pseudohypoparathyroidism. Skel Radiol 10:161, 1983.
355. Foley TP Jr, Harrison HC, Arnaud CD, et al: Familial benign hypercalcemia. J Pediatr 81:1060, 1972.
356. Marx SJ, Attie MF, Levine MA, et al: Familial hypocalciuric hypercalcemia: Recognition among patients referred after unsuccessful parathyroid exploration. Ann Intern Med 92:351, 1980.
357. Law WM Jr, Wahner HW, Heath H III: Bone mineral density and skeletal fractures in familial benign hypercalcemia (hypocalciuric hypercalcemia). Mayo Clin Proc 59:811, 1984.
358. Arnaud CD: Familial benign hypercalcemia: Nature's solution to neonatal hyperparathyroidism? Editorial. Mayo Clin Proc 59:864, 1984.
359. Auwerx J, Demedts M, Bouillon R: Altered parathyroid set point to calcium in familial hypocalciuric hypercalcemia. Acta Endocrinol (Kopenh) 106:215, 1984.
360. Matsuo M, Okita K, Takemine H, et al: Neonatal primary hyperparathyroidism in familial hypocalciuric hypercalcemia. Am J Dis Child 136:728, 1982.
361. Carney JA, Bianco AJ Jr, Sizemore GW, et al: Multiple endocrine neoplasia with skeletal manifestations. J Bone Joint Surg [Am] 63:405, 1981.
362. Carney JA, Go VLW, Gordon H, et al: Familial pheochromocytoma and islet cell tumor of the pancreas. Am J Med 68:515, 1980.
363. Wagener GWW, Sandler M, Hough FS: Advanced osteitis fibrosa cystica in the absence of phalangeal subperiosteal resorption. A case report and review of the literature. S Afr Med J 67:31, 1985.
364. Lachmann M, Kricun ME, Schwartz EE: Case report 310. Skel Radiol 13:248, 1985.
365. Lavalle C, Aparicio LA, Moreno J, et al: Bilateral avulsion of quadriceps tendons in primary hyperparathyroidism. J Rheumatol 12:596, 1985.
366. Richardson ML, Pozzi-Mucelli RS, Kanter AS, et al: Bone mineral changes in primary hyperparathyroidism. Skel Radiol 15:85, 1986.
367. Gilsanz V, Fernal W, Reid BS, et al: Nephrolithiasis in premature infants. Radiology 154:107, 1985.
368. Doppman JL: Multiple endocrine syndromes—a nightmare for the endocrinologic radiologist. Semin Roentgenol 20:7, 1985.
369. Dodds WJ, Wilson SD, Thorsen MK, et al: MEN I syndrome and islet cell lesions of the pancreas. Semin Roentgenol 20:17, 1985.
370. Dodd GD: The radiologic features of multiple endocrine neoplasia types IIA and IIB. Semin Roentgenol 20:64, 1985.
371. Law WM Jr, Heath H III: Familial benign hypercalcemia (hypocalciuric hyper-

calcemia). Clinical and pathogenetic studies in 21 families. Ann Intern Med *102*:511, 1985.

372. Brunt LM, Wells SA Jr: The multiple endocrine neoplasia syndromes. Invest Radiol *20*:916, 1985.
373. Meema HE, Oreopoulos DG, Murray TM: Periosteal resorption and periosteal neostosis: Comparison of normal subjects and renal failure patients on chronic ambulatory peritoneal dialysis using MOP-3 image analysis system and a grading method. Skel Radiol *15*:14, 1986.
374. Bone LB, Roach JW, Ward WT, et al: Slipped capital femoral epiphysis associated with hyperparathyroidism. J Pediatr Orthop *5*:589, 1985.
375. Meema HE, Oreopoulos DG: Morphology, progression, and regression of arterial and periarterial calcifications in patients with end-stage renal disease. Radiology *158*:671, 1986.
376. Bauer TW, Popowniak KL, Stulberg BN, et al: Osteomalacia associated with aluminum intoxication in a patient with chronic renal failure. Cleve Clin Q *52*:271, 1985.
377. Mudde AH, Roodvoets AP, van Groningen K: Hypercalcaemic osteomalacia and encephalopathy due to aluminum intoxication in haemodialysis patients. Neth J Med *28*:6, 1985.
378. Charhon SA, Chavassieux PM, Meunier PJ, et al: Serum aluminum concentration and aluminum deposits in bone in patients receiving haemodialysis. Br Med J *290*:1613, 1985.
379. Garrett P, McWade M, O'Callaghan J: Radiological assessment of aluminum-related bone disease. Clin Radiol *37*:63, 1986.
380. Chambers SE, Winney RJ: Periosteal new bone in patients on intermittent haemodialysis: An early indicator of aluminum-induced osteomalacia. Clin Radiol *36*:163, 1985.
381. Chan Y-L, Furlong TJ, Cornish CJ, et al: Dialysis osteodystrophy. A study involving 94 patients. Medicine *64*:296, 1985.
382. Sebert J-L, Fardellone P, Marie A, et al: Destructive spondylarthropathy in hemodialyzed patients: Possible role of amyloidosis. Arthritis Rheum *29*:301, 1986.
383. Bradish CF: Carpal tunnel syndrome in patients on haemodialysis. J Bone Joint Surg [Br] *67*:130, 1985.
384. Bardin T, Kuntz D, Zingraff J, et al: Synovial amyloidosis in patients undergoing long-term hemodialysis. Arthritis Rheum *28*:1052, 1985.
385. Fenves AZ, Emmett M, White MG, et al: Carpal tunnel syndrome with cystic bone lesions secondary to amyloidosis in chronic hemodialysis patients. Am J Kid Dis *7*:130, 1986.
386. Metselaar HJ, van Steenberge EJP, Bijnen AB, et al: Incidence of osteonecrosis after renal transplantation. Acta Orthop Scand *56*:413, 1985.
387. Bomalaski JS, Williamson PK, Goldstein CS: Infectious arthritis in renal transplant patients. Arthritis Rheum *29*:227, 1986.
388. Rosen RIA, Deshmukh SM: Growth arrest recovery lines in hypoparathyroidism. Radiology *155*:61, 1985.
389. de Carvalho A, Jurik AG, Illum F: Case report 335. Skel Radiol *15*:52, 1986.
390. Burnstein MI, Kottamasu SR, Pettifor JM, et al: Metabolic bone disease in pseudohypoparathyroidism: Radiologic features. Radiology *155*:351, 1985.
391. Firooznia H, Golimbu C, Rafii M: Case report 312. Skel Radiol *13*:310, 1985.
392. Schimke RN: Multiple endocrine neoplasia. Search for the oncogenic trigger. N Engl J Med *314*:1315, 1986.
393. Spencer JD: Bone and joint infection in a renal unit. J Bone Joint Surg [Br] *68*:489, 1986.
394. Goldman AB, Abrahams TG: Case report 356. Skel Radiol *15*:308, 1986.
395. Bergradá E, Montoliu J, Subías R, et al: Síndrome del túnel carpiano con depósito local y articular de sustancia amiloide en el hemodializado. Med Clin (Barcelona) *86*:319, 1986.
396. Cushner HM, Adams ND: Review: Renal osteodystrophy—pathogenesis and treatment. Am J Med Sci *29*:264, 1986.
397. Hardouin P, Flipo RM, Pouyol F, et al: Les discopathies érosives des hémodialysés chronique. Rev Rhum Mal Osteoartic *53*:301, 1986.
398. Gómez JM, Estrada-Laza P: Early radiologic manifestations of destructive spondyloarthropathy in hemodialyzed patients. Arthritis Rheum *29*:1171, 1986.
399. Kaplan P, Resnick D, Murphey M, et al: Destructive noninfectious spondyloarthropathy in hemodialysis patients: A report of four cases. Radiology *162*:241, 1986.
400. Huaux JP, DeDeuxchaisnes CN: Amyloid arthropathy in patients with chronic renal failure. Ann Rheum Dis *45*:878, 1986.
401. McClure J, Bartley CJ, Ackrill P: Carpal tunnel syndrome caused by amyloid containing β₂ microglobulin: A new amyloid and a complication of long term haemodialysis. Ann Rheum Dis *45*:1007, 1986.
402. Casey TT, Stone WJ, DiRaimondo CR, et al: Tumoral amyloidosis of bone of beta₂-microglobulin origin in association with long-term hemodialysis: A new type of amyloid disease. Hum Pathol *17*:731, 1986.
403. Andresen J, Nielsen HE: Quantitative metacarpal bone measurements before and after renal transplantation. Acta Radiol Diagn *27*:437, 1986.
404. Murphey MD: Digital skeletal radiography: Spatial resolution requirements for detection of subperiosteal resorption. AJR *152*:541, 1989.
405. Zamurovic D, Andry G, Lemort M, et al: Concomitant osteitis fibrosa cystica and ameloblastoma of the mandible. J Rheumatol *16*:397, 1989.
406. Samaan NA, Ouais S, Ordonez NG, et al: Multiple endocrine syndrome type I. Clinical, laboratory findings, and management in five families. Cancer *64*:741, 1989.
407. Larsson C, Skogseid B, Oberg K, et al: Multiple endocrine neoplasia type I gene maps to chromosome 11 and is lost in insulinoma. Nature *332*:85, 1988.
408. Sundaram M: Renal osteodystrophy. Skel Radiol *18*:415, 1989.

409. Wolfson BJ, Capitanio MA: The wide spectrum of renal osteodystrophy in children. CRC Crit Rev Diagn Imaging *27*:297, 1987.
410. Present D, Calderoni P, Bacchini P, et al: Brown tumor of the tibia as an early manifestation of renal osteodystrophy. A case report. Clin Orthop *231*:303, 1988.
411. Parnell AP, Simpson W, Ward MK: Periosteal new bone formation in chronic renal failure. Clin Radiol *40*:490, 1989.
412. Tarr RW, Kaye JJ, Nance EP Jr: Insufficiency fractures of the femoral neck in association with chronic renal failure. South Med J *81*:863, 1988.
413. Chalmers J, Irvine GB: Fractures of the femoral neck in elderly patients with hyperparathyroidism. Clin Orthop *229*:125, 1988.
414. Arvin M, White SJ, Braunstein EM: Growth plate injury of the hand and wrist in renal osteodystrophy. Skel Radiol *19*:515, 1990.
415. Reginato AJ, Kurnik B: Calcium oxalate and other crystals associated with kidney diseases and arthritis. Semin Arthritis Rheum *18*:198, 1989.
416. Schumacher HR Jr, Reginato AJ, Pullman S: Synovial fluid oxalate deposition complicating rheumatoid arthritis with amyloidosis and renal failure. Demonstration of intracellular oxalate crystals. J Rheumatol *14*:361, 1987.
417. Chen YM, Bohrer SP: Coracoclavicular and coracoacromial ligament calcification and ossification. Skel Radiol *19*:263, 1990.
418. de Waal Malefijt MC, Beeker TW: Avulsion of the triceps tendon in secondary hyperparathyroidism. A case report. Acta Orthop Scand *58*:434, 1987.
419. Babini SM, Arturi A, Marcos JC, et al: Laxity and rupture of the patellar tendon in systemic lupus erythematosus. Association with secondary hyperparathyroidism. J Rheumatol *15*:1162, 1988.
420. Duncan IJS, Hurst NP, Sebben R, et al: Premature development of erosive osteoarthritis in the hands in patients with chronic renal failure. Ann Rheumat Dis *49*:378, 1990.
421. Rault R, Carpenter B: Pseudoclubbing in chronic renal failure. Q J Med *271*:1063, 1989.
422. Wu AC, Gilula LA: Distal phalangeal brachydactyly secondary to healed renal osteodystrophy. Skel Radiol *16*:312, 1987.
423. Young W, Sevcik M, Tallroth K: Metaphyseal sclerosis in patients with chronic renal failure. Skel Radiol *20*:197, 1991.
424. Griffith TM, Fitzgerald E, Cochlin DL: Osteomesopyknosis: Benign axial osteosclerosis. Br J Radiol *61*:951, 1988.
425. Charhon SA, Chavassieux PM, Chapuy MC, et al: High bone turnover associated with an aluminum-induced impairment of bone mineralization. Bone *7*:319, 1986.
426. Milliner D, Malekzadeh M, Lieberman E, et al: Plasma aluminum levels in pediatric dialysis patients: Comparison of hemodialysis and continuous ambulatory peritoneal dialysis. Mayo Clin Proc *62*:269, 1987.
427. Kriegshauser JS, Swee RG, McCarthy JT, et al: Aluminum toxicity in patients undergoing dialysis: Radiographic findings and prediction of bone biopsy results. Radiology *164*:399, 1987.
428. Mjöberg B: Aluminum-induced hip fractures: A hypothesis. J Bone Joint Surg [Br] *71*:538, 1989.
429. Brem AS, DiMario C, Levy DL: Perceived aluminum-related disease in a dialysis population. Arch Intern Med *149*:2541, 1989.
430. Sundaram M, Dessner D, Ballal S: Solitary, spontaneous cervical and large bone fractures in aluminum osteodystrophy. Skel Radiol *20*:91, 1991.
431. Nebeker HG, Coburn JW: Aluminum and renal osteodystrophy. Ann Rev Med *37*:79, 1986.
432. Oppenheim WL, Namba R, Goodman WG, et al: Aluminum toxicity complicating renal osteodystrophy: A case report. J Bone Joint Surg [Am] *71*:446, 1989.
433. Langevitz P, Buskila D, Stewart J, et al: Osteonecrosis in patients receiving dialysis: Report of two cases and review of the literature. J Rheumatol *17*:402, 1990.
434. Mitrovic DR, Bardin T, Kuntz D: Osteonecrosis in a patient receiving longterm hemodialysis. J Rheumatol *18*:1270, 1991.
435. Deramond H, Sebert JL, Rosat P: Destructive spondyloarthropathy in chronic hemodialysis patients. Current data and radiological aspects. J Neuroradiol *14*:27, 1987.
436. Isaacs M, Bansal M, Flombaum CD, et al: Case report 772. Skel Radiol *22*:129, 1992.
437. Varga J, Fenves A: Destructive spondyloarthropathy in hemodialysis patients. Radiology *164*:584, 1987.
438. Naidich JB, Mossey RT, McHeffey-Atkinson B, et al: Spondyloarthropathy from long-term dialysis. Radiology *167*:761, 1988.
439. McCarthy JT, Dahlberg PJ, Kriegshauser JS, et al: Erosive spondyloarthropathy in long-term dialysis patients: Relationship to severe hyperparathyroidism. Mayo Clin Proc *63*:446, 1988.
440. Kerr R, Bjorkengren A, Bielecki DK, et al: Destructive spondyloarthropathy in hemodialysis patients. Report of four cases and prospective study. Skel Radiol *17*:176, 1988.
441. Rafto SE, Dalinka MK, Schiebler ML, et al: Spondyloarthropathy of the cervical spine in long-term hemodialysis. Radiology *166*:201, 1988.
442. Hurst NP, Van den Berg R: Destructive spondyloarthropathy and chronic renal failure. Arthritis Rheum *31*:1331, 1988.
443. Orzincolo C, Bedani PL, Scutellari PN, et al: Destructive spondyloarthropathy and radiographic follow-up in hemodialysis patients. Skel Radiol *19*:483, 1990.
444. Naito M, Ogata K, Nakamoto M, et al: Destructive spondylo-arthropathy during long-term haemodialysis. J Bone Joint Surg [Br] *74*:686, 1992.
445. Daly KE, Kavannagh TG: Bone cyst in the cervical spine due to secondary amyloidosis. A case report. Acta Orthop Scand *63*:221, 1992.

446. Alcalay M, Goupy M-C, Azais I, et al: Hemodialysis is not essential for the development of destructive spondylarthropathy in patients with chronic renal failure. Arthritis Rheum 30:1182, 1987.

447. Carruzzo PA, Gerster JC, Wauters JP, et al: Spondyloarthropathies de l'hemodialyse chronique: Étude de la charnière occipitale chez 23 patients. Rev Rhum Mal Osteoartic 55:847, 1988.

448. Gerster JC, Carruzzo PA, Ginalski JM, et al: Cervicooccipital hinge changes during longterm hemodialysis. J Rheumatol 16:1469, 1989.

449. Rousselin B, Helenon O, Zingraff J, et al: Pseudotumor of the craniocervical junction during long-term hemodialysis. Arthritis Rheum 33:1567, 1990.

450. Kessler M, Netter P, Grignon B, et al: Destructive β₂-microglobulin amyloid arthropathy of the cervico-occipital hinge in a hemodialyzed patient. Arthritis Rheum 33:602, 1990.

451. Patel B, Mistry CD, Kumar EN, et al: Magnetic resonance imaging in non-infective destructive spondyloarthropathy. Br J Radiol 61:511, 1988.

452. Stäbler A, Kröner G, Seiderer M, et al: MRT der dialyseassoziierten, destruierenden spondylarthropathie der Atlantoaxial region. ROFO 154:469, 1991.

453. Gilbert MS, Robinson A, Baez A, et al: Carpal tunnel syndrome in patients who are receiving long-term renal hemodialysis. J Bone Joint Surg [Am] 70:1145, 1988.

454. Ullian ME, Hammond WS, Alfrey AC, et al: Beta-2-microglobulin-associated amyloidosis in chronic hemodialysis patients with carpal tunnel syndrome. Medicine 68:107, 1989.

455. Cary NRB, Sethi D, Brown EA, et al: Dialysis arthropathy: Amyloid or iron? Br Med J 293:1392, 1986.

456. Netter P, Kessler M, Gaucher A, et al: Does aluminum have a pathogenic role in dialysis associated arthropathy? Ann Rheumatic Dis 49:573, 1990.

457. Bardin T: Dialysis related amyloidosis. J Rheumatol 14:647, 1987.

458. Muñoz-Gómez J, Solé M: Dialysis arthropathy of amyloid origin. J Rheumatol 17:723, 1990.

459. Bruckner FE, Burke M, Pereira RS, et al: Synovial amyloid in chronic haemodialysis contains β₂ microglobulin. Ann Rheumatic Dis 46:634, 1987.

460. Muñoz-Gómez J, Gómez-Pérez R, Solé-Arques M, et al: Synovial fluid examination for the diagnosis of synovial amyloidosis in patients with chronic renal failure undergoing haemodialysis. Ann Rheumatic Dis 46:324, 1987.

461. Bardin T, Zingraff J, Shirahama T, et al: Hemodialysis-associated amyloidosis and beta-2 microglobulin. Clinical and immunohistochemical study. Am J Med 83:419, 1987.

462. Gielen JL, van Holsbeeck MT, Hauglustaine D, et al: Growing bone cysts in long-term hemodialysis. Skel Radiol 19:43, 1990.

463. Westmark KD, Weissman BN: Radiologic vignette. Arthritis Rheum 34:1061, 1991.

464. Sargent MA, Fleming SJ, Chattopadhyay C, et al: Bone cysts and haemodialysis-related amyloidosis. Clin Radiol 40:277, 1989.

465. Mikawa Y, Watanabe R, Yamano Y: Hemodialysis-associated amyloidosis of bone of beta-2 microglobulin origin. Arch Orthop Trauma Surg 109:109, 1990.

466. Ross LV, Ross GJ, Mesgarzadeh M, et al: Hemodialysis-related amyloidomas of bone. Radiology 178:263, 1991.

467. Heller DS, Klein MJ, Gordon RE, et al: Intraosseous beta-2-microglobulin amyloidosis. J Bone Joint Surg [Am] 71:1083, 1989.

468. Tateishi H, Maeda M, Yoh K, et al: Pathologic fracture associated with amyloid deposition in the bone of a chronic hemodialysis patient. A case report. Clin Orthop 274:300, 1992.

469. Scheumann GFW, Holch M, Nerlich ML, et al: Pathologic fractures and lytic bone lesion of the femoral neck associated with β₂-microglobulin amyloid deposition in long-term dialysis patients. Arch Orthop Trauma Surg 110:93, 1991.

470. Kurer MHJ, Baillod RA, Madgwick JCA: Musculoskeletal manifestations of amyloidosis. A review of 83 patients on haemodialysis for at least 10 years. J Bone Joint Surg [Br] 73:271, 1991.

471. Campistol JM, Solé M, Muñoz-Gomez J, et al: Pathologic fractures in patients who have amyloidosis associated with dialysis. A report of five cases. J Bone Joint Surg [Am] 72:568, 1990.

472. Solé M, Muñoz-Gomez J, Campistol JM: Role of amyloid in dialysis-related arthropathies. A morphological analysis of 23 cases. Virchows Archiv A Pathol Anat 417:523, 1990.

473. Allieu Y, Bénichou M, Clémencet F, et al: Les arthropathies amyloïdes à la main chez les hémodialysés chroniques. Ann Chir Main 9:282, 1990.

474. Gaudin P, Juvin R, Sirajedine K, et al: Arthropathie des doigts chez l'insuffisant rénal chronique hémodialysé. Rev Rhum Mal Osteoartic 58:7, 1991.

475. Cary NRB: Clinicopathological importance of deposits of amyloid in the femoral head. J Clin Pathol 38:868, 1985.

476. Kokubo T, Takatori Y, Okutsu I, et al: MR demonstration of intraosseous beta-2-microglobulin amyloidosis. J Comput Assist Tomogr 14:1030, 1990.

477. Claudon M, Regent D, Gaucher A, et al: MR patterns of dialysis arthropathy. J Comput Assist Tomogr 14:968, 1990.

478. Cobby MJ, Adler RS, Swartz R, et al: Dialysis-related amyloid arthropathy: MR findings in four patients. AJR 157:1023, 1991.

479. Hurst NP, van den Berg R, Disney A, et al: "Dialysis related arthropathy": A survey of 95 patients receiving chronic haemodialysis with special reference to β₂ microglobulin related amyloidosis. Ann Rheumatic Dis 48:409, 1989.

480. Kessler M, Netter P, Azoulay E, et al: Dialysis-associated arthropathy: A multicentre survey of 171 patients receiving haemodialysis for over 10 years. Br J Rheumatol 31:157, 1992.

481. Mitrovic DR, Darmon N, Barbara A, et al: Chondrolysis of the hip joint in a patient receiving long-term hemodialysis: Histologic and biochemical evaluation. Arthritis Rheum 32:1477, 1989.

482. Naidich T, Karmel MI, Mossey RT, et al: Osteoarthropathy of the hand and wrist in patients undergoing long-term hemodialysis. Radiology 164:205, 1987.

483. Braunstein EM, Menerey K, Martel W, et al: Radiologic features of a pyrophosphate-like arthropathy associated with long-term dialysis. Skel Radiol 16:437, 1987.

484. Hardouin P, Flipo R-M, Foissac-Gegoux P, et al: Current aspects of osteoarticular pathology in patients undergoing hemodialysis: Study of 80 patients. Part 1. Clinical and radiological analysis. J Rheumatol 14:780, 1987.

485. Hardouin P, Lecomte-Houcke M, Flipo R-M, et al: Current aspects of osteoarticular pathology in patients undergoing hemodialysis: Study of 80 patients. Part 2. Laboratory and pathologic analysis. Discussion of the pathogenic mechanism. J Rheumatol 14:784, 1987.

486. Bardin T, Kuntz D: The arthropathy of chronic haemodialysis. Clin Exp Rheumatol 5:379, 1987.

487. Menerey K, Braunstein E, Brown M, et al: Musculoskeletal symptoms related to arthropathy in patients receiving dialysis. J Rheumatol 15:1848, 1988.

488. Schaab PC, Murphy G, Tzamaloukas AH, et al: Femoral neck fractures in patients receiving long-term dialysis. Clin Orthop 260:224, 1990.

489. Sundaram M, Seelig R, Pohl D: Vertebral erosions in patients undergoing maintenance hemodialysis for chronic renal failure. AJR 149:323, 1987.

490. Rillo OL, Babini SM, Basnak A, et al: Tendinous and ligamentous hyperlaxity in patients receiving longterm hemodialysis. J Rheumatol 18:1227, 1991.

491. Grinlinton FM, Vuletic JC, Gow PJ, et al: Rapidly progressive calcific periarthritis occurring in a patient with lupus nephritis receiving chronic ambulatory peritoneal dialysis. J Rheumatol 17:1100, 1990.

492. Schenkier SL, Gertner E: Massive soft tissue calcification causing complete loss of extensor tendon function in renal failure. J Rheumatol 19:1640, 1992.

493. Meltzer CC, Fishman EK, Scott WW Jr: Tumoral calcinosis causing bone erosion in a renal dialysis patient. Clin Imaging 16:49, 1992.

494. Cornélis F, Bardin T, Faller B, et al: Rheumatic syndromes and β₂-microglobulin amyloidosis in patients receiving long-term peritoneal dialysis. Arthritis Rheum 32:785, 1989.

495. Röckel A, Gilge U, Muller R, et al: Elimination of low molecular weight proteins during hemofiltration and CAPD. Trans Am Soc Artif Intern Organs 28:382, 1982.

496. Ménard H-A, Langevin S, Lévesque R-Y: Destructive spondyloarthropathy in short term chronic ambulatory peritoneal dialysis and hemodialysis. J Rheumatol 15:644, 1988.

497. Bicknell JM, Lim AC, Raroque HG Jr, et al: Carpal tunnel syndrome, subclinical median mononeuropathy, and peripheral polyneuropathy: Common early complications of chronic peritoneal dialysis and hemodialysis. Arch Phys Med Rehabil 72:378, 1991.

498. Kessler M, Grignon B, Renoult E, et al: Complete resolution of large periarticular calcifications after renal transplantation. J Rheumatol 16:854, 1989.

499. Lausten GS, Jensen JS, Ølgaard K: Necrosis of the femoral head after renal transplantation. Acta Orthop Scand 59:650, 1988.

500. Tervonen O, Mueller DM, Matteson EL, et al: Clinically occult avascular necrosis of the hip: Prevalence in an asymptomatic population at risk. Radiology 182:845, 1992.

501. Farge D, Remy Ph, Poignet JL, et al: Isolated bone-end sclerosis simulating osteonecrosis after renal transplantation. Arthritis Rheum 33:1444, 1990.

502. Spencer JD: Spontaneous rupture of tendons in dialysis and renal transplant patients. Injury 19:86, 1988.

503. Agarwal S, Owen R: Tendinitis and tendon ruptures in successful renal transplant recipients. Clin Orthop 252:270, 1990.

504. Lambert RGW, Becker EJ: Diffuse skeletal hyperostosis in idiopathic hypoparathyroidism. Clin Radiol 40:212, 1989.

505. Pagès M, Lassoued S, Fournie B, et al: Association d'une hypoparathyroïdie idiopathique au syndrome de Fahr (calcifications intra-crâniennes) et d'une maladie hyperostosante. Sem Hôp Paris 65:2928, 1989.

506. Van Dop C, Wang H, Mulaikal RM, et al: Pseudopseudohypoparathyroidism with spinal cord compression. Pediatr Radiol 18:429, 1988.

507. Hayes CW, Conway WF: Hyperparathyroidism. Radiol Clin North Am 29:85, 1991.

508. Chew FS, Huang-Hellinger F: Brown tumor. AJR 160:752, 1993.

509. Murase T, Kawai H: Carpal-tunnel syndrome in hemodialysis. Syndrome diagnosed in 8 of 60 patients. Acta Orthop Scand 64:475, 1993.

510. Tierney GS, Goulet JA, Greenfield ML, et al: Mortality after fracture of the hip in patients who have end-stage renal disease. J Bone Joint Surg [Am] 76:709, 1994.

511. Vande Berg BC, Malghem J, Goffin EJ, et al: Transient epiphyseal lesions in renal transplant recipients: Presumed insufficiency stress fractures. Radiology 191:403, 1994.

512. Mankin HJ: Metabolic bone disease. J Bone Joint Surg [Am] 76:760, 1994.

58

Disorders of Other Endocrine Glands and of Pregnancy

Donald Resnick, M.D.

Included in this chapter is a discussion of several additional endocrine disorders that may be associated with significant abnormalities of the skeleton. Some of these diseases may lead to bone and joint changes that are included more appropriately elsewhere in the book (e.g., diabetic neuropathic osteoarthropathy and infection; steroid-induced osteonecrosis) so that these changes will receive only limited attention here. In addition, musculoskeletal manifestations accompanying or occurring after pregnancy are discussed.

CUSHING'S DISEASE

General Features

Cushing's syndrome, first described by Cushing in 1932, is caused by the presence of excessive amounts of adrenocortical glucocorticoid steroids in the body. This excess may be induced by hyperplasia or hyperfunctioning tumors of the adrenal cortex (endogenous Cushing's disease) or by excessive administration of corticosteroid medication (exogenous Cushing's disease). Endogenous Cushing's disease usually results from adrenal hyperplasia (approximately 75 per cent), less commonly from adenoma or carcinoma of the adrenal gland, and rarely from neuroblastoma, anterior pituitary neoplasm, ectopic adrenal tissue, and ectopic adrenocorticotropic hormone–producing tumors.[1, 2] The disease can occur at any age but is most frequent in women between the ages of 20 and 60 years. Its onset is variable; in some patients, an insidious clinical picture is evident, whereas in others, symptoms and signs appear rapidly.[3] Easy bruisability and the development of purpura, especially in the hands and forearms, may be early manifestations. In women, menstrual abnormalities may herald the onset of the disease, with irregularity of menses or even amenorrhea. Generalized obesity, muscle weakness, emotional disturbance, and backache are additional common symptoms. On physical examination, patients may demonstrate moon face (increased fullness of the face and cheeks), buffalo hump (fatty deposition over the dorsal spine), increased transparency of the skin, abdominal and axillary purple striae, abnormal distribution of hair with hirsutism, hypertension, and bone tenderness. In children, growth arrest and short stature are observed.[4] Laboratory tests reveal leukocytosis and a glucose tolerance test with results characteristic of diabetes mellitus. Modest hypercalciuria is frequent. Abdominal radiographs coupled with special studies, including intravenous pyelography, nephrotomography, CT, and arteriography, outline enlarged adrenal glands and renal calculi (approximately 15 to 20 per cent of patients).

Osteoporosis

Reduced bone substance in Cushing's syndrome frequently is severe, reflecting decreased bony deposition associated with increased bony resorption.[5, 6] The histologic appearance is designated "smooth bone atrophy" by pathologists,[7] as it resembles osteoporosis accompanying the postmenopausal and senile states. It is most pronounced in the axial skeleton, particularly the vertebral column, pelvis, ribs, and cranial vault. Microscopic analysis delineates thin, sparse spongy trabeculae whose surfaces contain few osteoblasts or Howship's lacunae. Fatty infiltration of the marrow spaces can be identified.[8, 9] Cortical thinning and osseous deformity with fracture, particularly of the vertebral bodies, can be seen. Of interest is the appearance of endosteal callus, often exuberant in quantity, surrounding fracture sites, accounting for exaggerated radiodensity about compressed vertebrae. This excessive callus formation is observed not only in endogenous steroid excess (Cushing's syndrome) but also in exogenous excess from administration of steroid medication.[10] It is not a specific sign, as it is evident in other diseases, such as osteogenesis imperfecta.

Radiographic examination of patients with Cushing's syndrome reveals typical findings of osteoporosis. The changes predominate in the spine, where diminished bone density, biconcave deformities of vertebral bodies (fish vertebrae), compression fractures, and exaggerated kyphosis are apparent (Fig. 58–1). The appearance is not unlike that in other disorders associated with osteoporosis, although increased radiodensity of the superior and inferior margins of compressed or collapsed vertebral bodies allows specific diagnosis in some patients with Cushing's disease. Furthermore, as opposed to characteristics of postmenopausal and senile osteoporosis, the osteoporosis of Cushing's syndrome may involve the skull, creating peculiar patchy radiolucent areas in the cranial vault. The ribs also are involved, and rib fractures, which are frequent in Cushing's syndrome, may heal with abundant callus formation. Osteoporosis of the pelvis may be associated with protrusio acetabuli. Although osteopenia in the appendicular skeleton generally is not attributed to Cushing's syndrome, one or more pathologic fractures of the long tubular bones in the extremities has been noted on rare occasions in this condition.[11]

Osteoporosis, vertebral compression, and kyphosis also may occur with exogenous corticosteroid therapy.[12] The degree of osteoporosis may be influenced by the type and dose schedule of administered steroids. In addition, experimental evidence obtained from rabbits has indicated that corticosteroid administration may be associated with an initial phase of increased endosteal and trabecular resorption, which is not followed by bone formation. Although this phase may subside after a few months, significant bone loss will have occurred, a fact that may be important in patients who receive an initial high dose of corticosteroids.[13]

Osteonecrosis

Osteonecrosis is a well-recognized complication of exogenous hypercortisolism.[14–16] A similar occurrence in endogenous hypercortisolism is not commonly recorded.[17–23] Osteonecrosis in this latter situation most frequently involves the femoral head, although changes in the humeral head also have been noted and, rarely, osteonecrosis may be the initial manifestation of the disease.[18, 22] Considering that similar factors may be operational in both exogenous and endogenous steroid excess, such as subchondral osteoporosis, vascular occlusion due to peripheral fat infiltration or embolization, hypercoagulability, vasculitis, and joint anesthesia, it is surprising that osteonecrosis is not reported more frequently during the course of endogenous Cushing's syndrome. The factors leading to steroid-induced osteonecrosis are discussed in more detail elsewhere in the book. When osteonecrosis occurs in this syndrome, typical radiographic features are evident, with subchondral curvilinear radiolucent shadows, osteoporosis, osteosclerosis, bony collapse and fragmentation, and a relatively normal articular space (Fig. 58–2).

Other Musculoskeletal Abnormalities

Although systemically or locally administered steroid medication may lead to a variety of abnormalities, including a peculiar destructive arthropathy that simulates neuropathic osteoarthropathy,[24] articular infection,[25] and tendon injury and rupture[26] (Fig. 58–3), these features are not recorded in endogenous Cushing's disease. Delayed skeletal maturation, growth recovery lines, decreased osteophyte formation about abnormal articulations, and loss of the lamina dura rarely can be observed in this disease.

Soft tissue changes relate to redistribution of fat, leading to accumulation of fatty tissue in the trunks of adults and in the trunks and extremities of children.[2] Muscle atrophy and mediastinal and retroperitoneal fat deposition may be noted.[27] CT scanning in Cushing's disease has confirmed the predisposition of such deposition in the trunk and supraclavicular and posterior cervical regions, as well as a dramatic increase in intra-abdominal fat.[28] With quantitative CT, intravertebral fat content in patients with this disease does not differ from that in a control population.[29]

CONGENITAL ADRENAL HYPERPLASIA

This condition, originally called the adrenogenital syndrome, is related to a relative or absolute loss of one of the various enzymes that are involved in the conversion of cholesterol to normal hormonal steroids. This defect allows the accumulation of steroid intermediates and, as a result of the hypothalamic-pituitary feedback system, leads to the secretion of excessive amounts of ACTH, with resultant adrenal hyperplasia.[30] The clinical picture varies according to the precise enzymatic defect that is present, but the most

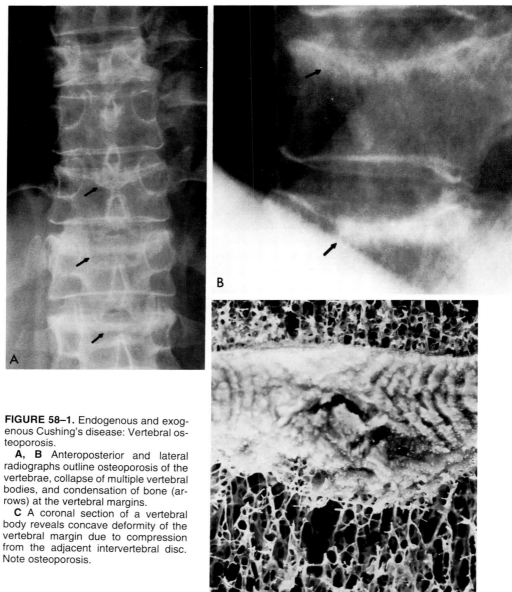

FIGURE 58–1. Endogenous and exogenous Cushing's disease: Vertebral osteoporosis.

A, B Anteroposterior and lateral radiographs outline osteoporosis of the vertebrae, collapse of multiple vertebral bodies, and condensation of bone (arrows) at the vertebral margins.

C A coronal section of a vertebral body reveals concave deformity of the vertebral margin due to compression from the adjacent intervertebral disc. Note osteoporosis.

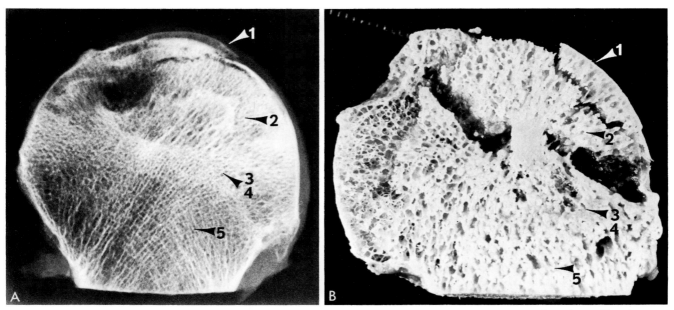

FIGURE 58–2. Exogenous Cushing's disease: Osteonecrosis. A radiograph and photograph of coronal sections of two femoral heads reveal osteonecrosis due to steroid medication. Observe a zone of articular cartilage with separated subchondral fragments (1), a zone of bone necrosis (2), zones of increased vascularity and new bone formation (3, 4), and a zone of normal bone (5). These zones are discussed in detail elsewhere in the book.

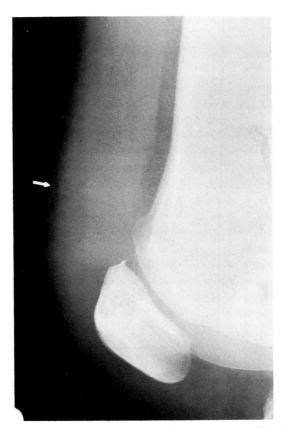

FIGURE 58–3. Steroid administration: Tendon rupture. After local injections of steroids, an acute (partial) quadriceps tendon rupture has occurred. Observe soft tissue swelling (arrow), effusion, and loss of normal tendinous anatomy.

frequent type of intersex problem is female pseudohermaphroditism. Virilization of the female usually is present at birth or, less frequently, in the first few months of life. Accelerated growth initially is seen, but premature physeal closure eventually may lead to short stature. Additional musculoskeletal manifestations include accelerated dental maturation, prominent musculature, and premature calcification of the costal cartilages.[2] The syndrome also may be observed in adults.

ADDISON'S DISEASE

Destruction of the adrenal cortex leading to Addison's disease can be attributed to a variety of processes, including infections such as tuberculosis or fungal diseases, and infiltrating neoplasms, although most commonly idiopathic atrophy of the adrenal glands, perhaps related to an autoimmune disorder,[31] is observed. The clinical manifestations usually are insidious and related to deficiencies of aldosterone (weight loss, weakness, hypovolemia, hypotension, decreased cardiac output, prerenal azotemia, acidosis, syncope, and shock) and cortisol (anorexia, nausea, vomiting, abdominal pain, lethargy, psychosis, hypotension, hypoglycemia, and hyperpigmentation). Musculoskeletal manifestations are not frequent or prominent; findings include migratory myalgias, back pain, and sciatica.[32–34] Additional abnormalities are the Guillain-Barré syndrome,[35] hyperkalemic neuromyopathy,[36] hyponatremic myopathy,[37] and flexion deformities (which may be severe and progressive and predominate in the lower limbs).[38] Radiographs in patients with Addison's disease may reveal calcification in the adrenal glands, external ear, periarticular areas, and costal cartilages, and skeletal maturation may be delayed.[2]

PHEOCHROMOCYTOMA

A pheochromocytoma arises from chromaffin elements, typically in the adrenal medulla but also in the para-aortic and thoracic sympathetic chains, the organs of Zuckerkandl, the carotid body, and the urinary bladder.[2] Adults between the ages of 30 and 50 years usually are affected, although the tumor may be seen in children. Familial cases and a bilateral distribution are recorded. Clinical abnormalities can result from the physical presence of the neoplasm itself but are related more frequently to the increased production of catecholamines, leading to hypertension, flushing or blanching, palpitations, excessive sweating, headache, anorexia, weight loss, decreased gastrointestinal motility, and psychosis.

With regard to the musculoskeletal system, osteolytic and osteosclerotic regions in the metaphyses of the tubular bones of children, presumably related to ischemia and infarction, have been reported (Fig. 58–4).[39, 40] The lesions regress after surgical treatment of the tumor.[41] A second osseous abnormality relates to sites of metastasis, which predominate in the axial skeleton.[42] Single or multiple, small or large, circular or oval osteolytic lesions are seen,

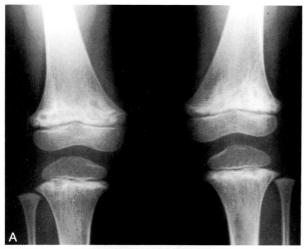
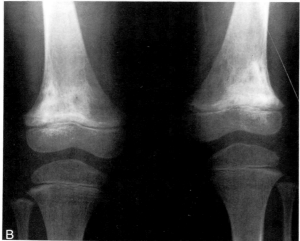

FIGURE 58–4. Pheochromocytoma: Metaphyseal abnormalities. Two examples demonstrate the type of metaphyseal alterations that have been described in children with pheochromocytoma. These lesions regress after surgical treatment of the tumor. (Courtesy of J. C. Hoeffel, M.D., Nancy, France.)

which may lead to bone expansion and fracture.[43] Irregularity of the epiphyses in the fingers of a child with pheochromocytoma also has been reported.[265]

NEUROBLASTOMA

Tumors of the sympathetic nervous system generally are classified as neuroblastoma, ganglioneuroblastoma, and ganglioneuroma.[2] Of these, neuroblastoma is most frequent and usually arises in the adrenal medulla. In common with pheochromocytoma, the tumor can be accompanied by excessive production of catecholamines and catecholamine metabolites; however, neuroblastoma is a very aggressive tumor characterized by rapid growth and widespread metastases.[30, 44] Approximately 80 per cent of patients are children less than 5 years of age, and most of these are younger than 2 years of age.[45] Boys and girls are affected in equal numbers. At the time that the neuroblastoma is discovered, skeletal metastases are frequent (see Chapter 85), especially in those instances in which the primary tumor is of adrenal medullary origin.[2] Bilateral and symmetric osseous lesions, especially in the metaphyseal segments, are typical (Fig. 58–5), although less widespread involvement can be evident. Osteolytic lesions with permeative bone destruction predominate, particularly in the femur and tibia; sclerosis is less common and is a late manifestation of the disease, but it may become extensive.[2] Mild to moderate periostitis is encountered.[46] In the skull, increased intracranial pressure (due to leptomeningeal involvement and leading to sutural diastasis), vertical osseous striations extending from the outer table, and soft tissue swelling are seen. Additional manifestations of the skeletal metastases include ''floating'' teeth related to mandibular involvement, vertebral collapse, rib alterations with extrapleural extension, and pelvic bone destruction with soft tissue masses compressing nearby viscera, such as the bladder. The differential diagnosis includes Ewing's sarcoma, lymphomas, leukemias, and metastases from other tumors, such as rhabdomyosarcoma, medulloblastoma, retinoblastoma, and Wilms' tumor.

DIABETES MELLITUS

General Features

Although numerous musculoskeletal disorders have been described in conjunction with diabetes mellitus, an association between diabetes and many of these other disorders has not been well documented (Table 58–1).[47] Much of the difficulty in associating diabetes and additional rheumatic conditions is related to the extreme frequency of this endocrine disease, so that its occurrence in combination with another disease process, such as gout, calcium pyrophosphate dihydrate crystal deposition disease, and diffuse idiopathic skeletal hyperostosis (ankylosing hyperostosis of the spine), may represent no more than the coincidental appearance of two diseases in the same patient. An exception to this is the association of diabetes mellitus with neuropathic osteoarthropathy, in which distinctive destructive and atrophic osseous changes may be apparent, particularly in the lower extremity, and in which septic arthritis and osteomyelitis may be additional features.

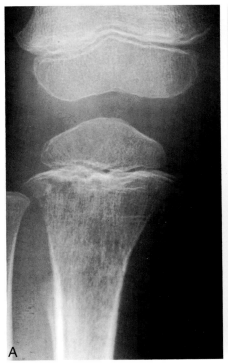
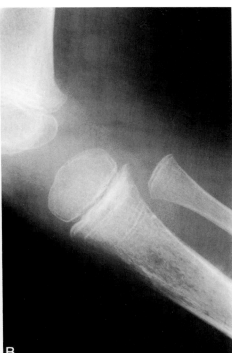

FIGURE 58–5. Neuroblastoma: Skeletal metastasis. In this 3 year old boy, observe permeative bone destruction and periostitis in the metaphysis of the tibia. Growth recovery lines also are evident.

Gouty Arthritis

The relationship between diabetes mellitus and gouty arthritis is not well defined. Patients with uncontrolled diabetes and ketoacidosis may develop hyperuricemia owing to inhibition of urate excretion by the kidney, increased protein catabolism, and dehydration.[48] Controversy exists regarding the associations of hyperuricemia and stable diabetes mellitus and of hyperglycemia and gout. Reports of elevated levels of serum glucose and diabetes mellitus in patients with hyperuricemia and gout[49–51] have conflicted with other investigations in which no such association was detected.[52, 53] When patients with gout are compared with age- and weight-matched control subjects, no significant difference is found in glucose metabolism between the two groups.[54] This evidence suggests that the prevalence of diabetes in patients with gout is related to the high frequency of obesity in hyperuricemic subjects.[55]

TABLE 58–1. Musculoskeletal Manifestations of Diabetes Mellitus

Gout*
CPPD crystal deposition disease*
Degenerative joint disease*
DISH
Soft tissue and muscle syndromes
  Periarthritis
  Diabetic cheiroarthropathy
  Dupuytren's contracture
  Flexor tenosynovitis
  Carpal tunnel syndrome
  Skeletal muscle infarction
Osteomyelitis
Septic arthritis
Neuropathic osteoarthropathy
Forefoot osteolysis

*Possible association.

Calcium Pyrophosphate Dihydrate (CPPD) Crystal Deposition Disease

The frequency of diabetes mellitus in patients with CPPD crystal deposition disease may be quite high, some reports indicating such an association in over 40 per cent of persons.[56] Similarly, the frequency of CPPD crystal accumulation in persons with diabetes mellitus has been found to be quite high (see Chapter 44), although some investigators have failed to demonstrate an increased frequency of CPPD crystal deposition in diabetic patients compared with matched control subjects.[57] Thus, a true association of diabetes mellitus and CPPD crystal deposition disease is not clear at this time.

Degenerative Joint Disease

A possible association between diabetes mellitus and degenerative joint disease has been suggested in some reports.[58, 59] Although this association is not well documented and additional factors, such as obesity, must be taken into account in any analysis, a greater frequency, earlier onset, and more severe form of the disease may characterize the occurrence of degenerative joint disease in diabetic patients.[60]

Diffuse Idiopathic Skeletal Hyperostosis (Ankylosing Hyperostosis of the Spine)

Diffuse idiopathic skeletal hyperostosis (DISH) is a common and characteristic disorder of spinal and extraspinal sites that is discussed in detail elsewhere in the book. This disorder is particularly frequent in diabetic and obese patients[61, 62] (Fig. 58–6). In one series, 13 per cent of 510 diabetic persons demonstrated DISH, and in patients between the ages of 60 and 69 years, a greater frequency of

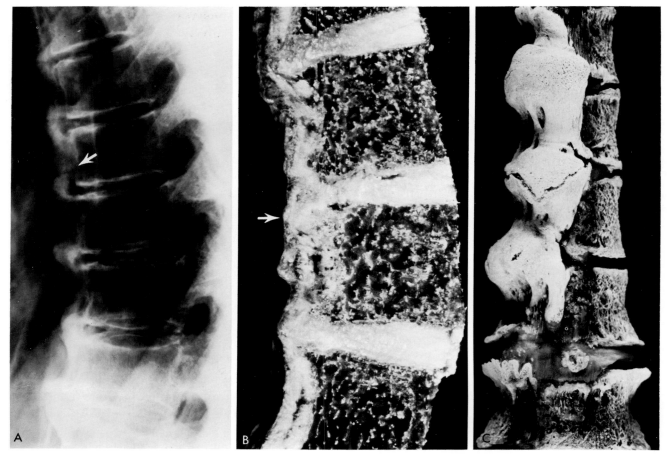

FIGURE 58–6. Diabetes mellitus and diffuse idiopathic skeletal hyperostosis (DISH).
A In a patient with diabetes, typical radiographic features of DISH are seen, with flowing ossification along the anterior aspect of the thoracic spine, a bumpy spinal contour, and a radiolucent area beneath the deposited bone (arrow).
B On a sagittal section of the spine, exuberant bone is apparent anteriorly (arrow), extending across multiple intervertebral discs.
C An anterior view of a macerated spine reveals the nature and extent of this flowing ossification and its predilection for the anterior aspect of the middle and lower thoracic spine.

DISH was detected in diabetic patients (21 per cent) than in nondiabetic patients (4 per cent).[63] Other series have arrived at similar conclusions.[64] Further evidence of an association between diabetes mellitus and DISH is a significant occurrence of glucose intolerance in patients with this ossifying diathesis.[65] In general, diabetes mellitus is mild in patients with DISH, and the severity of the disease does not correspond to the extent of DISH.[48]

Soft Tissue and Muscle Syndromes

Several syndromes involving soft tissues or skeletal muscle may be observed in patients with diabetes mellitus. Not included here is the increased frequency of soft tissue (as well as visceral) arterial calcification that may be seen in this disorder[66, 67] (see later discussion).

Periarthritis. Periarthritis produces a painful stiff shoulder characterized by loss of joint motion, particularly internal rotation and abduction, without evidence of intra-articular disease. The condition is more common in women and in those over the age of 40 years. It may be bilateral or unilateral in distribution, and in the latter case, there is a tendency for the nondominant extremity to be involved.[68] Periarthritis of the shoulder may be four or five times more

common in diabetic patients than in nondiabetic patients.[69] Periarthritis or bursitis in this region has been observed in 10 to 20 per cent of patients with diabetes mellitus, and abnormalities in serum glucose levels are reported to be frequent in persons with such shoulder abnormalities.[64] When associated with diabetes, the syndrome more commonly is bilateral in distribution and predominates in insulin-dependent patients whose disease is of long duration.

On radiographic examination, patients with periarthritis may reveal no abnormality, although calcific bursitis or tendinitis may be apparent.[70] Capsular fibrosis and thickening are pathologic findings in this condition.[71, 72]

Glenohumeral joint periarthritis can be accompanied by the shoulder-hand syndrome.[73, 74] Clinical findings include initial stiffness and pain of one or both hands, followed by diffuse swelling, warmth, erythema, tenderness, and hyperhidrosis of the hands. Subsequently, after several weeks or months, swelling decreases and atrophy of the skin and muscle, osteopenia, and thickening and contracture of the palmar fascia are noted. The syndrome may resolve spontaneously or be followed by permanent limb disability. As with periarthritis, this syndrome appears to be more common in patients with diabetes mellitus.

Diabetic Cheiroarthropathy. A condition sharing some

clinical features with the shoulder-hand syndrome has been described in as many as 40 per cent of patients with insulin-requiring juvenile diabetes.[75–86] Generally seen during the course of the diabetes or, rarely, preceding it,[80, 85] this condition may reflect an increased risk for microvascular disease,[83] a belief not shared by all investigators.[78] Characteristic findings of this syndrome, which is variously termed diabetic cheiroarthropathy and diabetic hand syndrome, are mild to moderately severe joint contractures of the fingers, particularly at the proximal interphalangeal joints and in the fourth and fifth digits, thickening and a waxy appearance of the skin on the dorsum of the hand, and short stature. There is no evidence of palmar fascial thickening or Dupuytren's contracture. Occasionally other joints may be involved, including the wrists, elbows, hips, knees, and toes.[87, 88] On rare occasions, cases of this syndrome have been identified in adults with insulin-dependent or non-insulin-dependent diabetes.[77, 81, 89–91]

The skin abnormalities resemble those of scleroderma, and biopsy reveals a marked increase in dermal thickness, an increase in connective tissue in the lower dermis, and a dearth of glands in hair follicles.[82] The pathogenesis of the syndrome is not certain, although an increase in cross linking of collagen is recognized in human and experimental diabetes mellitus; the scleroderma-like skin alterations in the disease may result from nonenzymatic glycosylation that may alter the packing, cross linking, and turnover of collagen.[76] Vascular abnormalities also may be an important pathogenetic factor. Neuropathy and myopathy could contribute to joint contracture.

Dupuytren's Contracture. A high frequency of Dupuytren's contracture has been recognized in patients with diabetes, with reports varying from 3 to 40 per cent.[92–95] Similarly, diabetes mellitus is not infrequent in patients who reveal Dupuytren's contracture; in a hospital survey of 90 patients with Dupuytren's contractures in a population of 900 patients, 47 per cent revealed overt diabetes.[96] In diabetic patients, the frequency of Dupuytren's contracture increases with long-standing disease, and involvement of the third finger is more common than in nondiabetic persons with similar contracture.[95] It generally is mild, rarely requiring surgery, and is somewhat more severe in men.[95]

This condition develops insidiously as nodular or plaque-like thickening of the palmar fascia, initially over the ulnar side of the hand.[73] Extension of the fibrous process to the metacarpophalangeal and proximal interphalangeal joints may result in finger contracture (Fig. 58–7). The overlying skin may be dimpled. Although the cause of this condition is unknown, genetic factors may be important, as a family history of Dupuytren's contracture may be apparent, and there is an ethnic and racial distribution of the disorder.[97]

Flexor Tenosynovitis. Flexor tenosynovitis (trigger finger, stenosing tenovaginitis) refers to a condition of one or more fingers associated with snapping, pain, locking, and limitation of motion of the interphalangeal joint due to obstruction of the flexor tendon in a constricted tendon sheath. The sheath is thickened, with local inflammatory changes, fibrous proliferation, and collagenous degeneration,[98, 99] which can be detected clinically as a node on the undersurface of the metacarpal head. Flexor tenosynovitis may be associated with the carpal tunnel syndrome due to concomitant involvement of the tendon sheaths of the hand and wrist.

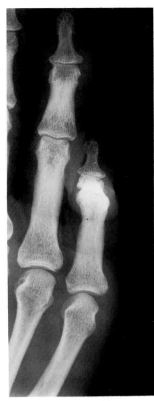

FIGURE 58–7. Diabetes mellitus and Dupuytren's contracture. Observe flexion contracture at the fifth proximal interphalangeal joint in this diabetic patient.

The condition has been described in a variety of clinical situations. In children, it may have a hereditary basis, with predilection for the first digit[100]; in adults, flexor tenosynovitis may be a manifestation of trauma, articular disorders, soft tissue tumors, and myxedema.[101] Some reports suggest that diabetes mellitus may be apparent in 10 to 30 per cent of patients with flexor tenosynovitis.[73, 102, 103] There is a marked female predominance and a modest predilection for involvement of the right hand.[103] Flexor tenosynovitis accompanying diabetes mellitus may occur in young adults and involve more than one digit.[104]

Carpal Tunnel Syndrome. The carpal tunnel syndrome results from entrapment of the median nerve within the carpal tunnel on the volar aspect of the wrist. Although 40 to 50 per cent of cases of carpal tunnel syndrome have no apparent cause, any process associated with a mass in and around the carpal tunnel can produce this syndrome. Tissue infiltration in leukemia, sarcoidosis, amyloidosis, and neoplasm; tissue edema in acromegaly and hypothyroidism; tissue hemorrhage occurring after trauma; and tissue inflammation in rheumatoid arthritis, systemic lupus erythematosus, dermatomyositis, gout, and CPPD crystal deposition disease are potential causes.[73] The frequency of diabetes mellitus in patients with the carpal tunnel syndrome has been reported as 5 to 17 per cent.[105, 106] It has been suggested that an increased occurrence of this syndrome in diabetes may be due to ischemic changes related to microvascular disease.[73, 107]

Skeletal Muscle Infarction. In diabetes mellitus, skeletal muscle infarction attributable to atherosclerosis obliterans may be observed.[267] This complication most typically is seen in patients with poorly controlled disease, and results in excruciating pain and tender swelling or a mass in the involved muscle. The muscles in the lower extremity, especially those in the thigh and calf, are involved most commonly, and multiple sites in one or both legs may be affected. Clinical manifestations may simulate those of myositis, abscess, neoplasm, deep venous thrombosis, or ruptured synovial cyst.[268] Open biopsy in cases of skeletal muscle infarction may be complicated by hemorrhage and slow healing, leading to an increased reliance on diagnostic imaging methods, especially scintigraphy and MR imaging.[268, 269] With the latter technique, involved muscles usually reveal little change in signal intensity or low signal intensity in T1-weighted images and hyperintensity in T2-weighted and short tau inversion recovery images.[268] Spontaneous resolution of the clinical and imaging abnormalities may occur with conservative treatment.

Osteomyelitis and Septic Arthritis

Soft tissue ulceration and infection, which are frequent in diabetes, may lead to contamination of contiguous bones and joints (see Chapter 64). This sequence is particularly frequent in the diabetic foot (Fig. 58–8). At this site, the presence of potential anatomic pathways in the soft tissues may lead to dissemination of contaminated fluid in patients with neglected infection, necessitating amputation of the lower leg.[108, 109] Initial soft tissue lesions in the diabetic foot are especially frequent beneath the first and fifth metatarsophalangeal joints and the calcaneus at pressure points. The soft tissue abnormalities may become severe, perhaps related to the presence of decreased host resistance to infection, small vessel angiopathy, and neuropathy.[110, 111] Diabetic foot infections usually involve mixed bacterial flora, including aerobic, facultatively anaerobic, and anaerobic microorganisms.[112, 113] The initial radiographic findings include defects in soft tissue contour, loss of tissue planes, and swelling.[114] As the infection reaches the bone, the radiographic findings of osteomyelitis and septic arthritis become evident. Although these findings (as well as the diagnostic role of scintigraphy, CT, and MR imaging) are discussed in more detail elsewhere (see Chapters 15 and 64), it should be noted that periosteal new bone formation

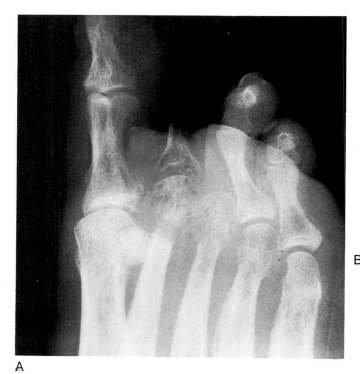

A

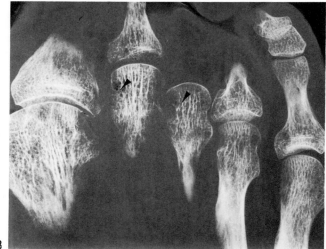

B

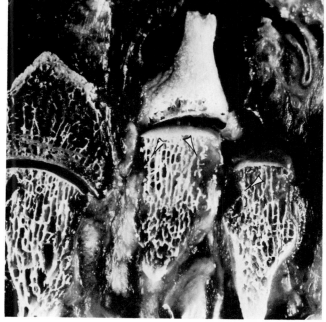

C

FIGURE 58–8. Diabetes mellitus: Association of osteomyelitis and septic arthritis.

A–C A clinical radiograph, transverse sectional radiograph, and sectional photograph illustrate soft tissue and osseous infection in a foot of a patient with diabetes, with associated skin ulceration. The second and third toes had been resected previously. The initial radiograph **(A)** outlines soft tissue swelling, radiolucency of the soft tissues, and osseous destruction of the second and third metatarsal heads. The bony changes are more readily apparent on the sectional radiograph **(B)** and photograph **(C)** of the gross specimen (arrowheads).

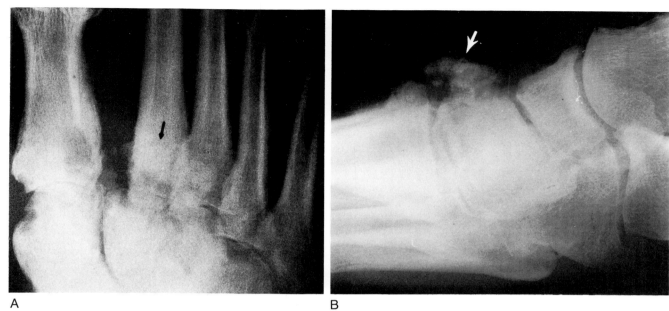

FIGURE 58–9. Diabetes mellitus: Association of neuropathic osteoarthropathy. In a patient with diabetes, neurologic deficit, and soft tissue infection, note the degree of sclerosis and fragmentation of the tarsometatarsal joints (arrows). Lateral displacement of the metatarsal bases is seen. These radiographs illustrate a common site of occurrence and appearance of neuropathic osteoarthropathy in diabetic patients.

and osteopenia may not be prominent in the diabetic foot, as bony proliferation and diffuse, patchy, or periarticular osteoporosis require an adequate vascular supply. The absence of resorptive changes in association with diabetic osteomyelitis is indicative of tissue ischemia. When present, osteoporosis may progress to cortical erosion, medullary destruction, loss of the subchondral bone plate, and joint space narrowing in association with continued infection of bone and joint. Spontaneous fracture, subluxation, and dislocation can be seen, frequently in association with neuropathic osteoarthropathy.

Osteomyelitis and septic arthritis in diabetic patients can occur in other locations, owing to contiguous spread of infection from contaminated soft tissues, and can be related to other mechanisms, such as hematogenous and postoperative infection. Furthermore, osteomyelitis commonly coexists with neuropathic osteoarthropathy in this disorder.

Neuropathic Osteoarthropathy

In recent years, diabetes has surpassed syphilis as the leading cause of neuropathic osteoarthropathy (see Chapter

FIGURE 58–10. Diabetes mellitus: Association of neuropathic osteoarthropathy. In a 63 year old man with diabetes mellitus, radiographs obtained 1 month apart reveal the spontaneous onset of dislocation involving the tarsometatarsal joints. Observe the displacement of the first and second metatarsals in a lateral direction with respect to the adjacent cuneiform bones, as well as diastasis between the medial and intermediate cuneiforms, an osseous fragment next to the medial cuneiform, and a previous fracture of the fifth metatarsal bone.

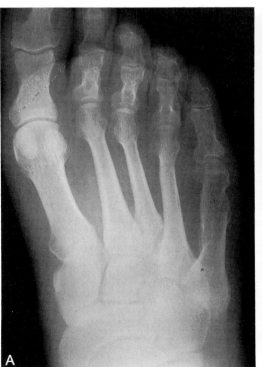 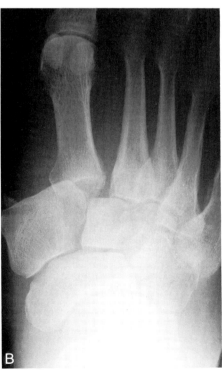

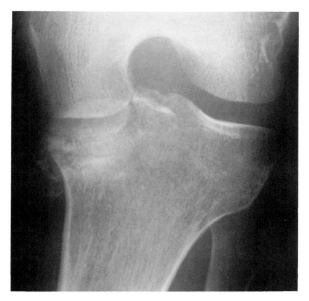

FIGURE 58–11. Diabetes mellitus: Association of neuropathic osteoarthropathy. In this 44 year old man with knee instability of 3 weeks' duration, depression of the medial tibial plateau is associated with a subchondral fracture and fragmentation.

78). This obviously relates to the larger number of patients with diabetes rather than a higher prevalence of diabetic patients who develop this articular complication.[115] The arthropathy appears to be a direct sequela of diabetic peripheral neuropathy, with loss of pain and proprioceptive sensations. Aggravating factors in the diabetic patient are ischemia, trauma, and infection.[116] Some of these factors, as well as the clinical, radiologic, and pathologic features of diabetic neuropathic osteoarthropathy, are common to all varieties of neuropathic bone and joint disease and are discussed elsewhere.

Diabetic neuropathic osteoarthropathy has a unique distribution. It frequently involves the tarsometatarsal, intertarsal, and metatarsophalangeal joints (Figs. 58–9 and 58–10). Abnormalities of the ankle and interphalangeal joints are less frequent. Occasionally changes occur at other sites, including the knee (Fig. 58–11), spine, and joints of the upper extremity. The radiographic and pathologic picture may be a composite of both neuropathic disease and infection. Osteolysis and resorptive changes may predominate over fragmentation and productive abnormalities. Spontaneous fractures and dislocations are not infrequent.[117–125] In this regard, diabetic neuropathic osteoarthropathy with findings resembling a Lisfranc fracture-dislocation at the tarsometatarsal joints is well recognized, and spontaneous fractures or dislocations at this location or elsewhere (such as the calcaneus[266]) can be the presenting manifestation of the disease.

A complete discussion of diabetic neuropathic osteoarthropathy and its evaluation with routine radiography and advanced imaging methods appears in Chapter 78.

Forefoot Osteolysis

A distinct osteolysis of the forefoot has been described in patients with diabetes mellitus,[126] characterized by patchy or generalized osteoporosis of the distal metatarsals and proximal phalanges, accompanied by a variable degree of pain. The articular surfaces initially are spared, although progressive osteolysis may become apparent with disappearance of adjacent bone. The process may terminate at any stage, and resolution may commence with partial or complete restoration of bony architecture. The cause of this condition is not clear, although a similar appearance may be seen in diabetic neuropathic osteoarthropathy. Although some diabetic patients with forefoot osteolysis do not have evidence of neurologic deficit, ischemia, or infection, it is probable that the condition is related to one or more of these factors. It also is possible that sympathetic nerve dysfunction is an important causative factor.

Osteopenia

Osteopenia, a decrease in the radiodensity of bone, is a well-recognized manifestation of insulin-treated diabetes mellitus in patients of all ages; its frequency in insulin-dependent disease is reported to be approximately 50 per cent of patients in many series. The loss of bone can be documented in a number of fashions, including radiogrammetry and photon absorption densitometry.[127–132] Although correlation of bone loss with the severity of the disorder is poor, bone loss is particularly marked initially and in the younger age groups and certainly is more severe in persons requiring insulin treatment.[48] In the early stages of the disease, bone loss appears to be more significant in women and girls than in men and boys and in whites than blacks.

The pathogenesis of diabetic osteopenia is not clear. Potential factors present in uncontrolled diabetes include glycosuria, calciuria, phosphaturia, systemic acidosis, and other hormonal aberrations.[133] Histologic data, although meager, indicate a state of low bone turnover. Experimentally induced diabetes mellitus is associated with an impairment of bone and matrix formation but does not disturb the maturation of osteoid or the initial phase of mineralization at sites of active bone formation.[133] In both human and experimental disease, the state of low bone formation and turnover develops early in the course of the disorder, is variable in severity, and may continue for a substantial period of time.

With regard to the clinical significance of osteopenia in diabetes mellitus, an increased risk for fractures in adults with this disease is controversial[134] and could be related to other factors, such as infection, ischemia, and neuropathic osteoarthropathy.

Vascular Calcification

Arterial calcifications, especially of the internal carotid and renal arteries, the aorta, and the arteries of the lower extremities and pelvis, commonly are observed during radiography in patients with diabetes mellitus.[67] In the leg, arterial calcifications of the media, rather than intimal calcifications, are the typical lesion of diabetes mellitus and lead to regular, diffuse, and fine-grained collections generally affecting the whole circumference of the vessel and accumulating in rings.[135, 136] Calcification in the interdigital arteries of the feet can aid in the diagnosis of clinically unsuspected diabetes as these vessels rarely exhibit calcification in nondiabetic persons.[67] Fractures of calcified vessels with callus formation may be noted.

Although common in diabetes mellitus, arterial calcifications generally do not impinge on the lumen of the vessel[135] and are regarded by some physicians as clinically insignificant.[137] Such calcifications are more frequent in diabetic patients with gangrene than in those without gangrene,[138] however, suggesting that arterial calcific deposits can lead to impaired circulation owing to increased rigidity of the vessel wall, with resultant inability to adjust to circulatory demands.[138–140] Some investigators have observed a distinctive diabetic macroangiopathy in the legs, characterized by uniform narrowing of the vessels and irregularity of the lumen, unrelated to calcification.[141] The severity of this angiopathy as well as the degree of arterial calcification of the media correlates with the duration of the disease.[141] The cause of the angiopathy is not clear, whereas the vascular calcification may be related to neuropathy, as similar alterations are observed in the vessels of patients with familial amyloidosis and neuropathy.[138]

LIPOATROPHIC DIABETES

General Features

Lipoatrophic diabetes was first noted by Ziegler[142] in 1928 and further described by Lawrence[143] in 1946. Its features include insulin-resistant diabetes, hepatosplenomegaly, hyperlipidemia, hypermetabolism, accelerated growth and maturation, muscular overdevelopment, hirsutism, hyperpigmentation, and progressive loss of adipose tissue without ketosis. Additional clinical features are cutaneous xanthomas, protuberant abdomen, corneal opacities, and mental retardation (Fig. 58–12A).

Lipoatrophic diabetes may be congenital or acquired. In the congenital form, there is paucity of fat at the time of birth, affected children are frequently the product of consanguineous marriages, and the patients may be of Norwegian, Portuguese, Spanish, or Negroid extraction.[144, 145] Diabetes commonly appears in the second decade of life. In acquired lipodystrophy, a relationship may exist with previous infections, such as pertussis and mumps. This form of the disease is more common in women than in men and may have its onset after difficult labor and delivery.

The cause of this disorder is unknown. Some reports suggest that the congenital form may be associated with abnormality of the hypothalamus or pituitary gland[146, 147] and concomitant gigantism and additional endocrine alterations may be apparent in these patients. The pathogenesis of the acquired variety of the disease may be related to brain damage after infection or trauma.

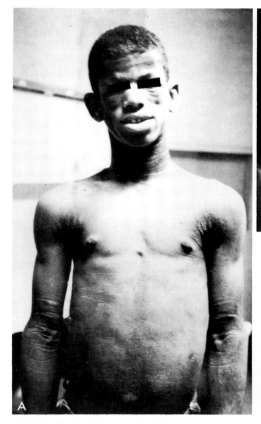
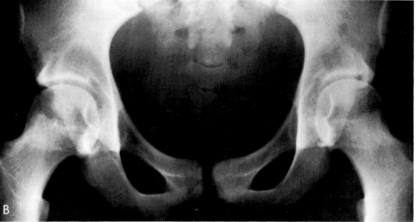
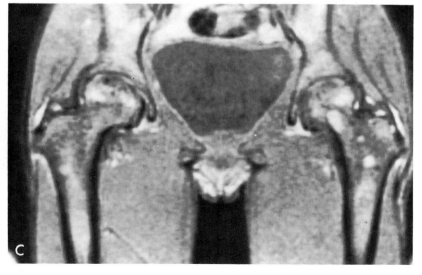

FIGURE 58–12. Lipoatrophic diabetes.

A In this 11 year old child, observe sunken cheeks, protuberant abdomen, skin creasing in areas of flexion, and phlebomegaly.

B In a brother of the patient in **A**, note increased radiodensity in the femoral necks.

(**A, B** From Gold RH, Steinbach HL: AJR *101*:884, 1967. Copyright 1967, American Roentgen Ray Society.)

C In a different patient with lipoatrophic diabetes, a coronal display of the pelvis using a T1-weighted (TR/TE, 600/20) spin echo MR sequence shows patchy areas of decreased signal intensity in the marrow of the proximal portion of the femora.

Radiographic Findings

The most striking radiographic finding is decrease or absence of body fat, manifested as loss of soft tissue planes. A markedly advanced bone age may be seen in children with this syndrome. Thickening of the diaphyseal cortices, metaphyseal sclerosis, and hypertrophy of the epiphyses have been described in the long bones. Small cystic lesions may appear in the metaphysis.[148] Changes in the skull may include dolichocephaly, brachycephaly, calcification of the falx cerebri, thickening of the calvarium, and advanced dentition. Pneumoencephalography, CT, or MR imaging may outline ventricular enlargement. Evidence of organomegaly may be seen in the chest and abdomen.

Cystic and sclerotic foci are particularly common in periarticular regions,[148, 149] and the findings may resemble those of osteonecrosis or osteopoikilosis (Fig. 58–12B). The regions of increased density may extend into the metaphysis and involve the margins of the vertebral bodies.[145] It has been suggested that the radiodense foci represent osteoblastic reaction to loss of fat in the bone marrow.[148] The marrow abnormalities are well demonstrated with MR imaging (Fig. 58–12C).[150]

As there are wide variations in the radiographic appearance of lipoatrophic diabetes, its differential diagnosis will depend on the distribution and severity of imaging findings in any particular person. The condition should be differentiated from partial lipodystrophy, in which loss of facial, trunk, and upper extremity fat is apparent in children between the ages of 5 and 15 years.[151] In this latter syndrome, radiography outlines the discrepancy in the amount of adipose tissue in the upper portion of the body compared with the lower portion. Decrease in subcutaneous fat may be seen in other conditions, such as hyperthyroidism, anorexia nervosa, progeria, and various other congenital and acquired disorders. The gigantism of lipoatrophic diabetes must be distinguished from pituitary and cerebral gigantism. In pituitary gigantism, increased subcutaneous fat and typical osseous changes are apparent, whereas in cerebral gigantism, there is excessive body fat and absence of hepatosplenomegaly. Additional skeletal manifestations of lipoatrophic diabetes are relatively nonspecific; advanced bone age and abnormalities of bone modeling are seen in many other diseases.

ANOMALIES IN INFANTS OF DIABETIC MOTHERS

Hyperinsulinemia in the fetus of a diabetic mother is presumed to be the result of maternal hyperglycemia, as insulin itself does not traverse the placental barrier. The elevated levels of insulin can promote abnormal growth, which is manifested in the newborn as visceromegaly and increased body fat. The frequency of more serious anomalies and even death in the infants of women with diabetes mellitus is difficult to define owing to wide variations in the criteria used to diagnose maternal diabetes.[152, 153] Furthermore, the frequency of such anomalies and other complications is influenced by the severity of the disease, being highest in insulin-dependent diabetic persons and in those with acetonuria, uncontrolled or long-standing disease, and vascular complications.[154] Despite such limitations, it generally is believed that the frequency of congenital anomalies in the offspring of diabetic mothers may be as high as 20 per cent but probably is far less.

As summarized by Dunn and collaborators,[155] a wide variety of congenital abnormalities is observed in such infants. These include respiratory anomalies (respiratory distress syndrome, wet lung syndrome, and persistence of the fetal circulation); cardiomyopathy and congenital heart disease; hyperviscosity, thrombosis, and hemorrhage; renal anomalies (hydronephrosis, duplications, cystic kidneys, renal agenesis, pseudohermaphroditism, and renal vein thrombosis); the small left colon syndrome; and alterations in the musculoskeletal system.

Sacrococcygeal agenesis, or the caudal regression syndrome, which is discussed elsewhere in this textbook, is one of the most specific anomalies in these infants.[156–159] Approximately 20 per cent of patients with this syndrome are the children of diabetic mothers and approximately 16 per cent of children born to diabetic mothers have sacral anomalies.[157] Agenesis varies in severity; in some cases, only minor coccygeal changes are present, whereas in others, aplasia of the lower thoracic and entire lumbar spine is combined with absence of one or more segments of the sacrum (Fig. 58–13). Associated abnormalities include meningocele, arthrogryposis, hip dislocations, flexion contractures of the knees and hips, foot deformities, and urinary tract anomalies.[155]

An additional skeletal malformation syndrome, consisting of unusual facies and femoral hypoplasia, has been identified in the infants of diabetic mothers.[160–162] Facial features include upslanting eyes, hypoplastic alae nasi with a broad nasal tip, a long philtrum with a thin upper lip, and a small mouth and mandible. Additional, less constant findings are Sprengel's deformity, radiohumeral or radioulnar synostosis, tapered, fused, or missing ribs, vertebral anomalies, and foot deformities.[162] The syndrome shares some characteristics with the caudal regression syndrome, but

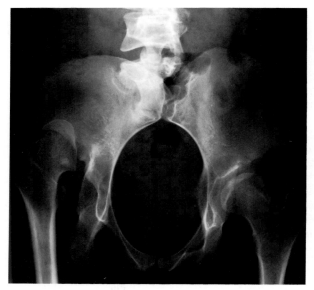

FIGURE 58–13. Anomalies in children of diabetic mothers: Caudal regression syndrome. In this 27 year old daughter of a diabetic mother, aplasia of the lower lumbar spine and sacrum is associated with pelvic and acetabular deformity and dislocation of the right hip. (Courtesy of S. Hilton, M.D., San Diego, California.)

femoral, facial, and upper extremity involvement is more typical in the former.

A specific cause for the association of congenital anomalies and diabetes mellitus has not been identified, and teratogenetic effects of insulin have not been defined precisely, although rump agenesis has been produced experimentally in fowl by injecting eggs with insulin.[155]

DISORDERS AND COMPLICATIONS OF PREGNANCY

The normal osseous architecture of the female pelvis differs from that of the male pelvis. In women, there is an increase in lumbar lordosis and angulation at the lumbosacral junction as well as an increase in obliquity of the pelvic bones themselves. During pregnancy, certain biomechanical changes occur that produce increased stress on the pelvic joints. In the pregnant woman, as a result of increased weight, the degree of lumbar lordosis increases and the center of mass is displaced. Sliding movement at the sacroiliac joint becomes accentuated owing to softening and relaxation of adjacent ligaments,[163, 164] and diastasis with gas in the symphysis pubis may be apparent during pregnancy.[165] On histologic examination by the second month of gestation, these articulations demonstrate cartilaginous fissuring, hypervascularity, and bony eburnation.[166] It generally is assumed that relaxation of the joints of the pelvis is an essential and normal accompaniment of pregnancy, which ensures the accommodation of the growing fetus and facilitates vaginal delivery. The changes are initiated during the first half of pregnancy, increase in the last trimester, and disappear within 3 to 5 months after delivery; they correlate with levels of the hormone relaxin and may be associated with generalized articular laxity, which involves sites in the appendicular skeleton as well.[167, 168]

These physiologic changes may be associated with clinical findings. Local tenderness and pain may be apparent over the sacroiliac joints and symphysis pubis and may be associated with a positive Trendelenburg sign and a hesitant, unstable gait. Low back pain may be an accompanying finding, and herniation of intervertebral discs can occur, which can be documented by myelography,[169, 170] and which has been attributed to tears of the fibers of the intervertebral disc related to the lithotomy position.[171] Whether or not pregnant women have an increased prevalence of discal abnormality, however, is not clear.[172]

The major radiographic findings associated with physiologic and pathologic changes during pregnancy occur at the sacroiliac joints and symphysis pubis. Bony eburnation about the sacroiliac joint is termed osteitis condensans ilii, whereas that at the symphysis pubis is termed osteitis pubis. Although either of the two conditions may be apparent in nulliparous women or even men, both are observed most frequently in multiparous women and most appropriately are discussed here.

Osteitis Condensans Ilii

Osteitis condensans ilii is a condition of the pelvis that involves predominantly the ilium adjacent to the sacroiliac joint. Usually, although not invariably, it is a bilateral and relatively symmetric process of women; rarely, men may be affected, and asymmetric or unilateral changes may be observed.[173–176] Its interest is mainly radiologic, as a characteristic radiographic appearance is required for diagnosis, which may be confused with that accompanying ankylosing spondylitis. Osteitis condensans ilii is associated with well-defined triangular sclerosis on the iliac aspect of the sacroiliac joint (Figs. 58–14 and 58–15). The bony eburnation involves the inferior portion of the bone, and the apex of the sclerosis extends into the auricular portion of the ilium. The subchondral bone generally is well defined, highlighted by the radiodensity of the involved osseous surface. Significant narrowing of the sacroiliac joint and extensive involvement of the sacrum are distinctly unusual. The size of the lesion is quite variable, although the sclerosis may be so widespread as to extend many centimeters from the joint margin. The condition may resolve or even disappear with time.[177, 178]

The frequency of osteitis condensans ilii has not been well delineated. In a review of 3260 radiographs of Japanese patients, some of whom had been exposed to atomic radiation, 1.6 per cent revealed changes compatible with this disorder.[179] A biopsy study of involved ilia using microradiographs and tetracycline fluorescence methods has revealed hypervascularity, thickened trabeculae, osteonecrosis, and signs of bony regeneration.[176] Additional histologic changes include hematopoietic, fatty, or fibrous bone marrow, mild inflammatory changes with round cell or eosinophilic cell infiltration, and cartilaginous alterations.[178]

The cause of osteitis condensans ilii is not clear. The predominant theory suggests that the condition is secondary to mechanical stress across the sacroiliac joint coupled with increased vascularity during pregnancy.[180] Its occurrence in nulliparous women and in men is inconsistent with this theory, although mechanical stress of different causation may be operational in these people. Dihlmann,[181] in a study of cadavers, stressed that osteitis condensans ilii was a reaction to abnormal stress in which a normal physiologic zone of hyperostosis on the anterior iliac margin became exaggerated.[178] He suggested that the condition was reversible and that in 50 per cent of cases, a simultaneous but variable sclerosis was evident in the sacrum. Additional radiographic manifestations of articular degeneration, such as osteophytosis and cyst formation, can be evident. Pathologically, degenerative changes in the cartilage have been observed.[178]

Urinary tract infections also have been implicated as a cause of this condition, renal or ureteral infection reaching the ilium via nutrient vessels.[182, 183] As many patients with osteitis condensans ilii do not relate a history of urinary tract infections, this theory does not have wide support.

A third theory suggests that osteitis condensans ilii is an inflammatory condition that is related to ankylosing spondylitis[184] (Table 58–2). Thompson noted that 7 of 20 women with an initial diagnosis of osteitis condensans ilii developed radiographic evidence of ankylosing spondylitis, two of whom revealed progressive stiffness of the spine.[175] This theory gained support from histologic studies indicating similar pathologic aberrations in osteitis condensans ilii and ankylosing spondylitis.[176] A search for the histocompatibility antigen HLA-B27 in patients with osteitis condensans ilii failed to document an increased occurrence of this antigen,[185, 186] however, although it is a well-known marker for ankylosing spondylitis. Although some authors have difficulty distinguishing between the sacroiliac joint

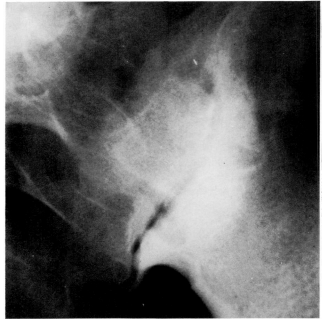

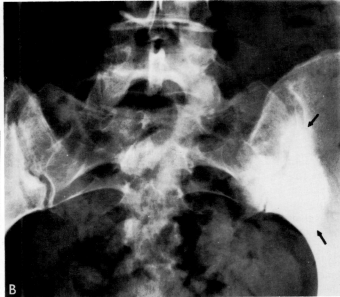

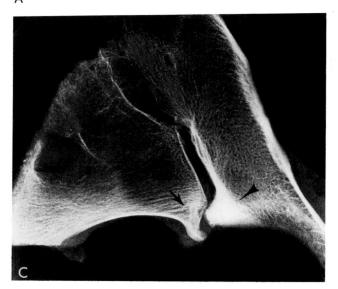

FIGURE 58–14. Osteitis condensans ilii.

A Typical radiographic features include well-defined sclerosis on the iliac aspect of the joint, triangular in shape. The articular space is relatively well defined.

B Although these changes usually are bilateral and symmetric, in this patient the findings are markedly asymmetric. On the left side, radiographic features are similar to those observed in **A.** Most, if not all, of the eburnated bone is located in the ilium (arrows).

C A radiograph of a transverse section through the midportion of the sacroiliac joint reveals typical findings of osteitis condensans ilii. The anterior aspect of the joint is located at the bottom of the illustration. Well-defined anterior iliac sclerosis is seen (arrowhead). Mild sclerosis and osteophytosis of the sacrum also are apparent (arrow).

FIGURE 58–15. Osteitis condensans ilii. A transverse T1-weighted (TR/TE, 550/20) spin echo MR image in a 34 year old woman with typical routine radiographic findings of bilateral disease shows regions of low signal intensity (arrows) in both ilia. The joints are normal. These regions corresponded to sites of bone sclerosis and remained of low signal intensity on T2-weighted images (not shown). Focal deposits of fat, characterized by areas of high signal intensity, are apparent in the right ilium and adjacent sacrum.

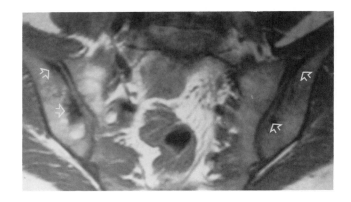

TABLE 58–2. Osteitis Condensans Ilii (OCI) Versus Ankylosing Spondylitis (AS)

	OCI	AS
Age	Young adults	Young adults
Sex	Women > men	Men > women
Clinical symptoms, signs	Absent or mild	Mild to severe
HLA-B27	Present in 8% (same as controls)	Present in 90%
Sacroiliac joint abnormalities		
Distribution	Bilateral, symmetric; iliac	Bilateral, symmetric; iliac > sacral
Sclerosis	Well defined	Poorly defined
Joint space	Normal	Narrowed
Erosion	Absent	Common
Bony ankylosis	Absent	Common
Spinal abnormalities	Absent	Common
Symphysis pubis abnormalities	Less common	More common

changes of osteitis condensans ilii and ankylosing spondylitis,[175] a difficulty that is accentuated by the mild and atypical clinical and radiographic findings that may accompany ankylosing spondylitis in women,[187] generally it is easy to differentiate the two conditions. Both conditions are characterized by bilateral, symmetric sacroiliac joint abnormalities; however, osseous erosion, indistinctness of subchon-

dral bone, joint space narrowing, sacral involvement, and ligamentous ossification are features that usually are prominent in ankylosing spondylitis and absent in osteitis condensans ilii (Fig. 58–16).

The occurrence of osteitis condensans ilii in association with extensive and premature calcification of costal cartilage due to hydroxyapatite crystal deposition has been identified in a familial distribution, suggesting still one more potential cause of some cases of the disorder.[188]

The presence and significance of symptoms and signs accompanying osteitis condensans ilii also are debated. A "low back" syndrome consisting of morning pain, stiffness, and limitation of motion may be seen in patients with this disease.[186] Polyarthralgia in peripheral joints and synovial effusion also can occur, although significant inflammatory articular findings generally are absent. A "fibrositis" syndrome also has been recognized. These clinical findings usually are mild; if the clinical findings are marked, another source for these manifestations must be sought before they are attributed to osteitis condensans ilii, which more typically is an incidental radiographic abnormality. Support for the clinical insignificance of osteitis condensans ilii in most patients with this finding includes the following: The disorder frequently is discovered in patients without low back or buttock pain; other abnormalities that may cause such pain commonly are found in patients with osteitis condensans ilii; patients with unilateral involvement frequently report pain on the contralateral side; and fibrositis is an associated finding in a significant number of affected persons.[189]

Differential diagnostic considerations in cases of osteitis

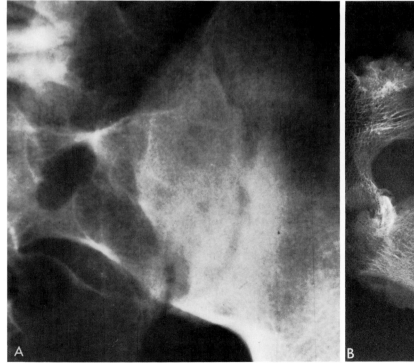
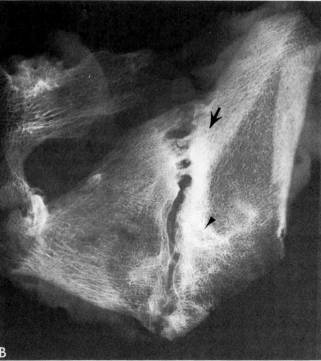

FIGURE 58–16. Ankylosing spondylitis.

A Ankylosing spondylitis differs from osteitis condensans ilii in its radiographic appearance. Observe irregular articular surfaces, poorly defined sclerosis, and blurring of the ligamentous space above the true joint.

B A coronal section through the sacroiliac joint reveals erosions of ilium and sacrum, poorly defined iliac sclerosis (arrowhead), and ligamentous ossification and hyperostosis above the true joint cavity (arrow).

condensans ilii include seronegative spondyloarthropathies, renal osteodystrophy and primary hyperparathyroidism, lymphoma, Paget's disease, and skeletal metastasis.[190]

Osteitis Pubis

Osteitis pubis is a painful condition of the symphysis pubis, which may become apparent within one or more months after delivery or other pelvic operations.[191–194] In men, osteitis pubis particularly is frequent after prostatic (or bladder) surgery.[195] Clinical findings are characterized by local pain and tenderness, muscle spasm, and unstable gait.[196] Laboratory evaluation generally is unremarkable.

The disorder should be distinguished from the normal symphyseal separation[197, 198] and hypermobility that may occur during pregnancy. In this normal situation, widening of the symphysis can be detected radiographically and can be accentuated by the patient's standing on one leg at a time. The width of the articulation usually is less than 7 mm,[199] and the symphyseal changes regress within a few months in the postpartum period (see later discussion). It is in the unusual circumstance in which the pubic changes do not regress and are associated with bony erosion, resorption, and eburnation that osteitis pubis may be diagnosed.

As noted previously, this abnormal condition occurs not only in women after pregnancy but also in men and women after pelvic surgery and, rarely, without any apparent precipitating event.[200–203] A similar lesion has been described in male and female athletes.[204–208] In some of these athletes, the irregularity of the symphysis pubis may have been due not to chronic stress across the articulation but rather to an acute avulsion at the sites of attachment of the adductor brevis, adductor longus, and gracilis muscles to the symphysis pubis[207, 209] (Fig. 58–17).

The radiographic appearance of osteitis pubis includes mild to severe subchondral bony irregularity of the symphysis pubis with resorption (Figs. 58–18 and 58–19). The condition usually involves both pubic bones in a symmetric fashion, although asymmetric or unilateral findings occasionally are encountered. The degree of resorption or sclerosis rarely may become striking, with osteolysis of a large segment of the pubic bones. Restoration of the osseous surface with disappearance of the sclerosis may be associated with bony ankylosis of the joint (Fig. 58–20).

Local aspiration occasionally has revealed an abscess cavity, and antibiotics can produce some relief of symptoms, observations that have led some investigators to speculate that the condition represents a low-grade infection. Cases of definite pubic osteomyelitis may reveal similar radiographic features.[210–213] Predisposing factors include parenteral drug abuse and pelvic surgery.[214–218] Clinical findings simulate those of "sterile" osteitis pubis, with distal anterior pelvic pain, spasm of the adductor and rectus abdominis muscles, and a waddling gait.[214] A more aggressive and progressive course is characteristic of some instances of infective osteitis pubis, but it cannot be denied that sterile and infective inflammatory changes of the symphysis pubis are similar (Fig. 58–21).

The cause of osteitis pubis in most cases remains speculative. In addition to low grade infection and trauma, venous congestion due to injury or inflammation is a proposed etiologic factor.[192] In support of the last theory, anticoagulant therapy has been used successfully by some investigators[219] but unsuccessfully by others.[220]

The differential diagnosis of osteitis pubis includes not only trauma and infection but also a variety of articular disorders characterized, in part, by inflammation of the symphysis pubis. Thus, ankylosing spondylitis and psoriatic arthritis, conditions that may involve synovial and cartilaginous joints as well as entheses, can produce erosion, sclerosis, and resorption of the pubis, combined with more typical abnormalities at other sites (Fig. 58–22). Subchondral resorption of bone in primary and secondary hyperparathyroidism and stress or insufficiency fractures in this condition as well as osteomalacia and osteoporosis can produce abnormalities that simulate osteitis pubis.

Symphyseal Diastasis and Rupture

As noted previously, symphyseal separation is a known complication seen during pregnancy. It generally is asymptomatic and appears to be related to an increase in the degree of elasticity of the pubic ligaments occurring in response to the hormones progesterone and relaxin. The

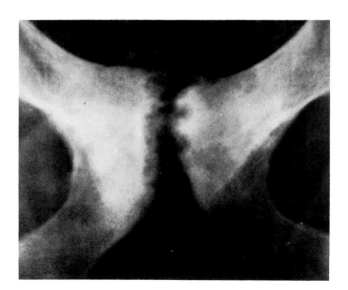

FIGURE 58–17. Ligamentous injury: Symphysis pubis. In this young man, avulsive injury of one or more of the adductors (adductor longus, adductor brevis, gracilis muscles) has created irregularity and sclerosis of apposing margins of the symphysis pubis. (From Schneider R, et al: Radiology 120:567, 1976.)

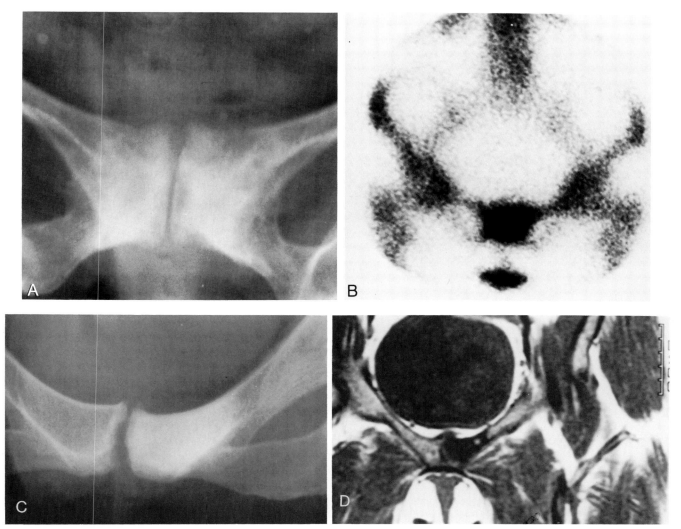

FIGURE 58–18. Osteitis pubis.

A, B In a 61 year old woman, local pain and tenderness about the symphysis pubis were the major clinical abnormalities. The radiograph **(A)** reveals considerable bone sclerosis on both sides of the symphysis with narrowing of the joint space. Marked increased accumulation of the bone-seeking radiopharmaceutical agent **(B)** is observed. (Courtesy of M. Austin, M.D., Newport Beach, California.)

C, D In this 34 year old woman, a routine radiograph **(C)** shows unilateral osteitis pubis. A coronal T1-weighted (TR/TE, 633/17) spin echo MR image **(D)** shows low signal intensity in the involved bone. (Courtesy of S. Eilenberg, M.D., San Diego, California.)

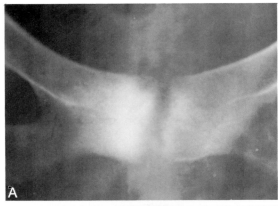

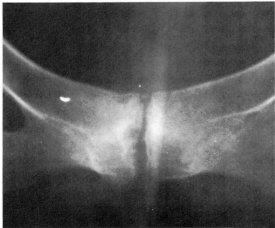

FIGURE 58–19. Osteitis pubis. Resolution of symphyseal abnormalities. In this 26 year old woman who developed pain and tenderness about the symphysis pubis during the third trimester of pregnancy, radiographs obtained 2 years apart reveal partial resolution of the abnormalities of osteitis pubis. (Courtesy of V. Vint, M.D., San Diego, California.)

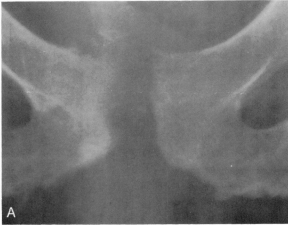

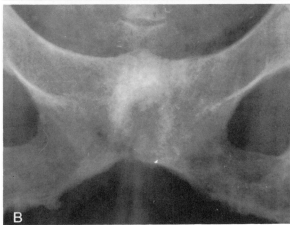

FIGURE 58–20. Osteitis pubis. Sequential abnormalities in a 65 year old man after transurethral resection of the prostate gland.

   A Initial findings include resorption of parasymphyseal bone, more prominent on the right side. Adjacent bone sclerosis is evident.

   B Nineteen months later, intra-articular bone ankylosis is evident.

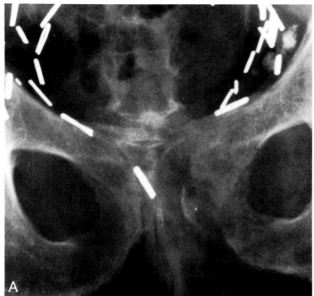

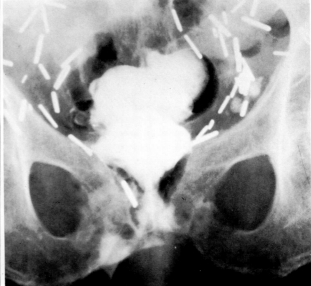

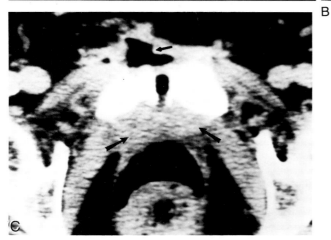

FIGURE 58–21. Infective osteitis pubis. This 71 year old man with bladder carcinoma underwent cystectomy, urinary diversion with the establishment of an ileal conduit, and radiation therapy. Five years later, he developed lower abdominal pain, fever, leukocytosis, and tenderness over the symphysis pubis.

A The radiograph shows widening of the symphysis pubis with indistinctness of the neighboring bone, especially on the left.

B An abscess was drained percutaneously and its opacification shows communication with the rectum. Cultures of the fluid documented the presence of many different types of gram-negative organisms.

C A transaxial CT image shows an abscess, containing gas, both anterior and posterior to the symphysis pubis (arrows). Gas also is present in the symphysis itself.

FIGURE 58–22. Ankylosing spondylitis. Pubic sclerosis is not infrequent in ankylosing spondylitis, nor is it infrequent in related disorders, such as psoriasis. The process generally is symmetric. Although not evident here, the joint space may be widened. In other instances, bony ankylosis of this joint is seen.

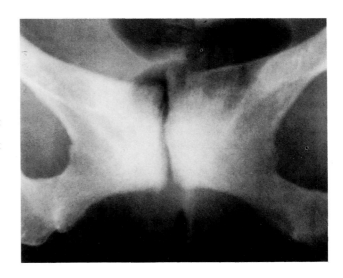

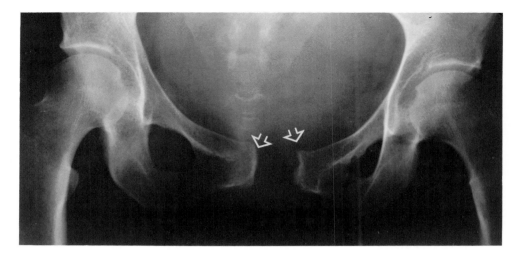

FIGURE 58–23. Symphyseal diastasis after pregnancy. In this 38 year old woman, continued symphyseal pain and tenderness occurred in the postpartum period. The radiograph reveals abnormal widening (>10 mm) of the symphysis pubis (arrows).

frequency of this finding in pregnant women has been estimated to be approximately 30 per cent,[221] although some investigators believe it is rare[222] or is evident in all pregnancies.[223] The width of the symphysis pubis may change progressively throughout the course of pregnancy, without a marked increase during labor or delivery.[224] The width of the symphysis pubis in this physiologic condition usually is less than 7 mm.[199]

In rare circumstances, rupture of the symphysis pubis occurs during the final stages of pregnancy and, particularly, during labor and delivery.[224, 225] Potential etiological factors include difficult and precipitous labor, complicated forceps delivery, abnormal fetal presentation, cephalopelvic disproportion, multiparity, forceful stress on the mother's thighs during delivery, and preexisting traumatic or metabolic changes of the pelvic bones.[224] The reported prevalence of such rupture has varied from 1 in about 500 deliveries to 1 in 30,000 deliveries.[224] Clinical findings include local pain, tenderness and a symphyseal gap; back, thigh and leg discomfort; and an abnormal gait. Radiographs reveal symphyseal separations varying from 1 cm to as much as 12 cm (Fig. 58–23), and diastasis of one or both sacroiliac joints may be an associated feature.[224, 225] Nonoperative treatment generally is sufficient, and functional recovery should be complete.[224]

Disseminated Intravascular Coagulation

Disseminated intravascular coagulation is a recognized complication of pregnancy, which may be related, in part, to amnionic fluid embolization in which amnionic fluid and its contaminants enter the maternal bloodstream during parturition, leading to hypofibrinogenemia. Hypofibrinogenemia also has been recognized in patients with premature separation of the placenta, septic abortion, and prolonged retention of a dead fetus. In rare instances, ischemic necrosis of bone marrow may be associated with disseminated intravascular coagulation.[226] Although such necrosis generally is patchy in distribution, it may become widespread, a phenomenon that has been identified in combination with postpartum toxemia.[227] Radiographic examination typically is unremarkable; however, progressive myelofibrosis may lead to generalized osteosclerosis of the skeleton.[228]

Ischemic Necrosis of Bone

Although infrequent, well-documented instances of ischemic necrosis of bone related to pregnancy have been reported,[229-232] transient osteoporosis of pregnancy (see later discussion) has been misinterpreted as bone infarction in some instances. Ischemic necrosis of bone usually is identified in close association with childbirth, and the femoral head or, less commonly, the humeral head is the principal target area. Identification of the abnormality close to or after parturition may reflect, in some cases, a general reluctance of physicians to obtain radiographs during the first few months of pregnancy, although the lack of earlier symptoms, the presence of initial radiographic signs of necrosis, and an increasing mechanical load suggest that the complication has its onset or is aggravated during the later stages of pregnancy.

Most of the prior reports of pregnancy-related ischemic necrosis of bone have been anecdotal, so that a meaningful association between the two has yet to be proved. Hormonal factors in the mother, such as an increase in adrenocortical activity[233-235] and hyperplasia of the parathyroid glands,[236] conceivably could be important in the pathogenesis of this complication. Furthermore, cases of osteonecrosis have been related to the use of oral contraceptives.[237]

Transient Osteoporosis of the Hip

As is discussed in Chapter 51, periarticular osteoporosis of the hip has been identified in women during the third trimester of pregnancy[238, 239] and, occasionally, inappropriately described as ischemic necrosis.[240] Affected women reveal joint pain, an antalgic limp, and restricted hip motion. The left side is involved almost exclusively (Fig. 58–24), although changes in the right hip, both hips, and other joints have been noted. The cause of the condition is unknown. Factors present in the pregnant woman, such as endocrine alterations and local compression of vessels and nerves by the enlarging fetus, have been implicated in some reports; however, the identification of transient osteoporosis of the hip in early pregnancy,[241] in nonpregnant women, and in men makes unlikely some of these proposed factors.

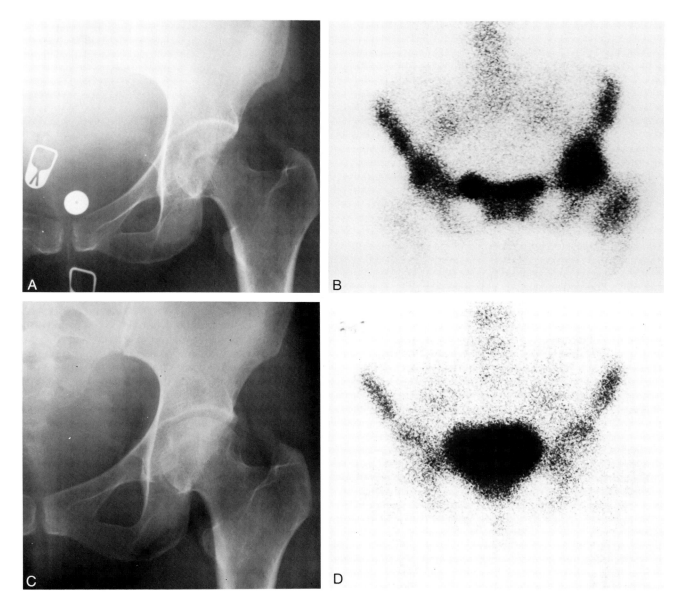

FIGURE 58–24. Transient osteoporosis of the hip. This 36 year old Indian woman developed left hip pain during the eighth month of pregnancy.

A, B After delivery of a normal infant, a radiograph reveals osteopenia in the left femoral head with a normal joint space. Accumulation of the bone-seeking radiopharmaceutical agent is observed in the left hip. The patient refused joint aspiration.

C, D Over the next 2 months, the symptoms decreased in intensity. A repeat radiograph and bone scan reveal resolution of the abnormal findings.

(Courtesy of G. Greenway, M.D., Dallas, Texas.)

Generalized Osteopenia

Osteopenia associated with pregnancy and lactation was described initially as a syndrome by Nordin and Roper in 1955[242] and reported subsequently by other investigators.[243, 244] Histologic data suggest that the decrease in bone mass is related principally to low-turnover osteoporosis.[245] Laboratory analysis generally is unremarkable. Fractures, especially in the spine, are detected during the time(s) of pregnancy and lactation and generally are not apparent over subsequent periods of observation.

This syndrome of generalized osteopenia is infrequent, as most pregnant women adjust well to the large placental transfer of calcium and phosphorus to the developing fetus and to the calcium demands during lactation.[245] Certain changes in maternal levels of serum calcium, parathyroid hormone, thyrocalcitonin, and vitamin D metabolites are considered physiologic and are not accompanied by a propensity to fracture. Why things go wrong in some women, leading to significant osteopenia in pregnancy and lactation, is not clear.

Stress Fractures

Stress fractures have been observed in the later stages of pregnancy[246] and in the postpartum period.[247] Pelvic sites such as the parasymphyseal bone and sacrum typically are involved. A potential cause of such fractures in the pubic rami in the final stages of pregnancy is the forceful descent of the fetal head against a pelvic ring that contains lax ligaments.[224] Stress fractures in the postpartum period may relate to increased body weight and increased levels of physical activity.

MISCELLANEOUS DISORDERS

Osteitis Condensans (Condensing Osteitis) of the Clavicle

Although this relatively newly described condition is not a complication of pregnancy, it does share morphologic and radiologic features with osteitis condensans ilii and osteitis pubis. In 1974, Brower and collaborators[248] reported two young women with pain and swelling over the medial end of the clavicle associated with bony eburnation and an intact articular space (Fig. 58–25). Histologic examination delineated thickening of trabeculae within the cancellous bone and periosteal reaction resembling an osteophyte. The pathologic changes were interpreted as a response to mechanical stress, as both patients had carried out strenuous activity involving this joint, and there was no evidence of inflammation or infection. In 1976, Solovjev[249] further described this entity, and in 1978, Teates and coworkers,[250] examining two other patients with bone-seeking agents, demonstrated that the lesions revealed increased accumulation of radionuclide activity. Additional cases of osteitis condensans of the clavicle have been reported subsequently.[251–259] Patients are women with an average age of 40 years (range, 20 to 50 years) and with a history of stress to the region of the sternoclavicular joint, usually associated with heavy lifting or sports activity. Pain most commonly is referred to the ipsilateral shoulder and is accentuated with abduction of the arm. No definite association with osteitis pubis or osteitis condensans ilii has been reported.

Radiographs reveal bone sclerosis and mild enlargement of the inferomedial aspect of the clavicle, as well as osteophytes in the inferior margin of the clavicular head (Fig. 58–26). The sternoclavicular joint space is not narrowed, and adjacent soft tissue and osseous structures are not affected. In addition to scintigraphy, which demonstrates increased accumulation of bone-seeking radiopharmaceutical agents, CT scanning and MR imaging can be used to document the extent of bone involvement.[242] Areas of low signal intensity within the clavicle on both T1-weighted and T2-weighted spin echo MR imaging sequences are typical, and these findings are indicative of the presence of sclerotic bone.[256] (Figs. 58–27 and 58–28). The author has noted recurrent pain about the clavicular remnant after surgical removal of the lesion, although radiographs have been normal.

The cause of condensing osteitis of the clavicle is unknown. Its occurrence in women of childbearing age suggests a common etiologic agent with osteitis condensans ilii, and stress-induced changes are most likely. Reports of similar clavicular abnormalities in young, physically active men support a stress-related causation.[260] The predilection for the medial end of the clavicle is noteworthy, although the author has seen a similar lesion in the upper sternum. Histologic analysis, which shows normal but thickened bone, has excluded an infectious cause. Such analysis has revealed marrow fibrosis associated with findings of osteonecrosis in some cases.[258]

The differential diagnosis of this clavicular lesion is limited. The most difficult entity to exclude is ischemic necrosis of the medial clavicular epiphysis (Friedrich's disease).[261] This rare disorder typically occurs in children and adolescents and is believed to be due to direct trauma or to an embolic event that results in obliteration of the vascular supply to the medial clavicular epiphysis. Clinically there is soft tissue swelling with tenderness to palpation of the medial aspect of the clavicle. Radiographs reveal osteosclerosis of the entire clavicular head, often with a notchlike defect in the middle of the medial articular surface. Necrotic bone may be recognized on biopsy. The disease appears to be a benign, self-limited process that responds well to conservative therapy.

Sternocostoclavicular hyperostosis is a second disease that affects the medial end of the clavicle.[262, 263] Hyperostosis of the clavicle, sternum, and upper anterior ribs with ossification of intervening soft tissues is observed. In contrast to condensing osteitis of the clavicle, this condition is more common in older patients and in men, is usually bilateral, and often is accompanied by pustular lesions of the palms and soles (pustulosis palmaris et plantaris).

Pyarthrosis of the sternoclavicular joint, especially the type seen in intravenous drug abusers, may mimic condensing osteitis of the clavicle, although laboratory values and radiographic evidence of narrowing of the sternoclavicular joint and osseous destruction assist in the differential diagnosis. Osteoarthritis of the sternoclavicular joint also may resemble condensing osteitis; however, joint space narrowing, osteophytosis, and subchondral cysts are seen on both sides of the articulation.

Chronic recurrent multifocal osteomyelitis (CRMO), also referred to as cleidometaphyseal or plasma cell osteomyelitis, is an unusual syndrome, seen in children and adolescents, leading to symmetric lesions of tubular bones and

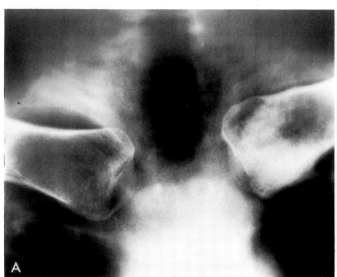
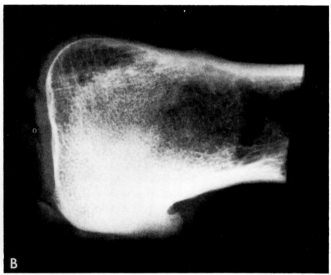
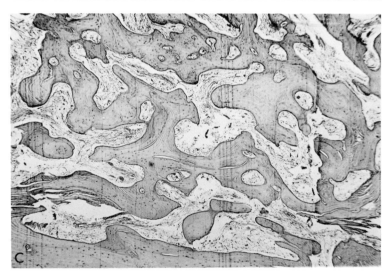

FIGURE 58–25. Condensing osteitis of the clavicle.

   A Note amorphous sclerosis of the proximal end of the left clavicle. The joint space appears relatively normal.

   B A specimen radiograph of the proximal end of the left clavicle demonstrates increase in number and thickness of the trabeculae.

   C On a photomicrograph (30×), the extent of bony sclerosis within the cancellous bone is well defined.

   (From Brower AC, et al: AJR *121*:17, 1974. Copyright 1974, American Roentgen Ray Society.)

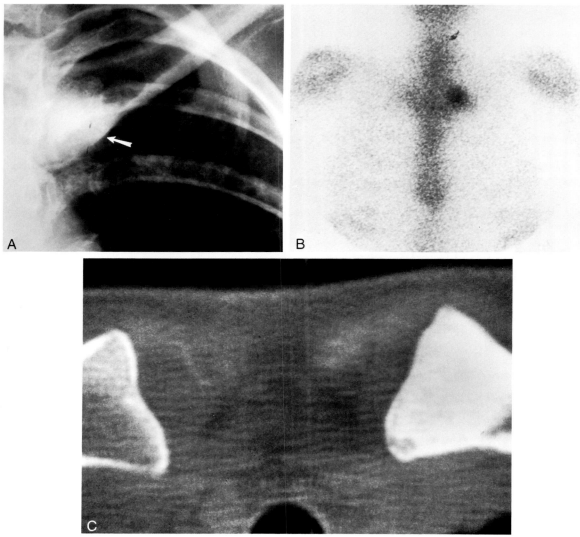

FIGURE 58–26. Condensing osteitis of the clavicle. A 36 year old woman developed left shoulder pain over a period of many years. The pain recently had increased in severity and was associated with tenderness to palpation of the medial end of the left clavicle.
    A The radiograph reveals increased density and enlargement of the inferomedial aspect of the left clavicle (arrow).
    B Increased accumulation of the bone-seeking radiopharmaceutical agent is evident.
    C A transaxial CT image documents the increased radiodensity of the medial end of the left clavicle.
    (Courtesy of W. Murray, M.D., Boise, Idaho.)

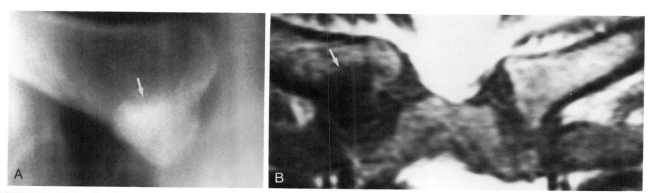

FIGURE 58–27. Condensing osteitis of the clavicle. A 40 year old woman developed pain and tenderness over the the medial end of the right clavicle.
    A Conventional tomography reveals bone sclerosis involving the inferomedial aspect of the bone (arrow).
    B A coronal T1-weighted (TR/TE, 300/11) spin echo MR image shows low signal intensity in this area (arrow). The diminished signal intensity persisted on T2-weighted spin echo and gradient echo images (not shown).
    (Courtesy of G. Greenway, M.D., Dallas, Texas.)

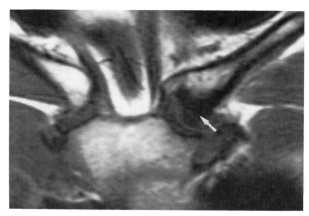

FIGURE 58–28. Condensing osteitis of the clavicle. A 37 year old woman developed persistent pain and swelling about the left sternoclavicular joint. A coronal T1-weighted (TR/TE, 450/11) spin echo MR image shows low signal intensity (arrow) in the medial portion of the left clavicle. Compare with the opposite uninvolved clavicle. (Courtesy of G. Applegate, M.D., Van Nuys, California.)

clavicles. Hyperostosis is a prominent feature of clavicular involvement,[264] producing enlargement of the bone that resembles the findings in sternocostoclavicular hyperostosis.[177] Furthermore, pustulosis palmaris et plantaris may be observed in both of these disorders, suggesting a relationship between the two. In CRMO, plasma cells are reported during histologic examination in some persons. CRMO and potentially related disorders such as sternocostoclavicular hyperostosis and the synovitis-acne-pustulosis-hyperostosis-osteitis (SAPHO) syndrome are discussed in Chapters 64 and 93.

Other causes of clavicular sclerosis and enlargement, such as Paget's disease, fibrous dysplasia, syphilis, and osteoid osteoma, do not realistically enter into the differential diagnosis of condensing osteitis.

SUMMARY

Various musculoskeletal manifestations may accompany endocrine disorders such as Cushing's syndrome, congenital adrenal hyperplasia, Addison's disease, pheochromocytoma, neuroblastoma, and diabetes mellitus. Furthermore, certain complications are apparent in women during and after pregnancy. In Cushing's disease, osteoporosis is most typical and, although osteonecrosis is seen occasionally, it is not as frequent as in cases of exogenous hypercortisolism. In diabetes mellitus, reports have indicated an increased occurrence of many disorders, although a conclusive relationship between diabetes and some of these diseases is lacking. The list of disorders that may be associated with diabetes includes crystal-induced arthropathy (gout and CPPD crystal deposition disease), degenerative joint disease, diffuse idiopathic skeletal hyperostosis, soft tissue contractures, osteomyelitis, septic arthritis, and neuropathic osteoarthropathy. Musculoskeletal anomalies, including the caudal regression syndrome and the combination of unusual facies and femoral hypoplasia, are identified in some infants born of diabetic mothers. After normal pregnancy, osteitis condensans ilii and osteitis pubis may be apparent, and a similar-appearing abnormality of the clavicle has been described. Other conditions associated with pregnancy include osteonecrosis, transient osteoporosis of the hip, disseminated intravascular coagulation, symphyseal diastasis and rupture, and stress fractures.

References

1. Bondy PK: The adrenal cortex. *In* PK Bondy, LE Rosenberg (Eds): Metabolic Control and Disease. 8th Ed. Philadelphia, WB Saunders Co, 1980, p 1427.
2. McAlister WH, Lester PD: Diseases of the adrenal. Med Radiogr Photogr *47*:62, 1971.
3. Ross EJ, Marshall-Jones P, Friedman M: Cushing's syndrome: Diagnostic criteria. Q J Med *35*:149, 1966.
4. Bessler W: Vertebral growth arrest lines after Cushing's syndrome. Diagn Imaging *51*:311, 1982.
5. Riggs BL, Jowsey J, Kelly PJ: Quantitative microradiographic study of bone remodelling in Cushing's syndrome. Metabolism *15*:773, 1966.
6. Molinatti GM, Camanni F, Olivetti M: A study on metabolism of calcium in the hyperadrenocortical syndrome. Acta Endocrinol *34*:323, 1960.
7. Jaffe HL: Metabolic, Degenerative and Inflammatory Diseases of Bones and Joints. Philadelphia, Lea & Febiger, 1972, p 353.
8. Sissons HA: The osteoporosis of Cushing's syndrome. J Bone Joint Surg [Br] *38*:418, 1956.
9. Mooser H: Ein Fall von endogener Fettsucht mit hochgradiger Osteoporose. Virchows Arch (Pathol Anat) *229*:247, 1920–1921.
10. Rosenberg EF: Rheumatoid arthritis, osteoporosis and fractures related to steroid therapy. Acta Med Scand *162*(Suppl 341):211, 1958.
11. Kaplan FS, Leone VJC, Fallon MD, et al: Multiple pathologic fractures of the appendicular skeleton in a patient with Cushing's disease. Clin Orthop *216*:171, 1987.
12. Curtiss PH, Clark WS, Herndon CH: Vertebral fractures resulting from prolonged cortisone and corticotropin therapy. JAMA *156*:467, 1954.
13. Parfitt AM, Duncan H: Metabolic bone disease affecting the spine. *In* RH Rothman, FA Simeone (Eds): The Spine. Philadelphia, WB Saunders Co, 1975, p 599.
14. Fisher DE, Bickel WH: Corticosteroid induced avascular necrosis. J Bone Joint Surg [Am] *53*:859, 1971.
15. Solomon L: Drug induced arthropathy and necrosis of the femoral head. J Bone Joint Surg [Br] *55*:246, 1973.
16. Cruess RL, Ross D, Crawshaw E: The etiology of steroid induced avascular necrosis of bone. Clin Orthop *113*:178, 1975.
17. Madell SH, Freeman LM: Avascular necrosis of bone in Cushing's syndrome. Radiology *83*:1068, 1969.
18. Cerletty JM, Ziebert AP, Mueller KH: Avascular necrosis of the femoral head as the presenting manifestation of Cushing's disease. Clin Orthop *97*:69, 1973.
19. Patterson RJ, Bickel WH, Dahlin DC: Idiopathic avascular necrosis of head of femur; study of 52 cases. J Bone Joint Surg [Am] *46*:267, 1964.
20. Sharon P, Kaplinsky N, Leiba S, et al: Aseptic necrosis of head of femur: Presenting manifestation in Cushing's disease. J Rheumatol *4*:73, 1977.
21. Phillips KA, Nance EP Jr, Rodriguez RM, et al: Avascular necrosis of bone: A manifestation of Cushing's disease. South Med J *79*:825, 1986.
22. Wicks IP, Calligeros D, Kidson W, et al: Cushing's disease presenting with avascular necrosis of the femoral heads and complicated by pituitary apoplexy. Ann Rheum Dis *46*:783, 1987.
23. Alexakis PG, Wallack M: Idiopathic osteonecrosis of the femoral head associated with a pituitary tumor. Report of a case. J Bone Joint Surg [Am] *71*:1412, 1989.
24. Miller WT, Restifo RA: Steroid arthropathy. Radiology *86*:652, 1966.
25. Tondreau RL, Hodes PJ, Schmidt ER Jr: Joint infections following steroid therapy: Roentgen manifestations. AJR *82*:258, 1959.
26. Halpern AA, Horowitz BG, Nagel DA: Tendon ruptures associated with corticosteroid therapy. West J Med *127*:378, 1977.
27. Gilsanz V, Brill PW, Wolf BS: Increased retroperitoneal fat: A sign of corticosteroid therapy. Radiology *123*:147, 1977.
28. Mayo-Smith W, Hayes CW, Biller BMK, et al: Body fat distribution measured with CT: Correlations in healthy subjects, patients with anorexia nervosa, and patients with Cushing's syndrome. Radiology *170*:515, 1989.
29. Mayo-Smith W, Rosenthal DI, Goodsitt MM, et al: Intravertebral fat measurement with quantitative CT in patients with Cushing disease and anorexia nervosa. Radiology *170*:835, 1989.
30. Bondy PK: The adrenal cortex. *In* PK Bondy, LE Rosenberg (Eds): Metabolic Control and Disease. 8th Ed. Philadelphia, WB Saunders Co, 1980, p 1427.
31. Blizzard RM, Kyle M: Studies of the adrenal antigens and antibodies in Addison's disease. J Clin Invest *42*:1653, 1963.
32. Calabrese LH, White CS: Musculoskeletal manifestations of Addison's disease. Arthritis Rheum *22*:558, 1979.
33. Zaleske DJ, Bode HH, Benz R, et al: Association of sciatica-like pain and Addison's disease. J Bone Joint Surg [Am] *66*:297, 1984.
34. Daupleix D, Dreyfus P, Sebaoun J, et al: Manifestations rhumatologiques des insuffisances surrenales. Ann Med Interne *136*:316, 1985.
35. Abbas PH, Schlagenhauff RE, Strong HE: Polyradiculoneuropathy in Addison's disease. Neurology *27*:94, 1977.
36. Pollen RH, Williams RH: Hyperkalemic neuromyopathy in Addison's disease. N Engl J Med *263*:273, 1960.
37. Mor F, Green P, Wysenbeek AJ: Myopathy in Addison's disease. Ann Rheum Dis *46*:81, 1987.

38. Harper WM, Wray CC, Burden AC: An unusual cause of flexion deformity of the hips and knees. A case report. J Bone Joint Surg [Am] 71:1416, 1989.

39. Becker MH, Redisch W, Messina EJ: Bone and microcirculatory changes in a child with benign pheochromocytoma. Radiology 88:487, 1967.

40. Delgoffe C, Bretagne MC, Hoeffel JC, et al: Phéochromocytomes bénins et lésions osseuses métaphysaires chez l'enfant. Arch Fr Pediatr 39:259, 1982.

41. Hoeffel JC, Diard F, Loirat C, et al: Bone lesions secondary to benign phaeochromocytoma. Four cases in childhood. J Bone Joint Surg [Br] 73:158, 1991.

42. James RE, Baker HL, Scanlon PW: The roentgenologic aspects of metastatic pheochromocytoma. AJR 115:783, 1972.

43. Lynn MD, Braunstein EM, Wahl RL, et al: Bone metastases in pheochromocytoma: Comparative studies of efficacy of imaging. Radiology 160:701, 1986.

44. Miraldi FD, Nelson AD, Kraly C, et al: Diagnostic imaging of human neuroblastoma with radiolabeled antibody. Radiology 161:413, 1986.

45. Kincaid OW, Hodgson JR, Dockerty MB: Neuroblastoma: A roentgenographic and pathologic study. AJR 78:420, 1957.

46. David R, Eftekhari F, Lamki N, et al: The many faces of neuroblastoma. RadioGraphics 9:859, 1989.

47. Lipinski JK, McCreath GT, Ireland JT: Diagnostic imaging in diabetes mellitus. J Can Assoc Radiol 30:249, 1979.

48. Holt PJL: Rheumatological manifestations of diabetes mellitus. Clin Rheum Dis 7:723, 1981.

49. Weiss TE, Segaloff A, Moore C: Gout and diabetes. Metabolism 6:103, 1957.

50. Herman JB: Gout and diabetes. Metabolism 7:703, 1958.

51. Whitehouse FW, Cleary WJ Jr: Diabetes mellitus in patients with gout. JAMA 197:73, 1966.

52. Mikkelson WM, Dodge HJ, Valkenburg H: The distribution of serum uric acid values in a population unselected as to gout or hyperuricemia: Tecumseh, Michigan, 1959–1960. Am J Med 39:242, 1965.

53. Hall AP, Barry PE, Dawber TR, et al: Epidemiology of gout and hyperuricemia: A long-term population study. Am J Med 42:27, 1967.

54. Boyle JA, McKiddie M, Buchanan KD, et al: Diabetes mellitus and gout. Blood sugar and plasma insulin responses to oral glucose in normal weight, overweight and gouty patients. Ann Rheum Dis 28:374, 1969.

55. Bluestone R: Rheumatological complications of some endocrinopathies. Clin Rheum Dis 1:95, 1975.

56. McCarty DJ Jr: Pseudogout: Articular chondrocalcinosis. In JL Hollander, DJ McCarty Jr (Eds): Arthritis and Allied Conditions. 8th Ed. Philadelphia, Lea & Febiger, 1972, p 1151.

57. McCarty DJ Jr, Silcox DC, Coe F, et al: Diseases associated with calcium pyrophosphate dihydrate crystal deposition: A controlled study. Am J Med 56:704, 1974.

58. Ghanem MH, Said M: Diabetes mellitus and osteoarthritis. Egypt Rheum 4:1, 1967.

59. Bianchi V, Ricci G: The role of various factors in the etiology of osteoarthritis: Observations on 500 subjects. Reumatismo (Milano) 19:146, 1967.

60. Waine H, Nevinny D, Rosenthal J, et al: Association of osteoarthritis and diabetes mellitus. Tufts Folia Med 7:13, 1961.

61. Forestier J, Lagier R: Ankylosing hyperostosis of the spine. Clin Orthop 74:65, 1971.

62. Forgács SS: Diabetes mellitus and rheumatic disease. Clin Rheum Dis 12:729, 1986.

63. Julkunen H, Karava R, Viljanen V: Hyperostosis of the spine in diabetes mellitus and acromegaly. Diabetologia 2:123, 1966.

64. Forgacs S: Bone and Joints in Diabetes Mellitus. Budapest, Akademiai Kiado, 1982.

65. Harris J, Carter AR, Glick EN, et al: Ankylosing hyperostosis. I. Clinical and radiologic features. Ann Rheum Dis 33:210, 1974.

66. Fisher MS, Hamm R: Uterine artery calcification: Its association with diabetes. Radiology 117:537, 1975.

67. Baum JK, Comstock CH, Joseph L: Intramammary arterial calcifications associated with diabetes. Radiology 136:61, 1980.

68. Connolly J, Regen E, Evans OB: The management of the painful stiff shoulder. Clin Orthop 84:97, 1972.

69. Bridgman JF: Periarthritis of the shoulder and diabetes mellitus. Ann Rheum Dis 31:69, 1972.

70. Mavrikakis ME, Drimis S, Kontoyannis DA, et al: Calcific shoulder periarthritis (tendinitis) in adult onset diabetes mellitus: A controlled study. Ann Rheum Dis 48:211, 1989.

71. Neviaser JS: Adhesive capsulitis of the shoulder: A study of the pathological findings in periarthritis of the shoulder. J Bone Joint Surg 27:211, 1945.

72. Lundberg BJ: The frozen shoulder. Acta Orthop Scand (Suppl)119:1, 1969.

73. Gray RG, Gottlieb NL: Rheumatic disorders associated with diabetes mellitus: Literature review. Semin Arthritis Rheum 6:19, 1976.

74. Morén-Hybbinette I, Moritz U, Scherstén B: The painful diabetic shoulder. Acta Med Scand 219:507, 1986.

75. Grgic A, Rosenbloom AL, Weber FT, et al: Joint contracture in childhood diabetes. N Engl J Med 292:372, 1975.

76. Buckingham BA, Uitto J, Sandborg C, et al: Scleroderma-like changes in insulin-dependent diabetes mellitus: Clinical and biochemical studies. Diabetes Care 7:163, 1984.

77. Fitzcharles MA, Duby S, Waddell RW, et al: Limitation of joint mobility (cheiroarthropathy) in adult noninsulin-dependent diabetic patients. Ann Rheum Dis 43:251, 1984.

78. Costello PB, Tambar PK, Green FA: The prevalence and possible prognostic importance of arthropathy in childhood diabetes. J Rheumatol 11:62, 1984.

79. Garza-Elizondo MA, Diaz-Jouanen E, Franco-Casique JJ, et al: Joint contractures and scleroderma-like skin changes in the hands of insulin-dependent juvenile diabetics. J Rheumatol 10:797, 1983.

80. Rosenbloom AL: Joint contractures preceding insulin-dependent diabetes mellitus. Arthritis Rheum 26:931, 1983.

81. Leden I, Svensson B, Sturfelt G, et al: "Rheumatic" hand symptoms as a clue to undiagnosed diabetes mellitus. Scand J Rheumatol 9:127, 1980.

82. Knowles HB Jr: Joint contractures, waxy skin, and control of diabetes. N Engl J Med 305:217, 1981.

83. Rosenbloom AL, Silverstein JH, Lezotte DC, et al: Limited joint mobility in childhood diabetes mellitus indicates increased risk for microvascular disease. N Engl J Med 305:191, 1981.

84. Seibold JR: Digital sclerosis in children with insulin-dependent diabetes mellitus. Arthritis Rheum 25:1357, 1982.

85. Sherry DD, Rothstein RRL, Petty RE: Joint contractures preceding insulin-dependent diabetes mellitus. Arthritis Rheum 25:1362, 1982.

86. Buckingham B, Perejda AJ, Sandborg C, et al: Skin, joint, and pulmonary changes in Type I diabetes mellitus. Am J Dis Child 140:420, 1986.

87. Choulot JJ, Saint-Martin J: Contractures articulaires evolutives. Une complication méconnue du diabète insulinodépendant. Nouv Presse Med 9:515, 1980.

88. Campbell RR, Hawkins SJ, Maddison PJ, et al: Limited joint mobility in diabetes mellitus. Ann Rheum Dis 44:93, 1985.

89. Jung Y, Hohmann TC, Gerneth JA, et al: Diabetic hand syndrome. Metabolism 20:1008, 1971.

90. Dorwart BB, Schumacher HR: Hand deformities resembling rheumatoid arthritis. Semin Arthritis Rheum 4:53, 1974.

91. Rossi P, Fossaluzza V: Diabetic cheiroarthropathy in adult non-insulin-dependent diabetes. Ann Rheum Dis 44:141, 1985.

92. Davis JS, Finesilver EM: Dupuytren's contraction: With a note on the incidence of the contraction in diabetes. Arch Surg 24:933, 1932.

93. Spring M, Fleck H, Cohen BD: Dupuytren's contracture: Warning of diabetes? NY State J Med 70:1037, 1970.

94. Ricci N, Tovanella B: Malattia di Dupuytren e diabete mellito. Minerva Med 54:3272, 1963.

95. Noble J, Heathcote JG, Cohen H: Diabetes mellitus in the aetiology of Dupuytren's disease. J Bone Joint Surg [Br] 66:322, 1984.

96. Revach M, Cabilli C: Dupuytren's contracture and diabetes mellitus. Isr J Med Sci 8:774, 1972.

97. Ling RSM: The genetic factor in Dupuytren's disease. J Bone Joint Surg [Br] 45:709, 1963.

98. Lapidus PW: Stenosing tenovaginitis. Surg Clin North Am 33:1317, 1953.

99. Lapidus PW, Guidotti FP: Stenosing tenovaginitis of the wrist and fingers. Clin Orthop 83:87, 1972.

100. Gharib R: Stenosing tenovaginitis (trigger-finger). J Pediatr 69:294, 1966.

101. Kellgren JH, Ball J: Tendon lesions in rheumatoid arthritis: A clinicopathologic study. Ann Rheum Dis 9:48, 1950.

102. Mackenzie AH: Final diagnoses in 63 patients presenting with multiple palmar flexor tenosynovitis (MPFT). Arthritis Rheum 18:415, 1975.

103. Rosenbloom AL: Skeletal and joint manifestations of childhood diabetes. Pediatr Clin North Amer 31:569, 1984.

104. Yosipovitch G, Yosipovitch Z, Karp M, et al: Trigger finger in young patients with insulin dependent diabetes. J Rheumatol 17:951, 1990.

105. Phalen GS: Reflections on twenty-one years' experience with the carpal tunnel syndrome. JAMA 212:1365, 1970.

106. Frymoyer JW, Bland J: Carpal tunnel syndrome in patients with myxedematous arthropathy. J Bone Joint Surg [Am] 55:78, 1973.

107. Phalen GS: The carpal tunnel syndrome. Seventeen years' experience in diagnosis and treatment of six hundred and fifty-four hands. J Bone Joint Surg [Am] 48:211, 1966.

108. Feingold ML, Resnick D, Niwayama G, et al: The plantar compartments of the foot: A roentgen approach. I. Experimental observations. Invest Radiol 12:281, 1977.

109. Sartoris DJ, Devine S, Resnick D, et al: Plantar compartmental infection in the diabetic foot. The role of computed tomography. Invest Radiol 20:772, 1985.

110. Meltzer AD, Skversky N, Ostrum BJ: Radiographic evaluation of soft tissue necrosis in diabetics. Radiology 90:300, 1968.

111. Pedersen J, Olsen S: Small vessel disease of the lower extremity in diabetes mellitus. On the pathogenesis of the foot lesions in diabetics. Acta Med Scand 171:551, 1962.

112. Wheat LJ, Allen SD, Henry M, et al: Diabetic foot infections. Bacteriologic analysis. Arch Intern Med 146:1935, 1986.

113. Bamberger DM, Daus GP, Gerding DN: Osteomyelitis in the feet of diabetic patients. Long-term results, prognostic factors, and the role of antimicrobial and surgical therapy. Am J Med 83:653, 1987.

114. Mendelson EB, Fisher MR, Deschler TW, et al: Osteomyelitis in the diabetic foot: A difficult diagnostic challenge. RadioGraphics 3:248, 1983.

115. Sinha S, Munichoodappa CS, Kozak GP: Neuro-arthropathy (Charcot joints) in diabetes mellitus (clinical study of 101 cases). Medicine 51:191, 1972.

116. Parsons H, Norton WS: Management of diabetic neuropathic joints. N Engl J Med 244:935, 1951.

117. El-Khoury GY, Kathol MH: Neuropathic fractures in patients with diabetes mellitus. Radiology 134:313, 1980.

118. Newman JH: Spontaneous dislocation in diabetic neuropathy. A report of six cases. J Bone Joint Surg [Br] 61:484, 1979.

119. Harper MC: Bilateral spontaneous avulsion fractures of the calcaneus in a diabetic patient. A case report. Orthopedics 7:869, 1984.

120. Raju UB, Fine G, Partamian JO: Diabetic neuroarthropathy (Charcot's joint). Arch Pathol Lab Med 106:349, 1982.
121. Hennessy O: Case report 264. Skel Radiol 11:155, 1984.
122. Kristiansen B: Ankle and foot fractures in diabetics provoking neuropathic joint changes. Acta Orthop Scand 51:975, 1980.
123. Lesko P, Maurer RC: Talonavicular dislocations and midfoot arthropathy in neuropathic diabetic feet. Natural course and principles of treatment. Clin Orthop 240:226, 1989.
124. Clohisy DR, Thompson RC Jr: Fractures associated with neuropathic arthropathy in adults who have juvenile-onset diabetes. J Bone Joint Surg [Am] 70:1192, 1988.
125. Slowman-Kovacs SD, Braunstein EM, Brandt KD: Rapidly progressive Charcot arthropathy following minor joint trauma in patients with diabetic neuropathy. Arthritis Rheum 33:412, 1990.
126. Pognowska MJ, Collins LC, Dobson HL: Diabetic osteopathy. Radiology 89:265, 1967.
127. Levin ME, Boisseau VC, Avioli LV: Effect of diabetes mellitus on bone mass in juvenile and adult-onset diabetes. N Engl J Med 294:291, 1976.
128. Rosenbloom AL, Lezotte DC, Weber FT, et al: Diminution of bone mass in childhood diabetes. Diabetes 26:1052, 1977.
129. Santiago JV, McAlister WH, Ratzan SK, et al: Decreased cortical thickness and osteopenia in children with diabetes mellitus. J Clin Endocrinol Metab 45:845, 1977.
130. Frazer TE, White NH, Hough S, et al: Alterations in circulating vitamin D metabolites in the young insulin dependent diabetic. J Clin Endocrinol Metab 53:1154, 1981.
131. McNair P, Madsbad S, Christiansen C, et al: Osteopenia in insulin treated diabetes mellitus. Diabetologia 15:87, 1978.
132. Wiske P, Wentworth SM, Norton JA Jr, et al: Evaluation of bone mass and growth in young diabetics. Metabolism 31:848, 1982.
133. Goodman WG, Hori MT: Diminished bone formation in experimental diabetes. Relationship to osteoid maturation and mineralization. Diabetes 33:825, 1984.
134. Heath H, Melton LJ, Chu C: Diabetes mellitus and risk of skeletal fracture. N Engl J Med 303:567, 1980.
135. Lindblom A: Arteriosclerosis and arterial thrombosis in the lower limb. A roentgenological study. Acta Radiol Diagn (Suppl) 80:38, 1950.
136. Ferrier TM: Radiologically demonstrable arterial calcification in diabetes mellitus. Aust Ann Med 13:222, 1964.
137. Lithner F: Cutaneous erythema, with or without necrosis, localized to the legs and feet—a lesion in elderly diabetics. Acta Med Scand 196:333, 1974.
138. Lithner F, Hietala S-O, Steen L: Skeletal lesions and arterial calcifications of the feet in diabetics. Acta Med Scand (Suppl) 687:47, 1984.
139. Edmonds ME, Roberts VC, Watkins RJ: Blood flow in the diabetic neuropathic foot. Diabetologia 22:9, 1982.
140. Edmondson ME, Morrison N, Laws JW, et al: Medial arterial calcification and diabetic neuropathy. Br Med J 284:928, 1982.
141. Neubauer B, Gundersen HJG: Calcifications, narrowing and rugosities of the leg arteries in diabetic patients. Acta Radiol Diagn 24:401, 1983.
142. Ziegler LH: Lipodystrophies: Report of 7 cases. Brain 51:147, 1928.
143. Lawrence RD: Lipodystrophy and hepatomegaly with diabetes, lipemia, and other metabolic disturbances: Case throwing new light on action of insulin. Lancet 1:724, 1946.
144. Wesenberg RL, Gwinn JL, Barner GR: The roentgenographic findings in total lipodystrophy. AJR 103:154, 1968.
145. Gold RH, Steinbach HL: Lipoatrophic diabetes mellitus (generalized lipodystrophy): Roentgen findings in two brothers with congenital disease. AJR 101:884, 1967.
146. Seip M: Lipodystrophy and gigantism with associated endocrine manifestations: New diencephalic syndrome? Acta Paediatr 48:555, 1959.
147. Zarafonetis CJ, Seifter J, Baeder DH, et al: Current clinical status of lipid-mobilizer hormone. Arch Intern Med 104:974, 1959.
148. Griffiths HJ, Rossini AA: A case of lipoatrophic diabetes. Radiology 114:329, 1975.
149. Lejeune E, Tourniarire J: Altérations osseuses et diabète lipo-atrophique (à propos d'une observation). Lyon Med 222:789, 1969.
150. Sebrechts C, Garvey WT, Sartoris DJ, et al: Case report 417. Skel Radiol 16:320, 1987.
151. Senior B, Gellis SS: Syndromes of total lipodystrophy and of partial lipodystrophy. Pediatrics 33:593, 1964.
152. Amankwah KS, Prentice RL, Fleury FJ: The incidence of gestational diabetes. Obstet Gynecol 49:497, 1977.
153. O'Sullivan JB, Mahan CM, Charles D, et al: Screening criteria for high risk gestational diabetic patients. Am J Obstet Gynecol 116:895, 1978.
154. Pedersen LM, Tygstrup I, Pedersen J: Congenital malformation in newborn infants of diabetic women. Correlation with maternal diabetic vascular complications. Lancet 1:1124, 1964.
155. Dunn V, Nixon GW, Jaffe RB, et al: Infants of diabetic mothers: Radiographic manifestations. AJR 137:123, 1981.
156. Blumel J, Evans EB, Eggers GWN: Partial and complete agenesis or malformation of the sacrum with associated anomalies. J Bone Joint Surg [Am] 41:497, 1959.
157. Stanley JK, Owen R, Koff S: Congenital sacral anomalies. J Bone Joint Surg [Br] 61:401, 1979.
158. Abraham E: Sacral agenesis with associated anomalies (caudal regression syndrome): Autopsy case report. Clin Orthop 145:168, 1979.
159. Guidera KJ, Raney E, Ogden JA, et al: Caudal regression: A review of seven cases, including the mermaid syndrome. J Pediatr Orthop 11:743, 1991.
160. Hurst D, Johnson DF: Femoral hypoplasia—unusual facies syndrome. Am J Med Genet 5:255, 1980.
161. Daentl DL, Smith DW, Scott CI, et al: Femoral hypoplasia—unusual facies syndrome. J Pediatr 86:107, 1975.
162. Johnson JP, Carey JC, Gooch WM III, et al: Femoral hypoplasia—unusual facies syndrome in infants of diabetic mothers. J Pediatr 102:866, 1983.
163. Thorp DJ, Fray WE: The pelvic joints during pregnancy and labor. JAMA 111:1162, 1938.
164. Abramson D, Roberts SM, Wilson PD: Relaxation of the pelvic joints in pregnancy. Surg Gynecol Obstet 58:595, 1934.
165. Russell JG: Moulding of the pelvic outlet. J Obstet Gynaecol Br Commw 76:817, 1969.
166. Loeschcke H: Untersuchungen über Entstehung und Bedeutung der spaltbildungen in der Symphyse, sowie über physiologische Erweiterugsvorgänge am Becken Schwangerer und Gebarender. Arch Gynaek 96:525, 1912.
167. Calguneri M, Bird HA, Wright V: Changes in joint laxity occurring during pregnancy. Ann Rheum Dis 41:126, 1982.
168. Zarrow M, Holmstrom EG, Salhanick HA: The concentration of relaxin in the blood serum and other tissues of women during pregnancy. J Clin Endocrinol 15:22, 1955.
169. Walde J: Obstetrical and gynaecological back and pelvic pain, especially those contracted during pregnancy. Acta Obstet Gynecol Scand 41 (Suppl 2):11, 1962.
170. Hagen R: Pelvic girdle relaxation from an orthopaedic point of view. Acta Orthop Scand 45:550, 1974.
171. Schmorl G: Über die an den Wirbelbandsch einen vorkommenden Aussehnungs und Zerreissungsvorgange und die dadurch an ihnen und der Wirbelspongiosa hervorg Veränderungen. Verh Deutsch Ges Pathol 22:250, 1927.
172. Weinreb JC, Wolbarsht LB, Cohen JM, et al: Prevalence of lumbosacral intervertebral disk abnormalities on MR images in pregnant and asymptomatic nonpregnant women. Radiology 170:125, 1989.
173. Gillespie HW, Lloyd-Roberts G: Osteitis condensans. Br J Rad 26:16, 1953.
174. Segal G, Kellogg DS: Osteitis condensans ilii. AJR 71:643, 1954.
175. Thompson M: Osteitis condensans ilii and its differentiation from ankylosing spondylitis. Ann Rheum Dis 13:147, 1954.
176. Julkunen H, Rokkanen P: Ankylosing spondylitis and osteitis condensans ilii. Acta Rheum Scand 15:224, 1969.
177. Appell RG, Oppermann HC, Becker W, et al: Condensing osteitis of the clavicle in childhood: A rare sclerotic bone lesion. Review of the literature and report of seven patients. Pediatr Radiol 13:301, 1983.
178. Dihlmann W: Diagnostic Radiology of the Sacroiliac Joints. New York, Georg Thieme Verlag, 1980, p 104.
179. Numaguchi Y: Osteitis condensans ilii, including its resolution. Radiology 98:1, 1971.
180. Berent F: Zur Atiologie der Ostitis condensans ilii. ROFO 49:263, 1934.
181. Dihlmann W: Die Hyperostosis triangularis ilii—das sakroiliakale knöcherne Stressphänomen. ROFO 124:1, 154, 1976.
182. Wells J: Osteitis condensans ilii. AJR 76:1141, 1956.
183. Szabados MD: Osteitis condensans ilii, report of 3 cases associated with urinary tract infection. J Fla Med Assoc 34:95, 1947.
184. Borak J: Significance of the sacroiliac findings in Marie-Strumpell's spondylitis. Radiology 47:128, 1946.
185. Singal DP, deBosset P, Gordon DA, et al: HLA antigens in osteitis condensans ilii and ankylosing spondylitis. J Rhematol (Suppl 3) 4:105, 1977.
186. DeBosset P, Gordon DA, Smythe HA, et al: Comparison of osteitis condensans ilii and ankylosing spondylitis in female patients: Clinical, radiological and HLA typing characteristics. J Chron Dis 31:171, 1978.
187. Resnick D, Dwosh I, Goergen TG, et al: Clinical and radiographic abnormalities in ankylosing spondylitis. A comparison of men and women. Radiology 179:293, 1976.
188. Arturi AS, Marcos JC, Maldonado-Cocco JA, et al: Osteitis condensans ilii in apatite crystal deposition disease. Arthritis Rheum 26:567, 1983.
189. Olivieri I, Gemignani G, Camerini E, et al: Differential diagnosis between osteitis condensans ilii and sacroiliitis. J Rheumatol 17:1504, 1990.
190. Parhami N, DiGiacomo R, Jouzevicius JL: Metastatic bone lesions of leiomyosarcoma mimicking osteitis condensans ilii. J Rheumatol 15:1035, 1988.
191. Coventry MB, Mitchell WC: Osteitis pubis. Observations based on a study of 45 patients. JAMA 178:898, 1961.
192. Steinbach L, Petrakis NL, Gilfillan RS, et al: The pathogenesis of osteitis pubis. J Urol 74:840, 1955.
193. Pizzarello LD, Golden GT, Shaw A: Acute abdominal pain caused by osteitis pubis. Am J Surg 40:660, 1974.
194. Huaux JP, Maldague B, Malghem J, et al: L'Ostéite pubienne. A propos de quatre observations vues en milieu rhumatologique. Louvain Med 105:283, 1986.
195. Barnes WC, Malament M: Osteitis pubis. Surg Gynaecol Obstet 117:277, 1963.
196. Grace JN, Sim FH, Shives TC, et al: Wedge resection of the symphysis pubis for the treatment of osteitis pubis. J Bone Joint Surg [Am] 71:358, 1989.
197. Walheim GG, Selvik G: Mobility of the pubic symphysis. In vivo measurements with an electromechanic method and a roentgen stereophotogrammetric method. Clin Orthop 191:129, 1984.
198. Walheim G, Olerud S, Ribbe T: Mobility of the pubic symphysis. Measurements by an electromechanical method. Acta Orthop Scand 55:203, 1984.

199. Williams JL: Gas in the symphysis pubis during and following pregnancy. AJR 73:403, 1955.
200. Olerud S, Grevsten S: Chronic pubis symphysiolysis, a case report. J Bone Joint Surg [Am] 56:799, 1974.
201. Harris NH: Lesions of the symphysis pubis in women. Br Med J 4:209, 1974.
202. Eickelmann HJ: Beitrag zur Atio-Pathogenese der Osteitis pubis. Zentralbl Chir 101:1184, 1976.
203. Mynors JM: Osteitis pubis. J Urol 112:664, 1974.
204. Harris NH, Murray RO: Lesions of the symphysis in athletes. Br Med J 4:211, 1974.
205. Rolland JJ, Menou P, LeBourg M, et al: Pubic pain and position of the pelvis. Anat Clin 4:69, 1982.
206. Koch RA, Jackson DW: Pubic symphysitis in runners. A report of two cases. Am J Sports Med 9:62, 1981.
207. Wiley JJ: Traumatic osteitis pubis: The gracilis syndrome. Am J Sports Med 11:360, 1983.
208. Fricker PA, Taunton JE, Ammann W: Osteitis pubis in athletes. Infection, inflammation or injury? Sports Med 12:266, 1991.
209. Schneider R, Kaye JJ, Ghelman B: Adductor avulsive injuries near the symphysis pubis. Radiology 120:567, 1976.
210. Burns JR, Gregory JG: Osteomyelitis of the pubic symphysis after urologic surgery. J Urology 118:803, 1977.
211. Bouza E, Winston DJ, Hewitt WL: Infectious osteitis pubis. Urology 12:663, 1978.
212. Gilbert DN, Azorr M, Gore R, et al: The bacterial causation of postoperative osteitis pubis. Surg Gynecol Obstet 141:195, 1975.
213. López-Guerra N, García-Moncó JC, Lario BA, et al: Osteomyelitis pubis in athletes. J Rheumatol 15:530, 1988.
214. Rosenthal RE, Spickard WA, Markham RD, et al: Osteomyelitis of the symphysis pubis: A separate disease from osteitis pubis. Report of three cases and review of the literature. J Bone Joint Surg [Am] 64:123, 1982.
215. del Busto R, Quinn EL, Fisher EJ, et al: Osteomyelitis of the pubis. Report of seven cases. JAMA 248:1498, 1982.
216. Sequeira W, Jones E, Siegel ME, et al: Pyogenic infections of the pubic symphysis. Ann Intern Med 96:604, 1982.
217. Arlet J, Bouteiller G, Durroux R, et al: Ostéites pubiennes et ischiopubiennes. Etude bactériologique et histopathologique de l'os pubien. Rev Rhum Mal Osteoartic 48:101, 1981.
218. Jenkins FH, Raff MJ, Florman LD, et al: Pubic osteomyelitis due to anaerobic bacteria. Arch Intern Med 144:842, 1984.
219. Mynors JM: Osteitis pubis. J Urol 112:664, 1974.
220. Nissenkorn I, Servadio C, Lubin E: The treatment of osteitis pubis with heparin. J Urol 125:528, 1981.
221. Barnes JM: The symphysis pubis in the female. AJR 30:797, 1933.
222. Reis RA, Baer JL, Arens RA, et al: Traumatic separation of the symphysis pubis during spontaneous labor with a clinical and x-ray study of the normal symphysis pubis during pregnancy and the puerperium. Surg Gynecol Obstet 55:336, 1932.
223. Heyman J, Lundqvist A: The symphysis pubis in pregnancy and parturition. Acta Obstet Gynecol Scand 12:191, 1932.
224. Lindsey RW, Leggon RE, Wright DG, et al: Separation of the symphysis pubis in association with childbearing. A case report. J Bone Joint Surg [Am] 70:289, 1988.
225. Dhar S, Anderton JM: Rupture of the symphysis pubis during labor. Clin Orthop 283:252, 1992.
226. Harigaya K, Watanabe Y, Kageymak, et al: Multiple bone marrow necrosis and disseminated intravascular coagulation. Arch Pathol Lab Med 101:652, 1977.
227. Rose MS: Apparent necrosis of bone marrow in a patient with disseminated intravascular coagulation, postpartum. Lancet 2:730, 1973.
228. Knickerbocker WJ, Quenville NF: Widespread marrow necrosis during pregnancy. Skel Radiol 9:37, 1982.
229. Pellicci PM, Zolla-Pazner S, Rabhan WN, et al: Osteonecrosis of the femoral head associated with pregnancy. Report of three cases. Clin Orthop 185:59, 1984.
230. Cheng N, Burssens A, Mulier JC: Pregnancy and post-pregnancy avascular necrosis of the femoral head. Arch Orthop Trauma Surg 100:199, 1982.
231. McGuigan L, Fleming A: Osteonecrosis of the humerus related to pregnancy. Ann Rheum Dis 42:597, 1983.
232. Lausten GS: Osteonecrosis of the femoral head during pregnancy. Arch Orthop Trauma Surg 110:214, 1991.
233. Bayliss RIS, Browne JC, Round BP, et al: Plasma-17-hydroxycorticosteroids in pregnancy. Lancet 1:607, 1955.
234. Burke CW, Roulet F: Increased exposure of tissue to cortisol in late pregnancy. Br M J 1:657, 1970.
235. Calvao-Teles A, Burke CW: Cortisol levels in toxemia and normal pregnancy. Lancet 1:737, 1973.
236. Cushard WG Jr, Creditor MA, Canterbury JM, et al: Physiologic hyperparathyroidism in pregnancy. J Clin Endocrinol Metab 34:767, 1972.
237. Jacobs B: Epidemiology of traumatic and nontraumatic osteonecrosis. Clin Orthop 130:51, 1978.
238. Curtiss PH Jr, Kincaid WE: Transient demineralization of the hip in pregnancy. J Bone Joint Surg [Am] 41:1327, 1959.
239. Longstreth PL, Malinak LR, Hill CS: Transient osteoporosis of the hip in pregnancy. Obstet Gynecol 41:563, 1973.
240. Zolla-Pazner S, Pazner SS, Lanyi V, et al: Osteonecrosis of the femoral head during pregnancy. JAMA 244:689, 1980.
241. Karasick D, Edeiken J: Case report 19. Skel Radiol 1:181, 1977.
242. Weiner SN, Levy M, Bernstein R, et al: Condensing osteitis of the clavicle. A case report. J Bone Joint Surg [Am] 66:1484, 1984.
243. Nordin BEC, Roper A: Post-pregnancy osteoporosis—a syndrome? Lancet 1:431, 1955.
244. Jowsey J, Kelly PJ: Effect of fluoride treatment in patient with osteoporosis. Mayo Clin Proc 43:435, 1968.
245. Gruber HE, Gutteridge DH, Baylink DJ: Osteoporosis associated with pregnancy and lactation: Bone biopsy and skeletal features in three patients. Metab Bone Dis Rel Res 5:159, 1984.
246. Mikawa Y, Watanabe R, Yamano Y, et al: Stress fracture of the body of pubis in a pregnant woman. Case report. Arch Orthop Trauma Surg 107:193, 1988.
247. Hoang T-A, Nguyen TH, Daffner RH, et al: Case report 491. Skel Radiol 17:364, 1988.
248. Brower AC, Sweet DE, Keats TE: Condensing osteitis of the clavicle: A new entity. AJR 121:17, 1974.
249. Solovjev M: Osteitis condensans claviculae. ROFO 125:375, 1976.
250. Teates CD, Brower AC, Williamson BRJ, et al: Bone scans in condensing osteitis of the clavicle. South Med J 71:736, 1978.
251. Duro JC, Estrada P, Ribas D, et al: Condensing osteitis of the clavicle. Arthritis Rheum 24:1454, 1981.
252. Cone RO, Resnick D, Goergen TG, et al: Condensing osteitis of the clavicle. AJR 141:387, 1983.
253. Jurik AG, DeCarvalho A, Graudal H: Sclerotic changes of the sternal end of the clavicle. Clin Radiol 36:23, 1985.
254. Hamilton-Wood C, Hollingworth P, Dieppe P, et al: The painful swollen sternoclavicular joint. Br J Radiol 58:941, 1985.
255. Kruger GD, Rock MG, Munro TG: Condensing osteitis of the clavicle. A review of the literature and report of three cases. J Bone Joint Surg [Am] 69:550, 1987.
256. Vierboom MAC, Steinberg JDJ, Mooyaart EL, et al: Condensing osteitis of the clavicle: Magnetic resonance imaging as an adjunct method for differential diagnosis. Ann Rheum Dis 51:539, 1992.
257. Abdelwahab IF, Hermann G, Ramos R, et al: Case report 623. Skel Radiol 19:387, 1990.
258. Greenspan A, Gerscovich E, Szabo RM, et al: Condensing osteitis of the clavicle: A rare but frequently misdiagnosed condition. AJR 156:1011, 1991.
259. Outwater E, Oates E: Condensing osteitis of the clavicle: Case report and review of the literature. J Nucl Med 29:1122, 1988.
260. Apter S, Hertz M, Salai M, et al: Post-traumatic reactive and resorptive lesions of the medial end of the clavicle. Clin Imaging 16:40, 1992.
261. Levy M, Goldberg I, Fischel RE, et al: Friedrich's disease: Aseptic necrosis of the sternal end of the clavicle. J Bone Joint Surg [Br] 63:539, 1981.
262. Köhler H, Uehlinger E, Kutzner J, et al: Sternocostoclavicular hyperostosis: Painful swelling of the sternum, clavicles, and upper ribs. Report of two new cases. Ann Intern Med 87:192, 1977.
263. Sonozaki H, Azuma A, Okai K, et al: Clinical features of 22 cases with ''inter-sterno-costo-clavicular ossification.'' A new syndrome. Arch Orthop Trauma Surg 95:13, 1979.
264. Jones MW, Carty H, Taylor JF, et al: Condensing osteitis of the clavicle: Does it exist? J Bone Joint Surg [Br] 72:464, 1990.
265. Hoeffel JC, Worms AM, Marcon F, et al: Acro-osteolysis of the phalanges and phaeochromocytoma. ROFO 157:100, 1992.
266. Kathol MH, El-Khoury GY, Moore TE, et al: Calcaneal insufficiency avulsion fractures in patients with diabetes mellitus. Radiology 180:725, 1991.
267. Chester CS, Banker BQ: Focal infarction of muscle in diabetics. Diabetes Care 9:623, 1986.
268. Nunez-Hoyo M, Gardner CL, Motta AO, et al: Skeletal muscle infarction in diabetes: MR findings. J Comput Assist Tomogr 17:986, 1993.
269. Reich S, Wiener SN, Chester S, et al: Clinical and radiologic features of spontaneous muscle infarction in the diabetic. Clin Nucl Med 10:876, 1985.

SECTION

XII

Diseases of the Hematopoietic System

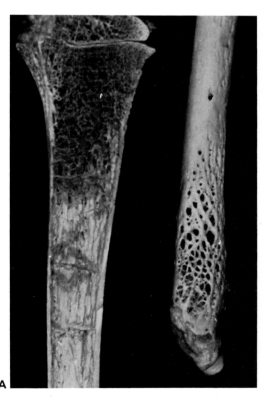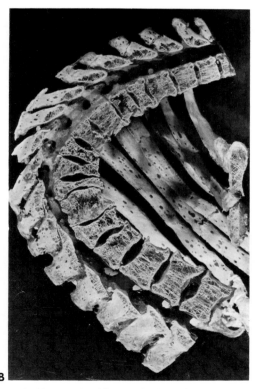

A Thalassemia major: A coronal section of the tibia (left) reveals diffuse thinning of the cortex with widening of the medullary canal; the external surface of the distal portion of the radius (right) demonstrates a lacelike appearance of the metaphyseal cortex.
B Plasma cell myeloma: Findings include trabecular resorption, compression fractures of vertebral bodies, exaggerated kyphosis, and multiple osteolytic lesions in the spinous processes and ribs.
(From Ortner DJ, Putschar WGJ: Identification of Pathological Conditions in Human Skeletal Remains. Washington, DC, Smithsonian Institution Press, 1981.)

59

Hemoglobinopathies and Other Anemias

Donald Resnick, M.D.

Anemia should be regarded as a clinical finding rather than as a specific disease. It is characterized by a reduction in the blood's capacity to transport oxygen. Oxygen combined with hemoglobin is transported by the red cell; therefore, anemia occurs when the circulating red cell mass is abnormally low. As the red cell mass generally is correlated with the concentration of hemoglobin or the hematocrit value, anemia usually is accompanied by a decrease in hemoglobin concentration (below 13.5 gm/dl in men and 12.0 gm/dl in women) and a fall in hematocrit; exceptions to this rule occur in a patient who is actively bleeding (in which there is a decrease in red cell mass without a dramatic change in hemoglobin concentration) and in a patient with an abnormal plasma volume (as in congestive heart failure or pregnancy).

Hemoglobin represents approximately one third of the wet weight of the red blood cell and 95 per cent of its dry weight. Ninety-seven per cent of the molecule consists of the polypeptide chains of globin and 3 per cent of the heme groups. The structure of 97 per cent of the hemoglobin in the normal adult, consisting of two pairs of coiled polypeptide chains (two alpha chains composed of 141 amino acids and two beta chains composed of 146 amino acids) is termed Hb A. A smaller fraction of hemoglobin (approximately 2 per cent) termed Hb A2 also may be found; this fraction contains a different second set of polypeptide chains. In the fetus, another type of hemoglobin is found, termed Hb F. This hemoglobin is present in infants at birth, varying in concentrations from 60 per cent to 90 per cent. It generally decreases in concentration during the neonatal period and, in most infants, it has almost disappeared by 4 months of age, by which time Hb A becomes predominant. In the adult, Hb F makes up the remaining 1 per cent of the hemoglobin. With Pauling's milestone discovery of a second adult human hemoglobin in certain persons with sickle cell anemia, Hb S,[1] considerable attention was focused on disease states associated with abnormal hemoglobins (the hemoglobinopathies), many of which produce significant musculoskeletal abnormalities. This chapter is devoted to a discussion of the skeletal effects of these and related hematologic disorders.

The clinical manifestations of anemia are variable, being influenced by its rate of development and the status or function of the cardiovascular, cerebrovascular, and renal systems. Mild or slowly developing anemias may be unaccompanied by significant symptoms and signs in the absence of heavy physical exertion. Fatigue, weakness, palpitations, and anorexia represent early and nonspecific clinical findings. More characteristic abnormalities include exertional dyspnea, tachycardia, claudication, vertigo, and angina, indicating the inadequate supply of oxygen to the body's tissues. Specific types of anemia, of which there are many, sometimes are associated with typical clinical clues, including the cholelithiasis seen in chronic hemolytic states and the bone pain and tenderness accompanying osseous metastasis with compromise of the bone marrow. Findings during physical examination supplemented with results of appropriate laboratory and imaging studies commonly allow a precise diagnosis of the disease responsible for the anemia.

The hypoxia of anemia represents a stimulus for increased erythropoiesis through the action of the hormone erythropoietin, formed principally in the kidneys. This hormone is responsible for increased cellular activity in the bone marrow, leading to an augmented rate of formation of red blood cells from precursor cells. In the presence of bone marrow compromise, which may relate to marrow infiltration with tumor or myelofibrosis, extramedullary sites, such as the liver and the spleen, become actively involved in hematopoiesis. Hepatosplenomegaly and even paravertebral masses are radiographic findings consistent with such hematopoiesis.

SICKLE CELL ANEMIA
General Features

Sickle cell disease is a term that describes all conditions characterized by the presence of Hb S. These conditions include sickle cell anemia (Hb S-S), sickle cell trait (Hb A-S), and diseases in which Hb S is combined with another abnormal hemoglobin. Hb S is characterized by a normal alpha chain and an abnormal beta chain, in which valine has replaced glutamic acid.

It has been estimated that the sickle cell trait exists in approximately 7 per cent of North American blacks and perhaps in 40 to 50 per cent of members of some African tribes.[1, 2] Sickle cell anemia occurs in approximately 0.3 to 1.3 per cent of North American blacks.[3] The disease first was noted by Herrick[4] in 1910 when he observed "a large number of thin, elongated, sickle-shaped and crescent-shaped forms" when the blood smear of an ailing black student was placed in a low oxygen environment. Hahn and Gillespie[5] in 1927 related the phenomenon of sickling to the removal of oxygen and noted the reversibility of the process. Hahn[6] later proposed the term *sickle cell trait* to describe the disorder in nonanemic persons whose cells could sickle in vitro. Osseous changes were found in sickle cell anemia[7, 8] prior to Pauling's discovery in 1949 of a specific hemoglobin molecular change as the basis for this disorder.[1]

Clinical Features

The clinical manifestations of sickle cell anemia have been well delineated.[9-13] Symptomatic, painful crises affecting the bones and joints of the extremities usually commence during the second or third year of life.[14] These crises are characterized by gradual or rapid worsening of anemia due to erythrocyte destruction and are associated with fever, icterus, nausea, vomiting, abdominal pain, and prostration. The basic pathogenesis of the sickle crisis appears to be deformation of red blood cells, which produces vaso-occlusion and tissue death; it is not clear if sickle cells are more likely to occlude capillaries because of their shape or if they are excluded from vessels because of this shape (Fig. 59–1).[15] The consensus however, is that the microcirculatory disturbance in sickle cell anemia is related to the abnormal rheologic properties of the sickle cell red blood cells. In homozygous sickle cell disease, deoxygenation of the erythrocytes causes the polymerization of Hb S and transformation of the intracellular fluid into a viscoelastic gel, a process that is most prominent in particularly dense red cells that possess a high concentration of Hb S.[16] These cells, therefore, are the most rigid, are the ones that accumulate at the entrance of narrow capillaries, and have the greatest effect on resistance to blood flow through the microcirculation.[16] Ischemia is the clinical (as well as radiologic and pathologic) consequence of these cellular characteristics. Osseous and articular pain and tenderness frequently are related to infarction of bone marrow. Indeed, such pain and tenderness appear to be the only clinical findings that consistently and specifically can be related to bone marrow necrosis; other associated abnormalities, which may include malaise, weight loss, and fever, more likely are manifestations of the underlying disease.[17] The sickle cell crisis can resolve, and the patient may be free of clinical manifestations for a long period of time prior to the onset of a second crisis. In patients with sickle cell trait, painful crises usually are not apparent unless the patient is exposed to an atmosphere low in oxygen.

Although sickle cell anemia rarely has its clinical onset in infants prior to the age of 6 months because of the persistence of Hb F, which reduces the sickling properties of the red blood cell, fever, pallor, and swelling of the hands are observed in children with this disease, apparently related in part to infarction of the small tubular bones. This "hand-foot" syndrome or dactylitis is most frequent between the ages of 6 months and 2 years.[18-21] It is the initial manifestation of the disease in approximately 30 per cent of cases.

Other clinical manifestations that may be apparent in sickle cell anemia are hepatosplenomegaly, cardiac enlargement, chronic leg ulcers, particularly over the malleoli, osteomyelitis, septic arthritis, pulmonary abnormalities including pneumonia and infarction, abdominal pain, cholelithiasis, jaundice, peptic ulcer disease, hematuria, priapism, neurologic findings, and lymphadenopathy. Death may result from infection, cardiac decompensation related to severe anemia, or thrombosis and infarction of various organs. In recent years, better nutrition and earlier and more adequate treatment of infections have contributed to in-

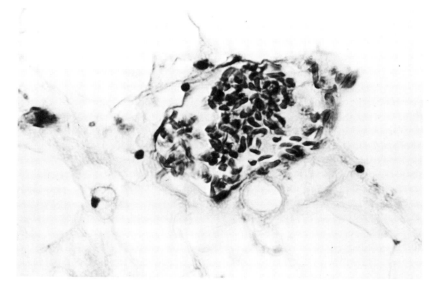

FIGURE 59–1. Sickle cells. Sludging of the abnormally shaped erythrocytes within a blood vessel is seen. (Courtesy of A. Norman, M.D., Valhalla, New York.)

creasing longevity of the patient with sickle cell anemia, so that many affected persons live past the age of 50 years.

Radiographic and Pathologic Features

The radiographic and pathologic findings that occur in sickle cell anemia relate to marrow hyperplasia, vascular occlusion, and miscellaneous findings.

Marrow Hyperplasia (Fig. 59–2). Hypercellularity of the bone marrow (erythrocytic, granulocytic, and megakaryocytic systems) in this disease is a response to anemia of long duration. In infants with sickle cell anemia, red marrow extends into all of the bones, including those of the

hands and feet; in older children and adults, red marrow recedes from some of these small bones but persists in the ankles, wrists, and shafts of the long bones.[22, 23] Marrow hyperplasia produces widening of the medullary cavities and intertrabecular spaces and rarefaction of remaining trabeculae in the spongiosa and cortex. These pathologic findings are associated with radiographic abnormalities, including increased radiolucency of osseous tissue, fewer and more accentuated bony trabeculae, and cortical thinning. The osseous changes are evident in many areas, particularly in the axial skeleton.

In the skull, diffuse widening of the diploic space is associated with thinning of both the outer and inner tables

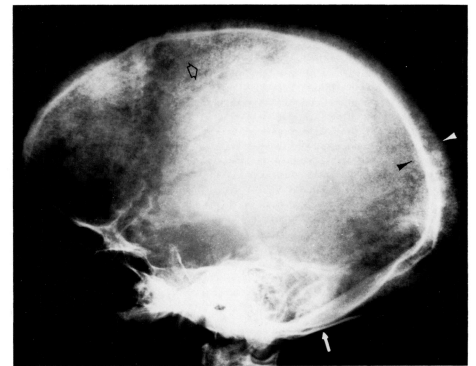

FIGURE 59–2. Sickle cell anemia: Marrow hyperplasia. A lateral view of the skull demonstrates widening of the diploic space (arrowheads). The base of the occiput is spared (arrow). Focal areas of increased radiodensity (open arrow) may represent myelofibrosis or healing infarcts.

of the skull.[24, 25] The appearance is that of a coarse granular osteoporosis involving the entire cranial vault except for the base of the occiput, which is relatively spared. Localized areas of hyperplastic marrow (or infarcts) lead to focal radiolucent areas simulating metastasis or myeloma.[26] In rare instances, focal or diffuse osteosclerosis of the cranium is observed, perhaps related to myelofibrosis. The facial bones, with the exception of the mandible, generally are not involved in sickle cell anemia, which differs from severe abnormalities in this location that may accompany thalassemia major. Rarely, patients with sickle cell anemia may have facial swelling, presumably related to bone infarcts.[22] Furthermore, brushlike new bone formation on the outer aspect of the cranial vault (hair-on-end appearance) is much more frequent in thalassemia than in sickle cell anemia.[27]

Mandibular involvement in sickle cell anemia is common.[28] Increased radiolucency and a coarsened trabecular pattern are characteristic. Prominence of the lamina dura may be observed. Some investigators note focal radiodense areas in the jaws consistent with healing or healed bone infarcts,[29] although others question the reliability of this finding.[28, 30] Pathologic examination of the teeth may reveal structural abnormalities of the enamel, dentin, and pulp cavity.[31]

Osteoporosis of vertebrae commonly is noted in patients with sickle cell anemia. This is manifested as increased radiolucency of the vertebral bodies, prominence of vertical trabeculae, and smooth deformity of the contour of the vertebral bodies (fish vertebrae) due to compression by the adjacent intervertebral discs. Collapse of vertebrae and exaggerated dorsal kyphosis and lumbar lordosis are observed. These changes are not specific, although another vertebral sign, squared-off indentations of the vertebral bodies, is virtually diagnostic of sickle cell anemia or related disorders. This abnormality of vertebral contour apparently relates to bone infarction and arrested growth and is discussed later in this chapter.

Marrow hyperplasia in bones of the thorax and extremities also may lead to osteoporosis and cortical thinning. The findings in the appendicular skeleton are not so prominent in the adult as in the child because of the normal fatty conversion of the marrow of the extremities that occurs with advancing age. In addition, associated findings, including bone infarcts, may obscure the abnormality related to marrow expansion.

Vascular Occlusion. Osteonecrosis is a well-recognized and significant complication of sickle cell anemia and its variants.[3, 22, 32–35] It is the sequela of the sickling phenomenon in which sequestration of cells occurs. With stasis and congestion of blood flow, anoxia results, which further increases the sickling process. Bone cell death with necrosis is the eventual outcome. Clinically, patients with osteonecrosis reveal fever, soft tissue swelling, bone pain and tenderness, and leukocytosis. Other clinical manifestations depend upon the site of osteonecrosis.

Sickle Cell Dactylitis (Figs. 59–3 and 59–4). In children between the ages of 6 months and 2 years, osteonecrosis may involve the small tubular bones of the hands and feet. This localization is related to the persistence of hematopoietic marrow in peripheral skeletal sites in this age group and the presence of vasoconstriction or arteriovenous shunt-

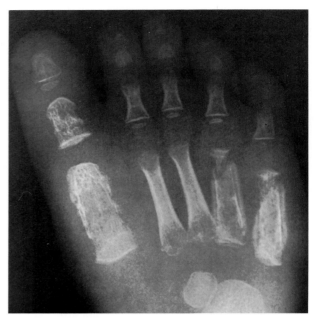

FIGURE 59–3. Sickle cell anemia: Vascular occlusion—sickle cell dactylitis. Observe soft tissue swelling, small osteolytic lesions (especially in the proximal phalanx of the great toe and the first, fourth, and fifth metatarsal bones), areas of more prominent osteolysis (including the distal portions of the fourth and fifth metatarsals), focal osteosclerosis, and periostitis. (Courtesy of P. Kaplan, M.D., Charlottesville, Virginia.)

ing due to cold.[22] Osteonecrosis in this clinical setting is termed the "hand-foot" syndrome or dactylitis.[18–21, 36–40] The syndrome may be present in as many as 20 to 50 per cent of children with sickle cell anemia.[41] Clinical manifestations, which are more frequent in the colder months of the year,[42, 43] include soft tissue swelling of the hands and feet, pain, tenderness, elevated temperature, and limitation of motion. These findings in a black child should arouse suspicion of this diagnosis.

Histologic changes are consistent with osteonecrosis.[39, 44] Infarction of marrow, of medullary trabeculae, and of the inner aspect of the cortex is observed. Circumferential periosteal elevation and subperiosteal new bone formation occur on a viable outer cortex.[39] In addition, alterations in the growth zone at the osteochondral junction are seen. This distribution of necrosis is consistent with interruption of the medullary blood flow and with sparing of the periosteal blood supply. Pathologic examination generally reveals absence of significant vascular thrombosis, supporting the concept that infarction in sickle cell anemia is due to capillary stasis caused by mechanical sequestration of sickled erythrocytes.[45] Within several months, subperiosteal bone may become consolidated with cortical bone, producing a widened osseous shadow. Subsequent remodeling can lead to a normal-appearing bone, although modeling defects and epiphyseal deformities may persist (see discussion later in this chapter).

In the early stages of sickle cell dactylitis, histologic changes may appear without radiographic findings, although soft tissue swelling frequently is seen. Within 1 to 2 weeks, patchy radiolucency of the shaft with surrounding periostitis is observed in the metacarpals, metatarsals, and

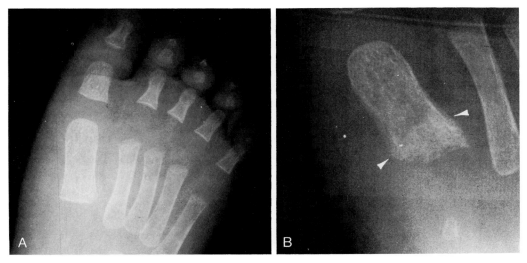

FIGURE 59–4. Sickle cell anemia: Vascular occlusion—sickle cell dactylitis. The patient was a 16 month old girl with sickle cell anemia with painful soft tissue swelling and tenderness of both hands and both feet.
  A Initial frontal radiograph of the foot reveals extensive soft tissue swelling without apparent osseous abnormalities.
  B A radiograph obtained 5 weeks later (at age 17 months) outlines metaphyseal destruction and periostitis of the first metatarsal bone (arrowheads). A bone biopsy confirmed the presence of osteonecrosis without osteomyelitis.

Illustration continued on following page

phalanges. Carpal and tarsal bones also may be involved. These findings are relatively symmetric in distribution in most persons and may affect the hands and feet simultaneously. Focal osteosclerosis also is seen, and the osseous outline may be lost. The findings resemble those of osteomyelitis, and differentiation of these two conditions is extremely difficult. Eventually, during a period of several months, bone reconstitution may lead to a completely normal osseous shadow, although growth recovery lines and abnormalities of the epiphyseal and diaphyseal shape may persist, marking the site of previous necrosis.[37]

The hand-foot syndrome is rare after the age of 6 years because the red marrow recedes from the distal bones of the extremities, being replaced by fibrous tissue whose oxygen demands are less rigid. In older children, however, similar infarction may occur in the shafts of the long tubular bones.

The differential diagnosis of the clinical and radiologic manifestations of this syndrome includes tuberculosis, syphilis, yaws, smallpox, other types of infection, leukemia, and fat necrosis.

Diaphyseal Infarction of Larger Tubular Bones (Fig. 59–5). Acute infarction of the skeleton may occur at all ages in patients with sickle cell anemia and may involve any bone, including those of the spine, thorax, face, or skull. The long tubular bones are common sites of such infarction, and involvement of the diaphysis or one or both epiphyses can occur. The most frequent site of infarction is the proximal aspect of the femur, although the proximal humerus, distal femur, proximal tibia, and other locations may be affected.

Extensive infarction of the shaft is associated with patchy lucency and sclerosis of the medullary bone. In addition, the diaphysis may be broadened or enlarged by the appearance and incorporation of subperiosteal new bone. This subperiosteal bone proliferation is the result of infarction of a large segment of cortical bone, followed by periosteal

inflammatory reaction, edema, exudation, and bone formation. On radiographic examination, such bone appears initially as a linear radiodense area adjacent to the cortex, which may extend along the entire shaft. Subsequently, the bone is incorporated into the cortex, producing cortical thickening. Within the bone along the inner surface of the cortex, laminated new bone formation in response to infarction can produce concentric cylinders of bone paralleling the cortical surface.[22, 30, 46] On radiographs, discrete linear bands beneath the cortical bone produce a bone-within-bone appearance, which is diagnostic of osteonecrosis.

Infarction of Other Bones (Fig. 59–6). Osteosclerosis in association with medullary infarction of bone can reach extreme proportions in sickle cell anemia, simulating the appearance of osteoblastic metastasis or Paget's disease.[46] These sclerotic findings are particularly common in the pelvis, spine, thorax, tibia, and fibula, producing increased radiodensity of bone and a coarsened trabecular pattern. Pathologically, necrosis of medullary bone is associated with fibrosis and granulation tissue, dystrophic calcification, metaplastic woven bone, and appositional new bone on dead trabeculae.[7, 33]

Ischemic necrosis in the small bones of the wrist and hindfoot is observed in sickle cell anemia but is less common than osteonecrosis in the tubular bones. Ischemic changes in the talus, calcaneus, and lunate have been described.[47, 48]

Sclerosis in the terminal phalanges of the hand, similar to that described in patients with various collagen vascular diseases, has been observed to occur with increased frequency in patients with sickle cell anemia (Fig. 59–7) compared with controls and may relate to ischemic necrosis.[49]

Sternal abnormalities, presumably related to infarction, also have been noted in patients with sickle cell anemia. Specifically, "cupping" of the inferior margins of one or more of the sternal segments has been observed in 8 per cent of children with homozygous sickle disease (and in 10

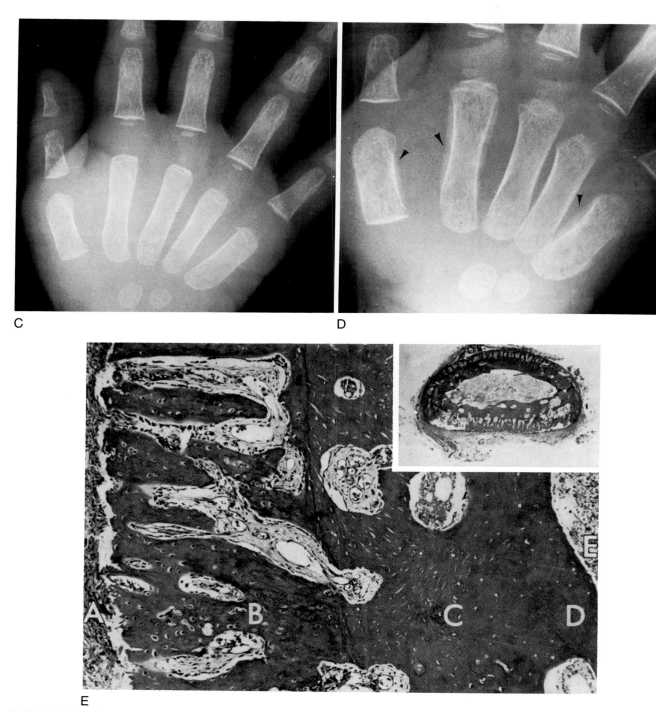

FIGURE 59–4 *Continued*

C Initial radiograph of the hand at 16 months of age reveals soft tissue swelling without bony alterations.

D A radiograph of the same hand at 18 months of age delineates medullary lytic defects with periostitis (arrowheads) of multiple metacarpal bones.

E On a photomicrograph (110×) of the midshaft of an involved proximal phalanx in a different child with sickle cell dactylitis, observe five distinct zones: *A,* periosteum; *B,* subperiosteal new bone; *C,* viable old cortex; *D,* dead cortex; *E,* necrotic marrow. The inset represents a lower magnification (7.5×) of the same bone.

(**E,** From Weinberg AG, Currarino G: Am J Clin Pathol *58*:518, 1972.)

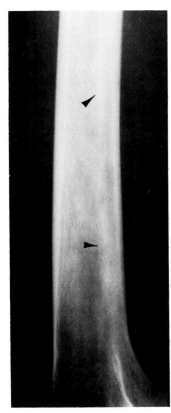

FIGURE 59–5. Sickle cell anemia: Vascular occlusion—diaphyseal infarction of larger tubular bones. A typical example is shown of a bone-within-bone appearance due to diaphyseal infarction. Observe linear sclerosis beneath the cortex (arrowheads) on this lateral view of the femur.

per cent of those with sickle cell-hemoglobin C disease).[50] The presence of acute anterior chest pain and the absence of accumulation of bone-seeking radiopharmaceutical agents in portions of the sternum in such children[51] support an ischemic pathogenesis of the radiographic finding, although a similar abnormality has been seen in juvenile chronic arthritis,[52] which clouds somewhat the issue of its pathophysiology.

Chest pain in patients with sickle cell anemia also may accompany osteonecrosis in the ribs.[312] Edema or fibrosis may lead to extrapleural masses in this situation.[53] Furthermore, hypoventilation related to the pain associated with the bone infarcts may contribute to the development of pulmonary infiltrates.[312]

Epiphyseal Infarction (Fig. 59–8). Epiphyseal infarcts in sickle cell anemia are frequent, although they may be even more common in certain sickle variants, such as sickle cell-hemoglobin C disease,[34, 54, 55] and less frequent in sickle cell trait and sickle cell-thalassemia disease.[56, 57] They are more prevalent in adults than in children, perhaps related to the fact that the large amount of cartilaginous epiphyseal tissue in a child gains much of its nutrition from the adjacent synovial fluid and is relatively independent of epiphyseal vascular supply.[33] Furthermore, other avenues of blood supply in children, such as a patent artery in the ligamentum teres and relatively large capsular arteries, may provide additional protection against bone infarction. Occasionally in older children, infarction of the capital femoral epiphysis leads to an appearance simulating that of Legg-Calvé-Perthes disease, with irregularity of the lateral two thirds of the epiphysis or the entire epiphysis.[58–60] Children with sickle cell anemia and necrosis of the proximal part of the femur are older than those with Legg-Calvé-Perthes dis-

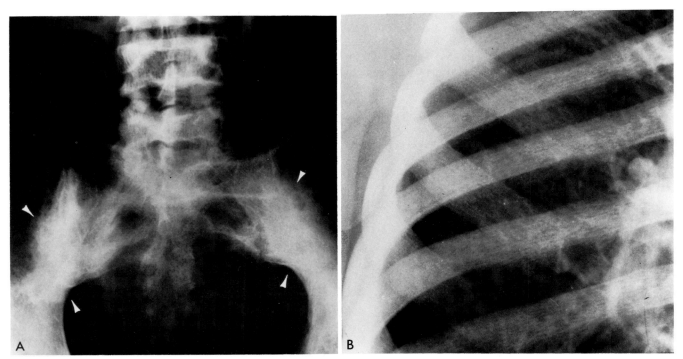

FIGURE 59–6. Sickle cell anemia: Vascular occlusion—infarction of other bones.
   A Osteosclerosis of the pelvis is particularly prominent about the sacroiliac joints (arrowheads), simulating the findings of ankylosing spondylitis.
   B In the ribs, diffuse sclerosis has resulted in a coarsened trabecular pattern.

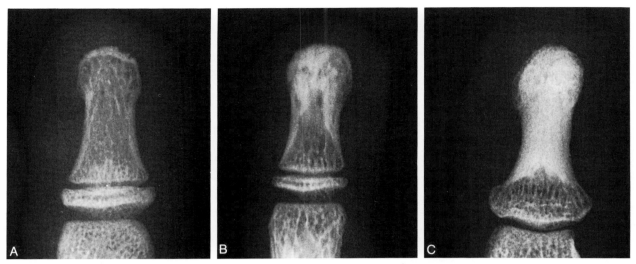

FIGURE 59–7. Sickle cell anemia: Probable vascular occlusion—phalangeal sclerosis. Different patterns of acrosclerosis are shown in a 15 year old boy **(A)**, a 10 year old girl **(B)**, and a 50 year old woman **(C)**. (From Sebes JI, Brown DL: AJR *140:*763, 1983. Copyright 1983, American Roentgen Ray Society.)

ease, however. In addition, bilaterality of femoral involvement and occurrence in blacks are two other features suggestive of sickle cell anemia or its variants. Epiphyseal infarction commonly is bilateral in distribution, with predilection for the capital femoral and proximal humeral epiphyses.[32, 59, 61, 304, 313] Occasionally, other sites are affected, including the distal femur, proximal tibia, and distal humerus.

Osteonecrosis of the epiphysis in the adult with sickle cell anemia mimics the necrosis and collapse of epiphyses that accompany other processes, including steroid-induced and fracture-related conditions. Focal lucency and sclerosis, subchondral linear or curvilinear radiolucent shadows, collapse, and fragmentation are evident in involved epiphyses. Revascularization of a partially necrotic femoral head is incomplete, associated with deposition of new bone on existing trabeculae. Detachment and displacement of articular cartilage result in exposure of granulation or fibrous tissue containing necrotic bone fragments. Subchondral and intraarticular hemorrhage provokes a chronic synovitis with ingrowth of pannus from hypertrophied synovium.[33]

Although collapse and disintegration of epiphyses, followed by the development of osteoarthritis,[59] may be observed in weight-bearing areas such as the hip, epiphyseal necrosis in non–weight-bearing sites may lead to osteosclerosis without significant loss of epiphyseal contour. This is frequent in the proximal part of the humerus, where alternating areas of lucency and sclerosis produce a "snow-capped" appearance. Symptoms and signs related to humeral involvement are less frequent and severe than those associated with femoral abnormalities.[62] Deterioration of the epiphysis in sickle cell anemia may necessitate surgical intervention with total joint replacement.[63, 64]

Acetabular abnormalities accompanying ischemic necrosis of the femoral head in this disease may occur in the absence of secondary osteoarthritis.[59] Osteophytes in the lateral aspect of the acetabulum may represent a stress-related phenomenon due to abnormal lateral mobility of the collapsed femoral head.

Growth Disturbances (Fig. 59–9). Numerous growth disturbances occur in sickle cell anemia, presumably related to bone infarction. These include epiphyseal shortening, deformities and delay in physeal closure, epiphyseal-metaphyseal abnormalities, and changes in spinal contour.

Damage to epiphyseal circulation may produce arrested or decreased cartilage proliferation in the growth plate, leading to shortening of the bone.[65, 66] Ingrowth of blood vessels from the metaphysis may cause osseous fusion, particularly in the central portion of the growth plate. This localization appears to relate to the fact that the central aspect of the plate is supplied by diaphyseal vessels, whereas the peripheral aspects are nourished by periosteal vessels.[39] A variety of epiphyseal-metaphyseal growth disturbances also have been emphasized in this disease.[67] These are particularly frequent in the hands and feet, although they may occur elsewhere, including the long tubular bones. Cone-shaped epiphyses and inverted V, "cup," or "channel" deformities of the adjacent metaphyses are observed in sickle cell anemia, although similar changes occur in many other disorders, including congenital diseases, infection, trauma, and radiation injury. In sickle cell anemia, channel deformity of the metaphysis may be due to ischemia with altered osteogenesis and chondrogenesis as well as revascularization with resorption of necrotic trabeculae.[67] Radiographically, relative radiolucency is seen in the central portion of the metaphysis.

When osteonecrosis affects the femoral head in children, a variety of growth deformities about the hip may develop later. These include coxa plana, shortening of the femoral neck, varus deformity of the proximal portion of the femur, acetabular dysplasia, and acetabular protrusion.[68]

Tibiotalar deformity has been mentioned as a radiographic finding in sickle cell anemia.[69] This deformity, which consists of slanting of the articular surfaces of the distal portion of the tibia and the talus, had previously been emphasized as a characteristic abnormality of hemophilia, juvenile-onset rheumatoid arthritis, and multiple epiphyseal dysplasia.[70–72] Shaub and associates[69] noted a similar abnor-

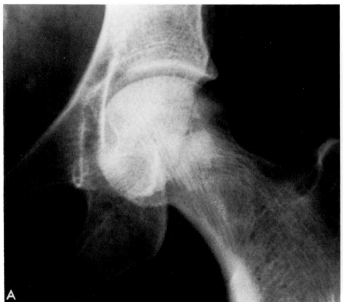

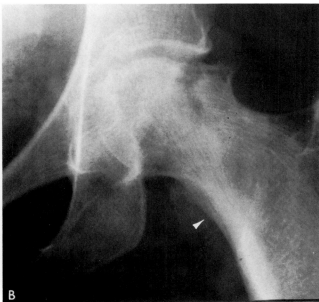

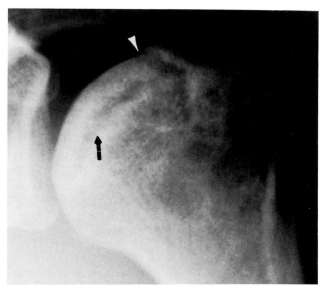

FIGURE 59–8. Sickle cell anemia: Vascular occlusion—epiphyseal infarction.

A, B Progressive changes of osteonecrosis of the femoral head are characterized by initial focal areas of sclerosis and subsequent collapse, with irregularity of the articular surface. On the later film (which is taken in a frog-leg position), observe lateral femoral osteophytes and buttressing (arrowhead) of the femoral neck.

C A "snow-capped" appearance of the humeral head is due to patchy sclerosis. Collapse of the articular surface (arrowhead) and subchondral fractures (arrow) are evident.

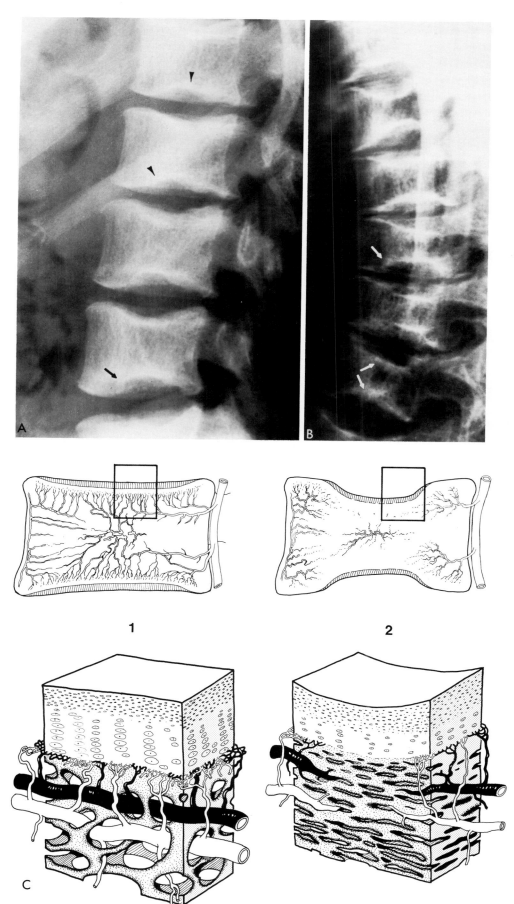

FIGURE 59–9. Sickle cell anemia: Growth disturbance—H vertebrae.

A, B Two examples are shown of H vertebrae characterized by central indentations of the vertebral bodies. Initially the abnormalities may simulate cartilaginous nodes or fish vertebrae (arrowheads), although eventually typical squared-off indentations are observed (arrows).

C Diagrammatic representation of the normal discovertebral junction (1) and that in sickle cell anemia (2). In the latter situation, ischemia of the central portions of the cartilaginous endplates results in abnormality of osteogenesis with steplike depressions of the vertebral endplate.

mality in 39 per cent of 36 patients with sickle cell anemia. As this was a retrospective study that did not exclude patients with positioning artifacts,[73] it was challenged by Leichtman and collaborators.[74] These latter investigators noted tibiotalar slant in only 1 of 28 patients with sickle cell anemia (3.6 per cent) in a prospective study. Thus, although tibiotalar slant in this disease may relate to premature fusion of the lateral portion of the distal growth plates secondary to local ischemia, it appears to be a relatively infrequent sign.

Central depression of the vertebral bodies may represent an additional growth disturbance of sickle cell anemia.[75] The resulting deformity of the vertebra consists of squared-off endplate depressions, the ''H'' vertebra. This deformity has been postulated to result from ischemia of the central portion of the vertebral growth plate, paralleling the vulnerability of the central aspect of the growth plate in the peripheral skeleton. The radiographic picture is characteristic and easily distinguished from the smooth biconcave contour defects of vertebral bodies that characterize many metabolic disorders. Although H vertebrae occasionally are described in other conditions, including thalassemia, Gaucher's disease, congenital hereditary spherocytosis, and osteoporosis,[76–79] their appearance is very suggestive of the diagnosis of sickle cell anemia. In addition, exaggerated anterior vertebral notching, perhaps related to venous stasis, has been described in sickle cell disease as well as other disorders.[80, 81]

Miscellaneous Findings

Fractures. Fractures in the appendicular and axial skeleton in patients with sickle cell anemia can occur spontaneously or after minor trauma. In the long tubular bones, marrow hyperplasia produces cortical thinning, which predisposes to this complication. New bone formation by subperiosteal osteoblasts may reinforce the cortex, however, diminishing the frequency of spontaneous fracture.[22] In addition, decreased physical activity due to bone pain at the time of sickle crisis may represent another reason why these fractures of long bones are relatively uncommon. When they are apparent, they generally are horizontal or transverse in appearance and diaphyseal in location. In the spine, marrow hyperplasia results in diffuse weakening of the entire vertebral body, which subsequently can undergo partial or complete collapse.[82] Typical deformities result from compression of the bone by the adjacent intervertebral discs (fish vertebrae) or from intraosseous displacement of portions of the intervertebral disc (cartilaginous or Schmorl's nodes).

Osteomyelitis and Septic Arthritis (Fig. 59–10). Patients with sickle cell anemia are susceptible to bacterial infection; the frequency of osteomyelitis related to a variety of organisms is reported to be more than 100 times that seen in normal persons.[83, 84] Infection represents a very common cause of hospitalization of such patients, particularly children.[85] The susceptibility of these patients to infections relates to a variety of causes: tissue injury from vascular insult with infarction; increased exposure to infection because of multiple hospitalizations; impaired phagocytosis at low oxygen tensions; and decreased splenic function attributable to fibrosis.[83] Bone and joint infections in sickle cell anemia are caused by salmonellae in over 50 per cent of cases.[305] It is suggested that these organisms gain entry to the bloodstream as a result of intestinal infarction produced by sickling within mesenteric vessels; typically, Salmonella

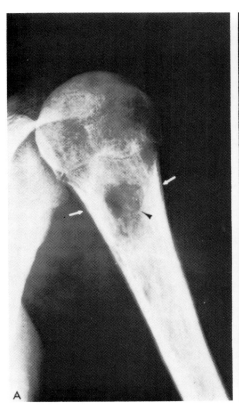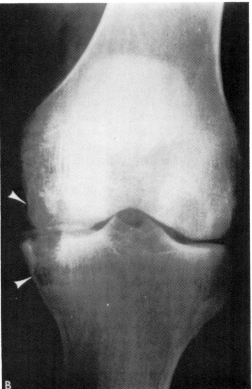

FIGURE 59–10. Sickle cell anemia: Osteomyelitis and septic arthritis.

A Salmonella infection of the humerus has led to lytic lesions (arrowhead) with surrounding periostitis (arrows). This organism may produce symmetric diaphyseal osteomyelitis of long tubular bones in patients with sickle cell anemia.

B Staphylococcal septic arthritis has resulted in lytic lesions of the femur and tibia (arrowheads) and joint space narrowing.

bacteremia precedes osteomyelitis, and the organisms then lodge in the bone marrow, presumably at sites of necrosis. Decreased serum bactericidal activity against Salmonella also has been observed in patients with sickle cell anemia,[86] perhaps explaining further the frequency of Salmonella osteomyelitis in such persons. Salmonella osteomyelitis appears to be particularly characteristic of sickle cell anemia occurring in African patients and in children.[88] Indeed, Salmonella osteomyelitis may complicate sickle cell dactylitis in the pediatric patient.[88] Staphylococci represent a second common cause of osteomyelitis in sickle cell anemia and, in some series, are implicated more frequently than salmonellae.[87, 88] Additional organisms that may be implicated in these infections are pneumococci, Serratia, Haemophilus, and *Escherichia coli,* as well as some unusual agents.[83–95]

Osteomyelitis is most frequent in the long tubular bones. Other bones, including those in the face[96] and the vertebrae,[97] may be infected, however. Infection, particularly that associated with salmonellae, although also that associated with other organisms, may produce symmetric involvement with diaphyseal localization. Clinically and radiographically the findings of osteomyelitis in patients with sickle cell anemia may simulate those of osteonecrosis, with fever, bone pain, and leukocytosis on clinical evaluation, and with osteolysis and periostitis on radiographic evaluation. Persistent fever and continued osseous destruction with involucrum formation, cortical sequestration, fracture, soft tissue abscesses, and sinus tracts are later manifestations of infection.[98–100]

Osteomyelitis in these patients may be due not only to hematogenous dissemination of infection to bone but also to direct spread from a contiguous soft tissue infection. Intractable leg ulcers are particularly common in this disease, and underlying periostitis and cortical destruction can indicate adjacent osseous infection.

Septic arthritis complicating sickle cell anemia is less frequent than osteomyelitis.[83, 89, 101–103] Implicated organisms have included staphylococci, *E. coli,* Enterobacter, salmonellae, and, rarely, anaerobic species.[104] It has been suggested that intravascular sickling in synovial capillaries can cause hyperviscosity and plugging, leading to increased susceptibility to joint infection. Furthermore, articular inflammation can cause hypoxia, acidosis, and hyperthermia, factors that can accelerate sickling, leading to further stasis.[105] Impaired synovial capillary flow in this clinical setting also may explain poor response to therapy.

The clinical diagnosis of septic arthritis complicating sickle cell anemia may be difficult because its manifestations may be confused with those of nonseptic arthropathy of a sickle crisis. In addition, joint manifestations associated with Salmonella osteomyelitis in patients with or without sickle cell anemia may occur without being an indication of joint infection.[106–108] Radiographic findings are typical of septic arthritis: soft tissue swelling, joint space narrowing, variable osteoporosis, and osseous destruction.[109]

Crystal Deposition. Hyperuricemia occurs in some patients with sickle cell anemia.[89, 110–115] The reported frequency of this laboratory finding in adults with this disease has varied from 20 to 40 per cent. The frequency of clinical attacks of gout and successful recovery of urate crystals from inflamed joints in patients with sickle cell anemia is lower.[116] Affected persons have included a high proportion

of young women.[117] The cause of hyperuricemia and gouty arthritis in these patients may be both overproduction[113, 118, 119] and diminished excretion[113, 119] of uric acid.

Although repeated blood transfusions in patients with thalassemia, spherocytosis, and hypoplastic and sideroblastic anemias may lead to secondary hemochromatosis with calcium pyrophosphate dihydrate (CPPD) crystal deposition,[102, 120, 121] this complication is not a manifestation of sickle cell anemia.

Hemarthrosis. Although hemarthrosis may accompany osteonecrosis with epiphyseal collapse in patients with sickle cell anemia, this is not a common complication of the disease.[122–125] Rarely, hemarthrosis has been recorded in patients with sickle cell trait.[126] Soft tissue hematomas may appear following minor trauma in persons with sickle cell anemia (Fig. 59–11).

Joint Effusions (Fig. 59–12). Schumacher and coworkers[102] have emphasized the relatively common occurrence of joint effusions in sickle cell anemia that are not associated with infection, crystal deposition, or hemarthrosis. Others have confirmed this observation.[127, 128] These effusions, which most frequently involve the knee and elbow, commonly are associated with clinical manifestations of crises, including fever, leukocytosis, pain, warmth, and tenderness. Fluid production generally is confined to one or two joints and subsides in 2 to 14 days. Radiographic examination may demonstrate osteonecrosis of adjacent bones, and radionuclide study using technetium sulfur colloid may show decreased marrow uptake in periarticular regions.[122] Joint aspiration usually will document the non-inflammatory nature of the joint fluid,[102] although occasionally a patient with inflammatory synovial fluid has been

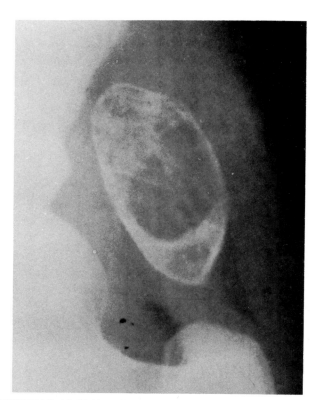

FIGURE 59–11. Sickle cell anemia: Soft tissue hematoma. An enlarging mass about the hip occurred after minor trauma in this patient. A calcified hematoma is evident.

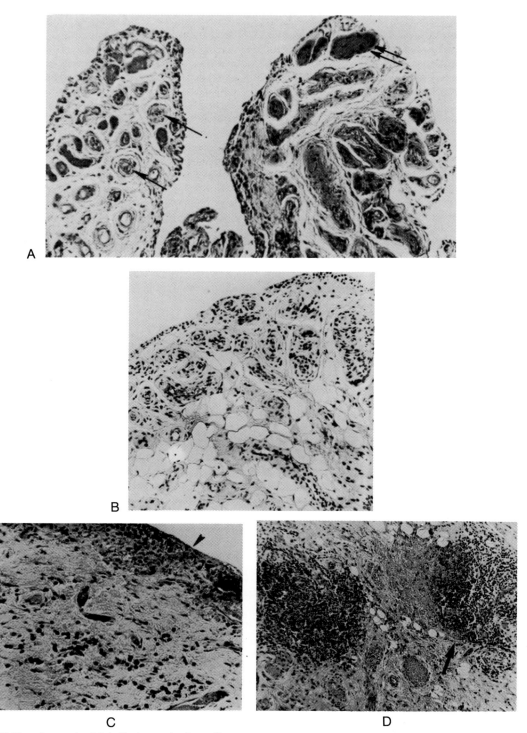

FIGURE 59–12. Sickle cell anemia: Joint effusion and arthropathy.

A, B Synovial membrane biopsy specimens from two patients with sickle cell anemia outline obliteration (arrows) and congestion (double arrows) of small vessels. Scattered mononuclear cells appear in the superficial synovial layers.

(**A, B,** From Schumacher HR, et al: Ann Intern Med *78:*203, 1973.)

C, D Synovial membrane biopsy specimen from a 33 year old man with sickle cell disease who had had progressive right hip pain and restricted motion outlines mildly hyperplastic synovial lining cells (arrowhead), scattered deep mononuclear cells, and intense deep chronic inflammatory cell infiltration (arrow).

(**C, D,** From Schumacher HR, et al: Ann Rheum Dis *36:*413, 1977.)

noted.[22, 111, 125, 127, 128] Effusions, which may be dark in color, reflecting the patient's hyperbilirubinemia,[102] also have been described in patients with sickle cell-thalassemia disease and sickle cell-hemoglobin C disease. Synovial biopsy during joint effusion has outlined mild focal proliferation of synovial lining cells, a few chronic inflammatory cells, vascular congestion, and perivascular fibrosis, findings that are consistent with antecedent synovial microvascular obstruction.[89, 102] The possibility of synovial ischemia is further supported by the association of arthritis and effusion in the ankle, with deterioration of leg ulcers related to skin infarction.

Other Abnormalities. Chronic synovitis leading to cartilaginous destruction with progressive loss of joint space has been described in patients with sickling disorders who have neither infection nor osteonecrosis.[130] Synovial biopsies in these patients document intense plasma and lymphocytic cellular infiltration. Radiographs may outline adjacent osteonecrosis and articular findings consistent with those of rheumatoid or septic arthritis. The mechanism for this pattern of joint destruction is not clear.

The occurrence of bony bridging of the spine and ankylosis of the hip in sickle cell disease has been noted,[22, 131] but these findings may represent the sequelae of infection or some other process. Sclerosis about the sacroiliac joints in this disease may result from bone infarction.[102, 132, 133] Careful evaluation will reveal an intact articular space, allowing differentiation from sacroiliitis.

Protrusio acetabuli was observed in approximately 20 per cent of adults with sickle cell anemia in one report.[134] The cause of this finding is not clear, although the occurrence of acetabular ischemia with disturbance of the growth of the triradiate cartilage may be an important etiologic factor.[68] Diffuse chondrolysis leading to narrowing of one or both hips also has been noted in patients with sickle cell anemia.[306]

A peculiar variety of osseous erosion involving the superior surface of the calcaneus was described in 9 per cent of patients with sickle cell anemia.[135] Its pathogenesis is not clear.

Two children, one with sickle cell anemia and one with sickle cell trait, were described who developed polyarthritis in association with a positive LE cell preparation, suggesting that patients with sickle cell hemoglobinopathy and arthritis should be evaluated for immunologic causes of articular disease.[136]

Radionuclide Findings

Alavi and others, in a series of articles, have outlined the role of radionuclide investigation in patients with sickle cell anemia.[122, 137–139] Both bone marrow scans using ^{99m}Tc sulfur colloid and bone scans using a variety of bone-seeking pharmaceutical agents may be useful in the detection of infarction.

As outlined with bone marrow scanning, reticuloendothelial activity corresponds to erythroblastic activity.[140, 141] In normal adults, bone marrow is located predominantly in the axial skeleton and proximal portions of femora and humeri; in patients with various anemias, the marrow expands symmetrically to occupy long bones and skull.[142, 143] During asymptomatic periods, patients with sickle cell anemia and

related disorders may reveal focal areas of decreased uptake, which can probably be attributed to sites of previous infarction.[144] During a crisis, additional areas are found that are without radionuclide activity, surrounded by active marrow.[35] After a crisis, the infarcted marrow may return to normal in 1 to 12 months or progress to permanent fibrosis,[137, 145] with corresponding changes in radionuclide activity. The sensitivity of this examination is greater than that of radiography, in which infarcts do not produce early detectable alterations. In addition, the presence of a normal marrow scan in a patient with joint symptoms usually indicates a cause other than infarction for the clinical findings.[122]

Bone scanning agents such as ^{99m}Tc polyphosphate demonstrate uptake related to the integrity of blood flow and the presence of new bone formation. In patients with sickle cell anemia and related diseases, marrow expansion is associated with increased blood flow and an increased accumulation of radionuclide in the skeleton, particularly in the lower extremities.[35] Immediately after a crisis, an area of infarction may demonstrate decreased or absent radionuclide activity (Fig. 59–13). The size of this defect in activity generally is smaller on bone scans than on bone marrow scans. One to 2 weeks after the crisis, increased activity by bone scanning is due to reactive bone formation about the area of infarction.[138] This abnormal activity may persist for several months.

It has been suggested that scanning with both bone- and bone-marrow–seeking radionuclides allows differentiation of osteomyelitis and osteonecrosis in patients with sickle cell anemia.[35] The combination of a large defect on the bone marrow scan and a smaller defect on the bone scan is typical of osteonecrosis. It also has been suggested that the combined use of bone imaging and gallium imaging is effective in the differentiation of osteomyelitis and other processes,[146] and the results of such a technique in distinguishing bone infarction and infection in patients with sickle cell anemia have been promising,[147–149] although not without controversy.[150] Proponents of this diagnostic method report that osteomyelitis is more probable when the intraosseous localization of gallium is increased relative to the uptake of the bone-seeking radiopharmaceutical agent, and that infarction is more likely when gallium scans reveal either no accumulation or less accumulation than the bone scan at symptomatic sites.[148]

Marrow scans with ^{99m}Tc sulfur colloid also may outline sites of extramedullary hematopoiesis in sickle cell anemia or related disorders.[141, 151, 152] In some patients, particularly those with thalassemia, the accumulation of radionuclide activity within paravertebral masses will differentiate extramedullary hematopoiesis accurately from neurogenic tumors or abscesses.

Magnetic Resonance Imaging Findings

Normal Findings. An understanding of the role of MR imaging in the assessment of patients with sickle cell anemia, as well as other types of anemia, requires a brief review of the anatomy and physiology of bone marrow.[153, 154] As summarized by Vogler and Murphy,[155] the bone marrow represents one of the largest and most important organs of the human body, providing those cells and elements (eryth-

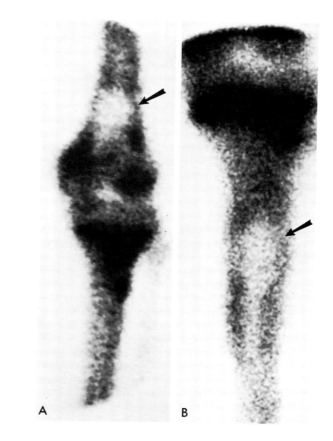

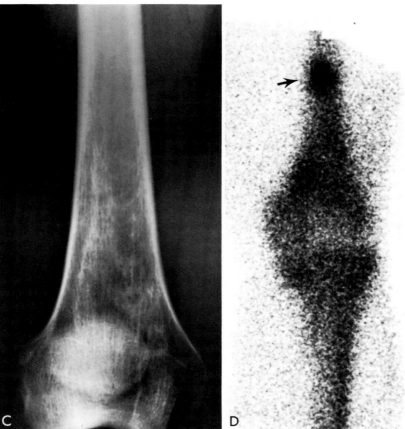

FIGURE 59–13. Sickle cell anemia: Radionuclide abnormalities—technetium polyphosphate bone scanning.

A, B Examples are shown of diaphyseal infarctions of the distal portion of the femur **(A)** and proximal end of the tibia **(B)** associated with focal decreased accumulation of radionuclide (arrows). Increased metaphyseal activity is apparent.

C, D In a different patient (with sickle cell–hemoglobin C disease), increasing leg pain resulted from a new area of bone infarction. Although the radiograph revealed medullary calcification of the distal portion of the femur consistent with previous bone infarction, no new abnormalities were detected. The bone scan reveals a new focal area of augmented radionuclide activity in the distal part of the femur (arrow).

rocytes, platelets, and leukocytes) that are fundamental to the processes of oxygenation, coagulation, and immunity. Cellular marrow constituents include erythrocytes and leukocytes in all stages of development as well as fat cells and reticulum cells.

From a functional viewpoint, bone marrow often is divided into "red marrow" and "yellow marrow," although components of both types of marrow frequently are encountered at any particular anatomic site. Red marrow is considered hematopoietically active, involved in the production of red cells, white cells, and platelets; yellow marrow is considered hematopoietically inactive and is composed predominantly of fat cells.[155] The chemical composition of red marrow consists of approximately 40 per cent water, 40 per cent fat, and 20 per cent protein; that of yellow marrow consists of approximately 15 per cent water, 80 per cent fat, and 5 per cent protein.[155] The precise amount of red and yellow marrow is dependent on a number of factors, including anatomic site, age of the person, and hematopoietic demand of the body. Under normal circumstances, a well-documented, orderly, and predictable transition, or conversion, of red to yellow marrow takes place during the growth and development of the human body. This conversion begins in the immediate postnatal period, generally progressing from appendicular to axial sites and, in the tubular bones, from diaphyseal to metaphyseal locations.[155, 156] The process shows individual variation, is not entirely symmetric in distribution, and is not uniform at all skeletal sites. The most dramatic changes occur in the tubular bones and in the first two decades of life.[157–159] Typically, histologic conversion of red to yellow marrow begins in the bones of the hands and feet, progresses to the distal and then the proximal long tubular bones, and finally occurs in the flat bones and vertebral bodies until the adult pattern of proximal femoral, proximal humeral, and axial hematopoietic marrow results.[158] The adult pattern generally is achieved by the age of 25 years[155] (Fig. 59–14). Once this pattern is established, additional but less dramatic changes in marrow content may occur with advancing age, characterized by an even further conversion of red to yellow marrow.[155] At any age, the apophyses and epiphyses of the skeleton contain predominantly yellow marrow.

The MR imaging appearance of normal bone marrow depends on its composition. Each of the marrow's components, fat, water, and mineral, contributes to this appearance. As the precise concentration of these three components varies from one skeletal site to another and, as indicated previously, is influenced by the age of the person, what is considered to be a normal MR imaging appearance at one location or in the immature skeleton may clearly be abnormal at a different site or in the adult. Furthermore, the specific MR imaging sequence that is used to examine the marrow has a significant and sometimes dramatic influence on this appearance. In regions of yellow marrow, fat is the tissue that contributes most heavily to the MR imaging signal. The short T1 relaxation time and the long T2 relaxation time of adipose tissue are the factors most responsible for the MR imaging characteristics of yellow marrow. The contribution of fat to the MR imaging signal pattern of red marrow also is significant, although the increased cellularity, water, and protein content in hematopoietic tissue lead to differences in the T1 and T2 characteristics of hematopoietic marrow when compared with yellow marrow.[155] The

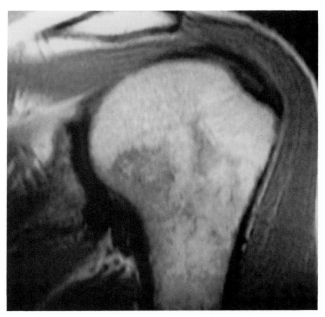

FIGURE 59–14. Normal bone marrow: Adult pattern in a 38 year old man. On this coronal oblique T1-weighted (TR/TE, 700/18) spin echo MR image, hematopoietic marrow with signal intensity similar to that of muscle is present in the metaphyseal region of the humerus. Fatty marrow with high signal intensity occupies the humeral head and greater tuberosity of the humerus.

short T1 and relatively long T2 relaxation times of fat are averaged with the longer T1 and T2 relaxation times of protein and water to produce a final signal intensity of red marrow; this final intensity, therefore, is characterized by T1 relaxation times that are longer than those of yellow marrow and by T2 relaxation times that vary according to the concentrations of fat, water, and protein that are present.[155] Adding to the complexity of the MR imaging representation of red and yellow marrow is its mineral content. Trabecular and cortical bone, which varies in content and distribution throughout the skeleton, is characterized by the absence of mobile proteins and, therefore, by little or no MR imaging signal. Furthermore, local magnetic field inhomogeneities are produced by mineralized matrix, which may influence the MR imaging appearance of adjacent bone marrow, especially in anatomic regions with more trabecular bone and on gradient echo sequences.[160] Resulting alterations in MR imaging signal patterns may lead to similarities in appearance of red and yellow marrow.

With spin echo imaging, T1-weighted sequences generally allow differentiation of regions of yellow marrow from those of red marrow (as well as many pathologic processes). Yellow marrow appears as areas of high signal intensity in such sequences; owing to the variability of the T1 value of hematopoietic marrow, however, its appearance on T1-weighted spin echo MR images is more variable.[158] Such marrow may have a signal intensity ranging from less than that of muscle to greater than that of muscle but less than that of fat (in hematopoietic marrow that contains a greater proportion of fat).[158] With more heavily T2-weighted spin echo MR images, differences in T2 relaxation times dictate the resulting appearance of the bone marrow. Discrimination between red and yellow marrow, which may be characterized by relatively small differences in T2 relaxation times, generally is poorer.[155]

Short tau inversion recovery (STIR) imaging provides a method in which the MR imaging signal derived from fat can be eliminated. Thus, the signal intensity of yellow marrow is nulled, and it appears black, allowing its differentiation from red marrow. STIR imaging also is an effective technique in accentuating pathologic processes that replace yellow marrow, although discrimination between these and hematopoietic marrow may be difficult. Chemical shift imaging also can be used to produce selective elimination of the fat signal and shares with STIR imaging the benefit of accentuating differences between red and yellow marrow.[161, 314]

A family of gradient echo imaging sequences has been introduced as one method of shortening the MR imaging examination time. These sequences are characterized by the use of a partial flip angle excitation pulse, typically less than 90 degrees, followed by a gradient reversal to refocus the echo and generate the signal.[160] Individual gradient echo sequences differ in a number of ways, including the manner in which any residual transverse magnetization is handled (e.g., steady state versus "spoiled"). The contrast of the image is dependent on many factors including T1, T2, T2*, or effective transverse relaxation time, flip angle, repetition time, echo time, magnetic field inhomogeneities, and susceptibility effects. The benefit of gradient echo imaging sequences in the analysis of bone marrow abnormalities is not clear, although the appearance of normal marrow on such sequences differs from that on spin echo sequences.[160, 307] In many types of gradient echo images, similarities exist in the appearance of red and yellow marrow.

It is apparent from this discussion that many factors, not the least of which is the pulse sequence, contribute to the MR imaging signal pattern of normal bone marrow, making identification of sites of abnormal marrow difficult in some cases. As indicated previously, fundamental to such identification is knowledge of the normal sequence of conversion of red to yellow marrow with advancing age. Although this sequence is not entirely uniform, certain of its characteristics are well established and have been summarized effectively by Moore and associates.[162]

1. Tubular bones: Four MR imaging patterns have been documented.[162] The *infantile pattern,* occurring in the first year of life, is characterized by homogeneous low signal intensity in the diaphyseal and metaphyseal marrow. The *childhood pattern,* occurring from one to 10 years of age, is characterized by higher signal intensity in the diaphyseal marrow. The *adolescent pattern,* occurring between 11 and 20 years of age, is accompanied by an increase in signal intensity in the distal metaphysis, with some heterogeneity of the metaphyseal signal intensity. The *adult pattern,* established by approximately 25 years of age, is characterized by relatively homogeneous high signal intensity in the diaphyseal and metaphyseal marrow and, occasionally, by low signal intensity in regions of dense trabecular bone and the physeal scar.

2. Vertebrae: Four MR imaging patterns of signal intensity also have been described in the vertebral bodies.[159] In *pattern 1,* uniform low signal intensity, except for linear areas of high signal intensity superior and inferior to the basivertebral vein, is seen. In *pattern 2,* bandlike and triangular areas of high signal intensity are found near the vertebral endplates and anteriorly and posteriorly at the corners

of the vertebral bodies. In *pattern 3,* diffusely distributed areas of high signal intensity, either well marginated or indistinct, are evident. In *pattern 4,* a combination of patterns 2 and 3 is seen. In the cervical spine, pattern 1 usually is apparent in persons younger than 40 years and patterns 2 and 3, in older persons; in the thoracic spine, pattern 1 is again identified in young persons and pattern 2 in older persons, and the age distribution of pattern 3 is relatively uniform; and in the lumbar spine, pattern 1 once more is evident primarily in younger persons with the other patterns occurring in older age groups. In general, in any region of the spine, pattern 1 rarely is seen after the age of 50 years and patterns 3 and 4 dominate after the age of 30 or 40 years. Furthermore, on the basis of anecdotal evidence, the vertebral bone marrow should be of higher signal intensity than that of the adjacent intervertebral discs on T1-weighted spin echo MR images after the age of 10 years.[162]

3. Pelvic bones: The pelvic bone marrow is of low to intermediate signal intensity in the first year of life; in children between 1 and 10 years of age, areas of increased signal intensity appear in the anterior portion of the ilium and in the acetabulum; and in persons aged 11 to 20 years, further marrow signal heterogeneity is not uncommon.[162] In middle-aged and elderly persons, regions of high signal intensity become more numerous and widely scattered, with predilection for the acetabulum, ilium, and para-articular areas about the sacroiliac joint.[157, 159]

4. Cranium: Three patterns of marrow distribution are identified.[159] *Pattern 1* is characterized by bone marrow of uniformly low signal intensity or, at most, the presence of very small areas of high signal intensity in the frontal and occipital bones. In *pattern 2,* the frontal and occipital bones are of uniformly high signal intensity, and patchy areas of high signal intensity appear in the parietal bone. In *pattern 3,* the entire skull is of uniformly high signal intensity. Pattern 1 is found predominantly in persons below the age of 10 or 20 years; patterns 2 and 3 increase in frequency with advancing age.[159]

Marrow Reconversion. Reversal of the normal sequence of conversion of red to yellow marrow, a process termed reconversion, may occur when an increased demand for hematopoiesis exists, as in patients with various types of anemia and those with diseases such as plasma cell myeloma, myelofibrosis, or skeletal metastasis that infiltrate or replace normal bone marrow. Marrow reconversion commences in the spine and flat bones, after which the tubular bones in the extremities are affected in a proximal to distal sequence that is the reverse of marrow conversion.[155] Rao and coworkers[163] emphasized this process in patients with sickle cell anemia, indicating an expanded distribution of hematopoietic bone marrow. Diffuse or focal areas of diminished signal intensity are seen with T1-weighted spin echo sequences (see Fig. 59–16). The signal characteristics on T2-weighted sequences are more variable, dependent on the amounts of cellularity and tissue water, and abnormal regions of marrow may reveal signal intensity that is less, equal to, or slightly greater than that of subcutaneous fat on such sequences.[162] The extent of reconversion of marrow is proportional to the severity of the process; patients with profound and chronic anemia will reveal a greater amount of reconversion.[155, 164] Iron overload, due to recurrent hemolysis and frequent blood transfusions, in some patients with chronic disorders of erythropoiesis, leads to iron deposition in the liver, spleen, and bone marrow, resulting in regions of low signal intensity on both T1- and T2-weighted images[162] (Fig. 59–15). Differentiation between marrow reconversion and iron overload on the basis of findings in T1-weighted spin echo MR images may be difficult; such differentiation is accomplished more easily when heavily T2-weighted spin echo images, combined with fat suppression, are obtained.[315] In these images, iron deposition is characterized by persistent low signal intensity.

Reconversion of bone marrow leads to signal changes on MR imaging that lack specificity. Similar findings on MR images may characterize the process of marrow replacement or infiltration that is seen in patients with lymphoma, leukemia, plasma cell myeloma, myelofibrosis, or skeletal metastasis. Furthermore, foci of marrow reconversion may be simulated by regions of residual or reconverted hematopoietic marrow that have been observed in healthy persons. This clinically insignificant process appears to be more frequent and extensive in obese women of menstruating age[165, 166] and in athletes involved in sports demanding long endurance.[167] In most reports, this process has been described in the marrow of the distal portion of the femur and, to a lesser extent, proximal portion of the tibia, detected as an incidental finding during MR imaging examination of the knee. Sparing or minimal involvement of the epiphysis also has been emphasized as an MR imaging finding that occurs in this benign condition, whereas epiphyseal involvement may be seen in more significant bone marrow disorders.[165, 168, 308]

Marrow Ischemia. In sickle cell anemia, ischemia with infarction may occur in diametaphyseal or subchondral locations, or both (Figs. 59–16 and 59–17). Although the MR imaging features of osteonecrosis are detailed in Chapter 80, some comments related to these features in patients with sickle cell anemia are included here.

MR imaging changes in regions of marrow ischemia and infarction relate to alterations in fat cells and replacement of fat-containing marrow by cellular debris, granulation tissue, and fibrosis. Some variability is seen in the signal patterns, although a loss of signal intensity in areas of fatty marrow on T1-weighted spin echo MR images is most characteristic. With regard to epiphyseal locations as typified by the femoral head, homogeneous or inhomogeneous regions of low signal intensity as well as bandlike patterns of low signal intensity or ringlike patterns comprising low signal intensity borders surrounding areas of normal marrow signal intensity have been described on such T1-weighted images.[155] With more heavily T2-weighted sequences, variability in patterns of signal intensity again is noted, which is related to the presence of fat, edema, hemorrhage, or fibrosis, or combinations of these tissue changes. The sensitivity of MR imaging in the early detection of ischemic necrosis is well recognized, although the precise time during the evolution of osteonecrosis at which the MR imaging abnormalities appear initially is not clear. Although some reports would indicate otherwise,[169] MR imaging appears to be effective as a screening procedure for the detection of ischemic necrosis of bone in patients with sickle cell anemia.

MR imaging also has been employed in an attempt to define the duration of marrow necrosis and to differentiate between acute infarction and chronic infarction with fibrosis.[155] Preliminary evidence suggests that signal characteristics may change during the course of marrow ischemia.[163, 164] Areas of chronic ischemia and infarction appear to be characterized by low signal intensity on both T1-weighted and T2-weighted spin echo MR images, whereas acute infarction accompanying a sickle crisis appears to be characterized by a region of low signal intensity on T1-weighted images and homogeneous or peripheral high signal intensity on T2-weighted images (Fig. 59–17). These features of acute infarction may be depicted more readily in metadiaphyseal than in epiphyseal locations.[164]

As decreased signal intensity on T1-weighted spin echo MR images represents a component of the MR imaging features of marrow necrosis, detection of such necrosis in normal or converted areas of hematopoietic marrow may present a diagnostic challenge when these images are used alone. The MR imaging findings of areas of acute or chronic infarction are more conspicuous when adipose tissue represents the background on which the infarction is displayed. The value of MR imaging in the differentiation of marrow ischemia and infection in patients with sickle cell anemia is not established.

Osteomyelitis. The MR imaging characteristics of osteomyelitis relate to replacement or infiltration of the normal (or ischemic) marrow by inflammatory cells. Bacterial in-

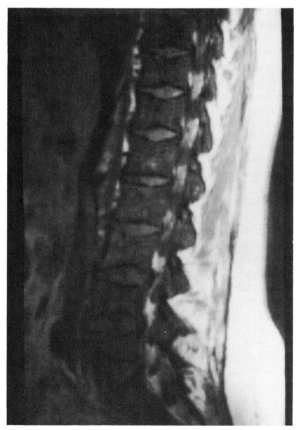

FIGURE 59–15. Sickle cell anemia: Iron overload. In this adolescent patient, a T1-weighted spin echo MR image of the spine shows diffuse decreased signal intensity in the bone marrow of the vertebrae. The signal intensity of the marrow remained low on T2-weighted images (not shown). (From Moore SG, et al: Radiology *179*:345, 1991.)

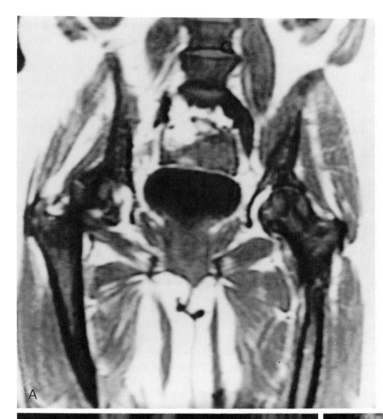

FIGURE 59–16. Sickle cell anemia: Marrow ischemia and reconversion.

A In this 26 year old woman, a T1-weighted (TR/TE, 600/20) spin echo MR image revealed an expanded distribution of hematopoietic marrow resulting in low signal intensity in all visualized bone marrow, including the diaphyses of the femora. Irregularity and collapse of both femoral heads are seen, consistent with osteonecrosis.

B, C In this 12 year old boy, sagittal proton density (TR/TE, 2000/30) **(B)** and T2-weighted (TR/TE, 2000/80)**(C)** spin echo MR images show marrow with diffusely low signal intensity in the diaphyses, metaphyses, and epiphyses of the femur and tibia.

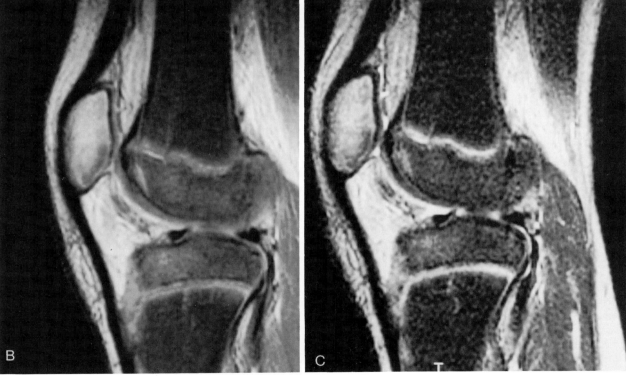

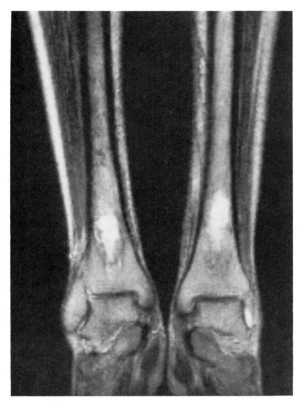

FIGURE 59–17. Sickle cell anemia: Marrow ischemia. On a T2-weighted coronal spin echo MR image, foci of increased signal intensity are seen in the bone marrow of the distal tibial metaphyses. The findings are consistent with acute medullary infarction. (From Moore SG, et al: Radiology *179*:345, 1991.)

fections of the marrow, which represent an important complication of sickle cell anemia, are accompanied by a rapid accumulation of fluid. As a result of the increased water content and cellularity, the affected region demonstrates decreased signal intensity on T1-weighted spin echo MR images and increased signal intensity on T2-weighted spin echo MR images.[155] The alterations on the T2-weighted sequences become more prominent as the time between the onset of the infection and the performance of the MR imaging examination increases.[162] Although the application of alternative MR imaging methods such as STIR or chemical saturation imaging or of intravenous injection of gadolinium-based compounds may enhance the sensitivity of the MR imaging examination in cases of osteomyelitis, specificity remains a problem. In patients with sickle cell anemia, differentiation of osteomyelitis and acute marrow ischemia and infarction using MR imaging may not be possible.

Marrow Heterotopia. Extramedullary hematopoiesis may be encountered in patients with chronic hemolytic anemias, especially thalassemia (see later discussion) but also sickle cell and other anemias. Resulting masses of hematopoietic tissue may be detected with MR imaging.[170, 171] On T1-weighted images, low signal intensity similar to that of hematopoietic marrow characterizes the masses, although a rim of higher signal intensity similar to that of fat has been emphasized as an MR imaging finding of paraspinal sites of extramedullary hematopoiesis.[170]

Muscle Abnormalities. Alterations in skeletal muscle occurring during sickle crises relate to hemorrhagic or ischemic changes that lead to inflammation and edema. Single or multiple foci in one or more extremities, particularly the legs, are affected, with resultant soft tissue swelling and pain. Early diagnosis may be provided by MR imaging, particularly T2-weighted spin echo sequences in which increased signal intensity in involved musculature can be detected.[316] Associated ischemic abnormalities in the nearby bone marrow are common but not invariable. Healing of infarcts in skeletal muscle may be accompanied by fibrosis with regions of low signal intensity in T1-weighted and T2-weighted spin echo images.[316]

SICKLE CELL TRAIT

Sickle cell trait is characterized by the presence of Hb AS. It can be associated with sickling if the blood is exposed to low oxygen tension. Patients with sickle cell trait are not jaundiced or anemic. Hyperplasia of bone marrow is not present. Occasionally, clinical problems may occur, such as infarction of the spleen or kidney. Musculoskeletal findings related to sickle cell trait are of low frequency. Osteonecrosis of the femoral head has been reported in some patients,[32, 57, 172–174] although the association may be only coincidental.[175] Infarction of the humeral head, fibula, and elbow region as well as osseous necrosis in the diaphyses of the tubular bones also has been described.[57, 176] Hemarthrosis has been reported in a patient with sickle cell trait and rheumatoid arthritis.[126] Osteomyelitis, related primarily to salmonellae, also has been identified in patients with this hemoglobin combination.[22, 88]

SICKLE CELL-HEMOGLOBIN C DISEASE

The observation that parents of atypical patients with sickle cell disease might not demonstrate sickling led to the discovery of hemoglobin C and of the hemoglobinopathy termed sickle cell-hemoglobin C disease.[177, 178] In this disease, which is the second most frequent sickling disorder, the S gene is inherited from one parent and the C gene from the other. The clinical disability is less severe than in homozygous sickle cell disease (sickle cell anemia) because hemoglobin S accounts for approximately 50 per cent of the total hemoglobin and, therefore, the diagnosis often is not established until adulthood. A typical complaint is musculoskeletal pain, which may localize in the joints. Splenomegaly commonly is apparent but icterus is absent.

Marrow hyperplasia in sickle cell-hemoglobin C disease may result in calvarial alterations in 25 per cent of patients.[30] The reported changes in the skull include granular osteoporosis, diploic widening, and thinning of the outer table. More severe changes in this location rarely are encountered. Spinal abnormality may be seen with biconcavity of the vertebral bodies and narrowing of the intervertebral discs.[22, 54]

Osteonecrosis of the femoral and humeral heads may be apparent.[54, 179–181] Some investigators have suggested that the frequency of bone necrosis is higher in this disease than in sickle cell anemia, perhaps related to a greater blood viscosity in SC hemoglobinopathy than in SS hemoglobinopathy[22] (Fig. 59–18). In this regard, Hill and collaborators[32] observed epiphyseal infarcts in 8 per cent of patients

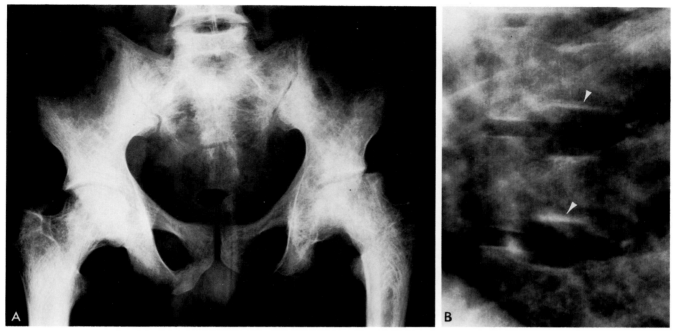

FIGURE 59–18. Sickle cell-hemoglobin C disease: Vascular occlusion.
  A Diffuse osteosclerosis of the pelvis and proximal long bones is associated with osteonecrosis of the femoral heads. Significant collapse of the left femoral head is apparent.
  B Observe H vertebrae with squared-off central depressions (arrowheads).

with sickle cell anemia and in 17 per cent of patients with sickle cell-hemoglobin C disease. Others have reported that 20 to 70 per cent of patients with SC hemoglobinopathy have hip involvement.[34, 54, 179, 181, 182] A higher frequency of ischemic necrosis in the epiphyses and diaphyses of tubular bones in SC disease than in SS disease is not uniformly found in the previous reports on this subject, however. Weinberg[46] observed that patients with severe long bone sclerosis were just as likely to have homozygous SS disease as they were to have SC (or sickle cell-thalassemia) disease; and Sebes and Kraus[61] noted ischemic necrosis of the femoral head in 19 per cent of patients with hemoglobin SS disease and in 9 per cent of those with hemoglobin SC disease. Furthermore, as patients with SC hemoglobinopathy reveal greater longevity than those with SS disease, the increased frequency of bone infarction noted in some reports of the former disease may represent an age-related phenomenon.[46]

SICKLE CELL-THALASSEMIA DISEASE

Sickle cell-thalassemia disease is caused by the inheritance of one gene for hemoglobin S and one gene for thalassemia.[183] The clinical and radiologic features of this disease vary: Some patients have manifestations that are almost identical to those associated with sickle cell anemia; other patients are entirely asymptomatic.[184] The clinical manifestations generally parallel the amount of hemoglobin A that is present.[15] Ischemic changes in the skeleton in sickle cell-thalassemia disease are common; Reynolds and coworkers[183] noted such changes in 68 per cent of 22 patients with the disease. Diaphyseal and epiphyseal infarcts are seen (Fig. 59–19). The former leads to patchy sclerosis and lucency and a bone-within-bone appearance, whereas the latter is most common in the proximal epiphyses of

femora and humeri, with lucency, sclerosis, collapse, and fragmentation.[185, 186] Epiphyseal infarcts are reported to occur at a later age in this disease than in sickle cell anemia.[32] H vertebrae also are encountered in sickle cell-thalassemia disease.[183]

Signs of marrow hyperplasia, which were reported by Reynolds and coworkers[183] in 14 per cent of their patients, consist of cortical thinning and osteoporosis of the long tubular bones (particularly in children),[187] increased radiolucency, trabecular coarsening, biconcave deformities of the spine,[188] thickening of the cranial vault with a mild hair-on-end appearance, and thinning of the outer table in the skull.[183, 189] The frequency of spinal abnormalities in this disease appears to be less than that in homozygous SS disease and greater than that in SC disease.

Osteomyelitis and septic arthritis may occur in sickle cell-thalassemia disease.[105, 183, 190] Salmonella frequently is the causative agent, and infection may occur in the appendicular or axial skeleton. Involvement of the spine is associated with disc space narrowing, vertebral body destruction, and paravertebral abscesses. A similar paravertebral soft tissue mass may indicate extramedullary hematopoiesis without infection in this condition.[191]

As in hemoglobin SS disease, hyperuricemia and gout have been identified in sickle cell-thalassemia hemoglobinopathy[192] (as well as in hemoglobin CC disease and sickle cell trait). The abnormalities are most frequent in sickle cell anemia.

OTHER HEMOGLOBINOPATHIES

Sickle cell-hemoglobin O Arab disease resembles sickle cell-hemoglobin C disease but is less common and more severe. *Sickle cell-hemoglobin D Punjab disease* resembles sickle cell anemia but is extremely rare and occurs in white

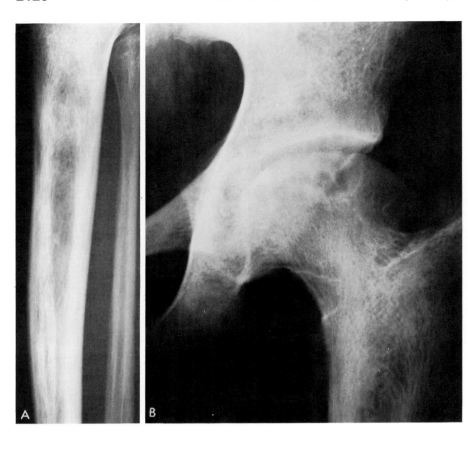

FIGURE 59–19. Sickle cell-thalassemia disease: Vascular occlusion.
A In the tibia, extensive bone infarction has resulted in a bone-within-bone appearance.
B Osteonecrosis of the femoral head is evident.

persons. It is associated with incapacitating vascular occlusive lesions. *Homozygous hemoglobin C disease (CC disease)* occurs in blacks, is associated with splenomegaly, and is without major symptoms.[193] *Hemoglobin C trait* is relatively common, perhaps affecting 2 per cent of American blacks, and is unassociated with anemia. *Homozygous hemoglobin E disease (EE disease)* is evident in Orientals[309] and is characterized by the presence of mild anemia and the absence of splenomegaly. *Homozyous hemoglobin D Punjab disease* is seen in India and less commonly in other countries, and it leads to an anemia of variable severity. The precise nature and frequency of musculoskeletal abnormalities in these hemoglobinopathies are not clear.

THALASSEMIA

General Features

In 1925, Cooley and Lee[194] described a form of severe anemia associated with splenomegaly and bone abnormalities, which they designated thalassemia, from the Greek word for "the sea," because their patients were of Mediterranean origin. It now is known that thalassemia is not a single disease but a group of disorders related to an inherited abnormality of globin production.[195, 196] These disorders differ from sickle cell anemia, which results from an inherited structural abnormality in one of the constituent globin chains; the thalassemias result from inherited defects in the rate of synthesis of one of the globin chains.[195] This leads to imbalanced globin-chain production contributing to ineffective erythropoiesis, hemolysis, and a variable degree of anemia.[196, 310]

There are two main groups of thalassemia: Alpha-thalassemia is characterized by a deficiency of alpha globin chain synthesis; beta-thalassemia is characterized by a deficiency of beta globin chain synthesis. As hemoglobin F contains alpha chains, the fetus is affected by alpha-thalassemia; beta-thalassemia becomes apparent after the newborn period as hemoglobin A replaces hemoglobin F. Several distinct disorders exist within these groups. Furthermore, thalassemia may exist in a homozygous form, called thalassemia major, or a heterozygous form, termed thalassemia minor or minima. Thalassemia intermedia represents a poorly defined intermediate variety of the disease. Although thalassemia has been denoted as "Mediterranean anemia" because of its peculiar geographic distribution with involvement of persons of Italian or Greek descent, this hemolytic anemia can be seen in people from other areas as well. Cases have been described in persons from Turkey, India, Syria, the Philippines, and Thailand. In addition, native Americans and blacks may be affected.

Clinical Features

Homozygous beta-thalassemia (thalassemia major), typically seen in persons of Mediterranean ancestry, is characterized by severe anemia, prominent hepatosplenomegaly, and early death, often in childhood. Anemia, which commonly begins shortly after the newborn period, leads to pallor, fatigability, jaundice, icterus, deficient growth, and significant osseous deformities, especially in the face. Cardiac enlargement and failure are frequent, owing to the severity of the anemia and the deposition of hemosiderin in the myocardium. Typical hematologic features are a hypochromic microcytic anemia with reticulocytosis, nucleated red blood cells, and "target" cells.

Heterozygous beta-thalassemia (thalassemia minor) generally is associated with mild clinical findings, including slight to moderate anemia, splenomegaly, and jaundice. It is observed throughout the world, most commonly in Mediterranean populations, and occurs in approximately 1 per cent of American blacks, most of whom are entirely asymptomatic.

With respect to alpha-thalassemia, the most severe form is hydrops fetalis with Bart's hemoglobin in which there is a complete absence of alpha chain production. The disease, which is seen almost exclusively in Southeast Asia, leads to death in utero or at birth.

A less severe variety of alpha-thalassemia is termed hemoglobin H disease. It is seen predominantly in the Mediterranean region, Asia, and the Middle East. Clinical manifestations include chronic hemolytic anemia, accentuated by the administration of sulfonamides, and splenomegaly.

Radiographic and Pathologic Features

Marrow Hyperplasia (Figs. 59–20 to 59–23). The radiographic and pathologic features of beta-thalassemia are due in large part to marrow hyperplasia. Initially, both the axial and the appendicular skeleton is altered, but as the patient reaches puberty, the appendicular skeletal changes diminish,[197] owing to normal regression of the hematopoietic marrow from the peripheral skeleton. The changes in thalassemia major are much more severe than those in thalassemia minor.

In the skull, the frontal bones reveal the earliest and most severe changes, and the inferior aspect of the occiput usually is unaltered. Findings include granular osteoporosis, widening of the diploic space, and thinning of the outer table. Bony proliferation on the outer table of the vault leads to a hair-on-end appearance.[27, 198] This appearance, which is more common in thalassemia major but which also may occur in thalassemia minor,[199] is characterized by dense radial striations traversing the thickened calvarium, which appear to extend beyond the outer table. Histologically, radiating bone spicules deposited by the pericranium on the outer table are seen.

The hair-on-end appearance is consistent with observations that indicate that the effect of pressure within the marrow space depends on the shape of the bone. According to physical laws, the force exerted by a semiliquid substance (marrow) enclosed between two curved parallel bones (as in the calvarium) is directed perpendicular to the enveloping surface. Thus, the outer table is subjected to a force that is diverging outward, resulting in radially oriented trabeculae, bone thinning, and perforation. The inner table, conversely, is subjected to a converging or compacting force and is not thinned.[200] Once the outer table is perforated, the expanding marrow may proliferate subperiosteally, resulting in reactive bone formation on the surface of the skull. The new bone would be subject to the same forces as those acting within the marrow space, forces directed at right angles to the bony surface, resulting in a perpendicular arrangement of the bone spicules.

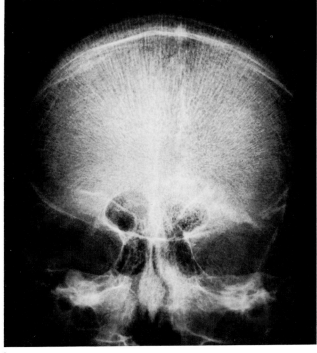
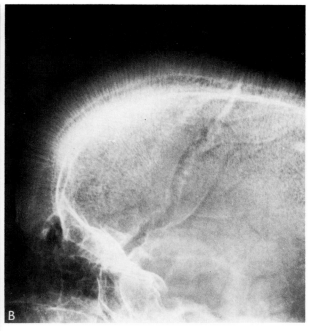

A

FIGURE 59–20. Thalassemia major: marrow hyperplasia—skull.
  A, B Frontal and lateral radiographs of the skull delineate striking abnormalities. Bony proliferation on the outer table of the vault has created a hair-on-end appearance, with dense radial striations traversing the thickened calvarium. Bony overgrowth in the face with decreased sinus aeration also is evident.

Illustration continued on following page

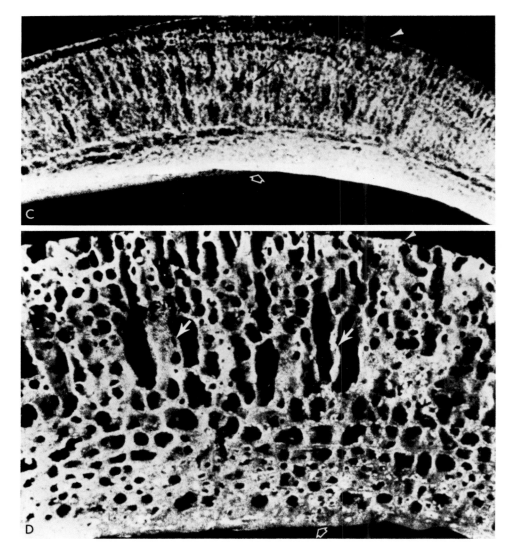

FIGURE 59–20 *Continued*
  C, D Hair-on-end appearance.
Section of diploë and tables. Bony
trabeculae extend in a radial fashion (arrows) across the tables. It
has been suggested that marrow
overgrowth causes abnormal pressure on the trabecular structure of
the cranial vault. This pressure is
directed perpendicularly to the enveloping bone. Tension is created in
the outer portions of the vault, resulting in rarefaction of bone (arrowheads). Compression of trabeculae
is evident on the inner portion of the
cranial vault (open arrows).
  (C, D, From Reimann F, Kuran S:
Virchows Arch [Pathol Anat]
358:173, 1973.)

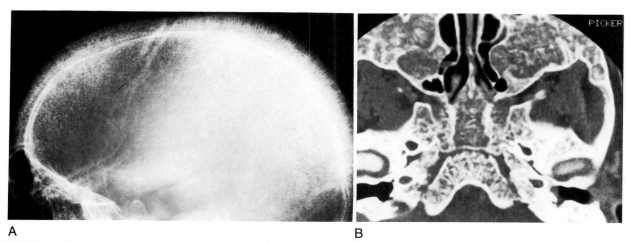

A   B

FIGURE 59–21. Thalassemia major: Marrow hyperplasia—skull and face. In this example, a hair-on-end appearance is well shown on the routine radiograph **(A)**, and the overgrowth of the facial bones is delineated with transaxial CT scanning **(B)**. (Courtesy of S. K. Brahme, M.D., San Diego, California.)

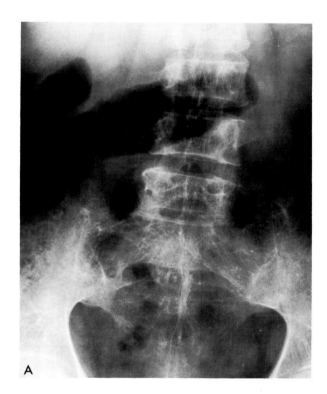

FIGURE 59–22. Thalassemia major: Marrow hyperplasia—axial and appendicular skeleton.
A Pelvis and spine. Osteoporosis of the pelvis and vertebrae is evident. Mild biconcave deformities of the vertebral bodies can be seen. The sacroiliac joints are poorly defined.
B Femur. Erlenmeyer flask deformity is apparent, with loss of normal concavity and straightening or convexity of the osseous contour, particularly along the medial aspect of the bone.
C Hands. Osteopenia, small cystic lesions, and bone reinforcement lines are apparent.
(**C,** Courtesy of S. K. Brahme, M.D., San Diego, California.)

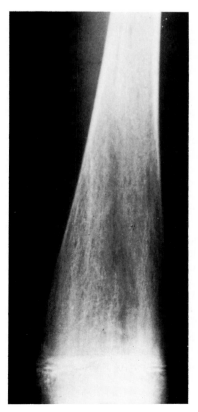

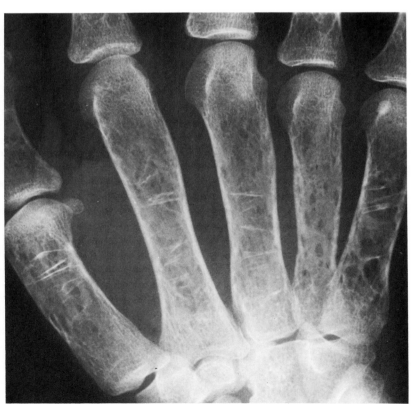

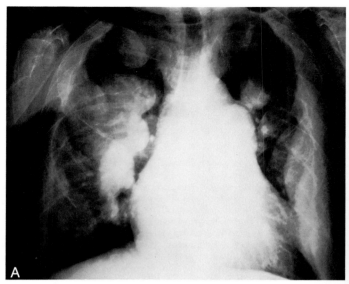

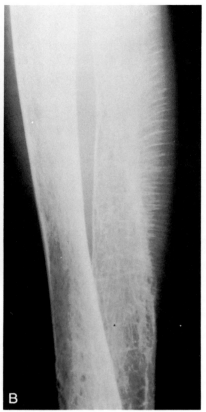

FIGURE 59–23. Thalassemia major: Marrow hyperplasia—axial and appendicular skeleton. Severe osseous abnormalities are observed in this 29 year old man.

A Widespread and marked involvement of the ribs is associated with osteopenia, cortical thinning, and bone expansion. The entire thorax and the humeri are affected.

B Both the tibia and the fibula reveal osteopenia, expansion, cortical thinning and small cystic lesions. A hair-on-end appearance of the posterior margin of the fibula is seen.

(Courtesy of A. Brower, M.D., Norfolk, Virginia.)

In thalassemia, marrow hyperplasia of the skull is not confined to the cranial vault but involves the facial bones as well. In infancy and early childhood, osseous expansion of the nasal and temporal bones leads to obliteration of the air spaces of the paranasal sinuses.[201] Maxillary alterations can produce lateral displacement of the orbits, leading to hypertelorism, malocclusion of the jaws, and displacement of dental structures, resulting in "rodent" facies (Fig. 59–21). The striking facial abnormalities accompanying this disease rarely are seen in other anemias and represent an important aspect in differential diagnosis. Furthermore, the extent and severity of cranial vault changes, including the hair-on-end appearance, are much greater in thalassemia than in other anemic disorders.

Osteoporosis of the vertebrae is most evident in the vertebral bodies. In this location, reduction in the number of trabeculae, thinning of the subchondral bone plates, accentuation of vertical trabeculation, and biconcave deformities (fish vertebrae) are evident. Rarely, central squared-off vertebral depressions or H vertebrae, characteristic of sickle cell anemia, are noted in thalassemia major.[78] As these changes have been related previously to vascular compromise, their occurrence in this latter disease is difficult to explain. Presumably they may be due to growth disturbance at the chondro-osseous junction of the vertebral body.

Medullary hyperplasia also is evident in other bones of the axial skeleton, including the ribs, pelvis, and clavicles, as well as the bones of the appendicular skeleton. The posterior aspects of multiple ribs frequently reveal significant expansion, cortical thinning, and osteoporosis. Additional rib changes include localized radiolucent lesions, subcortical radiolucency, a "rib-within-a-rib" appearance, and osteomas; they are more severe if the patient's hemo-

globin level cannot be maintained by transfusion.[202, 203] Similarly, the tubular bones reveal a widened marrow cavity, cortical thinning, and a coarse, trabeculated appearance.[204] The contour of some of the long bones is altered; normal concavity is lost, and the bones may have a straight or convex appearance. Widening of the metaphyses and epiphyses resembles an Erlenmeyer flask. Radionuclide studies in patients with thalassemia having diffuse marrow hyperplasia may reveal a generalized decrease in skeletal uptake of bone-seeking pharmaceutical agents.[205]

Growth Disturbances. Modeling deformity with an Erlenmeyer flask tubular bone is only one of the growth disturbances that may be encountered in patients with thalassemia. Near the ends of long bones, irregular transverse radiodense lines commonly can be detected in patients with this disorder. These dense shadows represent growth recovery lines and are an indication of a significant childhood illness that interfered, at least temporarily, with normal osseous growth and development. They are by no means specific, as they are encountered in innumerable other diseases.

Premature fusion of the physes (growth plates) in the tubular bones of the extremities represents a common finding in children with thalassemia major.[206] This finding, which has been noted in 10 to 15 per cent of patients, generally occurs after the age of 10 years and is most frequent in the proximal portion of the humerus and distal end of the femur.[206, 207] Such fusion occurs most commonly in patients who do not receive transfusions until late in childhood or adolescence, if they receive them at all.[208] It may be unilateral or bilateral. Shortening and deformity of the extremity may be apparent. In the humerus, varus deformity is characteristic and the pathogenesis of the finding appears to be marrow hyperplasia, cortical perforation, compression of the medial surface of the weakened osteopenic bone (a Salter-Harris Type V injury), and ultimately premature fusion of the physis.[208]

Fractures (Fig. 59–24). Infractions and spontaneous fractures are not uncommon in patients with thalassemia.[207] Dines and coworkers[207] noted one or more fractures in 33 per cent of 75 patients with homozygous beta-thalassemia, and Exarchou and associates[209] observed a similar frequency in 62 patients with beta-thalassemia. Multiple and recurrent fractures are not uncommon. Fractures are most frequent in the long bones of the lower extremity, particularly the femur, in the bones of the forearm, and in the vertebrae.[210, 211] They heal relatively slowly in most cases and may be associated with angulation and shortening of the extremities.[209]

Fractures are not unexpected in view of the severe osteopenia that is common in this condition and the increased life expectancy of patients as a consequence of more adequate transfusion therapy. Thalassemia patients have deficiencies in endocrine function and protein metabolism that contribute to weakening of bone. Shai and associates[212] demonstrated possible abnormal thyroid function, whereas Canale and colleagues[213] described altered parathyroid and gonadotropic hormone function due to pituitary dysfunction and hemochromatosis of the affected end organs in patients with thalassemia. Furthermore, increased catabolism of protein is evident in this condition, producing an increase in urinary excretion of hydroxyproline.[214]

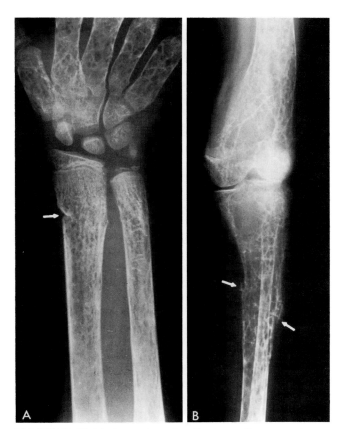

FIGURE 59–24. Thalassemia major: Fractures. Two examples are shown of extreme osteoporosis in the upper extremity **(A)** and lower extremity **(B).** The cortices are extensively thinned or absent. Fractures can be observed (arrows).

Crystal Deposition. Secondary hemochromatosis due to repeated transfusions can be seen in patients with thalassemia.[120, 121] Arthropathy in these patients resembles that of primary hemochromatosis, with joint space narrowing and sclerosis in the metacarpophalangeal joints, the knees, and the hips. Calcium pyrophosphate dihydrate (CPPD) crystal deposition may lead to chondrocalcinosis.

Hyperuricemia and acute gouty arthritis may appear during the clinical course of thalassemia.[215, 216]

Other Articular Abnormalities. A relationship of some forms of thalassemia, particularly thalassemia minor, with several additional articular abnormalities has been reported. Such abnormalities include septic arthritis and osteomyelitis, rheumatoid arthritis,[217] ischemic necrosis of bone,[218, 219] and a chronic seronegative arthritis.[220–222] The last-mentioned is characterized as a pauciarticular process with mild synovitis and small effusions. Affected joints have included the knees, ankles, wrists, elbows, and small joints of the hand. Osteopenia and joint space narrowing are the reported radiographic findings. The histologic appearance of the synovial tissue is normal or indicative of mild inflammation and does not resemble that of rheumatoid arthritis. Although a specific variety of seronegative polyarthritis in thalassemia minor is not supported by all observers,[223] the previous descriptions just cited indicate that such a possibility exists. Its potential cause and pathogenesis, including the importance of neighboring bone disease, are not certain.

Extramedullary Hematopoiesis. Extramedullary hematopoiesis represents the body's attempt to maintain erythrogenesis when there is an important alteration in blood cell population. It is observed in a variety of processes that have in common a change in bone marrow content. These processes include destruction of marrow by neoplasm or toxin, myeloproliferative disorders, and hemolytic anemias; extramedullary hematopoiesis is a well-recognized phenomenon in thalassemia.[151, 170, 171, 202, 203, 224–239] The mechanism, appearance, and location of extramedullary hematopoiesis vary somewhat among these disorders: in those instances in which the marrow is destroyed or is inefficient, focal areas of hematopoiesis appear in the liver, spleen, and lymph nodes, probably arising from multipotential stem cells; in hemolytic disorders, such as thalassemia, in which the marrow has accelerated activity, extraosseous herniation of medullary tissue is observed.[229, 240]

In thalassemia, posterior paravertebral mediastinal masses (Fig. 59–25), representing sites of extramedullary hematopoiesis, result from extraosseous extensions of medullary tissue derived from vertebral bodies[229] and ribs.[203] Marrow will proliferate into areas of least resistance; such tissue reaches the posterior mediastinum by violation of the anterior cortex of the ribs and extends into the spinal cord by expansion of the pedicles. The posterior margins of the ribs and pedicles, which are covered extensively by deep muscles, are protected.[208] Radiographs of the ribs in such cases document expanded and thinned cortices and cortical perforations with lobulated soft tissue masses; these findings are particularly well shown with CT[203, 233] or MR imaging.[170, 237] Spinal cord compression due to extradural hematopoietic tissue is best identified with myelography,[232] CT,[235] or MR imaging.[171, 238] In beta-thalassemia, this complication almost is universally seen in the thoracic region, a localization also noted in other hematologic diseases, such as sickle cell anemia and hereditary spherocytosis.[241]

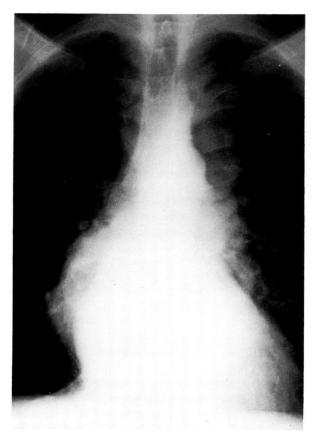

FIGURE 59–25. Thalassemia major: Extramedullary hematopoiesis. Bilateral lobulated posterior mediastinal masses can be seen. The heart is enlarged.

Extramedullary hematopoiesis in thalassemia as well as in other anemias can involve additional sites, including the retroperitoneal space and pelvis (Fig. 59–26).[231]

Miscellaneous Abnormalities. Enlargement of nutrient foramina in the phalanges of the hand has been identified in beta-thalassemia.[242, 243] The finding, which also is observed in Gaucher's disease,[243] presumably is related either to an increased arterial supply, an increased venous return, or both, to or from the hyperactive and hyperemic bone marrow.[242] In thalassemia, these foramina appear normal in those patients in whom transfusional therapy commenced at an early age and are largest in those who have never received such therapy or have a delay in the commencement of the transfusions to an older age; once enlarged, the foraminal size does not regress.[242]

Tortuous and widened vascular channels in the skull also have been seen in this disease.[242] These alterations, which are well documented with CT, usually correlate with the width of the calvarium and the enlargement of the nutrient foramina in the hands.

Three siblings have been described with both heterozygous beta-thalassemia and pyknodysostosis.[244]

Other Diagnostic Techniques

Although plain film radiography generally is adequate in defining the routine osseous abnormalities of thalassemia, xeroradiography has been used with some success to dem-

onstrate cortical thinning of tubular bones, alterations in trabecular pattern, and widening of the diploic space in the skull.[245] The routine use of xeroradiography is not required, however.

Iron overload resulting from repeated blood transfusions in thalassemia is associated with a reduction in skeletal uptake of phosphorus-containing bone-seeking radiopharmaceutical agents and an increase in renal and soft tissue radioactivity.[205, 246, 247] It is postulated that the mechanism explaining this phenomenon is bonding between the technetium-labeled phosphorus substances and the iron-containing compounds, which results in blood pool labeling.[247] Knowledge of this effect will allow more reasonable analysis of the patterns of altered osseous radionuclide activity during bone scintigraphy in patients with various anemias.

Similarly, analysis of sites of extramedullary hematopoiesis using radionuclide techniques can be accomplished if appropriate caution is exercised. The two general methods of imaging of the bone marrow are labeling of the reticuloendothelial system with radioactive colloids and use of isotopes of iron to image the erythropoietic system.[248] Indium-111 chloride originally was believed to be a pure erythropoietic agent; recent evidence suggests that indium-111 may localize in both reticuloendothelial and hematopoietic elements in the bone marrow. Technetium-99m sulfur colloid also has been used as a bone-marrow imaging agent (Fig. 59–26). Its advantages include a low radiation dose, an increased photon yield, and simultaneous imaging of the liver and spleen; its disadvantages include an uncertainty in interpretation, owing to the fact that the radiocolloid seeks only the reticuloendothelial marrow elements, and obscuration of lower thoracic and upper lumbar vertebral marrow activity related to hepatic uptake.[248]

CT scanning can document the abnormal deposition of iron that follows multiple blood transfusions in patients with thalassemia (or other anemias). This can be evident in the liver, spleen, bowel, pancreas, lymph nodes, and additional organs.[249, 250] Regions with high attenuation values are evident in the CT images. This technique also can be used to document sites of extramedullary hematopoiesis, particularly in the posterior mediastinum, spinal canal, and pelvis.[171, 203, 233, 235, 236, 238, 251]

MR imaging has been used as an additional diagnostic method in some patients with thalassemia. The intensity of the image obtained with MR provides a means of assessing the amount of iron that is deposited in the tissues of the body.[252] An observed depression of spin echo intensities in the liver and bone marrow and an elevation of these intensities in the kidneys and muscles correlate with changes in iron concentration and iron content per ferritin molecule. Other noninvasive techniques, such as dual-energy CT, can provide similar data.[253]

As discussed previously in this chapter, the ability of MR imaging to allow identification of fat owing to its strong signal is useful in the evaluation of various bone marrow diseases.[155, 162] Normal fatty marrow possesses a short T1 and a long T2 relaxation time, leading to an intense signal, irrespective of whether the pulse sequence has been chosen to emphasize T1 or T2.[254–256] A loss of signal intensity in the marrow indicates fat replacement by tumor or other tissue and can be seen in leukemia, neuroblastoma, osteosarcoma, and other neoplasms.[256] In various types of anemias, marrow reconversion from adipose to hematopoietic

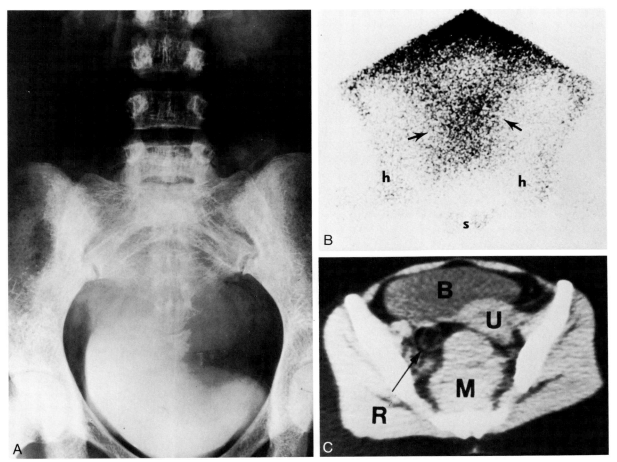

FIGURE 59–26. Thalassemia major: Extramedullary hematopoiesis. A 36 year old woman with beta thalassemia had a pelvic mass. A barium enema (not shown) documented that the mass displaced the rectum in an anterior direction.

A The intravenous pyelogram reveals pressure deformity in the superior surface of the bladder and bone changes consistent with thalassemia.

B A ⁹⁹ᵐTc sulfur colloid scan shows uptake in the pelvic mass (arrows). The radionuclide activity at the top of the image relates to hepatosplenomegaly. The symphysis pubis (*s*) and region of the hips (*h*) are identified.

C A transaxial CT image of the pelvis demonstrates the posterior mass (*M*), anterior displacement of the rectum (*R*), and the position of the bladder (*B*) and the uterus (*U*). At surgery, a 7 × 5 × 4 cm mass was the site of extramedullary hematopoiesis.

(Courtesy of J. Sebes, M.D., Memphis, Tennessee.)

tissue also alters significantly the signal characteristics derived from bone (see previous discussion). MR imaging will be useful in documenting the response of the bone marrow to therapeutic manipulation of various anemias[163] and tumors. MR imaging may be employed effectively in the assessment of marrow heterotopia, and it allows documentation of the effect of sites of extramedullary hematopoiesis on surrounding tissues and organs[155, 171, 238] (Fig. 59–27). A word of caution, however, is required. In one investigation, a magnetic field produced a striking perpendicular alignment of sickled erythrocytes, suggesting that MR imaging in patients with sickle cell anemia could result in worsening of vaso-occlusive complications.[257]

Effects of Therapeutic Modalities

Therapeutic methods that have been employed in patients with thalassemia have included repeated blood transfusions to maintain acceptable levels of hemoglobin and chelation to remove excessive amounts of iron that result from such transfusions. Although these methods have succeeded in prolonging the life span of some patients with various types

of thalassemia, complications related to the chelation therapy have been identified.

One of the chelation agents, deferoxamine, may lead to significant skeletal abnormalities when employed in the treatment of thalassemia major. In 1988, De Virgiliis and coworkers[259] observed growth retardation and metaphyseal abnormalities in children with thalassemia in whom chelation using subcutaneous infusion of deferoxamine was begun before the age of 3 years. Similar alterations occurred with lesser frequency in those children whose chelation therapy was initiated at an older age. The mean dosage of deferoxamine in these children varied from approximately 50 to 80 mg/kg/day. These investigators theorized that a direct toxic effect of the chelating agent on growing bone or mineral loss, or both, might be important in the pathogenesis of the skeletal changes and that initiation of such chelation at an early age was a significant risk factor. Brill and coworkers[260] in 1991 observed skeletal abnormalities simulating a bone dysplasia in two of five children with thalassemia major in whom a regimen of hypertransfusion and chelation with deferoxamine was begun before the age of 3 years; these abnormalities were not observed in 22

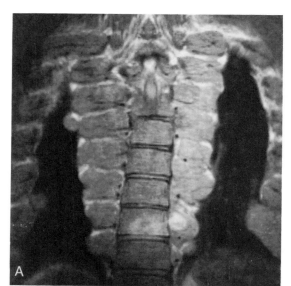
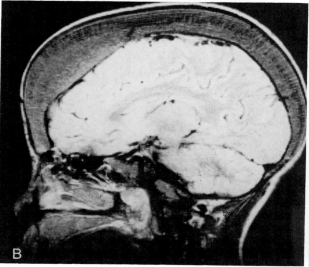
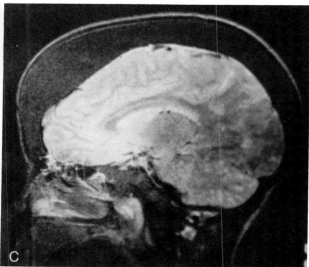

FIGURE 59–27. Thalassemia major: Marrow reconversion and heterotopia. In a 29 year old man, a T1-weighted (TR/TE, 700/20) coronal spin echo MR image of the thorax (**A**) and proton density (TR/TE, 2000/30) (**B**) and T2-weighted (TR/TE, 2000/90) (**C**) sagittal images of the skull reveal evidence of marrow reconversion and heterotopia. In **A**, note the presence of hematopoietic marrow in the vertebral bodies and ribs. The posterior portions of the ribs are expanded dramatically. In **B** and **C**, the hematopoietic marrow in the cranial vault is of intermediate or low signal intensity. Expansion of the diploic portion of the cranium is apparent. The facial bones also are involved. (Courtesy of M. Pathria, M.D., San Diego, California.)

other children whose chelation was started after the age of 3 years. These investigators were unable to determine whether the osseous abnormalities were related to the drug dose or to the age of onset of chelation, although improvement in the skeletal appearance was noted in one of the patients after the dose of deferoxamine was decreased. Orzincolo and colleagues[261] in 1992 further documented the detrimental effects of subcutaneous chelation therapy with deferoxamine in thalassemia in a description of 12 children between the ages of 3 and 16 years.

Clinically, affected patients have a short trunk with moderate sternal protrusion, genu valgum, generalized joint stiffness, and periarticular bone deformity.[259] Radiologically, both spinal and extraspinal abnormalities are seen (Fig. 59–28). Irregular flattening of the vertebral bodies in the thoracic and lumbar spine may be observed. More dramatic alterations affect the metaphyses of the tubular bones of the extremities, particularly those about the knees and wrists. Metaphyseal alterations typically begin at 2 to 4 years of age, consisting initially of concavity and widening with an intact metaphyseal line. Progressive changes subsequently occur, with metaphyseal irregularity and cupping as well as indistinctness and fraying of adjacent bone. Cystic and sclerotic regions in the metaphyses develop, and deformities such as genu valgum may appear. Premature closure of the physis does not appear to be a feature of this process. With a decrease in the dosage of deferoxamine, healing of the metaphyseal abnormalities with partial or complete obliteration of the cystic defects and increased bone sclerosis may be encountered. The bone changes typically are bilateral, and common sites of involvement include the distal femur, proximal tibia, and distal ulna. Other metaphyseal regions may be affected, however, including those in the proximal femur, proximal humerus, distal radius, and distal tibia.

Although the skeletal abnormalities resemble those encountered in spondylometaphyseal dysplasia, the findings do not correspond precisely to any of the recognized genetic dysplasias.[262, 311] The pattern of physeal widening simulates that seen in pseudoachondroplasia, spondyloenchondrodysplasia, and certain forms of multiple epiphyseal dysplasia.[260] Superficially, physeal widening, irregularity, and indistinctness in deferoxamine-induced disease simulate changes observed in rickets and scurvy as well.[261]

The precise relationship among the dose of deferoxamine, the age of the patient, and the severity of the skeletal alterations remains to be established. Furthermore, as chelation may lead to deficiencies of zinc and copper and, perhaps, other trace metals, the importance of these deficiencies and their contribution to the skeletal changes need to be defined.

THALASSEMIA VARIANTS

Thalassemia minor and thalassemia intermedia are associated with similar but less marked bony changes than thalassemia major.[195, 258] In addition, persons with thalassemia may have other abnormal hemoglobins, including C, S, H, E, Constant Spring, and Lepore; findings in these patients tend to be less striking. Homozygous states of some of these hemoglobinopathies, such as the Lepore disorder, can be associated with severe clinical manifestations.

IRON DEFICIENCY ANEMIA

In children, iron deficiency anemia results from insufficient intake or excessive loss of iron during the first 6 months of life, which depletes the iron that was stored during late prenatal life. This type of anemia is most frequent between 9 months and 2 years of age and is rare after the age of 3 years.[3]

Skeletal abnormalities generally are mild. Marrow hyperplasia may result in changes of the cranial vault[263–268] (Fig. 59–29). These changes, although usually observed in infants and young children, occasionally are encountered in older children and young adults. Thinning of the outer table and diploic widening are observed in the frontal, parietal, or occipital bone. As in cases of hemolytic anemia, the occipital squamosa inferior to the internal occipital protuberance is unaffected in this disease. Radial striations extending from the outer table are rare and usually are mild in iron deficiency anemia, allowing its distinction from thalassemia. Furthermore, facial involvement is not apparent in the former disease. Osteoporosis of other sites has been noted, including the long and short tubular bones.[265, 269, 270] Radiographic abnormalities are a poor index of the severity of the anemia, although they may regress under treatment and with advancing age.[271]

Paleopathologic investigations have uncovered a condition termed porotic hyperostosis of the skull, which probably is related to a variety of anemias, including iron deficiency anemia.[200, 266, 272–275] The lesion usually is distributed symmetrically and most commonly is seen in the posterior

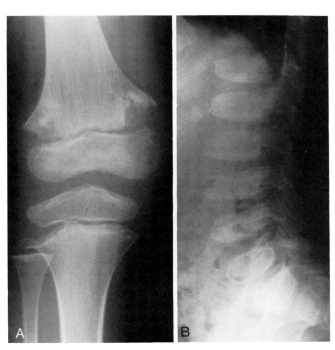

FIGURE 59–28. Thalassemia major: Deferoxamine-induced bone changes.

A In an anteroposterior radiograph of the knee, the metaphyses of the distal portion of the femur and proximal end of the tibia are deficient circumferentially. Note irregularity of the femoral metaphysis and, to a lesser extent, tibial and fibular metaphyses.

B In the lumbar spine, flattened vertebral bodies are evident.

(From Brill PW, et al: AJR *156*:561, 1991. Copyright 1991, American Roentgen Ray Society.)

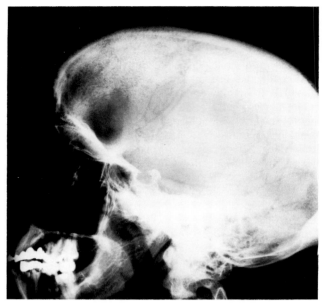

FIGURE 59–29. Iron deficiency anemia: Marrow hyperplasia—skull. Note the changes in the frontal region of the cranial vault. The tables are thinned and a reticulated appearance is evident.

portion of the parietal bone, in the occipital bone along the lambdoid suture, and on the orbital roof (Fig. 59–30).[200] Diploic widening, obliteration of the outer table, a hair-on-end appearance, and increased bone radiodensity are evident, particularly in children, and resemble the abnormalities observed in modern-day examples of anemia.

HEREDITARY SPHEROCYTOSIS

This hemolytic anemia, which is inherited as an autosomal dominant disorder, is worldwide in distribution but most common in northern Europeans. It is characterized by abnormally shaped red blood cells or spherocytes in the peripheral blood, which are hemolyzed in the spleen.

Spherocytes are formed because of a deficiency of spectrin, the largest and most abundant structural protein of the erythrocyte membrane, and they lack the strength, durability, and flexibility to withstand the stresses of the circulation; incapable of deforming adequately to traverse the splenic microcirculation, the relatively rigid spherocytes are trapped in the splenic red pulp and are destroyed.[276] The onset of disease varies from early infancy to adulthood, although the majority of cases become evident in late childhood and early adolescence.[277] Clinical features include anemia, jaundice, and splenomegaly. Gallstones and chronic leg ulcerations are two other potential manifestations of this disorder. Coincident syndromes, including unconjugated hyperbilirubinemia, familial myocardiopathy, and spinal cord dysfunction, are described.

As in other hemolytic diseases, compensatory hyperplasia of the bone marrow occurs with extension of red marrow into the diaphyses of long bones. In the cranial vault, diploic widening and thinning of the outer table are evident. Rarely, hair-on-end striations and medullary widening with osteoporosis in long bones are seen. Because anemia in this condition may not become manifest until late childhood or adolescence, at which time red cellular marrow is being converted to fatty marrow in the peripheral skeleton, significant long bone changes indeed are unusual. Occasionally, extramedullary hematopoiesis results in paravertebral masses simulating infection or tumor. Secondary hemochromatosis also has been noted in association with transfusional therapy for this condition.[121] The skeletal alterations may improve after splenectomy.[278]

HEREDITARY ELLIPTOCYTOSIS

In hereditary elliptocytosis, red cells are oval or elliptical in shape. The disorder is closely linked to hereditary spherocytosis, as some families contain persons with elliptocytosis and other persons with spherocytosis. Hemolysis occurs in the spleen. The bone abnormalities largely are undescribed.

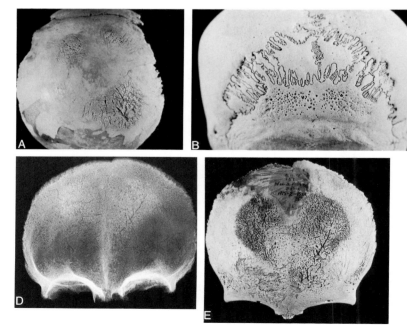

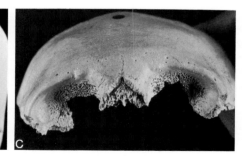

FIGURE 59–30. Porotic hyperostosis of the skull: Probable iron deficiency anemia. Paleopathologic specimens (pre-Columbian Peruvian Indians).

A–C Sites of porotic hyperostosis include the parietal and occipital bones **(A)**, the occipital bone **(B)**, and the orbital roof **(C)**.

D, E In this example, note striking porotic hyperostosis, symmetrically distributed in the frontal bone. A slight increase in radiodensity is seen about the porous regions.

NONSPHEROCYTIC HEMOLYTIC ANEMIA

Nonspherocytic hemolytic anemia is a designation that can be used for hereditary hemolytic processes not attributable to thalassemia, spherocytosis, elliptocytosis, or one of the hemoglobinopathies. Although several processes meet this criterion, the two most important disorders in this category are pyruvate kinase deficiency and glucose-6-phosphate dehydrogenase deficiency anemias. Radiographic changes have been documented in association with deficiency of pyruvate kinase.[279] Marrow hyperplasia producing osteoporosis, diploic widening, and thinning of the outer table in the cranial vault is a finding identical to that in other anemias. Unlike the case with thalassemia, the facial bones and sinuses are unaffected. Splenectomy may result in improvement of the anemia and in partial resolution of the skull changes.[280]

APLASTIC ANEMIA

An uncommon condition, aplastic anemia is characterized by an acellular or hypocellular bone marrow and is accompanied by pancytopenia, including anemia, neutropenia, and thrombocytopenia. Its causes are diverse, including drugs (chloramphenicol, phenytoin, gold, and benzene), radiation, paroxysmal nocturnal hemoglobinuria, Fanconi's anemia (see later discussion), viral hepatitis, pregnancy, and thymoma,[281] although many of the cases occur on an idiopathic basis. Patients with aplastic anemia have an impaired ability to incorporate iron into the marrow erythroid precursors.[281] Biopsy in untreated cases confirms the presence of marrow hypoplasia or aplasia, with a variable degree of fat replacement and degeneration. Various types of therapy, including repeated blood transfusions or marrow transplantation, can effect a partial or complete recovery of the bone marrow. Initially, after the onset of therapeutic measures, increased cellularity of the marrow in the form of clusters of hematopoietic precursors is a favorable response. Eventually, more complete recovery of the marrow may occur. Although repeated bone biopsies represent one method to monitor the therapeutic response in patients with aplastic anemia, sampling errors may occur and a more reliable and noninvasive technique is desirable.

MR imaging appears to have potential in the initial diagnosis of aplastic anemia and as a method of monitoring the therapeutic response. Data regarding the role of this imaging method in patients with aplastic anemia are preliminary and inconsistent, however. One initial report describing MR imaging abnormalities in untreated patients with aplastic anemia emphasized an augmentation of marrow signal intensity owing to the presence of fat[256] (Fig. 59–31). More recently, Kaplan and associates[282] employed spin echo MR imaging sequences in the evaluation of five adults and one child with aplastic anemia, all of whom had received some form of therapy for the disease. The signal characteristics of the pelvis and proximal femora in each case were consistent with the presence of marrow fat. Evaluation of the spine in these patients, however, revealed different MR imaging findings. In some instances, focal areas of low signal intensity interspersed with areas of high signal intensity were seen, and vertebral biopsy in one patient demonstrated evidence of islands of active hematopoietic cells scattered in otherwise fatty marrow. These

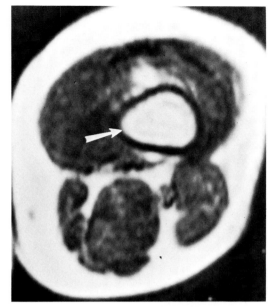

FIGURE 59–31. Aplastic anemia: Marrow aplasia. In a 10 year old girl, a transaxial T1-weighted (TR/TE, 250/24) spin echo MR image reveals a signal of high intensity from the marrow of the femur (arrow) suggesting a very high fat concentration in the marrow space. A marrow biopsy revealed extensive fat with few cellular elements and no tumor cells. (From Cohen MD, Klatte EC, Baehner R, et al: Radiology *151:*715, 1984.)

results support the concept that MR imaging may be valuable in assessing the response to therapy in patients with aplastic anemia.

MISCELLANEOUS ANEMIAS

Hemolytic disease of the newborn (erythroblastosis fetalis) is associated with excessive destruction of the erythrocytes beginning in fetal life, usually due to Rh incompatibility between the blood of the fetus and that of the mother. Clinical and radiographic findings include soft tissue edema ("halo sign"), loss of muscle and fat planes in the soft tissues, and metaphyseal lucency and sclerosis.[283–285] Periostitis is not apparent, allowing differentiation between this disorder and scurvy or congenital syphilis.

Fanconi's anemia consists of severe refractory hypoplastic anemia with pancytopenia, brown pigmentation of the skin, and multiple congenital anomalies.[286] The onset of the anemia frequently is delayed until the end of the first decade of life, although it may not appear until the third decade. Radiographic findings include anomalies of the radius and radial side of the hand, ranging from hypoplasia to aplasia of osseous structures, short stature, microcephaly, delayed ossification, developmental dislocation or subluxation of the hip, and renal anomalies[3, 287, 288] (Fig. 59–32).

The syndrome of thrombocytopenia and absent radius (TAR syndrome) resembles Fanconi's anemia.[289–291] It originally was described in 1969 by Hall and collaborators,[292] and it consists of congenital hypomegakaryocytic thrombocytopenia, severe hemorrhages, and skeletal anomalies. The anomalies include bilateral absence of the radius, shortening of the ulna, dysplasia of the knee, and osseous deformity. The presence of five digits in the hand in the TAR syndrome differs from the absence of the thumb in Fan-

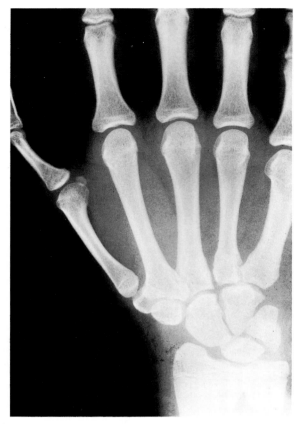

FIGURE 59–32. Fanconi's anemia: Skeletal anomalies. A hypoplastic first ray is evident. The scaphoid is absent. In many cases of this syndrome, the thumb also is absent.

coni's anemia. Furthermore, the TAR syndrome generally is evident in the first few years of life, whereas Fanconi's anemia has a later onset.[291]

Additional syndromes sharing features with Fanconi's anemia are trisomy 18, the Holt-Oram syndrome, and tha-

lidomide embryopathy.[291] Also, a rare X-linked disease, dyskeratosis congenita, associated with dermatologic manifestations, aplastic anemia, short stature, and malignancy, resembles Fanconi's anemia.[293] It can be differentiated from Fanconi's anemia by the skin changes, X-linked inheritance, and absence of both preaxial reduction anomalies and increased chromosomal breakage.[294] Skeletal changes in dyskeratosis congenita usually are mild but may include osteopenia, trabecular alterations, cysts, and fractures.[293]

DIFFERENTIAL DIAGNOSIS

Differentiation Among the Anemias
(Table 59–1)

Although there is considerable overlap in the radiographic features of the various anemic disorders, certain characteristics exist that may allow their differentiation.

Extensive thickening of the cranial vault associated with marked diploic expansion and a hair-on-end appearance is most characteristic of thalassemia. Its occurrence in patients with sickle cell anemia has been overemphasized, as this finding is evident in fewer than 5 per cent of patients with this disease.[295] Some thickening of the cranial vault can be apparent in sickle cell-hemoglobin C disease, sickle cell-thalassemia disease, iron deficiency anemia, hereditary spherocytosis, and pyruvate kinase deficiency, but widespread and severe skull alterations are rare in these disorders. Severe facial changes are limited to thalassemia.

Changes of marrow hyperplasia in the peripheral skeleton are most common and marked in thalassemia. In this disease, abnormality can occur in long and short tubular bones, although the changes may regress and disappear with advancing age. In children with sickle cell anemia, osteoporosis and cortical thinning in the small tubular bones of the hands and feet can be seen, although the findings generally are mild. In the adult with sickle cell anemia, the findings of marrow hyperplasia in the peripheral skeleton are overshadowed by findings of multiple bone infarcts. In iron deficiency anemia and sickle cell-thalassemia disease,

TABLE 59–1. Characteristic Skeletal Findings in the Anemias

Disease	Marrow Hyperplasia			Bone Infarction		Growth Disturbances		Fractures	Osteomyelitis and Septic Arthritis	Crystal Deposition	
	Cranial Vault	Facial Bones	Tubular Bones	Long Tubular Bones	Hands, Feet	H Vertebrae	Flaring of Tubular Bones			Calcium Pyrophosphate Dihydrate	Monosodium Urate
Sickle cell anemia	+		+	+	+	+		+	+		+
Sickle cell trait				+					+		
Sickle cell–hemoglobin C disease	+			+		+					
Sickle cell–thalassemia disease	+		+	+		+			+		
Thalassemia	+	+	+			+	+	+	+	+	+
Iron deficiency anemia	+		+								
Spherocytosis	+									+	
Nonspherocytic hemolytic anemia	+										

changes of marrow hyperplasia in the tubular bones are absent or mild.

Bone infarction is particularly common in sickle cell anemia and sickle cell-hemoglobin C disease. Ischemic skeletal changes are less frequent in sickle cell-thalassemia disease and sickle cell trait and are not characteristic of thalassemia or iron deficiency anemia. Osteonecrosis of epiphyses may be more frequent in sickle cell-hemoglobin C disease than in sickle cell anemia, although this point is debated. Diaphyseal infarction with surrounding sclerosis producing a bone-within-bone appearance is suggestive of sickle cell anemia or sickle cell-hemoglobin C disease, being rare in other anemias. Infarction of the small bones of the hands and feet in children, producing dactylitis and the hand-foot syndrome, almost is diagnostic of sickle cell anemia.

Growth disturbances can be seen in many of the anemias. Abnormalities of vertebral body contour with squared-off compressions of the vertebrae (H vertebrae) occur in sickle cell anemia, sickle cell-hemoglobin C disease, and sickle cell-thalassemia disease, although such abnormalities may be seen in thalassemia and in other conditions, such as Gaucher's disease. Flaring of the ends of the tubular bones, the Erlenmeyer flask appearance, is most suggestive of thalassemia. This finding, too, can be seen in disorders other than anemias. Premature fusion of the growth plate has been described in both sickle cell anemia and thalassemia.

Osteopenia, which may be found in many of the anemic disorders, leads to osseous weakening, predisposing to skeletal fractures. Pathologic fractures have been noted in sickle cell anemia and thalassemia, although they are to be expected in the other anemias as well.

Osteomyelitis, particularly that associated with Salmonella infection, is a known complication of sickle cell anemia, although infections of bones and joints can be observed in thalassemia and other hemoglobinopathies.

Secondary hemochromatosis with or without CPPD crystal deposition may complicate repeated blood transfusions in thalassemia, spherocytosis, and hypoplastic and sideroblastic anemias. Hyperuricemia and gouty arthritis occur with sickle cell anemia and thalassemia and, occasionally, in other anemias as well.[296]

Differentiation of Anemia from Other Conditions

In anemic disorders, diffuse skeletal abnormality characterized by decreased radiographic density (osteopenia) indicates marrow hyperplasia. This finding may be simulated by changes in additional disorders. Other primary marrow diseases, such as Gaucher's disease and Niemann-Pick disease, are associated with similar findings. Osteopenia also may accompany osteogenesis imperfecta, idiopathic juvenile osteoporosis, hyperparathyroidism, and leukemia as well as other diseases, although additional abnormalities usually are apparent that permit an accurate diagnosis. In sickle cell anemia, infarction in the long tubular bones of the appendicular skeleton and in portions of the axial skeleton may lead to increased radiodensity with a coarsened trabecular pattern simulating the changes of renal osteodystrophy, myelofibrosis, and osteomalacia.

Thickening of the cranial vault is a radiographic finding that is apparent in many disorders. In anemias, this thickening frequently involves the entire cranium with the exception of the inferior aspect of the occipital bone and base of the skull. Fibrous dysplasia and leontiasis ossea can lead to excessive hyperostosis of the skull, but changes usually predominate in the frontal regions and face. Hyperostosis frontalis interna generally (but not invariably) is confined to the anterior aspect of the cranial vault, whereas acromegaly, Paget's disease, and hypoparathyroidism may produce diffuse thickening of the cranium (Fig. 59–33). The hair-on-end appearance that is characteristic of thalassemia is virtually diagnostic of an anemic condition. It differs considerably from the thin radiolucent vertex striations that are seen in lateral radiographs of the normal skull.[297]

Epiphyseal and diaphyseal bone infarction occurs not only in anemia but also in other diseases. Epiphyseal ischemia, particularly of the femoral head, is noted in endogenous and exogenous corticosteroid excess, caisson disease, Gaucher's disease, Legg-Calvé-Perthes disease, collagen vascular disorders, alcoholism with pancreatitis, and radiation therapy, as well as after trauma and in many other processes. Diametaphyseal ischemia is seen in association with steroid administration, caisson disease, pancreatitis, and Gaucher's disease.

Abnormality of vertebral body contour characterized by steplike depressions of the osseous surface, the H vertebra, is a relatively specific radiographic sign of anemia. It has been noted rarely in other conditions, including Gaucher's disease, but its detection should initiate a thorough search for the presence of sickle cell anemia or a related condition. The H vertebra with its abrupt endplate indentations can be distinguished from the fish vertebra, which has a smooth biconcave appearance. Fish vertebrae may be observed in anemias, but the changes are not specific, as they appear in all forms of osteoporosis and in other conditions producing diffuse weakening of bone, including osteomalacia, hyperparathyroidism, Paget's disease, and neoplasm.

The findings of sickle cell dactylitis may simulate the changes of other disorders associated with destruction and

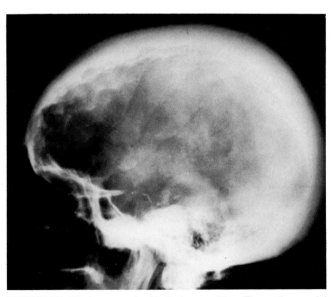

FIGURE 59–33. Acromegaly: Skull abnormalities. The entire cranial vault is thickened. Involvement of the occipital bone also is observed. The sella turcica is enlarged.

periostitis of small tubular bones in the hands and feet. Tuberculous dactylitis may occur in children[298, 299] or, less commonly, in adults.[300, 301] This form of tuberculosis has been termed spina ventosa (from Latin *spina,* "spinelike projection"; ventosa, "puffed full of air"). Soft tissue swelling, bone destruction, periostitis, and bone expansion are observed at single or multiple sites (Fig. 59–34). Dactylitis may be apparent in other infiltrative diseases, including syphilis, leprosy, and fungal and pyogenic disorders. Furthermore, periostitis of small tubular bones with or without bone destruction can accompany leukemia, scurvy, hypervitaminosis A, trauma, and infantile cortical hyperostosis. In most instances, differential diagnosis is not difficult.

The findings of bone infarction of long and short tubular bones in sickle cell anemia can simulate osteomyelitis. In fact, differentiation of infarction versus infection in a patient with sickle cell anemia can be extremely difficult, particularly as Salmonella involvement of bone, common in this disease, may localize in the diaphyses of multiple bones, producing osseous destruction and periostitis. Radionuclide examination with both bone- and bone marrow-seeking agents may allow differentiation of these two complications of the disease.[35, 147–150]

Extramedullary hematopoiesis accompanying thalassemia and, less commonly, other anemias leads to enlargement of the posterior portions of the ribs, simulating the findings in fibrous dysplasia, and lobulated posterior mediastinal masses resembling neoplasm. With regard to the rib lesions, multiplicity, bilaterality, and the known presence of an anemia generally allow differentiation of sites of extramedullary hematopoiesis from the other causes of rib expansion. It should be noted, however, that solitary or focal sites of hematopoietic hyperplasia in ribs have been encountered, even in the absence of an associated hematologic process.[302] Resulting masses are termed myelolipomas and are seen more frequently in extraosseous sites, such as the liver, stomach, adrenal gland, and presacral space, where they are referred to as bone marrow heterotopias.[303]

SUMMARY

The hemoglobinopathies are associated with characteristic abnormalities of the skeleton. In general, the abnormalities are related to marrow hyperplasia, vascular occlusion, and several additional problems, including fracture and infection. Although these features are apparent in almost all of the hemoglobin disorders, their severity varies from one to another, allowing, in some instances, differentiation among these disorders. Articular manifestations in hemoglobinopathies can be attributed to epiphyseal osteonecrosis, growth disturbances, osseous weakening, infection, crystal deposition, hemarthrosis, and synovial membrane microvascular obstruction. In some patients, these articular abnormalities overshadow other clinical manifestations of the disease.

References

1. Pauling L, Itano HA, Singer SJ, et al: Sickle cell anemia, a molecular disease. Science 110:543, 1949.
2. Scott RB: Sickle cell anemia—pathogenesis and treatment. Pediatr Clin North Am 9:649, 1962.
3. O'Hara AE: Roentgenographic osseous manifestations of the anemias and the leukemias. Clin Orthop 52:63, 1967.
4. Herrick JB: Peculiar elongated sickle-shaped red blood corpuscles in a case of severe anemia. Arch Intern Med 6:517, 1910.
5. Hahn EV, Gillespie EG: Sickle cell anemia: Report of a case greatly improved by splenectomy. Experimental study of sickle cell formation. Arch Intern Med 39:233, 1927.
6. Hahn EV: Sickle cell (drepanocytic) anemia with a report of a second case successfully treated by splenectomy and further observations on the mechanism of sickle cell formation. Am J Med Sci 175:206, 1928.
7. Graham GS: Case of sickle cell anemia with necropsy. Arch Intern Med 34:778, 1924.
8. Cooley TB, Lee P: The sickle cell phenomenon. Am J Dis Child 32:334, 1926.
9. Anderson WW, Ware RL: Sickle cell anemia. Am J Dis Child 44:1055, 1932.
10. Grover V.: The clinical manifestations of sickle cell anemia. Ann Intern Med 26:843, 1947.
11. Margolies MP: Sickle cell anemia: A composite study and survey. Medicine 30:357, 1951.
12. Henderson AB: Sickle cell anemia: Clinical study of fifty-four cases. Am J Med 9:757, 1950.
13. Karayalcin G., Rosner F, Kim KY, et al: Sickle cell anemia—clinical manifestations in 100 patients and review of the literature. Am J Med Sci 269:51, 1975.
14. Pearson HA, Diamond LK: The critically ill child: Sickle cell disease crises and their management. Pediatrics 48:629, 1971.
15. Winslow RM, Anderson WF: The hemoglobinopathies. In JG Stanbury, JB Wyngaarden, DS Fredrickson (Eds): The Metabolic Basis of Inherited Diseases. 4th Ed. New York: McGraw-Hill, 1978, p 1465.
16. Chien S: Rheology of sickle cells and the microcirculation. N Engl J Med 311:1567, 1984.
17. Davis S, Trubowitz S: Pathologic reactions involving the bone marrow. In S Trubowitz, S Davis (Eds): The Human Bone Marrow: Anatomy, Physiology, and Pathophysiology. Boca Raton, FL: CRC Press, 1982, p 243.
18. Burko H, Watson RJ, Robinson M: Unusual bone changes in sickle cell disease in childhood. Radiology 80:957, 1963.
19. Watson RJ, Burko H, Megas H, et al: Hand-foot syndrome in sickle cell disease in young children. Pediatrics 31:975, 1963.
20. Scott RB, Ferguson AD: Studies in sickle cell anemia: XXVII. Complications in infants and children in the United States. Clin Pediatr 5:403, 1966.
21. Booker CR, Scott RB, Ferguson AD: Studies in sickle cell anemia: XXII. Clinical manifestations of sickle cell anemia during the first two years of life. Clin Pediatr 3:111, 1964.
22. Diggs LW: Bone and joint lesions in sickle-cell disease. Clin Orthop 52:119, 1967.

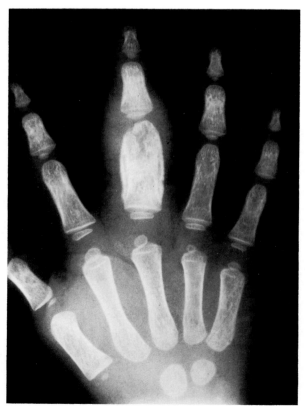

FIGURE 59–34. Tuberculosis: Dactylitis. Findings include soft tissue swelling of the third finger and destruction of the proximal phalanx with extensive periostitis.

23. Jaffe HL: Metabolic, Degenerative and Inflammatory Diseases of Bones and Joints. Philadelphia: Lea & Febiger, 1972, p 693.
24. Reimann F., Talasli U, Gökmen E: Zur röntgenologischen Bestimmung der Dicke der Schädelknochen und ihrer Verbreiterung bei Patienten mit schwerer Bluterkrankung und Hyperplasie des roten Knochenmarks. ROFO 125:540, 1976.
25. Sebes JI, Diggs LW: Radiographic changes of the skull in sickle cell anemia. AJR 132:373, 1979.
26. Carroll DS: Roentgen manifestations of sickle cell disease. South Med J 50:1486, 1957.
27. Reimann F, Kuran S: Ursache, Entstehung und Wesen des ''Bürstensymptoms'' am Schädel bei schweren erkrankungen des Blutes. VI. Untersuchungen über die Veränderungen des Skeletsystems bei schweren Bluterkrankungen. Virchows Arch (Pathol Anat) 358:173, 1973.
28. Mourshed F, Tuckson CR: A study of the radiographic features of the jaws in sickle cell anemia. Oral Surg 37:812, 1974.
29. Prowler JR, Smith EW: Dental bone changes occurring in sickle cell diseases and abnormal hemoglobin traits. Radiology 65:762, 1955.
30. Reynolds J: The Roentgenological Features of Sickle Cell Disease and Related Hemoglobinopathies. Springfield, IL: Charles C Thomas, 1965.
31. Soni NN: Microradiographic study of dental tissues in sickle cell anemia. Arch Oral Pathol 11:561, 1966.
32. Hill MC, Oh KS, Bowerman JW et al: Abnormal epiphyses in the sickling disorders. AJR 124:34, 1975.
33. Sherman M: Pathogenesis of disintegration of the hip in sickle cell anemia. South Med J 52:632, 1959.
34. Chung SMK, Ralston EL: Necrosis of the femoral head associated with sickle-cell anemia and its genetic variants. J Bone Joint Surg [Am] 51:33, 1969.
35. Chung SMK, Alavi A, Russell MO: Management of osteonecrosis in sickle cell anemia and its genetic variants. Clin Orthop 130:158, 1978.
36. Worrall VT, Butera V: Sickle cell dactylitis. J Bone Joint Surg [Am] 58:1161, 1976.
37. Cockshott WP: Dactylitis and growth disorders. Br J Radiol 36:19, 1963.
38. Victor AB, Imperiale LE: The pulmonary and small bone changes in infants with sickle cell anemia. NY State J Med 57:1403, 1957.
39. Weinberg AG, Currarino G: Sickle cell dactylitis: Histopathologic observations. Am J Clin Pathol 58:518, 1972.
40. Espinosa GA: Hand-foot roentgen findings in sickle cell anemia. J Natl Med Assoc 71:171, 1979.
41. Stevens MCG, Padwick GR, Serjeant GR: Observations on the natural history of dactylitis in homozygous sickle cell disease. Clin Pediatr 20:311, 1981.
42. Amjad H, Bannerman RM, Judisch JM: Sickling pain and season. Br Med J 2:54, 1974.
43. Redwood AM, Williams EM, Desai P, et al: Climate and painful crisis of sickle cell disease in Jamaica. Br Med J 1:66, 1976.
44. Carache S, Page DL: Infarctions of bone marrow in sickle cell disorders. Ann Intern Med 67:1195, 1967.
45. Kimmelstiel P: Vascular occlusion and ischemic infarction in sickle cell disease. Am J Med Sci 216:11, 1948.
46. Weinberg S: Severe sclerosis of the long bones in sickle cell anemia. Radiology 145:41, 1982.
47. Allen BJ, Andrews BS: Bilateral aseptic necrosis of calcanei in an adult male with sickle cell disease treated by a surgical coring procedure. J Rheumatol 10:294, 1983.
48. Lanzer W, Szabo R, Gelberman R: Avascular necrosis of the lunate and sickle cell anemia. A case report. Clin Orthop 187:168, 1984.
49. Sebes JI, Brown DL: Terminal phalangeal sclerosis in sickle cell disease. AJR 140:763, 1983.
50. Levine MS, Borden S IV, Gill FM: Sternal cupping: A new finding in childhood sickle cell anemia. Radiology 142:367, 1982.
51. Harcke HT, Capitanio MA, Naiman JL: Sternal infarction in sickle-cell anemia: Concise communication. J Nucl Med 22:322, 1981.
52. Keller MS: Sternal cupping. Radiology 145:854, 1982.
53. Cockshott WP: Rib infarcts in sickling disease. Eur J Radiol 14:63, 1992.
54. Barton CJ, Cockshott WP: Bone changes in hemoglobin SC disease. AJR 88:523, 1962.
55. Reynolds J: Roentgenographic and clinical appraisal of sickle cell hemoglobin C disease. AJR 88:512, 1962.
56. Hurwitz D, Roth H: Sickle cell thalassemia presenting as arthritis of the hip. Arthritis Rheum 13:422, 1970.
57. Ratcliffe RG, Wolf MD: Avascular necrosis of the femoral head associated with sickle cell trait. Ann Intern Med 57:299, 1962.
58. Golding JSR: Conditions of the hip associated with hemoglobinopathies. Clin Orthop 90:22, 1973.
59. Lee REJ, Golding JSR, Sergeant GR: The radiological features of avascular necrosis of the femoral head in homozygous sickle cell disease. Clin Radiol 32:205, 1981.
60. Iwegbu CG, Fleming AF: Avascular necrosis of the femoral head in sickle-cell disease. A series from the Guinea Savannah of Nigeria. J Bone Joint Surg [Br] 67:29, 1985.
61. Sebes JI, Kraus AP: Avascular necrosis of the hip in the sickle cell hemoglobinopathies. J Can Assoc Radiol 34:136, 1983.
62. Pollen AG: Bone changes in haemoglobin S-C disease. Proc R Soc Med 54:822, 1961.
63. Habermann ET, Grayzel AI: Bilateral total knee replacement in a patient with sickle cell disease. Clin Orthop 100:211, 1974.
64. Gunderson C, D'Ambrosia R, Shoji H: Total hip replacement in patients with sickle-cell disease. J Bone Joint Surg [Am] 59:760, 1977.
65. Siffert RS: The growth plate and its affections. J Bone Joint Surg [Am] 48:546, 1966.
66. Trueta J, Amato VP: The vascular contribution of osteogenesis. III. Changes in the growth cartilage caused by experimentally induced ischaemia. J Bone Joint Surg [Br] 42:571, 1960.
67. Bohrer SP: Growth disturbances of the distal femur following sickle cell bone infarcts and/or osteomyelitis. Clin Radiol 25:221, 1974.
68. Hernigou P, Galacteros F, Bachir D, et al: Deformities of the hip in adults who have sickle-cell disease and had avascular necrosis in childhood. A natural history of fifty-two patients. J Bone Joint Surg [Am] 73:81, 1991.
69. Shaub MS, Rosen R, Boswell W, et al: Tibiotalar slant: A new observation in sickle cell anemia. Radiology 117:551, 1975.
70. Leeds NE: Epiphysial dysplasia multiplex. AJR 84:506, 1960.
71. Fairbank T: Dysplasia epiphysialis multiplex. Br J Surg 34:225, 1947.
72. Brewer EJ Jr: Juvenile Rheumatoid Arthritis. Philadelphia: WB Saunders Co., 1970, p 65.
73. Bigongiari L: Pseudotibiotalar slant: A positioning artifact. Radiology 122:699, 1977.
74. Leichtman DA, Bigongiari LR, Wicks JD: The incidence and significance of tibiotalar slant in sickle cell anemia. Skel Radiol 3:99, 1978.
75. Reynolds J: A re-evaluation of the ''fish vertebra'' sign in sickle cell hemoglobinopathy. AJR 97:693, 1966.
76. Moseley JE: Skeletal changes in the anemias. Semin Roentgenol 9:169, 1974.
77. Hansen GC, Gold RH: Central depression of multiple vertebral endplates: A ''pathognomonic'' sign of sickle hemoglobinopathy in Gaucher's disease. AJR 129:343, 1977.
78. Cassady JR, Berdon WE, Baker DH: The ''typical'' spine changes of sickle cell anemia in a patient with thalassemia major (Cooley's anemia). Radiology 89:1065, 1967.
79. Rohlfing BM: Vertebral end-plate depression: Report of two patients with hemoglobinopathy. AJR 128:599, 1977.
80. Riggs W Jr, Rockett JF: Roentgen chest findings in childhood sickle cell anemia. A new vertebral body finding. AJR 104:838, 1968.
81. Mandell GA, Kricun ME: Exaggerated anterior vertebral notching. Radiology 131:367, 1979.
82. Henkin WA: Collapse of the vertebral bodies in sickle cell anemia. AJR 62:395, 1949.
83. Barrett-Connor E: Bacterial infection and sickle cell anemia. An analysis of 250 infections in 166 patients and a review of the literature. Medicine 50:97, 1971.
84. Engh CA, Hughes JL, Abrams RC, et al: Osteomyelitis in the patient with sickle-cell disease. Diagnosis and management. J Bone Joint Surg [Am] 53:1, 1971.
85. Landesman SH, Rao SP, Ahonkhai VI: Infections in children with sickle cell anemia. Special reference to pneumococcal and salmonella infections. Am J Pediatr Hematol Oncol 4:407, 1982.
86. Hand WL, King NL: Deficiency of serum bactericidal activity against Salmonella typhimurium in sickle cell anemia. Clin Exp Immunol 30:262, 1977.
87. Ali S, Kutty S, Kutty K: Recent observations on osteomyelitis in sickle-cell disease. Int Orthop (SICOT) 9:97, 1985.
88. Epps CH Jr, Bryant D'OD III, Coles MJM, et al.: Osteomyelitis in patients who have sickle-cell disease. Diagnosis and management. J Bone Joint Surg [Am] 73:1281, 1991.
89. Schumacher HR: Rheumatological manifestations of sickle cell disease and other hereditary haemoglobinopathies. Clin Rheum Dis 1:37, 1975.
90. Fonk J, Coonrod JD: Serratia osteomyelitis in sickle cell disease. JAMA 217:80, 1971.
91. Hughes J, Carroll D: Salmonella osteomyelitis complicating sickle-cell disease. Pediatrics 19:184, 1957.
92. Roberts AR, Hilburg L: Sickle cell disease with Salmonella osteomyelitis. J Pediat 52:170, 1958.
93. Rubin HM, Eardley W, Nichols BL: Shigella sonnei osteomyelitis and sickle cell anemia. Am J Dis Child 116:83, 1968.
94. Hruby MA, Honig GR, Lolekha S, et al: Arizona hinshawii osteomyelitis in sickle cell anemia. Am J Dis Child 125:867, 1973.
95. Barter SJ, Hennessy O: Actinomycetes as the causative organism of osteomyelitis in sickle cell disease. Skel Radiol 11:271, 1984.
96. Shroyer JV III, Lew D, Abreo F, et al: Osteomyelitis of the mandible as a result of sickle cell disease. Report and literature review. Oral Surg 72:25, 1991.
97. Martino AM, Winfield JA: Salmonella osteomyelitis with epidural abscess. Pediatr Neurosurg 16:321, 1990–1991.
98. Ebong WW, Lagundoye SB, Iyun KO: Sinography in chronic fistulating osteomyelitis in sickle-cell anemia. Clin Radiol 34:347, 1983.
99. Ebong WW: Pathological fracture complicating long bone osteomyelitis in patients with sickle cell disease. J Pediatr Orthop 6:177, 1986.
100. Ebong WW: Acute osteomyelitis in Nigerians with sickle disease. Ann Rheum Dis 45:911, 1986.
101. Palmer DW, Ellman MH, Jacobelli S: Septic arthritis in sickle-cell states: Pathophysiology of impaired response to infection and implications for management. Ann Intern Med 76:870, 1972.

102. Schumacher HR, Andrews R, McLaughlin G: Arthropathy in sickle cell disease. Ann Intern Med 78:203, 1973.
103. Palmer DW, Ellman MH: Septic arthritis and Reiter's syndrome in sickle cell disorders: Case reports and implications for management. South Med J 69:902, 1976.
104. Moxley GF, Owen DS Jr, Irby R: Septic arthritis due to *Fusobacterium varium* in a patient with sickle-cell anemia. J Rheumatol 10:161, 1983.
105. Palmer DW: Septic arthritis in sickle-cell thalassemia. Pathophysiology of impaired response to infection. Arthritis Rheum 18:339, 1975.
106. Warren CPW: Arthritis associated with Salmonella infections. Ann Rheum Dis 29:483, 1970.
107. Berglof FE: Arthritis and intestinal infection. Acta Rheumatol Scand 9:141, 1963.
108. Vartiainen J, Hurri L: Arthritis due to *Salmonella typhimurium*: Report of 12 cases of migratory arthritis in association with *Salmonella typhimurium* infection. Acta Med Scand 175:771, 1964.
109. Ebong WW: The treatment of severely ill patients with sickle cell anemia and associated septic arthritis. Clin Orthop 149:145, 1980.
110. Rodnan GP: Arthritis associated with hematologic disorders. Bull Rheum Dis 16:392, 1965.
111. Espinoza LR, Spilberg I, Osterland CK: Joint manifestations of sickle cell disease. Medicine 53:295, 1974.
112. Talbott JH: Gout and blood dyscrasias. Medicine 38:173, 1959.
113. Ball GV, Sorensen LB: The pathogenesis of hyperuricemia and gout in sickle cell anemia. Arthritis Rheum 13:846, 1970.
114. Aquilina JT, Moynihan JW, Bissell GW, et al: Gout in sickle cell anemia. Arch Interam Rheumatol 1:708, 1968.
115. Gold MS, Williams JC, Spivack M, et al: Sickle cell anemia and hyperuricemia. JAMA 206:1572, 1968.
116. Rothschild BM, Steinknecht CW, Kaplan SB, et al: Sickle cell disease associated with uric acid deposition disease. Ann Rheum Dis 39:392, 1980.
117. Reynolds MD: Gout and hyperuricemia associated with sickle-cell anemia. Semin Arthritis Rheum 12:404, 1983.
118. Walker BR, Alexander F: Uric acid excretion in sickle cell anemia. JAMA 215:255, 1971.
119. Diamond H, Sharon E, Holden D, et al: Renal handling of uric acid in sickle cell anemia. Clin Res 21:551, 1973.
120. Sella EJ, Goodman AH: Arthropathy secondary to transfusion hemochromatosis. J Bone Joint Surg [Am] 55:1077, 1973.
121. Abbott DF, Gresham GA: Arthropathy in transfusional siderosis. Br Med J 1:418, 1972.
122. Alavi A, Schumacher HR, Dowart B, et al: Bone marrow scan evaluation of arthropathy in sickle cell disorders. Arch Intern Med 136:436, 1976.
123. Dorwart BB, Alavi A, Schumacher HR, et al: Bone and bone marrow scans in evaluation of arthropathy of sickle cell disorders. J Rheumatol 1(Suppl 1):22, 1974.
124. Saheb F: Arthropathy in sickle cell disease. N Engl J Med 288:970, 1973.
125. Hanissian AS, Silverman A: Arthritis of sickle cell anemia. South Med J 67:28, 1974.
126. Casey DF, Cathcart ES: Hemarthrosis and sickle cell trait. Arthritis Rheum 13:882, 1970.
127. Goldberg MA: Sickle cell arthropathy: Analysis of synovial fluid in sickle cell anemia with joint effusion. South Med J 66:956, 1973.
128. Orozco-Alcala J, Baum J: Arthritis during sickle-cell crisis. N Engl J Med 288:420, 1973.
129. de Ceulaer K, Forbes M, Roper D, et al: Non-gouty arthritis in sickle cell disease: Report of 37 consecutive cases. Ann Rheum Dis 43:599, 1984.
130. Schumacher HR, Dorwart BB, Bond J, et al: Chronic synovitis with early cartilage destruction in sickle cell disease. Ann Rheum Dis 36:413, 1977.
131. Kanyerezi BR, Ndugwa C, Owor R, et al: The spinal column in sickle cell disease. J Rheumatol 1(Suppl 1):21, 1974.
132. Tanaka KR, Clifford GO, Axelrod AR: Sickle cell anemia (homozygous S) with aseptic necrosis of the femoral head. Blood 11:998, 1956.
133. Dihlmann W. Diagnostic Radiology of the Sacroiliac Joints. New York, George Thieme Verlag, 1980, p 38.
134. Martinez S, Apple JS, Baber C, et al: Protrusio acetabuli in sickle-cell anemia. Radiology 151:43, 1984.
135. Rothschild BM, Sebes JI: Calcaneal abnormalities and erosive bone disease associated with sickle cell anemia. Am J Med 71:427, 1981.
136. White LE, Reeves JD: Polyarthritis and positive LE preparation in sickle hemoglobinopathies: A report of two cases. J Pediatr 95:1003, 1979.
137. Alavi A, Bond JP, Kuhl DE, et al: Scan detection of bone marrow infarcts in sickle cell disorders. J Nucl Med 15:1003, 1974.
138. Lutzker LG, Alavi A: Bone and marrow imaging in sickle cell disease: Diagnosis of infarction. Semin Nucl Med 6:83, 1976.
139. Kim H, Alavi A, Russell MO, et al: Differentiation of bone and bone marrow infarcts from osteomyelitis in sickle cell disorders. Clin Nucl Med 14:249, 1989.
140. Van Dyke D, Shkurkin C, Price D, et al: Differences in distribution of erythropoietic and reticuloendothelial marrow in hematologic disease. Blood 30:364, 1967.
141. Datz FL, Taylor A Jr: The clinical use of radionuclide bone marrow imaging. Semin Nucl Med 15:239, 1985.
142. Van Dyke D, Anger HO: Patterns of marrow hypertrophy and atrophy in man. J Nucl Med 6:109, 1965.
143. Dibos PE, Judisch JM, Spaulding MB, et al: Scanning the reticuloendothelial system in hematological diseases. John Hopkins Med J 130:68, 1972.
144. Nelp WB, Bower RE: The quantitative distribution of the erythron and the RE cell in the bone marrow organ of man. Blood 34:276, 1969.
145. Charache S, Page DL: Infarction of bone marrow in sickle cell disorders. Ann Intern Med 67:1195, 1967.
146. Lisbona R, Rosenthall L: Observations on the sequential use of ^{99m}Tc-phosphate complex and ^{67}Ga imaging in osteomyelitis, cellulitis and septic arthritis. Radiology 123:123, 1977.
147. Armas RR, Goldsmith SJ: Gallium scintigraphy in bone infarction. Correlation with bone imaging. Clin Nucl Med 9:1, 1983.
148. Amundsen TR, Siegel MJ, Siegel BA: Osteomyelitis and infarction in sickle cell hemoglobinopathies: Differentiation by combined technetium and gallium scintigraphy. Radiology 153:807, 1984.
149. Koren A, Garty I, Katzuni E: Bone infarction in children with sickle cell disease: Early diagnosis and differentiation from osteomyelitis. Eur J Pediatr 142:93, 1984.
150. Keeley K, Buchanan GR: Acute infarction of long bones in children with sickle cell anemia. J Pediatr 101:170,1982.
151. Bronn LJ, Paquelet JR, Tetalman MR: Intrathoracic extramedullary hematopoiesis: Appearance on ^{99m}Tc sulfur colloid marrow scan. AJR 134:1254, 1980.
152. Parker LA, Vincent LM, Mauro MA, et al: Extramedullary hematopoiesis. Demonstration by transmission and emission computed tomography. Clin Nucl Med 11:1, 1986.
153. Trubowitz S, Davis S. The Human Bone Marrow: Anatomy, Physiology, and Pathophysiology. Boca Raton, FL:CRC Press, 1982.
154. Gordon MY, Barrett AJ: Bone Marrow Disorders. The Biological Basis of Clinical Problems. Oxford:Blackwell Scientific Publications, 1985.
155. Vogler JB III, Murphy WA: Bone marrow imaging. Radiology 168:679, 1988.
156. Kricun ME: Red-yellow marrow conversion: Its effects on the location of some solitary bone lesions. Skel Radiol 14:10, 1985.
157. Dawson KL, Moore SG, Rowland JM: Age-related marrow changes in the pelvis: MR and anatomic findings. Radiology 183:47, 1992.
158. Moore SG, Dawson KL: Red and yellow marrow in the femur: Age-related changes in appearance at MR imaging. Radiology 175:219, 1990.
159. Ricci C, Cova M, Kang YS, et al: Normal age-related patterns of cellular and fatty bone marrow distribution in the axial skeleton: MR imaging study. Radiology 177:83, 1990.
160. Sebag GH, Moore SG: Effect of trabecular bone on the appearance of marrow in gradient-echo imaging of the appendicular skeleton. Radiology 174:855, 1990.
161. Rosen BR, Fleming DM, Kushner DC, et al: Hematologic bone marrow disorders: Quantitative chemical shift MR imaging. Radiology 169:799, 1988.
162. Moore SG, Bisset GS III, Siegel MJ, et al: Pediatric musculoskeletal MR imaging. Radiology 179:345, 1991.
163. Rao VM, Fishman M, Mitchell DG, et al: Painful sickle cell crisis: Bone marrow patterns observed with MR imaging. Radiology 161:211, 1986.
164. Van Zanten TEG, Van Eps LWS, Golding RP, et al: Imaging the bone marrow with magnetic resonance during a crisis and in chronic forms of sickle cell disease. Clin Radiol 40:486, 1989.
165. Deutsch AL, Mink JH, Rosenfelt FP, et al: Incidental detection of hematopoietic hyperplasia on routine knee MR imaging. AJR 152:333, 1989.
166. Lang PH, Fritz R, Vahlensieck M, et al: Residuales und rekonvertiertes hämatopoetisches knochenmark im distalen Femur. ROFO 156:89, 1992.
167. Shellock FG, Morris E, Deutsch AL, et al: Hematopoietic bone marrow hyperplasia: High prevalence on MR images of the knee in asymptomatic marathon runners. AJR 158:335, 1992.
168. Schuck JE, Czarnecki DJ: MR detection of probable hematopoietic hyperplasia involving the knees, proximal femurs, and pelvis. AJR 153:655, 1989.
169. Ware HE, Brooks AP, Toye R, et al: Sickle cell disease and silent avascular necrosis of the hip. J Bone Joint Surg [Br] 73:947, 1991.
170. Papavasiliou C, Trakadas S, Gouliamos A, et al: Magnetic resonance imaging of marrow heterotopia in haemoglobinopathy. Eur J Radiol 8:50, 1988.
171. Papavasiliou C, Gouliamos A, Vlahos L, et al: CT and MRI of symptomatic spinal involvement by extramedullary haemopoiesis. Clin Radiol 42:91, 1990.
172. Blau S, Hamerman D: Aseptic necrosis of the femoral heads in sickle-A hemoglobin disease. Arthritis Rheum 10:397, 1967.
173. Keeling MM, Lockwood WB, Harris EA: Avascular necrosis and erythrocytosis in sickle cell trait. N Engl J Med 290:442, 1974.
174. Taylor PW, Thorpe WP, Trueblood MC: Osteonecrosis in sickle cell trait. J Rheumatol 13:643, 1986.
175. Jones JP Jr: Discussion. Arthritis Rheum 10:400, 1967.
176. Lally EV, Buckley WM, Claster S: Diaphyseal bone infarctions in a patient with sickle cell trait. J Rheumatol 10:813, 1983.
177. Neel JV, Kaplan E, Zuelzer WW: Further studies on hemoglobin C. I. A description of 3 additional families segregating for hemoglobin C and sickle cell hemoglobin. Blood 8:724, 1953.
178. Itano HA, Neel JV: A new inherited abnormality of human hemoglobin. Proc Natl Acad Sci USA 36:613, 1950.
179. Golding JSR, MacIver JE, Went LN: The bone changes in sickle cell anemia and its genetic variants. J Bone Joint Surg [Brit] 41:711, 1959.
180. Becker JA: Hemoglobin S-C disease. AJR 88:503, 1962.
181. Cockshott WP: Hemoglobin S-C disease. J Fac Radiol 9:211, 1958.
182. Smith EW, Krevans JR: Clinical manifestations of hemoglobin C disorders. Bull Johns Hopkins Hosp 104:17, 1959.

183. Reynolds J, Pritchard JA, Ludders D, et al: Roentgenographic and clinical appraisal of sickle cell beta-thalassemia disease. AJR *118*:378, 1973.

184. Reynolds WA: Benign sickle cell-thalassemia disease and cryptic thalassemia in a Negro family. Ann Intern Med *57*:121, 1962.

185. Hurwitz D, Roth H: Sickle cell-thalassemia presenting as arthritis of the hip. Arthritis Rheum *13*:422, 1970.

186. Reich RS, Rosenberg NJ: Aseptic necrosis of bone in Caucasians with chronic hemolytic anemia due to combined sickling and thalassemia traits. J Bone Joint Surg [Am] *35*:894, 1953.

187. Aksoy M, Lehmann H: Sickle cell-thalassemia disease in South Turkey. Br Med J *1*:734, 1957.

188. Brown DE, Ober WB: Sickle cell thalassemia (microdrepanocytic disease) in pregnancy. Am J Obstet Gynecol *75*:773, 1958.

189. Aksoy M: First observation of homozygous hemoglobin S-alpha thalassemia disease and two types of sickle cell thalassemia disease. Blood *22*:757, 1963.

190. Weiss H, Katz S: Salmonella paravertebral abscess and cervical osteomyelitis in sickle-thalassemia disease. South Med J *63*:339, 1970.

191. Hartfall SJ, Stewart MJ: Massive paravertebral heterotopia of bone marrow in case of acholuric jaundice. J Pathol Bacteriol *37*:455, 1933.

192. Leff RD, Aldo-Benson MA, Fife RS: Tophaceous gout in a patient with sickle cell-thalassemia: Case report and review of the literature. Arthritis Rheum *26*:928, 1983.

193. Ranney HM, Larson DL, McCormack GH Jr: Some clinical, biochemical and genetic observations on hemoglobin C. J Clin Invest *32*:1277, 1953.

194. Cooley TB, Lee P: A series of cases of splenomegaly in children with anemia and peculiar bone changes. Trans Am Pediatr Soc *37*:29, 1925.

195. Weatherall DJ: The thalassemias. *In* JB Stanbury, JB Wyngaarden, DS Fredrickson (Eds): The Metabolic Basis of Inherited Disease. New York:McGraw-Hill, 1978, p 1508.

196. Spritz RA, Forget BG: The thalassemias: Molecular mechanisms of human genetic disease. Am J Hum Genet *35*:333, 1983.

197. Caffey J: Cooley's anemia: A review of the roentgenographic findings in the skeleton. AJR *78*:381, 1957.

198. Hamperl H, Weiss P: Über die spongiöse Hyperostose an Schädeln aus Alt-Peru. Virchows Arch (Pathol Anat) *327*:629, 1955.

199. Sfikakis P, Stamatoyannopoulos G: Bone changes in thalassemia trait. Acta Haematol *29*:193, 1963.

200. Ponec DJ, Resnick D: On the etiology and pathogenesis of porotic hyperostosis of the skull. Invest Radiol *19*:313, 1984.

201. Fernbach SK: Case report 274. Skel Radiol *11*:307, 1984.

202. Lawson JP, Ablow RC, Pearson HA: The ribs in thalassemia. I. The relationship to therapy. Radiology *140*:663, 1981.

203. Lawson JP, Ablow RC, Pearson HA: The ribs in thalassemia. II. The pathogenesis of the changes. Radiology *140*:673, 1981.

204. Whipple GH, Bradford WL: Mediterranean disease—thalassemia (erythroblastic anemias of Cooley). Associated pigment abnormalities simulating hemochromatosis. J Pediatr *9*:279, 1936.

205. Valdez VA, Jacobstein JG: Decreased bone uptake of technetium-99m polyphosphate in thalassemia major. J Nucl Med *21*:47, 1980.

206. Currarino G, Erlandson ME: Premature fusion of epiphyses in Cooley's anemia. Radiology *83*:656, 1964.

207. Dines DM, Canale VC, Arnold WD: Fractures in thalassemia. J Bone Joint Surg [Am] *58*:662, 1976.

208. Lawson JP, Ablow RC, Pearson HA: Premature fusion of the proximal humeral epiphyses in thalassemia. AJR *140*:239, 1983.

209. Exarchou E, Politu C, Vretou E, et al: Fractures and epiphyseal deformities in beat-thalassemia. Clin Orthop *189*:229, 1984.

210. Finsterbush A, Farber I, Mogle P, et al: Fracture patterns in thalassemia. Clin Orthop *192*:132, 1985.

211. Finsterbush A, Farber I, Mogle P: Lower limb pain in thalassemia. J Rheumatol *12*:529, 1985.

212. Shai F, Wallach S, Cohen S, et al: Effects of chronic calcitonin administration on the bone disease of thalassemia. *In* B Frame et al (Eds): Clinical Aspects of Metabolic Bone Disease. International Congress Series No. 270. Amsterdam:Excerpta Medica, 1973.

213. Canale VC, Steinherz P, New M, et al: Endocrine function in thalassemia major. Ann NY Acad Sci *232*:333, 1974.

214. Liakakos D, Karpouzas M, Agathopoulos A: Hyperprolinemia and hyperprolinuria in thalassemia. J Pediatr *73*:419, 1968.

215. March H, Schlyen SM, Schwartz SE: Mediterranean hemopathic syndrome (Cooley's anemia) in adults. Study of a family with unusual complications. Am J Med *13*:46, 1952.

216. Middlebrook JE: Thalassemia in a family of pure German extraction. N Engl J Med *255*:815, 1956.

217. Marcolongo R, Trotta F, Scaramelli M: Beta-thalassemic trait and rheumatoid arthritis. Lancet *1*:1141, 1975.

218. Schlumpf U: Thalassemia minor and aseptic necrosis: A coincidence? Arthritis Rheum *21*:280, 1978.

219. Orzincolo C, Castaldi G, Scutellari PN, et al: Aseptic necrosis of femoral head complicating thalassemia. Skel Radiol *15*:541, 1986.

220. Dorwart BB, Schumacher HR: Arthritis in B thalassemia trait: Clinical and pathological features. Ann Rheum Dis *40*:185, 1981.

221. Gerster J-C, Dardel R, Guggi S: Recurrent episodes of arthritis in thalassemia minor. J Rheumatol *11*:352, 1984.

222. Schlumpf U: Arthritis in thalassemia minor. Arthritis Rheum *27*:1076, 1984.

223. Gorriz L, DeLeon C, Herrero-Beaumont G, et al.: Arthritis in beta-thalassemia minor. Arthritis Rheum *26*:1292, 1983.

224. Knoblich R: Extramedullary hematopoiesis presenting as intrathoracic tumors: Report of a case in a patient with thalassemia minor. Cancer *13*:462, 1960.

225. Pearson HA, Noyes WD: Thalassemia intermedia. Cases in Negro siblings with unusual differences in minor hemoglobin components. Blood *23*:829, 1964.

226. Korsten J, Grossman H, Winchester P, et al: Extramedullary hematopoiesis in patients with thalassemia anemia. Radiology *95*:257, 1970.

227. Winchester PH, Cerwin R, Dische R, et al: Hemosiderin laden lymph nodes. An unusual roentgenographic manifestation of homozygous thalassemia. AJR *118*:222, 1973.

228. Long JA Jr, Doppman JL, Nienhaus AW: Computed tomographic studies of thoracic extramedullary hematopoiesis. J Comput Assist Tomogr *4*:67, 1980.

229. Danza FM, Falappa P, Leone G, et al: Extramedullary hematopoiesis. AJR *139*:837, 1982.

230. Falappa P, Danza FM, Leone G, et al: Thoracic extramedullary hematopoiesis: Evaluation by conventional radiography and computed tomography. Diagn Imaging *51*:19, 1981.

231. Newton KL, McNeeley SG Jr, Novick M: Extramedullary hematopoiesis presenting as a pelvic mass in a patient with B-thalassemia intermedia. JAMA *250*:2178, 1983.

232. Ahmed F, Tobin MS, Cohen DF, et al: Beta thalassemia. Spinal cord compression. NY State J Med *81*:1505, 1981.

233. Gmeinwieser J, Gullotta U, Reiser M, et al: Extramedulläre Hämatopoese als Ursache paravertebraler Tumorbildungen in Thorax. ROFO *137*:68, 1982.

234. Luitjes WF, Braakman R, Ables J: Spinal cord compression in a new homozygous variant of beta-thalassemia. Case report. J Neurosurg *57*:846, 1982.

235. Rossi F, Pincelli G: Computed tomography diagnosis of spinal cord compression secondary to epidural extramedullary hematopoiesis. Diagn Imaging Clin Med *53*:255, 1984.

236. Sproat IA, Dobranowski J, Chen V, et al: Presacral extramedullary hematopoiesis in thalassemia intermedia. J Can Assoc Radiol *42*:278, 1991.

237. Chaljub G, Guinto FC Jr, Crow WN, et al: MR diagnosis of spinal cord compression in beta-thalassemia. Spine *16*:583, 1991.

238. Gouliamos A, Dardoufas C, Papailiou I, et al: Low back pain due to extramedullary hemopoiesis. Neuroradiology *33*:284, 1991.

239. Papavasiliou C, Gouliamos A, Andreou J: The marrow heterotopia in thalassemia. Eur J Radiol *6*:92, 1986.

240. Long JA Jr, Doppman JL, Nienhuis AW: Computed tomographic studies of thoracic extramedullary hematopoiesis. J Comput Assist Tomogr *4*:67, 1980.

241. Lewkow LM, Shah I: Sickle cell anemia and epidural extramedullary hematopoiesis. Am J Med *76*:748, 1984.

242. Lawson JP, Ablow RC, Pearson HA: Calvarial and phalangeal vascular impressions in thalassemia. AJR *143*:641, 1984.

243. Fink IJ, Pastakia B, Barranger JA: Enlarged phalangeal foramina in Gaucher disease and B-thalassemia major. AJR *143*:647, 1984.

244. Benz G, Schmid-Rüter E: Pycnodysostosis with heterozygous beta-thalassemia. Pediatr Radiol *5*:164, 1977.

245. Sculletari PN, Orzincolo C, Tamarozzi R: Xeroradiography in B-thalassemia. Skel Radiol *13*:39, 1985.

246. Parker JA, Jones AG, David MA, et al: Reduced uptake of bone-seeking radiopharmaceuticals related to iron excess. Clin Nucl Med *1*:267, 1976.

247. Choy D, Murray IPC, Hoschi R: The effect of iron on the biodistribution of bone scanning agents in humans. Radiology *140*:197, 1981.

248. Harnsberger HR, Datz FL, Knochel JQ, et al: Failure to detect extramedullary hematopoiesis during bone-marrow imaging with indium-111 or technetium-99m sulfur colloid. J Nucl Med *23*:589, 1982.

249. Mitnick JS, Bosniak MA, Megibow AJ, et al: CT in B-thalassemia: Iron deposition in the liver, spleen and lymph nodes. AJR *136*:1191, 1981.

250. Long JA Jr, Doppman JL, Nienhus AW, et al: Computed tomographic analysis of beta-thalassemic syndromes with hemochromatosis: Pathologic findings with clinical and laboratory correlations. J Comput Assist Tomogr *4*:159, 1980.

251. Price F, Bell H: Spinal cord compression due to extramedullary hematopoiesis. Successful treatment in a patient with long-standing myelofibrosis. JAMA *253*:2876, 1985.

252. Brasch RC, Wesbey GE, Gooding CA, et al: Magnetic resonance imaging of transfusional hemosiderosis complicating thalassemia major. Radiology *150*:767, 1984.

253. Goldberg HI, Cann CE, Moss AA, et al: Noninvasive quantification of liver iron in dogs with hemochromatosis using dual-energy CT scanning. Invest Radiol *17*:375, 1982.

254. Moon KL Jr, Genant HK, Helms CA, et al: Musculoskeletal applications of nuclear magnetic resonance. Radiology *147*:161, 1983.

255. Smith FW: The value of NMR imaging in pediatric practice: A preliminary report. Pediatr Radiol *13*:141, 1983.

256. Cohen MD, Klatte EC, Baehner R, et al: Magnetic resonance imaging of bone marrow disease in children. Radiology *151*:715, 1984.

257. Brody AS, Sorette MP, Gooding CA, et al: Induced alignment of flowing sickle erythrocytes in a magnetic field. A preliminary report. Invest Radiol *20*:560, 1985.

258. Steinberg MH, Adams JG: Thalassemic hemoglobinopathies. Am J Pathol *113*:396, 1983.

259. DeVirgiliis S, Congia M, Frau F, et al: Deferoxamine-induced growth retardation in patients with thalassemia major. J Pediatr *113*:661, 1988.

260. Brill PW, Winchester P, Giardina PJ, et al: Deferoxamine-induced bone dysplasia in patients with thalassemia major. AJR *156*:561, 1991.

261. Orzincolo C, Scutellari PN, Castaldi G: Growth plate injury of the long bones in treated beta-thalassemia. Skel Radiol *21*:39, 1992.

262. Kassner EG: Drug-related complications in infants and children: Imaging features. AJR *157*:1039, 1991.

263. Britton HA, Canby JP, Kohler CM: Iron deficiency anemia producing evidence of marrow hyperplasia in the calvarium. Pediatrics *25*:621, 1960.

264. Burko H, Mellins HZ, Watson J: Skull changes in iron deficiency anemia simulating congenital hemolytic anemia. AJR *86*:447, 1961.

265. Agarwal KN, Dhar N, Shar MM, et al: Roentgenologic changes in iron deficiency anemia. AJR *110*:635, 1970.

266. El-Najjar MY, Lozoff B, Ryan DJ: The paleoepidemiology of porotic hyperostosis in the American southwest: Radiological and ecological considerations. AJR *125*:918, 1975.

267. Eng LIL: Chronic iron deficiency anemia with bone changes resembling Cooley's anemia. Acta Haematol *19*:263, 1958.

268. Girdany BR, Gaffney PC: Skull changes in nutritional anemia in infancy. Proc Soc Pediatr Res 1952, p 49.

269. Prasad AS, Halsted JA, Nadimi M: Syndrome of iron deficiency anemia, hepatosplenomegaly, hypogonadism, dwarfism, and geophagia. Am J Med *31*:532, 1961.

270. Aksoy M, Camli N, Erdem S: Roentgenographic bone changes in chronic iron deficiency anemia. Blood *27*:677, 1966.

271. Lanzkowsky P: Radiological features of iron deficiency anemia. Am J Dis Child *116*:16, 1968.

272. Hrdlicka A: Anthropological work in Peru in 1913 with notes on the pathology of the ancient Peruvians. Smithsonian Misc Coll *16*:18, 1914.

273. Welcker H: Criba orbitalia ein ethnologische-diagnostisches Merkmal am Schadel mehrerer Menschenrassen. Arch Anthropol *17*:1, 1888.

274. Moseley JE: The paleopathologic riddle of "symmetrical osteoporosis." AJR *95*:135, 1965.

275. Von Endt DW, Ortner DJ: Amino acid analysis of bone from a possible case of prehistoric iron deficiency anemia from the American Southwest. Am J Phys Anthropol *59*:377, 1982.

276. Croom RD III, McMillan CW, Sheldon GF, et al: Hereditary spherocytosis. Recent experience and current concepts of pathophysiology. Ann Surg *203*:34, 1986.

277. Young LE, Izzo MJ, Platzer RF: Hereditary spherocytosis. I. Clinical, hematologic and genetic features in 28 cases with particular reference to the osmotic and mechanical fragility of incubated erythrocytes. Blood *6*:1073, 1951.

278. Snelling CE, Brown A: Case of hemolytic jaundice with bone changes. J Pediatr *8*:330, 1936.

279. Becker MH, Genieser NB, Piomelli S, et al: Roentgenographic manifestations of pyruvate kinase deficiency hemolytic anemia. AJR *113*:491, 1971.

280. Bowman HS, Procopio F: Hereditary non-spherocytic hemolytic anemia of the pyruvate kinase deficient type. Ann Intern Med *58*:567, 1963.

281. Davis S, Trubowitz S: Marrow aplasia. *In* S Trubowitz, S Davis (Eds): the Human Bone Marrow: Anatomy, Physiology, and Pathophysiology. Boca Raton, FL:CRC Press, 1982, p 211.

282. Kaplan PA, Asleson RJ, Klassen LW, et al: Bone marrow patterns in aplastic anemia: Observations with 1.5-T MR imaging. Radiology *164*:441, 1987.

283. Janus WL, Dietz MW: Osseous changes in erythroblastosis fetalis (21 cases). Radiology *53*:39, 1949.

284. Hellman LM, Irving FC: X-ray diagnosis of erythroblastosis. Surg Gynecol Obstet *67*:296, 1938.

285. Follis RH Jr, Jackson D, Carnes WH: Skeletal changes associated with erythroblastosis fetalis. J Pediatr *21*:80, 1942.

286. Fanconi G: Familiäre infantile perniziosa-artige Anämie (pernizioses Blutbild und Konstitution). Jahrb Kinderheilkd *117*:257, 1927.

287. Juhl JH, Wesenberg RL, Gwinn JL: Roentgenographic findings in Fanconi's anemia. Radiology *89*:646, 1967.

288. Dawson JP: Congenital pancytopenia associated with multiple congenital anomalies (Fanconi type). Review of literature and report of a 20-year-old female with 10-year follow up and apparently good response to splenectomy. Pediatrics *15*:325, 1955.

289. Dell PC, Sheppard JE: Thrombocytopenia, absent radius syndrome. Report of two siblings and a review of the hematologic and genetic features. Clin Orthop *162*:129, 1982.

290. Leclerc J, Toth J: Thrombocytopenia with absent radii. Can Med Assoc J *126*:506, 1982.

291. Schoenecker PL, Cohn AK, Sedgwick WG, et al: Dysplasia of the knee associated with the syndrome of thrombocytopenia and absent radius. J Bone Joint Surg [Am] *66*:421, 1984.

292. Hall JG, Levin J, Kuhn JP, et al: Thrombocytopenia with absent radius (TAR). Medicine *48*:411, 1969.

293. Kelly TE, Stelling CB: Dyskeratosis congenita: Radiologic features. Pediatr Radiol *12*:31, 1982.

294. Steier W, Van Voolen GA, Selmanowitz VJ: Dyskeratosis congenita: Relationship to Fanconi's anemia. Blood *39*:510, 1972.

295. Loiacono PJ, Reeder MM: An exercise in radiologic-pathologic correlation. Radiology *92*:385, 1969.

296. Liberman UA, Samuel R, Halabe A, et al: Juvenile metabolic gout caused by chronic compensated hemolytic syndrome. Arthritis Rheum *25*:1264, 1982.

297. Sarwar M, Virapongse C, Kier EL: Nature of vertex striations on lateral skull radiographs. Radiology *146*:90, 1983.

298. Hardy JB, Hartmann JR: Tuberculous dactylitis in childhood: Prognosis. J Pediatr *30*:146, 1947.

299. Herzfeld G, Tod MC: Tuberculous dactylitis in infancy. Arch Dis Child *1*:295, 1926.

300. Strenstrom B: Tuberculosis of phalanges in older individuals. Acta Radiol *16*:471, 1935.

301. Feldman F, Auerbach R, Johnston A: Tuberculous dactylitis in the adult. AJR *112*:460, 1971.

302. Edelstein G, Kyriakos M: Focal hematopoietic hyperplasia of the rib—a form of pseudotumor. Skel Radiol *11*:108, 1984.

303. Foster JBT: Primary thoracic myelolipoma. Arch Pathol *65*:295, 1958.

304. David HG, Bridgman SA, Davies SC, et al: The shoulder in sickle-cell disease. J Bone Joint Surg [Br] *75*:538, 1993.

305. Piehl FC, Davis RJ, Prugh SI: Osteomyelitis in sickle cell disease. J Pediatr Orthop *13*:225, 1993.

306. Schumacher HR Jr, Van Linthoudt D, Manno CS, et al: Diffuse chondrolytic arthritis in sickle cell disease. J Rheumatol *20*:385, 1993.

307. Lang PH, Fritz R, Majumdar S, et al: Hematopoietic bone marrow in the adult knee: Spin-echo and opposed-phase gradient-echo MR imaging. Skel Radiol *22*:95, 1993.

308. Mirowitz SA: Hematopoietic bone marrow within the proximal humeral epiphysis in normal adults: Investigation with MR imaging. Radiology *188*:689, 1993.

309. Katsanis E, Luke K-H, Hsu E, et al: Hemoglobin E: A common hemoglobinopathy among children of Southeast Asian origin. Can Med Assoc J *137*:39, 1987.

310. Forget BG: The pathophysiology and molecular genetics of beta-thalassemia. Mt Sinai J Med *60*:95, 1993.

311. Borenstein ZCF, Hyman CB, Rimoin DL, et al: Case report 744. Skel Radiol *21*:534, 1993.

312. Gelfand MJ, Daya SA, Rucknagel DL, et al: Simultaneous occurrence of rib infarction and pulmonary infiltrates in sickle cell disease patients with acute chest syndrome. J Nucl Med *34*:614, 1993.

313. Hernigou P, Bachir D, Galacteros F: Avascular necrosis of the femoral head in sickle-cell disease. Treatment of collapse by the injection of acrylic cement. J Bone Joint Surg [Br] *75*:875, 1993.

314. Mirowitz SA, Apicella P, Reinus WR, et al: MR imaging of bone marrow lesions: Relative conspicuousness on T1-weighted, fat-suppressed T2-weighted, and STIR images. AJR *162*:215, 1994.

315. Kaneko K, Humbert JH, Kogutt MS, et al: Iron deposition in cranial bone marrow with sickle cell disease: MR assessment using a fat suppression technique. Pediatr Radiol *23*:435, 1993.

316. Feldman F, Zwass A, Staron RB, et al: MRI of soft tissue abnormalities: A primary cause of sickle cell crisis. Skeletal Radiol *22*:501, 1993.

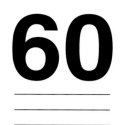

60

Plasma Cell Dyscrasias and Dysgammaglobulinemias

Donald Resnick, M.D.

Plasma cells are the functional unit of the immune defense system. They are found in various areas of the human body, particularly the lymph nodes, the spleen, the bone marrow, and the submucosa of the gastrointestinal tract, and they are responsible for antibody synthesis.[1] Plasma cells are derived from B lymphocytes and are the principal source of immunoglobulins, proteins of high molecular weight, which function as antibodies as they circulate throughout the tissues. In the normal bone marrow, plasma cells represent a small percentage of the nucleated cells. In the presence of infectious disease (as well as other disorders), the number of plasma cells in the bone marrow increases, resulting in a similar increase in the production of immunoglobulins. This response is termed plasmacytosis and is a normal consequence of infection or other processes that result in antigenic stimulation. In the normal adult, plasma cells are distributed strategically at the site of entry of antigens; their proliferation, resulting in plasmacytosis, occurs most typically in the tonsils, upper respiratory tract, mucosal surfaces of the gastrointestinal tract, and cervix and is accompanied by local inflammatory changes.[2] Criteria for the diagnosis of plasmacytosis are as follows: an increase of the plasma cell population in the bone marrow; the presence of a clinical disease that is known to be associated with an acute or chronic immune reaction; and no clinical evidence of a malignant plasma cell dyscrasia (see following discussion).[2] When plasma cell proliferation appears as an inappropriate or uncontrolled event, a disease state exists. Several diseases can be manifested in this fashion and are grouped together as plasma cell dyscrasias.[3, 4] The clinical manifestations of these diseases are attributable to the effects of expanding collections of cells or abnormal accumulations of substances produced by these cells. Plasma cell dyscrasias include multiple myeloma (in which there is an increase in plasma cells), Waldenström's macroglobulinemia (in which there is an increase in plasmacytoid lymphocytes), and amyloidosis (in which there is deposition in tissue of a specific immunoglobulin). Other plasma cell dyscrasias exist but most of these are not appropriately discussed here. Related conditions such as agammaglobulinemia and hypogammaglobulinemia are associated with a decrease in concentration of plasma gamma globulins and a concomitant impairment of antibody formation.

This chapter summarizes skeletal manifestations of certain plasma cell dyscrasias and dysgammaglobulinemias.

OVERVIEW

An understanding of the specific plasma cell dyscrasias that are described subsequently requires an initial review of some basic concepts and definitions. Following is a synopsis of such concepts, derived principally from a summary by Osserman.[5]

Plasma cell dyscrasias are characterized by the uncontrolled proliferation of plasma cells in the absence of an identifiable antigenic stimulus; the elaboration of electrophoretically and structurally homogeneous monoclonal, M type (plasma cell myeloma, macroglobulinemia) gamma globulins or excessive quantities of homogeneous polypeptide subunits of these proteins (Bence Jones proteins, H chains), or both; and a commonly associated deficiency in the synthesis of normal immunoglobulins.[5] Some of these dyscrasias, such as plasma cell myeloma, macroglobulinemia, amyloidosis, and heavy chain diseases, have a typical constellation of clinical manifestations that permits specific diagnosis, whereas others initially or ultimately defy precise classification. Disease states in the latter category include premyeloma, essential hypergammaglobulinemia, essential cryoglobulinemia, dysgammaglobulinemia, and idiopathic monoclonal gammopathy.[6]

Plasma cell dyscrasias result in the synthesis of large quantities of a single protein related to one of the major classes of immunoglobulins. Five antigenetically distinct, major classes of immunoglobulins are recognized: IgG, IgM, IgA, IgD, IgE. All of these consist of two identical heavy (H) chains linked to two identical light (L) chains. The type of immunoglobulin that is being elaborated abnormally can be identified by its electrophoretic pattern and varies among the plasma cell dyscrasias. For example, in patients with multiple myeloma, IgG predominates (approximately 55 per cent of cases), followed, in order of decreasing frequency, by IgA, IgD, IgM, and IgE. In Waldenström's macroglobulinemia, the elaboration of large amounts of IgM globulins is apparent. Furthermore, a subunit of one of these proteins may be identified in some of these dyscrasias; in multiple myeloma, large quantities of Bence Jones proteins (representing free light chains) are common and may be identified in the urine in approximately 50 per cent of cases.

In the pages that follow, attention is directed toward those plasma cell dyscrasias that possess distinctive clinical and pathologic features. Other dyscrasias that are clinically occult, transient, or associated with another chronic disease, such as infection, are not included.

PLASMA CELL MYELOMA

Background

Plasma cell myeloma (myelomatosis, Kahler's disease, plasmacytic myeloma, multiple myeloma, plasmacytoma) is a malignant disease of plasma cells that usually originates in the bone marrow but may involve other tissues as well.[7]

The first recorded patient with this disease was found in 1845 to have pain, and it was noted that his urine contained unusual ''animal'' matter that become soluble as the urine was heated.[8] The term multiple myeloma was originated in 1873 by Rustizky.[7] Subsequent steps in the history of this disease were the discovery of the plasma cell by Cajal in 1890, the recognition by Wright in 1900 that the myeloma tumor consisted of plasma cells, and the investigation of the disorder by electrophoretic techniques in 1939[9] and by immunoelectrophoresis in 1953.[10]

Clinical Features

Plasma cell myeloma is a common disease.[11] It has been estimated that this tumor represents approximately 1 per cent of all malignancies and 10 to 15 per cent of malignancies of the hematologic system. Its prevalence is underscored by the frequency of its appearance in tumor collections; at the Mayo Clinic, 43 per cent of all malignant bone tumors were myelomas.[12] The disease usually occurs between the ages of 25 and 80 years, predominantly in older patients.[7, 13] The average age of involved patients is 60 to 70 years. Myeloma is rare in childhood[14–16] and is unusual in persons below the age of 40 years.[17] It appears to be slightly more common in men than in women, although some series report a female predominance.[18] An even more striking male predilection may be seen in cases of solitary myeloma (single lesion).[19] Myeloma is particularly common in blacks.[20]

There are many symptoms and signs related to this disease,[21] although, infrequently, patients with multiple myeloma are asymptomatic (indolent or smoldering disease).[22] In large part, clinical manifestations are a consequence of excessive proliferation of abnormal plasma cells, creating a mechanical burden that compromises the skeleton by displacing and eroding bony trabeculae.[1] Symptoms include bone pain, particularly of the back and chest, which is sudden in onset and aggravated by movement, weakness, fatigue, and the presence of deformities such as exaggerated kyphosis and loss of height. Additionally, fever, weight loss, bleeding, and neurologic signs may be seen. Of these symptoms, bone pain represents the most persistent and incapacitating finding. Physical signs include fever, pallor, purpura, hepatosplenomegaly, bone tenderness, and extramedullary tumefaction, frequently in the nasopharynx, nasal fossa, and soft palate.[18, 23] With coexistent amyloidosis, additional clinical manifestations may be the result of macroglossia or cardiac and renal failure.

Laboratory investigation outlines moderate or severe anemia, elevated erythrocyte sedimentation rate, a normal or slightly elevated leukocyte count, a positive Coombs' test (10 per cent), thrombocytopenia (13 per cent), and a positive serologic test for rheumatoid factor (8 per cent).[7] Hypercalcemia (25 to 50 per cent) and hyperuricemia may be observed. Renal insufficiency[24] may lead to an elevated serum creatinine concentration.

Most patients with plasma cell myeloma demonstrate an increase in the total serum protein, usually due to an increase in the globulin fraction. Serum electrophoresis confirms the abnormality of the globulin fraction in 80 to 90 per cent of patients with multiple lesions. When patients with plasma cell myeloma are grouped according to the type of protein produced by the tumor, approximately 55 to 60 per cent have IgG myeloma, 20 per cent have IgA myeloma, and 1 to 2 per cent have IgD myeloma,[25] whereas IgE and IgM myelomas are rare. The IgM globulin contains cold agglutinins and rheumatoid factor and is associated with Waldenström's macroglobulinemia. Accumulation of a light chain protein may be observed in 20 to 25 per cent of patients. On rare occasions (approximately 1 per cent of cases), no abnormal protein is observed, a phenomenon called nonsecretory myeloma.[26–29] Some investigators have attempted to correlate the specific immunoglobulin production with radiologic manifestations and progress of the disease.[29, 30] IgD appears to represent a more severe form of the disease associated with decreased life expectancy. IgG myeloma may have a poorer prognosis than does IgA myeloma. Myeloma associated with light chain accumulation can have a fulminant course characterized by severe and widespread bone destruction and hypercalcemia.[1] Nonsecretory myeloma, which often is accompanied by hypogammaglobulinemia, has been characterized by sepsis, widespread osteolytic lesions, and the absence of renal complications.

Urinary electrophoresis is an important laboratory examination in patients with myeloma, as it may demonstrate abnormalities when the serum electrophoretic pattern is entirely normal. Bence Jones proteinuria is apparent in 40 to 60 per cent of patients with this disease. Excretion of these proteins (light chains) can lead to damage of the proximal renal tubules, which may be attributable to a toxic effect of the protein on renal tubular epithelium.[31] Fanconi's syndrome, characterized by urinary loss of sugar, amino acids, and phosphates[32, 33] and radiographic evidence of osteomalacia, can appear in patients with myeloma and amyloidosis.

Increased serum viscosity is a common feature in plasma cell myeloma.[7] This manifestation in general can be attributed to the large molecular size of certain immunoglobulins, such as IgG and IgM. As abnormal levels of IgM are characteristic of Waldenström's macroglobulinemia, it is not surprising that serum hyperviscosity is a frequent manifestation of this disease.[34] Symptoms and signs may become apparent when the viscosity of the serum increases to 5 or 6. The clinical manifestations include bleeding, particularly of the oronasal area, decrease of visual acuity, retinopathy, dizziness, confusion, neurologic symptoms, and congestive heart failure.[34, 35] Hyperviscosity can lead to bone infarction in patients with myeloma and macroglobulinemia.[1]

Additional laboratory studies that are important in establishing a diagnosis of plasma cell myeloma are bone biopsy and bone marrow aspiration. Plasmacytosis of the marrow is evident, which is associated with cellular immaturity, increased pleomorphism, and frequent mitoses. These features are important, as some degree of marrow plasmacytosis can accompany cases of carcinoma, connective tissue diseases, liver disorders, infection, and hypersensitivity states,[7, 36, 37] but additional cellular characteristics as noted previously usually are not prominent. Marrow involvement in myeloma is most frequent in the vertebrae, pelvis, ribs, and skull and less common in the sternum, clavicles, and proximal ends of the femora and humeri.[21] A negative bone marrow aspirate does not exclude the diagnosis of myeloma.[38] Furthermore, as indicated previously, the presence of plasma cell infiltration on marrow analysis does not, in itself, confirm the diagnosis of myeloma, although the presence of more than 10 per cent of plasma cells in a given specimen is suggestive and more than 40 per cent is indicative of plasma cell myeloma.[2]

The major causes of death in patients with myeloma are infection and renal failure.

Pathogenesis

The cause of the plasma cell proliferation in plasma cell myeloma is unknown. Although virus-like particles have been demonstrated in the cytoplasm of murine myeloma cells,[39] convincing evidence is lacking that an infectious agent is the cause of this disorder. It also has been shown that plasma cell proliferation can be induced by chronic inflammation: In C_3H mice, plasma cell collections can be seen adjacent to ileocecal ulcers; in this same rodent, plasma cell tumors in peritoneal or mediastinal lymph nodes can be produced by intraperitoneal injections of certain foreign substances.[40, 41] Another suggested etiologic factor in the development of plasma cell proliferation is that plasma cell myeloma may be related to chronic myeloproliferative disorders. Although this theory gains some credence from the observation of both myeloma and polycythemia vera in the same patient,[42] this association, which is indeed rare, may be purely coincidental.

Several instances of familial multiple myeloma have been documented,[11, 43, 44] perhaps indicating a genetic predisposition for the disease. An observed tendency for increased polyclonal immunoglobulin levels in close relatives of patients with myeloma[45] supports this concept, although familial clustering of cases does not eliminate the possible importance of environmental factors or infection in the causation of myeloma.

Whatever the cause of plasmacytosis in this disease, abnormal accumulation of plasma cells in myeloma is associated with single or multiple areas of bone lysis. Focal intraosseous collections of plasma cells are surrounded by areas of increased osteoclastic activity. Initially, this osteoclastosis was attributed to differentiation of plasma cells into osteoclasts, although it is now known that plasma cells can produce an osteoclastic stimulating factor (see Chapter 20) that may be responsible for the osteolytic lesions that are characteristic of myeloma.[46, 47] This factor also leads to inhibition of osteoblasts, although some investigators believe that another humeral factor, an osteoblast inhibiting factor, accounts for the poor or absent osteoblastic response that is characteristic of plasma cell myeloma.[48] Plasma cell infiltration is first apparent in the axial skeleton, at which site it leads to destruction of marrow. The body responds to this decrease in active marrow by reconversion of yellow to red marrow in the appendicular skeleton.[1] Eventually plasma cells invade peripheral skeletal sites as well. With increased cellular proliferation, extensive bone destruction, pathologic fractures, and hypercalcemia become evident.[49] The appearance of the lytic lesions may vary from well-defined to poorly defined areas, perhaps reflecting the relative virulence of the individual clone of plasma cells.[1] Patients with poorly defined lesions may have a poorer prognosis than those with well-defined lytic defects.[29]

Radiologic Features

General Abnormalities. The radiologic manifestations of plasma cell myeloma are well known.[13, 50–54] In almost all patients, the predominant pattern is osteolysis. Rarely, focal or diffuse sclerotic lesions are seen.[55–66] Although multiple sites of involvement are characteristic, solitary lesions, or plasmacytomas, may exist for prolonged periods of time.

Typically, the axial skeleton is the predominant site of abnormality (Fig. 60–1). Multiple lesions most commonly are apparent in the vertebral column, ribs, skull, pelvis, and femur, in descending order of frequency. Solitary plasmacytomas reveal a similar distribution, although well over 50 per cent of these lesions are localized in the vertebrae, followed by the pelvis, skull, sternum, and ribs.[50] Diffuse lesions of the appendicular skeleton have been described in plasma cell myeloma,[67, 68] usually accompanying extensive involvement of the axial skeleton. Rarely, plasma cell myeloma affecting exclusively the appendicular skeleton has been noted,[69, 70] almost invariably in association with lesions of central hematopoietic sites (myelofibrosis). Mandibular abnormalities are observed in approximately one third of patients with myeloma and may be the first bony manifestation of the disease.[71–73]

Because both myeloma and metastatic skeletal disease are associated with destructive bone lesions in middle-aged

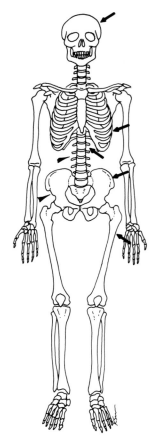

FIGURE 60–1. Plasma cell myeloma: Distribution of abnormalities. The most common sites of multiple lesions of myeloma are indicated on the right half of the diagram (arrows). These include the spine, the pelvis, the ribs, and the skull. The most common sites of solitary plasmacytoma are indicated on the left (arrowheads). These include the spine and the pelvis.

and elderly patients, differentiation between these two conditions may be difficult. Classically, multiple myeloma first is manifested as widespread osteolytic lesions with discrete margins, which appear uniform in size (Fig. 60–2). These characteristic morphologic features are seen much less frequently in bone metastasis. The more chronic and slowly progressive the myelomatous involvement, the more discrete and punched-out the areas of lysis. In unusual cases, a shell of bony condensation appears as a sclerotic rim about the lesion. Although smaller areas may coalesce into larger segments of destruction, such large foci more commonly are seen in skeletal metastasis.

Particularly distinctive in plasma cell myeloma is a subcortical circular or elliptical radiolucent shadow, most often observed in the long tubular bones. An associated mild periosteal proliferation may act as a buttress, preventing or resisting fracture. The subcortical defects cause erosion of the inner margins of the cortex and, when extensive, create a scalloped and wavy contour throughout the endosteal bone. This appearance is highly suggestive of plasma cell myeloma, is occasionally seen in cases of rapid and aggressive osteoporosis, and is unusual in skeletal metastasis, in which rapid cortical expansion and disruption are more characteristic. Expansile bony lesions of considerable size can be seen in both plasma cell myeloma and skeletal metastasis.

Diffuse skeletal osteopenia without well-defined areas of lysis also can be observed in plasma cell myeloma, a pattern of involvement that is infrequent with metastasis but that can simulate the appearance of osteoporosis (Fig. 60–3).

Sclerosis in plasma cell myeloma generally is seen after pathologic fracture, irradiation, or chemotherapy of lytic lesions, although occasionally it can be noted in conjunction with intact and untreated lesions (Fig. 60–4). Bone sclerosis may occur as a solitary focus or as multiple foci. Solitary sclerotic lesions are more common in the ribs, sternum, and ilium, although additional sites include the skull, long bones, and vertebrae. Diffuse sclerosis is apparent in fewer than 3 per cent of patients with plasma cell myeloma (Fig. 60–5). It can simulate the appearance of osteoblastic metastasis, lymphoma, mastocytosis, renal osteodystrophy, and myelofibrosis. Myeloma also has been described in association with other myeloproliferative disorders, including myelofibrosis,[74, 75] polycythemia vera, and myelogenous leukemia.[76] Sclerotic myeloma has been reported to occur in younger persons and is known to be associated with peripheral neuropathy. The cause of osteosclerosis in plasma cell myeloma is unknown, although it is attractive to postulate that the plasma cell, already known to secrete an osteoclast activating factor, may infrequently produce a factor that either inhibits osteoclasts or stimulates osteoblasts, or does both. On histologic examination, plasma cell infiltration and bone marrow fibrosis are observed. Markedly thickened trabeculae surrounding immature plasma cells[59] may reflect a bone-forming action of these cells. Although in most patients, the prognosis of "sclerotic" myeloma is identical to that of "lytic" myeloma, some reports have indicated a more favorable clinical course in patients with sclerotic myeloma as well as higher serum levels of alkaline phosphatase.[65]

Plasma cell myeloma involving bone, particularly in the ribs or vertebral column, often initiates the formation of an

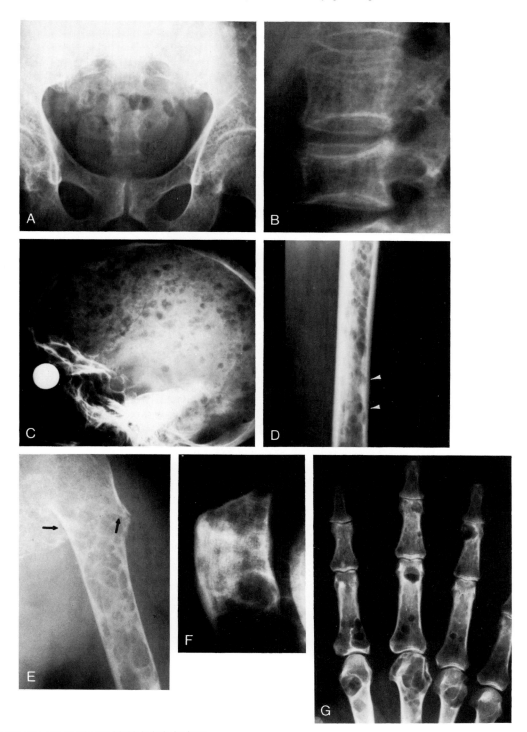

FIGURE 60–2. Plasma cell myeloma: Multiple lytic lesions.

A Pelvis. Although the major radiographic pattern is one of diffuse osteopenia, some lytic lesions can be identified, particularly in the ilium, the ischium, and the pubis.

B Spine. On a lateral radiograph of the lumbar spine, observe lytic lesions of multiple vertebral bodies with evidence of vertebral compression. Pediculate involvement is mild.

C Skull. Well-circumscribed radiolucent lesions without surrounding sclerosis are obvious. They are relatively uniform in size, a feature that is more suggestive of myeloma than skeletal metastasis. The radiodense area overlying the orbit represents an eye prosthesis.

D Femur. On this frontal radiograph, striking radiolucent lesions are seen throughout the diaphysis, producing scalloping of the endosteal margin of the cortex (arrowheads). This latter feature is particularly characteristic of plasma cell myeloma.

E Humerus. "Bubbly" bone lysis is evident. A pathologic fracture with deformity of the proximal humerus can be observed (arrows).

F Patella. Note the radiolucent lesions of the patella on this lateral radiograph.

G Hand. An unusual case in which lytic lesions predominated in the appendicular skeleton. Observe the well-defined lucent areas in the metacarpals and phalanges. A thin rim of sclerosis is evident about some of the lesions.

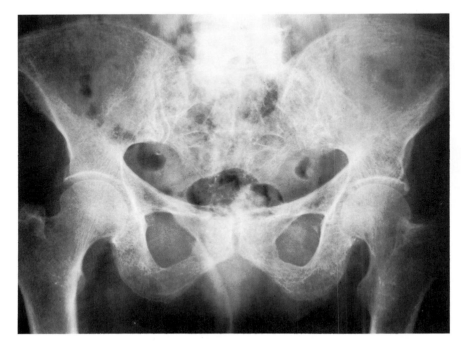

FIGURE 60–3. Plasma cell myeloma: Diffuse osteopenia. A radiograph of the pelvis reveals increased radiolucency of the skeleton and a coarsened trabecular pattern. There is no evidence of discrete lytic lesions. The pattern resembles that in osteoporosis or osteomalacia.

FIGURE 60–4. Plasma cell myeloma: Osteosclerosis.
   A Skull. A lytic lesion of the cranial vault is associated with a sclerotic rim.
   B Femur. A larger lesion of the proximal femur contains lucent and sclerotic areas.

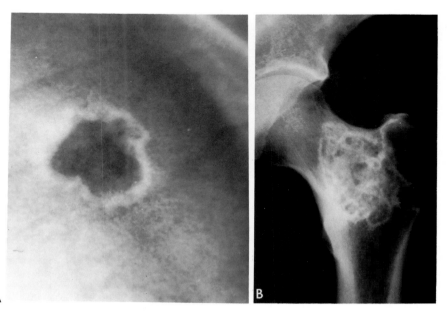

A   B

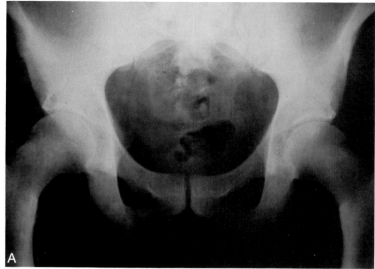
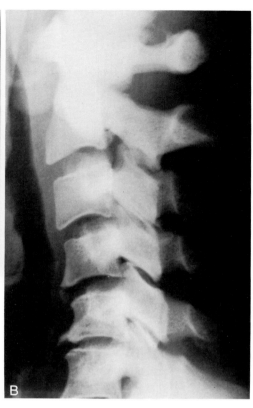

FIGURE 60–5. Plasma cell myeloma: Osteosclerosis. In this 70 year old man diffuse osteosclerosis is seen in the pelvis, proximal portion of the femora, and cervical spine.

adjacent soft tissue mass. Extensive paraspinal, intraspinal, or extrapleural masses are observed, which may seem out of proportion to the degree of bony disease, leading to an incorrect diagnosis of a primary pulmonary, mediastinal, or retroperitoneal neoplasm.

Specific Sites of Involvement. In the skull, numerous discrete lytic areas of uniform size are more common in plasma cell myeloma than in skeletal metastasis. Solitary cranial lesions do occur with plasma cell myeloma but are unusual. Myeloma may demonstrate a predilection for mandibular involvement (Fig. 60–6), an uncommon site for skeletal metastasis. Sternal involvement in myeloma is not infrequent and may lead to pathologic fracture.[77] Sternal fracture or collapse is associated with increasing thoracic

kyphosis related to vertebral compression in this disease (as well as in generalized osteoporosis).

In the spine, preferential destruction of the vertebral bodies with sparing of the posterior elements has been emphasized as a differential point favoring the diagnosis of myeloma rather than osteolytic metastasis.[78] Paraspinal and extradural extension of tumor is quite characteristic of myeloma. Scalloping of the anterior margins of the vertebral bodies is noted in both plasma cell myeloma and metastasis, perhaps related to osseous pressure from adjacent enlarged lymph nodes.

The frequency with which plasma cell myeloma involves the shoulder and elbow regions deserves emphasis (Fig. 60–7). Preferential involvement of the distal end of the clavicle,

FIGURE 60–6. Plasma cell myeloma: Mandibular involvement. Radiolucent lesions of the mandible (arrows) are distributed about the groove for the intraosseous nerves and vessels (arrowheads). Involvement of this bone is more common in plasma cell myeloma than in skeletal metastasis.

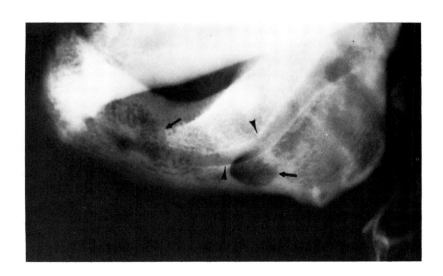

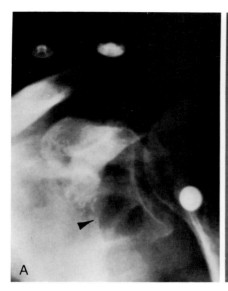

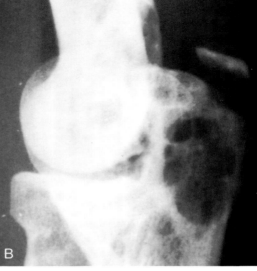

FIGURE 60–7. Plasma cell myeloma: Shoulder and elbow involvement.
  A Shoulder. Observe extensive destruction of the glenoid and adjacent scapula (arrowhead).
  B Elbow. Lytic lesions of the distal portion of the humerus, proximal part of the radius, and the ulna are seen. The largest lesion in the ulnar olecranon is associated with a pathologic fracture with displacement.

acromion, glenoid, and ulnar olecranon is seen, whereas this distribution is less common in metastatic disease involving the skeleton.

Pathologic Features

Myelomatous involvement of the skeleton is variable in extent, predominates in regions of red marrow but may affect areas of yellow marrow as well, and is manifested as discrete or homogeneous tumor masses, which are red or gray on gross pathologic examination[50] (Fig. 60–8). Such involvement may be observed in any bone of the human skeleton, even the laryngeal bones.[2] Smaller lesions are observed in cancellous bone, although they may be eccentric or subcortical in location. Larger lesions may involve the cortex, penetrate the periosteum, and extend into the surrounding soft tissues. This typically is seen in paracostal and paravertebral regions, although additional sites, including areas about the spinal cord, sometimes are affected. Pathologic documentation of such extraosseous extension is accomplished in approximately 50 per cent of cases.[21] Distant extraosseous involvement is most common in the spleen, liver, and lymph nodes, followed, in order of decreasing frequency, by the lungs, pleura, kidneys, adrenal glands, pancreas, and testes.[21] Pathologic fractures are frequent, especially in the vertebrae and ribs; other sites, such as the pelvis, sternum, clavicles, and tubular bones, are fractured less commonly.[77]

Histologically, myeloma is characterized by closely packed plasma cells ranging from undifferentiated to well differentiated[79] (Fig. 60–9). In well-differentiated lesions, the nuclei resemble normal plasma cells, whereas in poorly differentiated lesions, nuclear pleomorphism and cytoplasmic vacuolation may simulate the appearance of undifferentiated carcinoma.[50] Mitotic figures are unusual.[80] In general, less differentiated plasma cells are associated with

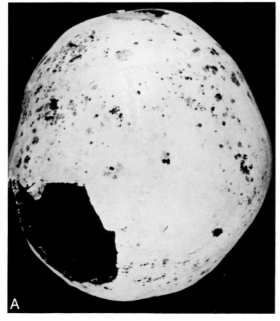

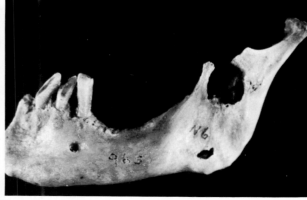

FIGURE 60–8. Plasma cell myeloma: Gross pathologic abnormalities.
  A, Discrete osteolytic lesions are scattered throughout the cranial vault. The larger area of bone dissolution is an artifact.
  B, Mandible. Several well-marginated lesions in the mandible are seen.

Illustration continued on opposite page

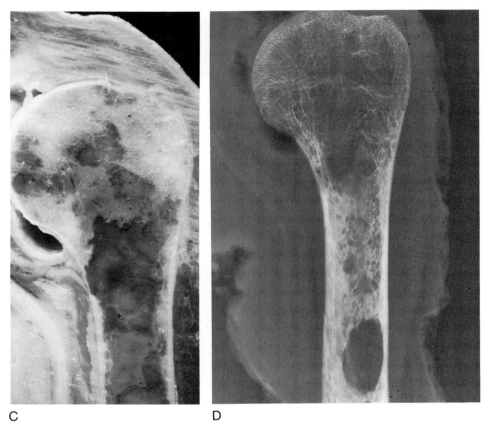

C   D

FIGURE 60–8 *Continued*
C–E Humerus. Osteolytic lesions, which are leading to endosteal erosion of the humeral cortex, are documented as multiple myeloma on photomicrography (4×).

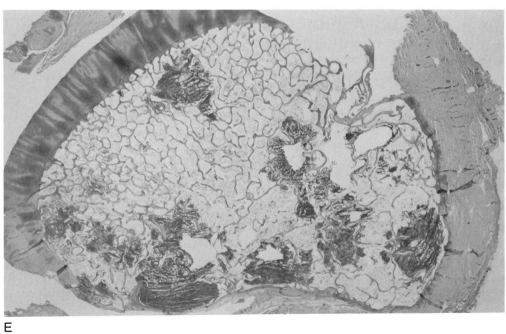

E

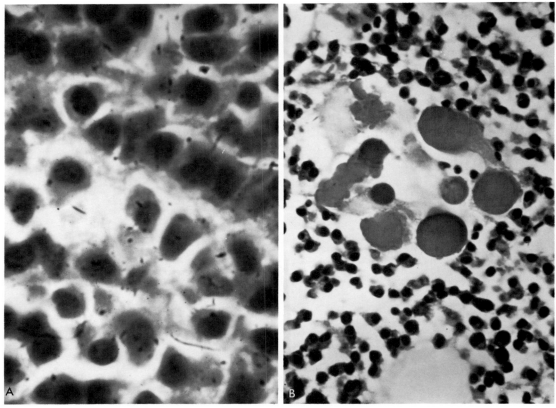

FIGURE 60–9. Plasma cell myeloma: Microscopic abnormalities.
A Typical closely packed plasma cells are evident.
B Amyloid deposits are apparent within sheets of plasma cells.

more widespread skeletal and extraskeletal involvement.[21] The absence of significant fibrovascular stroma in myeloma aids in its differentiation from an inflammatory process. Accompanying amyloid deposits are apparent histologically in approximately 10 per cent of patients.[50] These deposits may appear either in the neoplasm itself, perhaps replacing a large part of the lesion, or at distant sites, including the joint capsule, tongue, and renal parenchyma.

Radionuclide Examination

Although radionuclide examination using various technetium bone-seeking pharmaceutical agents is valuable in the early detection of most neoplastic processes of the skeleton, the results of this examination are less predictable in patients with myeloma (Fig. 60–10). False-negative scans are not uncommon in this disease, as the small, osteolytic lesions of myeloma may not concentrate the radionuclide.[81–86] In some patients myelomatous lesions can be detected at an early stage by scanning with ^{99m}Tc-polyphosphate[87] or ^{87m}Sr-citrate or carbonate.[88–91] In these cases, uptake of radionuclide is more pronounced in areas of osteoblastic activity with new bone formation. Rarely, in cases of diffuse osteosclerosis, a ''superscan,'' characterized by diffuse osseous uptake of the bone-seeking radiopharmaceutical agent and absence of renal activity, is seen.[64] In a study of patients with myeloma comparing the results of scintiscanning using bone-seeking and rare-earth radionuclides (^{67}Ga-citrate, ^{99m}Tc-polyphosphate, ^{99m}Tc-diphosphonate, ^{99m}Tc-sulfur colloid, ^{157}Dy, ^{167}Tm, and ^{171}Er), Hub-

ner and coworkers[92] noted that the lesions of myeloma were poorly visualized with most standard radionuclides and that rare-earth radiopharmaceutical agents offered little additional information. Other investigators,[93] although agreeing with the relative insensitivity of gallium scanning in myeloma, suggest that the finding of a high gallium uptake in osseous sites that are normal or only slightly abnormal on bone scan serves to identify a group of patients with this disease who have rapidly progressive abnormalities. Certainly, the current belief is that the radionuclide examination in patients with myeloma does not reveal all lesions, and that radiography is a more valuable technique in the assessment of the distribution of the lesions, with the possible exception of rib abnormalities, which may be seen more easily with scintigraphy. Furthermore, areas of increased uptake in some persons may indicate not the presence of tumor but amyloid deposition.[94] In fact, fractures account for augmented radionuclide uptake in a large percentage of patients with myeloma. No definite correlation is found between the extent of scintigraphic abnormality and the hematologic parameters of myeloma activity.[82] Rarely, soft tissue accumulation of radionuclides in patients with myeloma may correspond to sites of calcification[85] or of nodules containing amyloid.[95]

Although the radiographic examination appears to be more sensitive than scintigraphy in detecting the osseous alterations of plasma cell myeloma, it is far from ideal as an imaging method in monitoring the course of the disease. Clinical and laboratory evidence of patient improvement commonly is associated with unchanged alterations on se-

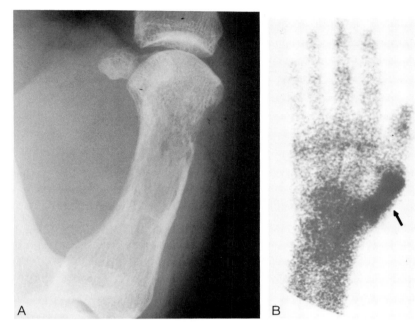

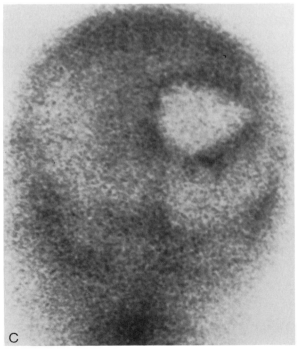

FIGURE 60–10. Plasma cell myeloma: Scintigraphic abnormalities.

A, B In a 69 year old man with diffuse skeletal involvement, a technetium phosphate bone scan reveals considerable accumulation of the radionuclide (arrow) at the site of an obvious lesion in the first metacarpal bone.

C In this 50 year old man with multiple myeloma, observe a large lesion of the cranial vault whose center shows a relative lack of accumulation of the bone-seeking radiopharmaceutical agent ("cold" lesion) with a peripheral rim of augmented radionuclide activity. This appearance is termed the doughnut sign.

rial radiologic studies.[96] Reports indicate that scintigraphy is a potential aid in following patients with myeloma who are receiving chemotherapy; remission is characterized by significant regression or disappearance of scintigraphic abnormalities in many of these patients.[97]

Computed Tomography

CT scanning, with its considerable ability to detect subtle changes in tissue density, is valuable in the delineation of lesions within the medullary canal, whether they be sites of metastasis, infection, or myeloma (Figs. 60–11 to 60–13). As opposed to plain film radiography, in which considerable osseous destruction is required before abnormalities become apparent, CT images may indicate minor alterations in radiodensity reflecting the presence of intramedullary myelomatous foci. The technique is well suited for the evaluation of patients in whom myeloma is suspected on the basis of clinical (back pain and tenderness) and laboratory (changes in serum electrophoresis) parameters and in whom radiographs are normal. In such persons, CT may outline typical spinal lesions of the disease.[98-101] One or two transaxial CT sections of the vertebrae may confirm the diagnosis. Furthermore, this technique can be used to detect the extent of osseous and soft tissue involvement in patients with well-documented myeloma, especially in areas of complicated anatomy such as the spine, pelvis, and face.[102]

Magnetic Resonance Imaging

MR imaging is effective in the analysis of a variety of disorders that lead to marrow reconversion, marrow infiltration or replacement, myeloid depletion, or marrow edema or ischemia (see Chapters 10, 59, 64, 70, 80, 83 and 85).[103]

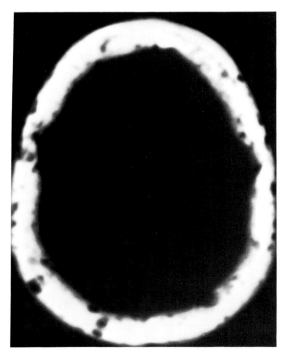

FIGURE 60–11. Plasma cell myeloma: CT abnormalities—skull. Observe well-defined radiolucent lesions involving the diploic portion and both tables of the skull.

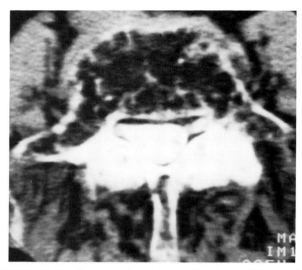

FIGURE 60–12. Plasma cell myeloma: CT abnormalities—spine. Osteolytic foci are apparent in the vertebral body, pedicles, and transverse and spinous processes.

In common with such processes as skeletal metastasis, leukemia, and lymphoma, plasma cell myeloma is characterized pathologically by infiltration or replacement of the cellular constituents of normal bone marrow by tumor cells. Microscopic studies of affected marrow in this disease document the occurrence of either diffuse infiltration or focal collections, or both, of plasma cells.[2] It is the hematopoietic compartment of the marrow that is replaced by tumorous infiltration in plasma cell myeloma. Indeed, there is no simple inverse relationship between the area of plasma cells and that of fat cells when random biopsy specimens of the marrow in patients with myeloma are examined histologically.[104, 105]

Although the general histopathologic abnormalities in plasma cell myeloma are irrefutable and form the basis of the MR imaging alterations that are seen in this disease, the population of plasma cells varies from one patient to another and the distribution of these cells is not uniform throughout the skeleton or, for that matter, in a single bone. Furthermore, therapeutic modification of the disease process will affect the cellular composition at sites of marrow involvement. These factors lead to some inconsistencies in the MR imaging findings in this disease that can produce diagnostic difficulty but, in some circumstances, also allow determination of disease activity. As the MR imaging abnormalities at any particular skeletal site are "painted on a canvas" (i.e., the bone marrow) whose normal signal pattern varies according to the distribution and extent of the hematopoietic or fatty elements that are present, such inconsistencies in the MR imaging appearance in plasma cell myeloma are to be expected. Finally, the choice of a specific imaging sequence and the use of ancillary methods such as the intravenous administration of gadolinium-based contrast agents will influence dramatically the manner in which myeloma is displayed on the MR imaging examination.

Most previous descriptions of the role of MR imaging in the assessment of patients with plasma cell myeloma have emphasized its spinal manifestations. As this disease typically occurs in middle-aged and elderly patients, the MR

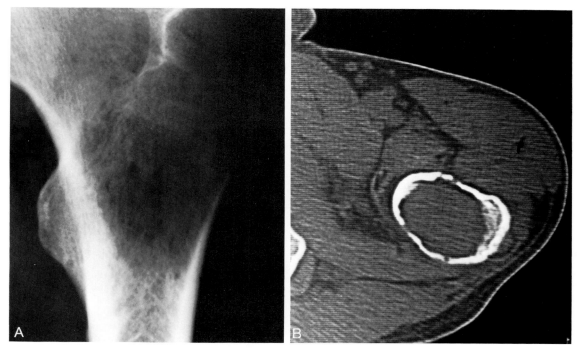

FIGURE 60–13. Plasma cell myeloma: CT abnormalities—femur. A radiograph **(A)** and a transaxial CT image **(B)** of a lesion in the intertrochanteric region of the femur in a 51 year old man show the severe degree of endosteal erosion as well as the extent of cortical perforation.

imaging appearance of uninvolved regions of bone marrow in the spine in this patient population is consistent with the presence of foci of yellow, or fatty, marrow of variable size located either peripherally or scattered throughout the vertebral body.[106] Irrespective of whichever MR imaging sequence is chosen, the detection of myeomatous involvement of the vertebral bodies (or elsewhere) is dependent on contrast differences between regions of tumor infiltration and background tissue composed of areas of either hematopoietic and fatty marrow, or both (Fig. 60–14).

One of the earliest MR imaging investigations related to the detection of vertebral abnormalities in patients with plasma cell myeloma was that of Fruehwald and coworkers.[107] A patient population consisting of 18 persons with and 21 persons without myeloma was studied with routine T1- and T2-weighted spin echo MR sequences. Two signal patterns were observed in the myeloma patients: (1) focal areas with reduced signal intensity in comparison to normal bone marrow on T1-weighted images and with enhanced signal intensity on T2-weighted images, a pattern observed predominantly in untreated patients; and (2) focal areas of decreased signal intensity on both T1-weighted and T2-weighted images, which were detected predominantly in those patients who had received radiation therapy. Diagnostic difficulties were encountered owing to the presence of signal inhomogeneity of the bone marrow without focal alterations; differentiation of a diffuse decrease in signal intensity of bone marrow caused by malignant infiltration from a similar signal pattern caused by the distance of the spine from the surface coil; the presence of focal intravertebral deposits of fat in the normal spine that lead to regions of increased signal intensity on the T1-weighted and T2-weighted images; and the lack of specificity of the MR imaging findings as other processes leading to vertebral infiltration may produce identical MR imaging findings.

Libshitz and colleagues[108] also employed standard T1-weighted and T2-weighted spin echo MR sequences in an analysis of the spine in 32 patients with multiple myeloma, and these investigators emphasized the variability of the findings in this disease related, in part, to the diffuse or focal nature of tumor infiltration and to the extent of fatty replacement of the hematopoietic bone marrow. On T1-weighted images, the signal intensity of affected vertebrae approximated that of muscle in 45 per cent of patients and was intermediate between the signal intensities of muscle and fat in 55 per cent of patients. On T2-weighted images, the signal intensity of such vertebrae approximated that of muscle in about 50 per cent of cases and was intermediate

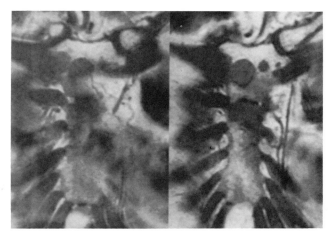

FIGURE 60–14. Plasma cell myeloma: MR imaging abnormalities—sternum. These sequential coronal T1-weighted (TR/TE, 600/20) spin echo MR images reveal multiple well-defined foci of tumor, appearing as regions of diminished signal intensity that are highlighted by the bright signal of the predominantly fatty bone marrow.

between the signal intensities of fat and muscle in the other 50 per cent of cases. Focal areas of myelomatous involvement produced regions of increased signal intensity on T2-weighted images in 53 per cent of patients. The authors concluded that focal areas of abnormality need not be seen in the spine in plasma cell myeloma; that, when present, such focal regions are more readily detected on T2-weighted images; that diffuse myelomatous involvement should be suspected when T1-weighted images fail to show evidence of any fatty bone marrow; and that difficulty arises in the differentiation of benign and malignant causes of vertebral collapse in patients with plasma cell myeloma.

In an analysis of 29 patients with plasma cell myeloma, Moulopoulos and coworkers[109] also encountered variability in the MR imaging characteristics of spinal involvement. Three patterns of abnormality were described: focal areas of marrow involvement (62 per cent of patients); total replacement of the bone marrow, the diffuse pattern (24 per cent of patients); and inhomogeneous marrow replacement, a variegated pattern (14 per cent of patients). Although all three patterns of marrow involvement could be seen on T1-weighted spin echo MR images, the variegated and diffuse patterns created diagnostic difficulties as they had to be differentiated from normal patterns of inhomogeneous distribution of fatty marrow often observed in older persons and from the persistent hematopoietic marrow pattern that occasionally is seen in younger persons with the disease. These authors emphasized that the focal myelomatous lesions could be of low signal or high signal intensity on T1-weighted images, the latter finding perhaps related to hemorrhagic areas.

These reported observations underscore some of the diagnostic limitations of standard spin echo imaging in the assessment of spinal involvement in plasma cell myeloma and have led to efforts to improve diagnostic accuracy through the use of additional MR imaging methods and sequences. Gadolinium-supplemented T1-weighted images are characterized by diffuse or inhomogeneous enhancement of diffuse or variegated marrow involvement[109] (Fig. 60–15). The pattern of enhancement of myelomatous foci differs from that typically encountered in regions of hematopoietic bone marrow. Although normal marrow may enhance markedly when a gadolinium-based contrast agent is administered intravenously to young children, such enhancement is subtle or absent in adults.[110, 111] In plasma cell myeloma, the intervertebral discs are isointense relative to spinal marrow in patients with diffuse marrow involvement; after intravenous administration of gadolinium agent, the discs become hypointense relative to marrow as the abnormal vertebral bodies enhance.[109] A potential drawback of the use of gadolinium enhancement in the assessment of spinal involvement in myeloma occurs in the setting of focal lesions in the vertebral body that, when enhanced with gadolinium contrast agent, may be masked because they become isointense relative to uninvolved marrow.[109, 112]

The use of gradient echo imaging in the evaluation of plasma cell myeloma has received limited attention.[109, 113] In most gradient echo sequences, magnetic susceptibility effects lead to signal intensity of bone that is markedly decreased in comparison to that of muscle. Therefore, although focal myelomatous lesions may appear as hyperintense foci with these sequences (Fig. 60–16), diffuse plasma cell infiltration may not produce a sufficient in-

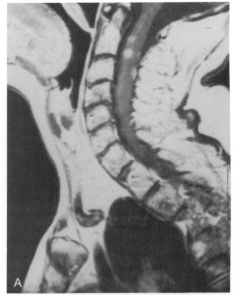

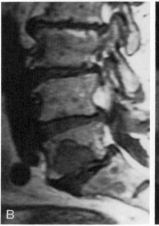
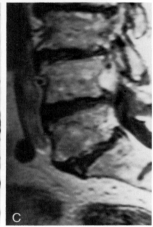

FIGURE 60–15. Plasma cell myeloma: MR imaging abnormalities—spine and spinal cord. Gadolinium enhancement.

A A sagittal T1-weighted (TR/TE, 600/20) spin echo MR image obtained immediately after the intravenous administration of gadolinium-based contrast agent reveals diffuse enhancement of signal in all of the cervical vertebral bodies. The resulting high signal intensity simulates that of fat. Leptomeningeal lesions of high signal intensity also are evident, as are myelomatous foci in the sternum. (Courtesy of K. Kortman, M.D., San Diego, California.)

B, C In this 65 year old woman, sagittal T1-weighted (TR/TE, 600/11) spin echo MR images obtained before (**B**) and after (**C**) the intravenous administration of gadolinium compound show vertebral lesions of low signal intensity with contrast enhancement of signal intensity. With regard to the large lesion in the fifth lumbar vertebral body, a rimlike pattern of enhancement is evident. (Courtesy of S. K. Brahme, M.D., La Jolla, California.)

crease in signal intensity to overcome these susceptibility effects.[109] In the posterior elements of the vertebrae, gradient echo sequences, by suppressing the signal of subcutaneous fat, may lead to an increase in lesion conspicuity, however.[109] Furthermore, preliminary data indicate that gadolinium-enhanced opposed-phase gradient echo techniques may be useful in the assessment of plasma cell myeloma[113] and other bone marrow disorders.[114]

Short tau inversion recovery (STIR) sequences have shown promise in the analysis of a variety of neoplastic and inflammatory processes involving bone marrow.[115, 116]

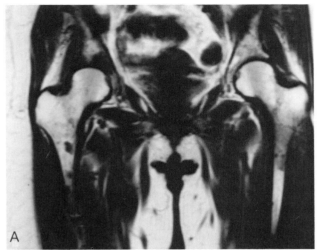

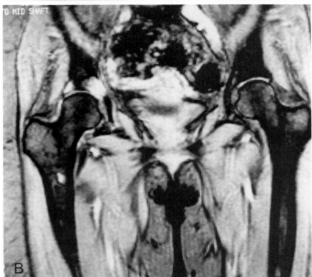

FIGURE 60–16. Plasma cell myeloma: MR imaging abnormalities—pelvis and femora.

A A coronal T1-weighted (TR/TE, 375/15) spin echo MR image shows myelomatous foci in both femora and the right acetabular region as areas of low signal intensity. Normal hematopoietic marrow is evident in the femoral necks and in the left acetabular region.

B A coronal gradient echo MR image (TR/TE, 400/10; flip angle, 20 degrees) reveals the lesions in the right femur and right acetabulum which are of high signal intensity.

Through the use of a short inversion time, fat-suppressed images can be generated with this technique. Signal intensity from tissue with long T1 and T2 relaxation times, such as neoplastic and inflammatory tissue, is enhanced. Disadvantages of the method when applied to assessment of neoplasms include lack of specificity and the vivid display of peritumoral edema, the latter making accurate staging of tumors more difficult.[116] Other general disadvantages of this method include a poor signal to noise ratio, susceptibility to motion and flow artifacts, and limitations in the number of slices that can be obtained. Chemical shift artifacts are reduced, however, and STIR imaging may allow detection of small focal collections of tumor that escape visualization with standard spin echo MR imaging methods. Other fat suppression techniques such as chemical shift imaging also can be employed in patients with plasma cell myeloma and

may be combined with the use of intravenous gadolinium-based contrast agent administration (Fig. 60–17), although the value of these modified MR imaging methods has yet to be proved in patients with this disease.[360] Preliminary data related to the comparison of fat-suppressed T2-weighted spin echo MR images and STIR images in the detection of a variety of marrow disorders have indicated practical advantages of the former technique, including acquisition of more slices per unit time and improved tissue specificity.[363]

Although existing data relate mainly to the assessment of spinal involvement in plasma cell myeloma, MR imaging also can be applied to the evaluation of disease presence and extent in extraspinal sites and to the analysis of solitary or multifocal plasmacytomas (see later discussion). Although the basic signal characteristics of the myelomatous process in these sites are similar to those in the vertebrae, lesion conspicuity will be influenced by the histologic composition of the adjacent bone marrow, which exhibits an increasing percentage of adipose tissue in an axial to appendicular skeletal direction.

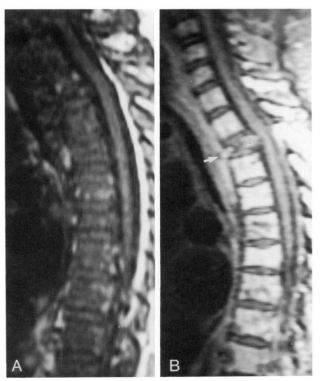

FIGURE 60–17. Plasma cell myeloma: MR imaging abnormalities—spine. Gadolinum enhancement and fat suppression.

A In a 62 year old woman, a sagittal T1-weighted (TR/TE, 500/12) spin echo MR image reveals diffuse areas of low signal intensity in the cervical and thoracic vertebral bodies, with scattered foci of higher signal intensity compatible with areas of fatty marrow. The resulting signal intensity of the vertebral bodies is lower than that of the intervertebral discs. Collapse of the second thoracic vertebral body is not well shown in this image.

B A similar T1-weighted (TR/TE, 800/20) spin echo MR image obtained after the intravenous administration of gadolinium contrast agent and with chemical shift fat suppression shows high signal intensity in all of the vertebral bodies, consistent with diffuse myelomatous involvement. Note collapse of the second thoracic vertebral body (arrow) with spinal cord compression. The degree of fat suppression is not uniform throughout the image.

The role of MR imaging in the assessment of therapeutic response in patients with plasma cell myeloma has been investigated.[361] Patterns of enhancement of signal intensity in myelomatous lesions of the spine are different before and after treatment when intravenous administration of gadolinium compounds is employed. Although preliminary in nature, reported data suggest that careful assessment of contrast-enhanced MR images may allow a means of effective monitoring of the response of focal bone lesions of myeloma to radiation therapy or chemotherapy.

Plasmacytoma

Myeloma can occur as a solitary lesion of bone.[117] Although laboratory analysis may reveal the same abnormalities as occur in disseminated myelomatosis, this is not always the case. In some patients with solitary plasmacytoma, serologic tests are negative or abnormal patterns of serum electrophoresis disappear after excision of the tumor.[118]

Many cases of apparently solitary plasmacytoma reveal multiple lesions if followed for a long period of time[119]; in fact, some investigators believe that all patients with plasmacytoma will eventually demonstrate multiple lesions, although such dissemination does not necessarily imply a poor prognosis.[120, 121] Although initial studies of bone marrow from other sites may reveal no abnormality in these cases, subsequent conversion from solitary to multiple myeloma suggests a definite relationship between the two processes.[122, 123] In other patients, solitary lesions may never demonstrate evidence of dissemination even when patients are followed for 20 to 30 years,[120, 121, 124, 125] although in some of these latter instances, the initial lesion could conceivably have been a benign plasmacytic focus (plasma cell granuloma) rather than a true plasmacytoma.[126] These varying results have led to a controversy regarding the very existence of solitary plasmacytoma. Griffiths[18] suggests that two strict criteria are prerequisites for the diagnosis of such a lesion: survival for longer than 12 years without evidence of dissemination and negative histologic examination of all bones at necropsy. In those cases in which plasmacytoma apparently has converted to multiple myeloma, dissemination usually occurs in the first 5 years of disease, although, rarely, it may occur after 20 years or more.[122] After dissemination, the clinical and pathologic features usually are typical of multiple myeloma, with a generally poor prognosis, although instances of patients developing multiple ''plasmacytomas'' are recorded, in whom long survival periods may be apparent.

Solitary plasmacytoma, as compared with multiple myeloma, is rare (representing less than 5 per cent of plasma cell dyscrasias), affects younger patients (the average age is about 50 years), commonly is accompanied by neurologic manifestations, and can simulate giant cell tumor on radiologic examination.[127] It is most frequent in the spine (especially the thoracic and lumbar segments) and pelvis[128-131] although it may occur at other skeletal sites[118-120, 124, 129, 132-134] or in extraskeletal locations, particularly the nasal cavities, paranasal sinuses, or upper airways[123, 135-137] (Figs. 60–18 to 60–22). The radiographic features are variable. A multicystic expansile lesion with thickened trabeculae or a purely osteolytic focus without expansion may be observed. Sclerotic lesions also have been identified and, in fact, solitary plasmacytoma may appear as a radiodense vertebral body, the ivory vertebra[138] (Fig. 60–23). Calcification in plasmacytomas may indicate amyloid deposition, and the resulting radiographic appearance can simulate that of a chondrosarcoma.[364]

Solitary plasmacytoma of the spine deserves special emphasis. This diagnosis must be considered in any middle-aged or elderly patient with a single osteolytic lesion of a vertebral body or, less commonly, a vertebral arch (Fig. 60–24). An involved vertebral body may collapse and disappear completely, or the lesion may extend into the spinal canal or across the intervertebral disc to invade the adjacent vertebral body[128] (Fig. 60–25), simulating the appearance of infection. In fact, plasmacytoma in any juxta-articular site can extend across the articular space and involve the adjacent bone (Fig. 60–26). This complication is especially characteristic in joints such as the discovertebral junction and sacroiliac joint that lack mobility.[139, 140] In patients with spinal plasmacytomas, clinical findings include backache, nerve root irritation, and paraplegia. The last complication is even more common in patients with solitary plasmacytoma than in those with multiple myeloma, perhaps related to longer survival rates in the former patients. Rarely, spinal cord compression in this disorder relates to a plasmacytoma developing in an epidural location.[142]

Rheumatologic Manifestations

Rheumatologic manifestations in association with plasma cell myeloma may reveal one of several patterns.

Bone Pain. Skeletal pain is a frequent finding in patients with myeloma.[143] This symptom is most prominent in the back, associated with destructive lesions and vertebral collapse, although it may be observed in articular sites, including the hip and shoulder, in conjunction with osteolytic foci (Fig. 60–27).

Neurologic Findings. Sciatica and brachial neuralgia are encountered in patients with spinal disease, related to nerve root pressure. In addition, patients with sclerotic plasma cell myeloma (or rarely osteolytic myeloma) may reveal an associated peripheral neuropathy.[62, 144] This first was recorded by Scheinker in 1938[145] and subsequently was confirmed by other investigators.[146-148] It has been suggested that peripheral neuropathy may be related to dysglobulinemia,[149] although protein abnormalities are not always detectable in patients revealing such neuropathy.[148] Peripheral neuropathy occurs in less than 1 per cent of plasma cell neoplasms, is more frequent in men, and is of a mixed sensorimotor type; it may be associated with osteosclerotic lesions and with three or fewer abnormal skeletal foci.[150] It is rare in solitary plasmacytoma.[151] Neuropathic osteoarthropathy is distinctly uncommon (Fig. 60–28).

POEMS Syndrome. A syndrome of plasma cell dyscrasia (plasma cell myeloma, extramedullary plasmacytoma, isolated monoclonal gammopathy, or isolated polyclonal gammopathy), chronic progressive polyneuropathy, and endocrine disturbances, including diabetes mellitus, has been recognized[6, 152-168] (Figs. 60–29 to 60–31). M protein abnormalities, if present, are lambda light chains, unlike the kappa light chains evident in classic myeloma.[165] Additional characteristics of this syndrome are thickening and pigmentation of the skin, edema, excess perspiration, hirsutism, impotence, gynecomastia or amenorrhea, and hepatosplenomegaly. Nodular regenerative hyperplasia of the liver and

Text continued on page 2172

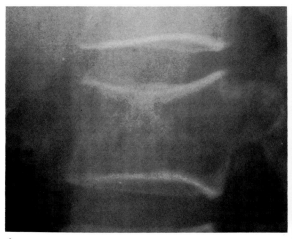

A

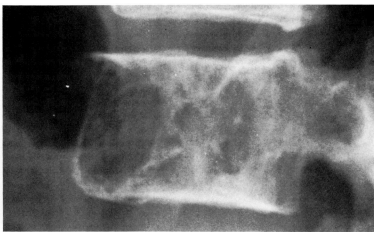

B

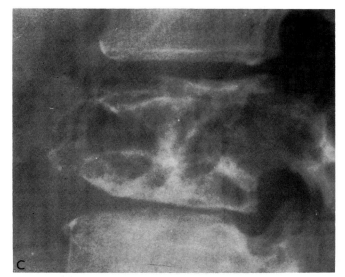

C

FIGURE 60–18. Plasmacytoma: Spine.

A–C Progressive changes in the spine in a 37 year old man with low back pain. The initial radiograph **(A)** demonstrates increased lucency of the third lumbar vertebral body with slight compression of its superior surface. Two years later **(B),** the lesion has progressed and appears "bubbly" or septated. **C,** Four months after **B,** further progression and vertebral collapse are evident. Following the study, a myelogram revealed extradural compression of the spinal cord. A bone biopsy documented the presence of a plasmacytoma.

D, E In a different patient with a plasmacytoma, the tomogram **(D)** delineates lysis of the third cervical vertebral body with complete collapse. The intervertebral disc spaces are not narrowed. A myelogram **(E)** outlines an extradural defect at the level of the collapsed vertebra.

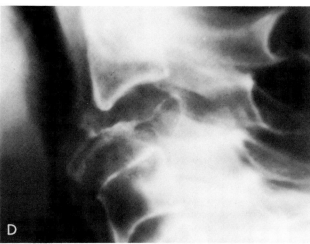

D

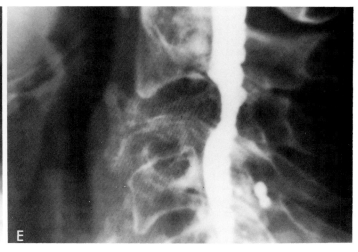

E

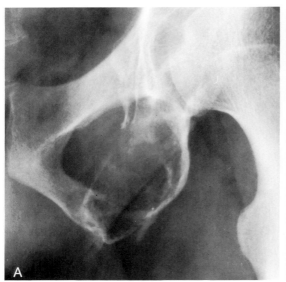
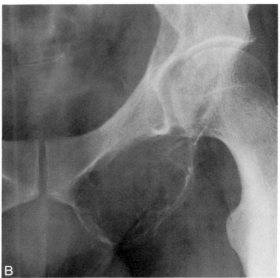
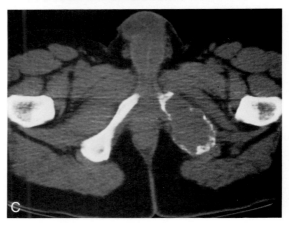

FIGURE 60–19. Plasmacytoma: Pelvis. A 34 year old man developed left hip pain, which progressed over a 2 year period.

A, B Radiographs obtained 16 months apart reveal an expansile trabeculated lesion of the ischium.

C A transaxial CT image at the level of the ischial tuberosity, obtained at the same time as **B,** reveals the expansile lesion, cortical thinning and perforation, and the absence of a soft tissue mass. An open biopsy confirmed the diagnosis of plasmacytoma.

(Courtesy of G. Greenway, M.D., Dallas, Texas.)

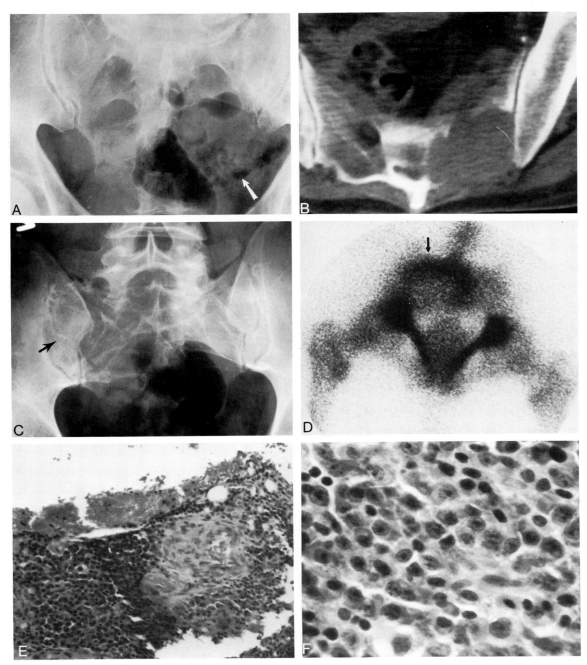

FIGURE 60–20. Plasmacytoma: Sacrum.

A, B A 74 year old man developed progressive pain in the lower back and left buttock over a 6 week period. The pain radiated into the left thigh and calf and was intensified when the leg was raised. The subtle osteolytic lesion of the sacrum (arrow), demonstrable on the plain film, is readily evident on a transaxial CT image. A closed biopsy of the lesion confirmed the presence of a plasmacytoma. (Courtesy of G. Greenway, M.D., Dallas, Texas.)

C–F A 45 year old man developed low back pain over a 2 year period. The radiograph **(C)** shows a destructive lesion in the sacrum (arrow), which on bone scan **(D)** is seen to be associated with increased accumulation of the radiopharmaceutical agent at its superior margin (arrow). Photomicrography **(E, F)** reveals a morphologic spectrum of cellular differentiation varying from poorly differentiated cells with vesicular nuclei and prominent nucleoli to relatively well differentiated cells with plasma cell features including dense, eccentric nuclei and a nuclear hof (10×, 40×).

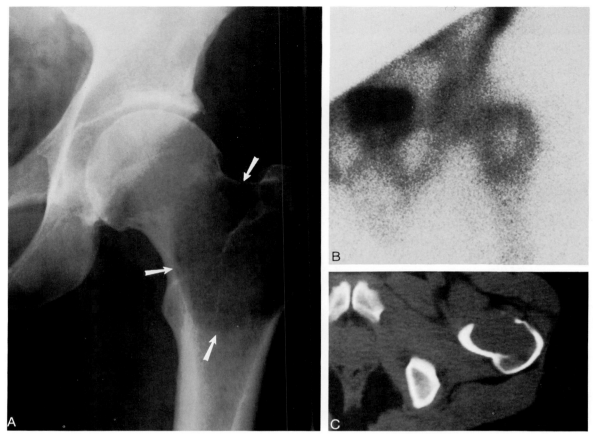

FIGURE 60–21. Plasmacytoma: Femur. A 37 year old man had a 4 month history of hip pain and a limp.
  A A large osteolytic lesion (arrows) is seen in the proximal portion of the femur.
  B On a bone scan, the periphery of the lesion reveals increased accumulation of the radiopharmaceutical agent.
  C The transaxial CT image shows cortical perforation and a soft tissue mass.
  (Courtesy of G. Greenway, M.D., Dallas, Texas.)

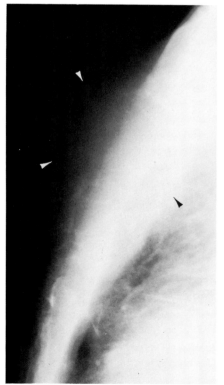

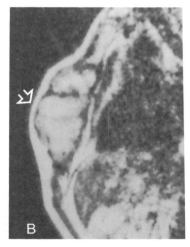

FIGURE 60–22. Plasmacytoma: Sternum.
  A Observe extensive destruction of the body of the sternum with a large soft tissue mass (arrowheads).
  B In a different patient, a sagittal T2-weighted (TR/TE, 1133/100) spin echo MR image reveals an expansile sternal lesion (arrow) of high signal intensity. (**B,** Courtesy of R. Kerr, M.D., Los Angeles, California.)

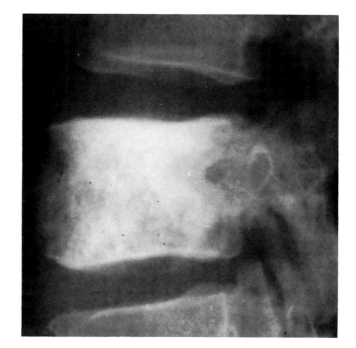

FIGURE 60–23. Plasmacytoma: Ivory vertebra. In a 33 year old man with a 1 month history of low back pain, laboratory evaluation revealed normal serum and urine electrophoresis. Osteosclerosis of the entire third lumbar vertebral body is observed, with areas of permeative bone destruction. The intervertebral disc spaces are normal. An open biopsy documented the presence of a plasmacytoma.

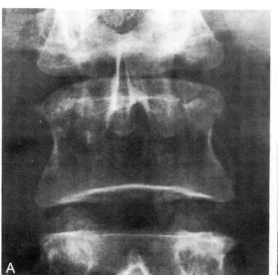

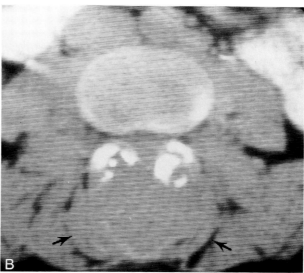

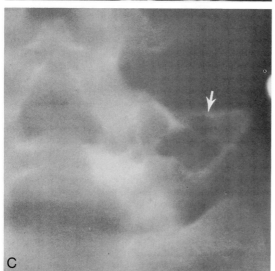

FIGURE 60–24. Plasmacytoma: Vertebral arch.
  A, B In this patient, the spinous process, laminae, articular processes, and pedicles are destroyed. Observe the soft tissue mass (arrows). (Courtesy of J. Slivka, M.D., San Diego, California.)
  C In a different patient, an expansile osteolytic lesion in the transverse process of the fifth lumbar vertebra (arrow) is evident. (Courtesy of J. A. Amberg, M.D., San Diego, California.)

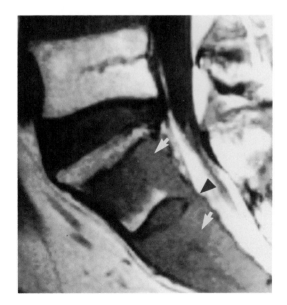

FIGURE 60–25. Plasmacytoma: Extension across the intervertebral disc space. In this 59 year old man, a plasmacytoma developed in a transitional type of lumbosacral junction. A sagittal T1-weighted (TR/TE, 750/15) spin echo MR image shows involvement of the transitional vertebral body and sacrum (arrows) as well as the posterior portion of the intervening disc (arrowhead). The tumor is of low signal intensity and was of high signal intensity on T2-weighted images (not shown). (Courtesy of G. S. Huang, M.D., Taipei, Taiwan.)

FIGURE 60–26. Plasmacytoma: Extension across the articular space. A 51 year old man had a plasmacytoma of the iliac crest, which was verified on biopsy. On radiographs, an enlarging lesion of the ilium adjacent to the sacroiliac joint eventually extended across the joint to involve the sacrum (arrows). Conventional tomograms verified abnormalities of both sacrum and ilium.

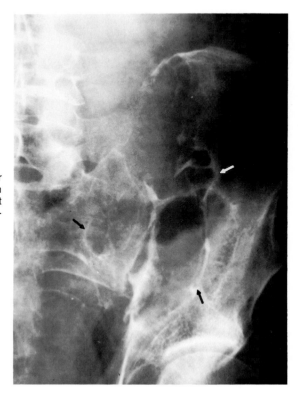

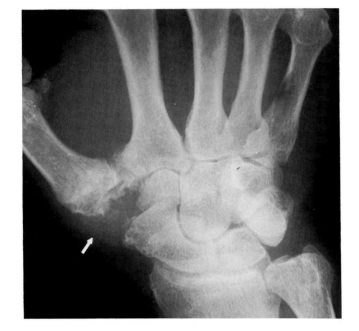

FIGURE 60–27. Plasma cell myeloma: Periarticular lesions. Wrist. The trapezium has been completely destroyed. Observe adjacent soft tissue swelling (arrow), proliferation at the base of the first and second metacarpals, and a lytic lesion of the fifth metacarpal.

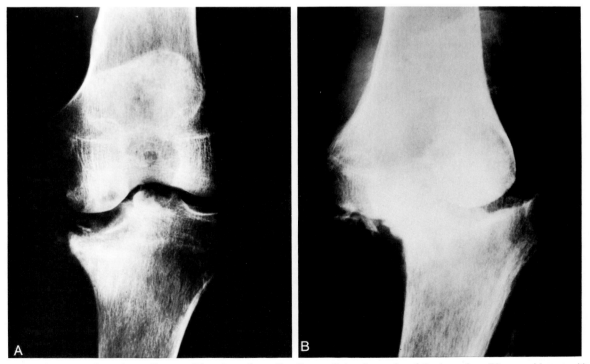

FIGURE 60–28. Plasma cell myeloma: Neuropathic osteoarthropathy. Sequential radiographs of the knee in a 70 year old man with plasma cell myeloma and peripheral neuropathy reveal characteristic and progressive features of neuropathic osteoarthropathy, including bone collapse, fragmentation and sclerosis, and subluxation. This patient had no evidence of diabetes mellitus, syphilis, or amyloidosis. (Courtesy of V. Vint, M.D., San Diego, California.)

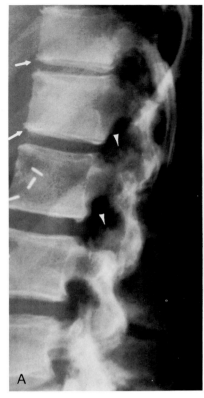

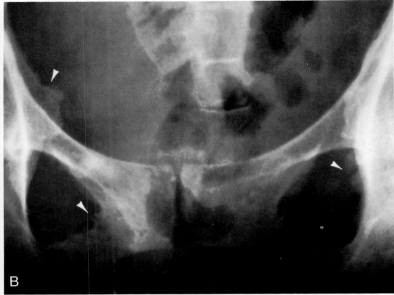

FIGURE 60–29. Syndrome of plasma cell dyscrasia, polyneuropathy, and endocrine disturbances (POEMS syndrome). A 43 year old woman developed skin abnormality, organomegaly, polyneuropathy, and plasma cell dyscrasia.

A On a lateral radiograph of the lumbar spine, observe peculiar proliferative changes about the apophyseal joints (arrowheads) and, to a lesser extent, the discovertebral junctions (arrows). The bones appear radiodense.

B A view of the symphysis pubis outlines similar bony proliferation in neighboring areas (arrowheads).

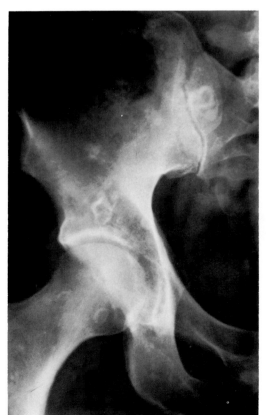

FIGURE 60–30. Syndrome of plasma cell dyscrasia, polyneuropathy, and endocrine disturbances (POEMS syndrome). A 50 year old man with clinical findings similar to those of the woman in Figure 60–29. The radiograph outlines many sclerotic lesions of the ilium, sacrum, and femur.

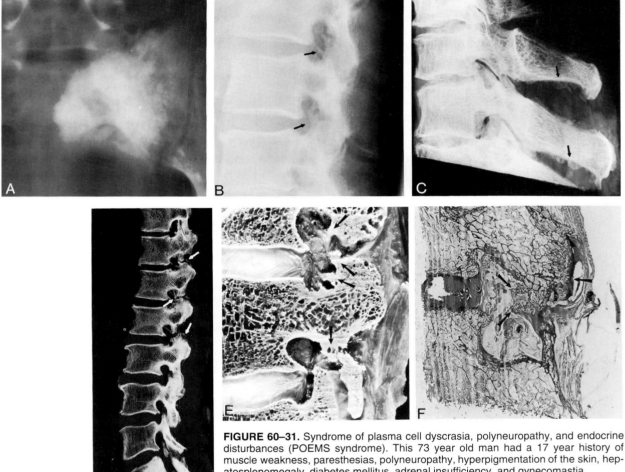

FIGURE 60–31. Syndrome of plasma cell dyscrasia, polyneuropathy, and endocrine disturbances (POEMS syndrome). This 73 year old man had a 17 year history of muscle weakness, paresthesias, polyneuropathy, hyperpigmentation of the skin, hepatosplenomegaly, diabetes mellitus, adrenal insufficiency, and gynecomastia.

A A frontal tomogram of the sacrum reveals a large sclerotic lesion extending to the region of the sacroiliac joint.

B A lateral radiograph of the lumbar spine shows a peculiar pattern of bone proliferation involving the articular processes of the vertebrae (arrows).

C In the cervical spine, similar bone proliferation affects the spinous processes (arrows). In this illustration and subsequent ones, sections of the spine after the patient's demise are shown.

D The radiograph of a sagittal section of the thoracolumbar spine shows the distinctive pattern of osseous proliferation (arrows) as well as the sclerotic lesion of the sacrum (arrowhead).

E The photograph of a macerated sagittal section of the spine documents bone spiculation (arrows) affecting the pedicles and articular processes.

F A low power photomicrograph illustrates areas of sclerotic bone and osseous proliferation (arrows) in the spine.

neuropathic osteoarthropathy have been identified in one patient.[159] Microangiopathic glomerulopathy has been recognized in another.[161] Affected patients do not have an increased incidence of amyloidosis (with rare exceptions[169]) and rarely reveal Bence Jones proteinuria.[165] The syndrome is more frequent in men and usually has its onset at a young age. Patients with disease onset in the sixth to eighth decades of life also have been identified, however. Sclerotic plasmacytomas are evident in most cases, particularly in the spine and pelvis. The lesions may be uniformly sclerotic or appear target-like, with a peripheral margin of bone sclerosis. Ivory vertebral bodies may be evident, and areas showing features similar to those of bone islands may be seen.[165] In the author's experience and that of others, proliferation is apparent at sites of tendon and ligament attachment to bone.[164, 165, 170, 171] Particularly characteristic are irregular bony excrescences involving the posterior elements of the spine, including the articular, transverse, and spinous processes.[170] Similar findings are observed about the sacroiliac and costovertebral joints. Bone pain is a rare clinical feature in this syndrome. Histologic analysis reveals areas of sclerotic cortical bone, cancellous trabeculae that possess irregular borders and moderate appositional new bone, and bone marrow generally free of plasma cell infiltration.[171] Amelioration of clinical and laboratory features may occur after a combination of chemotherapy and radiation has been employed, although the radiographic abnormalities usually remain unchanged.[165]

The cause of this syndrome is not known. Trentham and colleagues[155] considered that it was a unique connective tissue disorder because of its multisystem nature and because of microvascular abnormalities that suggested a vasculopathic process.[160] In addition, their patient had no evidence of an underlying plasma cell dyscrasia. The identification of paraproteins in the spinal fluid of patients with progressive polyneuropathy[172] as well as those with this peculiar syndrome[159, 173] suggests an increased permeability of the blood–cerebrospinal fluid barrier, allowing the influx of abnormal serum proteins into the cerebrospinal fluid, which may be important in the pathogenesis of the disorder. Furthermore, the association of this syndrome with giant lymph node hyperplasia (Castleman's disease) and with dermal mastocytosis may provide additional clues regarding its pathogenesis.[165, 167]

To facilitate recognition of the most constant features of this syndrome—polyneuropathy (P), organomegaly (O), endocrinopathy (E), M proteins (M), and skin changes (S)—the author and his colleagues have suggested the acronym POEMS.[157]

Polyarthritis and Amyloid Deposition. Plasma cell myeloma may be manifested as a polyarthritis that resembles rheumatoid arthritis superficially.[143, 174–182] Findings include pain, swelling, and limitation of motion of peripheral joints, particularly in the hands. Soft tissue nodules in periarticular locations, carpal tunnel syndrome, and macroglossia also may be apparent. These articular manifestations can precede any overt manifestation of myelomatosis or develop after the onset of this latter disease. Synovial fluid aspiration generally reveals the absence of inflammatory characteristics of rheumatoid arthritis, and, in some cases, the presence of M component and amyloid-containing material.[180] Radiographs can demonstrate soft tissue masses,

periarticular swelling, and osseous erosion. Synovial biopsy or autopsy examination outlines amyloid deposition within the synovium, the para-articular tissues including muscle, and the carpal tunnel as well as at distant sites.

Amyloidosis occurs in approximately 15 per cent of patients with plasma cell myeloma.[183, 184] The distribution of amyloid in these patients resembles that in primary amyloidosis. In fact, differentiation of myeloma with coexistent amyloidosis from primary amyloidosis may be extremely difficult because of the presence in the latter disease of various M components in the serum and urine, Bence Jones proteinuria, osteolytic lesions due to bone replacement by amyloid, and a rheumatoid arthritis–like polyarthritis due to amyloid deposition in the synovium.[180, 185–189] This difficulty in separating patients with primary and secondary amyloidosis is underscored by a case described by Goldberg and coworkers[178] in which a patient with multiple myeloma and arthropathy appeared to have had primary amyloidosis.[180, 190] To make evaluation of patients with plasma cell myeloma and polyarthritis even more troublesome, some investigators report that synovial biopsies in these patients may reveal findings indistinguishable from those of rheumatoid arthritis.[143] Furthermore, the occurrence of rheumatoid arthritis in association with serum M components without evidence of either myeloma or amyloidosis has been described.[143, 191–193] The appearance of a clone of neoplastic plasma cells in association with rheumatoid arthritis or other conditions, such as Paget's disease, Gaucher's disease, and histiocytosis, probably is related to prolonged stimulation of the reticuloendothelial system.[1, 194–196] In most patients with myeloma and polyarthritis, tests for serum rheumatoid factor are negative.[180]

Thus, it appears that the majority of patients with plasma cell myeloma and polyarthritis have coexistent amyloidosis. These patients must be differentiated, however, from those with plasma cell myeloma and coincidental rheumatoid arthritis, from those with primary amyloidosis with joint manifestations, and from those with rheumatoid arthritis and serum M components without myeloma or amyloidosis.

Rarely, a circumscribed mass of amyloid may be identified within a plasmacytoma in the skeleton.[197] Its presence can be suspected when areas of calcification are evident in the lesion.[364] The resulting radiographic abnormalities resemble those of chondrosarcoma (Fig. 60–32).

Gouty Arthritis. There are several reports of the association of plasma cell myeloma and gout[143, 198–201] (Fig. 60–33). In many of these patients, joint symptoms preceded the recognition of myeloma by a prolonged period of time.

Infection. Although the total serum globulin is increased in patients with myeloma because of the monoclonal spike, the concentrations of all other immunoglobulins are decreased. Hypogammaglobulinemia in this disorder results in impairment in humoral immunity and an increased susceptibility to infection.[202] The most frequent sites of infection are the lung and the urinary tract, although soft tissue involvement also is common[11] Osteomyelitis and septic arthritis may be seen. The organisms most typically implicated in cases of infection complicating myeloma are staphylococci, *Escherichia coli,* Pseudomonas, Klebsiella, and *Haemophilus influenzae,*[11] although other organisms, including *Neisseria meningitidis,*[203] may be responsible for such infection.

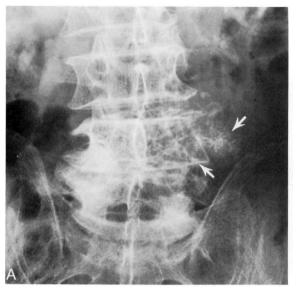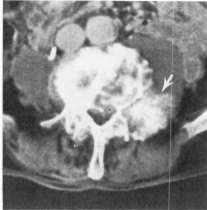

FIGURE 60–32. Plasmacytoma with amyloid deposition. Abdominal pain developed in a 70 year old man. A solitary lesion of the skeleton was biopsied, documenting the presence of a plasmacytoma with amyloid deposition.
   A Observe an osteolytic lesion with calcification (arrows) in the fourth lumbar vertebra.
   B A transaxial CT image shows the extent of bone destruction and the presence of calcification (arrow). (Courtesy of J. Castello, M.D., Madrid, Spain.)

Hemarthrosis and Myelomatous Infiltration of Synovium. Hemarthrosis may complicate myeloproliferative diseases,[204] including myeloma.[205] This clinical finding can be the initial manifestation of the disease, associated with thrombocytosis and platelet malfunction as well as myeloma cell infiltration of the synovium. Generalized hemorrhagic phenomena also can be associated with plasmacytomas. Extramedullary deposits may lead to spontaneous bleeding from the gastrointestinal, genitourinary, or respiratory tract, and massive bleeding may complicate biopsy of an osseous plasmacytoma.[206]

Miscellaneous Findings. Additional reported rheumatologic manifestations of plasma cell myeloma include tendon sheath abnormalities with or without amyloid deposition,[143] incidental degenerative joint disease,[143] fatal necrotizing polyarteritis of the coronary and renal vessels,[207] and osteonecrosis, perhaps related to hyperviscosity.[1]

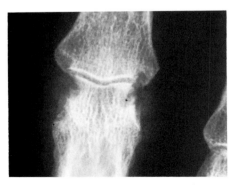

FIGURE 60–33. Plasma cell myeloma and secondary gout. Articular abnormalities at the third proximal interphalangeal joint consist of soft tissue swelling and marginal erosions, in the absence of both osteoporosis and severe joint space loss.

Differential Diagnosis

Widespread osteolytic lesions in a middle-aged or elderly patient should arouse suspicion of myeloma or skeletal metastasis. Differentiation of the radiographic features in these two disorders causes some difficulty (Table 60–1). Certain features favor the diagnosis of myeloma, including symmetrically distributed lesions of equal size without adjacent sclerosis; subcortical lucent areas with endosteal scalloping; involvement of the mandible, shoulder girdle, and elbow region; and spinal lesions with preservation of the pediculate shadow. None of these characteristics is pathognomonic of myeloma, however. Additional disorders also may be associated with widespread osteolysis, including macroglobulinemia, leukemia, histiocytosis, Gaucher's disease (Fig. 60–34), vascular tumors, infections such as tuberculosis and fungal disease, fibrous dysplasia, hyperparathyroidism, pancreatitis with fat necrosis, and Weber-Christian disease.

Diffuse osteosclerosis is unusual in plasma cell myeloma. When present, the pattern simulates that associated with myelofibrosis, osteoblastic metastasis, sickle cell anemia, Paget's disease, fibrous dysplasia, lymphoma, mastocytosis, tuberous sclerosis, renal osteodystrophy, and sarcoidosis.

Single (or several) lytic foci in myeloma are difficult to distinguish from many other primary and secondary skeletal neoplasms and infections. Expansile myelomatous lesions can simulate skeletal metastasis (particularly from thyroid and renal carcinoma), brown tumors of hyperparathyroidism, fibrous dysplasia, angiomatous lesions, hemophilic pseudotumors, and several primary bone tumors. In addition, single (or several) sclerotic foci in myeloma are not diagnostic. Osteoblastic metastasis, bone sarcomas, lymphoma, fibrous dysplasia, and infection can produce similar radiodense shadows. In the spine, an ivory vertebra, which occasionally is observed in myeloma, also is seen in scle-

TABLE 60–1. Plasma Cell Myeloma Versus Skeletal Metastasis

	Plasma Cell Myeloma	Skeletal Metastasis
Distribution and common sites	Symmetric Axial skeleton; proximal portions of long bones; shoulder and elbow region	Asymmetric Axial skeleton; proximal portions of long bones
Predominant pattern	Osteolyic lesions > osteosclerotic lesions Diffuse osteopenia (common) Diffuse osteosclerosis (rare)	Osteolytic or osteosclerotic lesions Diffuse osteopenia (rare) Diffuse osteosclerosis (common with prostatic carcinoma)
Morphology of lesions	Well-circumscribed lesions of uniform size Medullary or subcortical lucent lesions with cortical scalloping Expansile lesions or soft tissue mass or both (common in ribs, spine)	Poorly circumscribed lesions of varying size Medullary, subcortical, or cortical lucent lesions with cortical destruction Expansile lesions or soft tissue mass or both (common with thyroid and renal carcinoma)

rotic metastasis, Paget's disease, lymphoma, and rarely chordoma.

Radiographic abnormalities of joints in patients with myeloma and secondary amyloidosis resemble those of primary amyloidosis and are discussed in detail later in this chapter. Although the findings may simulate rheumatoid arthritis or other synovial disorders, the presence of atypical erosions (lacking a classic marginal distribution), bulky asymmetric periarticular masses, and diffuse osteolytic lesions allows differentation of myeloma with amyloidosis from these other disorders. The radiographic abnormalities of infection or gout in patients with myeloma essentially are the same as those accompanying these conditions in patients without myeloma.

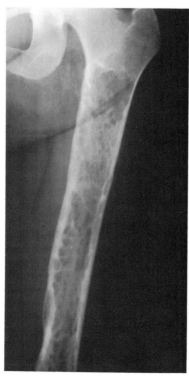

FIGURE 60–34. Gaucher's disease. Note osteolysis involving a long segment of the diaphysis of the femur. Endosteal erosion is prominent. (Courtesy of P. Kaplan, M.D., Charlottesville, Virginia.)

WALDENSTRÖM'S MACROGLOBULINEMIA

Background and Clinical Features

Macroglobulinemia is a disorder of middle-aged and elderly persons that initially was described by Waldenström in 1944.[208] It is a disease of differentiating B lymphocytes that is associated with the production of monoclonal macroglobulins.[2] Symptoms include weakness, weight loss, a bleeding diathesis, dyspnea, and personality changes; physical findings include retinal hemorrhages, hepatosplenomegaly, and lymphadenopathy. Laboratory analysis outlines anemia, elevated sedimentation rate, increased serum viscosity, hyperglobulinemia, and increased cerebrospinal fluid protein. Biopsy of bone marrow, liver, and spleen may reveal little abnormality, although lymphocytic infiltration, particularly about the portal tracts, is characteristic. Typical abnormalities related to microscopic inspection of biopsy specimens of the bone marrow include hypercellularity with a pleomorphic cellular infiltration that is composed, in varying degrees, of small or intermediate sized lymphocytes, lymphocytoid plasma cells, plasma cells, mast cells, and reticulum cells.[2] Bone marrow aspiration, however, may result in a "dry tap" related, in part, to the high viscosity of the blood.[2] Immunoelectrophoresis demonstrates globulins (IgM) with a large effective weight and size. Amyloidosis may be a complicating condition in approximately 10 per cent of cases.[209–211]

Cellular infiltration (lymphocytes, plasma cells, histiocytes, and mast cells) into various organs accounts for the clinical and radiologic manifestations of this disease. Involvement of the lung and gastrointestinal tract is well documented.[212, 213] Histologic abnormalities in osseous[214, 215] and synovial[216] tissue also are described.

Skeletal Manifestations

Skeletal findings in Waldenström's macroglobulinemia are similar to those of multiple myeloma. Osteopenia, widening of the marrow spaces, and endosteal erosion are evident.[213, 217] The remaining trabeculae may be coarsened, resulting in focal osteosclerosis.[218] Vertebral collapse is encountered.[219] Osteolytic lesions also can be observed, the reported frequency varying from 10 to 15 per cent[214, 220–224] (Fig. 60–35). These lesions can be solitary or multiple, and they may be small or large. Involvement of the pelvis,

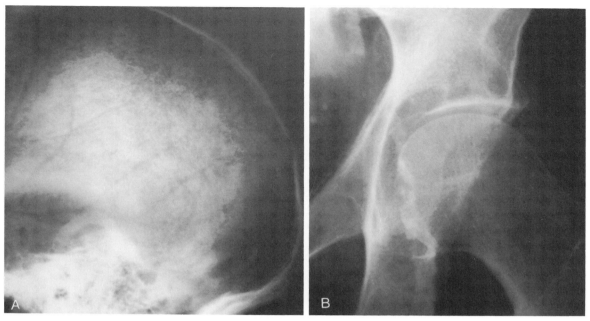

FIGURE 60–35. Waldenström's macroglobulinemia. In two different patients, observe osteolytic lesions of the skull **(A)** and para-acetabular region **(B)**.

perhaps with predilection for the para-acetabular regions, is not uncommon.[214] It has been suggested that osteolytic lesions predominate in those patients with Waldenström's macroglobulinemia who reveal plasmacytic cell morphology,[220] suggesting a close association between macroglobulinemia and myeloma. In fact, these two diseases may coexist in the same patient.[225] As is true in myeloma, the role of scintigraphy in the evaluation of bone lesions in Waldenström's macroglobulinemia is not clear.[226] MR imaging of spinal lesions in Waldenström's macroglobulinemia shows diffuse or patchy patterns of marrow involvement similar to those of plasma cell myeloma.[362] The extent of the disease and its response to therapy may be assessed with this imaging method.

Ischemic necrosis of the femoral or humeral head(s), which could be related to hyperviscosity of the blood, may be an additional manifestation of Waldenström's macroglobulinemia.[227, 228]

Rheumatologic Manifestations

Amyloid deposition in peri- and intra-articular locations in patients with macroglobulinemia has been described.[229] As in myeloma with secondary amyloidosis, the resulting arthropathy may simulate rheumatoid arthritis because of the presence of subcutaneous nodules, symmetric synovial thickening, and osseous erosions. In an additional patient with Waldenström's macroglobulinemia and amyloidosis, peripheral neuropathy and neuropathic osteoarthropathy were apparent.[230] Polyarticular involvement of a lower extremity led to radiographic findings identical to those in neuropathic osteoarthropathy from other causes. Secondary gouty arthritis can be observed in patients with Waldenström's macroglobulinemia.[131]

HEAVY CHAIN DISEASES

Heavy chain disorders consist of a heterogeneous group of conditions characterized by production of fragments of immunoglobulin molecules.[1, 231] Three separate syndromes have been recognized.

Gamma heavy chain disease (heavy chain of IgG) simulates malignant lymphoma. Patients reveal anemia, fever, hepatosplenomegaly, lymphadenopathy, and recurrent infections. Significantly, these persons may reveal historical evidence of tuberculosis or autoimmune diseases (rheumatoid arthritis, systemic lupus erythematosus, and Sjögren's disease). Abnormal cells found on tissue biopsy consist of lymphocytes, plasma cells, plasmacytoid cells, reticulum cells, and eosinophils. Radiographs may outline osteolytic lesions with predilection for the axial skeleton.[231, 232]

Alpha heavy chain disease (heavy chain of IgA)[1] is associated with alpha heavy chains in the serum and an illness whose major manifestations are gastrointestinal.[233]

Mu heavy chain disease (heavy chain of IgM) is the rarest of the three syndromes.[1] It is associated with synthesis of both light and heavy chains of IgM. Pathologic fractures have been reported in this heavy chain disease, perhaps related to steroid therapy.[234]

The heavy chain diseases merge imperceptibly with various lymphoproliferative disorders, including Mediterranean lymphoma, reticulum cell sarcoma, and chronic lymphatic leukemia.[235] Destructive bone lesions and hyperuricemia may be apparent in any of these disorders.

AMYLOIDOSIS

Background

In 1854, Virchow[236, 237] defined a peculiar substance, amyloid, that was capable of infiltrating and enlarging the liver and kidney in conjunction with certain inflammatory diseases. Five years later, Freidreich and Kekule[238] identified the proteinaceous nature of this substance. Sixty years passed before amyloid was studied with direct biopsy procedures[239] and the Congo red staining technique.[240] Subsequently, disorders characterized by amyloid deposition have been investigated in detail, revealing that amyloidosis is not a rare phenomenon. At present, a number of comprehensive reviews of the subject are available.[241–244]

Several systems for classification of cases of amyloidosis have been proposed.[241, 245] Reimann and coworkers[246] divided these cases into primary amyloidosis (no antecedent or coexistent disease), secondary amyloidosis (associated with a chronic disease), tumor-forming amyloidosis (single or multiple amyloid masses in the respiratory tract and genitourinary system), and amyloidosis associated with plasma cell myeloma. Dahlin[247] made use of a similar system, classifying amyloidosis as primary, secondary, and myeloma-associated types, whereas Symmers[248] divided the disorders into generalized amyloidosis without predisposing disease, generalized amyloidosis with predisposing disease, and localized amyloidosis. Although other investigators have used classification systems based on anatomic sites of amyloid deposition,[249] most authors still categorize the disorder as primary and secondary in type, indicating that additional cases must occasionally be placed in other categories, including various hereditary and familial types as well as senile amyloidosis.[250] Their classification system is as follows:

A. *Primary Amyloidosis.* The primary form of amyloidosis occurs without coexistent or antecedent disease. Most frequently it involves certain mesenchymal structures, such as the heart, muscle, tongue, synovial membrane, and perivascular connective tissue. In many patients, primary amyloidosis is associated with multiple myeloma, which generally is nearly simultaneous in onset.[251]

B. *Secondary Amyloidosis.* The secondary form is associated with various chronic diseases, including rheumatoid arthritis, sepsis, neoplasm, inflammatory disorders, and familial Mediterranean fever. It is an important complication of Crohn's disease and cystic fibrosis as well as of chronic drug abuse.[252] Amyloid deposition in the secondary type shows predilection for the liver, spleen, kidneys, and adrenals.

C. *Heredofamilial Amyloidosis.* An increasing number of heredofamilial amyloid syndromes have been described.[241, 253] Affected families have been found in Portugal, Japan, Sweden, Italy, Greece, Denmark, France, Israel, Brazil, and the United States. These syndromes can be classified by the site of predominant organ involvement. Thus, heredofamilial amyloidoses include neuropathies, nephropathies, cardiomyopathies, and miscellaneous types.

D. *Senile Amyloidosis.* Senile amyloidosis refers to a type that increases with age but is not more frequent in any age group in patients with chronic disorders, such as rheumatoid arthritis.[250, 254]

E. *Localized Amyloid Tumors.* In this type of amyloidosis, focal growths occur in the larynx, trachea, bronchi, and rarely skin (lichen amyloidosus).

The foregoing classification system is based primarily on clinical parameters. In recent years, supplementary data related to biochemical information have led to modifications

in the classification of amyloidosis that have been summarized by Cohen.[252] *Primary, or idiopathic, amyloidosis* is related to AL protein, consisting of a portion of the variable region of either kappa or lambda light chains or the whole molecule. *Secondary, or reactive, amyloidosis* is composed of protein AA. *Hereditary, or heredofamilial, amyloidosis* is associated with a variety of protein precursors including transthyretin (prealbumin), apolipoprotein AI, gelsolin, cystatin C, and others. *Amyloid of chronic hemodialysis* is composed of beta-2 microglobulin. This last type of amyloidosis is discussed in detail in Chapter 57 and is addressed further in the following pages.

General Clinical Features

Primary amyloidosis is more frequent in men than in women and its onset generally is between the ages of 40 and 80 years. Cardiac deposition of amyloid results in decompensation with dyspnea, edema, and pleural effusion. Macroglossia produces dysphagia and dysarthria. Additional manifestations are hypertension, lymphadenopathy, weight loss, purpura, scleroderma-like skin changes, and joint pain. If amyloid is deposited in the liver, spleen, and kidney, hepatosplenomegaly and renal abnormality become evident, although these organs are more frequently involved in secondary amyloidosis.

Secondary amyloidosis can develop at any age, depending on the underlying disease process. Amyloid deposition in the kidneys leads to the nephrotic syndrome with albuminuria, cylindruria, edema, hypoalbuminemia, and hypercholesterolemia. Hepatosplenomegaly and adrenal insufficiency may become apparent. Amyloidosis of the gastrointestinal tract may be manifested as obstruction, malabsorption, hemorrhage, protein loss, and diarrhea.

Amyloidosis occurring in association with plasma cell myeloma may be difficult to detect because of the presence of significant clinical findings related to this latter disease. Renal involvement and hepatosplenomegaly can be apparent.

Localized amyloid tumors of the respiratory tract may cause hoarseness, dyspnea, epistaxis, dysphagia, and hemoptysis.

Heredofamilial amyloidoses are associated with neurologic (including sensory neuropathies, autonomic nervous system symptoms and signs, and cranial nerve alterations), cardiac, and renal abnormalities.

Although no laboratory examination is pathognomonic of amyloidosis, the diagnosis can be substantiated by performance of the Congo red test. This test depends on the removal from the blood of injected dye by selective absorption by amyloid deposits. A positive test results in green birefringence when the sample is examined with polarization microscopy. Amyloid deposits can be classified further by treating the tissue with potassium permanganate; AA protein will lose Congo red affinity with such treatment whereas AL protein will not.[252] Both immunofluorescence and immunoperoxidase techniques can be used for precise typing of the amyloid protein. Although multiple organs and tissues, including the gingiva, rectum, liver, spleen, kidney, small intestine, and skin, have been used for diagnostic biopsy, an aspiration biopsy of the subcutaneous abdominal fat pad has become the method of choice.[252]

Musculoskeletal Features

Osseous and articular abnormalities can appear during the course of amyloidosis.[255] In many instances, the abnormalities are the result of amyloid deposition in bone, synovium, and soft tissue. Additionally, in some varieties of amyloidosis, musculoskeletal features are indicative of an underlying disease process. Thus, bone alterations in amyloidosis may relate to coexistent plasma cell myeloma and macroglobulinemia. Secondary amyloidosis may occur in other skeletal disorders,[242] such as chronic osteomyelitis (tuberculous or nontuberculous), and neoplasm.

Amyloidosis Complicating Rheumatologic Disorders. The association of rheumatoid arthritis and secondary amyloidosis is well established, and in many large series of patients with this type of amyloid deposition, rheumatoid arthritis is its leading cause. The reported frequency of amyloidosis in rheumatoid arthritis has varied, most investigations indicating an occurrence rate of 5 to 25 per cent.[256–259] Much of this variation relates to patient selection and diagnostic procedures used to establish amyloid disease. Amyloidosis rarely develops in patients with rheumatoid arthritis who have had their disease for less than 2 years. The clinical diagnosis of secondary amyloidosis in patients with rheumatoid arthritis is supported by the presence of proteinuria, although hepatosplenomegaly and gastrointestinal bleeding are other important diagnostic findings. Amyloidosis developing in children is most frequently secondary to juvenile-onset rheumatoid arthritis,[260–262] although it also may complicate chronic suppurative diseases and familial Mediterranean fever in this age group. The reported prevalence of amyloidosis in patients with juvenile-onset rheumatoid arthritis has varied from less than 1 per cent to more than 10 per cent.[252]

Amyloidosis may occur during the course of ankylosing spondylitis.[263] Jayson and coworkers[264] detected rectal amyloidosis in 9 per cent of patients with this disease. Amyloidosis also may occur during the course of other spondyloarthropathies, including Reiter's disease,[265–268] psoriatic arthritis,[269–271] and intestinal arthropathies.[272–274]

Amyloid deposition may be apparent in collagen vascular disorders such as systemic lupus erythematosus, dermatomyositis,[275, 276] polyarteritis nodosa,[277] and Gaucher's disease.[278, 279] Amyloid deposition may be recognized as an incidental finding in the articular capsule, cartilage, and synovial membrane of patients with osteoarthritis,[280–284] within joints of elderly asymptomatic persons,[285, 286] and in the herniated intervertebral discs of older patients.[287, 288] Widespread intervertebral discal calcification has been observed in primary amyloidosis.[289]

Although rare, amyloidosis has been reported in association with gout, generally preceding the acute attacks of this articular disease and accompanied by chronic infections.[290, 291] An association of amyloidosis with calcium pyrophosphate dihydrate crystal deposition disease is suggested by an increasing number of reports describing cartilage, synovial, and capsular calcification in the former disorder.[292–295] Some of these reports state that calcium pyrophosphate dihydrate crystals have been recovered during joint aspiration, and both local amyloid and calcium pyrophosphate dihydrate crystal deposits occasionally are observed in capsular tissues of patients with osteoarthritis or pyrophosphate arthropathy.[296]

Amyloidosis complicating familial Mediterranean fever deserves special emphasis.[297] This disorder, which was described by Siegal in 1945,[298] is characterized by fever, recurrent attacks of pleural and peritoneal pain due to serositis, and articular symptoms; occurs predominantly in childhood; and shows predilection for persons from eastern Mediterranean areas.[299] As many as 25 to 30 per cent of patients with this disorder may develop secondary amyloidosis,[300] and this complication ultimately can lead to the patient's death from renal failure. Additional patients may reveal splenomegaly and, rarely, hepatomegaly and malabsorption.

Bone Lesions. Although articular involvement is a known complication of amyloidosis, there are few descriptions of osseous changes in this disease[189, 255, 301–306] (Table 60–2). Osteoporosis, lytic lesions of bone, and pathologic fractures may be observed (Fig. 60–36).[307] Radiolucent areas of variable size are detected within medullary and cortical bone, particularly in the proximal portion of the femur and proximal end of the humerus. These lesions produce scalloping along the endosteal margin of the cortex, simulating the appearance of plasma cell myeloma. They are produced by focal deposits of amyloid, some of which may localize in subchondral bone.[302] In this latter location, secondary occlusion of blood vessels related to perivascular amyloidosis can lead to osteonecrosis of epiphyses with collapse. Subperiosteal deposits of amyloid have been described[306] but are rare. Elsewhere, amyloidosis of bone marrow can produce vertebral osteoporosis and collapse.[303, 305, 308, 309]

There are occasional reports of tumorous lesions of bone containing amyloid.[303, 307, 310–312] These lesions predominate in patients with plasma cell myeloma and coexistent amyloidosis and usually are associated with plasma cell infiltration as well.[313–315] As in cases of diffuse amyloidosis of bone, pathologic fractures, especially in the spine and proximal portion of the femur, complicate localized "amyloidomas." Calcification within these lesions may be evident.

Articular and Periarticular Lesions. The articular manifestations of amyloidosis are characterized by the accumulation of this substance in synovial tissue, other intra-articular structures, peritendinous areas, and surrounding soft tissue[316] (Figs. 60–37 to 60–39). Soft tissue amyloid deposition produces nodules resembling those of rheumatoid arthritis. Amyloid nodules are particularly prominent in the olecranon region and about joints of the hand and wrist. These masses as well as other soft tissue amyloid collections may accumulate bone-seeking radiopharmaceutical agents.[317] Extensive infiltration about the shoulders produces rubbery, hard masses that are accentuated by surrounding muscle atrophy, resembling the shoulder pads

TABLE 60–2. Radiographic Manifestations of Musculoskeletal Involvement in Amyloidosis

Osteoporosis
Lytic lesions
Pathologic fractures
Osteonecrosis
Soft tissue nodules and swelling
Subchondral cysts and erosions
Joint subluxations and contractures
Neuropathic osteoarthropathy

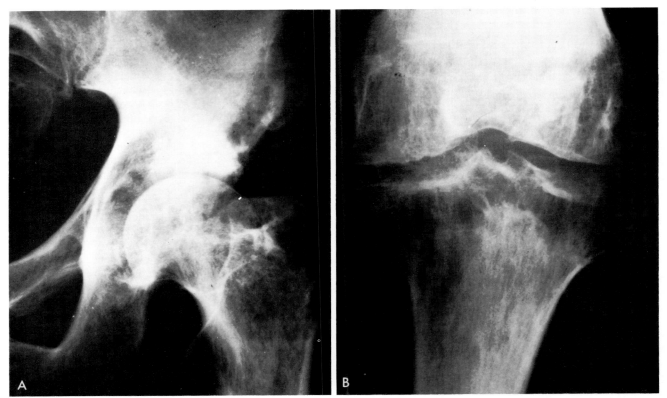

FIGURE 60–36. Amyloidosis: Lytic lesions and osteoporosis. A 48 year old black man developed a progressive neuropathy of the lower extremities and diarrhea. Amyloidosis was confirmed on biopsy of the muscle, stomach, and ilium. There was no clinical or laboratory evidence of myeloma.

A Osteolytic lesions with reactive sclerosis can be seen in the ilium and proximal portion of the femur.

B In the femur and tibia, there appears to be evidence of both osteoporosis and small lytic lesions.

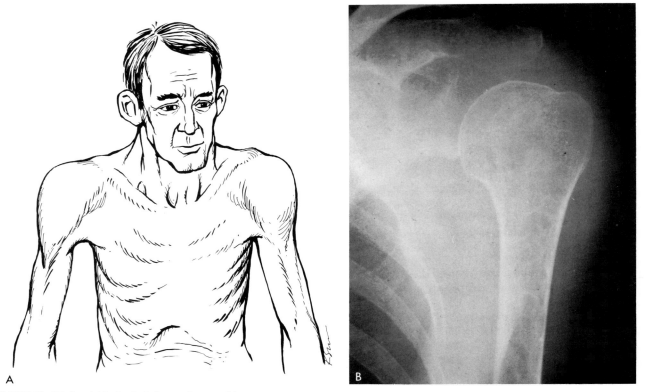

FIGURE 60–37. Amyloidosis: Soft tissue abnormalities.

A Patients with amyloidosis may have hard, rubbery masses about the shoulders resembling in appearance the shoulder pads worn by football players.

B Radiographs in such patients may indicate the degree of soft tissue swelling and associated osteoporosis of underlying bones.

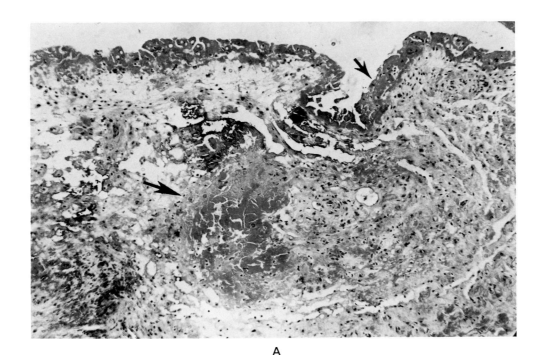

A

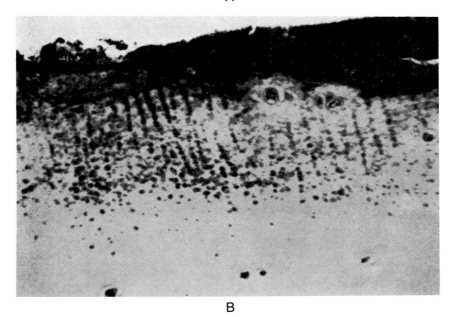

B

FIGURE 60–38. Amyloidosis: Articular abnormalities—pathologic alterations.
 A Amyloid deposition in the synovial membrane. On a photomicrograph (150×), amyloid deposition (arrows) is located predominantly superficially in the synovial lining cells and deeper in the subsynovial tissue.
 B Amyloid deposition in the cartilage. On a photomicrograph (300×), surface and deeper deposits of amyloid are apparent. This deposition has occurred both parallel to the surface and as strings of beads along parallel straight lines extending deeply from the surface.
 (**A,** From Copeman WS, 1969, by courtesy of E. G. L. Bywaters, M.D., London, England; **B,** From Bywaters EGL, Dorling J: Ann Rheum Dis *29:*294, 1970).

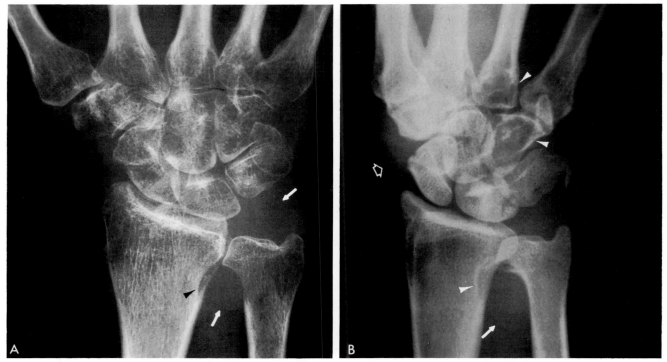

FIGURE 60–39. Amyloidosis: Articular abnormalities—radiographic alterations.

A A 47 year old woman with progressive pain and swelling in multiple joints developed the carpal tunnel syndrome. Complete workup revealed the presence of amyloidosis complicating plasma cell myeloma. Observe soft tissue swelling and osteoporosis. A distended inferior radioulnar joint can be seen (arrows) with associated osseous erosion (arrowhead).

B In a different patient, similar soft tissue swelling (open arrow) and distention of the inferior radioulnar joint are apparent (solid arrow). More extensive osseous erosions are evident (arrowheads). Wrist biopsy documented the presence of amyloid infiltration. This person, who also had plasma cell myeloma, died approximately 1 year later. (**B**, Courtesy of A. Brower, M.D., Norfolk, Virginia.)

worn by football players.[190, 318, 319] Similar deposits in the carpal canal lead to the carpal tunnel syndrome[320, 321]; in fact, 5 to 10 per cent of patients with this syndrome may reveal amyloid infiltration in the adjacent soft tissues.[322] Alternatively, 10 to 30 per cent of patients with primary amyloidosis reveal the carpal tunnel syndrome, and the prevalence of this syndrome may be even higher in persons with plasma cell myeloma and amyloidosis. Furthermore, amyloid deposition has been documented in the wrists of patients with chronic renal disease (requiring dialysis) and the carpal tunnel syndrome (see Chapter 57). Typically, in cases of this syndrome that result from amyloidosis, a bilateral distribution is seen, and symptoms and signs related to this complication commonly precede other manifestations of the disease, underscoring the advisability of biopsy of the synovium and flexor retinaculum at the time of carpal tunnel decompression.[320]

The clinical findings of amyloid joint disease resemble the manifestations of rheumatoid arthritis.[180, 181, 323–326] Bilateral symmetric arthritis of large and small joints characterized by pain, stiffness, swelling, and palpable nodules is seen in both disorders. This clinical difficulty in distinguishing patients with amyloidosis from those with rheumatoid arthritis is accentuated by the pathologic observation that rheumatoid arthritis frequently is associated with articular deposits of amyloid, although these deposits generally are microscopic and asymptomatic. The absence of fever, of joint tenderness to palpation, and of evidence of true inflammation as detected by synovial fluid analysis[185, 327] is a clinical and laboratory characteristic of amy-

loidosis that is not evident in rheumatoid arthritis. Furthermore, analysis of synovial fluid sediments with Congo red testing may represent a simple and sensitive diagnostic test of amyloid arthropathy.[328]

Amyloidosis may lead to joint contractures; these contractures usually are the result of muscle and nerve involvement, although articular and periarticular amyloid deposition may contribute to this clinical finding. Contractures can appear in any joint, including those of the fingers.[329]

In addition to localization in soft tissue, joint capsule, tendon, bone, and synovial membrane, amyloid deposition also occurs in the surface layers of articular cartilage.[330, 331] Although the mechanism by which amyloid becomes located within cartilage is not known, it has been suggested that these cartilaginous deposits result from the diffusion of a soluble amyloid precursor from the synovial fluid, or alternatively from the permeation of fine amyloid fibrils that have been cast into the synovial fluid from the synovial membrane.[331] An additional possibility is that amyloid may be secreted by chondrocytes into cartilage matrix.

The radiographic findings of joint involvement in amyloidosis reflect this intra-articular and periarticular distribution of amyloid[185, 316, 322, 326, 329–332] (Table 60–2). Asymmetric soft tissue masses, periarticular osteoporosis, widening of the articular space, subchondral cysts, and erosions are seen. Subluxation, lytic lesions of bone, and pathologic fractures are additional manifestations. These abnormalities may appear in any involved joint, particularly the wrists, hips, shoulders, elbows, and knees. Involvement frequently is bilateral in distribution. Although the radiographic appearance is reminiscent of that in rheumatoid arthritis, extensive soft tissue nodular masses, well-defined cystic lesions with or without surrounding sclerosis, and preservation of joint space are more characteristic of amyloid joint disease. These latter features can be observed in gout and xanthomatosis, disorders whose appearance may be quite similar to that of amyloidosis. Arthrography in patients with amyloid joint disease may reveal an enlarged joint cavity and numerous filling defects.[329]

Extensive joint destruction occasionally is encountered in amyloidosis. This may result from osteonecrosis of epiphyseal surfaces[333] or neuropathic osteoarthropathy.[230, 334] Neuropathy in amyloidosis is common in some of the hereditary forms of the disease, although it may be apparent in the primary and secondary forms as well. Sensory loss is particularly characteristic, perhaps attributable to amyloid infiltration within nerve tissue or the spinal canal[335] or to accompanying uremic neuropathy. Despite the frequency of amyloid neuropathy, only on rare occasions has neuropathic osteoarthropathy been encountered with typical radiographic characteristics, including soft tissue swelling, extreme sclerosis, bony fragmentation, and disorganization (Fig. 60–40).[336]

These descriptions of amyloid arthritis generally relate to primary amyloidosis or that associated with multiple myeloma. Rarely, erosive arthritis of the hands and wrists has been noted in patients with heredofamilial amyloidosis.[337, 338] In such cases, small bone erosions and cysts are observed, and scintigraphy reveals increased local accumulation of bone-seeking radiopharmaceutical agents (Fig. 60–41). As tissue biopsies have outlined evidence of only minimal amyloid deposition, the precise cause of articular disease in heredofamilial amyloidosis is not clear.[338]

Magnetic Resonance Imaging

The MR imaging features of amyloid arthropathy in patients with the primary or secondary type of disease have received little attention. In one report, Tagliabue and coworkers[339] emphasized that this imaging method allows analysis of cartilaginous and bone destruction accompanying this arthropathy and that a homogeneous intermediate signal intensity of amyloid deposition is evident on both T1-weighted and T2-weighted spin echo sequences. In this report, the soft tissue and capsular deposits of amyloid were demonstrated vividly on the T2-weighted images owing to their relatively low signal intensity in comparison to that of the adjacent joint effusion. The gradient echo and short tau inversion recovery (STIR) sequences that also were employed by these investigators proved useful in the assessment of the extent of joint involvement.

Metzler and coworkers[340] investigated the role of MR imaging in the evaluation of amyloid myopathy. Such myopathy, which is a rare manifestation of primary amyloidosis, leads to stiffness, weakness, generalized enlargement of muscles, and a woody consistency of the limbs. These investigators used spin echo and STIR MR imaging sequences in two patients with amyloid myopathy. With all sequences, signal intensity alterations in involved musculature were minimal, in contrast to a wide variety of other myopathies, in which focal collections of fat or edema, or both, produce dramatic changes in intramuscular signal intensity. In amyloidosis, enlargement of affected muscles and disappearance of normal muscle contour and boundaries may be evident, and a coarse reticulated pattern of decreased signal intensity within the subcutaneous tissue also may be encountered.[340]

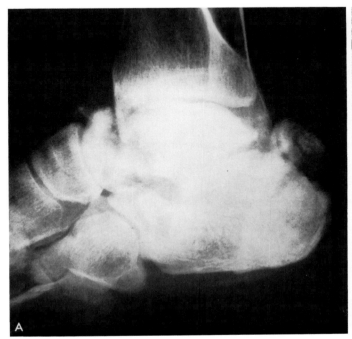 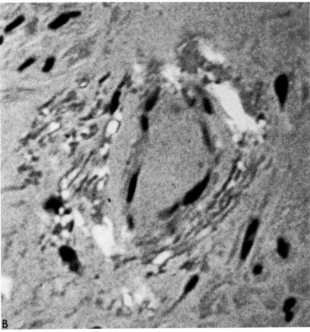

FIGURE 60–40. Amyloidosis: Articular abnormalities—neuropathic osteoarthropathy. A 50 year old man with primary amyloidosis developed progressive renal disease and sensory neuropathy of the legs.
  A Observe the extreme destruction of the talus and calcaneus, characterized by sclerosis and fragmentation.
  B A photomicrograph (1000×, Congo red) following a sural nerve biopsy reveals amyloid deposits in and around an arteriole of the nerve. (From Peitzman SJ, et al: JAMA 235:1345, 1976. Copyright 1976, American Medical Association.)

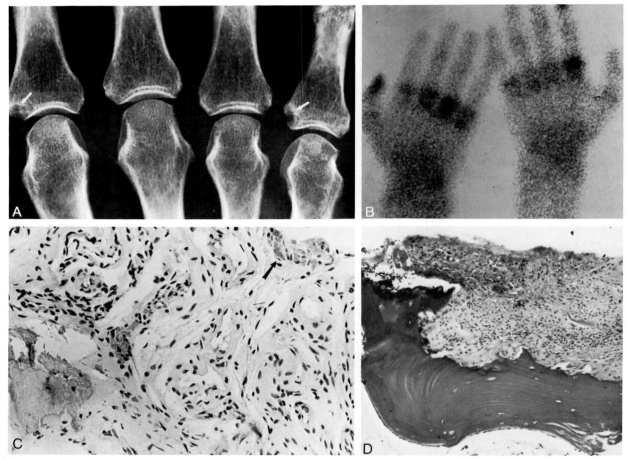

FIGURE 60–41. Heredofamilial amyloidosis: Articular erosions. This 57 year old man developed carpal tunnel syndrome, vitreous opacities, shortness of breath, and swelling in the lower extremities. He had a 10 year history of fullness and stiffness in the metacarpophalangeal joints and, to a lesser extent, wrists and metatarsophalangeal articulations. Biopsy of the skin and rectum revealed amyloid deposits. Other family members were affected similarly.

A The radiograph reveals small, discrete erosions, particularly in the proximal phalanges of the second and fifth digits (arrows).

B A radioisotope (^{99m}Tc methylene diphosphonate) study shows increased uptake of the radiopharmaceutical agent about the metacarpophalangeal joints.

C A histopathologic section (using Congo red stain) of tissue from an involved metacarpophalangeal joint indicates mild proliferation of the synovium and amyloid deposits (arrow).

D In a different patient (a 50 year old Swedish man) with the same disease, a photomicrograph of abnormal synovium in a distal interphalangeal joint of the hand shows synovial proliferation with erosion of cartilage and bone. No large deposits of amyloid were identified.

(From Eyanson S, Benson MD: Arthritis Rheum *26*:1145, 1983.)

A further discussion of MR imaging in the assessment of musculoskeletal involvement in amyloidosis is contained in Chapter 57 in which dialysis-related amyloid deposition is considered.

Differential Diagnosis

Bone Lesions. Diffuse lytic lesions in amyloidosis are indistinguishable from those accompanying more common disorders, particularly skeletal metastasis and plasma cell myeloma. Differentiation of amyloidosis from this latter disorder is especially difficult, as both myeloma and amyloidosis are associated with subcortical radiolucent shadows with scalloping of the adjacent cortex, and, in addition, both diseases may coexist in the same person. Bone lysis in Waldenström's macroglobulinemia also is virtually identical to that accompanying amyloidosis.

Localized destructive lesions of the skeleton in amyloidosis resemble sites of metastasis or a primary bone neoplasm. They generally are well marginated and located in the spine or the metaphyseal and diaphyseal regions of tubular bones, especially the femur. A soft tissue mass is common, but periostitis is rare.[326]

Articular Lesions. Articular lesions in amyloidosis are characterized by bulky soft tissue masses, well-defined erosions and cysts, and preservation of joint space. These features usually can be distinguished from those of rheumatoid arthritis, which is associated with symmetric soft tissue swelling, early joint space loss, and marginal erosions of bone, although in some patients, amyloidosis and rheumatoid arthritis can produce similar abnormalities on both radiographic and clinical examination. Amyloid joint disease shares many radiographic characteristics with gouty arthritis and xanthomatosis, although clinical and laboratory manifestations of these latter disorders usually ensure their accurate diagnosis. The arthropathy of amyloidosis also resembles pigmented villonodular synovitis; distinguishing features of the former include multiple sites of involvement, juxta-articular osteoporosis, and the older age of the patients.[326]

AGAMMAGLOBULINEMIA AND HYPOGAMMAGLOBULINEMIA

Background and General Features

Agammaglobulinemia and hypogammaglobulinemia are syndromes associated with considerable impairment of antibody formation and, in most instances, depressed levels of plasma gamma globulins. These disorders may arise from either a diminished rate of synthesis of gamma globulins (primary form) or an increased rate of catabolism or loss of gamma globulins (secondary form).[341–343] The primary form of agammaglobulinemia may be congenital or acquired and is associated with morphologic changes in the lymphoid tissue and with failure in the development of plasma cells in lymph nodes and bone marrow and of antibodies in the blood after antigenic stimulation. The secondary form of hypogammaglobulinemia results from gamma globulin loss in the intestine, urine, or skin. Histologically the lymphoid tissue in secondary hypogammaglobulinemia is normal, and the serum levels of plasma gamma globulins

generally are higher than those in the primary form of the disease.

The clinical manifestations of agammaglobulinemia and hypogammaglobulinemia are characterized by recurrent and severe infections, most commonly related to bacterial organisms. The age of onset of infection will vary, depending on the type of syndrome that is present. Congenital (primary) agammaglobulinemia may appear in infants, whereas acquired (primary) agammaglobulinemia and hypogammaglobulinemia secondary to nephrotic syndrome or exudative enteropathy may occur at any age. The types of infection encountered in these disorders include sinusitis, otitis media, conjunctivitis, pneumonia, meningitis, septic arthritis,[344] and furunculosis. Tuberculosis and fungal disorders also can be apparent. Lymphadenopathy and splenomegaly are seen. Repeated infections can lead to bronchiectasis, pulmonary scarring, and pleural thickening after thoracic disease, hydrocephalus after meningitis, and hearing loss from recurrent otitis media. In addition, certain connective tissue disorders appear with increased frequency in patients so affected; these disorders include systemic lupus erythematosus, scleroderma, polyarteritis nodosa, dermatomyositis, and a noninflammatory synovitis.[341–343, 345, 346]

Musculoskeletal Abnormalities

A chronic inflammatory polyarthritis that resembles rheumatoid arthritis is seen in patients with agammaglobulinemia and hypogammaglobulinemia[347–357] (Fig. 60–42). The reported frequency of this complication has varied from 10 to 30 per cent of patients.[348–351] It is more frequent in men than in women, in children than in adults, and in patients with very low levels or total lack of globulins.[354] Clinically, pain, tenderness, stiffness, and swelling in small and large joints resemble findings of rheumatoid arthritis, although asymmetric involvement is more characteristic of agammaglobulinemia than of rheumatoid arthritis. Symptoms and signs may be transient, disappearing spontaneously, or persistent, although permanent joint damage is uncommon. Subcutaneous nodules may appear in the elbows and elsewhere, which histologically resemble rheumatoid nodules except for the absence of plasma cells. Laboratory analysis usually reveals an elevated erythrocyte sedimentation rate and nonreactive serum rheumatoid factor. The joint aspirate reveals fluid that is noninflammatory in type. Although the polyarthritis is associated with extremely low or undetectable amounts of serum immunoglobulins, these substances can be detected in the synovial fluid and synovial membrane in some patients.[351, 352, 358]

Synovial histologic findings include lymphocytic infiltration and proliferation of blood vessels.[347, 352] Mononuclear cells containing immunoglobulins are seen, but plasma cells usually are not apparent. Other reports have indicated that synovial biopsy in these patients may reveal capillary proliferation and infiltration with macrophages but without lymphocytic infiltration. Rarely, rice bodies have been found.[359]

Illustrated radiographs in these earlier reports have shown soft tissue swelling, periarticular osteoporosis, joint space narrowing, and deformities without osseous erosions.[354] The radiographic appearance is reminiscent of Jac-

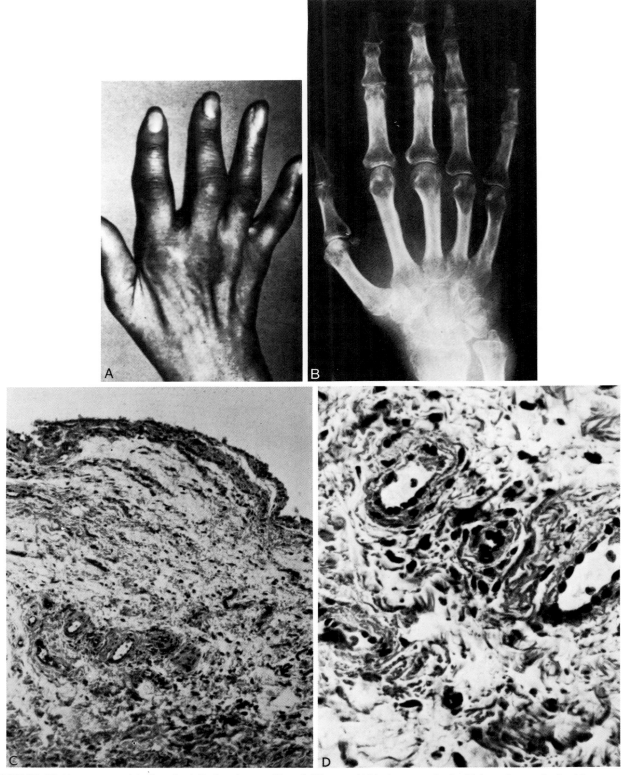

FIGURE 60–42. Hypogammaglobulinemia: Articular abnormalities. A 57 year old black woman had a history of a mediastinal thymoma and an inflammatory polyarthritis with symmetric involvement of the small joints of the hands, the wrists, the shoulders, the knees, and the ankles. Hypogammaglobulinemia was noted. The patient died several months later.

   A A clinical photograph reveals soft tissue swelling about interphalangeal and wrist joints. The opposite side was affected similarly.

   B A radiograph outlines soft tissue swelling, periarticular osteoporosis, and joint space narrowing of proximal interphalangeal, metacarpophalangeal, and wrist joints. No erosions are evident.

   C, D Low (110×) and high (400×) power photomicrographs after synovial biopsy of the right knee reveal hypertrophy of the subsynovial tissues and marked proliferation of new blood vessels, with endothelial cell hypertrophy and proliferation. Very few inflammatory cells are apparent within the synovium, no collections of lymphocytes are present, and the synovial lining cells are not hyperplastic.

   (From Grayzel AI, et al: Arthritis Rheum *20:*887, 1977.)

coud's arthropathy and that accompanying systemic lupus erythematosus.

The pathogenesis of these joint abnormalities in patients with hypogammaglobulinemia and agammaglobulinemia is not clear.[353, 354] Its variable nature may be related to the presence or absence of lymphocytic response and immunoglobulins within the involved joint.[357] The condition should be suspected clinically in either a child or an adult who historically has had recurrent infections and who develops polyarthritis that is characterized by asymmetry, osteoporosis, and joint deformity without the appearance of significant bony erosions.

SUMMARY

Musculoskeletal findings occur in various plasma cell dyscrasias and dysgammaglobulinemias. In plasma cell myeloma, such findings represent a predominant manifestation of the disease, which leads to characteristic pathologic and radiologic abnormalities. Widespread or localized osteolysis can be attributed, in large part, to plasma cell infiltration in the bone marrow. Accompanying amyloid deposition in some patients may become manifest as articular and periarticular alterations. Additional joint findings in plasma cell myeloma may be related to secondary gout, infection, and hemarthrosis. Skeletal and articular manifestations of Waldenström's macroglobulinemia, although less frequent and less well known, resemble those of plasma cell myeloma. Amyloidosis, which can occur in both plasma cell myeloma and Waldenström's macroglobulinemia, also can be apparent in a primary form without antecedent cause or in a secondary form in various other conditions. In both primary and secondary types, amyloid deposition can lead to significant bone and joint changes, including osteoporosis, osseous lytic lesions, and tumorous foci in both articular and extra-articular locations. Finally, syndromes related to antibody deficiency (agammaglobulinemia, hypogammaglobulinemia) are associated with recurrent and severe infections that may involve bones and joints and a rheumatoid arthritis-like chronic asymmetric polyarthritis.

References

1. Siegelman SS: Plasma cell dyscrasias. *In* RO Murray, HG Jacobson (Eds): The Radiology of Skeletal Disorders. 2nd Ed. Edinburgh, Churchill Livingstone, 1977, p 1824.
2. Park YK, Trubowitz S, Davis S: Plasma cell in the bone marrow. *In* Trubowitz S, Davis S (Eds): The Human Bone Marrow: Anatomy, Physiology, and Pathophysiology. Vol 2. Boca Raton, FL:CRC Press, 1982, p 187.
3. Osserman EF: Plasma cell dyscrasias. *In* PB Beeson, W McDermott, JB Wyngaarden (Eds): Cecil Textbook of Medicine. 15th Ed. Philadelphia, WB Saunders Co, 1979, p 1852.
4. Isobe, T, Osserman EF: Pathologic conditions associated with plasma cell dyscrasias: A study of 806 cases. Ann NY Acad Sci *190*:507, 1971.
5. Osserman EF: Plasma cell dyscrasias. *In* PB Beeson, W McDermott, JB Wyngaarden (Eds): Cecil Textbook of Medicine. 15th Ed. Philadelphia, WB Saunders Co, 1979, p 1852.
6. Moya-Mir MS, Martin-Martin F, Barbadillo R, et al: Plasma cell dyscrasia with polyneuritis and dermato-endocrine alterations. Postgrad Med J *56*:427, 1980.
7. Kyle RA: Multiple myeloma. Review of 869 cases. Mayo Clin Proc *50*:29, 1975.
8. Clamp, JR: Some aspects of the first recorded case of multiple myeloma. Lancet *2*:1354, 1967.
9. Longsworth LG, Shedlovsky T, MacInnes DA: Electrophoretic patterns of normal and pathological human blood serum and plasma. J Exp Med *70*:399, 1939.
10. Grabar P, Williams CA: Méthode permettant l'étude conjuguée des propriétes électrophoretiques et immunochimiques d'un mélange de protéines: Application au sérum sanguin. Biochim Biophys Acta *10*:193, 1953.
11. Oken MM: Multiple myeloma. Med Clin North Am *68*:757, 1984.
12. Dahlin DC: Plasma cell myeloma. *In* Bone Tumors. Springfield, Ill. Charles C Thomas, 1967, p 116.
13. Carson CP, Ackerman LV, Maltby JD: Plasma cell myeloma. A clinical, pathologic and roentgenologic review of 90 cases. Am J Clin Pathol *25*:849, 1955.
14. Jacoby P: Myelomatosis in a child of 8 years. Acta Radiol *11*:224, 1930.
15. Slavens JJ: Multiple myeloma in a child. Am J Dis Child *47*:821, 1934.
16. Porter FS: Multiple myeloma in a child. J Pediatr *62*:602, 1963.
17. Hewell GM, Alexanian R: Multiple myeloma in young persons. Ann Intern Med *84*:441, 1976.
18. Griffiths DL: Orthopedic aspects of myelomatosis. J Bone Joint Surg [Br] *48*:703, 1966.
19. Todd IDH: Treatment of solitary plasmacytoma. Clin Radiol *16*:395, 1965.
20. Goodman MA: Plasma cell tumors. Clin Orthop *204*:86, 1986.
21. Kapadia SB: Multiple myeloma: A clinicopathologic study of 62 consecutively autopsied cases. Medicine *59*:380, 1980.
22. Alexanian R, Barlogie B, Dixon D: Prognosis of asymptomatic multiple myeloma. Arch Intern Med *148*:1963, 1988.
23. Hellwig CA: Extramedullary plasma cell tumors as observed in various locations. Arch Pathol *36*:95, 1943.
24. Martinez-Maldonado M, Yium J, Suki WN, et al: Renal complications in multiple myeloma: Pathophysiology and some aspects of clinical management. J Chron Dis *24*:221, 1971.
25. De Waal A, Potgieter GM, Visser AE, et al: IgD myeloma. S Afr Med J *61*:407, 1982.
26. Mancilla R, Davis CL: Nonsecretory multiple myeloma. Am J Med *63*:1015, 1977.
27. Azar HA, Zarrico EC, Pham TD, et al: "Nonsecretory" plasma cell myeloma—observations on seven cases with electron microscopic studies. Am J Clin Pathol *58*:618, 1972.
28. Moehring HD: Nonsecretory myeloma. A case report. Clin Orthop *171*:196, 1982.
29. Gompels GM, Votaw ML, Martel W: Correlation of radiological manifestations of multiple myeloma with immunoglobulin abnormalities and prognosis. Radiology *104*:509, 1972.
30. Pruzanski W, Rother I: IgD plasma cell neoplasia: Clinical manifestations and characteristic features. Can Med Assoc J *102*:1061, 1970.
31. Clyne DH, Brendstrup L, First MR, et al: Renal effects of intraperitoneal kappa chain injection: Induction of crystals in renal tubular cells. Lab Invest *31*:131, 1974.
32. Maldanado JE, Velosa JA, Kyle RA, et al: Fanconi syndrome in adults. A manifestation of a latent form of myeloma. Am J Med *58*:354, 1975.
33. Harrison JF, Blainey JD: Adult Fanconi syndrome with monoclonal abnormality of immunoglobulin light chain. J Clin Pathol *20*:42, 1967.
34. Fahey JL, Barth WF, Solomon A: Serum hyperviscosity syndrome. JAMA *192*:464, 1965.
35. Mackenzie MR, Fudenberg HH, O'Reilly HA: The hyperviscosity syndrome. I. In IgG myeloma. The role of protein concentration and molecular shape. J Clin Invest *49*:15, 1970.
36. Fadem RS: Differentiation of plasmacytic responses from myelomatous diseases on the basis of bone-marrow findings. Cancer *5*:128, 1952.
37. Liu CT, Dahlke MB: Bone marrow findings of reactive plasmacytosis. Am J Clin Pathol *48*:546, 1967.
38. Buss DH, Prichard RW, Hartz JW, et al: Initial bone marrow findings in multiple myeloma. Significance of plasma cell nodules. Arch Pathol Lab Med *110*:30, 1986.
39. Pettengill OS, Sorenson GD, Elliott ML: Murine myeloma in tissue culture. Arch Pathol *82*:483, 1966.
40. Potter M: A resume of the current status of the development of plasma cell tumors in mice. Cancer Res *28*:1891, 1968.
41. Pilgrim HI: The relationship of chronic ulceration of the ileocecal junction to the development of reticuloendothelial tumors in C₃H mice. Cancer Res *25*:53, 1965.
42. Franzen S, Johansson B, Kaigas M: Primary polycythaemia associated with multiple myeloma. Acta Med Scand (Suppl 445) *179*:336, 1966.
43. Maldonado JE, Kyle RA: Familial myeloma. Report of eight families and a study of serum proteins in their relatives. Am J Med *57*:875, 1974.
44. Shoenfeld Y, Berliner S, Shaklai M, et al: Familial multiple myeloma. A review of thirty-seven families. Postgrad Med J *58*:12, 1982.
45. Festen JJ, Marrink J, Le Waard-Kuiper EH, et al: Immunoglobulins in families of myeloma patients. Scand J Immunol *6*:887, 1977.
46. Mundy GR, Raisz LG, Cooper RA, et al: Evidence for the secretion of an osteoclast stimulating factor in myeloma. N Engl J Med *291*:1041, 1974.
47. Durie BGM, Salmon SE, Mundy GR: Relation of osteoclast activating factor production to extent of bone disease in multiple myeloma. Br J Haematol *47*:21, 1981.
48. Evans CE, Galasko CB, Ward C: Does myeloma secrete an osteoblast inhibiting factor? J Bone Joint Surg [Br] *71*:288, 1989.
49. Salmon SE: Immunoglobulin synthesis and tumor kinetics of multiple myeloma. Semin Hematol *10*:135, 1973.
50. Spjut HJ, Dorfman HD, Fechner RE, et al: Tumors of Bone and Cartilage. Atlas of Tumor Pathology. Second Series. Fascicle 5. Washington DC, Armed Forces Institute of Pathology, 1971, p 201.
51. Meszaros WT: The many facets of multiple myeloma. Semin Roentgenol *9*:219, 1974.

52. Heiser S, Schwartzman JJ: Variation in the roentgen appearance of the skeletal system in myeloma. Radiology 58:178, 1952.
53. Osserman EF: Natural history of multiple myeloma before radiological evidence of disease. Radiology 71:157, 1958.
54. Yentis I: Radiological aspects of myelomatosis. Clin Radiol 12:1, 1961.
55. Wiedermann B, Krvč C, Soyka O, et al: Plasmozytome mit generalisierter Osteosklerose. Folia Haemat 86:47, 1966.
56. Clarisse PDT, Staple TW: Diffuse bone sclerosis in multiple myeloma. Radiology 99:327, 1971.
57. Himmelfarb E, Sebes J, Rabinowitz J: Unusual roentgenographic presentations of multiple myeloma. Report of three cases. J Bone Joint Surg [Am] 56:1723, 1974.
58. Evison G, Evans KT: Bone sclerosis in multiple myeloma. Br J Radiol 40:81, 1967.
59. Engels EP, Smith RC, Krantz S: Bone sclerosis in multiple myeloma. Radiology 75:242, 1960.
60. Lewin H, Stein JM: Solitary plasma cell myeloma with new bone formation. AJR 79:630, 1958.
61. Odelberg-Johnson O: Osteosclerotic changes in myelomatosis: Report of a case. Acta Radiol (Diagn) 52:139, 1959.
62. Rypins EL: An unusual roentgenologic finding in multiple myeloma. AJR 30:56, 1933.
63. Blaquiere RM, Guyer PB, Buchanan RB, et al: Sclerotic bone deposits in multiple myeloma. Br J Radiol 55:591, 1982.
64. Edelman RR, Kaufman H, Kolodny GM: Case report 350. Skel Radiol 15:160, 1986.
65. Hall FM, Gore SM: Osteosclerotic myeloma variants. Skel Radiol 17:101, 1988.
66. Quilichini R, Lafeuillade A, Albatro J, et al: Myélome ostéocondensant et neuropathie périphérique. Un nouveau cas. Sem Hôp Paris 67:227, 1991.
67. Farman J, Degnan TJ: Multiple myeloma with small-bone involvement. NY State Med 76:990, 1976.
68. Pobanz DM, Condon JV, Baker LA: Plasma-cell myelomatosis: Report of a case with multiple large tumors involving the digits of both hands. Arch Intern Med 96:828, 1955.
69. Uehlinger E: Case report 1. Skel Radiol 1:55, 1976.
70. Kouwenber JJ, Simons AJ: Case report 383. Skel Radiol 15:484, 1986.
71. Lewin RW, Cataldo E: Multiple myeloma discovered from oral manifestations: Report of a case. J Oral Surg 25:68, 1967.
72. Spitzer R, Price LW: Solitary myeloma of the mandible. Br Med J 1:1027, 1948.
73. Ramon Y, Oberman M, Horowitz I, et al: A large mandibular tumor with a distinct radiological "sun-ray effect" as the primary manifestation of multiple myeloma. J Oral Surg 36:52, 1978.
74. Coughlin C, Greenwald ES, Schraft WC, et al: Myelofibrosis associated with multiple myeloma. Arch Intern Med 138:590, 1978.
75. Brody JI, Beizer LH, Schwartz S: Multiple myeloma and the myeloproliferative syndromes. Am J Med 36:315, 1964.
76. Modan B: Inter-relationship between polycythemia vera, leukemia, and myeloid metaplasia. Clin Hematol 4:427, 1975.
77. Bowyer RC, Touquet VLR: Spontaneous sternal fracture—a misnomer. J R Soc Med 79:175, 1986.
78. Jacobson HG, Poppel MH, Shapiro JH, et al: The vertebral pedicle sign: A roentgen finding to differentiate metastatic carcinoma from multiple myeloma. AJR 80:817, 1958.
79. Bayrd ED: The bone marrow on sternal aspiration in multiple myeloma. Blood 3:987, 1948.
80. Erf LA, Herbut PA: Comparative cytology of Wright's stained smears and histologic sections in multiple myeloma. Am J Clin Pathol 16:1, 1946.
81. Bell EG: Nuclear medicine and skeletal disease. Hosp Pract 7:49, 1962.
82. Woolfenden JM, Pitt MJ, Durie BGM, et al: Comparison of bone scintigraphy and radiography in multiple myeloma. Radiology 134:723, 1980.
83. Leonard RCF, Owen JP, Proctor SJ, et al: Multiple myeloma: Radiology or bone scanning? Clin Radiol 32:291, 1981.
84. Ludwig H, Kumpan W, Sinzinger H: Radiography and bone scintigraphy in multiple myeloma: A comparative analysis. Br J Radiol 55:173, 1982.
85. Nilsson-Ehle H, Holmdahl C, Suurkula M, et al: Bone scintigraphy in the diagnosis of skeletal involvement and metastatic calcification in multiple myeloma. Acta Med Scand 211:427, 1982.
86. Valat JP, Eveleigh MC, Fouquet B, et al: La scintigraphic osseuse dans le myélome multiple. Rev Rhum Mal Osteoartic 52:707, 1985.
87. Goldberg ME: Scan conference: Painful ribs. Minn Med 57:403, 1974.
88. Puranen J, Salokannel J, Timonen T: Strontium-85 profile counting of spine in multiple myeloma. Blut 29:351, 1974.
89. Charkes ND, Durant J, Barry WE: Bone pain in multiple myeloma. Studies with radioactive 87mSr. Arch Intern Med 130:53, 1972.
90. Tong ECK, Ruberfeld S: The strontium-85 bone scan in myeloma. AJR 103:843, 1968.
91. DeNardo GL: The 85Sr scintiscan in bone disease. Ann Intern Med 65:44, 1966.
92. Hubner KF, Andrews GA, Hayes RL, et al: The use of rare-earth radionuclides and other bone-seekers in the evaluation of bone lesions in patients with multiple myeloma or solitary plasmacytoma. Radiology 125:171, 1977.
93. Waxman AD, Siemsen JK, Levine AM, et al: Radiographic and radionuclide imaging in multiple myeloma: The role of gallium scintigraphy: Concise communication. J Nucl Med 22:232, 1981.
94. VanAntwerp JD. O'Mara RE, Pitt MJ, et al: Technetium-99m-diphosphonate accumulation in amyloid. J Nucl Med 16:238, 1975.
95. Moyle JM, Spies SM: Bone scan in a case of amyloidosis. Clin Nucl Med 5:51, 1980.
96. Wahlin A, Holm J, Osterman G, et al: Evaluation of serial bone x-ray examination in multiple myeloma. Acta Med Scand 212:385, 1982.
97. Bataille R, Chevalier J, Rossi M, et al: Bone scintigraphy in plasma cell myeloma. A prospective study of 70 patients. Radiology 145:801, 1982.
98. Helms CA, Genant HK: Computed tomography in the early detection of skeletal involvement with multiple myeloma. JAMA 248:2886, 1982.
99. Solomon A, Rahamani R, Seligsohn U, et al: Multiple myeloma: Early vertebral involvement assessed by computerized tomography. Skel Radiol 11:258, 1984.
100. Schreiman JS, McLeod RA, Kyle RA, et al: Multiple myeloma: Evaluation by CT. Radiology 154:483, 1985.
101. Kyle RA, Schreman JJ, McLeod RA, et al: Computed tomography in diagnosis and management of multiple myeloma and its variants. Arch Intern Med 145:1451, 1985.
102. Price HI, Danziger A, Wainwright HC, et al: CT of orbital multiple myeloma. Am J Neuroradiol 1:573, 1980.
103. Vogler JB III, Murphy WA: Bone marrow imaging. Radiology 168:679, 1988.
104. Bartl R, Burkhardt R, Gierster P, et al: Significance of bone marrow biopsy in multiple myeloma. Rec Prog Cell Biol 45:81, 1978.
105. Hansen OP: Bone marrow studies in myelomatosis. Scand J Hematol 21:265, 1978.
106. Ricci C, Cova M, Kany YS, et al: Normal age-related patterns of cellular and fatty bone marrow distribution in the axial skeleton: MR imaging study. Radiology 177:83, 1990.
107. Fruehwald FX, Tscholakoff D, Schwaighofer B, et al: Magnetic resonance imaging of the lower vertebral column in patients with multiple myeloma. Invest Radiol 23:193, 1988.
108. Libshitz HI, Malthouse SR, Cunningham D, et al: Multiple myeloma: Appearance at MR imaging. Radiology 182:833, 1992.
109. Moulopoulos LA, Varma DG, Dimopoulos MA, et al: Multiple myeloma: Spinal MR imaging in patients with untreated newly diagnosed disease. Radiology 185:833, 1992.
110. Sze G, Bravo S, Baierl P, et al: Developing spinal column: Gadolinium-enhanced MR imaging. Radiology 180:497, 1991.
111. Breger RK, Williams AL, Daniels D, et al: Contrast enhancement in spinal cord imaging. AJR 153:387, 1989.
112. Sze G: Gadolinium-DTPA in spinal disease. Radiol Clin North Am 26:1009, 1988.
113. Hosten VN, Schörner W, Neumann K, et al: Magnetresonanztomographische Screening-untersuchungen des Knochenmarkes mit Gradientecho-Sequenzen. ROFO 157:53, 1992.
114. Hosten VN, Sander B, Schörner W, et al: Kernspintomographische Screeninguntersuchungen des Knochenmarkes mit Gradientecho-Sequenzen. ROFO 154:6, 1991.
115. Golfieri R, Baddeley H, Pringle JS, et al: The role of the STIR sequence in magnetic resonance imaging examination of bone tumours. Br J Radiol 63:251, 1990.
116. Munk PL: Recent advances in magnetic resonance imaging of musculoskeletal tumours. J Can Assoc Radiol 42:37, 1991.
117. Gootnick LT: Solitary myeloma: Review of sixty-one cases. Radiology 45:385, 1945.
118. Lane SL: Plasmacytoma of mandible. Oral Surg 5:434, 1952.
119. Pankovich AM, Griem ML: Plasma-cell myeloma. A thirty year followup. Radiology 104:521, 1972.
120. Carson CP, Ackerman LV, Maltby JD: Plasma-cell myeloma. A clinical, pathologic and roentgenologic review of 90 cases. Am J Clin Pathol 25:849, 1955.
121. Kaye RL, Martin WJ, Campbell DC, et al: Long survival in disseminated myeloma with onset as solitary lesions: Two cases. Ann Intern Med 54:535, 1961.
122. Woodruff RK, Malpas JS, White FE: Solitary plasmacytoma. II. Solitary plasmacytoma of bone. Cancer 43:2344, 1979.
123. Tong D, Griffin TW, Laramore GE, et al: Solitary plasmacytoma of bone and soft tissues. Radiology 135:195, 1980.
124. McLauchlan J: Solitary myeloma of the clavicle with long survival after total excision. Report of a case. J Bone Joint Surg [Br] 55:357, 1973.
125. Wright CJE: Long survival in solitary plasmacytoma of bone. J Bone Joint Surg [Br] 43:767, 1961.
126. Markel SE, Theros EG: RPC of the month from the AFIP. Plasma cell granuloma of the pelvis and femora. Radiology 95:679, 1970.
127. Bataille R, Sany J: Solitary myeloma: Clinical and prognostic features of a review of 114 cases. Cancer 48:845, 1981.
128. Valderrama JAF, Bullough PG: Solitary myeloma of the spine. J Bone Joint Surg [Br] 50:82, 1968.
129. Paul LW, Pohle EA: Solitary myeloma of bone: A review of the roentgenologic features with a report of four additional cases. Radiology 35:651, 1940.
130. Gordon R, Bonakdarpour A, Soulen R, et al: Case report 56. Skel Radiol 2:254, 1978.
131. Krull P, Holsten H, Seeberg A, et al: Klinische und röntgenologische Besonderheiten des solitären Plasmozytoms. ROFO 117:324, 1972.
132. Calle R, Graic Y, Mazabraud A, et al: Plasmocytome osseux solitaire: À propos de quatre case. Bull Cancer 59:395, 1972.

133. Woodring JH, Umer MA, Bernardy MO: Solitary plasmacytoma of the sternum: Diagnosis by computed tomography. CT 9:17, 1985.
134. Sprinkle RLB III, Santangelo L, De Ugarte R: Solitary plasmacytoma of bone in the calcaneus. J Am Podiatr Med Assoc 78:636, 1988.
135. Schabel SI, Rogers CI, Rittenberg GM, Bubanj R: Extramedullary plasmacytoma. Radiology 128:625, 1978.
136. Woodruff RK, Whittle JM, Malpas JS: Solitary plasmacytoma. I. Extra-medullary soft tissue plasmacytoma. Cancer 43:2340, 1979.
137. Meis JM, Butler JJ, Osborne BM, et al: Solitary plasmacytomas of bone and extramedullary plasmacytomas. A clinicopathologic immunohistochemical study. Cancer 59:1475, 1987.
138. Roberts M, Rinaudo PA, Vilinskas J, et al: Solitary sclerosing plasma-cell myeloma of the spine. Case report. J Neurosurg 40:125, 1974.
139. Abdelwahab IF, Miller TT, Hermann G, et al: Transarticular invasion of joints by bone tumors: Hypothesis. Skel Radiol 20:279, 1991.
140. Yasuma T, Yamauchi Y, Arai K, et al: Histopathologic study on tumor infiltration into the intervertebral disc. Spine 14:1245, 1989.
141. Delauche-Cavallier MC, Laredo JD, Wybier M, et al: Solitary plasmacytoma of the spine. Long-term clinical course. Cancer 61:1707, 1988.
142. Kim FM, Rosenblum J: Extramedullary plasmacytoma manifested as an epidural mass. AJR 159:904, 1992.
143. Hamilton EBD, Bywaters EGL: Joint symptoms in myelomatosis and similar conditions. Ann Rheum Dis 20:353, 1961.
144. Talerman A: Sclerotic bone deposits in multiple myeloma. Br J Radiol 56:691, 1983.
145. Scheinker I: Myelom und Nervensystem: Über eine bischer nicht beschriebene mit eigentümlichen Hautveränderungen einhergehende Polyneuritis bei einem plasmazellulären Myelom des Sternums. Dtsch Z Nervenheilkd 147:247, 1938.
146. Aguayo, A, Thompson DW, Humphrey JG: Multiple myeloma with polyneuropathy and osteosclerotic lesions. J Neurol Neurosurg Psychiatry 27:562, 1964.
147. Morley JB, Schwieger AC: The relation between chronic polyneuropathy and osteosclerotic myeloma. J Neurol Neurosurg Psychiatry 30:432, 1967.
148. Talerman A, Bateson EM: Multiple myeloma associated with bone sclerosis and peripheral neuropathy. Br J Radiol 43:698, 1970.
149. Simpson JA: The neuropathies. In D Williams (Ed): Modern Trends in Neurology. Series 3. London, Butterworths, 1962, p 245.
150. Driedger H, Pruzanski W: Plasma cell neoplasia with peripheral polyneuropathy. A study of five cases and a review of the literature. Medicine 59:301, 1980.
151. Hermann G, Sherry H, Rabinowitz JG: Case report 151. Skel Radiol 6:217, 1981.
152. Imawari M, Akatsuka N, Ishibashi M, et al: Syndrome of plasma cell dyscrasia, polyneuropathy and endocrine disturbances. Report of a case. Ann Intern Med 81:490, 1974.
153. Yodor J, Takatsuki K, Wakisaka K: Association of atypical myeloma, polyneuropathy, pigmentation and gynecomastia. A possible new syndrome. Acta Haematol Jpn 36:363, 1973.
154. Shimomori T, Kusumoto M: A case of solitary plasmacytoma with polyneuropathy, pigmentation and gynecomastia (Abstr). J Jpn Soc Intern Med 59:1008, 1970.
155. Trentham DE, Masi AT, Marker HW: Polyneuropathy and anasarca: Evidence for a new connective-tissue syndrome and vasculopathic contribution. Ann Intern Med 84:271, 1976.
156. Waldenstrom JG, Adner A, Gydell K, et al: Osteosclerotic "plasmocytoma" with polyneuropathy, hypertrichosis and diabetes. Acta Med Scand 203:297, 1978.
157. Bardwick PA, Zvaifler NJ, Gill GN, et al: Plasma cell dyscrasia with polyneuropathy, organomegaly, endocrinopathy, M protein, and skin changes: The POEMS syndrome. Medicine 59:311, 1980.
158. Tobin MJ, Fitzgerald MX: The Japanese plasma cell dyscrasia syndrome: Case report and theory of pathogenesis. Postgrad Med J 58:786, 1982.
159. Zea-Mendoza AC, Alonso-Ruiz A, Garcia-Vadillo A, et al: POEMS syndrome with neuroathropathy and nodular regenerative hyperplasia of the liver. Arthritis Rheum 27:1053, 1984.
160. Tanaka O, Ohsawa T: The POEMS syndrome: Report of three cases with radiographic abnormalities. Radiologe 24:472, 1984.
161. Fam AG, Rubenstein JD, Cowan DH: POEMS syndrome. Study of a patient with proteinuria, microangiopathic glomerulopathy, and renal enlargement. Arthritis Rheum 29:233, 1986.
162. Semble EL, Challa VR, Holt DA, et al: Light and electron microscopic findings in POEMS, or Japanese multisystem syndrome. Arthritis Rheum 29:286, 1986.
163. Meier C, Reulecke M, Kesselring J, et al: Polyneuropathie, Organomegalie, Endokrinopathie und Hautveränderungen bei einem Fall mit solitärem Myelom. Schweiz Med Wschr 116:1326, 1986.
164. Aggarwal S, Goulatia RK, Sood A, et al: POEMS syndrome: A rare variety of plasma cell dyscrasia. AJR 155:339, 1990.
165. Brandon C, Martel W, Weatherbee L, et al: Case report 572. Skel Radiol 18:542, 1989.
166. Bessler W, Antonucci F, Stamm B, et al: Case report 646. Skel Radiol 20:212, 1991.
167. Jackson A, Burton IE: A case of POEMS syndrome associated with essential thrombocythaemia and dermal mastocytosis. Postgrad Med J 66:761, 1990.
168. Gherardi RK, Amiel H, Martin-Mondiere C, et al: Solitary plasmacytoma of the skull revealed by a mononeuritis multiplex associated with immune complex vasculitis. Arthritis Rheum 32:1470, 1989.

169. Toyokuni S, Ebina Y, Okada S, et al: Report of a patient with POEMS/Takatsuki/Crow-Fukase syndrome associated with focal spinal pachymeningeal amyloidosis. Cancer 70:882, 1992.
170. Resnick D, Greenway GD, Bardwick PA, et al: Plasma-cell dyscrasia with polyneuropathy, organomegaly, endocrinopathy, M-protein, and skin changes: The POEMS syndrome. Radiology 140:17, 1981.
171. Resnick D, Haghighi P, Guerra J Jr: Bone sclerosis and proliferation in a man with multisystem disease. Invest Radiol 19:1, 1984.
172. Dalakas MC, Papadopoulos NM: Paraproteins in the spinal fluid of patients with paraproteinemic polyneuropathies. Ann Neurol 15:590, 1984.
173. Pruzanski W: Takatsuki syndrome: A reversible multisystem plasma cell dyscrasia. Arthritis Rheum 29:1534, 1986.
174. Magnus-Levy A: Multiple myeloma. Acta Med Scand 95:217, 1938.
175. Stewart A, Weber FP: Myelomatosis. Q J Med 7:211, 1938.
176. Tarr L, Ferris HW: Multiple myeloma associated with nodular deposits of amyloid in the muscle and joints and with Bence-Jones proteinuria. Arch Intern Med 64:820, 1939.
177. Davis JS, Weber FC, Bartfield H: Conditions involving the hematopoietic system resulting in a pseudorheumatoid arthritis: similarity of multiple myeloma and rheumatoid arthritis. Ann Intern Med 47:10, 1957.
178. Goldberg A, Brodsky C, McCarty D: Multiple myeloma with paramyloidosis presenting as rheumatoid disease. Am J Med 37:653, 1964.
179. Arkin CR, Ward LE: Multiple myeloma with amyloid in synovium. Postgrad Med 44:86, 1968.
180. Gordon DA, Pruzanski W, Ogryzlo MA, et al: Amyloid arthritis simulating rheumatoid disease in five patients with multiple myeloma. Am J Med 55:142, 1973.
181. Nashel DJ, Widerlite LW, Pekin TJ Jr: IgD myeloma with amyloid arthropathy. Am J Med 55:426, 1973.
182. Kavanaugh JH: Multiple myeloma, amyloid arthropathy and pathological fracture of the femur. A case report. J Bone Joint Surg [Am] 60:135, 1978.
183. Magnus-Levy A: Amyloidosis in multiple myeloma: Progress noted in 50 years of personal observation. J Mt Sinai Hosp 19:8, 1952.
184. Osserman EF, Fahey JL: Plasma cell dyscrasia. Current clinical and biochemical concepts. Am J Med 44:256, 1968.
185. Bernhard GC, Hensley GT: Amyloid arthropathy. Arthritis Rheum 12:444, 1969.
186. Osserman EF, Takatsuki N, Talal N: Multiple myeloma. I. The pathogenesis of amyloidosis. Semin Hematol 1:3, 1964.
187. Cathcart ES, Ritchie RF, Cohen AS, et al: Immunoglobulins and amyloidosis. Am J Med 52:93, 1972.
188. Abruzzo JL, Amante CM, Heimer R: Primary amyloidosis with "monoclonal" immunoglobulin. A proteinemia. Am J Med 45:460, 1968.
189. Grossman RE, Hensley GT: Bone lesions in primary amyloidosis. AJR 101:872, 1967.
190. McCarty DJ: Discussion of amyloid arthropathy. Arthritis Rheum 12:451, 1969.
191. Ogryzlo MA, MacLachlan M, Dauphinee JA, et al: The serum proteins in health and disease. Filter paper electrophoresis. Am J Med 27:596, 1959.
192. Michaux JL, Heremans JF: Thirty cases of monoclonal immuno-globulin disorders other than myeloma or macroglobulinemia. Am J Med 46:562, 1969.
193. Dryll A, Rousselot F, Ryckewaert A, et al: Rheumatismes inflammatoires et paraprotéine en dehors du myélome et de la maladie de Waldenström. Sem Hôp Paris 45:2135, 1969.
194. Zawadzki ZA, Benedek TG: Rheumatoid arthritis, dysproteinemic arthropathy, and paraproteinuria. Arthritis Rheum 12:555, 1969.
195. Pratt PW, Estren S, Kochwa S: Immunoglobulin abnormalities in Gaucher's disease. Report of 16 cases. Blood 31:633, 1968.
196. Ruestow PC, Levinson DJ, Catchatourian R, et al: Coexistence of IgA myeloma and Gaucher's disease. Arch Intern Med 140:1115, 1980.
197. Mulder JD, Van Rijssel TG: Case report 233. Skel Radiol 10:53, 1983.
198. Talbott JH: Gout and blood dyscrasias. Medicine 38:173, 1959.
199. Bronsky D, Berstein A: Acute gout secondary to multiple myeloma: a case report. Ann Intern Med 41:820, 1954.
200. Barr DP, Reader GG, Wheeler CH: Cryoglobulinemia: Report of two cases with discussion of clinical manifestations, incidence and significance. Ann Intern Med 32:6, 1950.
201. Foord, AG: Hyperproteinemia, autohemagglutination, renal insufficiency, and abnormal bleeding in multiple myeloma. Ann Intern Med 8:1071, 1935.
202. Fahey JL, Scoggins R, Utz JP, et al: Infection, antibody response and gamma globulin components in multiple myeloma and macroglobulinemia. Am J Med 35:698, 1963.
203. Miller MI, Hoppman RA, Pisko EJ: Multiple myeloma presenting with primary meningococcal arthritis. Am J Med 82:1257, 1987.
204. Harris BK, Ross HA: Hemarthrosis as the presenting manifestation of myeloproliferative disease. Arthritis Rheum 17:696, 1974.
205. Mintz G, Robles-Saavedra EJ, Enriquez RD, et al: Hemarthrosis as the presenting manifestation of true myeloma joint disease. Arthritis Rheum 21:148, 1978.
206. Rubins J, Qazi R, Woll JE: Massive bleeding after biopsy of plasmacytoma. Report of two cases. J Bone Joint Surg [Am] 62:138, 1980.
207. Skoog WA, Adams WS: Metabolic balance study of a patient with multiple myeloma treated with dexamethasone. Am J Med 34:417, 1963.
208. Waldenström J: Incipient myelomatosis or "essential" hyperglobulinemia with fibrinogenopenia—a new syndrome. Acta Med Scand 117:216, 1944.
209. Forget BG, Squires JW, Sheldon H: Waldenström's macroglobulinemia with generalized amyloidosis. Arch Intern Med 118:363, 1966.

210. Kobayashi S, Kaneko H, Oonishi Y, et al: An autopsy case of macroglobulinemia showing amyloid degeneration and endocarditis verrucosa (pathological aspect). Acta Haematol Jpn 26:751, 1963.

211. Nick J, Contamin F, Brion S, et al: Macroglobulinémie de Waldenström avec neuropathique amyloide: Observation anatomo-clinique. Rev Neurol 109:21, 1963.

212. Khilnani MT, Keller RJ, Cuttner J: Macroglobulinemia and steatorrhea: Roentgen and pathologic findings in the intestinal tract. Radiol Clin North Am 7:43, 1969.

213. Renner RR, Nelson DA, Lozner EL: Roentgenologic manifestations of primary macroglobulinemia (Waldenström). AJR 113:499, 1971.

214. Vermess M, Pearson KD, Einstein AB, et al: Osseous manifestations of Waldenström's macroglobulinemia. Radiology 102:497, 1972.

215. Burki F, Pitrou E, Bordessoule D, et al: Localisation osseuse de la maladie de Waldenström. Rev Rhum Mal Osteoartic 50:159, 1983.

216. Benoist M, Degott C, Bernard JF, et al: Les manifestations articulaires de la maladie de Waldenström. Rev Rhum Mal Osteoartic 47:369, 1980.

217. Kessler M, Bartl R, Küffer G: Röntgenologische und histobioptische Veränderungen des Skeletts bei hämatologischen Systemerkrankungren. ROFO 132:301, 1980.

218. Stanley P, Baker SL, Byers PD: Unusual bone trabeculation in a patient with macroglobulinemia simulating fibrogenesis imperfecta ossium. Br J Radiol 44:305, 1971.

219. Sundaram M, Heiberg E, Brown GO, et al: Case report 215. Skel Radiol 9:132, 1982.

220. Berman HH: Waldenström's macroglobulinemia with lytic osseous lesions and plasma-cell morphology. Report of a case. Am J Clin Pathol 63:397, 1975.

221. Adner PL, Wallenius G, Werner I: Macroglobulinemia and myelomatosis. Acta Med Scand 168:431, 1960.

222. Welton J, Walker S, Sharp G, et al: Macroglobulinemia with bone destruction. Am J Med 44:280, 1968.

223. Mackenzie MR, Fudenberg HH: Macroglobulinemia: An analysis of forty patients. Blood 39:874, 1972.

224. Youinou P, LeGoff P, Leroy JP, et al: Une forme ostéolytique de macroglobulinemie de Waldenström revelée par une tétraparesie. Sem Hôp Paris 52:2231, 1975.

225. McNutt DR, Fudenberg HH: IgG myeloma and Waldenström macroglobulinemia. Coexistence and clinical manifestations in one patient. Arch Intern Med 131:731, 1973.

226. Marks MA, Tow DE, Jay M: Bone scanning in Waldenström's macroglobulinemia. J Nucl Med 26:1412, 1985.

227. Ghozlan R, Dupuis M, Antebi L: Ostéonécrose de la tête femorale au cours d'une maladie de Waldenström. Rev Rhum Mal Osteoartic 48:721, 1981.

228. Siame JL: Maladie de Waldenström et ostéonécrose de la tête fémorale. Rev Rhum Mal Osteoartic 54:617, 1987.

229. Goldberg LS, Fisher R, Castronova EA, et al: Amyloid arthritis associated with Waldenström's macroglobulinemia. N Engl J Med 281:256, 1969.

230. Scott RB, Elmore SMcD, Brackett NC Jr, et al: Neuropathic joint disease (Charcot joints) in Waldenström's macroglobulinemia with amyloidosis. Am J Med 54:534, 1973.

231. Frangione B, Franklin EC: Heavy chain diseases: Clinical features and molecular significance of the disordered immunoglobulin structure. Semin Hematol 10:53, 1973.

232. Bloch KJ, Lee L, Mills JA, et al: Gamma heavy chain disease—an expanding clinical and laboratory spectrum. Am J Med 55:61, 1973.

233. Seligmann M, Danon F, Hurez D, et al: Alpha chain disease: A new immunoglobulin abnormality. Science 162:1396, 1968.

234. Renner RR, Smith JR: Plasma cell dyscrasias (except myeloma). Semin Roentgenol 9:209, 1974.

235. Marsh WL Jr, Worthman JW, Spiegelberg HL: The pathology of gamma heavy chain disease: Report of a case with morphologic progression from lymphocytic to plasmacytic proliferation. Cancer 47:2878, 1981.

236. Virchow R: Weitere Mittheilungen über das Vorkommen der pflanzlichen Cellulose beim Menschen. Virchows Arch (Pathol Anat) 6:268, 1854.

237. Virchow R: Zur Cellulose-frage. Virchows Arch (Pathol Anat) 6:416, 1854.

238. Freidreich N, Kekule A: Zur Amyloidfrage. Virchows Arch (Pathol Anat) 16:50, 1859.

239. Waldenstrom H: On the formation and disappearance of amyloid in man. Acta Chir Scand 63:479, 1928.

240. Bennhold H: Eine spezifische Amyloidfarbung mit Kongorot. Münch. Med Wochenschr 69:1537, 1922.

241. Cohen AS: Inherited systemic amyloidosis. In JB Stanbury et al (Eds): The Metabolic Basis of Inherited Diseases. 3rd Ed. New York, McGraw-Hill Book Co, 1972, p 1273.

242. Kyle RA, Bayrd ED: Amyloidosis: Review of 236 cases. Medicine 54:271, 1975.

243. Cohen AS: Amyloidosis, N Engl J Med 277:522, 574, 628, 1967.

244. Glenner GG, Terry WD, Isersky C: Amyloidosis: Its nature and pathogenesis. Semin Hematol 10:65, 1973.

245. Cohen AS, Wegelius O: Classification of amyloid: 1979–1980. Arthritis Rheum 23:644, 1980.

246. Reimann HA, Koucky RF, Eklund CM: Primary amyloidosis limited to tissue of mesodermal origin. Am J Pathol 11:977, 1935.

247. Dahlin DC: Classification and general aspects of amyloidosis. Med Clin North Am 34:1107, 1950.

248. Symmers WS: Primary amyloidosis. A review. J Clin Pathol 9:187, 1956.

249. Missmahl HP, Hartwig M: Polarisationsoptische Untersuchungen an der Amyloidsubstanz. Virchows Arch (Pathol Anat) 324:489, 1953.

250. Bywaters EGL: Amyloidosis. In JT Scott (Ed): Copeman's Textbook of the Rheumatic Diseases. 5th Ed. Edinburgh. Churchill Livingstone, 1978, p 746.

251. Brandt K, Cathcart ES, Cohen AS: A clinical analysis of the course and prognosis of forty-two patients with amyloidosis. Am J Med 44:955, 1968.

252. Cohen AS: Amyloidosis. Bull Rheum Dis 40:1, 1991.

253. Benson MD, Wallace MR, Tejada E, et al: Hereditary amyloidosis: Description of a new American kindred with late onset cardiomyopathy. Appalachian amyloid. Arthritis Rheum 30:195, 1987.

254. Ozdemir AI, Wright JR, Calkins E: Influence of rheumatoid arthritis on amyloidosis of aging. N Engl J Med 285:534, 1971.

255. Subbarao K, Jacobson HG: Amyloidosis and plasma cell dyscrasias of the musculoskeletal system. Semin Roentgenol 21:139, 1986.

256. Arapakis G, Tribe CR: Amyloidosis in rheumatoid arthritis investigated by means of rectal biopsy. Ann Rheum Dis 22:256, 1963.

257. Missen GAK, Taylor JD: Amyloidosis in rheumatoid arthritis. J Pathol Bacteriol 71:179, 1956.

258. Brun C, Olsen TS, Raaschou F, et al: Renal biopsy in rheumatoid arthritis. Nephron 2:65, 1965.

259. Calkins E, Cohen AS: Diagnosis of amyloidosis. Bull Rheum Dis 10:215, 1960.

260. Schnitzer TJ, Ansell BM: Amyloidosis in juvenile chronic polyarthritis. Arthritis Rheum 20(Suppl):245, 1977.

261. Smith ME, Ansell BM, Bywaters EGL: Mortality and prognosis related to amyloidosis of Still's disease. Ann Rheum Dis 27:137, 1968.

262. Harrington TM, Moran JJ, Davis DE: Amyloidosis in adult onset Still's disease. J Rheumatol 8:833, 1981.

263. Benedek TG, Zawadzki ZA: Ankylosing spondylitis with ulcerative colitis and amyloidosis: Report of a case and review of the literature. Am J Med 40:431, 1966.

264. Jayson MI, Salmon PR, Harrison W: Amyloidosis in ankylosing spondylitis. Rheumatol Phys Med 11:78, 1971.

265. Caughey DE, Wakem CJ: A fatal case of Reiter's disease complicated by amyloidosis. Arthritis Rheum 16:695, 1973.

266. Bleehen SS, Everall JD, Tighe JR: Amyloidosis complicating Reiter's syndrome. Br J Vener Dis 42:88, 1966.

267. Miller LD, Brown EC Jr, Arnett FC: Amyloidosis in Reiter's syndrome. J Rheumatol 6:225, 1979.

268. Stone G, Wolfe F: Collateral ligament calcification complicating amyloidosis and Reiter's syndrome. J Rheumatol 11:248, 1984.

269. Berger PA: Amyloidosis—a complication of pustular psoriasis. Br Med J 2:351, 1969.

270. Ferguson A, Downie WW: Gastrointestinal amyloidosis in psoriatic arthritis. Ann Rheum Dis 27:245, 1968.

271. Friedman R, Agus B, Ames E: Amyloid arthropathy in a patient with psoriasis and amyloidosis. Arthritis Rheum 24:1320, 1981.

272. Forshaw JWB, Moorhouse EH: Amyloidosis secondary to chronic ulcerative colitis. Br Med J 2:94, 1964.

273. Mir-Madjlessi SH, Brown CH, Hawk WA: Amyloidosis associated with Crohn's disease. Am J Gastroenterol 58:563, 1972.

274. Sander S: Whipple's disease associated with amyloidosis. Acta Pathol Microbiol Scand 61:530, 1964.

275. Mirouze J, Pages A, Mion C: Amyloid nephrosis in the course of an unusual recurring acute dermatomyositis. J Urol Nephrol 68:152, 1962.

276. Gelderman AH, Levine RA, Arndt KA: Dermatomyositis complicated by generalized amyloidosis. Report of a case. N Engl J Med 267:858, 1962.

277. Oppenheimer BS, Silver S: Recession of renal amyloidosis due to multiple skin gangrene associated with arteritis of the skin. J Mt Sinai Hosp 4:851, 1938.

278. Dikman SH, Goldstein M, Kahn T, et al: Amyloidosis. An unusual complication of Gaucher's disease. Arch Pathol Lab Med 102:460, 1978.

279. Hanash SM, Rucknagel DL, Heidelberger KP, et al: Primary amyloidosis associated with Gaucher's disease. Ann Intern Med 89:639, 1978.

280. Egan MW, Goldenberg DL, Segal D, et al: Unexpected amyloid and inflammatory synovial membranes in osteoarthritis (Abstr). Arthritis Rheum 23:668, 1980.

281. Goffin Y, De Doncker E: Altérations histologiques et histochimiques de la capsule articulaire dans l'arthrose et chez les sujets séniles. Rev Rhum Mal Osteoartic 47:15, 1980.

282. Ladefoged C: Amyloid in osteoarthritic hip joints. A pathoanatomical and histological investigation of femoral head cartilage. Acta Orthop Scand 53:581, 1982.

283. Ladefoged C, Christensen HE, Sorensen KH: Amyloid in osteoarthritic hip joints. Depositions in cartilage and capsule. Semiquantitative aspects. Acta Orthop Scand 53:587, 1982.

284. Ladefoged C: Amyloid deposits in the knee joint at autopsy. Ann Rheum Dis 45:668, 1986.

285. Goffin YA, Thoua Y, Potvliege PR: Microdeposition of amyloid in the joints. Ann Rheum Dis 40:27, 1981.

286. Mohr W, Kirkpatrick CJ: Articular amyloid. J Rheumatol 10:335, 1983.

287. Takeda T, Sanada H, Ishii M, et al: Age-associated amyloid deposition in surgically removed intervertebral discs. Arthritis Rheum 27:1063, 1984.

288. Ladefoged C, Fedders O, Petersen OF: Amyloid in intervertebral discs: A histopathological investigation of surgical material from 100 consecutive operations on herniated discs. Ann Rheum Dis 45:239, 1986.

289. Ballou SP, Khan MA, Kushner I: Diffuse intervertebral disk calcification in primary amyloidosis. Ann Intern Med 85:616, 1976.

290. Levo Y, Shalev O, Rosenmann E, et al: Gout and amyloidosis. Ann Rheum Dis 39:589, 1980.

291. Rubinow A, Sonnenblick M: Amyloidosis secondary to polyarticular gout. Arthritis Rheum 24:1425, 1981.

292. Ryan LM, Bernhard GC, Liang G, et al: Amyloid arthropathy in the absence of dysproteinemia: A possible association with chondrocalcinosis (Abstr). Arthritis Rheum 21:587, 1978.

293. Wilson DA, Irvin WS: Chondrocalcinosis and amyloidosis. J Rheumatol 8:355, 1981.

294. Sorensen KH, Teglbjaerg PS, Ladefoged C, et al: Pyrophosphate arthritis with local amyloid deposition. Acta Orthop Scand 52:129, 1981.

295. Ryan LM, Liang G, Kozin F: Amyloid arthropathy: Possible association with chondrocalcinosis. J Rheumatol 9:273, 1982.

296. Ladefoged C: Amyloid in osteoarthritic hip joints: Deposits in relation to chondromatosis, pyrophosphate, and inflammatory cell infiltrate in the synovial membrane and fibrous capsule. Ann Rheum Dis 42:659, 1983.

297. Meyerhoff J: Familial Mediterranean fever: Report of a large family, review of the literature, and discussion of the frequency of amyloidosis. Medicine 59:66, 1980.

298. Siegal S: Benign paroxysmal peritonitis. Ann Intern Med 23:1, 1945.

299. Sohar E, Pras M, Gafni G: Familial Mediterranean fever and its articular manifestations. Clin Rheum Dis 1:195, 1975.

300. Gafni J, Ravid M, Sohar E: The role of amyloidosis in familial Mediterranean fever. Isr J Med Sci 4:995, 1968.

301. Gardner H: Bone lesions in primary systemic amyloidosis: Report of a case. Br J Radiol 34:778, 1961.

302. Weinfeld A, Stern MH, Marx LH: Amyloid lesions of bone. AJR 108:799, 1970.

303. Axelsson U, Hallen A, Rausing A: Amyloidosis of bone. Report of two cases. J Bone Joint Surg [Br] 52:717, 1970.

304. Koletsky S, Stecher RM: Primary systemic amyloidosis: Involvement of cardiac valves, joints and bones with pathologic fractures of femur. Arch Pathol 27:267, 1939.

305. Brzeski M, Fox JG, Boulton-Jones JM, et al: Vertebral bony collapse due to primary amyloidosis. J Rheumatol 17:1701, 1990.

306. Yoshida SO, Karjoo R, Johnstone MR: Case report 480. Skel Radiol 17:226, 1988.

307. Lai KN, Chan KW, Siu DLS, et al: Pathologic hip fractures secondary to amyloidoma. Case report and review of the literature. Am J Med 77:937, 1984.

308. Gerber IE: Amyloidosis of bone marrow. Arch Pathol 17:620, 1934.

309. Bhate DV, Azar-kia B, Supan WAP: Case report 76. Skel Radiol 3:193, 1978.

310. Bauer WH, Kuzma JF: Solitary ''tumors'' of atypical amyloid (paramyloid). Am J Clin Pathol 19:1097, 1949.

311. Pawar S, Kay CJ, Anderson HH, et al: Primary amyloidoma of the spine. J Comput Assist Tomogr 6:1175, 1982.

312. Leeson MC, Rechtine GR, Makley JT, et al: Primary amyloidoma of the spine. A case report and review of the literature. Spine 10:303, 1985.

313. Fadell EJ, Morris HC: Amyloidoma presenting as primary sternal tumor. Am J Surg 108:75, 1964.

314. Lowell DM: Amyloid-producing plasmacytoma of pelvis. Arch Surg 94:899, 1967.

315. Rosenblum AH, Kirshbaum JD: Multiple myeloma with tumor-like amyloidosis: Clinical and pathologic study. JAMA 106:988, 1936.

316. Wiernik PH: Amyloid joint disease. Medicine 51:465, 1972.

317. Yood RA, Skinner M, Cohen AS, et al: Soft tissue uptake of bone seeking radionuclide in amyloidosis. J Rheumatol 8:760, 1981.

318. Katz GA, Peter JB, Pearson CM, et al: The shoulder-pad sign—a diagnostic feature of amyloid arthropathy. N Engl J Med 288:354, 1973.

319. Paige BH: A case of myeloma with unusual amyloid deposition. Am J Pathol 7:691, 1976.

320. Chapman RH, Cotter F: The carpal tunnel syndrome and amyloidosis. A case report. Clin Orthop 169:159, 1982.

321. Bjerrum OW, Rygaard-Olson C, Dahlerup B, et al: The carpal tunnel syndrome and amyloidosis. A clinical and histological study. Clin Neurol Neurosurg 86:29, 1984.

322. Mohr W: Amyloid deposits in the periarticular tissue. Z Rheumatol 35:412, 1976.

323. Bird HA: Joint amyloid presenting as ''polymyalgic'' rheumatoid arthritis. Ann Rheum Dis 37:479, 1978.

324. Hickling P, Wilkins M, Newman GR, et al: A study of amyloid arthropathy in multiple myeloma. Q J Med 50:417, 1981.

326. Goldman AB, Pavlov H, Bullough P: Case report 137. Skel Radiol 6:69, 1981.

327. Ropes M, Bauer W: Synovial Fluid Changes in Joint Disease. Cambridge, Mass. Harvard University Press, 1953.

328. Lakhanpal S, Li CY, Gertz MA, et al: Synovial fluid analysis for diagnosis of amyloid arthropathy. Arthritis Rheum 30:419, 1987.

329. Bussière JL, Missioux D, Champeyroux J, et al: Arthropathies amyloïdes. A propos d'un cas. Rev Rhum Mal Osteoartic 43:655, 1976.

330. Gamarski J, Baretto Neto MB: Osteoarticular manifestations in primary amyloidosis: Case presentation. Arch Interam Rheum 2:651, 1969.

331. Bywaters EGL, Dorling J: Amyloid deposits in articular cartilage. Ann Rheum Dis 29:294, 1970.

332. Dalziell H, Spencer D, Corrigan AB, et al: Amyloid arthropathy. Australas Radiol 21:76, 1977.

333. Deshayes P, Verdure J, Fondimare A, et al: Neuropathie amyloïde avec ostéonecrose du plateau tibial interne. Sem Hôp Paris 49:1233, 1973.

334. Peitzman SJ, Miller JL, Ortega L, et al: Charcot arthropathy secondary to amyloid neuropathy. JAMA 235:1345, 1976.

335. McAnena OJ, Feely MP, Kealy WF: Spinal cord compression by amyloid tissue. J Neurol Neurosurg Psychiatry 45:1067, 1982.

336. Pruzanski W, Baron M, Shupak R: Neuroarthropathy (Charcot joints) in familial amyloid polyneuropathy. J Rheumatol 8:477, 1981.

337. Evanson S, Benson MD: Erosive arthritis in heredofamilial amyloidosis (Abstr). Arthritis Rheum 28:671, 1980.

338. Eyanson S, Benson MD: Erosive arthritis in hereditary amyloidosis. Arthritis Rheum 26:1145, 1983.

339. Tagliabue JR, Stull MA, Lack EE, et al: Case report 610. Skel Radiol 19:448, 1990.

340. Metzler JP, Fleckenstein JL, White CL III, et al: MRI evaluation of amyloid myopathy. Skel Radiol 21:463, 1992.

341. Rosen FS, Janeway CA: The gamma globulins. III. The antibody deficiency syndromes. Part 1. N Engl J Med 275:709, 1966.

342. Rosen FS, Janeway CA: The gamma globulins. III. The antibody deficiency syndromes. Part 2. N Engl J Med 275:769, 1966.

343. Rosen FS, Merler E: Genetic defects in gamma globulin synthesis. In JB Stanbury et al (Eds): The Metabolic Basis of Inherited Disease. 3rd Ed. New York, McGraw-Hill, 1972, p 1643.

344. Johnston CLW, Webster ADB, Taylor-Robinson D, et al: Primary late-onset hypogammaglobulinaemia associated with inflammatory polyarthritis and septic arthritis due to Mycoplasma pneumoniae. Ann Rheum Dis 42:108, 1983.

345. Cook CD, Rosen FS, Banker BQ: Dermatomyositis and focal scleroderma. Pediatr Clin North Am 10:979, 1963.

346. Gelder DW van: Clinical significance of alterations in gamma globulin levels. South Med J 50:43, 1957.

347. Good RA, Rotstein J, Mazzitello WF: The simultaneous occurrence of rheumatoid arthritis and agammaglobulinemia. J Lab Clin Med 49:343, 1957.

348. Good RA, Rotstein J: Rheumatoid arthritis and agammaglobulinemia. Bull Rheum Dis 10:203, 1960.

349. Squire JR: Hypogammaglobulinemia in the United Kingdom 1956–61. Proc R Soc Med 55:393, 1962.

350. Webster AD: Thymoma, polyarthropathy and hypogammaglobulinaemia. Proc R Soc Med 69:58, 1976.

351. Chaouat Y, Faures B, Ginet CL, et al: Les manifestations rhumatismales de l'hypogammaglobulinemie primaire de l'adulte. Rev Rhum Mal Osteoartic 41:593, 1974.

352. Barnett EV, Winkelstein A, Weinberger HJ: Agammaglobulinemia with polyarthritis and subcutaneous nodules. Am J Med 48:40, 1970.

353. Romeyn JA: The relation of rheumatoid arthritis to hypogammaglobulinemia. J Rheumatol 5:245, 1978.

354. Grayzel AI, Marcus R, Stern R, et al: Chronic polyarthritis associated with hypogammaglobulinemia. A study of two patients. Arthritis Rheum 20:887, 1977.

355. Mozziconacci, P, Griscelli C, Sorin M: Les rhumatismes inflammatoires au cours des déficits immunitaires. Rev Rhum Mal Osteoartic 41:587, 1974.

356. Laravoire P, Ott H: Polyarthrite sévère chez un patient atteint d'une hypogammaglobulinemie. Rev Rhum Mal Osteoartic 47:571, 1980.

357. Sany J, Jorgenson CH, Anaya JM, et al: Arthritis associated with primary agammaglobulinemia: New clues to its immunopathology. Clin Ex Rheumatol 11:65, 1993.

358. Rawson AJ, Hollander JL, Abelson NM, et al: Immunoglobulins in the joint fluid and cells of arthritis with agammaglobulinemia (Abstr). Arthritis Rheum 9:534, 1966.

359. Taborn JD: Rice bodies in hypogammaglobulinemic arthritis. J Rheumatol 8:165, 1981.

360. Rahmouni A, Divine M, Mathieu D, et al: Detection of multiple myeloma involving the spine: Efficacy of fat-suppression and contrast-enhanced MR imaging. AJR 160:1049, 1993.

361. Rahmouni A, Divine M, Mathieu D, et al: MR appearance of multiple myeloma of the spine before and after treatment. AJR 160:1053, 1993.

362. Moulopoulos LA, Dimopoulos MA, Varma DGK, et al: Waldenström macroglobulinemia: MR imaging of the spine and CT of the abdomen and pelvis. Radiology 188:669, 1993.

363. Mirowitz SA, Apicella P, Reinus WR, et al: MR imaging of bone marrow lesions: Relative conspicuousness on T1-weighted, fat-suppressed T2-weighted, and STIR images. AJR 162:215, 1994.

364. Reinus WR, Kyriakos M, Gilula LA, et al: Plasma cell tumors with calcified amyloid deposition mistaken for chondrosarcoma. Radiology 189:505, 1993.

61

Lipidoses, Histiocytoses, and Hyperlipoproteinemias

Donald Resnick, M.D.

No uniform agreement exists regarding the classification of lipid storage and histiocytic disorders, related, in part, to a lack of clear understanding of the cause and pathogenesis of many of these processes. In fact, the precise derivation of the cellular elements that characterize such disorders is not certain, and this uncertainty has led to a system of nomenclature that is challenged by some investigators. For example, some investigators suggested that words beginning with *reticulo,* such as reticuloendotheliosis, reticulohistiocytosis, and reticulosis, should be avoided until such time as the origin, function, and specific characteristics of the reticulum cell are defined in a manner on which there could be general agreement.[163] It has been further suggested that activation of macrophages occurs in certain of the histiocytic disorders and that the interaction of such macrophages with surrounding normal tissue is fundamental to the pathophysiology of the disease process.[163] In this regard, evidence exists that a cooperative effort involving lymphocytes and activated macrophages leads to a release of osteolytic substances, including osteoclast-activating factor, which may be influential in the osseous destruction seen in eosinophilic granuloma and Hand-Schüller-Christian disease.[164–166]

Histiocytes are derived from cells that originate in the bone marrow. Two basic types of histiocytes can be identified: ordinary histiocytes, which are components of the mononuclear phagocytic system; and dendritic cells, which may represent specialized cells of this system or of separate lineage.[293] Because of their enormous capacity for morphologic and functional change, secretion of cytokines, and interaction with one another as well as other cells, histiocytes show extreme variability in appearance; they may appear as prosaic mononuclear cells, foam cells, phagocytic

TABLE 61–1. Lipid Storage and Histiocytic Disorders

Lipid Storage Diseases
Gaucher's disease (glycosylceramide lipidosis)
Niemann-Pick disease (sphingomyelin lipidosis)
Fabry's disease (glycolipidosis)
Refsum's disease (phytanic acid storage disease)
Krabbe's disease (galactosylceramide lipidosis)
Metachromatic leukodystrophy (sulfatide lipidosis)
Farber's lipogranulomatosis (ceramidase deficiency)
Gangliosidoses
Sea-blue histiocytosis
Tay-Sachs disease
Fucosidosis

Reactive Histiocytoses
Multicentric reticulohistiocytosis
Langerhans cell histiocytosis
Lipid granulomatosis (Erdheim-Chester disease)
Sinus histiocytosis with lymphadenopathy
Erythrophagocytic lymphohistiocytosis

Neoplastic Histiocytoses
Acute monocytic leukemia
Chronic myelomonocytic leukemia
Histiocytic lymphoma
Malignant histiocytosis (histiocytic medullary reticulosis)

Disorders of Lipoprotein Metabolism
Hyperlipoproteinemias
Hypolipoproteinemias

Miscellaneous Disorders
Membranous lipodystrophy

---

macrophages, plasmacytoid cells, and multinucleated giant cells of various types.[293] A classification system of lipid storage and histiocytic diseases, based on a composite of systems found in several reference sources,[163, 167, 168] is contained in Table 61–1. This chapter presents a summary of some of these diseases, particularly those with prominent musculoskeletal involvement. Any such discussion rapidly becomes outdated, as the number of disorders characterized by abnormal lipid metabolism is large and continually growing. Additional information regarding these and related diseases is given in Chapter 88.

GAUCHER'S DISEASE

Background and General Features

In 1882, Gaucher described a chronic progressive disorder characterized by enlargement of the liver and spleen.[1] As subsequent reports of this disorder appeared, theories of its causation abounded. Some investigators believed it was related to a primary neoplasm,[1] an abnormal connective tissue proliferation,[2] a manifestation of a toxic or foreign substance,[3, 4] and an abnormality of the lymphatic-hematopoietic system.[2] With further examination of the large cells that infiltrated the spleen in this disorder, a "lipoid" material was discovered.[5] In 1924, Lieb[6] documented the presence of large amounts of cerebrosides in the spleens of patients with Gaucher's disease, substances that subsequently have been defined in great detail.[7]

Gaucher's disease now is recognized as a rare familial disorder of cerebroside metabolism caused by a deficit of a specific enzyme (glucocerebroside hydrolase or beta glucosidase) that leads to abnormal accumulation of lipid material in the reticuloendothelial cells of the body. The disease affects both men and women and may develop at any age, although it is particularly frequent in childhood and early adult life. Many patients are Ashkenazic Jews; however, others may be affected, including members of Caucasian, Negroid, and Oriental groups.[157]

The manifestations of Gaucher's disease can be attributed to accumulation of Gaucher cells (a reticulum cell of 20 to 80 μm in diameter) in various tissues of the body, although the pathogenesis of cerebroside infiltration within these cells is not known.[8-10] Proliferation of Gaucher cells in the liver and spleen leads to hepatosplenomegaly. Similarly, accumulation of these cells in the lymph nodes produces lymphadenopathy, and, in the brain, glial cell proliferation and degenerative changes in the pyramidal cells of the cerebral cortex occur. Cellular infiltration also occurs in the lungs, kidneys, tonsils, thyroid, thymus, intestines, and adrenals, causing impairment of these organs. The bone marrow is not immune. Accumulation of Gaucher cells in this location may cause osseous destruction, hematologic abnormalities, and articular manifestations.

Clinical Features

Gaucher's disease has been divided into three clinical forms, types 1, 2, and 3.[11-16] Common to all three types are recessive inheritance, hepatosplenomegaly, deficient acid β-glucosidase activity, elevated nontartrate-inhibitable acid phosphatase activity, and characteristic Gaucher cells in the bone marrow. Type 1 disease, termed chronic non-neuronopathic or "adult" Gaucher's disease, is the most frequent, occurring in Ashkenazic Jewish persons and leading to clinical manifestations that initially may appear in childhood but subsequently worsen as the patient enters the second and third decades of life. Such manifestations include a protuberant abdomen and episodic pain, often severe, in the arms, legs, and back. Fever, growth disturbance, respiratory distress, pneumonia, and diffuse yellow-brown pigmentation on the lower legs and face also are seen. Laboratory findings include microcytic anemia, leukopenia, and a decreased number of platelets in association with easy bruisability and a bleeding diathesis. Bone involvement is common.

Type 2, acute neuronopathic Gaucher's disease, is a rare, fatal neurodegenerative disorder, with no particular ethnic predilection, which becomes manifest clinically shortly after birth or in the first few months of life. Neurologic manifestations include head retraction, spasticity, strabismus, mental retardation, loss of sensation, and seizures. Bone abnormalities are limited. The average time of survival is approximately 1 year.

Type 3, subacute neuronopathic (juvenile) Gaucher's disease, is uncommon and is characterized by hepatosplenomegaly appearing in the first few years of life. Neurologic and skeletal manifestations appear during childhood or adolescence, and the majority of the affected children have convulsions. Additional manifestations are hypertonicity, lack of coordination, strabismus, and alterations detectable on electroencephalography. Very rarely, a similar clinical pattern is observed in adults.

The presence of enlarged lipid-laden histiocytes, the Gaucher cells, represents the hallmark of all types of the disease. These cells are distributed in a variable fashion in the organs and tissues of the reticuloendothelial system. Gaucher cells are particularly prominent in the red pulp of

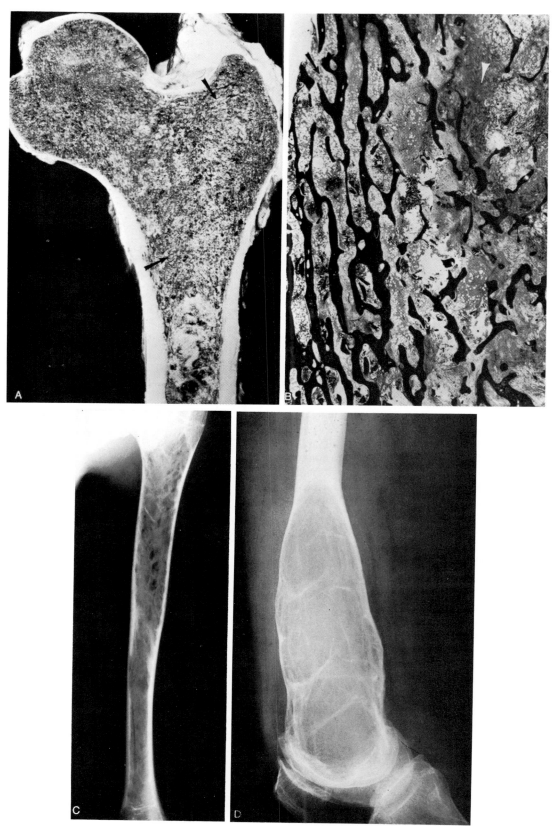

FIGURE 61–1 *See legend on opposite page*

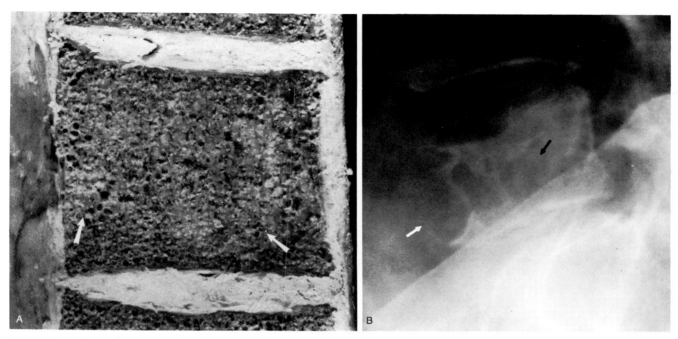

FIGURE 61–2. Gaucher's disease: Marrow infiltration in spine.

A A photograph of a sagittal section of a thoracic vertebral body in a 42 year old man with Gaucher's disease reveals infiltration of the marrow spaces of the spongiosa of the vertebral body with Gaucher cells (arrows), producing a grayish color.

B A lateral radiograph of the lower lumbosacral spine demonstrates a "bubbly" lytic lesion of the vertebral body (arrows) with partial vertebral collapse.

(**A,** From Jaffe HL: Metabolic, Degenerative and Inflammatory Diseases of Bones and Joints. Philadelphia, Lea & Febiger, 1972.)

the spleen, the bone marrow, and the sinusoids and medullary portions of the lymph nodes. They also may be evident in arterioles, veins, lymphatic vessels, and capillaries of the alveoli.

Musculoskeletal Abnormalities

Osteoarticular findings are well recognized in Gaucher's disease.[17–22] These findings may be minimal in young infants with the acute, fulminant variety of disease. They are more pronounced in older infants, children, and adults who suffer from the more chronic form of Gaucher's disease. In some patients, evidence of skeletal disease can be the earliest and most prominent feature and can occur before the onset of splenomegaly. Most observers believe that splenectomy has little or no effect on the occurrence or progression of skeletal lesion, although bone marrow transplantation has been reported to lead to an improvement in the skeletal abnormalities, particularly when evaluated with CT (see later discussion).

Marrow Infiltration (Figs. 61–1 and 61–2). Accumulation of Gaucher cells within the bone marrow is associated with cellular necrosis, fibrous proliferation, and resorption of spongy trabeculae.[169] Erosion of the endosteal surface of the cortex also is apparent. These pathologic skeletal changes become manifest on radiographs as increased radiolucency of bone and cortical scalloping and thinning. They predominate in the axial skeleton and proximal portions of the long bones, although abnormalities may be detected at other skeletal sites. The findings are particularly prominent in the distal portion of the femur. Abnormalities of the long bones usually are bilateral and frequently are symmetric. Even the small tubular bones of the hands and feet may reveal osteopenia and a coarsened trabecular pattern. In this location, enlargement of the nutrient foramina has been described.[172] Isolated focal destructive areas can create radiolucent shadows with geographic or motheaten patterns of destruction simulating the appearance of the pseudotumor of hemophilia, plasma cell myeloma, or skeletal metastasis.[257, 272] Adjacent reactive sclerosis may indicate accompanying osteonecrosis.

FIGURE 61–1. Gaucher's disease: Marrow infiltration in appendicular skeleton.

A A photograph of a cut section of the proximal end of the femur in a 29 year old woman with Gaucher's disease reveals infiltration of the marrow cavity with Gaucher cells (arrows), producing a grayish appearance to the spongiosa bone. Osteonecrosis of the femoral head is not apparent.

B A photomicrograph (7×) of the cortex and spongiosa in the distal metaphysis of the femur in the same woman illustrates Gaucher cellular infiltration in the marrow of rarefied cortical bone (arrow) and medullary bone (arrowhead). These cells reveal focal necrosis and replacement with connective tissue.

C The radiographic abnormalities of the humerus in a different patient with Gaucher's disease include osteopenia, osteolytic lesions, medullary widening, and cortical diminution. The resemblance to features of plasma cell myeloma is obvious.

D Observe the long expansile lesion of the distal end of the femur with a "ground glass" appearance, crossing trabeculae, and cortical diminution.

(**A, B,** From Jaffe HL: Metabolic, Degenerative and Inflammatory Diseases of Bones and Joints. Philadelphia, Lea & Febiger, 1972.)

In the spine, cellular infiltration results in loss of trabeculae with increased radiolucency of the vertebral bodies, accentuation of vertical trabeculae, and multiple compression fractures. Kyphosis, gibbus deformity, and bony ankylosis across the intervertebral disc eventually may become apparent. Spinal cord compression is a rare complication of vertebral collapse in this disease.[278]

In the calvarium, the marrow of the diploic space is replaced by Gaucher cells. Trabecular destruction and thinning of both the outer and inner tables can be seen. Mandibular involvement is not unusual.

Fractures (Fig. 61–3). Infiltration of the marrow spaces with Gaucher cells and trabecular resorption produce osseous weakening, which may result in pathologic fractures. Such fractures may develop rapidly after splenectomy.[173] Most frequently, fractures appear in the vertebral column. Intraosseous discal displacements (cartilaginous or Schmorl's nodes) and compression of the vertebral bodies are seen. Angular deformity may be evident.[171] The involved vertebral body may become completely flattened (vertebra plana).[278] This appearance, which is identical to that accompanying the histiocytoses, can be evident at multiple levels, associated with paravertebral soft tissue swelling.

Fractures also are observed in the ribs and in the long and short tubular bones of the appendicular skeleton, particularly the femur, the tibia, and the humerus.[17, 20, 21] These fractures may appear in the diaphyses or the epiphyses,[23] although in the latter location, their occurrence may reflect underlying osteonecrosis. Fracture of the femoral neck is associated with coxa vara deformity. It usually is seen in

children less than 10 years of age in the absence of significant trauma.[170] After fracture, ordinarily prompt callus formation and early osseous union occur.[17]

Modeling Deformities (Fig. 61–4). One of the most characteristic osseous manifestations of chronic Gaucher's disease is modeling deformities, particularly in the appendicular skeleton. Expansion of the contour of the long tubular bones is most frequent in the lower ends of both femoral shafts, particularly medially. It results in cortical thinning and loss of the normal concavity of the bony outline. The appearance of a straightened or convex osseous margin, which has been termed an Erlenmeyer flask deformity, is very suggestive of the diagnosis of Gaucher's disease, particularly if it is associated with epiphyseal osteonecrosis. Erlenmeyer flask deformities occasionally are encountered in other conditions as well (see discussion later in this chapter).

Peculiar steplike depressions of the superior and inferior margins of the vertebral bodies (Fig. 61–5) have been described in Gaucher's disease,[24] identical to those that are typical of sickle cell anemia and other hemoglobinopathies.[25, 26] This deformity, which has been termed the ''H'' vertebra because of its resemblance to this capital letter, has been attributed to growth disturbance at the chondro-osseous junction due to vessel occlusion by abnormal red blood cells in hemoglobinopathic disorders.[25] In Gaucher's disease, massive infiltration within the marrow by glucocerebroside-laden cells may lead to compression of intra-osseous blood vessels. Furthermore, the vascular walls themselves undergo infiltration by these cells.[27] Thus, H

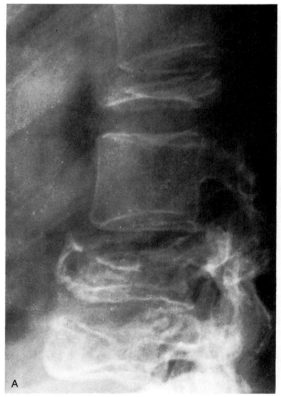
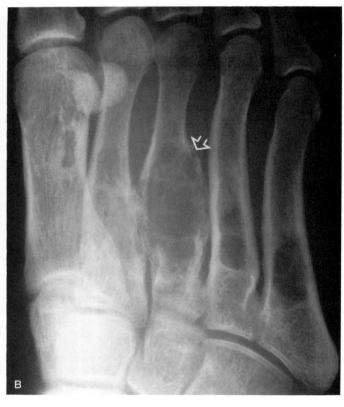

FIGURE 61–3. Gaucher's disease: Fractures.
   A Vertebral fracture and collapse in this disease are particularly frequent. In this case, marrow replacement has led to dramatic collapse of multiple vertebral bodies, some of which have been reduced to a flattened structure (vertebra plana).
   B Marrow infiltration has produced multiple osteolytic lesions of the metatarsal bones with a pathologic fracture (arrow) of one of the lesions.

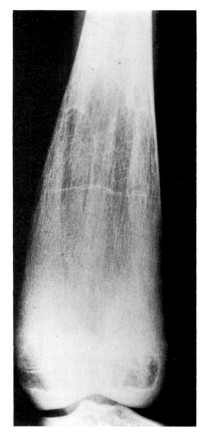

FIGURE 61–4. Gaucher's disease: Modeling deformities. An example of an Erlenmeyer flask deformity of the distal end of the femur. Note the expansion of the contour of the long tubular bone, with straightening and convexity of the osseous margin, particularly along the medial aspect of the metaphysis.

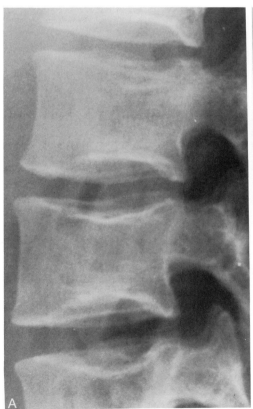

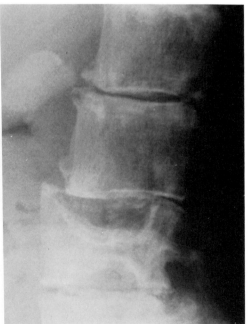

FIGURE 61–5. Gaucher's disease: Modeling deformities.

A Observe central depressions of the superior and inferior surfaces of multiple vertebral bodies in this 24 year old man.

B In a 46 year old woman, steplike deformity of a lumbar vertebral body and severe loss of height of multiple intervertebral discs are seen. The precise cause of these changes is not clear.

(**A, B,** Courtesy of V. Vint, M.D., San Diego, California.)

vertebrae in Gaucher's disease could possibly relate to ischemia resulting from both extrinsic compression and intrinsic abnormality of vessels. An alternative theory suggests that the "stepped" vertebral body in Gaucher's disease is caused by initial collapse of the vertebral body, with subsequent growth recovery peripherally.[154]

Osteonecrosis (Figs. 61–6 and 61–7). Osteonecrosis of epiphyses and diaphyses is well recognized in Gaucher's disease.[17–19, 22, 23, 28, 29] Episodes of bone crisis may appear with acute pain, tenderness, and elevated temperature, simulating the clinical findings of osteomyelitis.[187] In the shafts of long bones, alternating radiolucency and sclerosis appear with associated periostitis.[30] In the cortex, an inner layer of new bone formation, which does not merge with the overlying cortical bone, produces a bone-within-bone appearance[17] identical to that seen in sickle cell anemia.

Radiologic and pathologic evidence of epiphyseal bone

necrosis can be visualized in one or both femoral heads,[18, 19, 28, 29, 31, 32, 279] humeral heads,[33, 34] and tibial plateaus[23] in children and adults. Other skeletal sites also may be involved, including the distal femoral epiphyses[22] and small bones of the hands, wrists, and feet.[280] The pathogenesis of epiphyseal necrosis in Gaucher's disease apparently is related to compression of intraosseous sinusoids and lumina by masses of Gaucher cells and macrophages.[35] Cellular death leads to dense collagenous scarring of the marrow, which may aggravate osteonecrosis by subsequent vascular compression.[36–38] The resulting radiographic picture of osteonecrosis is identical to that accompanying many other diseases, although bony sclerosis may not be so prominent in Gaucher's disease. Secondary degenerative joint disease may appear, which can be attributed to osseous irregularity of the articular surfaces. Hip arthroplasty may be required in the treatment of osteonecrosis and osteoarthritis in pa-

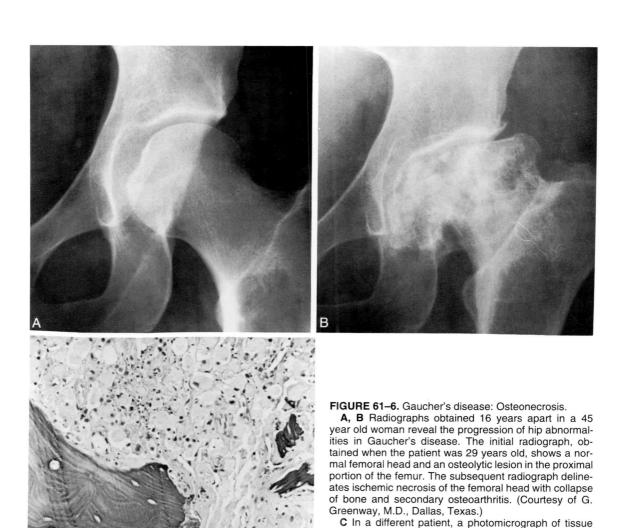

FIGURE 61–6. Gaucher's disease: Osteonecrosis.

A, B Radiographs obtained 16 years apart in a 45 year old woman reveal the progression of hip abnormalities in Gaucher's disease. The initial radiograph, obtained when the patient was 29 years old, shows a normal femoral head and an osteolytic lesion in the proximal portion of the femur. The subsequent radiograph delineates ischemic necrosis of the femoral head with collapse of bone and secondary osteoarthritis. (Courtesy of G. Greenway, M.D., Dallas, Texas.)

C In a different patient, a photomicrograph of tissue derived from the femoral head shows typical Gaucher's cells and osteonecrosis. (Courtesy of A. Norman, M.D., Valhalla, New York.)

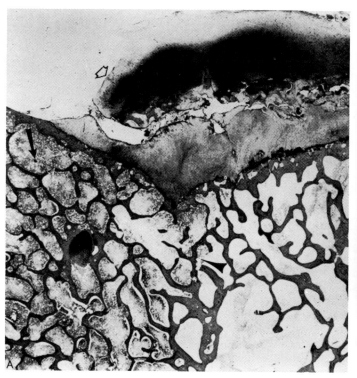

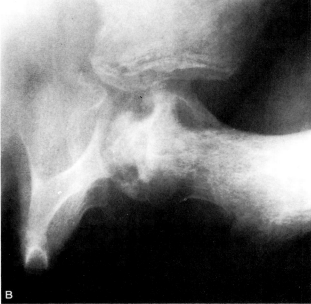

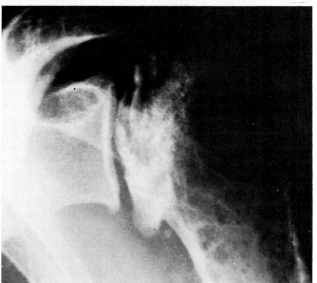

FIGURE 61–7. Gaucher's disease: Osteonecrosis.

A A photomicrograph (5×) of a femoral head in a 38 year old woman with Gaucher's disease reveals evidence of osteonecrosis. At the lower left of the picture, Gaucher cells can be seen within the marrow spaces of the spongiosa (arrow). Toward the right of the picture, the cells have undergone necrosis (arrowhead) and are surrounded by necrotic trabeculae. An osteochondral fragment is apparent (open arrow), which is partially attached to the parent bone.

B A radiograph of a hip in the frog-leg position reveals extensive changes of osteonecrosis with sclerosis, cystic lesions, and collapse. Surrounding osteoporosis is evident.

C Osteonecrosis is manifested as flattening and deformity of the humeral head, osteosclerosis, and joint space narrowing, the last representing secondary degenerative joint abnormalities. Observe lucency of the humeral shaft, reflecting the presence of Gaucher's disease.

(**A,** From Jaffe HL: Metabolic, Degenerative and Inflammatory Diseases of Bones and Joints. Philadelphia, Lea & Febiger, 1972.)

tients with Gaucher's disease,[279] although excessive intra-operative and postoperative bleeding is encountered.[174, 175]

Infection (Figs. 61–8 and 61–9). Although the clinical manifestations of osteonecrosis can simulate findings of osteomyelitis (pain, tenderness, swelling, warmth, decreased range of motion)[39–42] in Gaucher's disease, patients with this disease also have an increased susceptibility to development of bone infection.[19, 43, 273] The pathogenesis of infection in these patients is not clear, although it may be identical to that observed in sickle cell anemia and related disorders. Bone necrosis interspersed with areas of hemorrhage and lipid-containing marrow tissue produces an ideal environment for bacterial proliferation. Infection may involve any skeletal site, be caused by various organisms, including salmonellae, and be particularly prominent after bone and joint surgery.

Miscellaneous Articular Manifestations. In rare cases, Gaucher's disease is associated with a migratory polyarthritis, the nature of which is not clear.[44] More commonly, monoarticular or pauciarticular symptoms and signs in large and small joints are attributable to adjacent bone involvement.

Sclerosis of bone adjacent to the symphysis pubis and sacroiliac joint can be associated with apparent obliteration of the joint, simulating the findings of ankylosing spondylitis.[17, 18, 45] The cause of this abnormality is not known, although it also is seen in hemoglobinopathies and may relate to osteonecrosis of adjacent bone in both conditions.

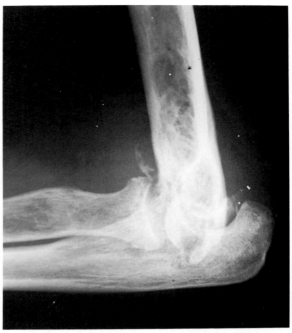

FIGURE 61–9. Gaucher's disease: Septic arthritis. In this 46 year old woman, septic arthritis of the elbow, resulting in severe bone destruction, was produced by *Listeria monocytogenes.* (Courtesy of V. Vint, M.D., San Diego, California.)

Although a hemorrhagic diathesis is a known manifestation of Gaucher's disease, bleeding other than in subperiosteal locations[46, 47] rarely is noted in descriptions of skeletal involvement. In one report, however, a large, expansile blood-filled cavity in the femur was observed as a complication of Gaucher's disease.[281] Hemarthrosis has not been emphasized; however, hemorrhaghic bursitis has been described.[176]

Degenerative joint disease is not unexpected considering the prevalence of osteonecrosis of the epiphyses. This complication is seen most commonly in the hip as a result of bone necrosis of the capital femoral epiphysis, although it also may be evident in the glenohumeral joint related to osteonecrosis of the humeral head.

The author has observed subperiosteal resorption of bone in several patients with Gaucher's disease (Fig. 61–10), although the pathogenesis of the finding is not certain.

A unique case of acro-osteolysis and a boot-shaped sella turcica has been described in Gaucher's disease.[48]

Advanced Imaging Methods

Radionuclide techniques, including bone scintigraphy (i.e., technetium diphosphonates) and bone marrow scintigraphy (i.e., technetium sulfur colloid) have been used to determine the extent and severity of skeletal involvement in patients with Gaucher's disease[282–284] (Fig. 61–11). Although some investigators have indicated the value of bone scintigraphy as a simple and sensitive test for assessment of the skeleton in this disease,[283] other studies employing a greater number of patients have indicated variability in the patterns of uptake of the bone-seeking radionuclides in Gaucher's disease.[282] Furthermore, in one investigation in which bone marrow scintigraphy and CT both were used in addition to bone scintigraphy, the former two methods were

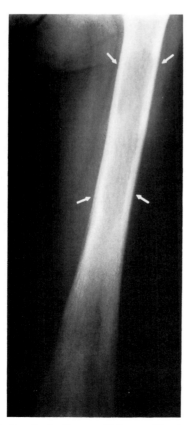

FIGURE 61–8. Gaucher's disease: Osteomyelitis. A poorly defined radiolucent shadow of the upper femoral shaft is associated with periosteal bone formation (arrows) in a patient with Gaucher's disease and documented Salmonella osteomyelitis. Observe the Erlenmeyer flask deformity of the distal end of the femur.

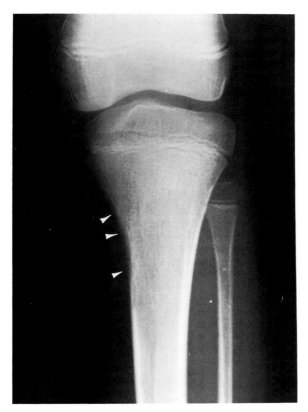

FIGURE 61–10. Gaucher's disease: Subperiosteal bone resorption. In this 12 year old girl, note resorption in the medial aspect of the tibia (arrowheads), resembling the abnormalities of hyperparathyroidism. (Courtesy of A. Brower, M.D., Norfolk, Virginia.)

ical and radiographic severity of skeletal involvement; peripheral marrow extension alone was associated with a lesser extent of skeletal involvement, whereas increasing loss, whether discrete or generalized, of radionuclide uptake by peripheral marrow was related to more extensive involvement. The most severely affected patients showed an almost total absence of radionuclide uptake. The authors speculated on the precise pathophysiologic events that caused the patterns of radionuclide uptake seen with bone marrow scintigraphy, indicating that a normal pattern may occur in an early stage of marrow infiltration with Gaucher cells; that the first of the three abnormal patterns suggests an increase in the number of Gaucher cells coincident with greater radionuclide uptake in the marrow; that the second of the three abnormal patterns corresponds to the development of foci of fibrotic or necrotic lesions in the bone marrow that prevent the appearance of uniform radionuclide activity; and that the last pattern, representing the most severe disease, results when decreased blood flow and necrosis preclude uptake of the radionuclide in viable reticuloendothelial cells in the bone marrow.

These same investigators as well as others[272, 285] have used *CT* as another method that allows assessment of the extent of marrow involvement in Gaucher's disease. The value of this technique lies in the observation that the attenuation properties of the Gaucher cell deposits are different from those of fat. Therefore, it is to be expected that marrow involved in this disease is denser than normal fatty marrow, a finding that has been confirmed.[277, 282] Rosenthal and coworkers[285] used quantitative CT to measure the trabecular bone density and bone marrow fat content in eight patients with Gaucher's disease. These investigators deter-

judged superior in the determination of the extent of skeletal involvement in patients with this disorder.[282]

Despite some difficulties that are encountered when bone scintigraphy is used to investigate patients with Gaucher's disease, the method has been reported to be valuable in the assessment of bone crises (perhaps related to hemorrhage or infarction) in this disease.[335] At the onset of a crisis, the bone scan typically shows decreased uptake of the radionuclide at the involved site: several weeks later, a margin of increase uptake surrounding a region of decreased uptake may be evident; and months later, the appearance of the radionuclide scan may be normal. Other investigators also have used the finding of decreased scintigraphic activity on a bone scan as a means to differentiate a crisis from osteomyelitis in patients with Gaucher's disease.[336]

Using technetium-99m sulfur colloid as a marrow-seeking radionuclide, Hermann and coworkers[282] defined three profiles of increasingly abnormal uptake of the radionuclide in 23 patients with Gaucher's disease: first, a pattern of bone marrow expansion with a uniformly dense uptake; second, a pattern of bone marrow expansion that was irregular and nonhomogeneous; and third, a pattern in which almost no uptake of the radionuclide was observed or in which such uptake was isolated to the midshaft of the femora and tibiae. In some patients who revealed the third of these patterns, the radionuclide was retained primarily in the vascular pool with additional accumulation in the reticuloendothelial cells in the lungs, liver, spleen, and lymph nodes. The extent of marrow involvement determined by bone marrow scintigraphy correlated directly with the clin-

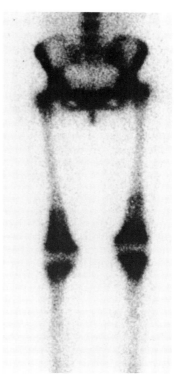

FIGURE 61–11. Gaucher's disease: Radionuclide abnormalities. Bone scintigraphy shows intense accumulation of the radionuclide in periarticular and metaphyseal regions, particularly about the knee. Note the Erlenmeyer flask deformities of the femora.

mined that the trabecular bone mass was moderately decreased and the bone marrow fat content was markedly decreased in these patients, presumably related to replacement of marrow fat by Gaucher cells. Although the presence of marrow fat in osteopenic patients without Gaucher's disease leads to lowering of attenuation values as determined by quantitative CT, similar bone density measurements in patients with Gaucher's disease reflect greater degrees of bone loss.[285] These data, although preliminary, indicate the potential of quantitative CT, by monitoring the levels of marrow fat, in assessing the severity of marrow involvement in this disease and its response to therapy.[334] In this regard, the report of Starer and colleagues[277] in which CT showed an improvement with a return of marrow attenuation to normal in children with Gaucher's disease treated successfully with bone marrow transplantation, is encouraging.

The expanding role of *MR imaging* in the analysis of bone marrow disorders is addressed in Chapter 59 and elsewhere in this textbook, and a summary of this role is provided in an article by Vogler and Murphey.[286] Little data have yet been accumulated on the value of MR imaging in the assessment of skeletal involvement in Gaucher's disease. Rosenthal and co-investigators[287] noted that regions of abnormal bone marrow in this disease were characterized by decreased signal intensity on T1- and T2-weighted spin echo MR images. This pattern of signal intensity, which also was observed by other investigators,[288] is consistent with marrow replacement by fibrosis and glucocerebroside-laden cells, may be homogeneous or inhomogeneous, progresses from proximal to distal sites in the appendicular skeleton, and generally spares the epiphyses unless extensive bone involvement is present.[286] The T1-weighted signal characteristics of affected bone marrow in Gaucher's disease are identical to those in other disorders characterized by marrow infiltration, such as metastatic disease, leukemia, lymphoma, and plasma cell myeloma, although the distribution and morphology of the process vary, to some extent, among these disorders. More helpful diagnostically in Gaucher's disease is persistent low signal intensity on T2-weighted spin echo MR images, which differs from the higher signal intensity on these images that may accompany skeletal metastasis, certain other tumors, and infection. The signal pattern, however, is not specific as the T2 values of tumors show considerable variability, the T2 values of hyperplastic normal marrow also are variable, and high signal intensity on T2-weighted spin echo MR sequences in the bone marrow of patients with Gaucher's disease has been encountered[288, 348] (Fig. 61–12). Bright signal on the T2-weighted images associated with acute bone pain in this disease may indicate fluid or blood within the medullary cavity occurring as a response to bone ischemia with reperfusion or venous obstruction.[288, 339] Osteomyelitis or intraosseous or subperiosteal hemorrhage complicating Gaucher's disease also may lead to high signal intensity on T2-weighted images[337] (Fig. 61–13).

As infiltration of the bone marrow by Gaucher cells leads to displacement of adipocytes, T1 values of the involved marrow increase owing to the higher T1 of water than of fat. This change forms the basis for the decreased signal intensity of the bone marrow that is evident on T1-weighted spin echo MR images and allows quantitative assessment

of the severity of the process using MR imaging. Johnson and coworkers[338] employed modified Dixon quantitative chemical shift imaging of the lumbar spine in 24 patients with Gaucher's disease and correlated the finding with results of quantitative analysis of marrow triglycerides and glucocerebrosides and with those of quantitative determination of splenic volume at MR imaging. Bulk T1 values were significantly longer, reflecting decreased marrow fat. Glucocerebroside concentrations were higher in diseased marrow and correlated inversely with triglyceride concentrations. The extent of marrow infiltration determined by fat fraction measurements correlated with the disease severity measured by splenic enlargement. These preliminary data suggest that quantitative chemical shift imaging may be a sensitive and noninvasive technique for evaluating bone marrow involvement in Gaucher's disease.

MR imaging also can be used effectively in the study of skeletal complications that occur in Gaucher's disease.[289, 340] Bone marrow ischemia and necrosis, osteomyelitis, and vertebral collapse are among the complications that may be assessed with MR imaging (Fig. 61–13). In the spine, the effect on the spinal cord at sites of vertebral fracture, deformity, or epidural mass is well shown with this imaging technique.[278]

Differential Diagnosis

Generalized increased radiolucency (osteopenia) in both the axial and the appendicular skeleton is not a specific sign of Gaucher's disease. This finding also is apparent in a variety of metabolic (osteoporosis, osteomalacia, and hyperparathyroidism), hematologic (sickle cell anemia and thalassemia), and neoplastic disorders (plasma cell myeloma and leukemia). In Gaucher's disease, localized lucent areas and cystic lesions producing a honeycomb appearance may simulate findings of plasma cell myeloma, amyloidosis, and skeletal metastasis. Furthermore, reports of coexistent Gaucher's disease and plasma cell myeloma indicate an additional source of diagnostic difficulty.[177]

Generalized or localized osteosclerosis likewise is not specific for Gaucher's disease. It is apparent in skeletal metastasis, tuberous sclerosis, mastocytosis, myelofibrosis, and Hodgkin's disease. In Gaucher's disease, the sclerosis includes a coarsened trabecular pattern and a bone-within-bone appearance, a finding that is not apparent in these other disorders. Similar changes can be seen in sickle cell anemia and its variants, however, the similarity being related to the occurrence of bone infarction and necrosis in these anemias and Gaucher's disease. Furthermore, epiphyseal osteonecrosis also is observed in both Gaucher's disease and hemoglobinopathies, complicating their differentiation. Epiphyseal osteonecrosis, particularly of the femoral head, which is seen in both Gaucher's disease and hemoglobinopathies, also is apparent in Cushing's syndrome and exogenous hypercortisolism, pancreatitis, caisson disease, collagen vascular disorders, and numerous other diseases. Diametaphyseal osteonecrosis is a manifestation of Gaucher's disease, hemoglobinopathies, pancreatitis, hypercortisolism, and caisson disease.

An Erlenmeyer flask appearance is seen in Gaucher's disease and other disorders (Table 61–2). These include certain anemias, fibrous dysplasia, Niemann-Pick disease,

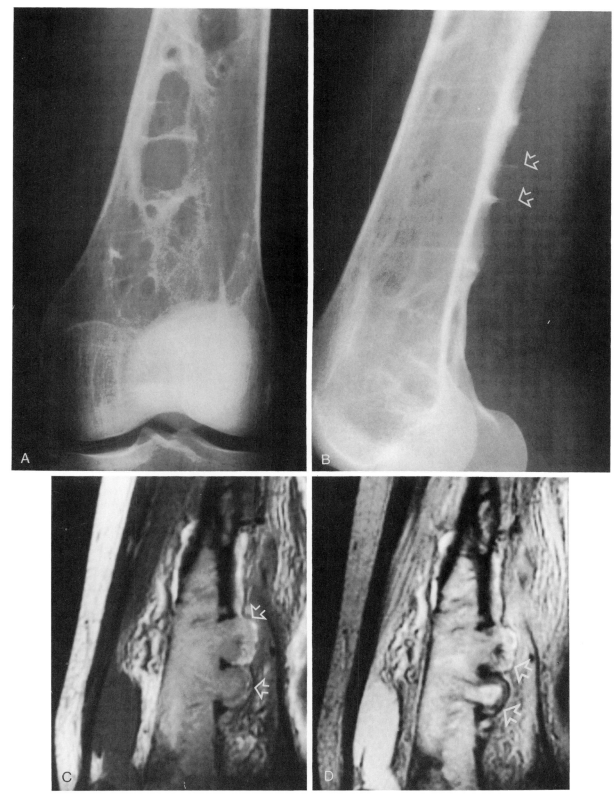

FIGURE 61–12. Gaucher's disease: MR imaging abnormalities. Marrow infiltration and cortical violation in a 40 year old woman.

A, B Routine radiographs reveal well-defined osteolytic lesions of the distal end of the femur. Note cortical thinning and erosion and the appearance of thick strands of bone extending from the posterior portion of the femur (arrows).

C A sagittal T1-weighted (TR/TE, 800/20) spin echo MR image shows tissue within the bone marrow replacing the normal fat. The tissue is of intermediate signal intensity and is violating the posterior cortex of the femur (arrows). A joint effusion is present in the knee.

D With T2 weighting (TR/TE, 1800/80), the abnormal tissue is inhomogeneous, displaying regions of both intermediate and high signal intensity. Cortical perforation is evident (arrows), and the joint effusion again is apparent.

(Courtesy of P. Kaplan, M.D., Charlottesville, Virginia.)

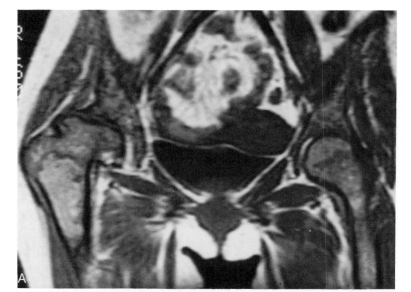

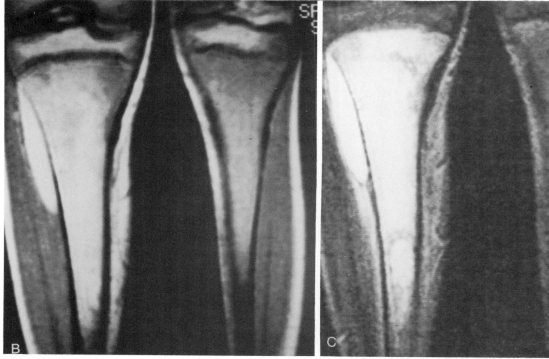

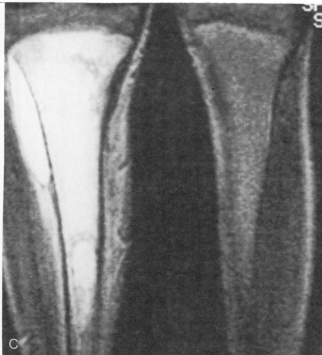

FIGURE 61–13. Gaucher's disease: MR imaging abnormalities.

A Marrow infiltration and osteonecrosis in a 31 year old woman. This coronal T1-weighted (TR/TE, 600/20) spin echo MR image shows abnormally low signal intensity in the marrow of the femora and innominate bones. Note deformity of the right femoral head indicative of osteonecrosis.

B, C Subperiosteal and intramedullary hemorrhage in a 12 year old girl. Coronal T1-weighted (TR/TE, 600/27) **(B)** and T2-weighted (TR/TE, 1800/100) **(C)** spin echo MR images show persistent high signal intensity in the tibia and adjacent soft tissues consistent with subacute hemorrhage.

(**B, C** From Horev G, et al: Skel Radiol *20*:479, 1991.)

**TABLE 61–2. Conditions Characterized
by Erlenmeyer Flask Deformity**

Gaucher's disease
Niemann-Pick disease
Anemias
Fibrous dysplasia
Metaphyseal dysplasia (Pyle's disease)
Osteopetrosis
Heavy metal poisoning

(cranio)metaphyseal dysplasia (Pyle's disease), heavy metal poisoning, and osteopetrosis. In many of these diseases, other findings allow accurate diagnosis.

It is obvious that the radiographic findings of Gaucher's disease reveal considerable overlap with those in other disorders, particularly the hemoglobinopathies. The diagnosis should be considered in a patient with hepatosplenomegaly who demonstrates widespread osteopenia with a coarsened trabecular pattern, focal osteosclerosis, ischemic necrosis of the proximal capital femoral epiphyses, and flaring or Erlenmeyer flask deformities of the distal portions of the femora.

NIEMANN-PICK DISEASE

Background and General Features

Niemann-Pick disease is a rare, genetically determined disorder characterized by the widespread accumulation of lipid, particularly sphingomyelin, in the body. It first was observed in 1914 by Niemann,[49] who, on noting abnormal cells in many organs during an autopsy of an 18 month old infant, falsely attributed the findings to Gaucher's disease. After additional cases of Gaucher's disease were reported,[50] Pick outlined the clinical features of this separate entity, calling it lipoid cell splenomegaly.[51] This disorder subsequently became known as Niemann-Pick disease. Further important contributions in the history of this disease were the discovery of increased tissue phospholipids,[52] specifically sphingomyelin,[53, 54] and deficient sphingomyelinase activity[55] in patients with Niemann-Pick disease. Sphingomyelin accumulations may be found in reticuloendothelial and parenchymal cells within many organs.

Niemann-Pick disease is not a single entity. Five types of sphingomyelin lipidoses are recognized[56]:

Type A. Acute neuronopathic form characterized by rapidly fatal disease of infancy with involvement of both viscera and nervous system and with a severe deficiency of sphingomyelinase.

Type B. Chronic form without nervous system involvement, characterized by visceral involvement in infants and a moderate to severe deficiency of sphingomyelinase.

Type C. Subacute (juvenile) form with neurologic abnormalities in childhood, usually leading to death by adolescence and with questionable sphingomyelinase deficiency.

Type D. Nova Scotia form, in which patients, other than having an ancestry in Nova Scotia, resemble those in Type C.

Type E. Indeterminate form, occurring in adults with visceral involvement and with questionable sphingomyelinase deficiency.

Clinical Features

The clinical manifestations vary with the specific type of the disease. The sex distribution is approximately equal, and many of the patients are of Jewish background. In general, symptoms and signs become apparent during infancy and progress rapidly, leading to the patient's demise. Findings in these infants may include jaundice, hepatosplenomegaly, abdominal enlargement, lymphadenopathy, emaciation, decreased visual acuity, and blindness. In some patients, clinical manifestations may not be detected until later in childhood, and affected children may live into adolescence. In these latter patients, gradual enlargement of the liver and spleen and mental and physical deterioration occur. A cherry-red spot in the macular region of each fundus is an important physical finding in this disease. Moderate anemia and thrombocytopenia commonly are apparent.

The diagnosis is suggested by identification of foam cells in marrow aspirates or tissue biopsy specimens and confirmed by the chemical determination of a predominant increase in sphingomyelin in abnormal tissue.

Musculoskeletal Abnormalities

Accumulation of lipid-containing foam cells occurs in the bone marrow, producing abnormality of adjacent bony trabeculae (Fig. 61–14). This is particularly frequent in children who have a type of Niemann-Pick disease that is compatible with longer life (type B). In tubular bones, decrease in size and number of trabeculae within the spongiosa is associated with cortical thinning.[57] On radiographs, this combination of spongiosa and cortical abnormalities results in increased osseous radiolucency and medullary widening with cortical diminution, findings that are similar to those of Gaucher's disease.[58] Modeling deformities in Niemann-Pick disease also are similar to those of Gaucher's disease, with straightening and convexity of the distal femoral contour.

Increased radiolucency, medullary widening, and a lace-like trabecular pattern may be seen in the tubular bones of the hands in patients with Niemann-Pick disease, particularly types B and C.[58] These changes are reminiscent of findings in mucopolysaccharidoses and thalassemia.

Additional findings that have been described in Niemann-Pick disease are coxa valga deformity (most prevalent in types A and C and probably related to decreased weight-bearing),[58] notched upper lumbar vertebrae (a nonspecific finding),[59] osseous defects of the proximal medial humerus (also described in glycogen storage disease, Gaucher's disease, and Hurler's syndrome and as a normal variant),[58] epiphyseal stippling,[58] and delayed ossification of various secondary centers (a finding that may be apparent in many chronic disorders).

Differential Diagnosis

The skeletal manifestations of Niemann-Pick disease are similar to those of Gaucher's disease, which is not surprising in view of their nearly identical pathogenesis (Table 61–3). Medullary widening, cortical thinning, and modeling deformities are seen in both disorders.[58, 60] Unlike Gaucher's disease, Niemann-Pick disease has not been associated with

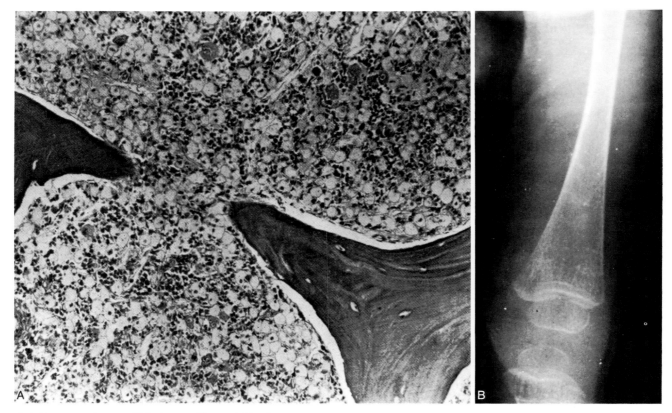

FIGURE 61–14. Niemann-Pick disease: Marrow infiltration.
A A photomicrograph (125×) of a section of a vertebral body in a 2 year old child with Niemann-Pick disease illustrates cellular infiltration of the marrow spaces of the spongiosa. The lipid-laden cells largely have replaced the myeloid cells.
B The distal femoral shaft is both osteopenic and expanded.
(**A**, From Jaffe HL: Metabolic, Degenerative and Inflammatory Diseases of Bones and Joints. Philadelphia, Lea & Febiger, 1972.)

epiphyseal osteonecrosis or with a high frequency of well-circumscribed radiolucent lesions. These differences facilitate the radiographic diagnosis of Niemann-Pick disease.

FABRY'S DISEASE

Background and General Features

Fabry's disease or glycosphingolipidosis is a hereditary, X-linked systemic disorder characterized by accumulation in various tissues of ceramide trihexoside. This birefringent lipid is deposited in endothelial, perithelial, and smooth muscle cells of blood vessels, in perineural cells and ganglion cells of the autonomic nervous system, in epithelial cells of the cornea, in reticuloendothelial, myocardial, and connective tissue cells, and in other viscera and tissues.[61]

TABLE 61–3. Musculoskeletal Manifestations of Gaucher's Disease and Niemann-Pick Disease

	Gaucher's Disease	Niemann-Pick Disease
Osteopenia	+	+
Cortical thinning or erosion	+	+
Coarsened trabecular pattern	+	+
Lytic lesions	+	−
Modeling deformity	+	+
Osteonecrosis	+	−

The disorder first was described by both Fabry[62] and Anderson[63] in 1898 and was termed angiokeratoma corporis diffusum because of a characteristic skin lesion that accompanies the disease. Because the skin manifestation is not always present, Fabry's disease has become the accepted name of the disorder.[64, 65]

The accumulation of lipid in Fabry's disease, which occurs as the result of an absence of a specific enzyme (ceramide trihexosidase) required for the proper catabolism of trihexosyl ceramide, may lead to the patient's death by the fifth or sixth decade of life because of renal failure and hypertension with cardiac and neurologic complications.

Initial clinical manifestations may involve multiple organ systems. These manifestations vary in men and women and in hemizygotic and heterozygotic patients. The characteristic skin lesion of this disease is bilaterally distributed in the lower abdomen and legs, with involvement of the back, thighs, buttocks, hips, pelvis, and scrotum. Additionally, patients reveal fever, pain, and paresthesias, particularly in the fingers and toes. Signs of renal impairment include proteinuria and azotemia. Hypertension, cardiomegaly, myocardial infarction, seizures, sensory deficits, dizziness, aphasia, and cerebral hemorrhage are additional clinical findings of Fabry's disease.

The diagnosis is established by the detection of a characteristic skin lesion, corneal epithelial dystrophy, and abnormal levels of birefringent lipid material in the skin or kidney.

Musculoskeletal Abnormalities

Periarticular swelling in the knees, elbows, and small joints of the fingers may appear in Fabry's disease. Abnormalities of the distal interphalangeal joints of the fingers may lead to limitation of extension and permanent deformity.[64, 66, 67] Osteonecrosis is observed at many sites, including the femoral head and talus[68, 69] (Fig. 61–15). Presumably, the pathogenesis of bone necrosis is similar to that in Gaucher's disease, with lipid infiltration in marrow and vessel walls.

Additional findings include osteoporosis of vertebrae of the thoracolumbar spine[70] and alterations in the metatarsals, metacarpals, and temporomandibular joints.[71] Periarticular soft tissue prominence and enthesopathic changes may be evident.[265]

A synovial and joint capsule biopsy of an involved joint in one patient with Fabry's disease revealed mild proliferation of the synovial lining and subsynovial foam cells unrelated to and surrounding blood vessels.[149] The findings suggest that neuroischemia may be responsible for the joint pain that can be encountered in this disease.

REFSUM'S DISEASE

This rare inherited disorder of phytanic acid metabolism first was described in 1946 by Refsum.[178] Consequently, the disorder often is designated Refsum's disease, although it also is referred to as heredopathia atactica polyneuritiformis. Although a wide variety of clinical manifestations have been recorded in this disease, and these manifestations

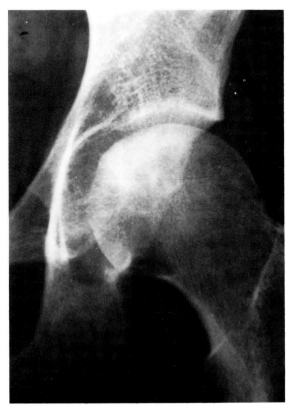

FIGURE 61–15. Fabry's disease: Osteonecrosis. In this patient, osteonecrosis of the femoral head is manifested as patchy sclerosis and radiolucency and minimal depression of the articular surface.

appear in various combinations, the features that are considered fundamental to its diagnosis are retinitis pigmentosa, peripheral polyneuropathy, cerebellar ataxia, and an elevated protein concentration (in the absence of pleocytosis) in the cerebrospinal fluid.[179, 180] The clinical onset of the disease usually is observed before the age of 20 years, although symptoms and signs beginning in childhood or in the fifth or sixth decade of life have been identified. A decrease in visual acuity, especially night blindness, and weakness are frequent early complaints. Clinical alterations generally progress, although periods of remission are encountered.

The basic pathologic alteration is accumulation of a 20-carbon branched chain acid, phytanic acid, in the body's tissues, such as the liver, kidney, heart, and peripheral nerves. The major source of phytanic acid is dietary, as it is present in chlorophyll-containing foods. Failure of conversion of phytanic acid to α-hydroxyphytanic acid, owing to absence of phytanic acid α-hydroxylase, represents the primary defect in Refsum's disease and accounts for the accumulation of phytanic acid in many organ systems. Thus, dietary control with elimination of exogenous phytanate provides therapeutic benefits, especially if treatment is begun early in the course of the disease.

There are few descriptions of the skeletal manifestations of Refsum's disease.[181, 182, 333] Reported findings include epiphyseal alterations resembling ischemic necrosis about the hips, shoulders, elbows, knees, hands, and feet; shortening of the metatarsals, metacarpals, and phalanges; and osseous irregularity in the vertebral bodies. These changes are similar to abnormalities occurring in Gaucher's disease, although osteopenia and modeling deformities, seen in the latter disorder, usually are not apparent in Refsum's disease. A distinctive skeletal abnormality of Refsum's disease, not seen in Gaucher's disease, is a short, conical terminal phalanx of the thumb.[333] As histologic analysis of the bone lesions has not been accomplished, the precise nature of the radiographic abnormalities is not known; examination of biopsy material derived from nerves and muscles indicates myelin degeneration and denervation, respectively.[182]

FARBER'S LIPOGRANULOMATOSIS

Farber's disease is a rare and progressive disorder of infancy and early childhood, transmitted as an autosomal recessive characteristic, which is accompanied by hoarseness, aphonia, painful and swollen joints, brownish desquamating dermatitis, subcutaneous and periarticular nodules, and pulmonary abnormalities.[183–186] The basic defect in this disease is a deficiency of acid ceramidase activity, leading to accumulation of ceramide in various tissues, including the kidneys, liver, lungs and lymph nodes. Subcutaneous nodules containing ceramide also are characteristic. Involved tissue reveals infiltration by macrophages and foam cells with granulomatous reaction.

Affected persons appear normal at birth, but symptoms and signs, especially those related to the joints, become evident in the first few weeks or months of life. Initially, generalized soft tissue swelling in the limbs is seen, which subsequently is transformed into nodular thickening about joints and tendons sheaths. These nodules increase in number and size as the disease progresses and are seen most frequently in the interphalangeal regions of the hands, wrists, elbows, and ankles. Additional sites of soft tissue nodules are the conjunctivae, nostrils, ears, skull (especially the occiput), and spine. Flexion contractures develop.

Histopathologically, the bones, cartilage, and soft tissues are observed to be infiltrated with macrophages, histiocytes, and foam cells containing lipid material that stains positively with periodic acid–Schiff (PAS) reagent. Granulomas are characterized by a central region of foam cells surrounded by giant cells, lymphocytes, and macrophages. Radiographic findings include soft tissue swelling, periarticular masses, and juxta-articular bone erosions.

No specific therapy has proved effective, so that rapid progression leading to the patient's demise in 1 or a few years is typical. Rarely, affected persons live into adolescence or early adulthood.

GENERALIZED (G_{M1}) GANGLIOSIDOSIS

Generalized gangliosidosis is an inherited liposomal storage disease caused by a deficiency of G_{M1}-ganglioside-β-galactosidase, leading to accumulation of ganglioside G_{M1} in various tissues, including the nervous system.[188] Several clinical varieties have been described, which differ principally in the time of onset of disease, the pattern of specific organic dysfunction, and the degree of neurologic deterioration. Common clinical manifestations of generalized (G_{M1}) gangliosidosis are mental retardation, a cherry-red spot in the macula, hepatomegaly, and osseous deformities.

Radiographic abnormalities related to the musculoskeletal system include diffuse osteopenia, a delay in bone maturation, thickening of the calvarium, horizontally oriented ribs, flattening and beaking of the vertebral bodies, flared iliac wings, acetabular dysplasia, epiphyseal fragmentation, and slender tubular bones.[189] Foam cells are present in the bone marrow.

Generally, prominent clinical manifestations appear in the first few months of life. Neurologic symptoms and signs dominate. Progression of these manifestations with early death is the rule. Rarely, patients with severe bony alterations and normal intelligence survive into adulthood.

FUCOSIDOSIS

Fucosidosis is an autosomal recessive disorder characterized by an absence of α-fucosidase activity, leading to accumulation of fucose-containing H-isoantigenic lipids and a decasaccharide in many tissues.[190, 191] Distinct clinical groups have been identified. In some cases, prominent abnormalities appear in the first few months or years of life and consist of hepatosplenomegaly, cardiomegaly, mental retardation, coarse facies, and skeletal changes resembling those seen in the mucopolysaccharidoses. In other cases, the disease is later in onset and slower in progression.

MULTICENTRIC RETICULOHISTIOCYTOSIS
Background and General Features

Multicentric reticulohistiocytosis is an uncommon systemic disease of unknown cause that becomes apparent in adult life and that is characterized by the proliferation of histiocytes in the skin, mucosa, subcutaneous tissues, syn-

ovia, and, on occasion, bone and periosteum. This name, which was used first by Goltz and Laymon,[72] is but one of many terms that have been applied to this disorder. Other names are lipoid dermatoarthritis,[73] reticulohistiocytoma,[74] lipoid rheumatism,[75] giant cell reticulohistiocytosis,[76] giant cell histiocytomatosis,[77] and giant cell histiocytosis,[78] as well as various other designations, which are summarized by Barrow and Holubar.[79] At this writing, multicentric reticulohistiocytosis is the most accepted name for the disease.

Targett in 1897[80] probably was the first physician to describe this condition, although his description of a 65 year old woman with "rheumatic and gouty habit" was vague and therefore was ignored by many later investigators. In 1952, Caro and Senear[74] proposed the term reticulohistiocytic granuloma to encompass the pathologic findings noted after biopsy of a patient with multiple cutaneous tumors. In 1937, Weber and Freudenthal[81] were the first to describe the entity adequately after observation of a 35 year old man with cutaneous nodules, polyarthritis, and tenosynovitis. In 1944, Portugal and coworkers[77] reported the second patient who clearly had this disease. After the report of Caro and Senear in 1952[74] of two additional patients, multicentric reticulohistiocytosis became recognized as a definite entity.

Clinical Features

Multicentric reticulohistiocytosis is a disease that demonstrates no particular geographic predilection. Its onset most frequently is in middle age (40 to 50 years), although cases occurring in childhood, adolescence, and senescence are known.[290] Women are affected more frequently than men.[79, 82–84] A familial predisposition has not been documented.

In approximately 60 to 70 per cent of patients, polyarthritis is the first manifestation of the disease, followed after months to years by a nodular eruption of the skin.[192] In the remainder of patients, skin nodules are present when the patient initially develops the disorder.[79] These nodules are pruritic, firm, yellow to red in color, and common in the ears, nose, scalp, face, dorsum of the hands, forearms, and elbows. Small tumefactions are characteristic about the nail folds, which may lead to alterations in nail growth.[85] Mucosal papules occur in 50 per cent of patients, involving the lips, buccal membrane, tongue, nasal septum, pharynx, and larynx.

Polyarticular manifestations are symmetric and involve, in descending order of frequency, the interphalangeal joints (including distal interphalangeal articulations) of the fingers, knees, shoulders, wrists, hips, ankles, feet, elbows, spine, and temporomandibular joints.[79] Clinical findings are soft tissue swelling, stiffness, and tenderness, resembling abnormalities of rheumatoid arthritis. Differences from this latter disease are the increased frequency of distal interphalangeal changes in multicentric reticulohistiocytosis and the severity of joint involvement that may occur in this disease. In fact, almost 50 per cent of patients with multicentric reticulohistiocytosis develop arthritis mutilans, although others may reveal spontaneous remission of symptoms and signs.

In addition to skin lesions and polyarthritis, patients with multicentric reticulohistiocytosis may reveal xanthelasmas. Xanthomas relate to the presence of hypercholesterolemia and involve predominantly the eyelids. Tendon sheath swelling, hypertension, lymphadenopathy, ganglia, erythema, joint hypermobility, and pathologic fractures, in descending order of frequency, are other clinical manifestations.[79] A variety of tumors also have been described in association with multicentric reticulohistiocytosis, including carcinomas in many different sites, such as the colon, bronchus, breast, and cervix. Sjögren's syndrome similarly has been associated with multicentric reticulohistiocytosis.[266] It is not certain if these associations are meaningful.

Some characteristics of laboratory examination in this disease are anemia, hypercholesterolemia, and elevated erythrocyte sedimentation rate. An increased frequency of positive tuberculin skin tests has been reported, but active mycobacterial infection is rare.[163]

Radiologic Abnormalities

The radiologic features of musculoskeletal involvement in multicentric reticulohistiocytosis have been well described[86–89] (Table 61–4). In general this disorder is characterized by the following features[86]: bilateral symmetric involvement; predilection for the interphalangeal joints of the hand and foot; early and severe involvement of the atlantoaxial articulation; erosive arthritis beginning at the margins of the joint and spreading centrally, producing separation of osseous surfaces; lack of significant periarticular osteoporosis or periosteal bone formation; and uncalcified nodules of skin, subcutaneous tissues, and tendon sheaths. These radiographic features may become severe and destructive, although associated clinical findings may be mild.[193]

The most characteristic site of involvement is the interphalangeal joints of the hands, which may be altered in as many as 75 per cent of patients with this disease (Figs. 61–16 and 61–17). Soft tissue swelling and marginal erosions, distributed symmetrically, are the initial features in this location. Associated involvement of the metacarpophalangeal joints and wrists can be apparent, with nodularity of the adjacent soft tissues. The erosions are well circumscribed (Fig. 61–18), resembling the defects of gouty arthritis. The articular space may be widened or narrowed. Progression of disease leads to dramatic resorption of the phalanges, foreshortening of the fingers, telescoping of the digits, and an end-stage arthritis mutilans.[89]

Abnormalities of the feet resemble those of the hands (Fig. 61–19). Symmetric involvement of interphalangeal joints, including the first, and of the metatarsophalangeal joints is apparent. Marginal and central erosions can be seen with or without narrowing of the articular space. The presence of soft tissue nodules and the absence of periosteal proliferation and periarticular osteoporosis are additional characteristics.

TABLE 61–4. Radiographic Characteristics of Multicentric Reticulohistiocytosis

Bilateral symmetric involvement
Predilection for the interphalangeal joints of hand, foot
Atlantoaxial subluxation
Marginal erosions
Absence of osteoporosis
Soft tissue nodules

Changes may be evident in other joints of the appendicular skeleton (Fig. 61–20), including the glenohumeral and acromioclavicular joints, hip, knee, elbow, and ankle.[150, 291] In each location, the severity of the process may vary, beginning with osseous defects and progressing to severe joint destruction. For example, in the hips, resorption of the femoral head and acetabular protrusion eventually can appear. Involvement usually is bilateral and symmetric.

The joints of the axial skeleton also can be affected (Fig. 61–21). The changes in the sacroiliac joint include erosion and obliteration, with bony ankylosis of the articular space.[86, 89, 90] Although this process may be bilateral and symmetric, the absence of adjacent sclerosis aids in distinguishing multicentric reticulohistiocytosis from ankylosing spondylitis. In the thoracic spine, erosion of costotransverse joints may be evident[86]; syndesmophytes are not seen. In the cervical spine, apophyseal joint erosions may be encountered.[150]

Severe destructive abnormalities in the cervical spine have been emphasized in multicentric reticulohistiocytosis. Subluxation at the atlantoaxial joint can be an early manifestation of the disease (Fig. 61–21). Osseous destruction of the atlas, the axis (including the odontoid process), and the base of the skull eventually can occur. The findings resemble those of rheumatoid arthritis, although they may be even more severe.

Pathologic Abnormalities (Fig. 61–22)

The skin lesions can be located in any layer of the dermis. They consist of a granulomatous infiltration of histiocytic multinucleated giant cells, which contain large amounts of PAS-positive material, which probably is a mixture of lipids, phospholipids, and cholesterol esters.[79, 91] The lesions of the mucous membrane resemble the skin nodules.[92] Similar nodules may be seen in other tissues, including the liver, kidney, lymph nodes, muscle, subcutaneous tissue, nail bed, and endocardium.

In the synovial tissues, histiocytic and giant cell proliferation is evident in the edematous and highly vascular stroma.[79, 86, 91] Lymphocytes and plasma cells also are evident, and vessels exhibit intimal thickening.[92] Villous hypertrophy of the synovial lining may be seen, and the synovial fluid may contain foamy giant cells.[91] Although the pathologic aberrations resemble those of rheumatoid arthritis, rheumatoid disease is characterized by more severe inflammation, more extensive villous hypertrophy, and many giant cells that do not contain foamy or granular cytoplasm.

Examination of bone reveals cellular infiltration similar to that in skin and synovium with histiocytes and giant cells.[93, 94]

In multicentric reticulohistiocytosis, immunohistochemical staining of tissue derived from involved synovium and skin has revealed that the histiocytes react positively to interleukin-1 β and platelet derived growth factor B, leading to the speculation that these cytokines may play a role in synovial proliferation in this disorder.[292]

Differential Diagnosis

The articular manifestations of multicentric reticulohistiocytosis must be distinguished from those of other conditions (Table 61–5). The early erosive changes at the mar-

Text continued on page 2214

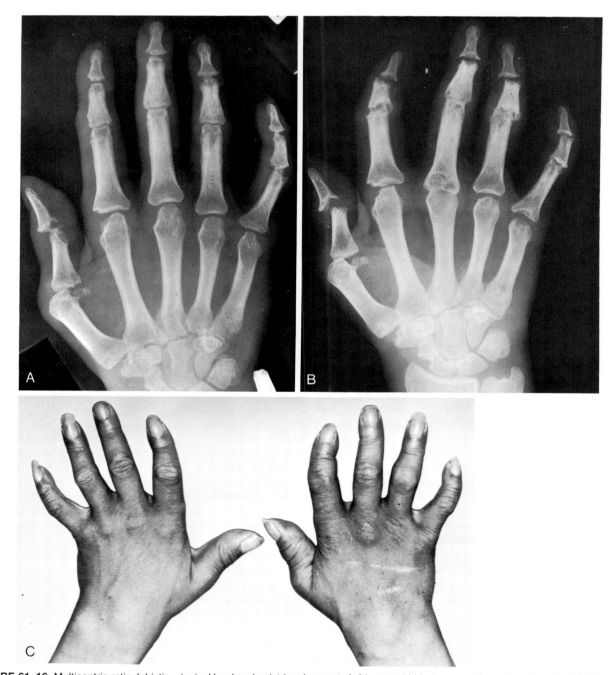

FIGURE 61–16. Multicentric reticulohistiocytosis: Hand and wrist involvement. A 31 year old black man with multicentric reticulohistiocytosis documented by biopsy of subcutaneous nodules.

A Radiograph of the right hand demonstrates well-circumscribed marginal erosions accompanied by nodular soft tissue swelling affecting all metacarpophalangeal and interphalangeal joints. In addition, erosions can be observed in several of the carpal bones, including the scaphoid and trapezium. The opposite side was affected similarly.

B, C A radiograph **(B)** of the right hand and a clinical photograph **(C)** of both hands several years later demonstrate progression of the osseous and articular changes. Ulnar deviation of the fingers is evident. The erosions are well circumscribed. The interphalangeal joints are severely eroded, with separation of the osseous margins.

(A–C, From Gold RH, et al: AJR *124*:610, 1975. Copyright 1975, American Roentgen Ray Society.)

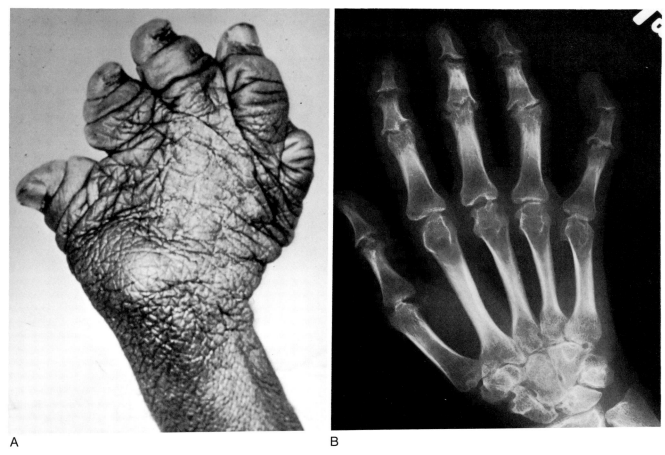

A   B

FIGURE 61–17. Multicentric reticulohistiocytosis: Hand and wrist involvement.
   A End-stage arthritis mutilans in a patient with multicentric reticulohistiocytosis. Note the "accordion hand," with shortening of the fingers and severe wrinkling of the skin.
   B In a different patient, a radiograph reveals well-defined erosions of interphalangeal and metacarpophalangeal joints as well as throughout the wrist.
   (**B,** Courtesy of A. Brower, M.D., Norfolk, Virginia.)

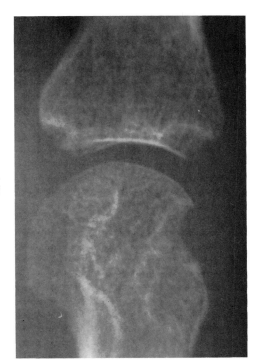

FIGURE 61–18. Multicentric reticulohistiocytosis: Metacarpophalangeal joint involvement. Note the well-circumscribed erosions, with sclerotic margins, resembling those of gouty arthritis. (Courtesy of M. Pathria, M.D., San Diego, California.)

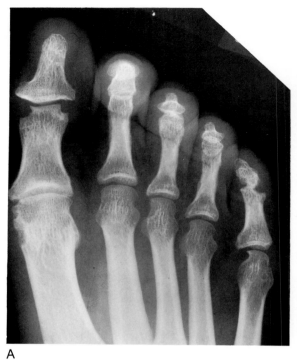

A

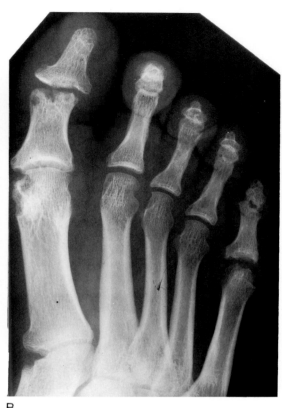

B

FIGURE 61–19. Multicentric reticulohistiocytosis: Foot involvement. Radiographs of the foot in a 31 year old black man (same patient as in Figure 61–16).

A In the right foot, nearly all joints manifest well-circumscribed marginal erosions. Osteoporosis and periostitis are not evident. Soft tissue swelling is apparent. The opposite foot was affected similarly.

B Several years later more extensive abnormalities are evident. Observe involvement of metatarsophalangeal and interphalangeal joints, relative preservation of joint space in some articulations, soft tissue swelling, well-circumscribed erosions, and lack of osteoporosis and periostitis.

(From Gold RH, et al: AJR *124*:610, 1975. Copyright 1975, American Roentgen Ray Society.)

TABLE 61–5. Differential Diagnosis of Multicentric Reticulohistiocytosis

	Symmetric Involvement	Involvement of DIP Joints*	Marginal Erosions	Osteo-porosis	Intra-articular Bony Ankylosis	Atlantoaxial Subluxation	Soft Tissue Nodules
Multicentric reticulohistiocytosis	+	+	+	−	−	+	+
Rheumatoid arthritis	+	−	+	+	−	+	+
Psoriatic arthritis	±	+	+	−	+	+	−
Inflammatory (erosive) osteoarthritis	+	+	±	−	+	−	−
Gouty arthritis	±	+	+	−	−	−	+

*DIP, distal interphalangeal.

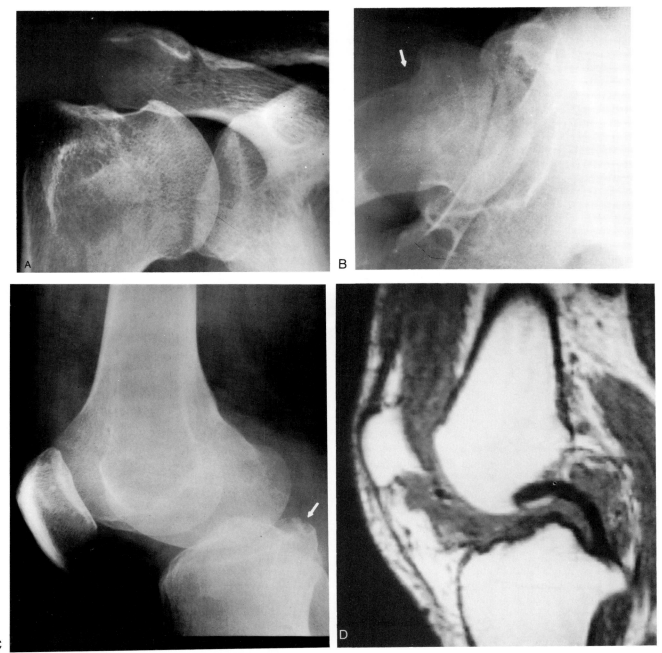

FIGURE 61–20. Multicentric reticulohistiocytosis: Involvement of other joints of the appendicular skeleton.
   A Extensive osseous erosions on the lateral aspect of the right humeral head can be seen. The erosions are well defined. The joint space is not narrowed.
   B In the hip, erosions of the femoral neck (arrow) have produced an "apple core" appearance.
   C In the knee, a well-circumscribed erosion is evident (arrow).
   D In another patient, a sagittal T1-weighted (TR/TE, 700/15) spin echo image reveals a distended knee joint filled with fluid and synovial inflammatory tissue of low signal intensity.
   (**A–C,** From Gold RH, et al: AJR *124*:610, 1975. Copyright 1975. American Roentgen Ray Society; **D,** Courtesy of M. Pathria, M.D., San Diego, California.)

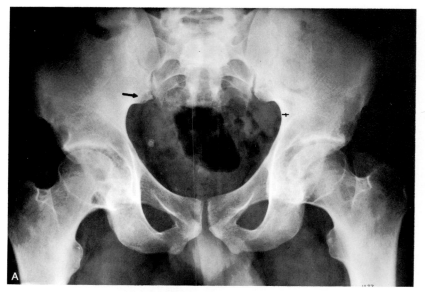

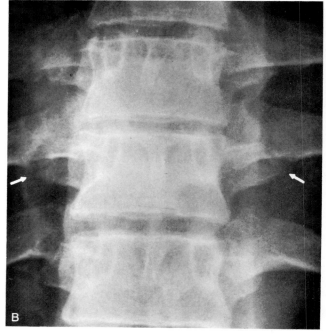
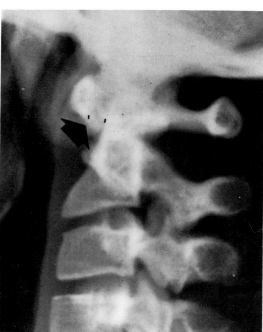

FIGURE 61–21. Multicentric reticulohistiocytosis: Involvement of articulations of the axial skeleton. Same patient as in Figures 61–16 and 61–19.

  A An anteroposterior radiograph of the pelvis discloses an erosion (arrow) along the inferior surface of the iliac bone about the right sacroiliac joint. Large acetabular erosions also are evident.

  B An anteroposterior view of the thoracic spine reveals erosions of the costotransverse joints of the ninth thoracic vertebra (arrows).

  C A lateral radiograph of the cervical spine discloses atlantoaxial subluxation of 6 mm (arrow).

  (From Gold RH, et al: AJR *124*:610, 1975. Copyright 1975, American Roentgen Ray Society.)

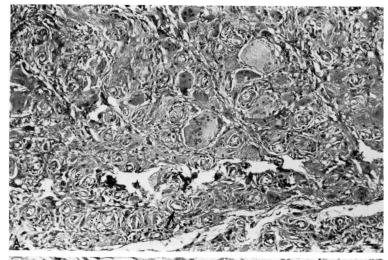

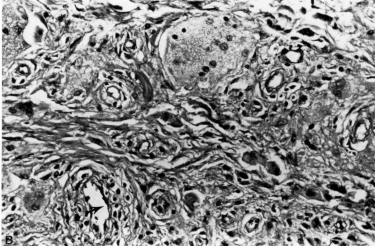

FIGURE 61–22. Multicentric reticulohistiocytosis: Pathologic abnormalities.

A, B Subcutaneous nodules. A photomicrograph (125×) **(A)** indicates dense fibrous connective tissue, large histiocytes containing multiple small round nuclei and granular cytoplasm, and numerous capillaries surrounded by concentric onionskin layers of fibrous tissue between which are lymphocytes (arrow). At higher magnification (350×) **(B)**, the histiocytes are seen to contain distinctive foamy cytoplasm, and concentrically layered capillaries are infiltrated by lymphocytes (arrow).

C Synovial membrane. A photomicrograph (360×) indicates extensive infiltration by large "foamy" cells. Increased vascularity and inflammatory cellular infiltration are observed (arrow).

D Synovial fluid. A smear reveals a giant cell, 60 μm in diameter, with three nuclei and granular cytoplasm.

(**A, B,** From Gold RH, et al: AJR *124*:610, 1975. Copyright 1975, American Roentgen Ray Society; **C, D,** From Crey PR, et al: Arthritis Rheum *17*:615, 1974.)

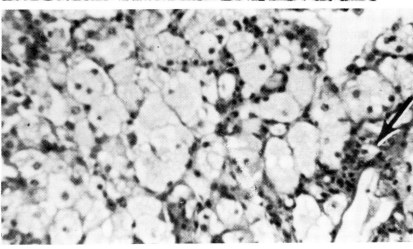

C

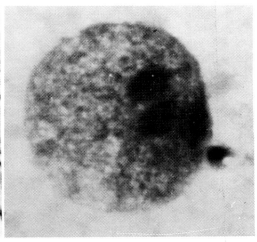

D

gins of joints resemble the erosions in a variety of synovial diseases, such as rheumatoid arthritis, psoriasis, ankylosing spondylitis, and Reiter's syndrome. Although symmetry of involvement and absence of new bone formation are seen in both multicentric reticulohistiocytosis and rheumatoid arthritis, periarticular osteoporosis and early joint space loss are characteristic of rheumatoid arthritis but may be absent in multicentric reticulohistiocytosis. In addition, significant destructive changes of distal interphalangeal joints are not common in rheumatoid arthritis but represent an important finding in multicentric reticulohistiocytosis. Atlantoaxial subluxation may be seen in both conditions. Certain findings in psoriatic arthritis resemble changes in multicentric reticulohistiocytosis, including predilection for interphalangeal joints, marginal and central erosions with separation of osseous surfaces, and lack of osteoporosis. Distinguishing features in psoriasis are asymmetric involvement, new bone formation and proliferation with poorly defined erosive alterations, and intra-articular bony ankylosis. The character of erosions in Reiter's syndrome and ankylosing spondylitis resembles that of psoriasis (poorly defined erosive change with proliferation), differing from the erosions in multicentric reticulohistiocytosis. In addition, the distribution of articular involvement in both Reiter's syndrome and ankylosing spondylitis is characteristic.

Inflammatory (erosive) osteoarthritis and scleroderma are two other diseases that may be associated with osseous erosion of interphalangeal joints. In the former disease, erosive changes may predominate in the central portion of the joint, a distinctive characteristic, and may be associated with osteophytosis and intra-articular bony ankylosis. These latter features are not part of the radiographic picture of multicentric reticulohistiocytosis. Distal interphalangeal joint erosions in scleroderma are unusual, and, when present, are associated with more typical findings, such as tuftal resorption and soft tissue calcification.

Gouty arthritis is characterized by soft tissue nodular masses, sharply marginated erosions, and lack of osteoporosis, radiographic findings that are identical to those of multicentric reticulohistiocytosis. Preservation of articular space is noted in gout and may be apparent in multicentric reticulohistiocytosis, particularly in the early phases of the disease. An asymmetric distribution, partially calcified soft tissue masses, and bone production with overhanging edges are findings of gout that are not apparent in multicentric reticulohistiocytosis.

LANGERHANS CELL HISTIOCYTOSIS (HISTIOCYTOSIS X)

Background and General Features

As histiocytic infiltration of tissues is the predominant pathologic characteristic of the histiocytoses, it is most appropriate to include this discussion in juxtaposition to that of other disorders characterized by histiocytic proliferation. It should be stressed, however, that lipid accumulation within histiocytes is a secondary phenomenon in the histiocytoses.

The three major conditions in the category of Langerhans cell histiocytosis are eosinophilic granuloma, Hand-Schüller-Christian disease, and Letterer-Siwe disease. In 1953, Lichtenstein[95] introduced the term histiocytosis X as

a comprehensive designation for these three conditions. The concept that eosinophilic granuloma, Hand-Schüller-Christian disease, and Letterer-Siwe disease are expressions of the same basic pathologic process has been supported by other investigators,[96-100] although some authors regard these disorders as unrelated.[101, 163] On the assumption that the histiocytoses are indeed a single entity, the three forms are divided according to the following scheme: eosinophilic granuloma—the mildest form, which may be manifested as single or multiple lesions of bone; Hand-Schüller-Christian disease—the most varied form, with chronic dissemination of osseous lesions; and Letterer-Siwe disease—the acute form, with rapid dissemination and poor clinical prognosis.

A clear distinction among these entities is not always possible on the basis of clinical and radiologic manifestations. Some patients initially reveal solitary bone lesions consistent with eosinophilic granuloma and subsequently develop more widespread skeletal and extraskeletal involvement, consistent with Hand-Schüller-Christian disease.[158] Other patients have a fulminant onset consistent with Letterer-Siwe disease, which progresses to a more chronic form involving bone and other organ systems. In a study of 43 patients with histiocytosis, McCullough[158] noted that approximately 85 per cent demonstrated a solitary focus on initial evaluation. Of these patients with solitary lesions, approximately 20 per cent later developed multiple lesions, and in some of these persons, features of Hand-Schüller-Christian disease appeared. A feature of prognostic significance was an increase in size of the presenting lesion after biopsy and curettage, which indicated that other bone or soft tissue lesions might appear.

Clear separation among these three forms of histiocytosis also is difficult on the basis of histologic manifestations. Proliferation of histiocytes, eosinophilic granulocytes, and other inflammatory cells is characteristic of each of these disorders. The aggressive phagocytic activity of the histiocytes is evidenced by the intracellular accumulation of blood pigment, or hemosiderin, and lipid, leading to their designation as foam or xanthomatous cells. Specific histologic features vary during the course of the disease: Initial lesions are characterized by an abundance of eosinophils or histiocytes; intermediate lesions show the preponderance of foam cells; and advanced lesions are characterized by fibrous reaction. These changing phases of the pathologic process, coupled with cellular variations within different portions of the lesion or different lesions developing simultaneously in a single person, create problems in the accurate appraisal of biopsy material and further hinder efforts to distinguish clearly among the forms of histiocytosis.

Additional evidence supporting the intimate relationship of eosinophilic granuloma, Hand-Schüller-Christian disease, and Letterer-Siwe disease is the identification in all three entities of specific histiocytic cells (Langerhans cells) containing cytoplasmic inclusion bodies (Langerhans granules or X bodies).[194, 195] Although similar granules have been found in normal persons and in patients with unrelated disorders, the Langerhans cells are believed by many investigators to be of histiocytic origin and virtually diagnostic of the histiocytoses. Furthermore, such cells reveal intense phagocytic activity and mobility, features that may account for the proclivity of the histiocytoses to disseminate widely in the body's tissues. Despite such histologic evidence, many other observers maintain that the three disorders are unrelated, emphasizing the differing clinical manifestations of the processes. Early and diffuse organ involvement and rapid patient demise, characteristics of Letterer-Siwe disease, support its classification as a malignant lymphoma, although the Langerhans cells, which are unreactive with antilymphocytes, appear to be of other than lymphatic or myelocytic origin. On the other side of the spectrum, eosinophilic granuloma certainly is benign in its clinical characteristics, resembling more an inflammatory process than a neoplasm. Hand-Schüller-Christian disease is believed by some investigators to be a multifocal variety of eosinophilic granuloma.

Owing to the increasing body of evidence that indicates the importance of the Langerhans cell as the common and distinct histologic component of the three disorders, eosinophilic granuloma, Hand-Schüller-Christian disease, and Letterer-Siwe disease, the designation of Langerhans cell histiocytosis for these disorders was proposed by the Histiocyte Society in 1987.[294] Currently, Langerhans cell histiocytosis is believed to be the preeminent form of the dendritic cell histiocytoses.[293]

The precise cause and pathogenesis of Langerhans cell histiocytosis remain unclear, however. Evidence exists that the disorder is a manifestation of, or is associated with, immunologic aberrations.[295] The stimulus to the immunologic system that causes poorly regulated activation of histiocytes in patients with Langerhans cell histiocytosis may be a virus.[293] Viruses appear to be the best candidates for being both activators and modifiers of host control of the resulting aberrations in histiocytes that characterize the various forms of Langerhans cell histiocytosis.[293]

Eosinophilic Granuloma

Eosinophilic granuloma, first described by Jaffe and Lichtenstein in 1944,[98] is characterized by single or multiple skeletal lesions occurring predominantly in children, adolescents, or young adults, although occasionally in older persons.[341] It represents approximately 70 per cent of the total number of cases of Langerhans cell histiocytosis, and it is more common in men than in women and in whites than in blacks. As with all forms of Langerhans cell histiocytosis, localized osseous involvement is uncommon in the nonwhite population.[296] Clinical manifestations include local pain, tenderness, and swelling related to adjacent skeletal lesions. A palpable soft tissue mass is common. Fever and leukocytosis also may be apparent. Eosinophilia occasionally is noted when the blood is examined. Moderate elevation of the erythrocyte sedimentation rate and a normochromic anemia sometimes are found.

Solitary lesions predominate over multiple lesions.[159] Although it has been estimated that only about 10 per cent of patients with a solitary lesion eventually will develop multifocal osseous (and extraosseous) disease,[296] the asymptomatic nature of many of the bone abnormalities suggests that the frequency of additional bone lesions may be underestimated.[297] In general, new skeletal lesions occur within 1 or 2 years after the initial solitary lesion is identified, although longer intervals (up to 5 years) between the diagnosis of the first and the subsequent skeletal lesions have been documented.[297] Any skeletal site can be affected, although abnormality of the small bones of the hands and feet is uncommon.[196, 197] The most common sites of involve-

ment are the skull, mandible, spine, ribs, and long bones, particularly the femur and the humerus. In older patients, changes in the flat bones are more common than changes in the tubular bones. Involvement of the sternum[199] and clavicles[298] is encountered. When tubular bones are affected, diaphyseal and metaphyseal localization is more frequent than epiphyseal localization, although occasionally a subchrondral lesion of a long tubular bone may simulate a cystic lesion associated with articular disease.[102] Epiphyseal lesions may occur in children.[103, 104] These may cross the open physeal plate.[198, 258]

The radiographic characteristics of eosinophilic granuloma vary with its skeletal location.[299] In long bones, the lesions appear as relatively well defined radiolucent areas, particularly in the medullary cavity (Fig. 61–23). With further growth, they encroach on the cortical bone, with endosteal erosion of the cortex and periosteal new bone formation. Lesions arising in the cortex itself, however, are rare.[300] Osseous expansion is seen.[301] The appearance can simulate that of osteomyelitis or malignant neoplasm, such as Ewing's sarcoma and lymphoma.[267] In ribs, single or multiple lesions can lead to pathologic fractures (Fig. 61–24). In the skull and pelvis, the lytic areas may be particularly well defined with or without surrounding sclerosis (Fig. 61–25). A radiodense focus within a lytic cranial lesion (or, rarely, in another location[300]) has been termed a ''button'' sequestrum (Fig. 61–26). Extension to the dura or into the brain substance is described. Skull lesions are especially prevalent in the frontal and parietal bones. The temporal bone, particularly the petrous ridges and mastoids, is the most commonly affected site in the base of the skull.[296] Infrequently, lesions may extend across sutural lines.[296] Nonuniform growth of the lesion leads to beveled bone margins and unequal destruction of the inner and outer tables of the vault. In the mandible, radiolucent lesions about the teeth may lead to loss of supporting bone and a ''floating teeth'' appearance.[105]

Soft tissue masses may accompany lesions in the tubular bones, skull, or other sites. Such masses may occur with or without associated pathologic fractures and, rarely, they may calcify. In some instances, soft tissue calcification may represent a secondary effect of corticosteroid injection into the lesion.[302]

Of all of the radiographic manifestations of eosinophilic granuloma, it is the changes of the spine that have received greatest attention.[106–111, 268, 303] Vertebral destruction can lead to a flattened vertebral body, termed vertebra plana, a finding that is much more frequent in children than in adults (Fig. 61–27).[201] In 1925, Calvé[112] first described vertebra plana, but not until later, after descriptions of the radiographic findings of eosinophilic granuloma, was it realized that most cases of vertebra plana were due to this condition. It should be realized, however, that eosinophilic granuloma can produce bubbly, lytic, expansile lesions of both the vertebral bodies and posterior osseous elements[200, 304, 342] without significant collapse. Thoracic and lumbar spine involvement predominates, and involvement of adjacent vertebrae sometimes is seen. In the latter situation, the height of the intervening intervertebral disc usually is normal. A paraspinal mass can be evident, simulating a soft tissue abscess related to vertebral osteomyelitis. Rarely, neurologic manifestations ensue.[202]

The gross pathologic abnormalities of eosinophilic gran-

SECTION XII—Diseases of the Hematopoietic System

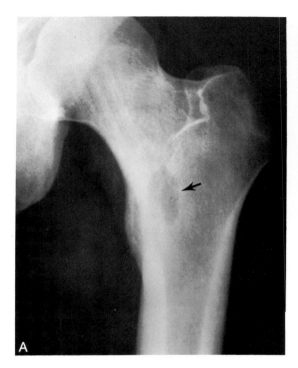

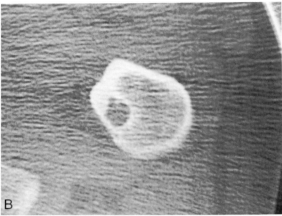

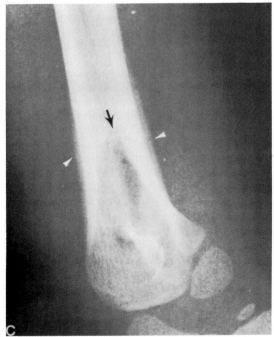

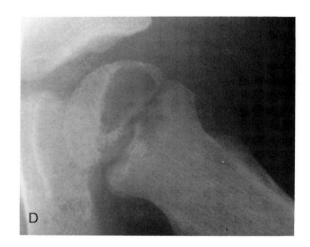

FIGURE 61–23. Eosinophilic granuloma: Radiographic abnormalities—tubular bones of appendicular skeleton.

A, B In this 33 year old man, pain in the thigh developed that was worse at night and relieved by aspirin. The radiograph reveals an eccentric, osteolytic lesion (arrow) with a sharp zone of transition between the abnormal and normal bone. A transaxial CT section through the lesion demonstrates its radiolucent center and sclerotic margin. Biopsy confirmed the presence of an eosinophilic granuloma. (Courtesy of P. Ellenbogen, M.D., Dallas, Texas.)

C A typical lesion of the distal end of the humerus in this child consists of an area of osteolysis (arrow) and thick, linear periosteal bone formation (arrowheads).

D In this patient, a lesion has violated the growth plate with involvement of both the epiphysis and the metaphysis. (**D,** Courtesy of M. Murphey, M.D., Washington, D.C.)

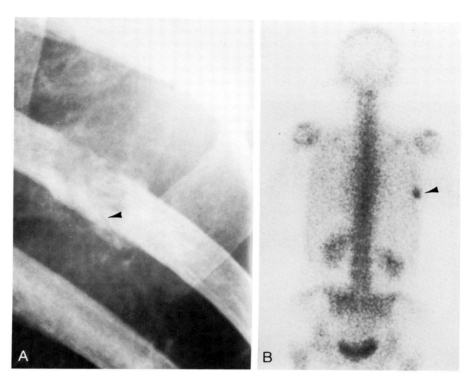

FIGURE 61–24. Eosinophilic granuloma: Radiographic abnormalities—ribs. This 44 year old woman had pleuritic chest pain of 1 month's duration.

A A poorly defined osteolytic lesion is evident. A pathologic fracture (arrowhead) extends across the lesion.

B After the injection of a bone-seeking radiopharmaceutical agent, an area of increased uptake of the agent (arrowhead) is apparent. An eosinophilic granuloma was found on examination of the resected rib.

(Courtesy of G. Greenway, M.D., Dallas, Texas.)

uloma include a soft, faintly yellow, hemorrhagic lesion consisting of reticulum cells, multinucleated giant cells, eosinophils, lymphocytes, and plasma cells (Fig. 61–28).[203]

Hand-Schüller-Christian Disease

The classic triad of Hand-Schüller-Christian disease is diabetes insipidus, unilateral or bilateral exophthalmos, and single or multiple areas of bone destruction. The finding of diabetes insipidus is attributable to extensive destruction of bone at the base of the skull and is not universally present in this disease.[113] In fact, the triad of this disease may be apparent in fewer than 10 per cent of patients. Hand-Schüller-Christian disease predominates in children (approximately two thirds of patients are less than 5 years of age at the time of clinical presentation[296]), although it may be observed in adolescents and, rarely, in older patients. The fundamental pathologic lesion is a histiocytic granuloma in which the histiocytes are filled with cholesterol.

Clinical characteristics are otitis media; cutaneous involvement with eczema, xanthomatosis, and soft tissue nodules; ulceration of the gums; lymphadenopathy; and hepatosplenomegaly. Visceral involvement of the lungs, kidneys, brain, liver, and spleen is observed. Anemia, when present, is a grave prognostic sign. In general, the disease runs a protracted course, sometimes extending over 10 to 20 years.

The skeletal lesions of Hand-Schüller-Christian disease may be widely disseminated (Fig. 61–29). The radiographic manifestations of individual lesions are similar to those of eosinophilic granuloma. In the skull, which is involved in over 90 per cent of patients, confluent areas of destruction may isolate islands of bone, creating the geographic skull. Similar findings in the mandible with isolation of teeth are termed the ''floating teeth'' appearance. The diagnosis of Hand-Schüller-Christian disease or a related histiocytosis

should be considered in any infant or child with osteolytic lesions of the pelvis or skull. Rapid expansion and destruction of bone are not infrequent in this disorder.[114]

Initially, the histologic picture of Hand-Schüller-Christian disease may closely resemble that of eosinophilic granuloma, with predominantly eosinophils and, also, inflammatory cells, leukocytes, lymphocytes, plasma cells, and neutrophils (Fig. 61–30). At this early stage, the histiocytes may not contain abundant lipid material. With time, the lesions undergo necrosis and contain some mature histiocytes with decrease in the number of inflammatory cells. Eventually the lipogranulomatous stage occurs, marked by histiocytic multinucleated giant cells, hemosiderin, necrosis, and cholesterol crystals. Scarring with proliferation of fibroblasts and collagen bundles may represent the end stage of the disease.

The outcome in cases of Hand-Schüller-Christian disease is variable. In some instances, bone lesions resolve gradually.[115] In other instances, bone lesions progress and, in fact, cases with initial involvement identical to that of eosinophilic granuloma may be associated with increased osseous dissemination and visceral involvement.[305] The prognosis worsens with involvement of multiple organ systems,[116] and the disease is fatal in 10 to 30 per cent of cases. Causes of death include anemia, pneumonia, transverse myelitis, cor pulmonale, and biliary cirrhosis.[296]

Letterer-Siwe Disease

Letterer-Siwe disease is a relatively acute syndrome that is most frequent in children below the age of 3 years, although occasionally cases are encountered in patients in late childhood or young adulthood. This disorder is characterized by histiocytic proliferation in multiple visceral organs. The designation Letterer-Siwe disease originated with Abt and Denenholz[117] in 1936, who recognized Letter-

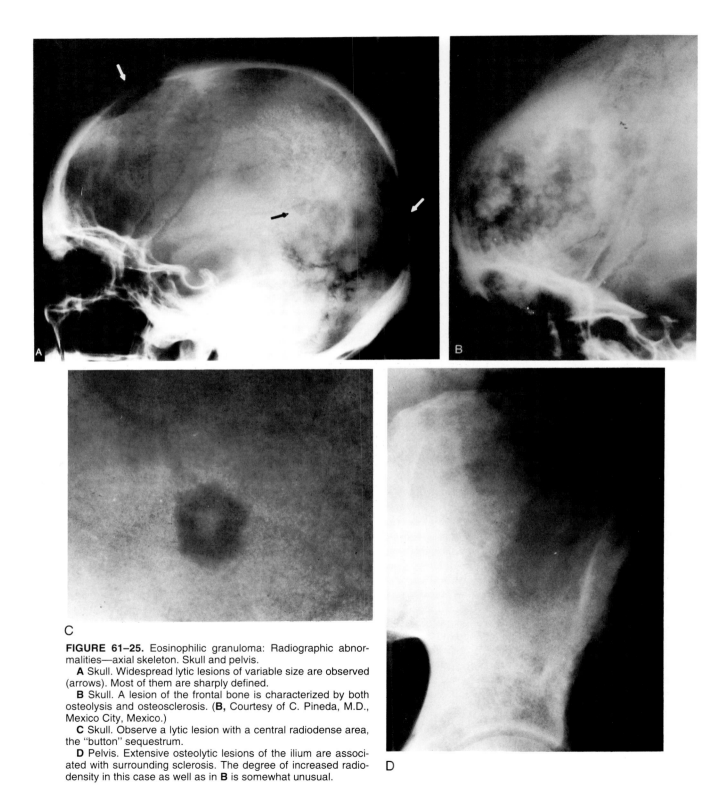

FIGURE 61–25. Eosinophilic granuloma: Radiographic abnormalities—axial skeleton. Skull and pelvis.

A Skull. Widespread lytic lesions of variable size are observed (arrows). Most of them are sharply defined.

B Skull. A lesion of the frontal bone is characterized by both osteolysis and osteosclerosis. (**B,** Courtesy of C. Pineda, M.D., Mexico City, Mexico.)

C Skull. Observe a lytic lesion with a central radiodense area, the "button" sequestrum.

D Pelvis. Extensive osteolytic lesions of the ilium are associated with surrounding sclerosis. The degree of increased radiodensity in this case as well as in **B** is somewhat unusual.

FIGURE 61–26. Eosinophilic granuloma: Radiographic abnormalities—"button" sequestrum. In this 23 year old man, a plain film **(A)** and CT scan **(B)** show an osteolytic lesion (arrows) with a radiodense sequestrum (arrowheads). The latter is more evident with CT. Soft tissue prominence also is seen.

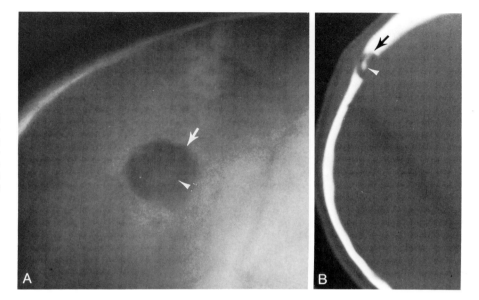

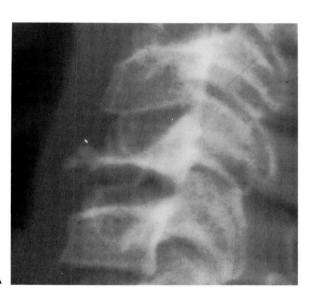

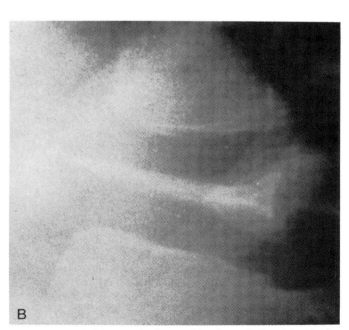

FIGURE 61–27. Eosinophilic granuloma: Radiographic abnormalities—vertebra plana. **A** Observe the flattened fourth cervical vertebral body. (Courtesy of T. Yochum, D.C., Denver, Colorado.)
B One additional example of vertebra plana in the thoracolumbar spine is shown.

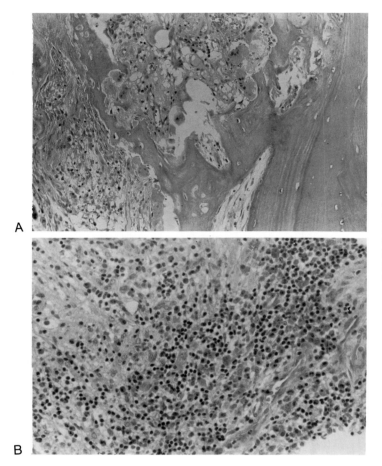

A

B

FIGURE 61–28. Eosinophilic granuloma: Pathologic abnormalities. In a 33 year old man with an eosinophilic granuloma of a rib, photomicrographs (215×) reveal bone resorption due to osteoclastosis and large areas of granulation tissue containing histiocytes admixed with eosinophils and occasional neutrophils and ringed with lymphocytes. Reactive fibroblasts are seen.

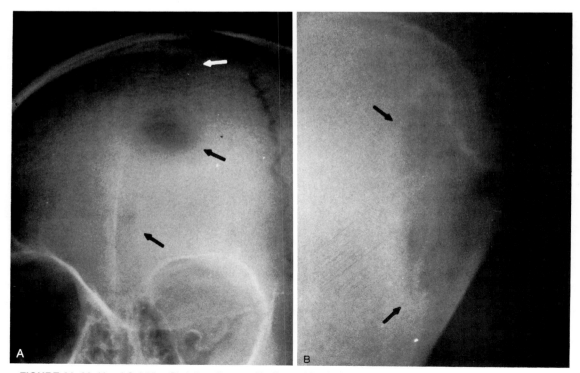

FIGURE 61–29. Hand-Schüller-Christian disease: Radiographic abnormalities.
A Skull. Several well-defined lytic lesions of the skull are apparent (arrows). Some of these have beveled margins.
B Pelvis. A large lytic lesion of the lateral aspect of the ilium is surrounded by a thin rim of sclerosis (arrows).

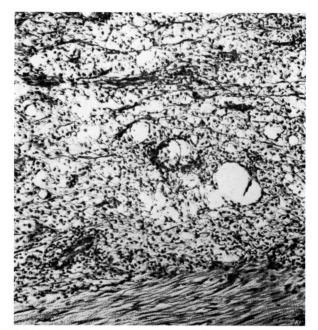

FIGURE 61–30. Hand-Schüller-Christian disease: Pathologic abnormalities. A photomicrograph (225×) of a rib in a 29 year old woman with Hand-Schüller-Christian disease outlines infiltration of marrow with foam cells that stain orange-red with sudan, indicating their cholesterol content. Fibrous tissue is evident at the bottom of the picture. (From Jaffe HL: Metabolic, Degenerative and Inflammatory Diseases of Bones and Joints. Philadelphia, Lea & Febiger, 1972.)

er's previous description of the pathologic changes and Siwe's previous account of the clinical features in patients with this disease. The frequency of this form is lower than that of eosinophilic granuloma and Hand-Schüller-Christian disease, composing approximately 10 per cent of all the histiocytoses.[114]

Clinical manifestations include febrile episodes, cachexia, hepatosplenomegaly, lymphadenopathy, purpuric skin eruption, hyperplasia of the gums, and progressive anemia. The course generally is rapidly progressive, most patients dying within 1 or 2 years, although occasionally patients develop a more prolonged clinical course, with features of Hand-Schüller-Christian disease. Terminally, findings may include ascites, subcutaneous edema, pleural effusion, and hemorrhage. In the preterminal stage, secondary bacterial infections are common, with otitis media, mastoiditis, and lymphadenitis. Diagnosis is established by biopsy of bone marrow or lymph nodes.

Nodular foci or diffuse areas of proliferating histiocytes are seen in this disease. These histiocytic collections mixed with lymphocytes, plasma cells, and eosinophils occur at multiple sites, including the lymph nodes, spleen, liver, thymus, tonsils, skin, lymphoid tissue of the gastrointestinal tract, bone marrow, lung, pancreas, kidney, heart, and endocrine glands.

Single or multiple areas of bone destruction are observed, particularly in the calvarium, base of the skull, and mandible (Fig. 61–31). More diffuse skeletal involvement can be encountered, although the hands and feet usually are spared. Histologically and radiologically, the bone lesions simulate those in eosinophilic granuloma (Fig. 61–31). Osteolytic lesions, which are relatively well defined, without significant surrounding bony eburnation, represent sites of histio-

cytic proliferation. Rarely, foam cells occur as a result of secondary precipitation of cholesterol esters in the histiocytes.

Disease Prognosis and Evolution of Osseous Abnormalities

As the distinction among the various forms of Langerhans cell histiocytosis is regarded by some authors as nonexistent or indistinct, disease characteristics can be found that are common to all three conditions. Each can affect tissues other than those of the musculoskeletal system, although this pattern of involvement is most typical of Hand-Schüller-Christian disease and Letterer-Siwe disease; with regard to eosinophilic granuloma, extraosseous localization is best exemplified by pulmonary involvement leading to diffuse micronodular and interstitial infiltrates and to a honeycomb appearance. In general, the prognosis of any of the types of histiocytosis is related to the location and the extent of organ involvement, so that clinical, radiologic, and laboratory evaluation of the patient must include an examination of all potential target areas of disease. The greater the number of tissues or systems that are affected, the poorer is the prognosis, especially if abnormalities of the liver, lung, or hematopoietic system are identified. Although the prognosis of Letterer-Siwe disease is guarded, in view of its propensity for rapid progression, as has already been noted cases have been documented in which clinical characteristics typical of one form of histiocytosis, such as Letterer-Siwe disease, are transformed into those typical of another, such as Hand-Schüller-Christian disease. The prognosis of the histiocytoses also is related to the age of the patient at the time of onset of clinical abnormalities; generally, the younger the patient, the poorer the prognosis.

Complicating any analysis of disease prognosis of the histiocytoses and the choice of appropriate therapeutic agents is the documentation that osseous as well as extraosseous lesions may resolve spontaneously at a rate unaffected by the mode of therapy; therefore, reports of the effectiveness of treatment regimens, such as partial or complete surgical excision, radiotherapy or chemotherapy, or corticosteroid administration, alone or in combination, must be interpreted cautiously. The healing of skeletal lesions, whether it be initiated through aggressive intervention or complete neglect, is accompanied by characteristic radiographic changes. Osteolytic lesions in extraspinal locations typically develop bone sclerosis during resolution and may divide into smaller isolated areas owing to septation.[204, 205, 306] Additional findings at these sites during the healing process include periosteal reaction, cortical thickening, and pathologic fracture,[204] and the changes may resemble those of Paget's disease. As sclerosis appears to represent the hallmark of the healing response, its appearance in the form of a partial or complete rim of increased radiodensity or patchy or diffuse bone reaction in untreated lesions may indicate spontaneous resolution and should be regarded as a favorable prognostic sign. Alternatively, enlargement of foci of osseous destruction or the appearance of new areas of lysis is a finding indicative of an unfavorable prognosis (Fig. 61–32).

The typical healing response of those spinal lesions that have produced vertebra plana is partial reconstitution of vertebral height,[204, 206, 207, 274, 299, 303] which is accompanied by

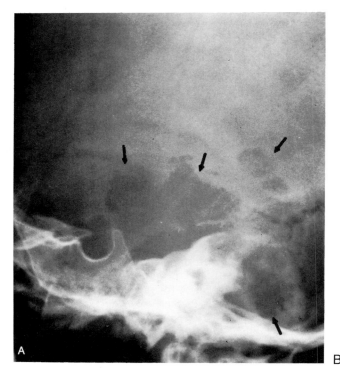

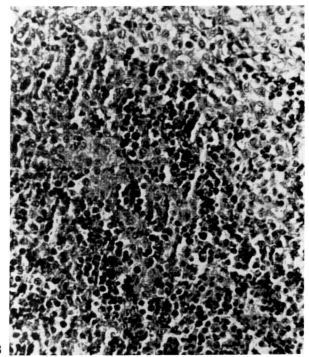

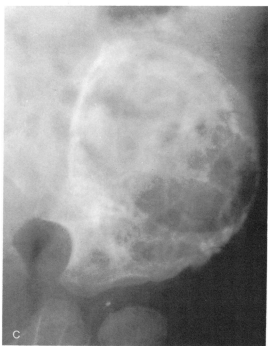

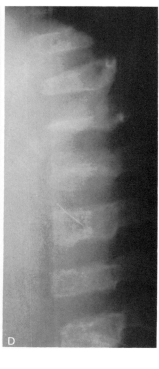

FIGURE 61–31. Letterer-Siwe disease: Radiographic and pathologic abnormalities.

A Note the confluent areas of bone destruction (arrows) at the base of the skull in a child with Letterer-Siwe disease.

B In a female infant of 10 months of age with Letterer-Siwe disease, a photomicrograph (150×) of a radial lesion reveals findings similar to those of eosinophilic granuloma. The lighter cells are histiocytes and the smaller and darker cells are eosinophils.

C, D In this child of 3 years of age, osteolytic lesions of the ilium and vertebrae are seen. Collapse of multiple vertebral bodies is evident.

(**B,** From Jaffe HL: Metabolic, Degenerative and Inflammatory Diseases of Bones and Joints. Philadelphia, Lea & Febiger, 1972.)

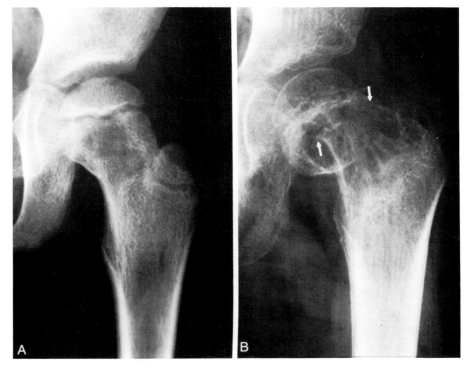

FIGURE 61–32. Eosinophilic granuloma: Course of the disease. A 6 year old boy developed back pain after a fall. A radiograph revealed a fracture of the ninth thoracic vertebral body. Two weeks later, the child developed partial paraplegia, and a myelogram indicated spinal cord compression adjacent to the collapsed vertebral body. Surgical confirmation of an eosinophilic granuloma was obtained. One year later, left hip pain was noted.

A A radiograph shows an osteolytic lesion in the metaphysis of the femur.

B Eight months later, the area of lysis has progressed and a pathologic fracture is seen (arrows). Periostitis is apparent. Open reduction with internal fixation of the fracture was accomplished, and biopsy of the femoral lesion indicated a second area of eosinophilic granuloma.

(Courtesy of G. Greenway, M.D., Dallas, Texas.)

residual bone sclerosis and coarsening of the trabecular pattern and, rarely, by a bone-within-bone appearance or interbody osseous fusion. The degree of recovery of the height of the vertebral body potentially is greater when the patient is young; in older children and adolescents who have almost completed their growth, reconstitution of vertebral height is more limited. When narrowing of the intervertebral disc space has accompanied the bone lesion, its recovery generally parallels that of the vertebral body.[206]

Intralesional injection of methylprednisolone sodium succinate after bone biopsy has become a popular method of treatment of the histiocytoses in recent years,[205, 208, 209] and it has been extended to the therapy of solitary bone cysts as well.[210] The dosage of methylprednisolone that has been used in patients with histiocytosis has ranged from 60 mg to 165 mg, delivered through a spinal, Ackerman, or Turkel needle.[205, 208, 209] Rarely, a second or third injection is required.[208, 259] Progressive healing of the osseous lesions generally becomes detectable radiographically after 2 to 4 months, as evidenced by a decrease in size, sclerosis of marginal bone, and increasing trabeculation. Clinical improvement, manifested as diminution of pain, accompanies the radiographic changes. The mechanism of action of the corticosteroid preparation after intralesional administration is not clear, and the possibility that similar resolution of the process occurs spontaneously or after biopsy alone further complicates the interpretation of the benefits of the therapeutic procedure.

Scintigraphy

Although radionuclide studies using bone-seeking radiopharmaceutical agents are an important and accepted method for documenting the presence and extent of skeletal involvement in a variety of disease processes, their benefit in the evaluation of patients with Langerhans cell histiocy-tosis is disputed.[211–218, 307] In general, bone scintigraphy has proved to be less sensitive than radiography in the detection of osseous lesions, with falsely negative radionuclide studies commonly being reported. The purely lytic nature of the lesions and their localization to complicated areas such as metaphyseal regions of tubular bones, sites that normally concentrate bone-seeking radionuclide agents, are reasons cited by some investigators for the disappointing results of bone scintigraphy in the histiocytoses. Use of ^{67}Ga-citrate and ^{99m}Tc-sulfur colloid bone marrow scanning offers no additional advantages.[214] When bone scanning findings are present, osseous lesions in histiocytosis demonstrate a spectrum of radionuclide abnormalities ranging from ''cold'' areas with decreased or absent accumulation of the radionuclide to areas of augmented activity (Figs. 61–24 and 61–33).

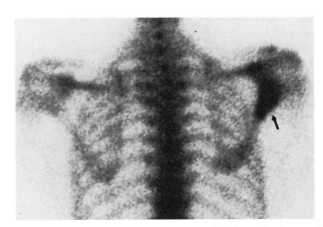

FIGURE 61–33. Eosinophilic granuloma: Scintigraphic abnormalities. An area of increased uptake (arrow) of a bone-seeking radiopharmaceutical agent is indicative of a lesion in the scapula.

The possibility that bone scintigraphy is more helpful than routine radiography in following the therapeutic response of the disease is suggested in some reports.[216]

Magnetic Resonance Imaging

In common with other disorders that infiltrate and replace normal bone marrow, Langerhans cell histiocytosis is suited to evaluation with MR imaging. Preliminary data indicate that spin echo imaging of the skeleton in patients with histiocytosis reveals one or more foci of decreased signal intensity on T1-weighted images and of increased signal intensity on T2-weighted images[296] (Figs. 61–34 and 61–35). Lesional enhancement after the intravenous injection of gadolinium contrast agent also has been noted.[296, 343]

The MR imaging abnormalities of the musculoskeletal system in Langerhans cell histiocytosis include features that simulate those of aggressive tumors and infection,[308, 344] underscoring again the nonspecific nature of many of the findings demonstrated with this imaging method.[309] As cortical perforation, periostitis, and soft tissue extension are known radiographic manifestations of eosinophilic granuloma and the other histiocytoses, the documentation of similar features with MR imaging (or CT) in these diseases is not unexpected. The large size, poor definition, and signal inhomogeneity of the soft tissue component accompanying skeletal involvement in the histiocytoses require emphasis, however (Fig. 61–36). The physician who employs MR imaging as a means to distinguish eosinophilic granuloma (and other histiocytoses) from more sinister processes such as Ewing's sarcoma, lymphoma, and osteosarcoma will be disappointed in most instances. The use of intravenous injection of gadolinium-based contrast agent offers no solution to this diagnostic dilemma owing to the occurrence of tissue enhancement in the histiocytoses as well. Furthermore, other conditions such as osteomyelitis and stress fractures have the same MR imaging features as the histiocytoses. More important in the differentiation among these processes is careful analysis of data provided by clinical and laboratory examination and routine radiography.

The value of MR imaging of the musculoskeletal system in patients with Langerhans cell histiocytosis lies in the sensitivity, rather than the specificity, of the technique. Although MR imaging cannot be considered to be practical when employed as a screening method for skeletal involvement in these diseases, its importance in defining the extent of involvement at one or a few skeletal sites, such as the spine,[310] is established. Problems exist, however, even in this regard owing to difficulties in determining the degree of cortical violation (a task better accomplished with CT) and in distinguishing between histiocytic tissue and surrounding edema.

Differential Diagnosis

The predominant pattern of the histiocytoses is osteolysis. Osteolytic lesions may be single or multiple. Single lytic defects must be differentiated from neoplastic and inflammatory lesions as well as fibrous dysplasia. Multiple lytic lesions may simulate infection, skeletal metastasis, leukemia, lymphoma, hyperparathyroidism with brown tumors, and Gaucher's disease. The morphologic characteristics of the osteolytic defect (well-defined contour, endosteal scalloping, and periosteal buttressing) and their predilection for certain sites (pelvis and skull) usually provide important clues in the diagnosis of the histiocytoses.

LIPID GRANULOMATOSIS (ERDHEIM-CHESTER DISEASE)

In 1930, Chester[151] described two patients with a distinctive and unusual lipidosis that differed from other known conditions. Additional cases later were reported by Sorensen[152] and Jaffe,[27] and more recently, by Simpson and coworkers[153] as well as others.[219–221, 260, 269, 275, 311–315] The clinical manifestations are not well defined, although men and women in the fifth through seventh decades appear to be affected. Cardiac and pulmonary manifestations due to liberation of cholesterol from foam cells and xanthomatous patches in the eyelids may be seen. Chronic lipogranulomatous pyelonephritis has been reported. Mild local pain and tenderness over areas of skeletal abnormality are noted, although patients may be entirely asymptomatic.

Radiographic abnormalities are distinctive[160] (Figs. 61–37 and 61–38). The major long bones of the limbs invariably are affected, whereas axial skeletal involvement, which has been documented in the skull, ribs, and innominate bone, is unusual. A patchy or diffuse increase in density, coarsened trabecular pattern, medullary sclerosis, and cortical thickening appear in the diaphysis and metaphysis, with minor changes or sparing of the epiphysis. Symmetry is the rule. In one case, a focal area of cortical destruction with adjacent periostitis has been related to the presence of a sinus tract discharging xanthogranulomatous material from bone.[161] Radionuclide studies using bone-seeking radiopharmaceutical agents demonstrate increased accumulation of isotope in areas of radiographic abnormality.[219, 312, 313, 315] Gallium imaging may reveal a similar distribution.[220] Bone marrow scanning using technetium sulfur colloid may show an expanded bone marrow pattern and decreased radionuclide activity at sites of the most intense uptake on the bone scan, and indium chloride scanning may demonstrate a similar distribution of bone marrow.[312] Although data regarding MR imaging findings in this disease are limited, replacement of normal marrow fat by lipid infiltration has been accompanied by a decrease of signal intensity on T1-weighted spin echo MR images and regions of low and high signal intensity on T2-weighted images.[315, 316]

Pathologic findings in the skeleton resemble those in extraskeletal sites, where extensive lipogranulomatous changes in internal organs (kidneys, liver, spleen, pancreas, lung, and heart) and even retroperitoneal xanthogranulomas may be observed (Fig. 61–39). The original spongiosa is replaced by sclerotic bone, especially in the metaphyseal regions. Yellowish areas representing cholesterol-laden cells and lipid granulomas are seen. On microscopic examination, swollen cells rich in cholesterol, interspersed with lymphocytes and plasma cells within the cortex, and connective tissue cells intermingled with foam cells within the spongiosa (Fig. 61–40) are evident.[27, 221] In both areas, osteosclerosis is detected. The pathologic aberrations in bone most resemble those of Hand-Schüller-Christian disease. Histologic abnormalities in the muscles in Erdheim-Chester disease have included nonspecific atrophy, and those in the synovium have included mild villous proliferation of the

Text continued on page 2230

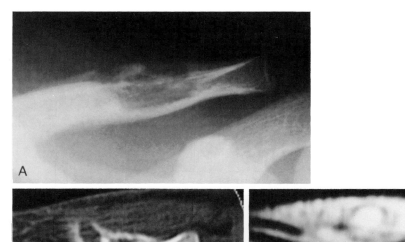

FIGURE 61–34. Eosinophilic granuloma: MR imaging abnormalities. Clavicle. This 9 year old boy developed progressive shoulder pain.

A Routine radiography reveals an expansile osteolytic lesion of the clavicle.

B Transaxial CT scan further documents the extent of the clavicular lesion. It appears osteolytic, septated, and expansile.

C A transaxial T2-weighted (TR/TE, 2000/80) spin echo MR image shows intense high signal in the clavicle. The anterior cortex appears violated. With T1 weighting (not shown), the lesion's signal intensity was slightly higher than that of muscle.

(**A–C,** Courtesy of G. Greenway, M.D., Dallas, Texas.)

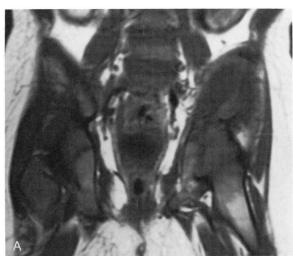

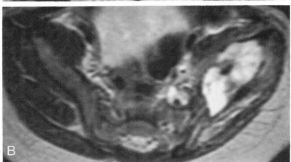

FIGURE 61–35. Eosinophilic granuloma: MR imaging abnormalities. Ilium. A 20 month old infant developed tenderness about the left hip with a limp. A routine radiograph (not shown) revealed a large osteolytic lesion of the ilium.

A A coronal T1-weighted (TR/TE, 600/15) spin echo MR image reveals low signal intensity of hematopoietic marrow in the spine, innominate bones, and proximal ends of the femora. Deformity of the left ilium is seen, with signal intensity similar to that of muscle and lower than that on the opposite side.

B A transaxial T2-weighted (TR/TE, 2000/80) spin echo MR image reveals the expansile lesion of the ilium with inhomogeneous but generally high signal intensity. The adjacent musculature also shows increased signal intensity.

(**A, B,** Courtesy of S. Wootton, M.D., Denver, Colorado.)

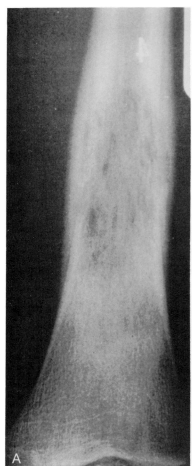

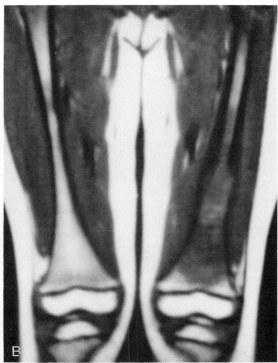

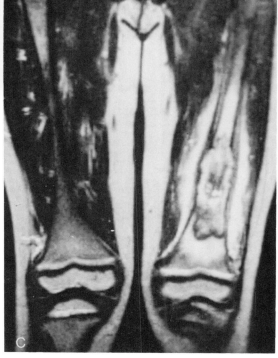

FIGURE 61–36. Eosinophilic granuloma: MR imaging abnormalities. Femur. Pain and swelling in the thigh occurred in this 4 year old girl.

A The routine radiograph shows an osteolytic lesion with motheaten bone destruction and thick periosteal reaction in the diaphysis of the femur.

B On a coronal T1-weighted (TR/TE, 500/20) spin echo MR image, low signal intensity is evident in the diaphyseal and distal metaphyseal portions of the femur. Periosteal new bone also exhibits low signal intensity.

C With T2 weighting (TR/TE, 2000/90), the femoral lesion is inhomogeneous but generally of high signal intensity. Note the elevated periosteum with new bone formation and the irregular and extensive soft tissue component with very high signal intensity. Differentiation of the lesion itself and adjacent edema is impossible.

(**A–C,** Courtesy of M. Pathria, M.D., San Diego, California.)

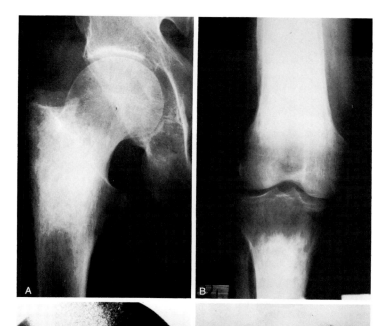

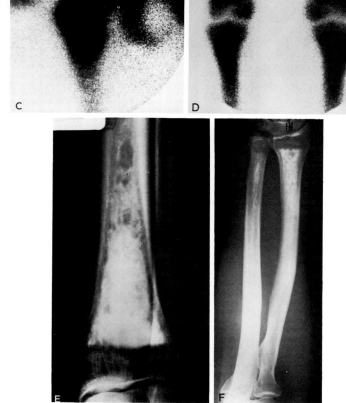

FIGURE 61–37. Erdheim-Chester disease.

A–D This 57 year old man had proteinuria, edema, and peripheral neuropathy. Extensive evaluation revealed, in addition to abnormal radiographs of the bones, retroperitoneal xanthogranulomas and xanthogranulomatous pyelonephritis. Bone biopsy confirmed the diagnosis of Erdheim-Chester disease. Observe the sclerotic lesion of the proximal portion of the right femur **(A)** and distal ends of the femur and tibia **(B).** The epiphyses are spared, and the opposite side was involved similarly. Radionuclide studies reveal increased uptake of bone-seeking agents **(C, D).** (Courtesy of G. Greenway, M.D., Dallas, Texas.)

E, F In a different patient, note the characteristic sclerosis of the diaphyses of tibia, radius, and ulna. (Courtesy of A. Brower, M.D., Norfolk, Virginia.)

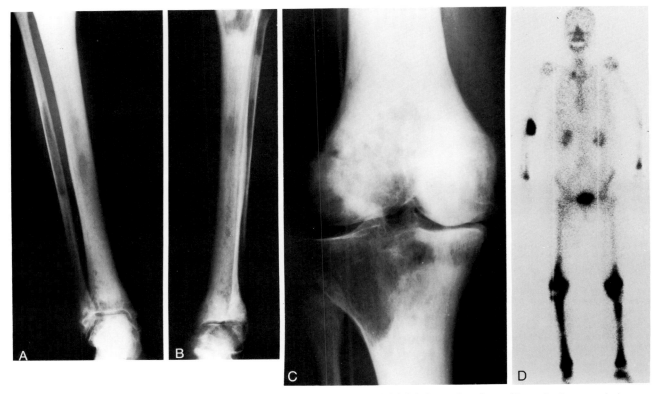

FIGURE 61–38. Erdheim-Chester disease. A 64 year old woman developed a painful right knee. A radiographic evaluation revealed osseous abnormalities (shown here), indicating need for a more extensive radiographic survey and scintigraphy. Laboratory values were normal. At the time of total knee replacement, histologic examination of the distal portion of the femur demonstrated dense, sclerotic, and thickened trabeculae with areas of intense osteoblastic activity and, to a lesser extent, osteolytic activity. Marrow fibrosis and lymphoid infiltration were evident. Subsequently, pericardial and renal abnormalities appeared. Pericardial fluid contained cells of mesothelial origin, and a nephrectomy was required. On microscopic examination, the kidney revealed marked chronic interstitial inflammation with lymphocytes and histiocytic foam cells.

A, B Frontal radiographs of the lower legs demonstrate widespread osteosclerosis and focal osteolytic lesions involving the diaphyseal, metaphyseal, and epiphyseal portions of the tibiae and fibulae. The tarsal bones also are affected.

C About the knee, a similar process involves the distal portion of the femur.

D A bone scan documents increased accumulation of the radioisotope in the distal ends of the femora, tibiae, and fibulae and in the proximal tarsal bones. Minimally abnormal accumulation also is evident in the distal portion of both radii.

(From Resnick D, et al: Radiology *142*:289, 1984.)

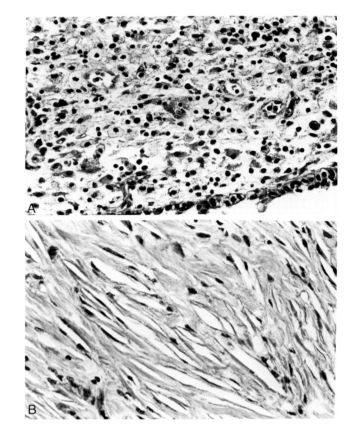

FIGURE 61–39. Erdheim-Chester disease: Pathologic findings in extraskeletal sites. In the same patient as in Figure 61–38, pathologic abnormalities in the kidney **(A)** consist of cellular infiltration with lymphocytes, plasmacytes, and foam cells (100×); in the perirenal fat **(B),** cholesterol clefts are apparent (100×). (From Resnick D, et al: Radiology *142*:289, 1984.)

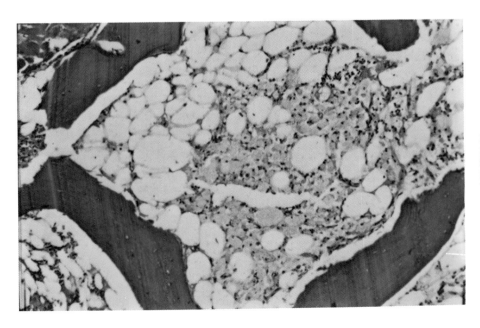

FIGURE 61–40. Erdheim-Chester disease: Pathologic findings in bone. Note intertrabecular fibrosis and foam cells. (From Resnick D, et al: Radiology *142*:289, 1984.)

lining cells, dilation of subsynovial vessels, and the absence of inflammatory cells and foamy histiocytes.[314]

The precise relationship of Erdheim-Chester disease to the histiocytoses is not known. The identification in one patient with Erdheim-Chester disease of an osteolytic lesion in the tibia (Fig. 61–41) that pathologically appeared to be an eosinophilic granuloma certainly suggests that lipid granulomatosis is part of the spectrum of Langerhans cell histiocytosis.[222] Reports of other patients have indicated similarities between the clinical, radiologic, and pathologic features of Erdheim-Chester disease and other histiocytoses,[315, 316] especially Hand-Schüller-Christian disease.[311] Indeed, when patients with Erdheim-Chester disease have been followed for a long time, some eventually have revealed findings more compatible with an aggressive systemic process.[311] Furthermore, the documentation of expansile and sclerotic lesions, confined to the ribs (Fig. 61–42), that pathologically are indistinguishable from those of Erdheim-Chester disease may indicate that lipid granulomatosis of bone encompasses a wide spectrum of abnormalities, ranging from local deposition of lipids to the widespread involvement previously reported as Erdheim-Chester disease.[223, 261, 313]

SINUS HISTIOCYTOSIS WITH LYMPHADENOPATHY

Sinus histiocytosis with massive lymphadenopathy, or Rosai-Dorfman disease, is a non-neoplastic, self-limited

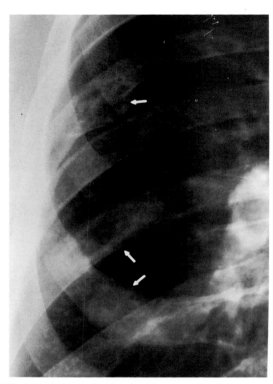

FIGURE 61–42. Erdheim-Chester disease: Focal involvement of ribs. A 62 year old man with low back pain had rib abnormalities detectable on a chest radiograph. Observe expansile lesions of the posterior portions of the sixth and eighth ribs and the anterior aspect of the fifth rib (arrows). A biopsy of one of the lesions confirmed the presence of lipid-laden histiocytes and reactive new bone formation, findings consistent with Erdheim-Chester disease. (From Dalinka MK, et al: Radiology *142*:297, 1982.)

disease occurring predominantly in the first three decades of life, especially in black patients, that is characterized by painless bilateral cervical adenopathy, adenopathy in other lymph node chains, fever, elevated erythrocyte sedimentation rate, neutrophilic leukocytosis, occasional eosinophilia, and hypergammaglobulinemia.[163, 224–228] Involved lymph nodes reveal distinctive microscopic abnormalities, including a marked proliferation of sinus histiocytes, which often contain phagocytized lymphocytes. Extranodal sites of involvement include the upper respiratory tract, salivary glands, orbits, eyelids, testes, and bone.[317, 318] Involvement of the kidney, lower respiratory tract, or liver is a poor prognostic sign.[319]

Osseous manifestations of this disease generally are restricted to multiple or, less frequently, solitary osteolytic lesions (Fig. 61–43) involving principally the long tubular bones but also the skull, pelvis, sternum, vertebral bodies, phalanges, metacarpals, and ribs.[229–231, 262, 270, 271, 276, 317] The lesions usually are asymptomatic, although spinal involvement may be associated with paresis.[271, 319] The epiphysis, diaphysis, or metaphysis is affected singly or in any combination. Of variable size, the lesions usually are medullary in location, although an occasional cortical focus is encountered,[229] which in some instances is related to extension from an adjacent soft tissue lesion.[319] Intralesional calcification and periostitis are absent. Surrounding sclerosis sometimes is apparent. Serial radiographs may reveal a continuous decrease in the size of the lytic defects with eventually their complete disappearance. Microscopically,

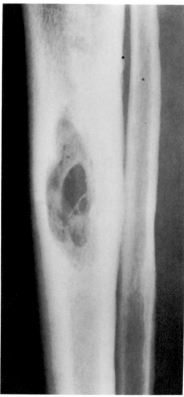

FIGURE 61–41. Erdheim-Chester disease and eosinophilic granuloma. This 66 year old man with biopsy-proved Erdheim-Chester disease developed an osteolytic lesion of the tibia. Note its large size and lobulated appearance. A biopsy of this lesion revealed tissue characteristics of an eosinophilic granuloma. (Courtesy of A. Brower, M.D., Norfolk, Virginia.)

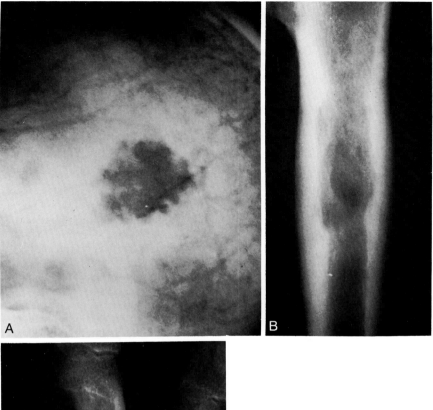

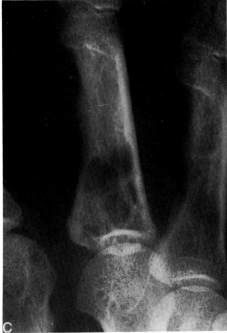

FIGURE 61–43. Sinus histiocytosis with lymphadenopathy. In a 55 year old woman, cervical lymphadenopathy, weight loss, and weakness developed over a 6 month period. Osteolytic foci are apparent in the skull, femur, and small tubular bones of the hand. (Courtesy of D. Sartoris, M.D., San Diego, California.)

an inflammatory infiltrate composed of mature histiocytes and accompanied by plasma cells and lymphocytes is seen.[229]

The cause of this disease is not known. Although certain pathologic features are consistent with a lymphoreticular malignant neoplasm, the benign clinical course makes this possibility unlikely. Cultures and serologic tests for a variety of pathogens almost uniformly are negative, although several patients have revealed significant antibody titers to *Klebsiella ozaenae* or *Klebsiella rhinoscleroma* antigens.[226, 318] Various viral serologic tests, particularly those related to the Epstein-Barr virus, also have been reported to be positive.[319] Morphologically and clinically, considerable overlap exists between this disease and Langerhans cell histiocytosis.

MALIGNANT HISTIOCYTOSIS

Malignant histiocytosis, which also is termed histiocytic medullary reticulosis, was first described clearly in 1939 by Scott and Robb-Smith.[232] Its major features are a variable age of onset (affecting both children and adults), fever, weight loss, hepatosplenomegaly, jaundice, and progressive pancytopenia.[163, 232–235] Histiocytic infiltration in lymph nodes, liver, spleen, and bone marrow is observed. Radiographically evident bone lesions are not common but have been described, appearing as osteolytic foci with sclerotic margins or, less commonly, areas of osteosclerosis.[236, 237] The pelvis, spine, and tubular bone are involved. These lesions may disappear during treatment. The prognosis of the disease is poor, as most patients die within 6 months of the onset of symptoms and signs. Rarely, partial or complete remissions are seen.

The cause of this disease is unknown. An apparently high rate of occurrence of cases in certain areas of Africa and Asia has generated speculation that malignant histiocytosis may be related to the transmission of an oncogenic virus by an arthropod vector.[163] Furthermore, examples of the disorder have appeared within several months of induction of chemotherapy with vincristine and prednisone for acute lymphoblastic leukemia.[163, 238, 239]

HYPERLIPOPROTEINEMIAS

Background and General Features

Primary familial hyperlipoproteinemias comprise a group of heritable diseases associated with an increase in plasma concentrations of cholesterol or triglycerides.[118] Currently, these diseases are subdivided into five major types according to the plasma lipoprotein pattern, although historically, familial hyperlipoproteinemia was first discovered because of one of its secondary and inconstant characteristics, the deposition of lipids in skin and tendons, called xanthomas. Early descriptions of patients with xanthomas were those of Rayer in 1827[119] and Addison and Gull in 1851.[120] Initially, most of the identified patients had xanthomas and hyperlipoproteinemias secondary to biliary obstruction, although subsequently it became obvious that these clinical and laboratory manifestations could occur in the absence of jaundice and might arise from hyperlipidemia.[121]

The five major types of hyperlipoproteinemias that are currently recognized have been well summarized[122, 123, 240] (Table 61–6):

Type I Hyperlipoproteinemia. In type I, massive amounts of chylomicrons are apparent while the patient is on a normal diet and disappear within a few days when the patient is placed on a fat-free diet. Primary type I hyperlipoproteinemia is related to a hereditary (autosomal recessive) abnormality in chylomicron removal in which there is a deficiency in plasma postheparin lipoprotein lipase activity. The plasma appears milky, plasma cholesterol levels are normal or slightly increased, and plasma triglyceride levels are elevated. Type I hyperlipoproteinemia may occur in a secondary form in diabetes mellitus, pancreatitis, and alcoholism. Most patients with primary type I hyperlipoproteinemia are diagnosed in the first or second decade of life. Clinical findings include lipemia retinalis, hepatosplenomegaly, abdominal pain, and pancreatitis.

Type II Hyperlipoproteinemia (Familial Hypercholesterolemia). Type II, the most common type, is related to an increase in the plasma concentration of low density lipoproteins or beta-lipoproteins. Type II is further divided into two subgroups, types IIA and IIB; the former is characterized by an excess of beta-lipoproteins and the latter by an excess of both beta- and prebeta-lipoproteins. In its primary form, type II hyperlipoproteinemia is an autosomal dominant hereditary abnormality associated with a clear plasma appearance, increased plasma cholesterol, and normal or slightly increased plasma triglyceride levels. It also may be secondary to many disorders, including hypothyroidism, plasma cell myeloma, macroglobulinemia, and obstructive liver disease. The diagnosis of primary type II hyperlipoproteinemia usually is established in early childhood. The findings include xanthomas and premature coronary, cerebral, and peripheral vascular disease.

Type III Hyperlipoproteinemia ("Broad-Beta" Disease). Type III, an uncommon type, is associated with beta- or prebeta-lipoprotein abnormality. In its primary form, type III hyperlipoproteinemia may be an autosomal recessive disorder resulting in a turbid plasma appearance and in elevated plasma cholesterol and triglyceride levels. Rarely

TABLE 61–6. Hyperlipoproteinemias

Type	Lipoprotein Abnormality	Primary Form	Secondary Forms	Xanthomas	Arthralgia or Arthritis	Hyper-uricemia
I	Chylomicrons	Autosomal recessive	Diabetes mellitus Pancreatitis Alcoholism	Skin		
II	Beta-lipoprotein	Autosomal dominant	Hypothyroidism Myeloma Macroglobulinemia Obstructive hepatic disease	Skin Tendinous Tuberous Subperiosteal	+	
III	Beta- or prebeta-lipoprotein	Autosomal recessive (?)	Diabetes mellitus Hypothyroidism	Skin Tendinous Tuberous Subperiosteal		+
IV	Prebeta-lipoprotein	Autosomal recessive	Diabetes mellitus Pancreatitis Alcoholism Hypothyroidism Glycogen storage disease Gaucher's disease Gout Hypercalcemia	Skin Tuberous Intraosseous	+	+
V	Prebeta-lipoprotein, chylomicrons	Autosomal dominant (?)		Skin		+

it is secondary to severe insulinopenic diabetes and hypothyroidism. Primary type III hyperlipoproteinemia may not be detected until the third, fourth, or fifth decade of life or even later. It rarely is observed below 25 years of age. Xanthomas and premature peripheral vascular disease are apparent.

Type IV Hyperlipoproteinemia. Type IV is characterized by the presence of increased low density lipoproteins or prebeta-lipoproteins without chylomicronemia. In its primary form, the disease appears to be an autosomal recessive disorder associated with a turbid plasma appearance, elevated plasma triglyceride levels, and normal or slightly elevated plasma cholesterol levels. Type IV hyperlipoproteinemia may be secondary to many diseases, including diabetes mellitus, pancreatitis, alcoholism, hypothyroidism, glycogen storage disease, Gaucher's diseases, gout, and hypercalcemia. In its primary form, the disease rarely is detected below the age of 20 years. Xanthomas, hyperuricemia, and coronary vascular disease may be evident.

Type V Hyperlipoproteinemia. Type V is similar to type IV, with an increase in low density lipoproteins and chylomicrons. The plasma appears turbid, and cholesterol and triglyceride levels are increased. In its primary form, it probably is an autosomal dominant hereditary disease that rarely is manifested clinically in childhood. Xanthomas, hyperuricemia, abdominal pain, hepatosplenomegaly, paresthesias, and lipemia retinalis can be detected.

Musculoskeletal Abnormalities

Xanthoma. Xanthomas may be apparent in all five types of hyperlipoproteinemia and in primary and secondary forms of the disease, although their appearance and location vary. Xanthomas can be classified as follows:

1. Eruptive xanthomas: Yellow papules containing triglycerides with surrounding erythema on the knees, buttocks, back, and shoulders.

2. Tendinous xanthomas: Localized deposits in the tendons of the palm and dorsum of the hand, the patellar tendon, the Achilles tendon, the plantar aponeurosis, the peroneal tendons, around the elbow, and the fascia and periosteum overlying the lower tibia.[124] These deposits are situated within the tendon fibers and not on the tendon sheath. They occur at sites of trauma, direct pressure, or stretching.

3. Tuberous xanthomas: Soft subcutaneous masses, which occur over extensor surfaces, including the elbows, knees, and hands as well as the buttocks.[125]

4. Subperiosteal and osseous xanthomas: Lipid deposits, which occur beneath the periosteum or replace trabeculae within the spongiosa, leading to osteolytic defects, periosteal or endosteal erosion of the cortex, and even pathologic fracture or osteonecrosis from vascular occlusion.[126–131, 242, 243, 263, 320] Lesions of subchondral bone may lead to osseous weakening and collapse.[128]

In type I hyperlipoproteinemia, xanthomas are of the eruptive type; they may appear at times of severe hyperlipidemia and disappear when the triglyceride level is reduced with low fatty intake.

In type II hyperlipoproteinemia, xanthomas may occur in as many as 80 per cent of patients before death. In those persons who are homozygous with respect to the abnormal gene, xanthomatosis occurs in childhood and may be extensive. Xanthomas can even be present at birth. In heterozygotes, tendinous xanthomas usually do not appear until the age of 30 years.[132] In both groups, palpebral, tendinous, tuberous, and subperiosteal xanthomas occur.[118, 345] Tendinous and tuberous xanthomas also may accompany type II hyperlipoproteinemia that is secondary to obstructive liver disease or, rarely, dysglobulinemia or myxedema.[133]

In type III hyperlipoproteinemia, tuberous, tendinous, and subperiosteal xanthomas may be manifest. In addition, lipid deposition (planar xanthoma) may produce yellowish elevation on the palmar surface of the hands and fingers, providing a distinctive clinical manifestation that also may be seen in homozygous type II and possibly in type IV hyperlipoproteinemia.[134] The frequency of planar xanthomas in type III patients may reach 65 to 70 per cent.[118, 135]

In approximately 15 per cent of patients with type IV hyperlipoproteinemia, eruptive xanthomas can be detected.[118] Tuberous, planar, and intraosseous xanthomas also have been described.[127, 134] In type V hyperlipoproteinemia, eruptive (45 per cent) xanthomas may appear.[118]

The radiographic features of these xanthomatous lesions have been outlined[127, 128, 131, 155, 156] (Figs. 61–44 and 61–45). Tuberous and tendinous xanthomas produce nodular masses in soft tissue and tendons. These rarely calcify. Subtle thickening of the tendon may be the only radiographic abnormality.[244, 245] Subperiosteal xanthomas are associated with scalloping of the external cortical surface. This reflects pressure erosion or cortical extension of the lipid-rich material. Intramedullary lipid deposition leads to lytic defects, endosteal erosion, subchondral collapse, juxta-articular erosive changes, and pathologic fractures (Fig. 61–46). In general, the bony defects are well defined, with a sharp zone of transition between abnormal and normal bone. In the hands and feet, they may reveal a symmetric distribution and "ground glass" appearance, bearing some resemblance to the lesions of fibrous dysplasia and neurofibromatosis.

The diagnosis of soft tissue xanthomas, particularly those of the Achilles tendon, can be accomplished with ultrasonography,[321, 322, 325, 346, 347] CT,[326] and MR imaging.[323–325, 347] The signal intensity of xanthomas, when studied with MR imaging, is variable, depending in part on the chemical constituents of the lesions. In vitro studies have documented that triglycerides may lead to high signal intensity on some MR imaging sequences, whereas cholesterols do not.[325] Although tendinous xanthomas may contain both triglycerides and cholesterols, most reports of MR imaging features of such lesions have documented persistent low to intermediate signal intensity on T1-weighted and T2-weighted spin echo MR images and signal inhomogeneity[323, 324] (Fig. 61–47). Focal areas of high signal intensity occasionally may be encountered on T2-weighted images, however, perhaps indicating a high percentage of triglyceride deposition.[325] Alternatively, such high signal intensity may relate to inflammatory changes in the tendon. A diffuse speckled or reticulated pattern of intratendinous signal intensity, most obvious on transaxial images and fat-suppressed T1-weighted images, is evident in some cases[347] and may have diagnostic significance. This appearance differs from the typical features of acute or chronic tendinitis and partial tears (see Chapter 70).

Histologically, lipid accumulations are encountered at various sites (Fig. 61–48). Inflammatory reaction usually is

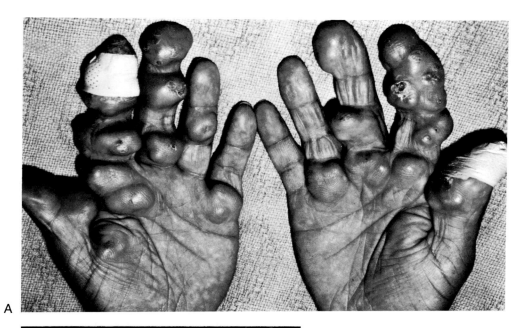

A

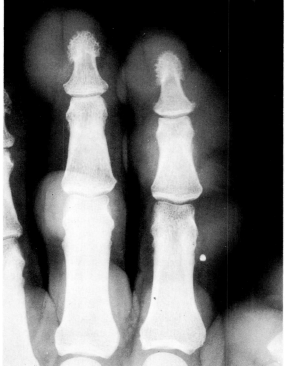

B

FIGURE 61–44. Hyperlipoproteinemia: Xanthomas without bony abnormalities.

A A clinical photograph of a patient with widespread tendinous and tuberous xanthomas. In the hand, note the large asymmetric soft tissue masses, particularly of the digits. Some of the lesions have ulcerated.

B A radiograph reveals asymmetric soft tissue masses in periarticular and periosseous locations. Neither soft tissue calcification nor significant osseous erosions are evident.

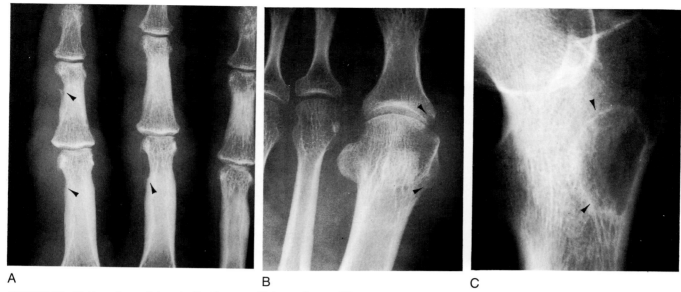

FIGURE 61–45. Hyperlipoproteinemia: Xanthomas with bony abnormalities.
A Observe nodular soft tissue masses with subjacent osseous erosion (arrowheads). The osseous defects are eccentric and well defined. Osteoporosis and joint space narrowing are not apparent.
B Involvement of the first metatarsophalangeal joint is characterized by soft tissue swelling and well-defined eccentric osseous erosions (arrowheads). The findings are reminiscent of those in gout.
C An intraosseous xanthoma has produced a well-defined lytic lesion of the proximal femur with a sclerotic rim (arrowheads).

mild, although a few giant cells may be seen. The lesions have been examined chemically. In most cases they contain phospholipids, cholesterol, cholesteryl esters, and triglycerides.[136–138] Rarely, small foci of calcification also may be identified, although these foci are not demonstrable with routine radiography.[326]

Gout. Hyperuricemia and clinical gout have been reported in association with types III, IV, and V hyperlipoproteinemias[118, 139, 140, 241] but not with type I or II hyperlipoproteinemia.[118, 141] Typical radiographic findings of gout may be encountered in patients with hyperuricemia[142] (Fig. 61–49).

Arthralgias and Arthritis. In type II hyperlipoproteinemia, a migratory polyarthritis may be detected affecting large and small peripheral joints.[124, 143, 264, 327, 328] Involved sites include the ankles, knees, hips, elbows, wrists, and, rarely, hands. Attacks, which generally are of a few days' duration, consist of pain, tenderness, redness, and swelling and are associated with fever and leukocytosis. Tendinous xanthomas commonly are apparent, and these may produce concomitant mechanical defects or tendinitis. Symptoms and signs may migrate from one joint to another, simulating the findings of rheumatic fever. The distribution is either unilateral or bilateral, and the articular symptoms may recur over prolonged periods of time. Soft tissue swelling may be observed on radiographs of involved joints. Of interest is the report of two patients with type II hyperlipoproteinemia and arthralgias in whom a biopsy of the synovial membrane of the knees revealed monosodium urate crystals.[162] In fact, it has been suggested that articular inflammation occurring in association with this type of hyperlipoproteinemia as well as other types is related to abnormal deposition of crystals, including urates or cholesterol.[241]

Arthralgias may occur in patients with type IV hyperlipoproteinemia.[144] Women are affected more frequently than men. Joint pain, tenderness, and stiffness may be evident,

but synovitis is not detectable. An additional syndrome in this type of hyperlipoproteinemia consists of synovitis in large and small joints.[145] On radiographs, lucent areas may be observed in epiphyses and metaphyses. Joint aspiration reveals fluid with an increased number of mononuclear leukocytes, and histologic examination of synovium demonstrates villous proliferation. Hyperuricemia and positive serologic tests for rheumatoid factor have been described in these patients.

Cerebrotendinous Xanthomatosis

Xanthomatous disorders may occur without hyperlipidemia. Cerebrotendinous xanthomatosis is one such disorder. It is a rare disease characterized by xanthomas, cataracts, progressive cerebellar ataxia, and dementia.[146, 147, 326, 329] Accumulation of cholesterol and cholesterol-like crystals occurs in the white matter of the brain and in xanthomas. Serum cholesterol levels are normal or low and cholestanol levels are elevated markedly. Synthesis of bile acids is defective, resulting in the virtual absence of chenodeoxycholic acid in the bile and the excretion of large amounts of bile alcohols conjugated with glucoronic acid in the bile and urine.[329] Cerebrotendinous xanthomatosis is an autosomal recessive disorder whose biochemical basis is not known. Disability is progressive, although patients may survive until the sixth or seventh decade of life. Initial clinical manifestations, which may be apparent by 10 to 15 years of age, include dementia, cataracts, tendinous xanthomas, spasticity, and ataxia. Additional clinical findings are atherosclerosis, myocardial infarction, and paroxysmal atrial tachycardia. Treatment with chenodeoxycholic acid has been reported to normalize serum cholestanol levels and to improve the neurologic status in a majority of treated patients.[326, 329]

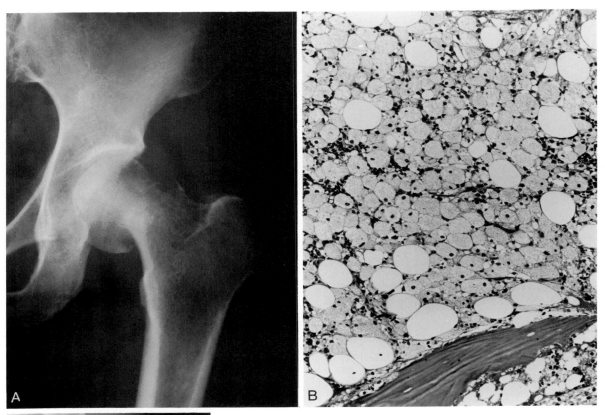

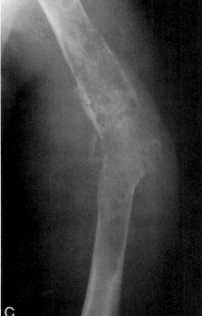

FIGURE 61–46. Hyperlipoproteinemia: Xanthomas with bony abnormalities. Pathologic fracture.

A, B A 48 year old woman with type II hyperlipoproteinemia developed spontaneous onset of left hip pain. A routine radiograph **(A)** shows patchy osteolysis of the proximal end of the femur with a pathologic fracture. Histologic analysis **(B)** of a specimen derived from the femoral head reveals dense aggregates of lipid-laden macrophages, a few normal blood-forming elements, and a reduced number of normal trabeculae. (Hematoxylin and eosin, ×100.)

C In a different patient with a similar type of hyperlipoproteinemia, biopsy-proved xanthomas developed in both humeri. A radiograph of the left humerus shows a large osteolytic lesion with a pathologic fracture.

(**A, B,** From Yokoyama K, et al: Clin Orthop 236:307, 1988; **C,** Courtesy of M. Pathria, M.D., San Diego, California.)

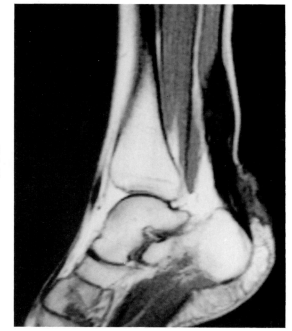

FIGURE 61–47. Hyperlipoproteinemia: Xanthomas. On a sagittal T1-weighted (TR/TE, 550/30) spin echo MR image, observe the thickened and irregular Achilles tendon of low signal intensity. (From Liem MSL, et al: Skel Radiol *21*:453, 1992.)

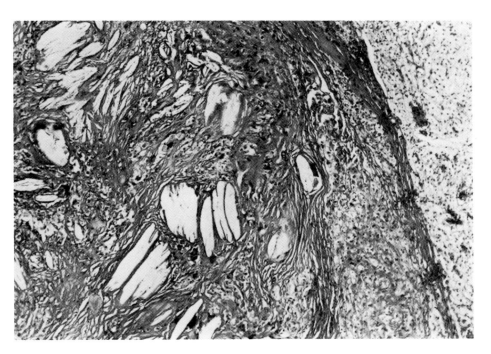

FIGURE 61–48. Hyperlipoproteinemia: Xanthoma—histologic features. Photomicrograph (55×) of a tissue section from a subcutaneous xanthoma about the elbow illustrates numerous cholesterol slits, many of which have foreign body giant cells bordering upon them. Interspersed between the cholesterol slits are foam cells and thick collagenous fibers. At the upper right, intact cholesterol-bearing foam cells are evident. (From Jaffe HL: Metabolic, Degenerative and Inflammatory Diseases of Bones and Joints. Philadelphia, Lea & Febiger, 1972.)

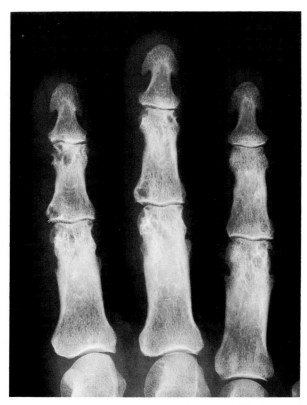

FIGURE 61–49. Hyperlipoproteinemia: Gouty arthritis. In a patient with type IV hyperlipoproteinemia and documented hyperuricemia and gout, typical findings of gouty arthritis include soft tissue swelling, eccentric, well-circumscribed osseous erosions of proximal and distal interphalangeal joints, mild joint space narrowing, and absence of osteoporosis. Intraosseous xanthomas could have a similar appearance.

Tendinous xanthomas are most frequent in the Achilles tendon but also may involve the triceps tendon, extensor tendons of the fingers, and tibial tuberosities. Palpebral xanthomas also may be apparent. The xanthomas show increased proportions of cholestanol in comparison to those in other types of hyperlipoproteinemia.[329] The radiographic features are similar to those of other disorders characterized by xanthomas, although a case of cerebrotendinous xanthomatosis with peculiar increased bone density has been described[148] (Fig. 61–50). Furthermore, osteoporosis and frequent fractures have been observed in some patients with this disorder, apparently related to depressed serum levels of 25-hydroxyvitamin D_3 and 24,25-dihydroxyvitamin D_3.[329] Additional musculoskeletal findings include joint hypermobility (similar to that occurring in other hereditary diseases such as Marfan's syndrome, Ehlers-Danlos syndrome, pseudoxanthoma elasticum, homocystinuria, and myotonia congenita) and pes cavus deformity.[330]

Differential Diagnosis

One radiographic characteristic of the hyperlipoproteinemias consisting of eccentric masses without calcification can be simulated by changes in other diseases, particularly gouty arthritis. This similarity is accentuated by the localization of masses to periarticular soft tissues, tendons, and subperiosteal and osseous areas, by the adjacent bone lysis,

and by the simultaneous occurrence of both hyperlipidemia and hyperuricemia. Secondary gout may complicate hyperlipidemia and may be accentuated by lipid-lowering agents; alternatively, elevated plasma triglyceride levels are common in gout and are not necessarily corrected by maintaining normouricemia.[142] The osseous erosions in both disorders share common features, including well-defined margins, eccentricity, and intra- and extra-articular distribution. Similar joints are involved. The soft tissue swelling of gout may contain radiographically evident calcification, a finding that is not characteristic of xanthoma. Erosions in hyperlipoproteinemia also may resemble the defects in multicentric reticulohistiocytosis, although large soft tissue masses are not characteristic of this latter disorder.

Subperiosteal xanthomas in hyperlipoproteinemias produce subjacent bone erosion. This appearance resembles subperiosteal erosion of hyperparathyroidism. Additional patterns of erosion in this latter disease allow accurate diagnosis.

The synovitis that occasionally is observed in types II and IV hyperlipoproteinemias produces periarticular swelling, which is a nonspecific finding that can be observed in numerous other inflammatory articular disorders.

MEMBRANOUS LIPODYSTROPHY

Membranous lipodystrophy, also termed polycystic lipomembranous osteodysplasia, is a rare hereditary disorder of adipose tissue affecting several organ systems but especially the bones and brain. Many of the original cases were described in Japan,[246–250] with additional reports appearing from Finland,[251, 252] Sweden,[253] Norway,[254] and the United States.[255, 256] Prominent neuropsychiatric manifestations relating to sclerosing leukoencephalopathy accounted for the frequent discovery of membranous lipodystrophy in patients in mental hospitals. Strong evidence exists that the disease is of autosomal recessive inheritance,[331] affecting both sexes and occurring in isolation or in siblings with normal parents.

Clinical characteristics include an uneventful childhood with the appearance of painful bones and joints in the second or third decade of life. By the age of 30 years, most affected persons have developed pathologic fractures of bone. Subsequently, neuropsychiatric symptoms and signs resembling those of Alzheimer's disease appear and progress rapidly to total dementia, often culminating in death by the fourth or fifth decade of life.

Histologic abnormalities are observed in the fat cells throughout the body. Convolution of the membranes of these cells and accumulation of lipid vesicles in extracellular spaces are seen. In the brain, pathologic findings have included atrophy of subcortical white matter with marked gliosis, degeneration of myelin, vascular calcification, and sudanophilic leukodsytrophy with an increase in free fatty acids and a decrease in unsaturated fatty acids.

Osseous alterations are distinctive and dominate the early phases of the disease. The osseous lesions occur as early as infancy, although they are seen more typically in childhood. Symmetric radiolucent lesions appear in the tubular bones of the extremities, carpus, tarsus, metacarpals, metatarsals, and phalanges (Fig. 61–51). The axial skeleton is spared. A metaphyseal and epiphyseal localization is typical. The cystic areas have poorly defined margins, possess trabecula-

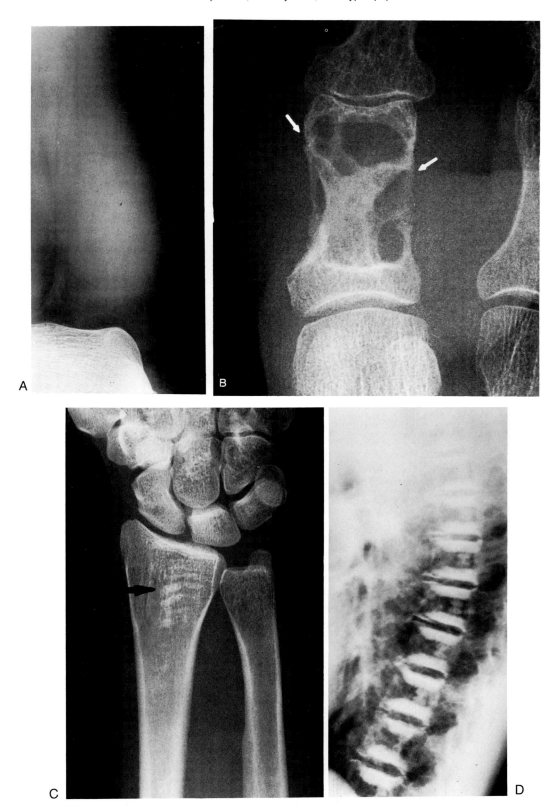

FIGURE 61–50. Cerebrotendinous xanthomatosis.
    A A 28 year old woman with cerebrotendinous xanthomatosis had ataxia, low intelligence, cataracts, and progressive enlargement of the Achilles tendons. The lateral radiograph of the ankle reveals xanthomatous infiltration in the Achilles tendon.
    B A 47 year old woman had an unsteady gait for 5 years. She had had xanthomas removed from the quadriceps and Achilles tendons. Physical examination revealed multiple xanthomas, hyperactive reflexes, and cerebellar ataxia. An anteroposterior radiograph of the great toe reveals a soft tissue mass and osseous erosions (arrows) creating a lucent lesion with residual trabeculae.
    C, D A 49 year old woman had multiple xanthomas. Radiographs reveal dense radiopaque bands and patchy sclerosis of the distal end of the radius (arrow) and superior and inferior margins of the vertebral bodies.
    (From Pastershank SP, et al: J Can Assoc Radiol 25:282, 1974.)

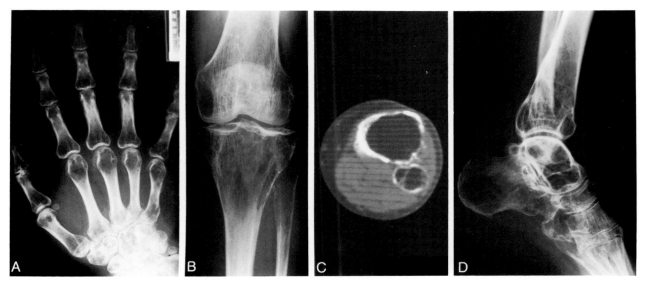

FIGURE 61–51. Membranous lipodystrophy: Radiographic abnormalities.

A Observe symmetric radiolucent lesions involving virtually all of the bones of the hand and wrist. The opposite side was affected similarly.

B Poorly defined osteolytic areas in the metaphyseal and epiphyseal regions of the femur, tibia, and fibula are associated with mild expansion of the bone. Similar lesions were present on the opposite side.

C A transaxial CT scan through the proximal portions of the tibia and fibula demonstrates the radiolucent lesions in the medullary space and cortical thinning.

D Similar radiographic abnormalities are present in the bones about the ankle, including the tarsus.

(Courtesy of I. Sugiura, M.D., Nagoya, Japan.)

tions, and are unassociated with sclerotic reaction. Bone deformities result from pathologic fractures and consist also of an Erlenmeyer flask appearance. Serial radiographic examinations document either little change in the size of the lesions or slow progression. Pathologically, cystic areas in the bone contain fatty material and convoluted membranes (Fig. 61–52). The jellylike material in the cyst is PAS-positive, suggesting a glycoprotein structure. The membranes themselves have a complex microvillous appearance.

The cause of membranous lipodystrophy is unknown. The process does not appear to be neoplastic or metabolic, but, rather, may represent a metaplastic disorder leading to the replacement of bone by a distinctive type of lipomembranous tissue. The tissue itself may represent the remnants of necrotic cells, either stromal fibroblasts or cells derived from the mild inflammatory infiltrate that is observed around blood vessels.[332] The diffuse nature of the process is underscored by documentation of cases involving, in addition to the brain and bones, the pericardium, mesentery, thymus, adrenal glands, testes, and perineal and perilymphoid tissues.

The differential diagnosis of the radiographic changes in the bones includes fibrous dysplasia, hyperparathyroidism, neurofibromatosis, sarcoidosis, lymphangiomatosis, and hemangiomatosis. Knowledge of accompanying neuropsychiatric symptoms and signs combined with radiographic features consisting of symmetric osseous lesions confined to the appendicular skeleton aids in correct diagnosis of this unusual disease.

SUMMARY

Musculoskeletal findings are a significant part of the lipidoses, histiocytoses, and hyperlipoproteinemias. In Gauch-

er's disease, cellular accumulation in the bone marrow leads to replacement of trabeculae, endosteal erosion of the cortex, cortical thinning, lytic defects, and fractures. Osteonecrosis and modeling deformities of long bones are characteristic. The findings in Niemann-Pick disease may resemble those of Gaucher's disease, although osteonecrosis is not encountered. This latter abnormality is detected in Fabry's disease.

Multicentric reticulohistiocytosis is characterized by proliferation of histiocytes in various tissues. Skeletal involvement can lead to a symmetric destructive polyarthritis with predilection for the interphalangeal joints of the hands and feet, early and severe abnormalities of the atlantoaxial joints, and changes in other articulations of the appendicular skeleton.

The Langerhans cell histiocytoses consist of three disorders: eosinophilic granuloma, Hand-Schüller-Christian disease, and Letterer-Siwe disease. These disorders share numerous radiologic and pathologic features, although classic clinical characteristics lead to their separation into discrete entities. Eosinophilic granuloma is considered the mildest form, Hand-Schüller-Christian disease is the most varied in its manifestations, and Letterer-Siwe disease represents an acute form with rapid dissemination and poor prognosis. Single or multiple osteolytic lesions may be apparent in any of these three disorders.

Erdheim-Chester disease is an unusual lipidosis leading to characteristic skeletal abnormalities. Its relationship to the histiocytoses is not clear. Sinus histiocytosis with massive lymphadenopathy is a self-limited disease associated with osteolytic lesions. Malignant histiocytosis, on the other hand, produces similar bone abnormalities but has a poor prognosis.

The hyperlipoproteinemias are divided into five types according to the predominant lipoprotein pattern. Similar

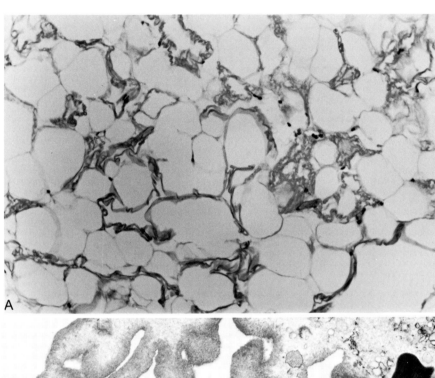

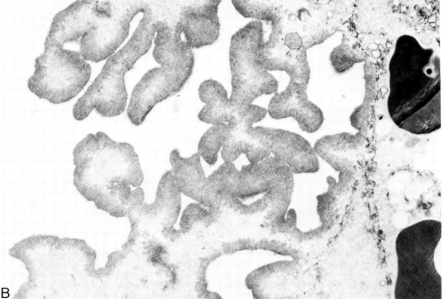

FIGURE 61–52. Membranous lipodystrophy: Pathologic abnormalities.

A Normal fat cells have been replaced by numerous membranous structures.

B The membranous structures are composed of an outer, more dense layer containing microtubular structures and an inner layer containing a fatlike substance.

(Courtesy of I. Sugiura, M.D., Nagoya, Japan.)

clinical and radiologic manifestations are observed in these disorders, which may include xanthomatous collections in soft tissue, tendon, subperiosteal and intra-osseous locations, gout, arthralgias, and arthritis.

Membranous lipodystrophy is a rare disorder characterized by neuropsychiatric manifestations and symmetrically distributed osteolytic areas in the appendicular skeleton.

References

1. Gaucher P: De l'epithelioma primitif de la rate, hypertrophie idiopathique de la rate sans leucémie. Thése de Paris, 1882.
2. Schlaugenhaufer F: Uber meist familiar vorkommende histologische, characterische splenomegallen (typus Gaucher). Virchows Arch Pathol Anat 87:125, 1907.
3. Bovaird D Jr: Primary splenomegaly. Am J Med Sci 120:377, 1900.
4. Marchand F: Uber sogenannte idiopathische splenomegalie—typus Gaucher. Münch Med Wochenschr 54:1102, 1907.
5. Epstein E: Beitrag zur chemie der Gaucherschen Krankheit. Biochem Z 145:398, 1924.
6. Lieb H: Cerebrosidspeicherung bei Splenomegalie typus Gaucher. Z Physiol Chem 140:305, 1924.
7. Carter HE, Johnson P, Weber EJ: Glycolipids. In JM Juch, PD Boyer (Eds): Annual Review of Biochemistry. Vol 34, Palo Alto, Calif, Annual Reviews, 1965, p 109.
8. Statter M, Shapiro B: Studies on the etiology of Gaucher's disease. Isr J Med Sci 1:514, 1965.
9. Kennaway NG, Woolf LI: Splenic lipids in Gaucher's disease. J Lipid Res 9:755, 1968.
10. Patrick AD: A deficiency of glucocerebrosidase in Gaucher's disease. Biochem J 97:17c, 1965.
11. Medolf AS, Bayrd ED: Gaucher's disease in 29 cases: Hematologic complications and effect of splenectomy. Ann Intern Med 40:481, 1954.
12. Reich C, Seife M, Kessler BJ: Gaucher's disease: A review and discussion of twenty cases. Medicine 30:1, 1951.
13. Hsia DY, Naylor J, Bigler JA: Gaucher's disease: Report of two cases in father and son and review of the literature. N Engl J Med 261:164, 1959.
14. Fredrickson DS, Sloan HR: Glucosyl ceramide lipidoses: Gaucher's disease. In JB Stanbury et al (Eds): The Metabolic Basis of Inherited Disease. 3rd Ed. New York, McGraw-Hill, 1972, p 730.
15. Tuchman LR, Swick M: High acid phosphatase level indicating Gaucher's disease in patients with prostatism. JAMA 164:2034, 1957.
16. Tuchman LR, Suna H, Carr JJ: Elevation of serum acid phosphatase in Gaucher's disease. J Mt Sinai Hosp 23:227, 1956.
17. Greenfield GB: Bone changes in chronic adult Gaucher's disease. AJR 110:800, 1970.
18. Katz M, Dorfmann H, Hubault A, et al: Maladie de Gaucher. A propos d'une observation à manifestations osteoarticulaires dominantes. J Radiol Electrol Med Nucl 54:61, 1973.
19. Amstutz HC, Carey EJ: Skeletal manifestations and treatment of Gaucher's disease. Review of twenty cases. J Bone Joint Surg [Am] 48:670, 1966.
20. Strickland B: Skeletal manifestations of Gaucher's disease with some unusual findings. Br J Radiol 31:246, 1958.
21. Silverstein MN, Kelly PJ: Osteoarticular manifestations of Gaucher's disease. Am J Med Sci 253:569, 1967.
22. Gordon EJ: Gaucher's disease in adults. South Med J 69:664, 1976.
23. Seinsheimer F III, Mankin HJ: Acute bilateral symmetrical pathologic fractures of the lateral tibial plateaus in a patient with Gaucher's disease. Arthritis Rheum 20:1550, 1977.
24. Hansen GC, Gold RH: Central depression of multiple vertebral endplates: A "pathognomonic" sign of sickle hemoglobinopathy in Gaucher's disease. AJR 129:343, 1977.
25. Reynolds J: A re-evaluation of the "fish vertebra" sign in sickle-cell hemoglobinopathy. AJR 97:693, 1966.
26. Cassady JR, Berdon WE, Baker DH: The "typical" spine changes of sickle-cell anemia in a patient with thalassemia major (Cooley's anemia). Radiology 89:1065, 1967.
27. Jaffe HL: Metabolic, Degenerative and Inflammatory Diseases of Bones and Joints. Philadelphia, Lea & Febiger, 1972, p 506.
28. Schein AJ, Arkin AM: Hip joint involvement in Gaucher's disease. J Bone Joint Surg 24:396, 1942.
29. Arkin AM, Schein AJ: Aseptic necrosis in Gaucher's disease. J Bone Joint Surg [Am] 30:631, 1948.
30. Windholz F, Foster SE: Sclerosis of bones in Gaucher's disease. AJR 60:246, 1948.
31. Todd RM, Keidan SE: Changes in the head of the femur in children suffering from Gaucher's disease. J Bone Joint Surg [Br] 34:447, 1952.
32. Amstutz HC: The hip in Gaucher's disease. Clin Orthop 90:83, 1973.
33. James NE: Gaucher's disease; report of a case. J Bone Joint Surg [Br] 34:464, 1952.
34. Rourke JA, Heslin DJ: Gaucher's disease. Roentgenologic bone changes over 20 years interval. AJR 94:621, 1965.
35. Johnson LC: Histogenesis of avascular necrosis. In Proceedings of the Conference on Aseptic Necrosis of the Femoral Head. St Louis, National Institute of Health, 1964, p 55.
36. Cushing EH, Stout AP: Gaucher's disease with report of a case showing bone disintegration and joint involvement. Arch Surg 12:539, 1926.
37. Melamed S, Chester W: Osseous form of Gaucher's disease. Arch Intern Med 61:798, 1938.
38. Battaglia L, Chiandussi D: Manifestazioni ossee della lipoidosi cerebrosidica di Gaucher. Chir Organi Mov 54:151, 1965.
39. Capper A, Epstein H, Schless RA: Gaucher's disease, report of case with presentation of a table differentiating the lipoid disturbances. Am J Med Sci 188:84, 1934.
40. Kroboth FJ Jr, Johnson EW Jr: Osseous Gaucher's disease, report of a case with pathologic fracture of the left humerus. Surg Clin North Am 32:1141, 1952.
41. Levin B: Gaucher's disease. Clinical and roentgenologic manifestations. AJR 85:685, 1961.
42. Reiss O, Kato K: Gaucher's disease. A clinical study with special reference to the roentgenography of bones. Am J Dis Child 43:365, 1932.
43. Noyes FR, Smith WS: Bone crisis and chronic osteomyelitis in Gaucher's disease. Clin Orthop 79:132, 1971.
44. Rodnan GP: Arthritis associated with hematologic disorders. Bull Rheum Dis 16:392, 1965.
45. Kulowski J: Gaucher's disease in bone. AJR 63:840, 1950.
46. Moschcowitz E: A case of Gaucher's disease. Proc NY Pathol Soc 24:18, 1924.
47. Yossipovitch ZH, Herman G, Makin M: Aseptic osteomyelitis in Gaucher's disease. Isr J Med Sci 1:531, 1965.
48. Taubman J, MacKeith M: Gaucher's disease with acro-osteolysis. Proc R Soc Med 56:294, 1963.
49. Niemann A: Ein unbekanntes Krankheitsbild. Jahrb Kinderheilkd 29:1, 1914.
50. Knox JHM Jr, Wahl HR, Schmeisser HC: Gaucher's disease: A report of two cases in infants. Bull Johns Hopkins Hosp 27:1, 1916.
51. Pick L: II. Niemann-Pick's disease and other forms of so-called xanthomatosis. Am J Med Sci 185:601, 1933.
52. Wahl HR, Richardson ML: A study of lipid content of a case of Gaucher's disease in an infant. Arch Intern Med 17:238, 1916.
53. Klenk E: Über die Natur der Phosphatide der Milz bei der Niemann-Pickschen Krankheit. Z Physiol Chem 229:151, 1934.
54. Klenk E: Über die Natur der Phosphatide und anderer Lipoide des Gehirns und der Leber bei der Niemann-Picksehen Krankheit. 12. Mitteilung über LeBer Phosphatide. Z Physiol Chem 235:24, 1935.
55. Brady RO, Kanfer JN, Mock MB, et al: The metabolism of sphingomyelin. II. Evidence of an enzymatic deficiency in Niemann-Pick disease. Proc Natl Acad Sci 55:366, 1966.
56. Fredrickson DS, Sloan HR: Sphingomyelin lipidoses: Niemann-Pick disease. In JB Stanbury et al (Eds): The Metabolic Basis of Inherited Disease. 3rd Ed. New York, McGraw-Hill, 1972, p 783.
57. Baumann T, Klenk E, Scheidegger S: Die Niemann-Picksche Krankheit. Ein klinische, chemische und histopathologische Studie. Ergeb Allg Pathol 30:183, 1936.
58. Lachman R, Crocker A, Schulman J, et al: Radiological findings in Niemann-Pick disease. Radiology 108:659, 1973.
59. Swischuk LE: The beaked, notched or hooked vertebra. Its significance in infants and young children. Radiology 95:661, 1970.
60. Gildenhorn HL, Amromin GD: Report of a case with Niemann-Pick disease: Correlation of roentgenographic and autopsy findings. AJR 85:680, 1961.
61. Sweeley CC, Klionsky B, Krivit W, et al: Fabry's disease: Glycosphingolipid lipidosis. In JB Stanbury et al (Eds): The Metabolic Basis of Inherited Disease. 3rd Ed. New York, McGraw-Hill, 1972, p 663.
62. Fabry J: Ein Beitrag zur Kenntnis der Purpura haemorrhagica nodularis (Purpura papulosa hemorrhagica Hebrae). Arch Dermatol Syphilol 43:187, 1898.
63. Anderson W: A case of angiokeratoma. Br J Dermatol 10:113, 1898.
64. Johnston AW, Weller SD, Warland BJ: Angiokeratoma corporis diffusum. Some clinical aspects. Arch Dis Child 43:73, 1968.
65. Von Gemmingen G, Kierland RR, Opitz JM: Angiokeratoma corporis diffusum (Fabry's disease). Arch Dermatol 91:206, 1965.
66. Wise D, Wallace HJ, Jellinck EH: Angiokeratoma corporis diffusum: A clinical study of eight affected families. J Med 31:177, 1962.
67. Lilis M, Vulcan P, Peresecenschi G: Notes on a case of angiokeratoma corporis diffusum (Fabry's disease). Rum Med Rev 20:29, 1966.
68. Pittelkow RB, Kierland RR, Montgomery H: Angiokeratoma corporis diffusum. Arch Dermatol 72:556, 1955.
69. Fone D, King WE: Angiokeratoma corporis diffusum (Fabry's syndrome). Australas Ann Med 13:339, 1964.
70. Bethune JE, Landrigan PL, Chipman CD: Angiokeratoma corporis diffusum universale (Fabry's disease in two brothers). N Engl J Med 264:1280, 1961.
71. Spaeth GL, Frost P: Fabry's disease: Its ocular manifestations. Arch Ophthalmol 74:760, 1965.
72. Goltz RW, Laymon CW: Multicentric reticulohistiocytosis of the skin and synovia; reticulohistiocytoma or ganglioneuroma. Arch Dermatol Syphilol 69:717, 1954.
73. Albert J, Bruce W, Allen AC, et al: Lipoid dermatoarthritis. Reticulohistiocytoma of the skin and joints. Am J Med 28:661, 1960.
74. Caro MR, Senear FE: Reticulohistiocytoma of the skin. Arch Dermatol Syphilol 65:701, 1952.

75. Weber FP: Lipoid rheumatism. Br J Dermatol Syphilol 60:106, 1948.
76. Granelli V, Bignami A, Nazzaro P: Giant cell reticulohistiocytosis (lipoid dermatoarthritis). G Ital Derm 104:285, 1963.
77. Portugal H, Fialho F, Miliano A: Generalized giant-cell histiocytomatosis. Rev Argent Dermatol 28:121, 1944.
78. Holubar K, Mach K: Giant cell histiocytosis. A contribution to the clinical and histological aspects. Hautarzt 17:440, 1966.
79. Barrow MV, Holubar K: Multicentric reticulohistiocytosis. A review of 33 patients. Medicine 48:287, 1969.
80. Targett JH: Giant cell tumors of the integuments. Trans Pathol Soc Lond 48:230, 1897.
81. Weber FP, Freudenthal W: Nodular nondiabetic cutaneous xanthomatosis with hypercholesterolemia and atypical histological features. Proc R Soc Med 30:522, 1937.
82. Bortz AI, Vincent M: Lipoid dermato-arthritis and arthritis mutilans. Am J Med 30:951, 1961.
83. Melton JW III, Irby R: Multicentric reticulohistiocytosis. Arthritis Rheum 15:221, 1972.
84. Ehrlich GE, Young I, Nosheny SZ, et al: Multicentric reticulohistiocytosis (lipoid dermatoarthritis). A multisystem disorder. Am J Med 52:830, 1972.
85. Barrow MV: The nails in multicentric reticulohistiocytosis (lipoid dermatoarthritis). Arch Dermatol 95:200, 1967.
86. Gold RH, Metzger AL, Mirra JM, et al: Multicentric reticulohistiocytosis (lipoid dermatoarthritis). An erosive polyarthritis with distinctive clinical, roentgenographic, and pathologic features. AJR 124:610, 1975.
87. Brodey PA: Multicentric reticulohistiocytosis: A rare cause of destructive polyarthritis. Radiology 114:327, 1975.
88. Schwartz E, Fish A: Reticulohistiocytoma. A rare dermatologic disease with roentgen manifestations. AJR 83:692, 1960.
89. Martel W, Abell MR, Duff IF: Cervical spine involvement in lipoid dermatoarthritis. Radiology 77:613, 1961.
90. Johnson HM, Tilden IL: Reticulohistiocytic granulomas of skin associated with arthritis mutilans: Report of a case followed fourteen years. Arch Dermatol 75:405, 1957.
91. Krey PR, Comerford FR, Cohen AS: Multicentric reticulohistiocytosis. Fine structural analysis of the synovium and synovial fluid cells. Arthritis Rheum 17:615, 1974.
92. Orkin M, Goltz RW, Good RA, et al: A study of multicentric reticulohistiocytosis. Arch Dermatol 89:640, 1964.
93. Montgomery H, Polley HF, Pugh DG: Reticulohistiocytoma (reticulohistiocytic granuloma). Arch Dermatol 77:61, 1958.
94. Warin RP, Evans CD, Hewitt M, et al: Reticulohistiocytosis (lipoid dermatoarthritis). Br Med J 1:1387, 1957.
95. Lichtenstein L: Histiocytosis X. Integration of eosinophilic granuloma of bone, "Letterer-Siwe Disease" and "Schüller-Christian" disease as related manifestations of a single nosologic entity. Arch Pathol 56:84, 1953.
96. Avery ME, McAfee JG, Guild HG: The course and prognosis of reticulendotheliosis (eosinophilic granuloma, Schüller-Christian disease and Letterer-Siwe disease). Am J Med 22:636, 1957.
97. Acromano JP, Bartnett JC, Wunderlich HO: Histiocytosis X. AJR 85:663, 1961.
98. Jaffe HL, Lichtenstein L: Eosinophilic granuloma of bone. A condition affecting one, several or many bones, but apparently limited to the skeleton and representing the mildest clinical expression of the peculiar inflammatory histiocytosis also underlying Letterer-Siwe disease and Schüller-Christian disease. Arch Pathol 37:99, 1944.
99. Schajowicz F, Slullitel J: Eosinophilic granuloma of bone and its relationship to Hand-Schüller-Christian and Letterer-Siwe syndromes. J Bone Joint Surg [Br] 55:545, 1973.
100. Enriquez P, Dahlin DC, Hayles AB, et al: Histiocytosis X. Mayo Clin Proc 42:88, 1967.
101. Lieberman PH, Jones CR, Dargeon HWK, et al: A reappraisal of eosinophilic granuloma of bone, Hand-Schüller-Christian syndrome and Letterer-Siwe syndrome. Medicine 48:375, 1969.
102. Ochsner SF: Eosinophilic granuloma of bone. AJR 97:719, 1966.
103. Stern MB, Cassidy R, Mirra J: Eosinophilic granuloma of the proximal tibial epiphysis. Clin Orthop 118:153, 1976.
104. Fevre M, Bertrand P: Existence de granulomes eosinophiles epiphysaires. Rev Chir Orthop 56:345, 1970.
105. Keusch KD, Poole CA, King DR: The significance of "floating teeth" in children. Radiology 86:215, 1966.
106. Cheyne C: Histiocytosis X. J Bone Joint Surg [Br] 53:366, 1971.
107. Kaye JJ, Freiberger RH: Eosinophilic granuloma of the spine without vertebra plana. A report of two unusual cases. Radiology 92:1188, 1969.
108. Sherk HH, Nicholson JT, Nixon JE: Vertebra plana and eosinophilic granuloma of the cervical spine in children. Spine 3:116, 1978.
109. Poulsen JO, Thommesen P: An unusual case of histiocytosis X in the spine. Acta Orthop Scand 47:59, 1976.
110. Ferris RA, Pettrone FA, McKelvie AM, et al: Eosinophilic granuloma of the spine: An unusual radiographic presentation. Clin Orthop 99:57, 1974.
111. Fowles JV, Bobechko WP: Solitary eosinophilic granuloma in bone. J Bone Joint Surg [Br] 52:238, 1970.
112. Calvé J: Localized affection of spine suggesting osteochondritis of vertebral body with clinical aspects of Pott's disease. J Bone Joint Surg 7:41, 1925.
113. Takahashi M, Martel W, Oberman HA: The variable roentgenographic appearance of idiopathic histiocytosis. Clin Radiol 17:48, 1966.
114. Mickelson MR, Bonfiglio M: Eosinophilic granuloma and its variations. Orthop Clin North Am 8:933, 1977.
115. Ponseti I: Bone lesions in eosinophilic granuloma, Hand-Schüller-Christian disease, and Letterer-Siwe disease. J Bone Joint Surg [Am] 30:811, 1948.
116. Lahey ME: Prognosis in reticuloendotheliosis in children. J Pediatr 60:664, 1962.
117. Abt AF, Deneholz EJ: Letterer-Siwe's disease: Splenohepatomegaly associated with widespread hyperplasia of nonlipoid-storing macrophages; discussion of the so-called reticulo-endotheliosis. Am J Dis Child 51:499, 1936.
118. Fredrickson DS, Levy RI: Familial hyperlipoproteinemia. In JB Stanbury et al (Eds): The Metabolic Basis of Inherited Disease. 3rd Ed. New York, McGraw-Hill, 1972, p 545.
119. Rayer PFO: Traite theorique et pratiques des maladies de la peau. Paris, JB Bailliere, 1827.
120. Addison T, Gull W: On a certain affection of the skin, vitiligoidea a. plana b. tuberosa with remarks. Guys Hosp Rev 7:265, 1851.
121. Chauffard A, LaRoche G: Pathogenie du xanthelasma. Sem Med 30:241, 1910.
122. Rifkind BM: The hyperlipoproteinemias. Br J Hosp Med 4:683, 1970.
123. Fredrickson DS, Levy RI, Lees RS: Fat transport in lipoproteins—an integrated approach to mechanisms and disorders. N Engl J Med 276:34, 94, 148, 215, 273, 1967.
124. Glueck CJ, Levy RI, Fredrickson DS: Acute tendinitis and arthritis—a presenting symptom of familial type II hyperlipoproteinemia. JAMA 206:2895, 1968.
125. Fleischmajer R: Cutaneous and tendon xanthomas. Dermatologica 128:113, 1964.
126. Siegelman SS, Schlossberg I, Becker NH, et al: Hyperlipoproteinemia with skeletal lesions. Clin Orthop 87:228, 1972.
127. Freiberg RA, Air GW, Glueck CJ, et al: Multiple intraosseous lipomas with Type-IV hyperlipoproteinemia. A case report. J Bone Joint Surg [Am] 56:1729, 1974.
128. Ansell BM, Bywaters EGL: Histiocytic bone and joint disease. Ann Rheum Dis 16:503, 1957.
129. Whelton MJ: Arthropathy and liver disease. Br J Hosp Med 3:243, 1970.
130. Whelton MJ: Arthropathy and liver disease. J Ir Med Assoc 65:456, 1972.
131. O'Connell DJ, Marx WJ: Hand changes in primary biliary cirrhosis. Radiology 129:31, 1978.
132. Harlan WR Jr, Graham JB, Estes EH: Familial hypercholesterolemia: A genetic and metabolic study. Medicine 45:77, 1966.
133. Beaumont JL, Jacotot B, Beaumont V: L'hyperlipidemie par autoanticorps une cause d'atherosclerose. Presse Med 75:2315, 1967.
134. Jepson EM, Fahmy MFI, Torrens PE, et al: Treatment of essential hyperlipidaemia. Lancet 2:1315, 1969.
135. Borrie P: Type III hyperlipoproteinemia. Br Med J 2:665, 1969.
136. Wilson JD: Studies on the origin of the lipid components of xanthomata. Circ Res 12:472, 1963.
137. Fletcher RF, Gloster J: The lipids in xanthomata. J Clin Invest 43:2104, 1964.
138. Baes H, Van Gent CM, Pries C: Lipid composition of various types of xanthoma. J Invest Dermatol 51:286, 1968.
139. Berkowitz D: Blood lipid and uric acid inter-relationships. JAMA 190:856, 1964.
140. Berkowitz D: Gout, hyperlipidiemia and diabetes interrelatioships. JAMA 197:77, 1966.
141. Jensen J, Blankenhorn DH, Kornerup V: Blood uric-acid levels in familial hypercholesterolaemia. Lancet 1:298, 1966.
142. Bluestone R: Hyperlipoproteinaemia and arthritis (two cases). Proc R Soc Med 64:669, 1971.
143. Khachadurian AK: Migratory polyarthritis in familial hypercholesterolaemia (Type II hyperlipoproteinaemia). Arthritis Rheum 11:385, 1968.
144. Goldman JA, Glueck CJ, Abrams NR, et al: Musculoskeletal disorders associated with Type IV hyperlipoproteinaemia. Lancet 2:449, 1972.
145. Buckingham RB, Bole GG, Bassett DR: Polyarthritis associated with Type IV hyperlipoproteinaemia. Arch Intern Med 135:286, 1975.
146. Sloan HR, Fredrickson DS: Rare familial diseases with neutral lipid storage: Wolman's disease, cholesteryl ester storage disease and cerebrotendinous xanthomatosis. In JB Stanbury et al (Eds): The Metabolic Basis of Inherited Disease. 3rd Ed. New York, McGraw-Hill, 1972, p 808.
147. Menkes JH, Schimschock JR, Swanson PD: Cerebrotendinous xanthomatosis: The storage of cholestanol within the nervous system. Arch Neurol 19:47, 1968.
148. Pastershank SP, Yip S, Sodhi HS: Cerebrotendinous xanthomatosis. J Can Assoc Radiol 25:282, 1974.
149. Sheth KJ, Bernhard GC: The arthropathy of Fabry disease. Arthritis Rheum 22:781, 1979.
150. Freyschmidt J, Wilmowsky H, Krmpotic L: Multizentrische Retikulo-histiozytose als ursache einer erosiv-destruktiven Arthropathie. ROFO 129:605, 1978.
151. Chester H: Uber lipoidgranulomatose. Virchows Arch (Pathol Anat Phys) 279:561, 1930–1931.
152. Sorensen EW: Hyperlipemia: A report of an unusual case complicated by bone lesions, macrocytic anaemia and leukemoid bone marrow. Acta Med Scand 175:207, 1964.
153. Simpson FG, Robinson PJ, Hardy GJ, et al: Erdheim-Chester disease associated with retroperitoneal xanthogranuloma. Br J Radiol 52:232, 1979.
154. Schwartz AM, Homer MJ, McCauley RGK: "Step-off" vertebral body: Gaucher's disease versus sickle cell hemoglobinopathy. AJR 132:81, 1979.
155. Bjersand AJ: Bone changes in hypercholesterolemia. Radiology 130:101, 1979.
156. Merril AS: Case of xanthoma showing multiple bone lesions. AJR 7:480, 1920.

157. Novy SB, Natelson E, Stuart L, et al: Gaucher's disease in a black adult. AJR *133*:947, 1979.
158. McCullough CJ: Eosinophilic granuloma of bone. Acta Orthop Scand *51*:389, 1980.
159. Balducci L, Dreiling B, Steinberg MH, et al: Multifocal eosinophilic granuloma: Description of an unusual case. South Med J *72*:884, 1979.
160. Bohne WHO, Goldman AB, Bullough P: Case report 96. Skel Radiol *4*:164, 1979.
161. Dee P, Westgaard T, Langholm R: Erdheim-Chester disease: Case with chronic discharging sinus from bone. AJR *134*:837, 1980.
162. Zoppini A, Teodori S, Taccari E: Valeur de la biopsie synoviale dans le diagnostic des arthropathies associées au hyperlipoprotéinémies. Rev Rhum Mal Osteoartic *47*:111, 1980.
163. Groopman JE, Golde DW: The histiocytic disorders: A pathophysiologic analysis. Ann Intern Med *94*:95, 1981.
164. Koeffler HP, Mundy GR, Golde DW, et al: Production of bone resorbing activity in poorly differentiated monocytic malignancy. Cancer *41*:2438, 1978.
165. Mergenhagen SE, Wahl SM, Wahl LM, et al: The role of lymphocytes and macrophages in the destruction of bone and collagen. Ann NY Acad Sci *256*:132, 1975.
166. Mundy GR, Altman AJ, Gondek MD, et al: Direct resorption of bone by human monocytes. Science *196*:1109, 1977.
167. Bokkerink JPM, de Vaan GAM: Histiocytosis X. Eur J Pediatr *135*:129, 1980.
168. Brady RO: The sphingolipidoses. *In* PK Bondy, LE Rosenberg (Eds): Metabolic Control and Disease. 8th Ed. Philadelphia, WB Saunders Co, 1980, p 523.
169. Matsubara T, Yoshiya S, Maeda M, et al: Histologic and histochemical investigation of Gaucher cells. Clin Orthop *166*:233, 1982.
170. Goldman AB, Jacobs B: Femoral neck fractures complicating Gaucher disease in children. Skel Radiol *12*:162, 1984.
171. Ruff ME, Weis LD, Kean JR: Acute thoracic kyphosis in Gaucher's disease. A case report. Spine *9*:835, 1984.
172. Fink IJ, Pastakia B, Barranger JA: Enlarged phalangeal nutrient foramina in Gaucher disease and B-thalassemia major. AJR *143*:647, 1984.
173. Rose JS, Grabowski GA, Barnett SH, et al: Accelerated skeletal deterioration after splenectomy in Gaucher type I disease. AJR *139*:1202, 1982.
174. Lau MM, Lichtman DM, Hamati YI, et al: Hip arthroplasties in Gaucher's disease. J Bone Joint Surg [Am] *63*:591, 1981.
175. Lachiewicz PF, Lane JM, Wilson PD Jr: Total hip replacement in Gaucher's disease. J Bone Joint Surg [Am] *63*:602, 1981.
176. Gelfand G, Bienenstock H: Hemorrhagic bursitis and bone crises in chronic adult Gaucher's disease: A case report. Arthritis Rheum *25*:1369, 1982.
177. Miller W, Lamon JM, Tavassolli M, et al: Multiple myeloma complicating Gaucher's disease. West J Med *136*:122, 1982.
178. Refsum S: Heredopathia atactica polyneuritiformis. Acta Psychiatr Scand *38*(Suppl):9, 1946.
179. Steinberg D, Vroom FQ, Engel WK, et al: Refsum's disease—a recently characterized lipidosis involving the nervous system. Ann Intern Med *66*:365, 1967.
180. Try K: Heredopathia atactica polyneuritiformis (Refsum's disease): The diagnostic value of phytanic acid determination in serum lipids. Eur Neurol *2*:296, 1969.
181. Wall WJH, Worthington BS: Skeletal changes in Refsum's disease. Clin Radiol *30*:657, 1979.
182. Lovelock J, Griffiths H: Case report 175. Skel Radiol *7*:214, 1981.
183. Farber S, Cohen J, Uzman LL: Lipogranulomatosis: A new lipoglycoprotein "storage" disease. J Mt Sinai Hosp *24*:816, 1957.
184. Schultze G, Lang EK: Disseminated lipogranulomatosis: Report of a case. Radiology *74*:428, 1960.
185. Schanche AF, Bierman SM, Sopher RL, et al: Disseminated lipogranulomatosis: Early roentgenographic changes. Radiology *82*:675, 1964.
186. Bierman SM, Edgington T, Newcomber VD, et al: Farber's disease: A disorder of mucopolysaccharide metabolism with articular, respiratory, and neurologic manifestations. Arthritis Rheum *9*:620, 1966.
187. Davidson A, Kalff V, Ryan PFJ: Bone crisis of Gaucher's disease due to bone ischemia: A case report. Arthritis Rheum *28*:218, 1985.
188. Okada S, O'Brien JS: Generalized gangliosidosis: β-galactosidase deficiency. Science *160*:1002, 1968.
189. Owman T, Sjoblad ST, Gothlin J: Radiographic skeletal changes in juvenile GM₁-gangliosidosis. ROFO *132*:682, 1980.
190. Durand P, Borrone C, Della Cella G: Fucosidosis. J Pediatr *75*:665, 1969.
191. Van Hoof F, Hers HG: Mucopolysaccharidosis by absence of α-fucosidase. Lancet *1*:1198, 1968.
192. Lesher JL Jr, Allen BS: Multicentric reticulohistiocytosis. J Am Acad Dermatol *11*:713, 1984.
193. Doherty M, Martin MFR, Dieppe PA: Multicentric reticulohistiocytosis associated with primary biliary cirrhosis: Successful treatment with cytoxic agents. Arthritis Rheum *27*:344, 1984.
194. Nezelof C, Basset F, Rousseau MF: Histiocytosis X. Histogenetic arguments for a Langerhans cell origin. Biomedicine *18*:365, 1973.
195. Cutler LS, Krutchkoff D: An ultrastructural study of eosinophilic granuloma: The Langerhans cell—its role in histiogenesis and diagnosis. Oral Surg *44*:246, 1977.
196. Jennings CD, Stelling CB, Powell DE: Case report 199. Skel Radiol *8*:229, 1982.
197. Palmer RE: Eosinophilic granuloma of the hand: Case report. J Hand Surg [Am] *9*:283, 1984.
198. Usui M, Matsuno T, Kobayashi M, et al: Eosinophilic granuloma of the growing epiphysis. A case report and review of the literature. Clin Orthop *176*:201, 1983.
199. Gugliantini P, Barbuti D, Rosati D, et al: Histiocytosis X: Solitary localization in the sternum of a 2-year-old child. Pediatr Radiol *12*:102, 1982.
200. Bonakdarpour A, Mayer DP, Clancy M, et al: Case report 208. Skel Radiol *8*:319, 1982.
201. Casson IR, Blair D, Gerard G, et al: Eosinophilic granuloma of the cervical spine in an adult. NY State J Med *81*:1102, 1981.
202. Green NE, Robertson WW Jr, Kilroy AW: Eosinophilic granuloma of the spine with associated neural deficit. Report of three cases. J Bone Joint Surg [Am] *62*:1198, 1980.
203. Katz RL, Silva EG, DeSantos LA, et al: Diagnosis of eosinophilic granuloma of bone by cytology, histology, and electron microscopy of transcutaneous bone-aspiration biopsy. J Bone Joint Surg [Am] *62*:1284, 1980.
204. Sartoris DJ, Parker BR: Histiocytosis X: Rate and pattern of resolution of osseous lesions. Radiology *152*:679, 1984.
205. Nauert C, Zornoza J, Ayala A, et al: Eosinophilic granuloma of bone: Diagnosis and management. Skel Radiol *10*:227, 1983.
206. Ippolito E, Farsetti P, Tudisco C: Vertebra plana. Long-term follow up in five patients. J Bone Joint Surg [Am] *66*:1364, 1984.
207. Seimon LP: Eosinophil granuloma of the spine. J Pediatr Orthop *1*:371, 1981.
208. Cohen M, Zornoza J, Cangir A, et al: Direct injection of methylprednisolone sodium succinate in the treatment of solitary eosinophilic granuloma of bone. A report of 9 cases. Radiology *136*:289, 1980.
209. Ruff S, Chapman GK, Taylor TKF, et al: The evolution of eosinophilic granuloma of bone: A case report. Skel Radiol *10*:37, 1983.
210. Scaglietti O, Marchetti PG, Bartolozzi P: The effects of methylprednisolone acetate in the treatment of bone cysts. Results of three years follow-up. J Bone Joint Surg [Br] *61*:200, 1979.
211. Eil C, Adornato BT: Caution on bone scans in eosinophilic granuloma (Letter). Ann Intern Med *89*:289, 1978.
212. Antonmattei S, Tetalman MR, Lloyd TV: The multiscan appearance of eosinophilic granuloma. Clin Nucl Med *4*:53, 1979.
213. Parker BR, Pinckney L, Etcubanas E: Relative efficacy of radiographic and radionuclide bone surveys in the detection of the skeletal lesions of histiocytosis X. Radiology *134*:377, 1980.
214. Siddiqui AR, Tashjian JH, Lazarus K, et al: Nuclear medicine studies in the evaluation of skeletal lesions in children with histiocytosis X. Radiology *140*:787, 1981.
215. Kumar R, Balachandran S: Relative roles of radionuclide scanning and radiographic imaging in eosinophilic granuloma. Clin Nucl Med *5*:538, 1980.
216. Crone-Munzebrock W, Brassow F: A comparison of radiographic and bone scan findings in histiocytosis X. Skel Radiol *9*:170, 1983.
217. Schaub T, Eissner D, Hahn K, et al: Bone scanning in the detection and follow-up of skeletal lesions in histiocytosis X. Ann Radiol *26*:407, 1983.
218. Benz-Bohm G, Georgi P: Szintigraphische und radiologische Befunde beim eosinophilen Granulom. Radiologe *21*:195, 1981.
219. Resnick D, Greenway G, Genant H, et al: Erdheim-Chester disease. Radiology *142*:289, 1982.
220. Martin W III, Klein A, Buss D: Case report 213. Skel Radiol *9*:69, 1982.
221. Poehling GG, Adair DM, Haupt HA: Erdheim-Chester disease. A case report. Clin Orthop *185*:241, 1984.
222. Brower AC, Worsham GF, Dudley AH: Erdheim-Chester disease: A distinct lipidosis or part of the spectrum of histiocytosis? Radiology *151*:35, 1984.
223. Dalinka MK, Turner ML, Thompson JJ, et al: Lipid granulomatosis of the ribs: Focal Erdheim-Chester disease. Radiology *142*:297, 1982.
224. Rosai J, Dorfman RF: Sinus histiocytosis with massive lymphadenopathy. A newly recognized benign clinicopathological entity. Arch Pathol *87*:63, 1969.
225. Rosai J, Dorfman RF: Sinus histiocytosis with massive lymphadenopathy: A pseudolymphomatous benign disorder. Analysis of 34 cases. Cancer *30*:1174, 1972.
226. Lampert F, Lennert K: Sinus histiocytosis with massive lymphadenopathy. Fifteen new cases. Cancer *37*:783, 1976.
227. Foucar E, Rosai J, Dorfman RF: Sinus histiocytosis with massive lymphadenopathy. Ear, nose, and throat manifestations. Arch Otolaryngol *104*:687, 1978.
228. Sanchez R, Rosai J, Dorfman RF: Sinus histiocytosis with massive lymphadenopathy: An analysis of 113 cases with special emphasis on its extranodal manifestations. Lab Invest *36*:349, 1977.
229. Walker PD, Rosai J, Dorfman RF: The osseous manifestations of sinus histiocytosis with massive lymphadenopathy. Am J Clin Pathol *75*:131, 1981.
230. Delauche M-C, Clauvel J-P, Tricot G, et al: Sinus histiocytosis with massive lymphadenopathy: One further case with osteoarticular presentation. J Rheumatol *11*:83, 1984.
231. Ramos CV: Widespread bone involvement in sinus histiocytosis. Arch Pathol Lab Med *100*:606, 1976.
232. Scott RB, Robb-Smith AHT: Histiocytic medullary reticulosis. Lancet *2*:194, 1939.
233. Warnke RA, Kim H, Dorfman RF: Malignant histiocytosis (histiocytic medullary reticulosis). I. Clinicopathologic study of 29 cases. Cancer *35*:215, 1975.
234. Hammoudeh M, Khan MA: Cranial arteritis as the initial manifestation of malignant histiocytosis. J Rheumatol *9*:443, 1982.
235. Huhn D, Meister P: Malignant histiocytosis: Morphologic and cytochemical findings. Cancer *42*:1341, 1978.
236. Vanel D, Couanet D, Piekarski JD, et al: Radiological findings in 23 pediatric cases of malignant histiocytosis (MH). Eur J Radiol *3*:60, 1983.

237. Dunnick NR, Parker BR, Warnke RA, et al: Radiographic manifestations of malignant histiocytosis. AJR 127:611, 1976.
238. Griffin JD, Ellman L, Long JC, et al: Development of a histiocytic medullary reticulosis-like syndrome during the course of acute lymphocytic leukemia. Am J Med 64:851, 1978.
239. Karcher DS, Head DR, Mullins JD: Malignant histiocytosis occurring in patients with acute lymphocytic leukemia. Cancer 41:1967, 1978.
240. Zech LA, Gregg RE, Schwartz D, et al: Type III hyperlipoproteinemia: Diagnosis, molecular defects, pathology, and treatment. Ann Intern Med 98:623, 1983.
241. Struthers GR, Scott DL, Bacon PA, et al: Musculoskeletal disorders in patients with hyperlipidaemia. Ann Rheum Dis 42:519, 1983.
242. Inserra S, Einhorn TA, Vigorita VJ, et al: Intraosseous xanthoma associated with hyperlipoproteinemia. A case report. Clin Orthop 187:218, 1984.
243. Palmer AK, Hensinger RN, Costenbader JM, et al: Osteonecrosis of the femoral head in a family with hyperlipoproteinemia. Clin Orthop 155:166, 1981.
244. Lehtonen A, Makela P, Viikari J, et al: Achilles tendon thickness in hypercholesterolaemia. Ann Clin Res 13:39, 1981.
245. Thomas D, Demange J, Hoeffel JC, et al: Mesure xérographique du tendon d'Achille dans l'hypercholestérolémie de type II. J Radiol 63:345, 1982.
246. Nasu T, Tsukahara Y, Terayama K: A lipid metabolic disease—"membranous lipodystrophy." An autopsy case demonstrating numerous peculiar membrane-structures composed of compound lipid in bone and bone marrow and various adipose tissues. Acta Pathol Jpn 23:539, 1973.
247. Akai M, Tateishi A, Cheng CH, et al: Membranous lipodystrophy. A clinico-pathological study of six cases. J Bone Joint Surg [Am] 59:802, 1977.
248. Nasu T: Membranous lipodystrophy. Nichi-Byori-Kaishi 67:57, 1978.
249. Tashiro Y, Koide O, Yatanabe Y, et al: "Membranous lipodystrophy" (NASU) as lipid metabolic disease. Rinsho Seikeigeka 11:614, 1976.
250. Hasegawa Y, Inagaki Y: Membranous lipodystrophy (lipomembranous polycystic osteodysplasia). Two case reports. Clin Orthop 181:229, 1983.
251. Hakola HPA: Neuropsychiatric and genetic aspects of a new hereditary disease characterized by progressive dementia and lipomembranous polycystic osteodysplasia. Acta Psychiatr Scand 232(Suppl):1, 1972.
252. Makela P, Jarvi O, Hakola P, et al: Radiologic bone changes of polycystic lipomembranous osteodysplasia with sclerosing leukoencephalopathy. Skel Radiol 8:51, 1982.
253. Adolfsson R, Forsell A, Johansson G: Hereditary polycystic osteodysplasia with progressive dementia in Sweden. Lancet 1:1209, 1978.
254. Edvardsen P, Halvorsen TB, Nesse O: Lipomembranous osteodysplasia: A case report. Int Orthop (SICOT) 7:99, 1983.
255. Wood C: Membranous lipodystrophy of bone. Arch Pathol Lab Med 102:22, 1978.
256. Bird TD, Koerker RM, Leaird BJ, et al: Lipomembranous polycystic osteodysplasia (brain, bone, and fat disease): A genetic cause of presenile dementia. Neurology 33:81, 1983.
257. Watanabe M, Yanagisawa M, Sonobe S, et al: An adult form of Gaucher's disease with a huge tumour formation of the right tibia. Int Orthop (SICOT) 8:195, 1984.
258. Leeson MC, Smith A, Carter JR, et al: Eosinophilic granuloma of bone in the growing epiphysis. J Pediatr Orthop 5:147, 1985.
259. Capanna R, Springfield DS, Ruggieri P, et al: Direct cortisone injection in eosinophilic granuloma of bone: A preliminary report on 11 patients. J Pediatr Orthop 5:339, 1985.
260. Palmer FJ, Talley NJ: Erdheim-Chester disease with bilateral exophthalmus and liver cell adenoma. Australas Radiol 28:305, 1984.
261. Cozzutto C: Xanthogranulomatous osteomyelitis. Arch Pathol Lab Med 108:973, 1984.
262. Puczynski MS, Demos TC, Suarez CR: Sinus histiocytosis with massive lymphadenopathy: Skeletal involvement. Pediatr Radiol 15:259, 1985.
263. Fink IJ, Lee MA, Gregg RE: Radiographic and CT appearance of intraosseous xanthoma mimicking a malignant lesion. Br J Radiol 58:262, 1985.
264. Mathon G, Gagne C, Brun D, et al: Articular manifestations of familial hypercholesterolaemia. Ann Rheum Dis 44:599, 1985.
265. Fischer E: Morbus Fabry, eine Erkrankung mit Rheumaaspekten: Radiologie der Weichteil-und Knochenveränderungen an der Hand. Z Rheumatol 45:36, 1986.
266. Carey RN, Blotzer JW, Wolfe ID, et al: Multicentric reticulohistiocytosis and Sjögren's syndrome. J Rheumatol 12:1193, 1985.
267. Schlesinger AE, Glass RBJ, Young S, Fernbach SK: Case report 342. Skel Radiol 15:57, 1986.
268. Makley JT, Carter JR: Eosinophilic granuloma of bone. Clin Orthop 204:37, 1986.
269. Rozenberg I, Wechsler J, Koenig F, et al: Erdheim-Chester disease presenting as malignant exophthalmos. Br J Radiol 59:173, 1986.
270. Puczyski MS, Demos TC, Suarez CR: Sinus histiocytosis with massive lymphadenopathy: Skeletal involvement. Pediatr Radiol 15:259, 1985.
271. Chan KW, Chow YYN, Ghadially FN, et al: Rosai-Dorfman disease presenting as spinal tumor. A case report with ultrastructural and immunohistochemical studies. J Bone Joint Surg [Am] 67:1427, 1985.
272. Tabas JH, Daffner RH, Hartsock RJ, et al: Case report 387. Skel Radiol 15:499, 1986.
273. Bell RS, Mankin HJ, Doppelt SH: Osteomyelitis in Gaucher's disease. J Bone Joint Surg [Am] 68:1380, 1986.
274. Canadell J, Villas C, Martinez-Denegri J, et al: Vertebral eosinophilic granuloma. Long-term evolution of a case. Spine 11:767, 1986.
275. Freyschmidt J, Ostertag H, Lang W: Case report 365. Skel Radiol 15:316, 1986.
276. Sartoris DJ, Resnick D: Osseous involvement in sinus histiocytosis with massive lymphadenopathy (Rosai-Dorfman disease). Eur J Pediatr 145:238, 1986.
277. Starer F, Sargent JD, Hobbs JR: Regression of the radiological changes of Gaucher's disease following bone marrow transplantation. Br J Radiol 60:1189, 1987.
278. Hermann G, Wagner LD, Gendal ES, et al: Spinal cord compression in Type I Gaucher disease. Radiology 170:147, 1989.
279. Goldblatt J, Sacks S, Dall D, et al: Total hip arthroplasty in Gaucher's disease. Long-term prognosis. Clin Orthop 228:94, 1988.
280. Wounlund J, Lohmann M: Aseptic necrosis of the capitate secondary to Gaucher's disease: A case report. J Hand Surg [Br] 14:336, 1989.
281. Springfield DS, Landfried M, Mankin HJ: Gaucher hemorrhagic cyst of bone. A case report. J,Bone Joint Surg [Am] 71:141, 1989.
282. Hermann G, Goldblatt J, Levy RN, et al: Gaucher's disease Type I: Assessment of bone involvement by CT and scintigraphy. AJR 147:943, 1986.
283. Israel O, Jerushalmi J, Front D: Scintigraphic findings in Gaucher's disease. J Nucl Med 27:1557, 1986.
284. Zanzi I, Taylor S, Gould E, et al: Scintigraphic and magnetic resonance studies in a patient with Gaucher's disease. Clin Nucl Med 13:491, 1988.
285. Rosenthal DI, Mayo-Smith W, Goodsitt MM, et al: Bone and bone marrow changes in Gaucher disease: Evaluation with quantitative CT. Radiology 170:143, 1989.
286. Vogler JB III, Murphey WA: Bone marrow imaging. Radiology 168:679, 1988.
287. Rosenthal DI, Scott JA, Barranger J, et al: Evaluation of Gaucher disease using magnetic resonance imaging. J Bone Joint Surg [Am] 68:802, 1986.
288. Lanir A, Hadar H, Cohen I, et al: Gaucher disease: Assessment with MR imaging. Radiology 161:239, 1986.
289. Cremin BJ, Davey H, Goldblatt J: Skeletal complications of type I Gaucher disease: The magnetic resonance features. Clin Radiol 41:244, 1990.
290. Omdal R, Laerdal A, Kjellevold KH: Multicentric reticulohistiocytosis in a 9-year-old boy. Arthritis Rheum 31:1588, 1988.
291. Amor B, Kahan A, Laoussadi S, et al: Réticulo-histiocytose multicentrique. Un cas avec asec aspects cliniques, radiologiques et ultrastructuraux inhabituels. Rev Rhum Mal Osteoartic 54:113, 1987.
292. Nakajima Y, Sato K, Morita H, et al: Severe progressive erosive arthritis in multicentric reticulohistiocytosis: Possible involvement of cytokines in synovial proliferation. Arthritis Rheum 19:1643, 1992.
293. Favara BE: Langerhans' cell histiocytosis: Pathobiology and pathogenesis. Semin Oncol 18:3, 1991.
294. Chu T, D'Angio GJ, Favara B, et al: Histiocytosis syndromes in children. Lancet 1:208, 1987.
295. Leiken SL: Immunobiology of histiocytosis X. Hematol Oncol Clin North Am 1:49, 1987.
296. Stull MA, Kransdorf MJ, Devaney KO: Langerhans cell histiocytosis of bone. RadioGraphics 12:801, 1992.
297. Dimentberg RA, Brown KLB: Diagnostic evaluation of patients with histiocytosis X. J Pediatr Orthop 10:733, 1990.
298. Gabaudan P, Troussier B, Saragaglia D, et al: Granulome éosnophile à localsation osseouse claviculaire et sous-cutanée. Rev Rhum Mal Osteoartic 57:899, 1990.
299. David R, Oria RA, Kumar R, et al: Radiologic features of eosinophilic granuloma of bone. AJR 153:1021, 1989.
300. Mayo-Smith W, Rosenthal DI, Kattapuram SV, et al: Case report 542. Skel Radiol 18:245, 1989.
301. Thijn CJP, Martijn A, Postma A, et al: Case report 615. Skel Radiol 19:309, 1990.
302. Shenouda NF, Azouz EM: Case report 702. Skel Radiol 20:620, 1991.
303. Robert H, Dubousset J, Miladi L: Histiocytosis X in the juvenile spine. Spine 12:167, 1987.
304. Baber WW, Numaguchi Y, Nadell JM, et al: Eosinophilic granuloma of the cervical spine without vertebrae plana. J Comput Tomogr 11:346, 1987.
305. Adler C-P, Schaefer HE: Case report 508. Skel Radiol 17:531, 1988.
306. De Camargo OP, Oliveira NRB, Andrade JS, et al: Eosinophilic granuloma of the ischium: Long-term evaluation of a patient treated with steroids. A case report. J Bone Joint Surg [Am] 74:445, 1992.
307. Schaub T, Ash JM, Gilday DL: Radionuclide imaging in histiocytosis X. Pediatr Radiol 17:397, 1987.
308. Hayes CW, Conway WF, Sundaram M: Misleading aggressive MR imaging appearance of some benign musculoskeletal lesions. RadioGraphics 12:1119, 1992.
309. Daffner RH: Invited commentary. RadioGraphics 12:1135, 1992.
310. Haggstrom JA, Brown JC, Marsh PW: Eosinophilic granuloma of the spine: MR demonstration. J Comput Assist Tomogr 12:344, 1988.
311. Miller RL, Sheeler LR, Bauer TW, et al: Erdheim-Chester disease. Case report and review of the literature. Am J Med 80:1230, 1986.
312. Molnar CP, Gottschalk R, Gallagher B, et al: Lipid granulomatosis: Erdheim-Chester disease. Clin Nucl Med 13:736, 1988.
313. Lantz B, Lange TA, Heiner J, et al: Erdheim-Chester disease. A report of three cases. J Bone Joint Surg [Am] 71:456, 1989.
314. Brown R, van den Berg R, Hurst NP, et al: Erdheim-Chester disease associated with hydrocalycosis and arthropathy. Arthritis Rheum 31:1215, 1988.
315. Strouse PJ, Ellis BI, Shifrin LZ, et al: Case report 710. Skel Radiol 21:64, 1992.

316. Waite RJ, Doherty PW, Liepman M, et al: Langerhans cell histiocytosis with the radiographic findings of Erdheim-Chester disease. AJR *150*:869, 1988.
317. Unni KK: Case report 457. Skel Radiol *17*:129, 1988.
318. Miettinen M, Paljakka P, Haveri P, et al: Sinus histiocytosis with massive lymphadenopathy. A nodal and extranodal proliferation of S-100 protein positive histiocytes? Am J Clin Pathol *88*:270, 1987.
319. Foucar E, Rosai J, Dorfman R: Sinus histiocytosis with massive lymphadenopathy (Rosai-Dorfman disease): Review of the entity. Semin Diagn Pathol *7*:19, 1990.
320. Yokoyama K, Shinohara N, Wada K: Osseous xanthomatosis and a pathologic fracture in a patient with hyperlipidemia. A case report. Clin Orthop *236*:307, 1988.
321. Blei CL, Nirschl RP, Grant EG: Achilles tendon: US diagnosis of pathologic conditions. Work in progress. Radiology *159*:765, 1986.
322. Fornage BD: Achilles tendon: US examination. Radiology *159*:759, 1986.
323. Burnstein M, Buckwalter KA, Martel W, et al: Case report 427. Skel Radiol *16*:346, 1987.
324. Kenan S, Abdelwahab IF, Klein MJ, et al: Case report 754. Skel Radiol *21*:471, 1992.
325. Liem MSL, Leuven JAG, Bloem JL, et al: Magnetic resonance imaging of Achilles tendon xanthomas in familial hypercholesterolemia. Skel Radiol *21*:453, 1992.
326. Hertzanu Y, Berginer J, Berginer VM: Computed tomography of tendinous xanthomata in cerebrotendinous xanthomatosis. Skel Radiol *20*:99, 1991.
327. Wysenbeek AJ, Shani E, Beigel Y: Musculoskeletal manifestations in patients with hypercholesterolemia. J Rheumatol *16*:643, 1989.
328. Rimon D, Cohen L: Hypercholesterolemic (Type II hyperlipoproteinemic) arthritis. J Rheumatol *16*:703, 1989.
329. Berginer VM, Salen G, Shefer S: Cerebrotendinous xanthomatosis. Neurologic Clin *7*:55, 1989.
330. Sukenik S, Horowitz J, Berginer VM: Joint hypermobility in patients with cerebrotendinous xanthomatosis. J Rheumatol *16*:1611, 1989.
331. Araki T, Ohba H, Monzawa S, et al: Membranous lipodystrophy: MR imaging appearance of the brain. Radiology *180*:793, 1991.
332. Pazzaglia UE, Benazzo F, Byers PD, et al: Pathogenesis of membranous lipodystrophy. Case report and review of the literature. Clin Orthop *225*:279, 1987.
333. Plant GR, Hansell DM, Gibberd FB, et al: Skeletal abnormalities in Refsum's disease (heredopathia atactica polyneuritiformis). Br J Radiol *63*:537, 1990.
334. Rosenthal DI, Barton NW, McKusick KA, et al: Quantitative imaging of Gaucher disease. Radiology *185*:841, 1992.
335. Katz K, Mechlis-Frish S, Cohen IJ, et al: Bone scans in the diagnosis of bone crisis in patients who have Gaucher disease. J Bone Joint Surg [Am] *73*:513, 1991.
336. Bilchik TR, Heyman S: Skeletal scintigraphy of pseudo-osteomyelitis in Gaucher's disease. Clin Nucl Med *17*:279, 1992.
337. Horev G, Kornreich L, Hadar H, et al: Hemorrhage associated with "bone crisis" in Gaucher's disease identified by magnetic resonance imaging. Skel Radiol *20*:479, 1991.
338. Johnson LA, Hoppel BE, Gerard EL, et al: Quantitative chemical shift imaging of vertebral bone marrow in patients with Gaucher disease. Radiology *182*:451, 1992.
339. Hermann G, Shapiro R, Abdelwahab IF, et al: MR imaging in adults with Gaucher disease type I: Evaluation of marrow involvement and disease activity. Skel Radiol *22*:247, 1993.
340. Bisagni-Faure A, Dupont A-M, Chazerain P, et al: Magnetic resonance imaging assessment of sacroiliac joint involvement in Gaucher's disease. J Rheumatol *19*:1984, 1992.
341. DeCandido P, Resnik CS, Aisner SC: Case report 792. Skel Radiol *22*:371, 1993.
342. Johnson S, Klostermeier T, Weinstein A: Case report 768. Skel Radiol *22*:63, 1993.
343. De Schepper AMA, Ramon F, Van Marck E: MR imaging of eosinophilic granuloma: Report of 11 cases. Skel Radiol *22*:163, 1993.
344. Beltran J, Aparisi F, Bonmati LM, et al: Eosinophilic granuloma: MRI manifestations. Skel Radiol *22*:157, 1993.
345. Tomita T, Ochi T, Fushimi H, et al: Reconstruction of the Achilles tendon for xanthoma: Findings at operative re-exploration. A case report. J Bone Joint Surg [Am] *76*:444, 1994.
346. Bude RO, Adler RS, Bassett DR, et al: Heterozygous familial hypercholesterolemia: Detection of xanthomas in the Achilles tendon with US. Radiology *188*:567, 1993.
347. Bude RO, Adler RS, Bassett DR: Diagnosis of Achilles tendon xanthoma in patients with heterozygous familial hypercholesterolemia: MR vs sonography. AJR *162*:913, 1994.
348. Hermann G, Shapiro R, Abdelwahab IF, et al: Extraosseous extension of Gaucher cell deposits mimicking malignancy. Skeletal Radiol *23*:253, 1994.

62

Myeloproliferative Disorders

Donald Resnick, M.D., and Parviz Haghighi, M.D.

Certain myeloproliferative disorders are associated with definite skeletal manifestations, which at times can constitute an initial or dominant part of the entire clinical picture. In some instances, articular symptoms and signs are the result of intra- or periarticular abnormalities related to the primary disease process; in other instances, the metabolic consequences of the primary disease are responsible for these clinical findings. In this chapter, attention will be directed toward skeletal alterations in leukemias, lymphomas, Sjögren's syndrome, systemic mastocytosis (urticaria pigmentosa), polycythemia vera, and myelofibrosis.

LEUKEMIAS

General Features

The leukemias represent diffuse lesions of the bone marrow and, as such, produce osseous changes in almost all cases. These changes generally can be recognized during careful postmortem examination, although they may not be detectable on antemortem radiographs. The more significant bony abnormalities are associated with the more aggressive varieties of leukemias and with the younger age groups.

It is convenient to divide the leukemias into acute and chronic forms (Table 62–1). Acute leukemias are accompanied by the accumulation of immature, or blast, cells owing to a defect in the production of mature hemic cells; chronic leukemias are accompanied by a massive overgrowth of mature cells.[293] Although the different types of granulocytes and their precursors can readily be distinguished morphologically, functionally distinct subpopulations of lymphocytes and lymphoid precursors cannot be

TABLE 62–1. Skeletal Alterations in the Leukemias*

	Acute Childhood Leukemia	Acute Adult Leukemia	Chronic Leukemia
Osteopenia	+ +	+ +	+
Metaphyseal abnormalities	+ +	+	–
Osteolysis	+ +	+ +	+
Periostitis	+ +	+	+
Osteosclerosis	+	+	+
Articular abnormalities	+ +	+	+

*+ +, Common; +, uncommon; –, absent.

separated in this fashion. Rather, the determination of phenotypes of lymphoid and myeloid cells can be accomplished using monoclonal antibodies that generally are directed against surface membrane proteins.[299] Two broad populations of lymphocytes involved in the immune response can be identified: thymus-derived lymphocytes (T cells), which require the thymus for normal differentiation; and bone marrow–derived lymphocytes (B cells), which undergo initial differentiation in the bone marrow.[300] Thus, leukemias can be classified not only on the basis of the acute or chronic nature of the disorder but also on their predominant cellular morphology and their T cell or B cell constituency.

Acute leukemia can affect both children and adults. In children, acute leukemia almost always is lymphoblastic in cell origin, and the survival time is limited to approximately 1 year; in adults, acute leukemia frequently is myeloid in cell origin.[1] Chronic leukemia may be granulocytic or lymphocytic; chronic lymphocytic leukemia is closely related to lymphosarcoma. The chronic types of leukemia have a peak age of onset of 35 to 55 years and an average survival time of approximately 3 years.[2]

The general clinical manifestations of the leukemias are a consequence of the distribution of abnormal cells in the various organs and tissues of the body.[294] Anemia, neutropenia, and thrombocytopenia result from suppression of normal hematopoiesis by the proliferation of leukemic cells in the bone marrow and lead to bleeding episodes and recurrent infections. Increased cellular breakdown accompanies leukemic cell production in the bone marrow; gout and renal failure occur owing to increased production of uric acid by the catabolism of nucleic acids. As leukemic cells accumulate and expand in the confined space of the marrow cavity, bone pain, fractures and osteonecrosis are encountered.[294] Marked leukocytosis causes hyperviscosity of blood with resultant neurologic and cardiac complications.

Acute Childhood Leukemia

Acute leukemia represents the commonest form of childhood malignancy. Acute leukemia in children is a disease of the first few years of life, the peak prevalence occurring between 2 and 5 years of age. Approximately 80 per cent of cases are lymphoblastic in origin, 10 per cent are myeloblastic, and 10 per cent are of other cellular origin.[157] The early manifestations of acute leukemia are extremely variable.[1–5] In some children, acute leukemia has a paucity

of clinical signs, but this is more typical of acute myeloblastic leukemia than of acute lymphoblastic leukemia, in which numerous clinical findings may be encountered, including lymphadenopathy and splenomegaly. Bone and joint pain, tenderness, and swelling, common findings in children with leukemia, may cause confusion with rheumatic fever, juvenile chronic polyarthritis, or osteomyelitis.[279] Arthralgias and arthritis are common, having been reported in 12 to 65 per cent of patients.[6–14] These joint manifestations frequently are symmetric in distribution, with predilection for the large joints of the appendicular skeleton, although small joints also may be involved. They are attributable to hemorrhage or to leukemic masses in metaphyseal periosteum, subarticular bone, and synovium. The disappearance of joint complaints is recognized as an early indication of improvement after therapy with antileukemic agents.[12]

Radiographic changes in the skeleton are frequent in acute leukemia. The reported frequency of these changes has varied from 50 to 70 per cent in most series.[1, 15–17] Higher[3, 12, 18] and lower[19, 20] rates of occurrence occasionally are noted. Several radiographic findings may be observed.

Diffuse Osteopenia (15 to 100 Per Cent). Diffuse decrease in radiodensity of the skeleton may result from an alteration in mineral metabolism (i.e., parathyroid hormone abnormalities) or from leukemic infiltration of the bone marrow.[3, 4, 12, 295] Medullary widening and cortical thinning in tubular bones and vertebral compression are encountered.[21, 295, 296] Osteopenia may progress slowly without treatment or improve with therapy. Osteopenia occurring in leukemic patients who are being treated with steroids can be related to this therapeutic technique.

Although other radiographic findings are more specific, the occurrence of unexplained generalized osteopenia in a child should initiate a search for clinical and laboratory manifestations of leukemia.

Radiolucent and Radiodense Metaphyseal Bands (10 to 55 Per Cent) (Fig. 62–1). Symmetric metaphyseal bandlike radiolucent areas are observed in leukemia and other chronic childhood illnesses. This nonspecific finding probably reflects a nutritional deficit that interferes with proper osteogenesis. As a consequence, it most commonly is seen at sites of rapid bone growth, including the distal femur, the proximal tibia, the proximal humerus, and the distal radius. After the age of 2 years, radiolucent metaphyseal bands are more characteristic of leukemia than of these other conditions.[17] Histologically, the radiolucent lesions of the metaphysis are not associated with leukemic cell infiltration. Osseous weakening at radiolucent zones in the metaphysis can lead to fracture or epiphyseal separation and displacement.[4, 12] These findings are most common at the capital femoral and proximal humeral epiphyses, although they are observed elsewhere as well, such as about the knees, wrists, and ankles. Insufficiency fractures between the metaphyseal and diaphyseal segments of the tubular bones are distinctive.[297] Epiphyseal destruction may be an associated finding.[22]

Radiodense metaphyseal bands may be noted adjacent to the areas of increased radiolucency.[3–5, 16] In some cases, the entire metaphysis is radiodense. Abnormally large and coarse trabeculae with areas of unresorbed calcified cartilaginous matrix are evident on histologic examination, reflecting altered osteogenesis. Parallel radiodense growth re-

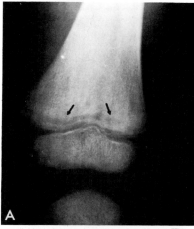

FIGURE 62–1. Acute childhood leukemia: Metaphyseal abnormalities.

A Observe a transverse band of radiolucency (arrows) in the metaphysis of the distal end of the femur. Adjacent minimal sclerosis and epiphyseal radiolucency are evident.

B, C A 10 year old boy with acute leukemia. The initial film **(B)** indicated a lytic lesion in the medial metaphysis of the proximal portion of the humerus (arrow). This appearance can be simulated by a normal developmental irregularity of the humerus. Six weeks later **(C)** further lysis has developed in the metaphysis (arrow), and diaphyseal periostitis is observed (arrowhead).

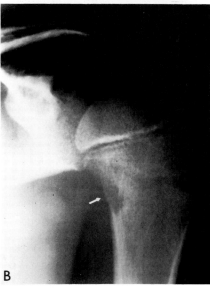

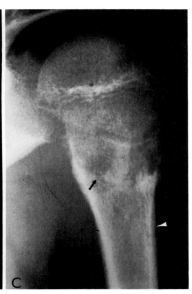

covery lines (of Harris) presumably are related to alternating periods of arrest and acceleration of bone growth. They may be observed in 50 per cent of children with leukemia.[3]

Transverse radiolucent bands also may be observed under the vertebral endplates.[23, 24] Growth disturbances in the spine may lead to platyspondyly, brachyspondyly, and wedge-shaped vertebrae.[25, 26]

Osteolytic Lesions (30 to 50 Per Cent) (Figs. 62–2 and 62–3). Multiple (or solitary) radiolucent lesions related to bone destruction are encountered in tubular and flat bones.[146] In the long bones of the extremities, radiolucent lesions of a metaphysis can extend into the diaphysis. Similar lesions are seen in the cranial vault, pelvis, ribs, and shoulder girdle. The medial cortex of the proximal portion of the humerus is a characteristic site of involvement.[164] Larger areas of bone destruction may represent a combination of leukemic infiltration in the bone marrow, hemorrhage, and osteonecrosis.[4, 165]

Periostitis (10 to 35 Per Cent) (Figs. 62–2 and 62–3). Periosteal bone formation can be associated with lytic lesions. Proliferating leukemic cells in the marrow invade the cortex via haversian canals and extend to subperiosteal locations, causing elevation of the periosteal membrane.[4,]

[16, 27–29] Subperiosteal hemorrhage may be an associated finding. Periostitis is particularly prominent in the long bones, although it may occur elsewhere. Single or multiple areas of involvement may be found.[5] Prominent symmetric periosteal new bone deposition in the tubular bones, evident in some leukemic children, simulates the appearance of secondary hypertrophic osteoarthropathy, syphilis, prostaglandin-induced periostitis, and other conditions.

Osteosclerosis (5 to 10 Per Cent). Osteosclerosis is a relatively infrequent finding in leukemia.[3, 5, 16] When apparent, it is particularly prominent in the metaphyses of long bones. Reactive bone formation in response to leukemic cell infiltration and infarction may be responsible for such sclerosis.

Other Skeletal Abnormalities. Sutural diastasis is common in infants and children with leukemia[5] (Fig. 62–4). It is produced by an increase in intracranial pressure due to leukemic cell infiltration of the meninges or cerebrum or to intracerebral hemorrhage. In older patients, sutural separations rarely is present except after chronic chemotherapy.[30]

Chloromas are greenish tumorous collections (see later discussion) that are observed in childhood myelogenous leukemia.[31, 280] They can be seen in acute or chronic varieties of the disease. Expansile lytic lesions with periostitis

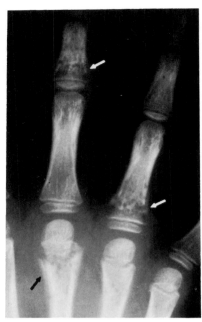

FIGURE 62–2. Acute childhood leukemia: Dactylitis. Soft tissue swelling, lytic foci, and periosteal bone formation are observed in the metacarpals, metatarsals, and phalanges (arrows).

are apparent in the long bones, calvarium, and periorbital tissues.

Course of the Skeletal Lesions. There is poor correlation between the extent of bone lesions and the progress of leukemia.[265, 266] During treatment, resolution of lytic defects is observed.[32] The disappearance of lucent metaphyseal bands during remission also has been noted[33] and may be associated with transient metaphyseal sclerosis.[32] Skeletal lesions may[34, 35] or may not[32, 36] reappear during relapse.

As the degree of osseous involvement has little influence on the prognosis of the disease and the response of bone lesions to therapy is highly variable, routine imaging studies during the course of acute childhood leukemia generally are not recommended. Such studies are more appropriately reserved for the evaluation of new or changing symptoms and signs that may indicate important complications, such as infection or fracture. Early reports of the role of MR imaging (Fig. 62–5) in the initial assessment of patients with leukemia and its subsequent response to therapy contained inconclusive data,[267, 287, 288] although the results of later investigations have been more promising (see later discussion).

Articular Abnormalities. The joint manifestations of acute leukemia that can lead to significant clinical findings are due to intra-articular leukemic cell infiltration and hemorrhage[12–14, 158–161, 278] and more commonly to periarticular bone lesions. Soft tissue swelling, effusion, and juxta-articular osteoporosis occasionally are seen.[10] Joint effusions are mildly inflammatory in character. The identification of leukemic involvement of the joint requires synovial biopsy, which reveals leukemic infiltration in the synovial membrane, or analysis of the synovial fluid using indirect immunofluorescence techniques and a panel of antibodies against leukemia-associated antigens.[161] These methods provide direct evidence that the tumor itself has involved the joint; indirect evidence of this phenomenon is the improve-

ment in or the disappearance of articular symptoms and signs after the initiation of chemotherapy.[160]

Patients with acute leukemia often develop hyperuricemia, and a few patients may reveal findings of secondary gout. This complication appears more frequent in chronic leukemia.[37, 38] On rare occasions, calcium pyrophosphate dihydrate crystals have been identified in the symptomatic joints of patients with acute leukemia.[159]

Epiphyseal osteonecrosis may occur in some patients, particularly those treated with steroid medication.[39, 298] It also has been documented in leukemic patients prior to such therapy,[162] leading to early onset of symptoms. In such cases, potential mechanisms include leukemic infiltration in the bone marrow or walls of the blood vessels and hyperviscosity of the blood. Bone marrow necrosis preceding the development of acute childhood leukemia also has been described.[163] Osteonecrosis occurring in association with leukemia typically affects the femoral epiphyses and condyles and the proximal portion of the humerus.

Septic arthritis and osteomyelitis can complicate the acute leukemias both in children and in adults.[152, 268]

Differential Diagnosis. The skeletal lesions of acute leukemia are similar to those in other disease processes. Metaphyseal radiolucency is a nonspecific finding that also may be encountered in systemic childhood illnesses, including transplacental infections (toxoplasmosis, rubella, cytome-

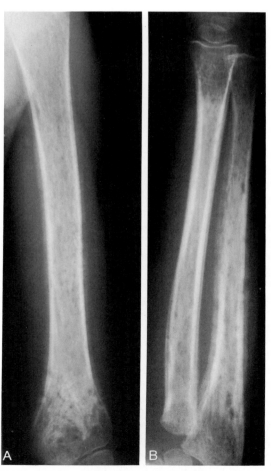

FIGURE 62–3. Acute childhood leukemia: Osteolysis and periostitis. Observe diffuse small osteolytic lesions in the humerus, radius, and ulna. Periostitis is apparent.

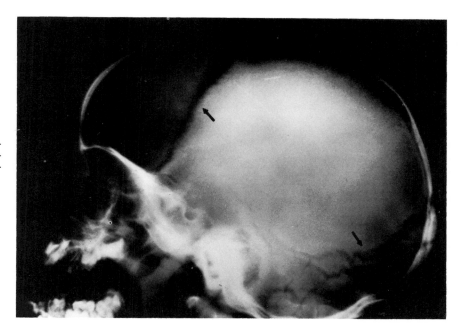

FIGURE 62–4. Acute childhood leukemia: Sutural diastasis. In an infant with leukemia, observe widening of the sutures in both the frontal and the occipital regions (arrows).

galic inclusion disease, herpes, syphilis), scurvy, juvenile chronic polyarthritis, healing rickets, and neuroblastoma. The last-mentioned disorder is associated with many of the radiographic findings that are seen in acute leukemia, including widespread osteolytic lesions and periostitis (Fig. 62–6). Similar findings also are observed in sickle cell anemia, skeletal metastasis (especially from retinoblastoma and embyronal rhabdomyosarcoma), infection, and syphilis (Fig. 62–6).

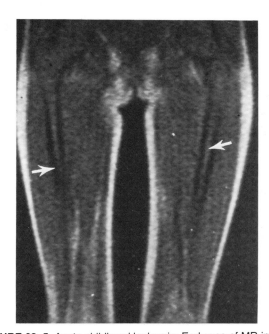

FIGURE 62–5. Acute childhood leukemia: Early use of MR imaging. A coronal T1-weighted (TR/TE,500/30) spin echo MR image of the femora in a 12 year old girl with leukemia shows a decrease in signal intensity from the bone marrow (arrows) consistent with fatty replacement by tumor cells. (From Cohen MD, et al: Radiology *151*:715, 1984.)

Acute Adult Leukemia

As a general rule, clinical and radiologic evidence of skeletal involvement in leukemia is less common in adults than in children. Acute leukemia in adults may be associated with bone pain and tenderness, however.[1, 394] Thomas and coworkers[12] reported that 5 per cent of such patients had bone pain initially and 50 per cent had this symptom sometime during their illness. Skeletal pain and tenderness are most frequent in the vertebral column and ribs. Articular symptoms and signs are less frequent than in children with acute leukemia.[278, 281] Adults with acute leukemia, however, may initially have articular findings simulating those of rheumatoid arthritis,[301] and proliferative synovitis may be documented on histologic analysis.[302]

The radiographic features in the skeleton in acute adult leukemia are diffuse osteopenia, discrete osteolytic lesions, and metaphyseal radiolucency. Diffuse osteopenia is a nonspecific finding simulating osteoporosis and other metabolic disorders. Lytic lesions (50 to 60 per cent) may be evident in the skull, pelvis, and proximal long bones.[1] Metaphyseal radiolucent bands (7 per cent) are not so frequent as in children with acute leukemia. Rare radiologic findings are large destructive lesions, periostitis, acro-osteolysis, discrete subperiosteal erosions, and focal or diffuse osteosclerosis.[303, 304]

The pathologic aberrations in the skeleton include medullary and subperiosteal leukemic infiltration with cortical destruction.

Chronic Leukemia

The osseous and articular manifestations of chronic leukemia are less common and less severe than those of acute leukemia. Marrow hyperplasia in some patients may become evident as nonspecific diffuse osteopenia, particularly in the axial skeleton.[150] Discrete osteolytic lesions are observed in fewer than 3 per cent of persons,[40, 167, 168] particularly in the femur and the humerus (Fig. 62–7). The lesions

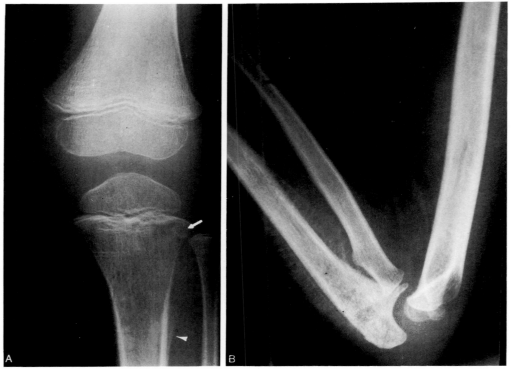

FIGURE 62–6. Differential diagnosis of acute childhood leukemia.

A Neuroblastoma. In this 3 year old boy with neuroblastoma and knee pain, observe metaphyseal radiolucency and destruction (arrow) and lytic lesions of the tibial diaphysis with periostitis (arrowhead).

B Retinoblastoma. A 3½ year old black girl with a retinoblastoma that required enucleation at age 2 years, who had had increasing pain in the right forearm for 3 to 4 months. Extensive bone lysis and periostitis are apparent in the proximal portion of the ulna.

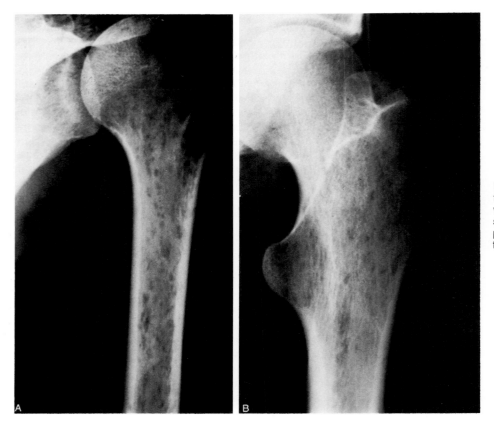

FIGURE 62–7. Chronic leukemia: Osteolytic lesions. A 27 year old woman with chronic leukemia demonstrates small focal radiolucent lesions of the proximal portions of the humerus and femur.

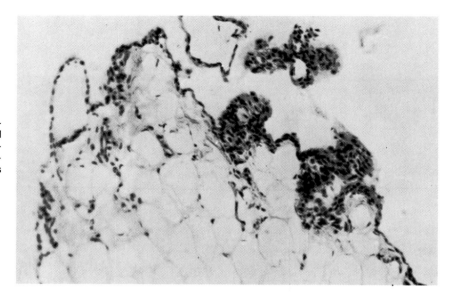

FIGURE 62–8. Chronic leukemia: Articular abnormalities. A photomicrograph of the synovial membrane in an adult patient with leukemia reveals clusters of myeloblasts infiltrating the synovium. (From Spilberg I, Meyer GJ: Arthritis Rheum *15*:630, 1972.)

are composed of myelocytes and histiocytes laden with foamy inclusions,[1] cells that are identical to Gaucher's cells.[41] Occasionally, larger and more aggressive lesions may be encountered.[42] Rarely, widespread or multifocal bone sclerosis is evident, perhaps related to diffuse marrow fibrosis.[166] Soft tissue accumulation of masses of leukemic cells (chloromas) can produce subjacent osseous erosion.

In adults (and in children), leukemic involvement of the small bones of the hand may be associated with soft tissue edema, clubbing, and bone destruction. This combination of findings is termed leukemic acropachy.[43, 44] Usually, metacarpal involvement is more frequent than phalangeal involvement, but in leukemic acropachy, symmetric destruction of terminal phalanges can occur in association with soft tissue masses.

Both the clinical and the radiographic manifestations of skeletal involvement in chronic leukemias can become more prominent during a blast crisis, in which large numbers of myeloblasts appear in the marrow and peripheral blood, and in which a downhill clinical course is characterized by anemia, myelofibrosis, and ultimately death.[151]

Articular findings in chronic leukemia have received little attention.[6, 10, 13] Spilberg and Meyer[10] noted arthritis related to the primary disease in 12 per cent of 62 patients with chronic leukemia. Polyarticular involvement is more frequent than monoarticular involvement. In some patients, joint alterations are migratory in type; in others, they are additive or involve multiple joints simultaneously. Clinical findings are commonly a late manifestation of the disease and show a predilection for the knees, the shoulders, and the ankles. Sternal pain and tenderness are common.[45] Radiographic findings are limited. Osteopenia and soft tissue swelling may be evident. Epiphyseal osteonecrosis has been described, usually, but not invariably,[305] related to steroid administration. As in acute leukemia, leukemic cellular infiltration of the synovium may be seen[10, 169, 306] (Fig. 62–8).

Secondary gout is a well known complication of chronic leukemia.[37, 38, 46, 47] Septic arthritis and osteomyelitis also may be evident (Fig. 62–9). Gallium scanning may be useful in detecting osseous (and extraosseous) sites of infection in patients with leukemia.[282]

Special Types of Leukemia

Hairy Cell Leukemia. Hairy cell leukemia, which also is termed leukemic reticuloendotheliosis, was first recognized in 1958 by Bouroncle and collaborators.[170] It appears to be a distinct entity, belonging to the lymphoproliferative diseases, and is responsible for approximately 2 per cent of all cases of leukemia.[171] Its name originated from the observations in 1966 of Schrek and Donnelly,[172] who described numerous short villi, resembling hairs, about the membrane of the lymphocytes (Fig. 62–10). The major clinical consequences of the disease relate to depressed bone marrow function and hypersplenism.[173]

Hairy cell leukemia typically develops in adults in the fourth, fifth, and sixth decades of life. Men are affected more commonly than women in a ratio of approximately 3 to 1. An insidious onset is characterized by fatigue, weakness, infectious episodes, abdominal pain (or, more rarely, hemorrhage), splenic rupture, and a pathologic fracture of bone.[174] Splenomegaly, hepatomegaly, and lymphadenopathy are present, in order of decreasing frequency. The disease is slowly progressive, but most patients die in the first 5 years. The most frequent complication and primary source of morbidity and mortality is infection, which commonly is related to unusual organisms.

Bone involvement is an infrequent feature of hairy cell leukemia.[175–177, 307, 308] When present, such involvement can lead to early and prominent clinical manifestations, especially pain. Solitary or, less commonly, multiple (usually two) osteolytic lesions are typical, with predilection for the spine and proximal portion of the femora (head and neck). Bone sclerosis is rare. Spontaneous fracture is a recognized complication of such lesions. Infrequent manifestations are osteoporosis and ischemic necrosis of the femoral head.[176] Radionuclide studies using technetium agents or gallium show exaggerated uptake of the radiopharmaceutical agent at the osseous sites of involvement.[177] Histologic examination of the bone documents infiltration with the abnormal leukemic cells.[176, 177] Radiation therapy and chemotherapy can lead to a decrease in symptoms and regression of the osteolytic process.[177]

Articular manifestations of hairy cell leukemia are ex-

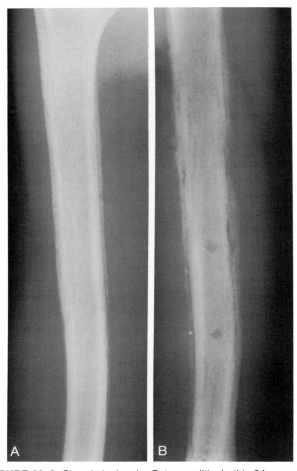

FIGURE 62–9. Chronic leukemia: Osteomyelitis. In this 34 year old woman, osteomyelitis due to Salmonella infection occurred in the humerus. As depicted in these radiographs obtained 2 weeks apart, findings include poorly defined osteolysis in the diaphysis associated with periostitis, abnormalities seen in uncomplicated leukemia as well. A biopsy of bone was undertaken in the interval between the two studies, explaining the circular osteolytic defects seen in **B.** Salmonella organisms were recovered from the biopsy material.

tremely rare.[178] Episodic, nonerosive, asymmetric arthropathy is associated with hairy cells in the synovial fluid.

Acute Megakaryoblastic Leukemia. This rare disorder, also termed malignant myelofibrosis, was described in 1963 by Lewis and Szur.[179] Both children and adults are affected, with an acute onset of symptoms and signs and a progressive course characterized by anemia, pancytopenia, and diffuse marrow fibrosis. Splenomegaly is absent or of mild degree. The proliferating cells in the bone marrow are variable in type, immature, and dominated by megakaryocytes.[180, 181]

In children, radiolucency in the metaphyseal regions of tubular bones and osteolytic lesions are seen. The degree of periosteal bone formation in both the appendicular and the axial skeleton can be profound.[182] In adults, focal or diffuse bone sclerosis is observed, which resembles the findings of myeloid metaplasia or skeletal metastatis.[183]

Granulocytic Sarcoma (Chloroma). Granulocytic sarcoma represents a localized tumor mass composed of immature cells of the granulocyte series. Its designation as chloroma stems from the frequently observed greenish color of the tumor, a phenomenon related to the presence of myeloperoxidase (verdoperoxidase) in the tumor cells.[184] Granulocytic sarcoma most commonly is associated with acute leukemia of the myeloid type, especially in children, although it also is observed in adults (Fig. 62–11) and in patients with additional varieties of leukemia, with other myeloproliferative disorders, or without obvious bone marrow dysfunction.[185–191, 269, 270] When accompanied by a myeloproliferative disorder, chloromas are associated with blast crisis; when occurring in the absence of a known disease, chloromas typically are followed in a period of months by acute leukemia.[184]

Granulocytic sarcomas are more common in children than in adults and may be single or multiple.[280] Frequent sites of involvement are bone, periosteum, soft tissue, orbit, lymph node, and skin.[184, 270, 309, 395] Lytic lesions characterize intraosseous involvement, which is especially prominent in the skull, spine, ribs, long tubular bones, and sternum.[157, 310, 311] Soft tissue tumors can lead to masses, as in a paraspinal location, that subsequently may erode the neighboring bone and lead to neurologic manifestations.

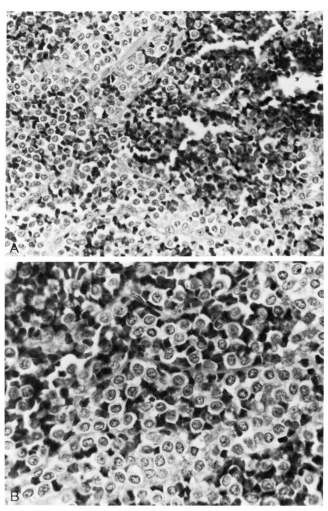

FIGURE 62–10. Hairy cell leukemia: Histologic abnormalities (spleen). Note the typical admixture of erythocytes and neoplastic cells, the latter being uniform, with fine, vesicular, generally round nuclei and clear cytoplasm, creating the so-called fried-egg appearance. (Hematoxylin and eosin stain, 100×, 160×.)

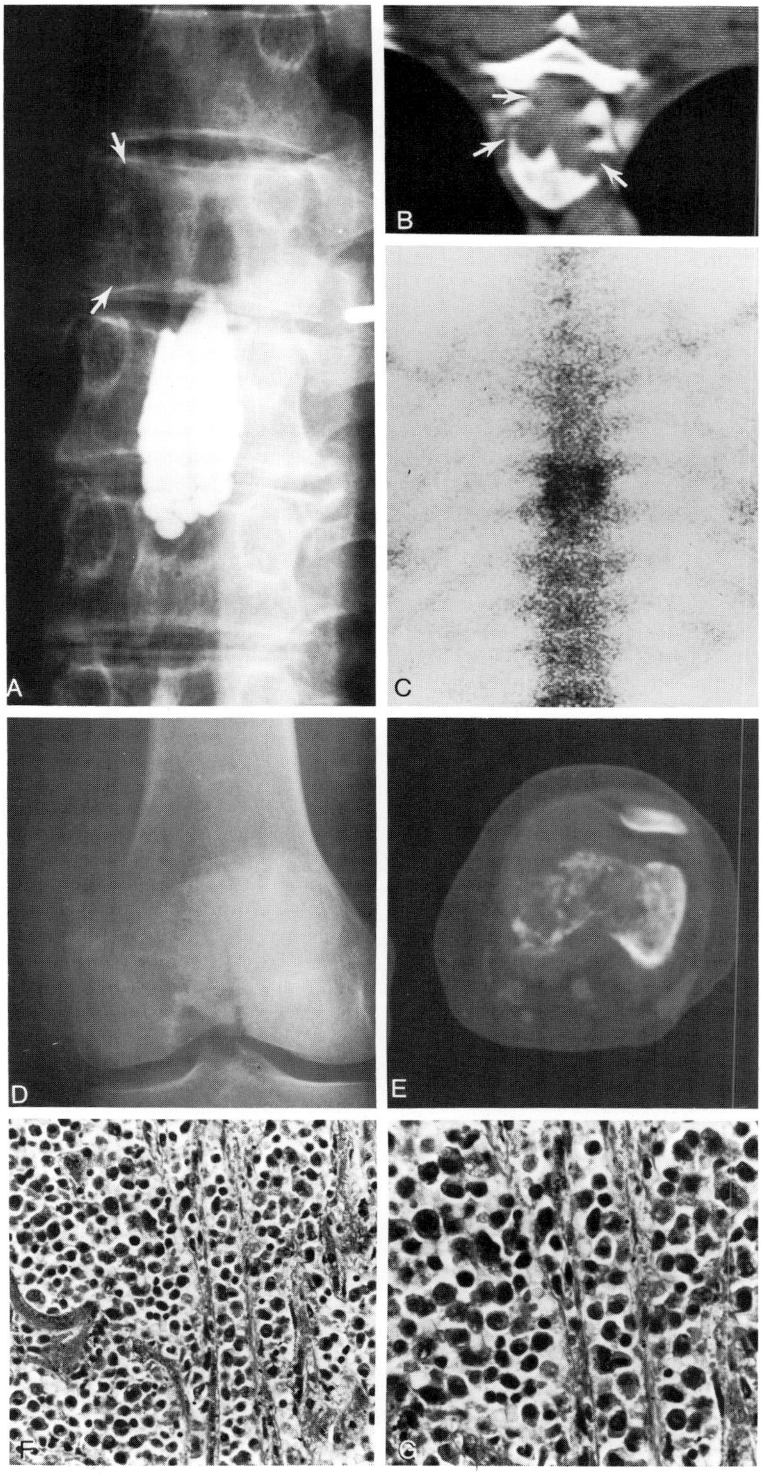

FIGURE 62–11. Granulocytic sarcoma (chloroma).

A–C A 50 year old man with chronic myelogenous leukemia developed the acute onset of upper thoracic pain. A frontal radiograph of the thoracic spine after a myelogram **(A)** reveals osteolysis in a midthoracic vertebral body and destruction of a pedicle (arrows). A partial obstruction to the flow of the contrast material is evident. In **B,** a transaxial CT scan (obtained with the patient in the prone position) shows the degree of bone destruction and intraspinal extension (arrows). Accumulation of the bone-seeking radiopharmaceutical agent is evident **(C).** Biopsy of the lesion, accomplished with CT monitoring, revealed findings consistent with granulocytic sarcoma.

D, E In this 61 year old woman with chronic myelogenous leukemia, a routine radiograph **(D)** and transaxial CT scan **(E)** show an osteolytic lesion with a soft tissue mass, which, on biopsy, was found to be a granulocytic sarcoma.

F, G In a third patient, the liver sinusoids are engorged with premature white blood cells. (Hematoxylin and eosin stain, 100×, 160×.)

(D, E, Courtesy of G. Greenway, M.D., Dallas, Texas.)

The histologic characteristics of granulocytic sarcoma include cellular proliferation that can be well differentiated or poorly differentiated. The morphologic features of the abnormal cells are highly variable, although granulocytic cells predominate, and, in some cases, can lead to a mistaken diagnosis of lymphoma.[184] Special staining procedures and electron microscopy aid in correct histologic interpretation.[184, 192, 283]

Magnetic Resonance Imaging

Broad applications of MR imaging to the analysis of musculoskeletal involvement in patients with leukemia include determination of the extent of alterations in the bone marrow prior to the initiation of therapy, assessment of the response of the disease to such therapy, detection of some of the skeletal complications of the disease or therapeutic regimen, and investigation of some special forms of leukemia, such as hairy cell leukemia and granulocytic sarcoma. Despite the nonspecific nature of many of the MR imaging findings in leukemia (as well as other disorders of the bone marrow) and the general absence of data regarding the clinical relevance or impact of such findings,[312] MR imaging does provide certain advantages over other diagnostic techniques and methods in the assessment of the bone marrow. As an example, although CT allows such assessment owing to the attenuation of the x-ray beam by both normal and abnormal constituents of the marrow, absolute attenuation of Hounsfield values are location dependent, influenced by the variable distribution of yellow and red marrow in the human skeleton, a distribution that also is dependent on the patient's age.[313] Comparison of marrow attenuation on one side of the body with the other may improve sensitivity, but this method is less valuable when a diffuse process such as leukemia is being investigated. Scintigraphy employing a wide range of radiopharmaceutical agents also has been used, in some instances successfully, to estimate the pattern and distribution of marrow involvement in a number of disorders; however, the technique lacks specificity and provides no morphologic information. Even bone marrow aspiration or biopsy, which still enjoys wide popularity, may lead to diagnostic difficulty owing to sampling errors created by inhomogeneous involvement of the marrow such that recovered tissue is not representative of the nature or extent of disease evident in other marrow locations.[312]

The MR imaging abnormalities accompanying leukemic infiltration of the bone marrow are similar or identical to those in a number of other infiltrative processes (e.g., plasma cell myeloma, lymphoma, and metastasis) (Fig. 62–12). Most commonly, leukemic marrow demonstrates a prolongation of the T1 relaxation value, leading to diminution of marrow signal intensity on T1-weighted spin echo MR images.[287, 288, 313–318] Diffuse or focal abnormalities are evident, the latter pattern being evident especially in acute myelogenous leukemia.[319] As many of the leukemias affect children, the resulting decrease in signal intensity at times is difficult to differentiate from the signal intensity of normal hematopoietic marrow. T2 changes are more variable and less dramatic and, in some studies, measured values of T2 relaxation times in leukemic marrow have not differed

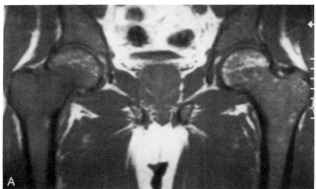
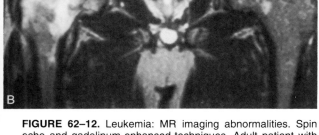
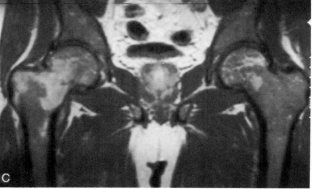

FIGURE 62–12. Leukemia: MR imaging abnormalities. Spin echo and gadolinum-enhanced techniques. Adult patient with pathologic fracture of femur.

A Standard coronal T1-weighted (TR/TE, 525/25) spin echo MR image reveals diffuse low signal intensity in the marrow of the diaphyses and metaphyses of the femora and of the innominate bones. The distribution of this signal intensity is too widespread to represent normal sites of hematopoietic marrow in an adult patient. Some fatty marrow, with high signal intensity, is seen in the femoral epiphyses and, on the left side, in the femoral metaphysis and diaphysis.

B With T2 weighting (TR/TE, 2200/90), regions of very high signal intensity are evident in the femoral necks, especially on the right side, and joint effusions in both hips are apparent. The remaining portions of the bone marrow are of moderately low signal intensity.

C A coronal T1-weighted (TR/TE, 525/25) spin echo MR image obtained after the intravenous administration of gadolinium contrast agent shows enhancement of signal intensity in the marrow, particularly in both femoral necks. The distribution of the abnormal signal changes in the femora is similar to that in **B**.

(Courtesy of J. Kramer, M.D., Vienna, Austria.)

with statistical significance from those of age-matched controls.[287] In one investigation, however, dramatic hyperintensity of the bone marrow on T2-weighted spin echo MR images was observed.[317] Indeed, as the marrow signal intensity on both T1- and T2-weighted images in the children with leukemia (as well as with neuroblastoma and rhabdomyosarcoma) was the reverse of that associated with normal fatty marrow, the authors of that investigation designated the findings as the "flip-flop" sign.

Quantitative chemical shift MR imaging has been used in patients with leukemia to determine the stage of the disease.[287, 320-322] This technique can help distinguish the individual contributions of fat and water to the total signal intensity, thus rendering a more quantitative assessment of the bone marrow than can be accomplished with conventional MR imaging techniques.[322] As T1 relaxation times of marrow are significantly longer in children with active leukemia than in children with leukemia in remission,[318, 326] quantitative chemical shift MR imaging may be useful in assessing the response of the disease to treatment.[323] Gerard and coworkers[322] employed this method in 10 patients with acute leukemia. They determined quantitative measures of fat fractions and the water and fat component T1 and T2 relaxation times, as well as average relaxation times. Their results showed sequential increases in fat fractions among patients responding to therapy, consistent with biopsy-confirmed clinical remission. In two patients who later developed disease relapses, decreases in fat fractions were noted. In two patients who failed to regenerate normal marrow, unchanging, low fat fractions were apparent.

With quantitative chemical shift imaging of bone marrow, fat fractions are the dominant influence on image contrast and are the best discriminator in differentiating between normal persons and those with leukemia.[320] The observed association between sequential increases in fat

fractions and favorable response to therapy in leukemic patients[322] is consistent with results derived from histologic studies of the bone marrow after chemotherapy for certain types of leukemia. Islam and coworkers[324] described three sequential stages of regeneration of the bone marrow after chemotherapy for acute leukemia: an initial acute edematous stage with hypocellularity and dilated sinuses; a second stage in which precursor multilocular fat cells are evident; and a third stage in which regenerating hematopoietic cells are evident particularly about aggregates of fat cells.[322] The close proximity of hematopoietic stem cells and fat cells suggests that the latter cells may be fundamental to proper hematopoietic regeneration[324] and that techniques that allow accurate measurement of marrow fat contents may be of great value in assessing therapeutic responses.[322] MR spectroscopy also may have potential in this assessment, allowing analysis of water and lipid content in the bone marrow.[325]

The role of other MR imaging techniques, such as gadolinium enhancement and short tau inversion recovery (STIR), in the evaluation of the therapeutic response of patients with leukemia (and other disseminated malignant disorders of the bone marrow) has received little attention to date (Fig. 62–13). Hanna and colleagues[327] used both of these methods and correlated the imaging findings with histologic analysis of bone marrow samples. Increased signal intensity was observed in the bone marrow on STIR images as well as on T1-weighted spin echo images after intravenous injection of gadolinium-based contrast agent; however, these methods, although sensitive, did not allow differentiation of tumor-containing and tumor-free regions of the bone marrow. Other techniques, such as chemical shift selective RF presaturation of fat, may prove useful in assessing leukemic involvement of the bone marrow.[399]

Although the value of MR imaging as a general screen-

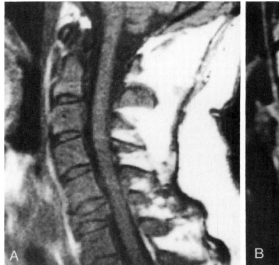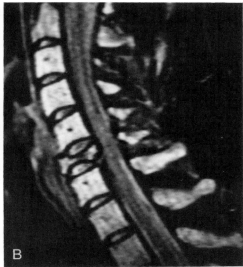

FIGURE 62–13. Leukemia: MR imaging abnormalities. Spin echo and short tau inversion recovery (STIR) techniques. Forty-one year old man with chronic lymphocytic leukemia and a pathologic vertebral fracture.
   A A sagittal T1-weighted (TR/TE, 500/15) spin echo MR image reveals low signal intensity in all of the cervical vertebral bodies. The signal intensity is similar to that of the intervertebral discs, and the resulting pattern is difficult to distinguish from normal. Collapse of the sixth cervical vertebral body is evident, with slight posterior displacement of bone into the spinal canal.
   B A sagittal STIR image (TR/TE, 1800/20; inversion time, 160 msec) reveals abnormally high signal intensity in all of the vertebral bodies and spinous processes. The collapsed vertebral body again is evident.

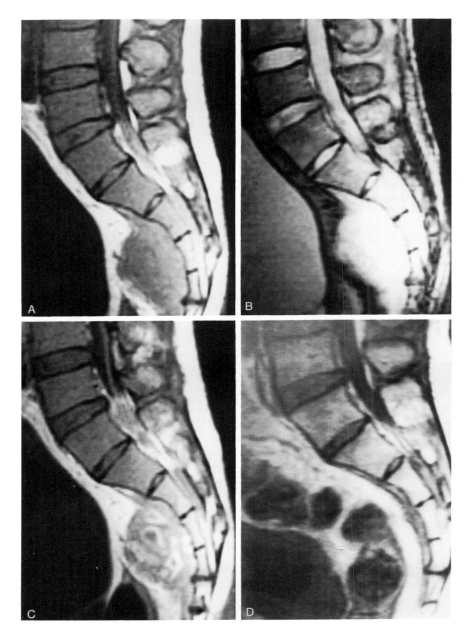

FIGURE 62–14. Leukemia: MR imaging abnormalities. Spin echo, gradient echo, and gadolinium-enhanced techniques. A 34 year old man with acute myelocytic leukemia and granulocytic sarcoma.

A A sagittal T-1 weighted spin echo MR image shows a large presacral mass with signal intensity similar to that of the bone marrow.

B A sagittal T2*-weighted gradient echo image reveals very high signal intensity in the mass.

C A sagittal gadolinium-enhanced T1-weighted spin echo MR image shows inhomogeneous signal intensity in the mass. When compared with **A,** areas of signal enhancement are evident.

D Three months after radiotherapy, a T1-weighted spin echo MR image shows dramatic resolution of the mass.

(Courtesy of H. S. Kang, M.D., Seoul, Korea.)

ing method in patients with suspected leukemia and as a technique allowing monitoring of disease activity requires further study, its value in defining local complications of musculoskeletal involvement is well established. Soft tissue extension of intraosseous lesions and compromise of the spinal cord accompanying vertebral involvement, especially in focal lesions associated with hairy cell leukemia[307, 308] and granulocytic sarcoma,[309, 395] are well shown with standard MR imaging techniques (Fig. 62–14). Furthermore, the assessment of complications resulting from chemotherapy, such as ischemic necrosis of bone, is accomplished with these techniques.[328, 329]

LYMPHOMAS

General Features

In addition to the leukemias, which represent myeloproliferative neoplasms of the reticuloendothelial system, lym-

phoreticular neoplasms of this system are well known, arising in lymphocytic cells, reticulum cells, or primitive precursor cells. A variety of diseases are grouped together as lymphoreticular neoplasms, including non-Hodgkin's lymphoma, Hodgkin's lymphoma, Burkitt's lymphoma, and mycosis fungoides. The classification of such diseases is complicated and debated, and it is made even more difficult because the terminology is continually undergoing modification (Fig. 62–15).[271, 289] As summarized by Carbone,[193] lymphoreticular tumors contain cells exhibiting different degrees of differentiation (i.e., well differentiated or poorly differentiated) and characteristics of lymphocytic or reticulum components, or both. Furthermore, the cell type and degree of differentiation may change with time, alterations that influence the prognosis and response to therapy. Adequate tissue sampling derived from substantial and, sometimes, repeated biopsies is fundamental to accurate diagnosis, and the standard histologic analyses commonly require

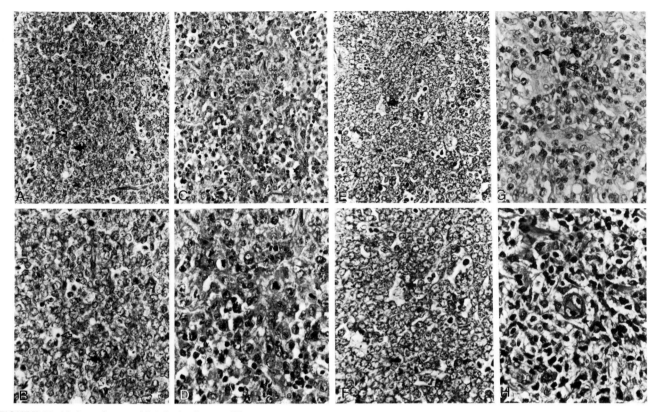

FIGURE 62–15. Lymphomas: Histologic abnormalities.

A, B Non-Hodgkin's lymphoma, lymphoblastic or convoluted lymphocytic type. This high turnover lymphoma shows irregular nuclear outlines with occasional small nucleoli near the nuclear membranes. Note nuclear debris, presumably reflecting high mitotic activity with consequent breakdown of tumor cell nuclei. (Hematoxylin and eosin stain, 100×, 160×.)

C, D Non-Hodgkin's lymphoma, histiocytic type. Although small lymphocytes are scattered in this field, the neoplastic cells generally are large, with abundant cytoplasm. Nuclei are variable in size and shape. Mitoses are noted in the center of the photographs. (Hematoxylin and eosin stain, 100×, 160×.)

E, F Non-Hodgkin's lymphoma, Burkitt's tumor. Tumor cells are closely packed and uniform, with round nuclei and small yet distinct central nucleoli and very little cytoplasm. A great deal of nuclear debris, some probably within a phagocyte, accounting for the frequently observed "starry sky" pattern, is seen. (Hematoxylin and eosin stain, 100×, 160×.)

G, H Hodgkin's disease, mixed cellularity type. Findings include a background of multiple cells, including eosinophils, plasma cells, and histiocytes; also, in **H**, a Reed-Sternberg cell is seen in the center of the photograph. (Hematoxylin and eosin stain, 160×, 160×.)

supplementation with imprint preparations, cytochemical studies, fluorescence techniques, and electron microscopy.

The lymphomas generally are divided into two broad categories—Hodgkin's disease and the malignant lymphomas. The malignant lymphomas occur about three times more commonly than Hodgkin's disease.[330] Non-Hodgkin's lymphomas have been classified further according to histologic characteristics into low grade, intermediate grade, and high grade categories, each of which can be divided still further according to specific cellular characteristics (Table 62–2).[330, 331] Common to all types of lymphoma are lymphadenopathy, mediastinal and abdominal masses, hepatomegaly or splenomegaly (or both), and, not uncommonly, constitutional symptoms that include fevers, night sweats, and weight loss.[330] Additional clinical manifestations vary among the lymphomas, related in part to the precise distribution of the lymphoreticular tumors in the body's tissues and organ systems. Some of these neoplasms arise in extraskeletal sites, appearing as single or multiple tumors in the lymph nodes, spleen, or gastrointestinal tract.[193] From these locations, abnormal cells may circulate in the blood and lodge in distant sites, such as the bone marrow, in which they may flourish. Lymphomatous involvement of the skel-

eton may result from such dissemination. Alternatively, lymphoreticular neoplasms may arise as a primary process of bone, an occurrence that accounts for approximately 5 per cent of all primary malignant osseous tumors.[157] Although virtually any type of lymphoreticular neoplasms on occasion may originate in the bone, the majority of cases result from histiocytic-type lymphomas. Such lymphomas originating in bone are observed in older patients (93 per cent of affected persons are over 20 years old and 50 per cent are beyond 40 years of age) and in men more frequently than in women.[157]

Owing to the process of initial localization in bone or of osseous dissemination from a tumor originating elsewhere in the body, skeletal changes are common in all of the lymphomas. Abnormalities may be identified in 5 to 50 per cent of cases, depending on the specific disease that is being investigated and the method of detection. For example, approximately 50 per cent of patients with Hodgkin's disease reveal bony abnormalities on adequate postmortem examination,[6] 10 to 25 per cent will have skeletal changes on radiographic examination,[1] and 15 per cent will reveal skeletal manifestations, such as pain, a palpable mass, or swelling, on clinical examination.[48] In histiocytic lympho-

TABLE 62–2. Classification of Non-Hodgkin's Lymphomas

New Classification	Old Classification
Low grade	
Small lymphocytic	Diffuse, lymphocytic, well differentiated
Follicular, small cleaved cell	Nodular lymphocytic, poorly differentiated
Follicular, mixed small cleaved and large cell	Nodular, mixed, lymphocytic and histiocytic
Intermediate grade	
Follicular, large cell	Nodular histiocytic
Diffuse, small cleaved cell	Diffuse lymphocytic, poorly differentiated
Diffuse, mixed small and large cell	Diffuse mixed, lymphocytic and histiocytic
Diffuse, large cell	Diffuse histiocytic
High grade	
Large cell immunoblastic	Diffuse histiocytic
Lymphoblastic	Lymphoblastic
Small noncleaved cell	Diffuse undifferentiated (Burkitt's and non-Burkitt's)

Modified with permission from Pond GD, et al: Radiology *170*:159, 1989.

mas, a 21 per cent frequency of bone involvement has been cited,[49] whereas in lymphocytic lymphomas, the frequency is approximately 12 per cent.[49] In general, it has been observed that the more immature the cell composing the lesion, the greater the frequency of bone involvement either by hematogenous spread or by direct invasion.[1] Histiocytic lymphomas metastasize to the skeleton quite commonly[153] and carry a poorer prognosis than do primary histiocytic lymphomas of bone.[153, 155]

As the prognosis of lymphoreticular neoplasms is intimately related to the extent of disease, initial evaluation must include a search for sites of involvement, a process called staging. Lower stages of disease are characterized by localization in a single lymph node or in a single extralymphatic site; or by involvement of lymph nodes, spleen, or extralymphatic sites confined to one side of the diaphragm. Higher stages of disease are characterized by transdiaphragmatic spread or by diffuse or disseminated involvement of extralymphatic sites (e.g., liver, lung, or bone marrow), with or without lymph node involvement.[330] A truly primary bone lesion is considered stage I non-Hodgkin's lymphoma, whereas a bone lesion associated with disease in other sites is considered stage IV.[157] To accomplish such staging, the clinical and laboratory examinations are supplemented with imaging and nonimaging techniques, including radioisotope studies, radiographs of the chest and abdomen, intravenous pyelograms, lymphography, bone marrow biopsy, and even laparoscopy and laparotomy with biopsy of the liver and other abdominal organs suspected of harboring neoplasm.[193, 331] The precise role of CT and MR imaging in this staging process is not yet clear, although both methods show promise in the detection of lymphadenopathy.[194, 195, 284, 331]

Skeletal Abnormalities

Non-Hodgkin's Lymphoma. Extraskeletal and skeletal findings in the lymphomas have been well described in various articles.[50–59, 153, 154, 157, 196–198, 202–205, 332, 334, 396] Involve-

ment of bone in non-Hodgkin's lymphoma more commonly is a manifestation of diffuse disease than a primary lesion. Estimates of the prevalance of skeletal alterations in widespread non-Hodgkin's lymphoma are 10 to 20 per cent in adults and 20 to 30 per cent in children. Such alterations generally appear after the presentation of the disease, although bone involvement may occur as part of the initial manifestations, especially in children. In the disseminated form, abnormalities of the axial skeleton predominate, with frequent involvement of the spine, pelvis, skull, ribs, and facial bones. Hematogenous spread of tumor is responsible for most of these lesions, although alterations can develop as a result of osseous invasion from surrounding soft tissues and lymph nodes. Multiple osteolytic lesions with moth-eaten or permeative bone destruction predominate (Figs. 62–16 and 62–17). Endosteal scalloping and cortical destruction are associated with spread to adjacent soft tissues. Periostitis occurs but is less frequent and severe than in Hodgkin's disease. On rare occasions, localized or diffuse osteosclerosis is evident,[60, 61, 333] although this finding, too, is more common in Hodgkin's disease.

Primary non-Hodgkin's lymphoma occurs at any age and affects men more frequently than women. Systemic symptoms and signs characteristically are absent; localized pain and swelling may be evident. The lesions predominate in the bones of the appendicular skeleton, especially those in the lower extremities (Figs. 62–18 to 62–20). An osteolytic lesion with poorly defined margins in the metaphyseal (or, rarely, epiphyseal[335–337] or diaphyseal) region of a long tubular bone is most typical, although short tubular bones and flat or irregular bones also can be affected (Figs. 62–21 and 62–22). Pathologic fractures and soft tissue masses are common. Detached pieces of bone, or sequestra, are reported to occur in approximately 10 per cent of cases.[397] Cases have been described in which disseminated osseous lesions have occurred in the absence of extraskeletal disease.[198] In such cases, differential diagnosis includes other processes, such as metastasis, leukemia, and Langerhans cell histiocytosis.

The frequency of skeletal involvement in non-Hodgkin's lymphoma is influenced by the precise histologic features of the lesions. Such involvement is more characteristic of histiocytic lymphomas than of lymphocytic lymphomas and of poorly differentiated or undifferentiated lymphomas than of well-differentiated lymphomas.[157] The prognosis of the disease has been related to morphologic variations in the abnormal cells[199, 334] and to specific radiographic signs,[200] although not without debate.[201]

Hodgkin's Disease. Although skeletal involvement in Hodgkin's disease is quite common, being detectable on radiographs in 10 to 25 per cent of cases, such involvement is infrequent at the time of clinical presentation.[157, 340] Bone abnormalities are more common in adults than in children. Tumor may reach the osseous tissue through either hematogenous dissemination or direct spread from contiguous involved lymph nodes; the former mechanism is associated with a poorer prognosis,[157] and the latter mechanism is especially common in the sternum, ribs, and spine.[208] Primary involvement of the skeleton in Hodgkin's disease is a debated issue, although reports have appeared of patients in whom solitary bone lesions were unassociated with disease elsewhere in the body.[207, 338, 339] The most common sites of involvement in Hodgkin's disease are the spine, pelvis, ribs,

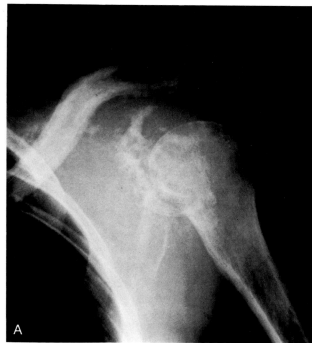

FIGURE 62–16. Non-Hodgkin's lymphoma: Histocytic type—disseminated disease.

A An extensive destructive lesion of the scapula in a 58 year old man is characterized by a soft tissue mass, osteolysis of the glenoid process and adjacent bone, and osteosclerosis. The humeral head appears involved and the shaft reveals osteoporosis.

B, C In this 22 year old man, osteolysis is observed in the femoral neck (**B**) and osteosclerosis is seen in the proximal portion of the humerus (**C**).

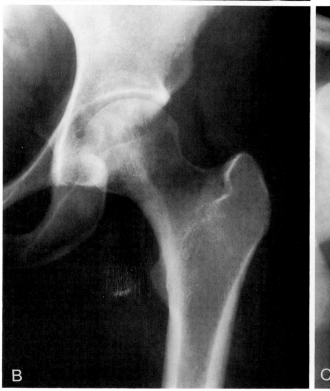

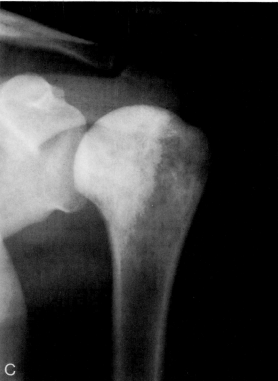

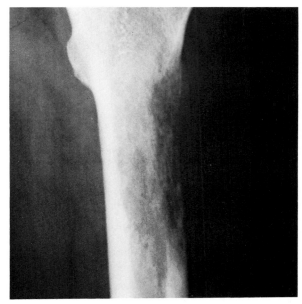

FIGURE 62–17. Non-Hodgkin's lymphoma: Histiocytic type—disseminated disease. In this 47 year old man, multiple organ systems were affected. Observe an eccentric diaphyseal lesion of the femur with motheaten bone destruction and cortical violation.

femora, and sternum.[206, 341, 342] Multiple lesions occur with a slightly greater frequency than solitary lesions. Clinical manifestations include significant local pain and tenderness.

With regard to the radiographic appearances, osteosclerosis alone, osteolysis alone, or osteosclerosis combined with osteolysis can be evident (Figs. 62–23 to 62–25). The

reported frequency of sclerotic lesions varies from 14 per cent to 45 per cent.[157] This bone response may accompany direct invasion from an adjacent lymph node, as occurs in the spine in the form of scalloping of the anterior surface of the vertebral body, in the sternum as a result of extension from affected internal mammary lymph nodes, and in the sacroiliac region owing to tumorous common iliac lymph nodes. Diffuse sclerosis of the vertebral body (an ivory vertebra) is similar to that observed in other lymphomas, skeletal metastasis, and Paget's disease. Widespread osteosclerosis may result from an osseous response to extensive bone marrow involvement or bone marrow fibrosis rather than from frank involvement of the bone itself.[157] Osteolytic lesions are poorly defined and associated with periostitis in approximately one third of cases. Similar periosteal bone formation may indicate associated hypertrophic osteoarthropathy.[6, 209, 332]

The prognosis of Hodgkin's disease depends on its histologic type.[210] Prognosis is favorable in cases in which lymphocytic predominance or nodular sclerosis is evident, less favorable in the presence of mixed cellularity, and even poorer in association with lymphocytic depletion.[211] The invasive nature of the more aggressive cell types of Hodgkin's disease is reflected in a higher frequency of skeletal involvement as well as of poorly defined or permeative bone destruction.[212]

Burkitt's Lymphoma. Burkitt's lymphoma is a stem cell lymphoma that is seen predominantly in children. It is the most common malignant disease of children in tropical Africa, although it also is recognized in other parts of the world. Involvement of facial bones is particularly characteristic,[62] especially in African patients. Such involvement is less common in North American patients, in whom the

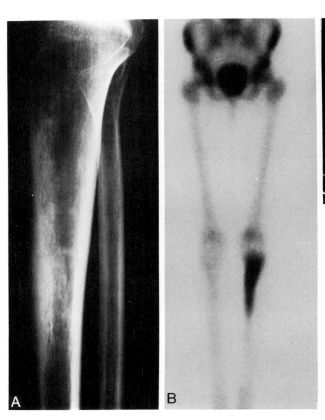

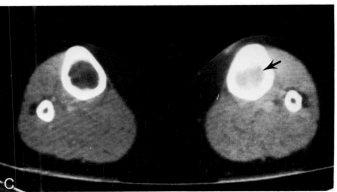

FIGURE 62–18. Non-Hodgkin's lymphoma: Histiocytic type—primary bone involvement. A 37 year old woman developed pain over the right tibia over a 2 year period. Initially, the diagnosis of a stress fracture was made.

A A lateral radiograph shows a lesion with both osteolysis and osteosclerosis in the diaphysis of the tibia.

B A bone scan documents increased accumulation of the radionuclide at the site of radiographic abnormality.

C On a transverse section through the lesion, CT shows increased radiodensity in the medullary canal of the affected tibia (arrow). Compare to the opposite side. Biopsy confirmed the presence of histiocytic lymphoma. No other organ systems were involved.

(Courtesy of G. Greenway, M.D., Dallas, Texas.)

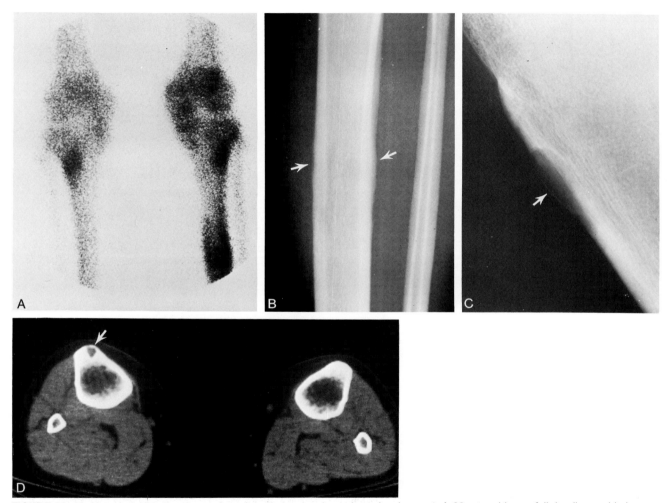

FIGURE 62–19. Non-Hodgkin's lymphoma: Lymphocytic type—primary bone involvement. A 20 year old man fell, landing on his knees, and developed pain that persisted for 6 months. On physical examination, exquisite tenderness to palpation of the right tibial tubercle and fusiform swelling and tenderness in the left lower leg were evident. A bone marrow aspiration was unrewarding.

A After the injection of a bone-seeking radiopharmaceutical, abnormal scintigraphic activity is evident in the right tibial tubercle, in the diaphysis and metaphysis of the left tibia, and about the left knee.

B A radiograph of the left tibia shows a poorly defined ostelytic process in the diaphyseal region, associated with periosteal bone formation (arrows).

C, D A lateral radiograph of the right tibia demonstrates a well-defined osteolytic lesion in the tibial tubercle, which also is evident on CT (arrows). A biopsy of the right tibial lesion revealed tissue consistent with lymphocytic lymphoma. The left tibial lesion was not biopsied. No other organ systems were affected.

(Courtesy of G. Greenway, M.D., Dallas, Texas.)

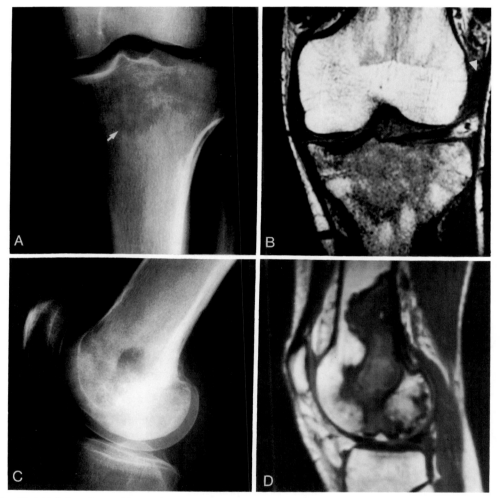

FIGURE 62–20. Non-Hodgkin's lymphoma: Histocytic type—primary bone involvement.

A, B This 20 year old man developed increasing pain in the knee. A routine radiograph **(A)** shows a poorly defined area of osteolysis (arrow) in the proximal portion of the tibia. A coronal T1-weighted (TR/TE, 667/16) spin echo MR image **(B)** reveals the epiphyseal and metaphyseal lesion, which is characterized by an irregular region of low signal intensity. A joint effusion is present (arrowhead). With T2 weighting (not shown) an inhomogeneous signal pattern, with areas of low and high signal intensity, was evident in the lesion. A biopsy confirmed the presence of a histiocyte-type lymphoma originating in bone.

(Courtesy of G. Greenway, M.D., Dallas, Texas.)

C, D In a different patient, patchy osteolysis in the distal end of the femur is evident on the radiograph **(C)**. A sagittal T1-weighted (TR/TE, 700/15) spin echo MR image **(D)** reveals the extent of the tumor, which is of low signal intensity. No enhancement of the lesion was evident on MR images obtained after intravenous administration of gadolinium contrast agent (not shown).

(Courtesy of J. Kramer, M.D., Vienna, Austria.)

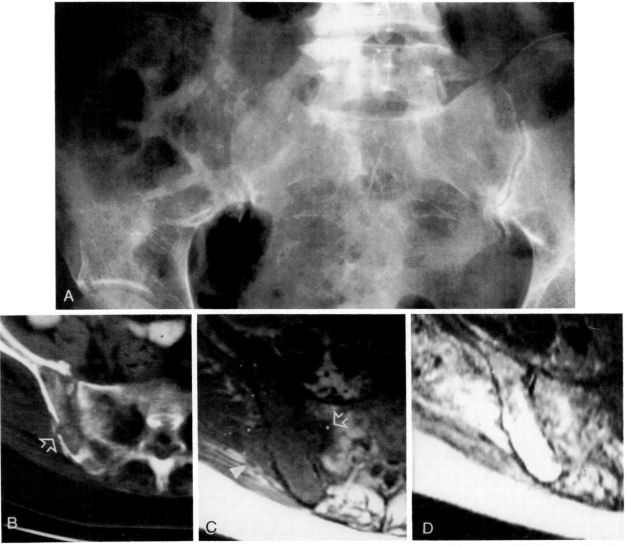

FIGURE 62–21. Non-Hodgkin's lymphoma: Histiocytic type—primary bone involvement. A 71 year old woman had low back and right buttock and lower extremity pain of 2 months' duration.

A A routine radiograph show poorly defined destruction of portions of the ilium and sacrum, about the sacroiliac joint.

B Transaxial CT scan shows the extent of the lesion, with involvement of both sides of the joint, and a pathologic fracture (arrow).

C On a transaxial T1-weighted (TR/TE, 600/20) spin echo MR image, low signal intensity is evident in the ilium and sacrum (arrow), with interruption of the lateral cortex of the ilium and an adjacent soft tissue mass (arrowhead).

D This transaxial T2-weighted (TR/TE, 2030/120) spin echo MR image reveals abnormally high signal intensity in the sacrum, ilium, and soft tissue.

(Courtesy of G. Greenway, M.D., Dallas, Texas.)

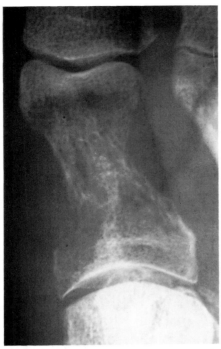

FIGURE 62–22. Non-Hodgkin's lymphoma: Histiocytic type—primary bone involvement. A 59 year old woman developed a mass in the great toe. A radiograph shows motheaten bone destruction in the proximal phalanx. A pathologic fracture is evident.
(Courtesy of M. Murphey, M.D., Washington, D.C.)

gastrointestinal tract may be affected.[157, 213, 343] Destruction of portions of the maxilla and, less frequently, the mandible can produce facial disfigurement.[156] Early radiographic changes include loss of the lamina dura, particularly around the molar teeth, and diminution and obscuration of trabeculae in the cancellous bone.[157, 344] With disruption of the cortex, a soft tissue mass may extend into the buccal cavity or maxillary antrum.[157]

Lesions in the tubular bones and pelvis have been described but are less frequent.[214, 215] The femur and the tibia are especially vulnerable. Osteolytic foci develop in the medullary portion of the bone, coalesce, penetrate the cortex, produce periostitis, and lead to a soft tissue mass.[214] They commonly are multiple, bilateral, and even symmetric in distribution. Diaphyseal, metaphyseal, or epiphyseal segments can be affected. Accurate diagnosis on the basis of the radiographic features is difficult, but clinical features, including the absence of severe pain and toxemia and the presence of tenderness or local inflammation and a soft tissue mass, are helpful diagnostic clues.[214]

Mycosis Fungoides. Mycosis fungoides is considered an unusual form of malignant (T cell) lymphoma with primary involvement of the skin.[63] It is uncommon but not rare. Its onset is in the fourth or fifth decade of life, affecting men more frequently than women. Initially mycosis fungoides may appear as nonspecific skin ulcerations. Subsequently its manifestations may be divided into three stages: erythema, plaque, and tumor. In any stage, cutaneous lesions may be associated with localized or generalized lymphadenopathy. In the tumor stage, extracutaneous manifestations with visceral involvement are evident. The lungs, spleen, liver, kidneys, thyroid gland, heart, brain, muscle,[219] and spinal cord[217] may be affected.[218] No tissue is immune to the disease. After the tumor stage, death commonly occurs within a few years, frequently due to septicemia. Skin biopsy generally is diagnostic, revealing evidence of a classic cellular infiltration, consisting of mycosis cells (resembling a histiocyte or reticulum cell) and similar-appearing cells (Fig. 62–26). Similar histologic findings have been documented in the synovial membrane in patients with monoarthritis or polyarthritis.[345, 346, 350]

Bone marrow involvement is rare. When present, bone lesions occur in the appendicular skeleton, with discrete or poorly defined medullary defects, cortical destruction, periostitis, and soft tissue swelling.[216] Although the skeletal abnormalities are similar to those accompanying other aggressive lesions such as metastasis and plasma cell myeloma, involvement of the peripheral skeleton including the hands may be a helpful clue in the diagnosis of mycosis fungoides.

The leukemic phase of this disease is termed Sézary syndrome.[64] It is a malignant syndrome characterized by generalized erythroderma, splenomegaly, lymphadenopathy, and leukocytosis, which may lead to death within 5 years of its onset. Destruction of terminal phalanges has been described in this syndrome[65] (Fig. 62–27). Polyarthritis is encountered related to cellular infiltration of the synovial membrane.[347]

Rheumatologic Abnormalities

In the malignant lymphomas, symptoms referable to bone lesions are seldom prominent, although localized pain, tenderness, and pathologic fractures may be an initial or significant part of the patient's clinical picture. Back pain and deformity relate to destructive vertebral lesions or, rarely, to severe generalized osteopenia.[66] Cellular infiltration in the synovium can lead to effusion and soft tissue swelling.[6, 220, 221, 348, 349] More frequently such infiltration is the result of intra-articular extension of a nearby osseous lesion.

Lymphomas may be associated with other rheumatologic disorders, including systemic lupus erythematosus,[222] rheumatoid arthritis, ataxia, telangiectasia, and the nephrotic syndrome.[67–70] A patient with relapsing polychondritis who subsequently developed lymphoma also has been described.[71]

Secondary gout is observed in some patients with malignant lymphomas.[37, 46, 47] Hypertrophic osteoarthropathy with its articular symptoms and signs also may be seen.[6, 332]

Muscle Abnormalities

Enlargement of muscles is a recognized manifestation of the lymphomas. Such enlargement can affect the musculature of the axial or the appendicular skeleton, or both. Lymphomatous infiltration of the muscle related either to primary involvement or to secondary extension from a contiguous tumor mass represents one mechanism for enlargement of the muscle.[351] Similar enlargement, however, can occur without histologic evidence of lymphomatous infiltration,[352] although the pathogenesis of the finding in this situation is not clear. CT or MR imaging represents an effective method in the analysis of muscle involvement in this disease.[351, 353]

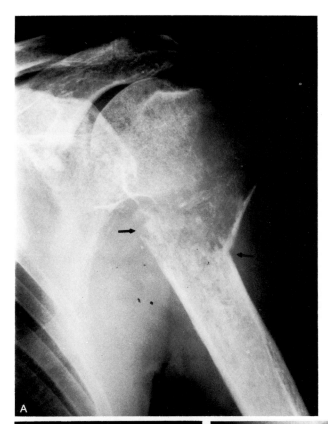

FIGURE 62–23. Hodgkin's disease: Extraspinal manifestations. Osteolysis.

A A large osteolytic lesion of the proximal end of the humerus has resulted in a pathologic fracture (arrows).

B Multiple large "cystic" osteolytic lesions of the proximal end of the humerus are associated with adjacent bony eburnation.

C In a 13 year old boy, several well-defined lytic lesions (arrows) of the proximal tibial metaphysis are surrounded by a sclerotic bony rim and are associated with adjacent periosteal bone formation (arrowhead).

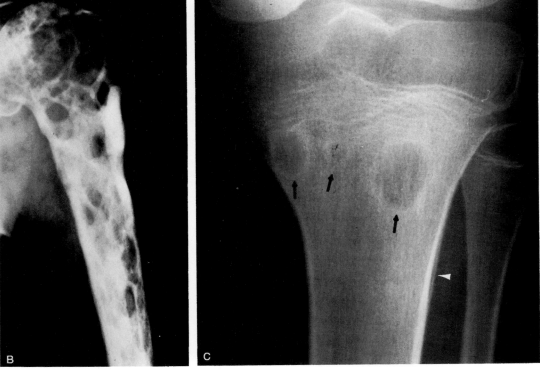

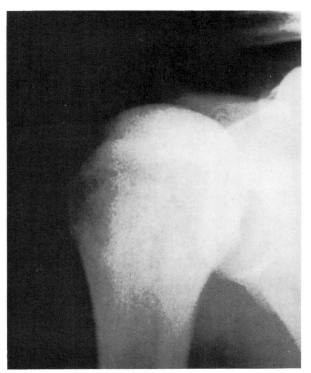

FIGURE 62–24. Hodgkin's disease: Extraspinal manifestations. Osteosclerosis. Sclerosis of the humeral epiphysis and diaphysis is associated with cortical thickening and periostitis.

Effects of Therapy

The association of ischemic necrosis of bone and the treatment of lymphoma with combination chemotherapy regimens that include intermittent corticosteroids has been reported on numerous occasions.[223–227, 290] The frequency of this complication in treated patients is approximately 1 to 3 per cent in Hodgkin's disease and somewhat lower in non-Hodgkin's lymphoma.[224, 225] Affected persons usually are physically active young men, although women may develop similar findings. Typically, ischemic necrosis of bone occurs 1 to 3 years after the initiation of the therapy (Fig. 62–28) with more unusual cases developing this complication after a shorter or longer interval of time. The femoral head (Fig. 62–29) and, less commonly, the humeral head are preferred sites of involvement, and multiple areas of necrosis have been described.[225, 272]

The precise cause of ischemic necrosis in these persons is not known. The almost constant association with corticosteroid administration suggests that these agents are important etiologic factors, although ischemic necrosis has been identified in patients with other malignant conditions treated with chemotherapy who did not receive corticosteroids.[228, 229, 285] The role of additional cytotoxic drugs, such as cyclophosphamide, vincristine, and procarbazine, in the production of ischemic necrosis of bone is unclear. Furthermore, radiation therapy to the axilla or pelvis, or both, commonly has been given to patients who subsequently develop this complication, suggesting that the inclusion of

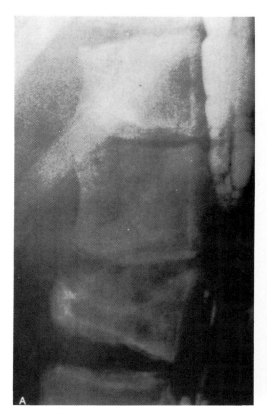
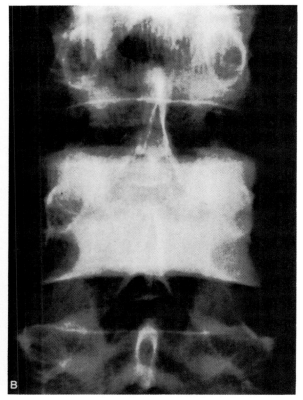

FIGURE 62–25. Hodgkin's disease: Spinal manifestations.

A On a lateral radiograph of the thoracolumbar junction, observe patchy sclerosis and lucency of multiple vertebral bodies with destruction and collapse. A myelogram had been accomplished previously.

B In a different patient, a frontal radiograph reveals an ivory vertebra. Note the homogeneous increase in radiodensity of the vertebral body without osseous enlargement.

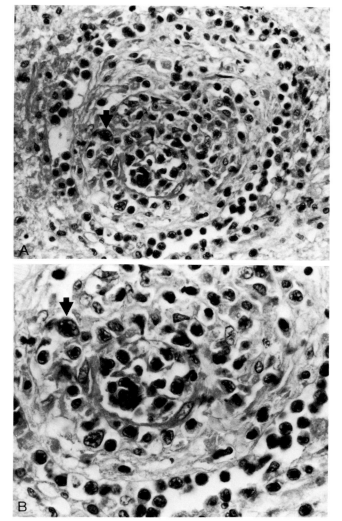

FIGURE 62–26. Mycosis fungoides: Histologic abnormalities. Note the pleomorphism of the cells within the infiltrate, including occasional cells with markedly convoluted nuclei (arrows). (Hematoxylin and eosin stain, 100×, 160×.)

the femoral or humeral head in the irradiation field is a significant factor in the development of ischemic necrosis.

A second complication of therapy in leukemia and, less typically, in lymphoma is related to the administration of methotrexate.[230–233] Skeletal changes usually occur 6 to 18 months after institution of the therapy. The abnormalities, which are termed methotrexate osteopathy,[233] are characterized by pain, osteopenia, growth recovery lines, dense metaphyseal bands, and fractures. Periostitis is either absent or localized. The bones of the lower extremities typically are affected, and the clinical and radiologic findings subside after withdrawal of the chemotherapeutic agent. The cause of methotrexate osteopathy is not known, although it may be related to the drug's interference with folic acid metabolism.[233]

Magnetic Resonance Imaging

The general applications of MR imaging to the assessment of musculoskeletal abnormalities in patients with lym-

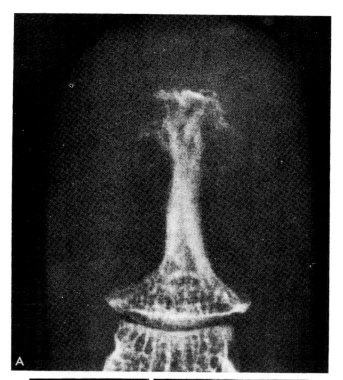

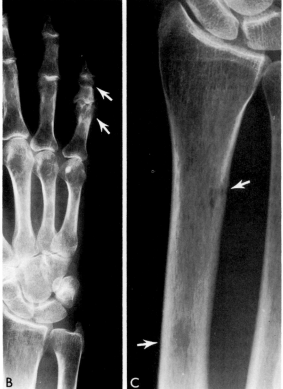

FIGURE 62–27. Mycosis fungoides: Sézary syndrome.

A A 63 year old woman with leukocytosis and swelling of the soft tissues of the fingers. The radiograph demonstrates bulbous soft tissue prominence, tuftal erosion, and concentric narrowing of the diaphysis of the distal phalanx. Other digits were involved similarly. (From McCormick CC: Skel Radiol *1*:183, 1977.)

B, C In a 62 year old woman, radiographic findings include destructive lesions of the phalanges and radius (arrows).

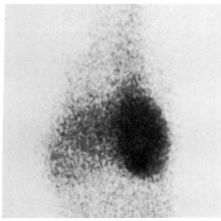

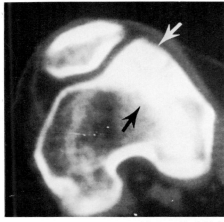

A   B

FIGURE 62-28. Non-Hodgkin's lymphoma: Ischemic necrosis of bone. A 47 year old woman with non-Hodgkin's lymphoma had been receiving combination chemotherapy, including corticosteroid preparations, for 3 years. Two months prior to the current evaluation, she developed knee pain and swelling. A lateral radiograph of the knee (not shown) revealed subtle permeative bone destruction and sclerosis in the anterior aspect of the femur.

A Increased accumulation of the bone-seeking radiopharmaceutical agent in this region is apparent.

B A transaxial CT image of the distal portion of the femur reveals bone sclerosis (arrows) consistent with ischemic necrosis. A biopsy of the region provided tissue that showed both lymphoma and osteonecrosis.

(Courtesy of G. Greenway, M.D., Dallas, Texas.)

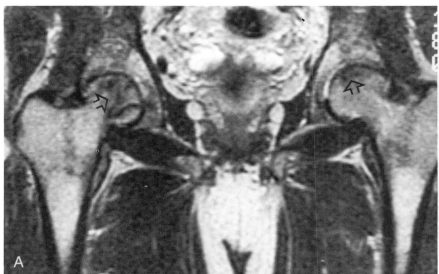

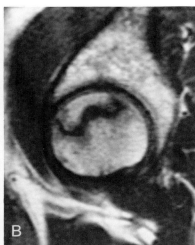

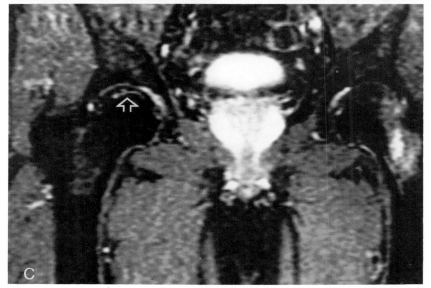

FIGURE 62-29. Non-Hodgkin's lymphoma: Ischemic necrosis of bone. This 58 year old man had been receiving combination chemotherapy, including corticosteroid preparations, for several years.

A A coronal T2-weighted (TR/TE, 2000,80) spin echo MR image shows evidence of osteonecrosis (arrows) in both femoral heads. Note the serpentine region of low signal intensity in the right femoral head, demarcating an area of osteonecrosis. The signal intensity in the metaphyseal regions of the proximal portion of the femora is inhomogeneous and asymmetric.

B A sagittal T1-weighted (TR/TE, 650/12) spin echo MR image of the right femoral head demonstrates the zone of osteonecrosis.

C, STIR imaging (TR/TE, 1800/30; inversion time, 160 msec) in the coronal plane shows high signal intensity in both femoral heads, with a crescentlike appearance on the right (arrow). On the left and, to a lesser extent, on the right, the femoral necks show areas of high signal intensity as well. Although the diagnosis of osteonecrosis of both femoral heads is clear, the cause of the changes in the femoral necks is not; tumor or ischemic necrosis, or both, as well as islands of hematopoietic marrow, may be present.

phoma are similar to those in patients with leukemia (see previous discussion). Despite interest in scintigraphic evaluation of the skeleton in lymphoma,[354] many investigators believe that MR imaging is a superior method in the analysis of bone marrow involvement in this disease. Previous reports have indicated, almost uniformly, that lymphomatous infiltration of the marrow leads to focal or diffuse regions of low signal intensity on T1-weighted spin echo MR images (Figs. 62–30 to 62–32).[313, 335–337, 340, 356–360] Furthermore, most descriptions of such infiltration have emphasized regions of high signal intensity on T2-weighted spin echo MR images[335–337, 340, 356] although this latter observation has not been entirely consistent. In an investigation of seven patients with non-Hodgkin's lymphoma of the skeleton and seven patients with other small cell bone tumors (primitive neuroectodermal tumor, or PNET), Stiglbauer and coworkers[361] found that the lymphomas demonstrated inhomogeneity in signal intensity on the T2-weighted images, with some regions of high signal intensity and others of intermediate signal intensity, whereas the PNET tumors were characterized by marked signal hyperintensity on these images. Histologic analysis confirmed the presence of fibrous tissue in the lymphomatous tumors, perhaps explaining their signal characteristics. In this same investigation, gadolinium contrast agent was given intravenously and regions of signal enhancement in lymphomas and PNET tumors were observed, probably corresponding to areas of cellularity. Stiglbauer and coworkers[361] also emphasized the epiphyseal or metaphyseal location of primary lymphoma of bone and the tendency of this tumor to spread beyond the bone into the joint.

Periosseous invasion of tissue such as muscle[337] in lymphoma can be shown with standard MR imaging, and the technique also can be applied to the analysis of cases in which the tumor initially involves soft tissue or muscle (Fig. 62–33).[353] In these instances, affected muscle is hypointense in comparison to fat on T1-weighted spin echo MR images, hypointense or isointense to fat on T2-weighted spin echo images, and hyperintense on STIR images.[353] MR imaging is particularly useful in the determination of the extent of bone and soft tissue involvement in

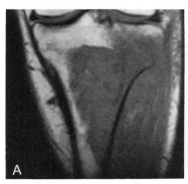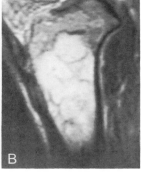

FIGURE 62–30. Non-Hodgkin's lymphoma—primary bone involvement. Spin echo MR imaging technique. Twenty year old man.

A This coronal T1-weighted (TR/TE, 500/20) MR image shows a lesion in the proximal portion of the tibia. Its signal intensity is similar to that of muscle.

B On a sagittal T2-weighted (TR/TE, 2000/80) MR image, the signal intensity of the lesion is inhomogeneous but mainly high. The tumor appears to be confined to bone.

(Courtesy of M. Schweitzer, M.D., Philadelphia, PA.)

patients who have spinal lymphoma (Fig. 62–34).[359, 360] In one study,[360] three types of spinal location of tumor were observed (paraspinal, vertebral, and epidural) either in isolation or in combination. Paraspinal tumors commonly extended over several vertebral levels and sometimes were accompanied by lymphadenopathy in mediastinal and retroperitoneal locations; the paraspinal lesions were hypo- or isotense with regard to signal characteristics relative to surrounding muscle tissue on T1-weighted spin echo MR images and were hyperintense to this tissue on T2-weighted spin echo images. Vertebral lymphoma led to changes in signal intensity in the vertebral bodies that were characterized by diffuse or focal regions of low signal intensity in comparison to uninvolved marrow on T1-weighted images and of homogeneous or inhomogeneous isointensity or higher signal intensity than marrow on T2-weighted images. Epidural lymphoma, in some instances, occurred in the absence of paravertebral or vertebral involvement, and the tumor spread over long segments of the spine. On T1-weighted images, the signal intensity of the epidural lymphoma was equal to or slightly lower than that of the cord or, rarely, higher than that of the spinal cord. Signal hyperintensity relative to that of the cord characterized the epidural tumor on the T2-weighted spin echo MR images.

The use of gradient echo sequences in the analysis of marrow involvement in lymphoma (as well as in other infiltrative processes) may lead to diagnostic difficulty.[362] Normal marrow exhibits a shortened effective transverse relaxation time (T2*) because of local magnetic field inhomogeneity and, therefore, low signal intensity with these sequences. This T2* effect is increased in regions with more trabecular bone (e.g., epiphysis) than regions with little trabecular bone (e.g., diaphysis).[362] Therefore, a low signal intensity on gradient echo images may characterize fatty marrow and resemble the signal intensity of hematopoietic marrow or infiltrative processes such as lymphoma. Erlemann and colleagues[363] used both spin echo and gradient echo (fast low-angle shot, FLASH) sequences, with and without intravenous administration of gadolinium based contrast agent, in the evaluation of patients with a variety of benign and malignant bone and soft tissue neoplasms, including five patients with intraosseous lymphoma. These investigators found that, in general, image contrast and contrast to noise ratios were lower with FLASH sequences than with spin echo sequences, although the image contrast usually was diagnostically sufficient for the differentiation of tumor from bone marrow or fatty tissue and insufficient for the differentiation of tumor from muscle. Furthermore, the selection of a suitable FLASH sequence for the differentiation of tumor from bone marrow depended on the predominating histologic tumor component. High contrast levels were obtained between tumors and bone marrow with the use of a flip angle of 90 degrees in sclerotic, calcified, and fibrotic lesions and a flip angle of 10 degrees in osteolytic lesions. These authors concluded that replacement of the T2-weighted spin echo sequences by FLASH sequences could not be recommended and that replacement of the T1-weighted spin echo sequences by FLASH sequences could be accomplished but does not significantly reduce examination time.

The precise role of MR imaging, as well as its advantages over CT and scintigraphy, in the analysis of the extent of marrow involvement in patients with lymphoma requires

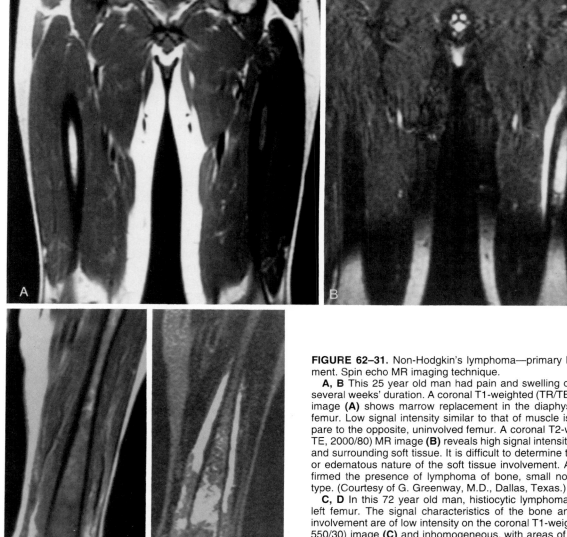

FIGURE 62–31. Non-Hodgkin's lymphoma—primary bone involvement. Spin echo MR imaging technique.

A, B This 25 year old man had pain and swelling of the thigh of several weeks' duration. A coronal T1-weighted (TR/TE, 700/16) MR image **(A)** shows marrow replacement in the diaphysis of the left femur. Low signal intensity similar to that of muscle is seen. Compare to the opposite, uninvolved femur. A coronal T2-weighted (TR/TE, 2000/80) MR image **(B)** reveals high signal intensity in the femur and surrounding soft tissue. It is difficult to determine the neoplastic or edematous nature of the soft tissue involvement. A biopsy confirmed the presence of lymphoma of bone, small noncleaved cell type. (Courtesy of G. Greenway, M.D., Dallas, Texas.)

C, D In this 72 year old man, histiocytic lymphoma involves the left femur. The signal characteristics of the bone and soft tissue involvement are of low intensity on the coronal T1-weighted (TR/TE, 550/30) image **(C)** and inhomogeneous, with areas of low and high intensity, on the coronal T2-weighted (TR/TE, 2300/200) image **(D).** (Courtesy of T. Mattsson, M.D., Riyadh, Saudi Arabia.)

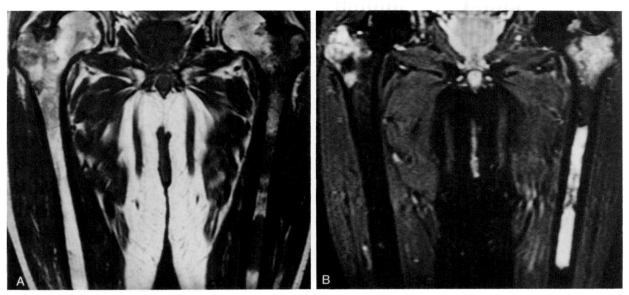

FIGURE 62–32. Non-Hodgkin's lymphoma—disseminated disease. Spin echo and STIR MR imaging techniques. Sixty-seven year old man.
   A The coronal T1-weighted (TR/TE, 800/20) spin echo MR image reveals bilateral femoral involvement, greater on the left side. Focal areas of low signal intensity in the bone marrow are evident.
   B With STIR imaging (TR/TE, 2000/30; inversion time, 160 msec), the lesions are of high signal intensity.

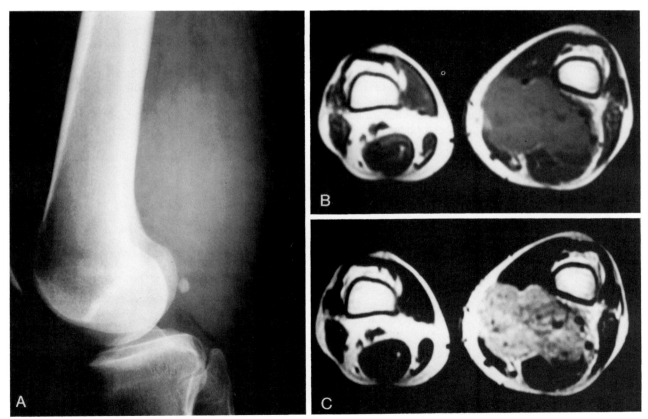

FIGURE 62–33. Non-Hodgkin's lymphoma—disseminated disease. Soft tissue involvement. Spin echo MR imaging technique. Sixty-six year old man.
   A A routine radiograph reveals a large mass posterior to the distal portion of the femur.
   B, C Transaxial proton density (TR/TE, 2000/20) **(B)** and T2-weighted (TR/TE, 2000/70) **(C)** MR images show the extent of the mass. The tumor is extramuscular and is involving the popliteal artery and vein and the adjacent nerve. It is of low signal intensity in **B** and inhomogeneous in signal intensity in **C**. The femur appears to be free of tumor.

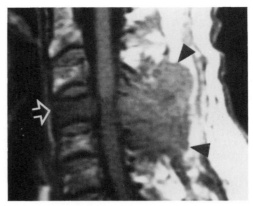

FIGURE 62–34. Non-Hodgkin's lymphoma—disseminated disease. Spinal involvement. Spin echo MR imaging technique. Sixty-five year old man with large cell lymphoma. A sagittal T1-weighted (TR/TE, 600/11) MR image reveals tumor involvement of the fourth cervical vertebral body (arrow) and posterior osseous elements (arrowheads). The spinal canal is narrowed with tumor about the cord. Its signal intensity is low. Inhomogeneous marrow signal intensity is evident in other cervical vertebral bodies. With T2-weighted images (not shown), the lymphomatous tissue was of high signal intensity, and the other cervical vertebral bodies were not involved.

further investigation.[355, 359] Some form of bone marrow imaging in combination with guided biopsy, however, appears to be superior to blind biopsy alone in the evaluation of bone marrow status in malignant lymphoma and in the staging of the disease.[355]

Other Lymphomas and Lymphoproliferative Disorders

Giant Follicle Lymphoma (Brill-Symmers Disease). Brill-Symmers disease is a type of lymphoma that is difficult to classify. It originally was described as a benign form of involvement leading to enlarged lymph nodes that usu-ally show numerous large follicles or germinal centers. Subsequently, it has become apparent that malignant transformation may occur, leading to the patient's demise, and that similar follicular involvement of lymph nodes occurs in patients with Hodgkin's disease, lymphocytic lymphoma, and, rarely, histiocytic lymphoma.[193] In fact, the histologic characteristics of Brill-Symmers disease may be evident in all forms of lymphoma except the Burkitt's tumor.

Although skeletal involvement is infrequent in the early, nonaggressive stage of the process, unusual osseous abnormalities have been described later in its course.[234] Grossly destructive osteolytic lesions are seen, especially in the hands and feet, associated with bone expansion, cortical disruption, and a peculiar lacelike trabecular pattern (Fig. 62–35). The latter may resemble the changes of other forms of lymphoma and leukemia[364] and of sarcoidosis.

Autoimmunoblastic Lymphadenopathy. Autoimmunoblastic lymphadenopathy is a systemic lymphoproliferative disease characterized by lymphadenopathy, hepatosplenomegaly, skin rash, anemia, lymphocytopenia, and polyclonal hypergammaglobulinemia.[193] Characteristic histologic findings in involved lymph nodes consist of prominent immunoblastic proliferation, the deposition of amorphous eosinophilic interstitial material, and proliferation of arborizing small blood vessels.[235, 236] Corticosteroid therapy or administration of cytotoxic agents may lead to remission, although the median survival is only 3 years.[193] The disease may be transformed into a malignant lymphoblastic lymphoma.

Articular involvement occurs in approximately 10 per cent of cases.[237, 238, 365] Arthralgias alone or mild, nondeforming arthritis is described. Joint effusions, soft tissue swelling, and, rarely, periarticular osteoporosis, joint space narrowing, and osseous erosions have been encountered.[238]

The cause and pathogenesis of autoimmunoblastic lymphadenopathy are not certain.[237] It has been suggested that the disease is an autoimmune disorder with defective T cell regulatory function, which may predispose to an abnormal

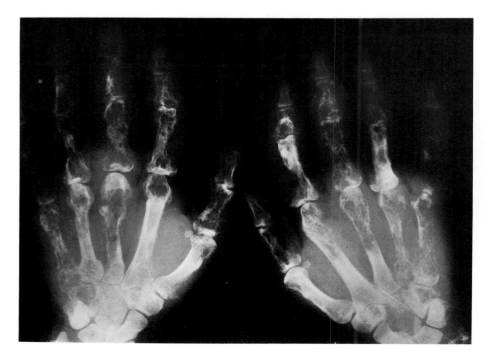

FIGURE 62–35. Giant follicle lymphoma (Brill-Symmers disease). In this unusual example, diffuse involvement in both hands is characterized by osteolysis, bone expansion, and soft tissue swelling. The findings resemble those of sarcoidosis. (Courtesy of R. Reichman, M.D., Los Angeles, California.)

proliferative reaction of B cells[239]; alternatively, it may be a hyperimmune entity with B cell proliferation that may be triggered by a hypersensitivity reaction to drugs.[240]

Angiofollicular Hyperplasia. In 1956, a group of patients with benign hyperplastic mediastinal adenopathy was described by Castleman and associates.[366] This disorder, which now is designated angiofollicular hyperplasia or Castleman's disease, has variable clinical features that depend on the precise histologic aberrations. Two distinct histologic subtypes of disease have been identified: the hyaline vascular form (90 per cent of cases), and the plasma cell form (10 per cent of cases).[367] Patients with the first subtype of disease generally are asymptomatic, whereas those with the plasma cell form may exhibit fever, anemia, and hypergammaglobulinemia. Widespread abnormalities and an aggressive clinical course may be associated with hepatosplenomegaly, lymphadenopathy, sepsis, and, in some instances, death.

An additional association of Castleman's disease is neoplasia,[368] including lymphoma, Kaposi's sarcoma, plasmacytoma, and colonic carcinoma. Skeletal lymphoma has been identified in one patient with angiofollicular hyperplasia.[368]

SJÖGREN'S SYNDROME

Background and General Features

The triad of keratoconjunctivitis sicca (dry eyes), xerostomia (dry mouth), and rheumatoid arthritis was first recorded by Hadden in 1888.[72] In 1892, Mikulicz[73] described a man with round cell infiltration in parotid and lacrimal glands producing enlargement of these structures. In 1927, Houwer[74] emphasized the relationship between filamentous keratitis and arthritis. Subsequently, in 1928, Betsch[75] and Albrich[76] further defined clinical and pathologic aspects of filamentous keratitis, including its relationship to hoarseness, dry mouth, rhinitis, parotid swelling, and lymphocytic infiltration in the lacrimal gland. The clinical and histologic manifestations of this syndrome were defined in detail by Sjögren[77] in 1933 in a study of 19 women with xerostomia and keratoconjunctivitis sicca, many of whom had chronic arthritis. This report stimulated numerous additional investigations of the syndrome. It later became evident that the articular disorder of Sjögren's syndrome was rheumatoid arthritis.[78] In some patients, the classic triad of the disease is not seen, rheumatoid arthritis being replaced by another disorder, such as systemic lupus erythematosus, periarteritis nodosa, progressive systemic sclerosis, or polymyositis.[79, 291] The diagnosis is established by the presence of two of the three major components.

Clinical Abnormalities

The disease is more common in women than in men. The average age at the time of presentation is 40 to 50 years. The two most common clinical patterns are the following[80]: the slowly progressive development of the sicca complex in a patient with chronic rheumatoid arthritis; and the more rapid development of oral and ocular dryness accompanied by episodic parotitis in an otherwise healthy person. Clinical manifestations of eye involvement include pain, a gritty sensation, redness, fatigue, photosensitivity, dryness with inability to cry, itching, decreased vision, and difficulties in

moving the eyelids. Corneal ulceration, opacification, and perforation may be evident. Oral and salivary gland involvement leads to dryness of the lips and mouth, difficulty with mastication and swallowing, ulcerations of the buccal membranes, lips, and tongue, and poor dentition. Parotid gland enlargement is evident in approximately 50 per cent of patients and may be accompanied by pain, tenderness, erythema, and fever.

Articular symptoms and signs may or may not be present. When apparent, the clinical manifestations almost invariably are those of rheumatoid arthritis. In fact, 10 to 15 per cent of patients with rheumatoid arthritis will develop keratoconjunctivitis sicca.[78] This latter condition develops after an average duration of arthritis of 9 years.[79] Subcutaneous nodules are apparent in approximately 60 per cent of patients with arthritis and histologically are typical of rheumatoid nodules.[79] Neither the onset nor the progression of the sicca complex can be related to the course or activity of articular disease. The eventual outcome of the joint disease is similar to that in uncomplicated rheumatoid arthritis. Occasionally patients with Sjögren's syndrome develop morning stiffness, fleeting arthralgias, joint swelling, and tenderness without deformity. Polyarticular involvement with predilection for the hands, wrists, elbows, ankles, and shoulders is observed.[241] This type of joint alteration is associated with synovitis but may be distinct from rheumatoid arthritis.

Additional manifestations of Sjögren's syndrome include Raynaud's phenomenon (20 per cent), splenomegaly and leukopenia suggestive of Felty's syndrome, infections (Fig. 62–36), vasculitis, peripheral neuropathy, glomerulonephri-

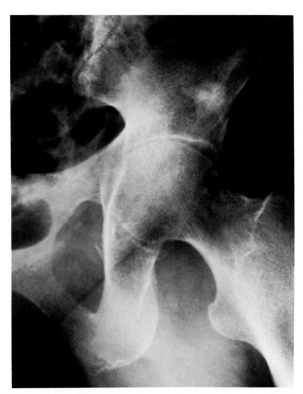

FIGURE 62–36. Sjögren's syndrome: Associated septic arthritis. In this 60 year old woman who drank unpasteurized milk, progressive hip pain was associated with radiographically evident loss of interosseous space. Salmonella organisms were aspirated from the joint. (Courtesy of V. Vint, M.D., San Diego, California.)

tis, and purpura. Myositis and muscle weakness, chronic thyroiditis of the Hashimoto type, adult celiac disease, biliary cirrhosis, and chronic active hepatitis have all been reported in association with Sjögren's syndrome.[80]

Radiologic Abnormalities

The extraskeletal radiographic manifestations of Sjögren's syndrome have been well described.[79, 81–84] The major articular findings are those of rheumatoid arthritis with soft tissue swelling, periarticular osteoporosis, marginal erosions, joint space narrowing, and intra-articular cystic lesions (Fig. 62–37). Typical target sites are affected, including the proximal interphalangeal and metacarpophalangeal joints of the hand, wrist, metatarsophalangeal joints of the foot, knee, and glenohumeral joint. Atlantoaxial subluxation and apophyseal, temporomandibular, and sacroiliac joint abnormalities have been noted. In addition, Silbiger and Peterson[84] observed psoriatic-like articular lesions with distal interphalangeal joint involvement and ungual tuft resorption. They also recorded chondrocalcinosis in one patient with Sjögren's syndrome. Additional reports have documented that, rarely, the erosive arthritis in the joints of the hand in patients with Sjögren's syndrome differs radiographically from typical rheumatoid arthritis.[286]

Pathologic Abnormalities

Pathologic examination reveals lymphocyte and plasma cell infiltration of salivary and lacrimal glands and other tissues, including the mucous glands of the respiratory tract, oral cavity, and upper esophagus.[79, 85] In joints, the findings are similar to those of rheumatoid arthritis.[86–88] Fibrous pannus with or without marked cellular infiltration of the synovium and cartilaginous and osseous erosion are seen. In muscle, perineural and perivascular foci of lymphocyte and plasma cell infiltration with some proliferation of fibrous tissue have been described.[85]

In some patients, the lymphoid infiltration in various tissues will be pleomorphic and immature, suggesting the presence of a malignancy. Lymph node architecture can be destroyed, with findings resembling those of a lymphoma.[80]

Relationship to Lymphoma and Other Malignancies

It is well known that lymphoma and leukemia can involve the lacrimal and salivary glands, producing abnormalities resembling Sjögren's syndrome. In addition, follow-up studies in patients with Sjögren's syndrome reveal that some persons develop malignant lymphoma[89–91] or other lymphoproliferative disease, or both.[242, 243] A patient with Sjögren's syndrome has been described whose illness terminated as a myeloproliferative disorder,[92] and patients with Sjögren's syndrome also may develop carcinomas.[91] In these patients with Sjögren's syndrome, the pathogenesis of this susceptibility to malignancy is not clear. In some instances, exposure to irradiation during therapy for enlarged lacrimal or parotid glands may be contributory, al-

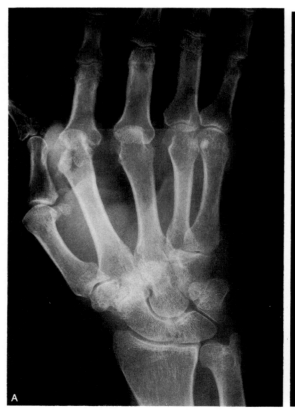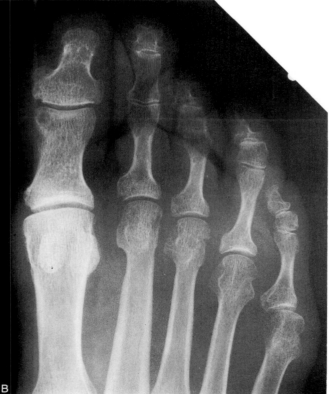

FIGURE 62–37. Sjögren's syndrome: Associated rheumatoid arthritis. In a patient with Sjögren's syndrome, typical abnormalities of the hand, wrist, and foot indicate the presence of rheumatoid arthritis. Observe marginal erosions in the wrist, metacarpophalangeal and proximal interphalangeal joints of the hand, metatarsophalangeal joints, and the interphalangeal joint of the great toe. Soft tissue swelling and subluxations also are evident. Changes at the trapezioscaphoid joint resemble degenerative joint disease.

though the radiation dose is relatively small.[79] Myeloproliferation may relate to a decreased cell-mediated immunity or to hematopoietic stem cell abnormality in some patients with Sjögren's syndrome.[92, 93] The anti-Ro (SS-A) antibody may be an immune marker of a lymphoproliferative clinical course.

SYSTEMIC MASTOCYTOSIS

General Features

The mast cell is a connective tissue cell that is widely distributed throughout the body.[369] Mast cells contain a large number of chemical mediators, including heparin, histamine, and serotonin; they are capable of responding to neural, chemical, and immunologic stimuli by releasing these mediators, which, when excessive, may lead to a variety of symptoms and signs, such as edema, bronchoconstriction, and anaphylaxis.[370] Disorders of mast cell proliferation include urticaria pigmentosa, systemic mastocytosis, and mast cell leukemia. Mast cells, however, have been observed in a wide variety of neoplastic, fibrotic, and inflammatory processes, including neurofibromas, synovial sarcomas, lymphoproliferative disorders, fibrotic lung disease, and adrenal cortical adenomas.[371, 372, 374]

Systemic mastocytosis is a rare proliferative disorder affecting both men and women, beginning in adult life. It was described as a skin disorder by Nettleship[94] in 1869 but now is recognized as a systemic process whose clinical manifestations resemble lymphoma or leukemia. Multiple organ systems may be altered, including the liver, the spleen, the lymph nodes, and the skeleton, although it is cutaneous involvement that is most common and characteristic.

Skin or mucous membrane lesions resemble urticaria pigmentosa of childhood.[95] This latter disease usually develops in infancy or early childhood, whereas systemic mastocytosis generally has an onset after puberty. Most typically, patients with systemic mastocytosis are in the fifth to eighth decades of life, although the disease may develop in the pediatric age groups as well. Men and women are affected with approximately equal frequency. The skin lesions of the systemic form of the disease consist of confluent macules, papules, and nodules (some of which resemble leukemia cutis) and chronic lichenified dermatitis. Skin pigmentation may be apparent. Progressive cutaneous change and extensive involvement of oral, nasal, and rectal mucosa are observed.

The clinical features relate, in part, to histamine release with local urticaria, flushing, shocklike episodes, diarrhea, and vomiting.[371, 373] In more severe cases, weight loss, weakness, malaise, hepatosplenomegaly, lymphadenopathy, and peptic ulcer disease are encountered. Hematologic abnormalities include anemia, leukopenia, thrombocytopenia, and eosinophilia. Hemorrhagic tendencies reflect the presence of both thrombocytopenia and prothrombin deficiency. Hepatic dysfunction occurs owing to mast cell proliferation and periportal fibrosis. The prognosis is variable, depending on the extent of systemic involvement. When the disease is confined to the skin and skeleton, it may run a mild, protracted course. With extensive abnormalities of the reticuloendothelial system, death may occur within a few years. Common causes of death are hemorrhage, infection, ca-

chexia, perforation of peptic ulcers, gastroenteritis, and leukemia.

The major pathologic characteristic of systemic mastocytosis is mast cell proliferation in any of the involved organs. The bone marrow represents the most commonly biopsied extracutaneous site used in establishing the diagnosis of systemic mastocytosis.[371] Mast cells may reveal a relatively normal appearance or, in some cases, a severe anaplasia, indicating malignant transformation. Mast cells have a significant effect on the skeleton, leading to a variety of clinical, pathologic, and radiologic manifestations.

Skeletal Abnormalities

Mast cell proliferation in skeletal tissue is a well-recognized and common manifestation of systemic mastocytosis[96–106] (Fig. 62–38). This proliferation may be silent clinically, although bone pain has been observed in as many as 28 per cent of patients.[371] Tenderness, soft tissue mass, and deformity secondary to pathologic fracture also can be ob-

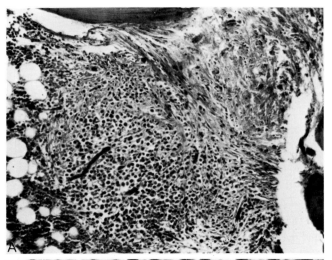

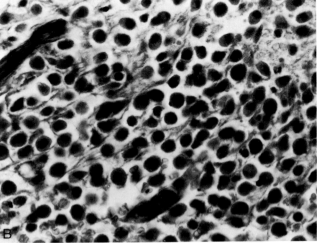

FIGURE 62–38. Mastocytosis: Histologic abnormalities. A nodule in the bone marrow is composed predominantly of mast cells, which are replacing most of the marrow elements **(A).** Fibrosis also is evident. At higher magnification **(B),** note that the mast cells possess centrally located dark nuclei and a relatively low nucleocytoplasmic ratio. (Hematoxylin and eosin stain, 40×, 160×.)

served. Such fractures are especially common in the spine,[247, 250] although they also are observed in the tubular bones of the extremities.[398] Mast cell infiltration into the bone marrow stimulates fibroblastic activity and granulomatous reaction, which lead to trabecular destruction and replacement with adjacent new bone formation.[249, 273] This infiltration accounts for significant radiographic abnormalities, which first were described by Sagher and coworkers[149] in 1952. These abnormalities, which occur in 70 per cent of patients,[371] can be classified into two types: (1) osteopenia and bone destruction and (2) osteosclerosis (Figs. 62–39 and 62–40). In either type, a focal or diffuse distribution may be seen. Diffuse lesions predominate in the axial skeleton, whereas focal lesions occur in both the axial and the appendicular skeleton. Progression of skeletal lesions is not uncommon, and initial focal lesions subsequently may become diffuse. Scintigraphy, which has been used to identify skeletal involvement in mastocytosis,[253–255] may be employed in the assessment of disease progression. Radionuclide patterns vary according to the distribution of the osseous lesions.[254, 274, 276]

Osteopenia and Bone Destruction. Diffuse osteopenia or multiple lytic lesions may be observed in systemic mastocytosis.[147, 370] Generalized rarefaction simulates the appearance of osteoporosis[107, 244, 375] and is most frequent in the skull, the pelvis, the spine, and the ribs. It may relate to malabsorption of calcium or changes in ground substance induced by heparin production.[108] Heparin is a potent in vitro bone resorbing agent; diffuse osteopenia may accompany long-term heparin therapy.[245, 246] Prostaglandins represent another by-product of mast cells and, owing to their known potent effect on bone resorption,[248] prostaglandins also may be important in causing the osteopenia of mastocytosis.[247, 275] Mast cell infiltration, in the form of

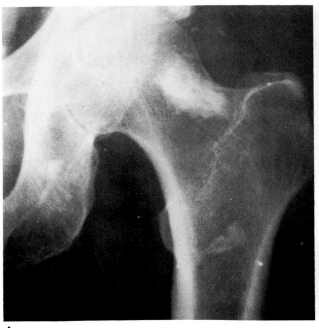

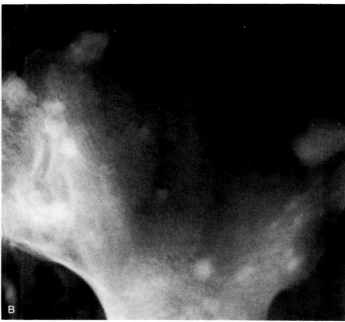

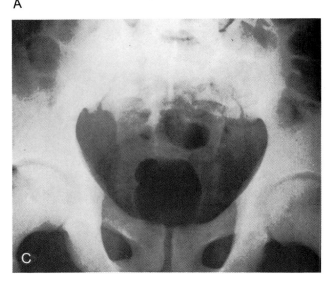

FIGURE 62–39. Mastocytosis: Radiographic abnormalities. Extraspinal sites.

A, B In this middle-aged woman, observe multiple focal, well-defined osteosclerotic lesions in the hemipelvis and femur.

C In a different patient, diffuse osteosclerosis of the entire pelvis and proximal femora is evident.

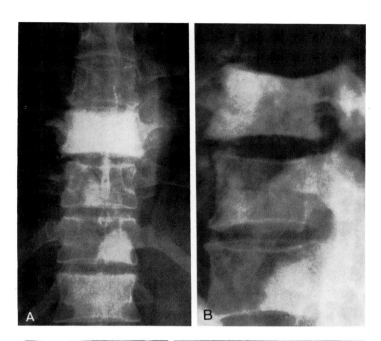

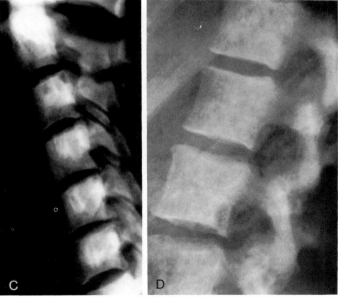

FIGURE 62–40. Mastocytosis: Imaging abnormalities. Spinal sites.

A, B In the same patient as in Figure 62–39 **A, B,** observe focal osteosclerotic lesions of the thoracic vertebrae with paravertebral swelling. An ivory vertebra has resulted.

C, D In a different patient, more widespread osteosclerosis of the cervical and lumbar spine is evident.

(**C, D,** Courtesy of B. Holtan, M.D., Rock Springs, Wyoming.)

Illustration continued on following page

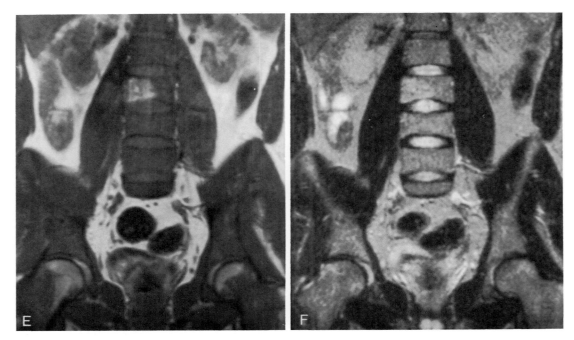

FIGURE 62–40. *Continued*
   E, F In a third patient, coronal T1-weighted (TR/TE, 550/25) **(E)** and T2-weighted (TR/TE, 2200/90) **(F)** spin echo MR images show marrow infiltration in the spine and osseous pelvis, as well as the proximal portion of the femora, manifest as low signal intensity in **E** and intermediate signal intensity (similar to that of fat) in **F.**
   (E, F, Courtesy of J. Kramer, M.D., Vienna, Austria.)

nodules, has been detected in patients with systemic mastocytosis and diffuse osteopenia, with additional histologic evidence of an increase in osteoclast surfaces and bone remodeling.[381] Furthermore, in mastocytosis, discrete lytic lesions represent areas of osseous resorption, perhaps related to pressure atrophy of trabeculae from adjacent mast cell accumulations. They tend to be small (less than 4 or 5 cm in diameter), poorly or well defined, and surrounded by a "halo" of sclerosis. The lesions can simulate the findings of cystic osteoporosis, Gaucher's disease, or thalassemia. These circumscribed lytic defects are most common in the pelvis, the skull, and the tubular bones. In tubular bones, lesions predominate in the metaphyseal regions.

Osteosclerosis. Focal or diffuse bone sclerosis is another radiographic pattern in systemic mastocytosis, which may appear in combination with osteolysis.[251, 292, 370, 376–380] Focal sclerotic lesions correspond to areas of prominent trabeculae with cortical thickening and narrowing of the marrow spaces, and these may be misinterpreted as skeletal metastases. In the axial skeleton, loss of delineation of bony trabeculae and the resulting homogeneous radiodense appearance resemble the abnormalities associated with myelofibrosis, fluorosis, sickle cell anemia, Paget's disease, and skeletal metastasis.[148]

In systemic mastocytosis, the cause of osteosclerosis is not known. Histologic studies confirm the presence of very extensive mast cell infiltration and fibrosis in the bone marrow in patients with such osteosclerosis.[381] It is suggested that bone formation may represent a response to the presence of abnormal cells in the marrow, perhaps mediated by the conversion of precursor cells to osteoblasts[252] or by prostaglandin or histamine.[275] Osteosclerosis also may reflect

bone infarction with osteonecrosis.[101] Osteonecrosis might be expected in this disease as mast cells can infiltrate the walls of blood vessels, proliferate in subendothelial layers, protrude into the lumen, and occlude blood flow partially or completely.[109]

Articular Abnormalities

Significant articular abnormalities are not a part of the clinical findings of systemic mastocytosis. Periarticular bone pain and tenderness can be observed in association with epiphyseal lesions. Similarly, back pain and tenderness can accompany spinal involvement in this disease. Articular inflammation with synovial effusion has been described. In one such patient, rheumatoid factor was present in the blood and the synovial fluid.[110]

Differential Diagnosis

The skeletal manifestations of systemic mastocytosis are nonspecific (Table 62–3). Diffuse osteopenia in this disease is nearly identical to that in osteoporosis, osteomalacia, hyperparathyroidism, and plasma cell myeloma. Diffuse cystic lesions in systemic mastocytosis can simulate the appearance of osteoporosis, sickle cell anemia, Gaucher's disease, and plasma cell myeloma. Diffuse osteosclerosis is observed not only in systemic mastocytosis but also in myelofibrosis, skeletal metastasis, fluorosis, Paget's disease, renal osteodystrophy, and numerous other conditions. Multiple focal osteosclerotic lesions in systemic mastocytosis resemble the findings in skeletal metastasis and tuberous sclerosis.

TABLE 62–3. Differential Diagnosis of Osteosclerosis*

	Skeletal Metastasis	Mastocytosis	Myelofibrosis	Lymphomas	Paget's Disease	Fluorosis	Renal Osteodystrophy	Axial Osteomalacia
Distribution	Axial > Appendicular	Axial > appendicular	Axial > appendicular	Axial > appendicular	Axial > appendicular	Axial > appendicular	Axial > appendicular	Axial
Diffuse sclerosis	+	+	+	+	+	+	+	+
Focal sclerosis	+	+	−	+	+	−	−	−
Osteopenia or bone lysis	+	+	+	+	+	−	+	−
Bony enlargement	−	−	−	−	+	−	−	−
Osteophytosis, ligament ossification	−	−	−	−	−	+	−	−
Splenomegaly	−	+	+	+	−	−	−	−

*+, Common; −, uncommon or rare.

POLYCYTHEMIA VERA

General Features

Polycythemia vera (primary polycythemia) is a disease of unknown cause that is characterized by hyperplasia of all of the cellular elements in the bone marrow (primarily erythrocytes), resulting in elevated red blood cell count, leukocytosis, and thrombocytosis.[111, 112] The relationship, if any, of this disorder to leukemia is not clear. Polycythemia vera occurs in middle-aged or elderly patients, predominantly men; however, it may be observed in children or young adults. Clinical complaints include headache, dizziness, weakness, fatigue, paresthesias, dyspnea, and visual disturbances. On physical examination, a ruddy complexion, hepatosplenomegaly, and systolic hypertension are seen. Vascular thrombosis is a recognized complication of the disease related to thrombocytosis and increased blood viscosity. Occlusion of hepatic veins (Budd-Chiari syndrome) and cirrhosis of the liver may be evident. Bleeding is another complication of polycythemia vera. In the later stages of the disease, myelofibrosis, progressive myeloid metaplasia, and anemia are encountered. The disorder is chronic and compatible with many years of life.

Musculoskeletal Abnormalities

The musculoskeletal manifestations of this disease are few. Vascular thrombosis can lead to osteonecrosis, particularly of the femoral head (Fig. 62–41),[113] and generalized marrow hyperplasia can produce patchy radiolucent lesions throughout the bone. Cranial abnormalities may resemble those of thalassemia major.[114] Myelofibrosis is associated with generalized increased radiodensity of the skeleton. An increased frequency of plasma cell myeloma has been observed.

Hyperuricemia is not infrequent in (primary) polycythemia vera or in secondary polycythemia. Gouty arthritis has been estimated to occur in 5 to 8 per cent of all cases.[115] The initial attack of gout usually is encountered in patients with active polycythemia,[6] in patients with thrombocytosis,[115] or in those in the transition period from polycythemia vera to myelofibrosis and myeloid metaplasia.[47] Occasionally, the first attack of gouty arthritis precedes the diagnosis of polycythemia vera by 1 to 10 years.[116]

The role of MR imaging in the assessment of patients with polycythemia vera is discussed later in this chapter.

MYELOFIBROSIS

Background and General Features

Myelofibrosis is an uncommon disease associated with fibrotic or sclerotic bone marrow and extramedullary hematopoiesis.[117–121] The combination of marrow fibrosis and a leukemoid hematologic picture first received attention in the 1870s.[122, 123] Since that time, a variety of names have been applied to this syndrome, including agnogenic myeloid metaplasia, aleukemic myelosis, leukoerythroblastic anemia, osteosclerosis, and myelosclerosis.[256] Its cause has not been determined precisely. In the past, it has been considered to be a variant of leukemia,[124] a primary bone abnormality,[125] a reaction to bone marrow injury or necrosis,[126, 127] and a myeloproliferative process of unknown cause.[118, 128] The association of myelofibrosis with exposure to benzene or other bone marrow toxins,[129] polycythemia vera,[130] chronic myelocytic leukemia,[131, 132] and refractory anemias[133] has been described.

It has been popular to divide myelofibrosis into two forms: primary or idiopathic and secondary. Difficulties arise in this classification as "secondary" causes of marrow fibrosis have subsequently appeared in some patients who initially were believed to have primary disease. For example, in one report, hairy cell leukemia became evident in approximately 8 per cent of cases of idiopathic myelofibrosis.[256] Whatever the associated disease or even in the absence of an underlying process, the basic pathologic finding is fibrosis of the bone marrow, which, in some instances, may replace almost the entire marrow tissue. Focal or diffuse areas of hypercellular marrow[134] may be combined with trabecular thickening and overgrowth.[126] Simultaneously, proliferation of potential bone marrow elements occurs in the spleen (Fig. 62–42), the liver, the lymph nodes, and the long bones (as well as the kidneys, the lungs, and other organs), and in these accessory sites, secondary fibrosis also may appear.[126, 127, 135]

The degree of bone marrow fibrosis generally is held to provide an indication of the severity of the disease process. The factor or factors leading to the fibrotic reaction are not known. It would appear that an insult to the marrow, in the form of a disease or exposure to irradiation or toxins, initiates a series of events culminating in fibrosis. One hypothesis indicates that excessive production of platelet-derived growth factor by abnormal megakaryocytes could be the cause of bone marrow fibrosis.[257]

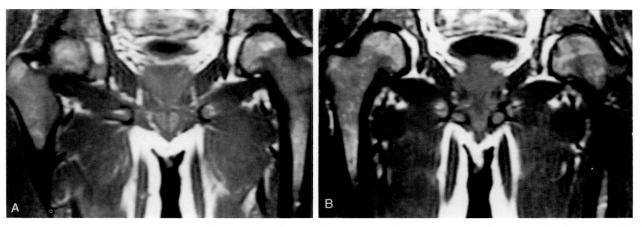

FIGURE 62–41. Polycythemia vera: Marrow cellular hyperplasia and osteonecrosis. MR imaging abnormalities, spin echo technique. This 44 year old man developed bilateral hip pain. Routine radiographs (not shown) revealed patchy osteosclerosis of the femoral heads, compatible with ischemic necrosis of bone. Two consecutive coronal T1-weighted (TR/TE, 600/20) MR images show diffuse low signal intensity in the marrow, especially in the femoral necks and shafts, consistent with cellular hyperplasia. Patchy regions of high signal intensity, representing areas of fat or hemorrhage, are evident in both femoral heads.

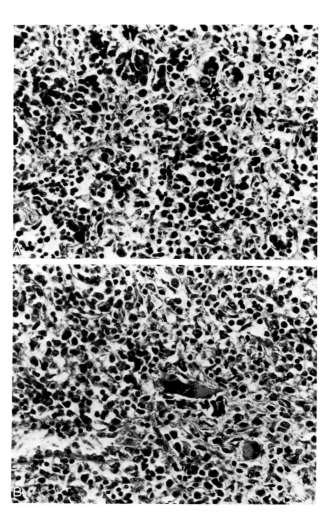

FIGURE 62–42. Myelofibrosis: Histologic abnormalities. Two photomicrographs of splenic involvement are shown. In **A,** observe the red pulp and white blood cell precursors, some appearing as fairly cohesive cell clusters. In **B,** note megakaryocytes in addition to the cells of the erythroid and myeloid series. (Hematoxylin and eosin stain, 100×, 100×.)

Clinical Abnormalities

Myelofibrosis generally is a disease of middle-aged and elderly men and women. Most affected patients are in the sixth or seventh decade of life. Despite reports that describe an acute form of the disease, characterized by minimal splenomegaly, leukoerythroblastosis, and short survival,[256, 258] the disease generally is insidious in onset. Symptoms include weakness, fatigue, weight loss, abdominal pain, anorexia, nausea, vomiting, and dyspnea. Physical signs may include abdominal swelling, hepatosplenomegaly, and purpura. Hematologic evaluation frequently reveals moderate to severe anemia, an increased number of nucleated red blood cells, leukocytosis or leukopenia, abnormal white blood cells, and elevated, normal, or low platelet counts. The diagnosis is established by bone marrow biopsy. The prognosis of the disease is variable. Some patients die within a few months of the initial diagnosis (malignant or acute myelofibrosis), whereas others survive for a prolonged period of time. Signs of poor prognosis are fever, weight loss, night sweats, anemia, and thrombocytopenia.[256] Myelofibrosis ultimately is fatal because of intramedullary and extramedullary marrow fibrosis.

Musculoskeletal Abnormalities

Characteristic pathologic abnormalities in the skeleton account for clinically evident bone pain and tenderness and radiographically detectable bone sclerosis. In the normal sites of active hematopoiesis in the adult (the vertebrae, the pelvis, and the ribs), focal areas of marrow fibrosis appear. This fibrosis progresses, and compensatory sites of marrow formation are detected within the fatty marrow of the proximal and distal ends of the femora, the humeri, and the tibiae. These accessory sites later demonstrate the same type of fibrosis that is evident in the axial skeleton. Osteoclastic activity results in spongy bone trabeculae, which are distorted and replaced by fibrous tissue; collagen fibers are interspersed with fibroblasts. Adjacent thickening and sclerosis of trabeculae lead to condensed and closely meshed bone.

The radiographic picture reflects these pathologic changes. In some instances, normal or osteopenic bone and osteolytic lesions are observed,[259, 260] but, in general, osteosclerosis is the predominant radiographic pattern, evident in both the axial skeleton and the proximal long bones (Fig. 62–43). This sclerosis is observed in 40 to 50 per cent of patients. The bones altered most commonly are the spine, the pelvis, the skull, the ribs, the proximal end of the humerus, and the proximal portion of the femur, although more peripheral skeletal sites occasionally are abnormal.[120] The osseous structures may be uniformly dense or demonstrate small areas of relative radiolucency. In the long bones, cortical thickening can be observed, due predominantly to endosteal sclerosis.[384] This results in obliteration of the normal demarcation between cortical and medullary bone. Periostitis generally is not prominent, although in a few reports, extensive periostitis simulating that of hypertrophic osteoarthropathy was evident in this disease (Fig. 62–44).[382, 383] In the spine, increased radiodensity or condensation of bone at the superior and inferior margins of the vertebral body (sandwich vertebrae) can be encountered. Focal or diffuse sclerosis in the skull may obscure the interface between the tables and diploë. Sclerosis may appear unchanged for long periods of time or progress slowly.

Extramedullary hematopoiesis in this condition can create lobulated, paravertebral intrathoracic masses.[136, 137, 261] In some instances, spinal cord compression from this abnormal tissue has been identified,[138–141, 262, 277] leading to neurologic dysfunction.

Articular Abnormalities

Bone and joint pain in both spinal and extraspinal sites can be evident. Hemarthrosis has been described in association with myeloproliferative disease and can be its presenting manifestation.[142, 143] Impaired platelet function presumably contributes to bleeding episodes.

The increased nucleoprotein turnover that accompanies this disease can lead to an increase in uric acid production. Fifty to 80 per cent of patients reveal elevated serum or urinary uric acid levels.[121] Secondary gout, which may antedate the diagnosis of myelofibrosis, occurs in 5 to 20 per cent of patients and may be associated with tophi and renal uric acid stones.[37, 47, 144] Uric acid levels may diminish after response to myelosuppressive therapy.

Polyarthralgias and polyarthritis in myelofibrosis may resemble rheumatoid arthritis[385] and also have been related to an immune pathogenesis[263] and to infiltration of the synovial membrane by bone marrow elements (Fig. 62–45).[264]

Magnetic Resonance Imaging

The basic histologic finding in the bone marrow in patients with myelofibrosis is fibrosis resulting from fibroblastic proliferation and increased production of collagen. Fibrotic replacement of the marrow, when examined with standard spin echo MR sequences, is characterized by decreased signal intensity on both T1-weighted and T2-weighted images.[313, 318] A focal or diffuse pattern of alteration in signal intensity may be encountered. As the initial sites of marrow fibrosis in this disease correspond to regions of active hematopoiesis in the adult, early MR imaging abnormalities are evident in the vertebrae, pelvis, and ribs (Fig. 62–46). Subsequent pathologic events, such as reconversion from fatty to hematopoietic marrow and marrow fibrosis, occur in the tubular bones, especially the femora, humeri, and tibiae, and they account for the same pattern of signal abnormality as is encountered in the axial skeleton (Fig. 62–47).

The most extensive MR imaging evaluation to date in patients with myelofibrosis (and with polycythemia) has been provided in a report from Kaplan and associates.[386] These investigators studied the spine, innominate bones, and proximal portions of the femora; correlated the imaging abnormalities with results provided by iliac crest biopsy; and established clinical parameters of disease severity (serum lactate dehydrogenase [LDH] and cholesterol levels) and chronicity (spleen size). They used in-phase and chemical shift opposed-phase spin echo MR sequences. On opposed-phase images, the phases of the echoes from water and fat are opposed such that the net signal intensity is the absolute difference between the water and triglyceride signals in each voxel.[387] To this imaging protocol, Kaplan and associates[386] added a hybrid fat suppression technique,

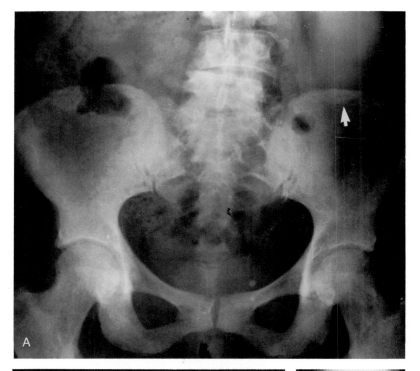

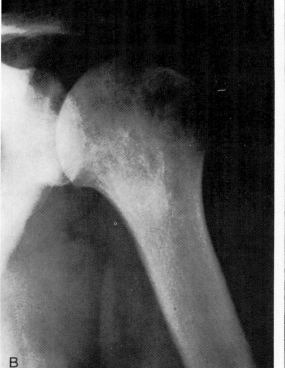

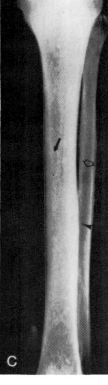

FIGURE 62–43. Myelofibrosis: Radiographic abnormalities. Osteosclerosis.

A In this case, patchy osteosclerosis of the entire pelvis is associated with small radiolucent areas. The spleen is enlarged (arrow).

B The proximal ends of the humerus and scapula demonstrate areas of focal and diffuse sclerosis.

C An anteroposterior radiograph of the tibia and fibula outlines increased radiodensity of bone caused predominantly by endosteal sclerosis (arrow), although there is evidence of periostitis as well (arrowhead). Focal lucent areas also are apparent (open arrow).

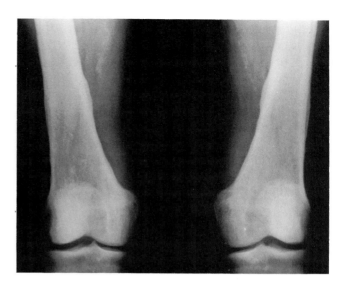

FIGURE 62–44. Myelofibrosis: Radiographic abnormalities. Periostitis. In this 71 year old woman with bilateral knee pain of 2 years' duration, note extensive periosteal bone formation in both femora. It was not present on a radiograph obtained 2 years previously. (Courtesy of G. Greenway, M.D., Dallas, Texas.)

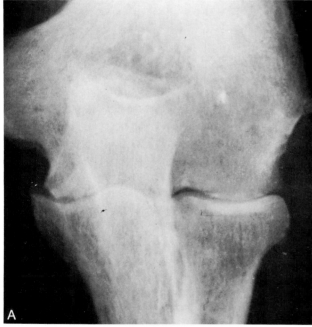

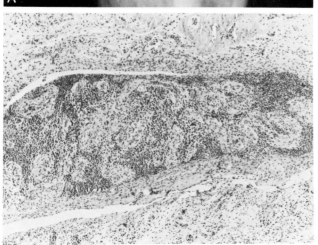

FIGURE 62–45. Myelofibrosis: Articular abnormalities. A 60 year old man developed polyarthralgias, a psoriasiform rash, and severe elbow pain. Peripheral blood smear and bone marrow biopsy established the diagnosis of myelofibrosis.

A A radiograph of the elbow shows diffuse loss of joint space, subchondral bone erosion, and patchy osteosclerosis.

B Synovectomy of the elbow performed because of the patient's progressive pain provided tissue for analysis. The synovial membrane was grossly thickened and hyperemic. Microscopically, a low grade diffuse inflammatory infiltrate and fibrovascular proliferation are evident (144×).

(From Heinicke MH, et al: Ann Rheum Dis *42*:196, 1983.)

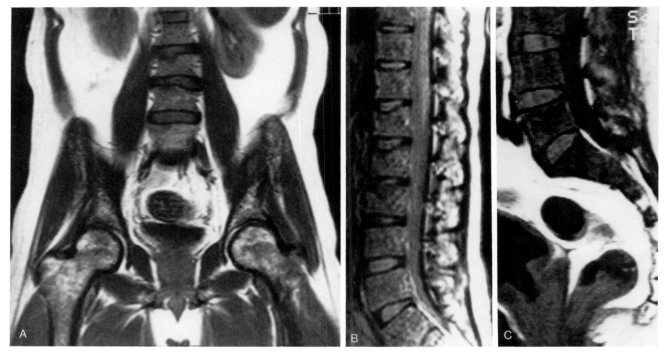

FIGURE 62–46. Myelofibrosis: MR imaging abnormalities. Axial skeleton. Spin echo MR imaging technique.
  A, B On a coronal T1-weighted (TR/TE, 650/30) spin echo MR image of the pelvis **(A)**, the marrow of the vertebral bodies, pelvic bones, and proximal femora is predominantly low in signal intensity. This pattern is consistent with the presence of hematopoietic marrow or fibrosis. Schmorl's nodes are evident, and the spleen is enlarged. On a sagittal T2-weighted (TR/TE, 1800/100) spin echo image of the thoracolumbar spine **(B)**, again note the low signal intensity in the bone marrow. (Courtesy of T. Mattsson, M.D., Riyadh, Saudi Arabia.)
  C In a different patient, a more dramatic decrease of signal intensity in the visualized bone marrow is evident on a sagittal T1-weighted (TR/TE, 500/22) MR image of the lumbosacral spine. (Courtesy of J. Rausch, M.D., Fort Wayne, Indiana.)

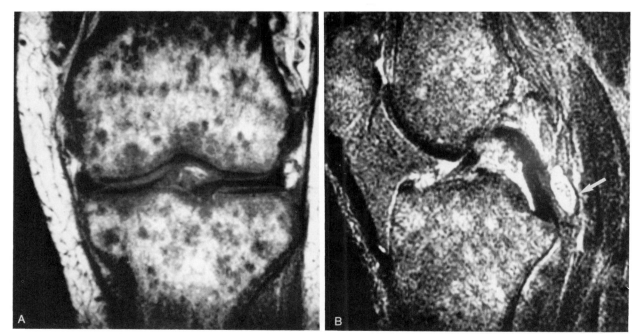

FIGURE 62–47. Myelofibrosis: MR imaging abnormalities. Appendicular skeleton, spin echo technique. This 71 year old woman had myelofibrosis and hepatosplenomegaly. Routine radiographs of the femora showed periostitis (see Figure 62–44). The coronal T1-weighted (TR/TE, 800/20) MR image **(A)** shows inhomogeneous signal intensity in the bone marrow of the distal femur and proximal tibia. The sagittal T2-weighted (TR/TE, 2000/80) MR image **(B)** again reveals inhomogeneous signal intensity in the bone marrow. The findings are consistent with hyperplastic red marrow, granulation tissue, and fibrosis. An incidental finding is a probable ganglion (arrow) arising near the posterior cruciate ligament. (Courtesy of G. Greenway, M.D., Dallas, Texas.)

which involved selective presaturation of the triglyceride signal followed by real-time subtraction of raw data from the in-phase and opposed-phase images.[388] They paid particular attention to the signal intensity patterns in the femoral capital epiphysis and greater trochanter. All patients revealed nonfatty marrow in the femoral neck and intertrochanteric region, findings considered abnormal in middle-aged and elderly adults, and many had nonfatty marrow in the apophyses or epiphyses, or both, findings considered abnormal in any person after the first few months of life. The apophyses were more resistant to reconversion of marrow than the epiphyses. Marrow patterns in the proximal ends of the femora in patients with polycythemia vera and myelofibrosis correlated with the clinical severity of the disorder (increased LDH and decreased cholesterol levels). Splenic volume, as determined by the MR images, was significantly greater in the myelofibrosis group of patients than in those with polycythemia vera. The authors concluded that MR imaging of the proximal portions of the femora is useful in both staging and evaluating the progression of these diseases, thereby circumventing the need for multiple blind bone marrow biopsies in most instances.[386]

Differential Diagnosis

The radiographic diagnosis of myelofibrosis should be suggested when axial skeleton osteosclerosis is combined with splenomegaly in a middle-aged or elderly patient (Table 62–3). Although lymphoma and leukemia can lead to splenomegaly, the extent of bone sclerosis is less in these conditions than in myelofibrosis. Systemic mastocytosis can produce diffuse or focal osteosclerosis and hepatosplenomegaly, and it may be difficult to differentiate from myelofibrosis.

Increased radiodensity of bone without splenic enlargement can be seen in some patients with myelofibrosis and is apparent in patients with this disorder who have had splenectomies. This combination of findings can be evident in other processes, including skeletal metastasis, fluorosis, Paget's disease, axial osteomalacia, and renal osteodystrophy. The differentiation of myelofibrosis and skeletal metastasis indeed can be difficult[145] (Fig. 62–48). In general,

the sclerosis observed in metastatic disease of the bone is less generalized, less symmetric, and associated more frequently with osteolytic lesions. In fluorosis, spinal osteophytosis, ligament calcification and ossification, and periostitis can be noted. In renal osteodystrophy, other changes, including those of hyperparathyroidism, are evident. In Paget's disease a characteristic coarsened trabecular pattern is present, whereas axial osteomalacia is confined to the axial skeleton and is associated with very prominent cervical spine abnormalities.

BONE MARROW TRANSPLANTATION

Bone marrow transplantation is a technique for replenishing the bone marrow with normal pluripotential stem cells. Allogeneic marrow transplantation is used for diseases caused by abnormalities in stem cell function (e.g., aplastic anemia, in which stem cells are deficient in numbers; and acute leukemia, in which stem cells are malignant).[389] Normal marrow cells from a histocompatible allogeneic donor are used to repopulate the diseased marrow, and such transplantation frequently is combined with intensive chemotherapy or immunosuppressive therapy.[389]

The major categories of disease that are indications for marrow transplantation include immunodeficiency states, nonmalignant disorders of hematopoiesis (aplastic anemia, thalassemia, other hereditary hemoglobinopathies, congenital aregenerative anemias), enzymatic disorders (mucopolysaccharidoses, Gaucher's disease), and malignant diseases (leukemias, lymphomas, myelofibrosis, plasma cell myeloma, neuroblastoma).[390] Three forms of transplantation are possible: autologous transplantation, in which a portion of the patient's own marrow is removed, the patient is treated with intensive chemotherapy or radiotherapy, or both, and the patient's marrow is reinfused; syngeneic transplantation, in which the marrow from a normal, genetically identical twin is used; and allogeneic transplantation in which the marrow from a normal, genetically different donor is employed.[390] Most allogeneic transplants have been performed between HLA identical siblings. The marrow usually is obtained from the donor's iliac crest. Radiographs obtained after the procedure may reveal multiple, small

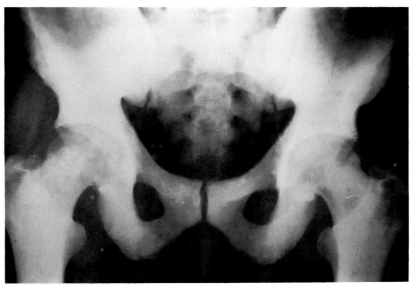

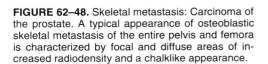
FIGURE 62–48. Skeletal metastasis: Carcinoma of the prostate. A typical appearance of osteoblastic skeletal metastasis of the entire pelvis and femora is characterized by focal and diffuse areas of increased radiodensity and a chalklike appearance.

radiolucent areas in the crest that, with healing, are surrounded by bone sclerosis.[391]

A variety of complications are related to bone marrow transplantations.[390–392] These may be categorized as pre-engraftment complications, immediate (within 3 months) postengraftment complications, and delayed (after 3 months) postengraftment complications.[391] The pre-engraftment, or peritransplantation, period is defined as the interval between the initiation of immunosuppressive treatment and the time of transplantation. Complications in this period include infections, tissue-damaging effects of therapy, hepatic veno-occlusive disease, and graft rejection.[391] Immediate postengraftment complications include infections, pneumatosis intestinalis, and acute graft-versus-host disease (GVHD). Delayed postengraftment complications include chronic GVHD and recurrence of the original marrow disorder.[391]

Infections developing immediately before or soon after bone marrow transplantation relate to the effects of chemotherapy and radiation therapy as well as of the transplantation itself. Pretransplantation therapy can lead to severe toxic effects, including cutaneous and mucosal disruption, pneumonitis, nausea, vomiting, and diarrhea. Bacterial (*Staphylococcus epidermidis*) and fungal (Candida and Aspergillus species) infections dominate in the pretransplantation period, and viral infections (herpes simplex virus) also may be encountered. During the first 2 or 3 weeks after transplantation, severe granulocytopenia, fever, and, in about 50 per cent of patients, at least one episode of bacteremia are seen.[390] Neutropenia at this time predisposes to infections caused by opportunistic organisms, including viral (cytomegalovirus, varicella-zoster virus, adenovirus, and herpes simplex virus), fungal (Candida and Aspergillus species), protozoal (*Pneumocystis carinii* and, rarely, *Toxoplasma gondii*), and bacterial agents.[391] Delayed posttransplantation infections usually are related to varicella-zoster virus or, in patients with chronic GVHD, recurrent bacterial or fungal infections.[380] T lymphocyte dysfunction and abnormal immunoregulation, amplified and prolonged by chronic GVHD, account for the infectious complications during this period.[392]

GVHD, which is discussed in detail in Chapter 34, is believed to be the result of allogeneic T cells that were transfused with the graft or developed from its reaction to targets of the genetically different host.[390] An immunologic attack on the recipient's tissues develops.[392] Acute GVHD occurs within the first 3 months after transplantation and is associated with lesions of the skin, liver, and gastrointestinal tract.[390] Specific clinical findings include an erythematous maculopapular skin rash on the face, trunk, and extremities, abdominal pain, diarrhea, nausea, and vomiting. Liver disease is characterized by elevation of serum levels of bilirubin, transaminases, and alkaline phosphatase. Chronic GVHD affects 20 to 40 per cent of patients who survive more than 6 months after transplantation.[390] It involves the skin, oral mucosa, serosal surfaces, skeletal muscle, gastrointestinal tract, liver, and lung, and its manifestations resemble those of a collagen vascular disorder, particularly scleroderma. Infections, which generally are bacterial and affect the upper respiratory tract, complicate chronic GVHD.

The cellular constituents of the bone marrow change dramatically immediately before and after transplantation

and, in the posttransplantation period, depend on the success or failure of the procedure. Chemotherapy and radiotherapy administered in the pretransplantation period are designed not only to induce immunologic suppression in the recipient but also to eliminate any residual malignant cell populations.[393] The initial response of the bone marrow to such therapy is congestion and edema. Subsequently, hematopoietic tissue disappears, the marrow becoming predominantly fatty.[313] High signal intensity on T1-weighted spin echo MR images and intermediate signal intensity on T2-weighted spin echo images, signal characteristics that are typical of adipose tissue, are observed. During transplantation, bone marrow cells are infused intravenously. After a transient residence in the lungs and spleen, the infused stem cells migrate to the bone marrow.[393] Hematologic engrafting typically takes 3 to 4 weeks and is heralded by a peripheral rise in granulocytes.[393]

Repopulation of the bone marrow in the spine after transplantation has been studied with MR imaging techniques by Stevens and coworkers.[393] A bandlike pattern of modification of signal intensity in the vertebral body was encountered in the first 6 months after marrow transplantation. On T1-weighted spin echo MR images, the superior and inferior margins of the vertebral bodies revealed low signal intensity, whereas the central portion of the vertebral bodies showed high signal intensity, consistent with fat. With STIR sequences, the opposite situation was apparent, with high signal intensity at the superior and inferior vertebral margins and low signal intensity centrally. At histologic examination, the marginal, or peripheral, regions of the vertebral body were found to contain a concentrated collection of repopulating cells, and the central region contained predominantly marrow fat. The authors speculated that the vascular supply of the vertebral body, which consists, in part, of branches of the nutrient arteries that terminate in capillaries near the endosteal surface of the cortex, explained the bandlike imaging and histologic characteristics after marrow transplantation. The bandlike MR imaging pattern persisted beyond 6 months after transplantation in all patients studied by Stevens and colleagues[393] except one patient in whom acute nonlymphocytic leukemia relapsed. In this last patient, a diffusely homogeneous area of abnormally low signal intensity in the vertebral bodies on T1-weighted spin echo images was seen. These investigators again speculated that MR imaging patterns and measurements of T1 relaxation times may prove useful in differentiating a fully reconstituted and healthy posttransplant marrow from one exhibiting disease relapse.

In some instances, the transplanted marrow graft functions only briefly. After a period of days or weeks, marrow function is lost, and myeloid elements are absent on marrow biopsy.[390] Graft rejection, in most cases, is believed to result from residual host immunity to the donor, and prior transfusions represent a definite risk factor for such rejection.

As total body irradiation, in combination with chemotherapy, may be employed prior to transplantation in the treatment of some disorders (such as childhood leukemia), it is not surprising that complications related to such irradiation may appear in long-term survivors. These complications include chronic restrictive and obstructive pulmonary disease, gonadal failure, cataracts, thyroid and adrenocortical dysfunction, deficiency of growth hormone with decreased longitudinal growth, and disturbed dental development.[400-402] Bone sequelae of total body irradiation include tumors and tumorlike lesions (osteochondromas, aneurysmal bone cysts, fibrous dysplasia, and sarcomas), osteonecrosis, slipped femoral capital epiphysis, and metaphyseal growth abnormalities.[403] Such bone sequelae may be less severe when total body irradiation is employed in children in the second (rather than the first) decade of life.

SUMMARY

Musculoskeletal abnormalities accompany a variety of myeloproliferative disorders. In leukemias, such abnormalities are particularly frequent in children. Osseous involvement from the primary disease leads to local symptoms and signs. Synovial involvement due to leukemic infiltration and hemorrhage can result in articular findings. Hyperuricemia and secondary gout can complicate this disease. Bone destruction and secondary gout also may be observed in the lymphomas. Sjögren's syndrome is associated with an arthritis that usually appears identical to rheumatoid arthritis. In systemic mastocytosis, characteristic skeletal abnormalities include focal or diffuse lytic or sclerotic lesions. In polycythemia vera, osteonecrosis, osteopenia, and hyperuricemia can appear. Myelofibrosis can be accompanied by osteosclerosis, particularly in the axial skeleton. In addition, hyperuricemia and secondary gout are relatively common in this disorder.

References

1. Van Slyck EJ: The bony changes in malignant hematologic disease. Orthop Clin North Am 3:733, 1972.
2. O'Hara AE: Roentgenographic osseous manifestations of the anemias and the leukemias. Clin Orthop 52:63, 1967.
3. Benz G, Brandeis WE, Willich E: Radiological aspects of leukemia in childhood. An analysis of 89 children. Pediatr Radiol 4:201, 1976.
4. Simmons CR, Harle TS, Singleton EB: The osseous manifestations of leukemia in children. Radiol Clin North Am 6:115, 1968.
5. Nixon GW, Gwinn JL: The roentgen manifestations of leukemia in infancy. Radiology 107:603, 1973.
6. Rodnan GP: Arthritis associated with hematologic disorders. Bull Rheum Dis 16:392, 1965.
7. Aisner M, Hoxie TB: Bone and joint pain in leukemia simulating acute rheumatic fever and subacute bacterial endocarditis. N Engl J Med 238:733, 1948.
8. Dresner E: The bone and joint lesions in acute leukemia and their response to folic acid antagonists. Q J Med 19:339, 1950.
9. Silverstein MN, Kelly PJ: Leukemia with osteoarticular symptoms and signs. Ann Intern Med 59:637, 1963.
10. Spilberg I, Meyer GJ: The arthritis of leukemia. Arthritis Rheum 15:630, 1972.
11. Cooke JV: Acute leukemia in children. JAMA 101:432, 1933.
12. Thomas LB, Forkner CE Jr, Frei E, et al: The skeletal lesions of acute leukemia. Cancer 14:608, 1961.
13. Bedwell GA, Dawson AM: Chronic myeloid leukemia in a child presenting as acute polyarthritis. Arch Dis Child 29:78, 1954.
14. Hindmarsh JR, Emslie-Smith D: Monocytic leukemia presenting as polyarthritis in an adult. Br Med J 1:593, 1953.
15. Baty JM, Vogt E: Bone changes of leukemia in children. AJR 34:310, 1935.
16. Silverman FN: The skeletal lesions of leukemia—clinical and roentgenographic observations in 103 infants and children with review of the literature. AJR 59:819, 1948.
17. Wilson JKV: The bone lesions of childhood leukemia. Radiology 72:672, 1959.
18. Landolt RF: Knochenveränderungen bei kindlichen Leukämien. Über rheumatoide leukämieformen. Ann Paediatr 167:293, 1946.
19. Somm P: Komplikationen der akuten Leukämie im Kindesalter unter kombinierter Steroid-Cytostatica-Therapie. Helv Pediatr Acta 20:75, 1965.
20. Aur RJA, Westbrook W, Riggs W Jr: Childhood acute lymphocytic leukemia. Am J Dis Child 124:653, 1972.
21. Epstein BS: Vertebral changes in childhood leukemia. Radiology 68:65, 1957.
22. Lichtenstein L: Bone Tumors. St. Louis, CV Mosby, 1952, p 253.
23. Reinberg SA: Clinico-roentgenological observations over a peculiar manifestation of leukemia in childhood. Pediatrics 41:15, 1962.
24. Eschenbach C: Über eine seltene Form der Wirbelsäulenbeteiligung au akuten Leukosen im Kindersalter. Monatsschr Kinderheilkd 113:68, 1965.
25. Gougleris K, Swoboda W, Wolf HG: Veränderungen der Wirbelsäuleim Verlauf der leukämie beim Kind. ROFO 88:309, 1958.
26. Kosenow W, Niederle J: Wirbelsäulenveränderungen im Röntgenbild bei malignen Geschwulsterkrankungen des Kindesalters. Monatsschr Kinderheikd 120:1, 1972.
27. Ehrlich JC, Forer S: Periosteal ossification in myelogenous leukemia: Report of a case associated with acute rheumatic fever. Arch Intern Med 53:938, 1934.
28. Kalayjian BS, Herbut PA, Erf LA: The bone changes of leukemia in children. Radiology 47:223, 1946.
29. Taylor HK: Periosteal changes in a case of lymphatic leukemia. Radiology 6:523, 1926.
30. Sullivan MP: Intracranial complications of leukemia in children. Pediatrics 20:757, 1957.
31. Austin JHM: Chloroma. Report of a patient with unusual rib lesions. Radiology 93:671, 1969.
32. Rosenfield NS, McIntosh S: Prospective analysis of bone changes in treated childhood leukemia. Radiology 123:413, 1977.
33. Karpinski FE Jr, Martin JF: The skeletal lesions of leukemic children treated with aminopterin. J Pediatr 37:208, 1950.
34. Dresner E: The bone and joint lesions in acute leukemia and their response to folic acid antagonists. Q J Med 19:339, 1950.
35. Brunner S, Gudbjerg CE, Iversen T: Skeletal lesions in leukemia in children. Acta Radiol 49:419, 1958.
36. Silverman FN: Treatment of leukemia and allied disorders with folic acid antagonists; effect of aminopterin on skeletal lesions. Radiology 54:665, 1950.
37. Talbott JH: Gout and blood dyscrasias. Medicine 38:173, 1959.
38. Shorvon LM: Gout in leukemia. Report of a case. Lancet 2:378, 1946.
39. Ansell BM: Case report 40. Skel Radiol 2:113, 1977.
40. Chabner BA, Haskell CM, Canellos GP: Destructive bone lesions in chronic granulocytic leukemia. Medicine 48:401, 1969.
41. Kattlove HE, Williams JC, Gaynor E, et al: Gaucher cells in chronic myelocytic leukemia: An acquired abnormality. Blood 33:379, 1969.
42. Spengler DM, Leiberg OU, Bailey RW: Rapid diaphyseal destruction. An unusual osseous manifestation of chronic granulocytic leukemia. Clin Orthop 115:231, 1976.
43. Glatt W, Weinstein A: Acropachy in lymphatic leukemia. Radiology 92:125, 1969.
44. Calvert RJ, Smith E: Metastatic acropachy in lymphatic leukemia. Blood 10:545, 1955.
45. Craver LF: Tenderness of the sternum in leukemia. Am J Med Sci 174:799, 1927.
46. Calabro JJ: Cancer and arthritis. Arthritis Rheum 10:553, 1967.
47. Yu TF: Secondary gout associated with myeloproliferative diseases. Arthritis Rheum 8:765, 1965.
48. Vieta JO, Friedell HL, Craver LF: A survey of Hodgkin's disease and lymphosarcoma in bone. Radiology 39:1, 1942.
49. Coles WC, Schulz MD: Bone involvement in malignant lymphoma. Radiology 50:458, 1948.
50. Martin DJ, Ash JM: Diagnostic radiology in non-Hodgkin's lymphoma. Semin Oncol 4:297, 1977.
51. Parker BR, Castellino RA, Kaplan HS: Pediatric Hodgkin's disease. I. Radiographic evaluation. Cancer 37:2430, 1976.
52. Castellino RA, Blank N, Cassady JR, et al: Roentgenologic aspects of Hodgkin's disease. II. Role of routine radiographs in detecting initial relapse. Cancer 31:316, 1973.
53. Schey WI, White H, Conway JJ, et al: Lymphosarcoma in children. A roentgenologic and clinical evaluation of 60 children. AJR 117:59, 1973.
54. Grossman H, Winchester PH, Bragg DG, et al: Roentgenographic changes in childhood Hodgkin's disease. AJR 108:354, 1970.
55. Castellino RA, Bellani FF, Gasparini M, et al: Radiographic findings in previously untreated children with non-Hodgkin's lymphoma. Radiology 117:657, 1975.
56. Cockshott WP: Radiology of Burkitt's tumor in young Nigerians. Symposium on Lympho-reticular Tumors in South Africa, Paris. 1963. Basel, S Karger, 1964, p 150.
57. Ferris RA, Hakkai HG, Cigtay OS: Radiologic manifestations of North American Burkitt's lymphoma. AJR 123:614, 1975.
58. Tefft M, Vawter GF, Mitus A: Paravertebral "round cell" tumors in children. Radiology 92:1501, 1969.
59. Dennis JM: The solitary dense vertebral body. Radiology 77:618, 1961.
60. Rosenberg SA, Diamond HD, Jaslowitz B, et al: Lymphosarcoma: A review of 1269 cases. Medicine 40:31, 1961.
61. Foley WD, Baum AM, Wheeler RH: Diffuse osteosclerosis with lymphocytic lymphoma. A case report. Radiology 117:553, 1975.
62. Burkitt D: A sarcoma involving the jaws in African children. Br J Surg 46:218, 1958.
63. O'Reilly GV, Clark TM, Crum CP: Skeletal involvement in mycosis fungoides. AJR 129:741, 1977.
64. Sézary A, Bouvrain Y: Erythrodermie avec présence de cellules monstreuses dan dermie et sang circulant. Bull Soc Fr Dermatol Syphiligr 45:254, 1938.
65. McCormick CC: Case report 20. Skel Radiol 1:183, 1977.
66. Child JA, Smith IE: Lymphoma presenting as "idiopathic" juvenile osteoporosis. Br Med J 1:720, 1975.
67. Cammarata RJ, Rodnan GP, Jensen WN: Systemic rheumatic disease and malignant lymphoma. Arch Intern Med 111:330, 1963.
68. Howqua J, Mackay IR: LE cells in lymphoma. Blood 22:191, 1963.
69. Miller DG: The association of immune disease and malignant lymphoma. Ann Intern Med 66:507, 1967.

70. Hench PK, Mayne JG, Kiely JM, et al: Clinical study of the rheumatic manifestations of lymphoma (Abstr). Arthritis Rheum 5:301, 1962.

71. Miller SB, Donlan CJ, Roth SB: Hodgkin's disease presenting as relapsing polychondritis. A previously undescribed association. Arthritis Rheum 17:598, 1974.

72. Hadden WB: On "dry mouth" or suppression of the salivary and buccal secretions. Trans Clin Soc London 21:176, 1888.

73. Mikulicz J: Concerning a peculiar symmetrical disease of the lacrimal and salivary glands. Med Classics 2:135, 1937.

74. Houwer AWM: Keratitis filamentosa and chronic arthritis. Trans Ophthalmol Soc UK 47:88, 1927.

75. Betsch A: Die chronische Keratitis filiformis. Folge mangelnder Tränensekretion. Kl Mbl Augenheilk 80:618, 1928.

76. Albrich K: Filiform keratitis due to insufficient secretion of lacrimal glands. 3 cases. Arch Ophthalmol 121:402, 1928.

77. Sjögren H: Zur Kenntnis der Keratoconjunctivitis sicca (Keratitis filiformis bei Hypofunktion der Tranendrusen). Acta Ophthalmol 11(Supp 2):1, 1933.

78. Stenstam T: On the occurrence of keratoconjunctivitis sicca in cases of rheumatoid arthritis. Acta Med Scand 127:130, 1947.

79. Bloch KJ, Buchanan WW, Whol MJ, et al: Sjögren's syndrome. A clinical, pathological and serological study of sixty-two cases. Medicine 44:187, 1965.

80. Talal N: Sjögren's syndrome and connective tissue disease with other immunologic disorders. In JL Hollander, DJ McCarthy Jr (Eds): Arthritis and Allied Conditions. 8th Ed. Philadelphia, Lea & Febiger, 1972, p 849.

81. Bunim JJ: Broader spectrum of Sjögren's syndrome and its pathogenetic implications. Ann Rheum Dis 20:1, 1961.

82. Rubin P, Besse BE Jr: Sialographic differentiation of Mikulicz's disease and Mikulicz's syndrome. Radiology 68:477, 1957.

83. Rubin P, Holt JF: Secretory sialography in disease of major salivary glands. AJR 77:575, 1957.

84. Silbiger ML, Peterson CC Jr: Sjögren's syndrome. Its roentgenographic features. AJR 100:554, 1967.

85. Reader SR, Whyte HM, Elmes PC: Sjögren's disease and rheumatoid arthritis. Ann Rheum Dis 10:288, 1951.

86. Cardell BS, Gurling KJ: Observations on the pathology of Sjögren's syndrome. J Pathol Bacteriol 68:137, 1954.

87. Ellman P, Weber FP, Goodier TEW: A contribution to the pathology of Sjögren's disease. Q J Med 20:33, 1951.

88. Szanto L, Farkas K, Gyulai E: On Sjögren's disease. Rheumatism 13:60, 1957.

89. Talal N, Bunim JJ: The development of malignant lymphoma in the course of Sjögren's syndrome. Am J Med 36:529, 1964.

90. Bunim JJ, Talal N: The association of malignant lymphoma with Sjögren's syndrome. Trans Assoc Am Physicians 76:45, 1963.

91. Anderson LG, Talal N: The spectrum of benign to malignant lymphoproliferation in Sjögren's syndrome. Clin Exp Immunol 10:199, 1972.

92. DeCoteau WE, Katakkar SB, Skinnider L, et al: Sjögren's syndrome terminating as a myeloproliferative disorder. J Rheumatol 2:331, 1975.

93. Leventhal BA, Waldorf DS, Talal N: Impaired lymphocyte transformation and delayed hypersensitivity in Sjögren's syndrome. J Clin Invest 46:1338, 1967.

94. Nettleship E: Rare forms of urticaria. Br Med J 2:323, 1869.

95. Finnerud CW: Urticaria pigmentosa (nodular type) with a summary of the literature. Arch Dermatol 8:344, 1923.

96. Bendel WL Jr, Race GJ: Urticaria pigmentosa with bone involvement. J Bone Joint Surg [Am] 45:1043, 1963.

97. Barer M, Peterson LFA, Dahlin DC, et al: Mastocytosis with osseous lesions resembling metastatic malignant lesions in bone. J Bone Joint Surg [Am] 50:142, 1968.

98. Poppel MH, Gruber WF, Silber R, et al: The roentgen manifestations of urticaria pigmentosa (mastocytosis). AJR 82:239, 1959.

99. Stark E, VanBuskirk FW, Daly JF: Radiologic and pathologic bone changes associated with urticaria pigmentosa. Arch Pathol 62:143, 1956.

100. Issrof SW, Cohen E: Systemic mastocytosis. South Afr Med J 47:1576, 1973.

101. Ting YM: Bone lesion in systemic mastocytosis. Australas Radiol 15:264, 1971.

102. Duriez J: L'atteinte osseuse au cours de la mastocytose cutanée. A propos de deux observations. Rev Rhum Mal Osteoartic 42:71, 1975.

103. Gagnon JH, Kalz F, Kadri AM, et al: Mastocytosis: Unusual manifestations: clinical and radiologic changes. Can Med Assoc J 112:1329, 1975.

104. Jensen WN, Lasser EC: Urticaria pigmentosa associated with widespread sclerosis of the spongiosa of bone. Radiology 71:826, 1958.

105. Asboe-Hansen G: Urticaria pigmentosa with bone lesions. Acta Dermatol Venereol 33:471, 1953.

106. Lees MH, Stroud CE: Bone lesions of urticaria pigmentosa in childhood. Arch Dis Child 34:205, 1959.

107. Prost A, Cottin S, Malkani K, et al: Etude d'une osteoporose diffuse dans un cas de mastocytose cutanée et osseuse. Rev Rhum Mal Osteoartic 41:277, 1974.

108. Zak FG, Covey JA, Snodgrass JJ: Osseous lesions in urticaria pigmentosa. N Engl J Med 256:56, 1957.

109. Loewenthal M, Schen RJ, Berlin C, et al: Urticaria pigmentosa with systemic mast cell involvement: Autopsy report. Arch Dermatol 75:512, 1957.

110. Ritz F, Geller M, Sims JL, et al: Systemic mastocytosis associated with presence of rheumatoid factor. JAMA 235:1586, 1976.

111. Wasserman LR, Bassen F: Polycythemia. J Mt Sinai Hosp 26:1, 1959.

112. Lawrence JH, Berlin NI, Huff RL: The nature and treatment of polycythemia. Medicine 32:323, 1953.

113. Murray RO, Jacobson HG: The Radiology of Skeletal Disorders. Edinburgh, Churchill Livingstone, 1971, p 1058.

114. Dykstra OH, Halbertsma T: Polycythaemia versa in childhood: Report of a case with changes in the skull. Am J Dis Child 60:907, 1940.

115. Gardner FH, Nathan DG: Secondary gout. Med Clin North Am 45:1273, 1961.

116. Denman AM, Szur L, Ansell BM: Joint complaints in polycythemia vera. Ann Rheum Dis 23:139, 1964.

117. Leigh TF, Corley CC Jr, Huguley CM Jr, et al: Myelofibrosis. The general and radiologic manifestations in 25 proven cases. AJR 82:183, 1959.

118. Bouroncle BA, Doan CA: Myelofibrosis, clinical, hematologic and pathologic study of 110 patients. Am J Med Sci 243:697, 1962.

119. Pitcock JA, Reinhard EH, Justus BW, et al: A clinical and pathological study of seventy cases of myelofibrosis. Ann Intern Med 57:73, 1962.

120. Pettigrew JD, Ward HP: Correlation of radiologic, histologic and clinical findings in agnogenic myeloid metaplasia. Radiology 93:541, 1969.

121. Gilbert HS: The spectrum of myeloproliferative disorders. Med Clin North Am 57:355, 1973.

122. Wood HC: On relations of leukocythaemia and pseudoleukemia. Am J Med Sci 62:373, 1871.

123. Heuck G: Zwei Falle von Leukämie mit eigenthümlichen Blut-resp. Knochenmarksbefund. Virchows Arch (Pathol Anat) 78:475, 1879.

124. Block M, Jacobson LO: Myeloid metaplasia. JAMA 143:1390, 1950.

125. Donhauser JL: Human spleen as haematoplastic organ, as exemplified in a case of splenomegaly with sclerosis of bone marrow. J Exp Med 10:559, 1908.

126. Wyatt JP, Sommers SC: Chronic marrow failure, myelosclerosis, and extramedullary hematopoiesis. Blood 5:329, 1950.

127. Peace RJ: Myelonecrosis, extramedullary myelopoiesis, and leukoerythroblastosis. Am J Pathol 29:1029, 1953.

128. Dameshek W: Some speculations on myeloproliferative syndromes. Blood 6:372, 1951.

129. Rawson R, Parker F Jr, Jackson H Jr: Industrial solvents as possible etiologic agents in myeloid metaplasia. Science 93:541, 1941.

130. Wasserman LR: Polycythemia vera—its course and treatment: Relation to myeloid metaplasia and leukemia. Bull NY Acad Med 30:343, 1954.

131. Mettier SR, Rusk GY: Fibrosis of bone marrow (myelofibrosis) associated with leukemoid blood picture. Am J Pathol 13:377, 1937.

132. Churg J, Wachstein M: Osteosclerosis, myelofibrosis and leukemia. Am J Med Sci 207:141, 1944.

133. Bomford RR, Rhoads CP: Refractory anaemia; clinical and pathological aspects. Q J Med 10:175, 1941.

134. Taylor HE, Simpson WW: Bone marrow fibrosis developing in aleukemic myelosis. Blood 5:348, 1950.

135. Korst DR, Clatanoff DV, Schilling RF: On myelofibrosis. Arch Intern Med 97:169, 1956.

136. Lowman RM, Bloor CM, Newcomb AW: Roentgen manifestations of thoracic extramedullary hematopoiesis. Dis Chest 44:154, 1963.

137. Ross P, Logan W: Roentgen findings in extramedullary hematopoiesis. AJR 106:604, 1969.

138. Close AS, Taira Y, Cleveland DA: Spinal cord compression due to extramedullary hematopoiesis. Ann Intern Med 48:421, 1958.

139. Appleby A, Batson GA, Lassman LT, et al: Spinal cord compression by extramedullary hematopoiesis in myelosclerosis. J Neurol Neurosurg Psychiatry 27:313, 1964.

140. Sorsdahl OS, Taylor PE, Noyes WD: Extramedullary hematopoiesis, mediastinal masses, and spinal cord compression. JAMA 189:343, 1964.

141. Cromwell LD, Kerber C: Spinal cord compression by extramedullary hematopoiesis in agnogenic myeloid metaplasia. Radiology 128:118, 1978.

142. Harris BK, Ross HA: Hemarthrosis as the presenting manifestation of myeloproliferative disease. Arthritis Rheum 17:969, 1974.

143. Gunz FW: Hemorrhagic thrombocythemia: A critical review. Blood 15:706, 1960.

144. Ward HP, Block MH: The natural history of agnogenic myeloid metaplasia (AMM) and a critical evaluation of its relationship with the myeloproliferative syndrome. Medicine 50:357, 1971.

145. Peison B, Benisch B: Malignant myelosclerosis simulating metastatic bone disease. Radiology 125:62, 1977.

146. Becker MH, Engler GL, Klein M: Case report 93. Skel Radiol 4:111, 1979.

147. Lucaya J, Perez-Candela V, Aso C, et al: Mastocytosis with skeletal and gastrointestinal involvement in infancy. Two case reports and a review of the literature. Radiology. 13:363, 1979.

148. Tubiana J-M, Dana A, Petit-Perrin D, Duperray B: Lymphographic patterns in systemic mastocytosis with diffuse bone involvement and hematological signs. Radiology 131:651, 1979.

149. Sagher F, Cohen C, Schorr S: Concomitant bone changes in urticaria pigmentosa. J Invest Dermatol 18:425, 1952.

150. Schabel SI, Tyminski L, Holland RD, et al: The skeletal manifestations of chronic myelogenous leukemia. Skel Radiol 5:145, 1980.

151. Braunstein EM, Hammond B, Schnitzer B: Bone destruction in myelogenous marrow crisis. J Can Assoc Radiol 31:69, 1980.

152. Shaikh BS, Appelbaum PC, Aber RC: Vertebral disc space infection and osteomyelitis due to Candida albicans in a patient with acute myelomonocytic leukemia. Cancer 45:1025, 1980.

153. Braunstein EM, White SJ: Non-Hodgkin lymphoma of bone. Radiology 135:59, 1980.

154. Solgaard S, Kristiansen B: Vertebra plana due to a malignant lymphoma. Acta Orthop Scand 51:267, 1980.

155. Mahoney JP, Alexander RW: Primary histiocytic lymphoma of bone. A light and ultrastructural study of four cases. Am J Surg Pathol 4:149, 1980.

156. Baker CG, Tishler JM: Malignant disease in the jaws. J Can Assoc Radiol 28:129, 1977.

157. Parker BR, Marglin S, Castellino RA: Skeletal manifestations of leukemia, Hodgkin disease and non-Hodgkin lymphoma. Semin Roentgenol 15:302, 1980.

158. Luzar MJ, Sharma HM: Leukemia and arthritis: Including reports on light, immunofluorescent, and electron microscopy of the synovium. J Rheumatol 10:132, 1983.

159. Weinberger A, Schumacher HR, Schimmer BM, et al: Arthritis in acute leukemia. Clinical and histopathological observations. Arch Intern Med 141:1183, 1981.

160. Costello PB, Brecher ML, Starr JI, et al: A prospective analysis of the frequency, course, and possible prognostic significance of the joint manifestations of childhood leukemia. J Rheumatol 10:753, 1983.

161. Harden EA, Moore JO, Haynes BF: Leukemia-associated arthritis: Identification of leukemic cells in synovial fluid using monoclonal and polyclonal antibodies. Arthritis Rheum 27:1306, 1984.

162. Muntean W, Zaunschirm A: Aseptic osteonecrosis in children with leukemia prior to institution of treatment. Eur J Pediatr 140:139, 1983.

163. Niebrugge DJ, Benjamin DR: Bone marrow necrosis proceding acute lymphoblastic leukemia in childhood. Cancer 52:2162, 1983.

164. Melhem RE, Saber TJ: Erosion of the medial cortex of the proximal humerus. A sign of leukemia on the chest radiograph. Radiology 137:77, 1980.

165. Hughes RG, Kay HEM: Major bone lesions in acute lymphoblastic leukaemia. Med Pediatr Oncol 10:67, 1982.

166. DeBoeck M, Peeters O, Van Camp B, et al: Monocytic leukaemia associated with myeloid metaplasia resembling metastatic bone disease. Skel Radiol 11:9, 1984.

167. Redmond J III, Stites DP, Beckstead JH, et al: Chronic lymphocytic leukemia with osteolytic bone lesions, hypercalcemia, and monoclonal protein. Am J Clin Pathol 79:616, 1983.

168. Junca-Piera J, Duran-Suarez JR, Triginer-Boixeda J: Lesiones osteoliticas en la leucemia mielode cronica. Presentacion de tres casos. Med Clin (Barcelona) 76:259, 1981.

169. Van Soesbergen RM, Feltkamp-Vroom TM, Feltkamp CA, et al: T cell leukemia presenting as chronic polyarthritis. Arthritis Rheum 25:87, 1982.

170. Bouroncle BA, Wiseman BK, Doan CA: Leukaemic reticulo-endotheliosis. Blood 13:609, 1958.

171. Bouroncle BA: Leukemic reticuloendotheliosis (hairy cell leukaemia). Blood 53:412, 1979.

172. Schrek R, Donnelly WJ: Hairy cells in blood lymphoreticular neoplastic disease and flagellated cells of normal lymph nodes. Blood 27:199, 1966.

173. Golomb HM, Catovsky D, Golde DW: Hairy cell leukemia. A clinical review based on 71 cases. Ann Intern Med 89:677, 1978.

174. Flandrin G, Sigaux F, Sebahoun G, et al: Hairy cell leukemia: Clinical presentation and follow-up of 211 patients. Semin Oncol 11:458, 1984.

175. Demanes DJ, Lane N, Beckstead JH: Bone involvement in hairy-cell leukemia. Cancer 49:1697, 1982.

176. Quesada JR, Keating MJ, Libshitz HI, et al: Bone involvement in hairy cell leukemia. Am J Med 74:228, 1983.

177. Arkel YS, Lake-Lewin D, Savopoulos AA, et al: Bone lesions in hairy cell leukemia. A case report and response of bone pains to steroids. Cancer 53:2401, 1984.

178. Sattar MA, Cawley MID: Arthritis associated with hairy cell leukaemia. Ann Rheum Dis 41:289, 1982.

179. Lewis S, Szur L: Malignant myelosclerosis. Br Med J 2:472, 1963.

180. Bearman R, Pangalis G, Rappaport H: Acute ("malignant") myelosclerosis. Cancer 43:279, 1979.

181. Habib A, Lee H, Chan M: Acute myelogenous leukemia with megakaryoblastic myelosis. Am J Clin Pathol 74:705, 1980.

182. Cronier J, Katz M, Flandrin G, et al: Les lésions osseuses au cours des leucémies à micromégacaryoblastes. Ann Radiol 23:495, 1980.

183. Karasick S, Karasick D, Schilling J: Acute megakaryoblastic leukemia (acute "malignant" myelofibrosis): An unusual cause of osteosclerosis. Skel Radiol 9:45, 1982.

184. Neiman RS, Barcos M, Berard C, et al: Granulocytic sarcoma: A clinicopathologic study of 61 biopsied cases. Cancer 48:1426, 1981.

185. Dock G: Chloroma and its relation to leukemia. Am J Med Sci 106:152, 1893.

186. Wiernick PH, Serpick AA: Granulocytic sarcoma (chloroma). Blood 35:361, 1970.

187. Brooks HW, Evans AE, Glass RM, et al: Chloromas of the head and neck in childhood. The initial manifestation of myeloid leukemia in three patients. Arch Otolaryngol 100:306, 1974.

188. Krause JR: Granulocytic sarcoma preceding acute leukemia. Cancer 44:1017, 1979.

189. Comings DE, Fayen AW, Carter P: Myeloblastoma preceding blood and marrow evidence of acute leukemia. Cancer 18:253, 1965.

190. Muss HB, Maloney WC: Chloroma and other myeloblastic tumors. Blood 42:721, 1973.

191. Ellman L, Hammond D, Atkins L: Eosinophilia, chloromas and a chromosome abnormality in a patient with a myeloproliferative syndrome. Cancer 43:2410, 1979.

192. McCarty KS Jr, Wortman J, Daly J, et al: Chloroma (granulocytic sarcoma) without evidence of leukemia: Facilitated light microscopic diagnosis. Blood 56:104, 1980.

193. Carbone PP: Introduction. Lymphoreticular neoplasms. In PB Beeson, W McDermott, JB Wyngaarden (Eds): Cecil Textbook of Medicine. 15th Ed. Philadelphia, WB Saunders Co, 1979, p 1829.

194. Heiberg E, Wolverson MK, Sundaram M, et al: CT findings in leukemia. AJR 143:1317, 1984.

195. Lee JKT, Heiken JP, Ling D, et al: Magnetic resonance imaging of abdominal and pelvic lymphadenopathy. Radiology 153:181, 1984.

196. Spagnoli I, Gattoni F, Viganotti G: Roentgenographic aspects of non-Hodgkin's lymphomas presenting with osseous lesions. Skel Radiol 8:39, 1982.

197. Klein RM, Thelmo W, Dorf D, et al: Case report 269. Skel Radiol 11:224, 1984.

198. Vanel D, Bayle C, Hartmann O, et al: Radiological study of two disseminated malignant non-Hodgkin's lymphomas affecting only the bones in children. Skel Radiol 9:83, 1982.

199. Dosoretz DE, Raymond AK, Murphy GF, et al: Primary lymphoma of bone. The relationship of morphologic diversity to clinical behavior. Cancer 50:1009, 1982.

200. Phillips WC, Kattapuram SV, Dosoretz DE, et al: Primary lymphoma of bone: Relationship of radiographic appearance and prognosis. Radiology 144:285, 1982.

201. Dalinka MK: Primary lymphoma of bone: Radiographic appearance and prognosis. Radiology 147:288, 1983.

202. Rodman D, Raymond AK, Phillips WC: Case report 201. Skel Radiol 8:235, 1982.

203. Raymond AK, Unni KK: Case report 194. Skel Radiol 8:153, 1982.

204. Sweet DL, Mass DP, Simon MA, et al: Histiocytic lymphoma (reticulum-cell sarcoma) of bone. J Bone Joint Surg [Am] 63:79, 1981.

205. Burgener FA, Hamlin DJ: Radiologic manifestations of histiocytic lymphoma in the skeletal and central nervous system. ROFO 134: 50, 1981.

206. Newcomer FA, Hamlin DJ: Radiologic manifestations of histiocytic lymphoma in the skeletal and central nervous system. ROFO 134:50, 1981.

207. Mills SE, Sloop FB Jr, Thiele AL, et al: Case report 251. Skel Radiol 10:287, 1983.

208. Appell RG, Oppermann HC, Brandeis WE: Skeletal lesions in Hodgkin's disease. Review of literature and case reports. Pediatr Radiol 11:61, 1981.

209. Kay CJ, Rosenberg MA, Burd R: Hypertrophic osteoarthropathy and childhood Hodgkin's disease. Radiology 112:177, 1974.

210. Butler JJ: Relationship of histological findings to survival in Hodgkin's disease. Cancer Res 31:1770, 1971.

211. Desser RK, Moran EM, Ultmann JE: Staging of Hodgkin's disease and lymphoma. Diagnostic procedures including staging laparotomy and splenectomy. Med Clin North Am 57:479, 1973.

212. Braunstein EM: Hodgkin disease of bone: Radiographic correlation with the histological classification. Radiology 137:643, 1980.

213. Levine PH, Cho BR: Burkitt's lymphoma: Clinical features of American cases. Cancer Res 34:1219, 1974.

214. Fowles JV, Olweny CLM, Katongole-Mbidde E, et al: Burkitt's lymphoma in the appendicular skeleton. J Bone Joint Surg [Br] 65:464, 1983.

215. Wright DH: Burkitt's tumor. A post-mortem study of 50 cases. Br J Surg 51:245, 1964.

216. Metzger H, Kurtz B, Ahlemann L: Osteolytische Knochenmanifestationen bei Mycosis fungoides. ROFO 133:331, 1980.

217. Ward JH, Kjeldsberg CR: Spinal cord compression in mycosis fungoides. Cancer 50:2510, 1982.

218. Rappaport H, Thomas LB: Mycosis fungoides: The pathology of extracutaneous involvement. Cancer 34:1198, 1974.

219. Shigeno C, Morita R, Fukunaga M, et al: Visualization of skeletal muscle involvement of mycosis fungoides on ^{67}Ga scintigraphy. Eur J Nucl Med 7:333, 1982.

220. Keller MS, Jackson DP, Breslow A, et al: Chronic knee pain in a 35 year-old man. Invest Radiol 16:1, 1981.

221. Rice DM, Semble E, Ahl ET, et al: Primary lymphoma of bone presenting as monoarthritis. J Rheumatol 11:851, 1984.

222. Agudelo CA, Schumacher HR, Glick JH, et al: Non-Hodgkin's lymphoma in systemic lupus erythematosus. Report of 4 cases with ultrastructural studies in 2. J Rheumatol 8:69, 1981.

223. Ihde DC, De Vita VT: Osteonecrosis of the femoral head in patient with lymphoma treated with intermittent combination chemotherapy (including corticosteroids). Cancer 36:1585, 1975.

224. Thorne JC, Evans WK, Alison RE, et al: Avascular necrosis of bone complicating treatment of malignant lymphoma. Am J Med 71:751, 1981.

225. Engel IA, Strauss DJ, Lacher M, et al: Osteonecrosis in patients with malignant lymphoma. A review of twenty-five cases. Cancer 48:1245, 1981.

226. Prosnitz LR, Lawson JP, Friedlaender GE, et al: Avascular necrosis of bone in Hodgkin's disease patients treated with combined modality therapy. Cancer 47:2793, 1981.

227. Mould JJ, Adam NM: The problem of avascular necrosis of bone in patients treated for Hodgkin's disease. Clin Radiol 34:231, 1983.

228. Harper PG, Trask C, Souhami RL: Avascular necrosis of bone caused by combination chemotherapy without corticosteroids. Br Med J 1:267, 1984.

229. Obrist P, Hartmann D, Obrecht JP: Osteonecrosis after chemotherapy. Lancet 1:1316, 1978.

230. O'Regan S, Melhorn DK, Newman AJ: Methotrexate-induced bone pain in childhood leukemia. Am J Dis Child 126:498, 1973.

231. Ragab AH, Frech RS, Vietti TJ: Osteoporotic fractures secondary to methotrexate therapy of acute leukemia in remission. Cancer 25:580, 1970.

232. Stanisaulge S, Babcock AL: Fractures in children treated with methotrexate for leukemia. Clin Orthop 125:139, 1977.
233. Schwartz AM, Leonidas JC: Methotrexate osteopathy. Skel Radiol 11:13, 1984.
234. Dihlmann W, Lotz W: Case report 167. Skel Radiology 7:82, 1981.
235. Moore SB, Harrison EG, Weiland LH: Angioimmunoblastic lymphadenopathy. Mayo Clin Proc 51:273, 1976.
236. Cullen MH, Stansfeld AG, Oliver RTD, et al: Angioimmunoblastic lymphadenopathy: Report of ten cases and review of the literature. Q J Med 48:151, 1979.
237. Davies PG, Fordham JN: Arthritis and angioimmunoblastic lymphadenopathy. Ann Rheum Dis 42:516, 1983.
238. Raskin RJ, Tesar JT, Lawless OJ: Polyarthritis in immunoblastic lymphadenopathy. Arthritis Rheum 25:1481, 1982.
239. Frizzera G, Moran EM, Rappaport H: Angioimmunoblastic lymphadenopathy: Diagnosis and clinical course. Am J Med 59:1, 1975.
240. Lukes RJ, Tindle BH: Immunoblastic lymphadenopathy: A hyperimmune entity resembling Hodgkin's disease. N Engl J Med 292:1, 1975.
241. Castro-Poltronieri A, Alarcón-Segovia D: Articular manifestations of primary Sjögren's syndrome. J Rheumatol 10:485, 1983.
242. Diaz-Jouanen E, Ruiz-Arguelles GJ, Vega-Ortiz JM, et al: From benign polyclonal to malignant monoclonal lymphoproliferation in a patient with primary Sjögren's syndrome. Arthritis Rheum 24:850, 1981.
243. Fye KH, Daniels TE, Zulman J, et al: Aplastic anemia and lymphoma in Sjögren's syndrome. Arthritis Rheum 23:1321, 1980.
244. Fallon MD, Whyte MP, Teitelbaum SL: Systemic mastocytosis associated with generalized osteopenia. Histopathological characterization of the skeletal lesion using undecalcified bone from two patients. Hum Pathol 12:813, 1981.
245. Goldhaber P: Heparin enhancement of factors stimulating bone resorption in tissue culture. Science 147:407, 1965.
246. Griffith GC, Nichols G, Asher JD, et al: Heparin osteoporosis. JAMA 193:91, 1965.
247. Rafii M, Firooznia H, Golimbu C, et al: Pathologic fracture in systemic mastocytosis. Radiographic spectrum and review of the literature. Clin Orthop 180:260, 1983.
248. Klein DC, Raisz LG: Prostaglandins: Stimulation of bone resorption in tissue culture. Endocrinology 86:1436, 1970.
249. Kermarec J, Canioni D, Zafisaona G: Pathologie estéo-médullaire dans cinq cas de mastocytose systématisée. Arch Anat Cytol Pathol 31:11, 1983.
250. Bojoly C, Bouvier M, Bonvoisin B, et al: Osteopathie fragilisante pseudomyelomateuse avec mastocytose medullaire (2 cas). Lyon Med 247:91, 1982.
251. Deramond H, Remond A, Grumbach Y, et al: Les localisations osseuses de la mastocytose systemique. Etude radiologique et scintigraphique. J Radiol 61:503, 1980.
252. Hills E, Dunstan CR, Evans RA: Bone metabolism in systemic mastocytosis. A case report. J Bone Joint Surg [Am] 63:665, 1981.
253. Ensslen RD, Jackson FI, Reid AM: Bone and gallium scans in mastocytosis: Correlation with count rates, radiography and microscopy. J Nucl Med 24:586, 1983.
254. Rosenbaum RC, Frieri M, Metcalfe DD: Patterns of skeletal scintigraphy and their relationship to plasma and urinary histamine levels in systemic mastocytosis. J Nucl Med 25:859, 1984.
255. Gupta SM, Gupta A, Spencer RP, et al: Bone and spleen lesions in systemic mastocytosis. Clin Nucl Med 8:34, 1983.
256. Varki A, Lottenberg R, Griffith R, et al: The syndrome of idiopathic myelofibrosis. A clinicopathologic review with emphasis on the prognostic variables predicting survival. Medicine 62:353, 1983.
257. Groopman JE: The pathogenesis of myelofibrosis in myeloproliferative disorders. Ann Intern Med 92:857, 1980.
258. Truong LD, Saleem A, Schwartz MR: Acute myelofibrosis. A report of four cases and review of the literature. Medicine 63:182, 1984.
259. Kosmidis PA, Palacas CG, Axelrod AR: Diffuse purely osteolytic lesions in myelofibrosis. Cancer 46:2263, 1980.
260. Ribera JM, Blade J, Cervantes F, et al: Lesiones osteoliticas en el curso de la mielofibrosis idiopatica: Presentacion de dos casos. Med Clin (Barcelona) 81:861, 1983.
261. Shaver RW, Clore FC: Extramedullary hematopoiesis in myeloid metaplasia. AJR 137:874, 1981.
262. Pile-Spellman J, Adelman L, Post KD: Extramedullary hematopoiesis causing spinal cord compression. Neurosurgery 8:728, 1981.
263. Connelly TJ, Abruzzo JL, Schwab RH: Agnogenic myeloid metaplasia with polyarthritis. J Rheumatol 9:954, 1982.
264. Heinicke MH, Zarrabi MH, Gorevic PD: Arthritis due to synovial involvement by extramedullary hematopoiesis in myelofibrosis with myeloid metaplasia. Ann Rheum Dis 42:196, 1983.
265. Appell RG, Bühler T, Willich E, et al: Absence of prognostic significance of skeletal involvement in acute lymphocytic leukemia and non-Hodgkin lymphoma in children. Pediatr Radiol 15:245, 1985.
266. Révész T, Kardos G, Kajtár P, et al: The prognostic significance of bone and joint manifestations in childhood leukemia. J Rheumatol 12:647, 1985.
267. Wismer GL, Rosen BR, Buxton R, et al: Chemical shift imaging of the bone marrow: Preliminary experience. AJR 145:1031, 1985.
268. Jones PG, Rolston K, Hopfer RL: Septic arthritis due to Histoplasma capsulatum in a leukaemic patient. Ann Rheum Dis 44:128, 1985.
269. Healey JH, Lane JM, Erlandson RA, et al: Solid leukemic tumor. An uncommon presentation of a common disease. Clin Orthop 194:248, 1985.
270. Pomeranz SJ, Hawkins HH, Towbin R, et al: Granulocytic sarcoma (chloroma): CT manifestations. Radiology 155:167, 1985.
271. Ultmann JE, Jacobs RH: The non-Hodgkin's lymphomas. CA 35:66, 1985.
272. Blijham GH, Vermeulen A, De Leon DEM: Osteonecrosis of sternum and rib in a patient treated for Hodgkin's disease. Cancer 56:2292, 1985.
273. Horny H-P, Parwaresch MR, Lennert K: Bone marrow findings in systemic mastocytosis. Hum Pathol 16:808, 1985.
274. Brinkley AB, O'Brien MW: Case report 320. Skel Radiol 14:68, 1985.
275. McKenna MJ, Frame B: The mast cell and bone. Clin Orthop 200:226, 1985.
276. Bieler EU, Wohlenberg H, Utech Ch: Die ossären manifestationen bei der generalisierten Mastozytose im Skelettszintigramm im Vergleich zum Rötgenbefund. ROFO 142:552, 1985.
277. Price F, Bell H: Spinal cord compression due to extramedullary hematopoiesis. Successful treatment in a patient with long-standing myelofibrosis. JAMA 253:2876, 1985.
278. Monsees B, Destouet JM, Totty WG, et al: Case report 349. Skel Radiol 15:154, 1986.
279. Rogalsky RJ, Black GB, Reed MH: Orthopaedic manifestations of leukemia in children. J Bone Joint Surg [Am] 68:494, 1986.
280. Stork JT, Cigtay OS, Schellenger D, et al: Recurrent chloromas in acute myelogenous leukemia. AJR 142:777, 1984.
281. Marsh WL Jr, Bylund DJ, Heath VC, et al: Osteoarticular and pulmonary manifestations of acute leukemia. Case report and review of the literature. Cancer 57:385, 1986.
282. Miller JH, Ettinger LJ: Gallium citrate Ga 67 scintigraphic detection of chronic osteomyelitis in children with leukemia. Am J Dis Child 140:230, 1986.
283. Welch P, Grossi C, Carroll A, et al: Granulocytic sarcoma with an indolent course and destructive skeletal disease. Tumor characterization with immunologic markers, electron microscopy, cytochemistry, and cytogenetic studies. Cancer 57:1005, 1986.
284. Holtś SL, Kido DK, Simon JH: MR imaging of spinal lymphoma. J Comput Assist Tomogr 10:111, 1986.
285. Marymount JV, Kaufman EE: Osteonecrosis of bone associated with combination chemotherapy without corticosteroids. Clin Orthop 204:150, 1986.
286. Shuckett R, Russell ML, Gladman DD: Atypical erosive osteoarthritis and Sjögren's syndrome. Ann Rheum Dis 45:281, 1986.
287. Moore SG, Gooding CA, Brasch RC, et al: Bone marrow in children with acute lymphocytic leukemia: MR relaxation times. Radiology 160:237, 1986.
288. Olson DO, Schields AF, Scheurich CJ, et al: Magnetic resonance imaging of the bone marrow in patients with leukemia, aplastic anemia, and lymphoma. Invest Radiol 21:540, 1986.
289. Wang Y: Classification of non-Hodgkin's lymphoma. AJR 147:205, 1986.
290. Rossleigh MA, Smith J, Straus DJ, et al: Osteonecrosis in patients with malignant lymphoma. A review of 31 cases. Cancer 58:1112, 1986.
291. Fox RI, Robinson CA, Curd JG, et al: Sjögren's syndrome. Proposed criteria for classification. Arthritis Rheum 29:577, 1986.
292. Rodenberg JC, Maegaard KK, Svanholm H: Case report 369. Skel Radiol 15:334, 1986.
293. Altman AJ: Chronic leukemias of childhood. Pediatr Clin North Am 35:765, 1988.
294. Gordon MY, Barrett AJ: Bone Marrow Disorders. The Biological Basis of Clinical Problems. Oxford, Blackwell Scientific Publications. 1985.
295. Cohn SL, Morgan ER, Mallette LE: The spectrum of metabolic bone disease in lymphoblastic leukemia. Cancer 59:346, 1987.
296. Ribeiro RC, Pui C-H, Schell MJ: Vertebral compression fracture as a presenting feature of acute lymphoblastic leukemia in children. Cancer 61:589, 1988.
297. Manson D, Martin RF, Cockshott WP: Metaphyseal impaction fractures in acute lymphoblastic leukemia. Skel Radiol 17:561, 1989.
298. Bömelburg T, von Lengerke H-J, Ritter J: Aseptic osteonecrosis in the treatment of childhood acute leukemias. Eur J Pediatr 149:20, 1989.
299. Hutton JJ: Evaluation of leukocytes. In JH Stein (Ed): Internal Medicine. 3rd Ed. Boston, Little, Brown and Company. 1990, p 983.
300. Stobo JD: The human immune response. In JH Stein (Ed): Internal Medicine. 3rd Ed. Boston, Little, Brown and Company. 1990, p 1624.
301. Eguchi K, Aoyagi T, Nakashima M, et al: A case of adult T cell leukemia complicated by proliferative synovitis. J Rhematol 18:297, 1991.
302. Taniguchi A, Takenaka Y, Noda Y, et al: Adult T cell leukemia presenting with proliferative synovitis. Arthritis Rheum 31:1076, 1988.
303. Aoki J, Yamamoto I, Hino M, et al: Case report 429. Skel Radiol 16:412, 1987.
304. Austin CB, Young JWR, Park HJ, et al: Massive acroosteolysis in adult T cell leukemia/lymphoma. Radiology 164:787, 1987.
305. Salimi Z, Vas W, Sundaram M: Avascular bone necrosis in an untreated case of chronic myelogenous leukemia. Skel Radiol 17:353, 1988.
306. Gagnerie F, Taillan B, Euller-Ziegler L, et al: Arthritis of the knees in B cell chronic lymphocytic leukemia: A patient with immunologic evidence of B lymphocytic synovial infiltration. Arthritis Rheum 31:815, 1988.
307. Peterson C, Kaplan PA, Lorenzen KM: Case report 410. Skel Radiol 16:82, 1987.
308. Herold CJ, Wittich GR, Schwarzinger I, et al: Skeletal involvement in hairy cell leukemia. Skel Radiol 17:171, 1988.
309. Turner RM, Peck WW, Prietto C: MR of soft tissue chloroma in a patient presenting with left pubic and hip pain. J Comput Assist Tomogr 15:700, 1991.
310. Hermann G, Feldman F, Abdelwahab IF, et al: Skeletal manifestations of granulocytic sarcoma (chloroma). Skel Radiol 20:509, 1991.
311. Xipell JM, Beamish MR, Clark D: Case report 432. Skel Radiol 16:425, 1987.

312. Jones RJ: The role of bone marrow imaging. Radiology *183*:321, 1992.
313. Vogler JB III, Murphy WA: Bone marrow imaging. Radiology *168*:679, 1988.
314. Nyman R, Rehn S, Glimelius B, et al: Magnetic resonance imaging in diffuse malignant bone marrow diseases. Acta Radiol (Diagn) *28*:199, 1987.
315. Thomsen C, Sorensen PG, Karle H, et al: Prolonged bone marrow T1-relaxation in acute leukemia. Magn Reson Imaging *5*:251, 1987.
316. Kanal E, Burk L Jr, Brunberg JA, et al: Pediatric musculoskeletal magnetic resonance imaging. Radiol Clin North Am *26*:211, 1988.
317. Ruzal-Shapiro C, Berdon WE, Cohen MD, et al: MR imaging of diffuse marrow replacement in pediatric patients with cancer. Radiology *181*:587, 1991.
318. Moore SG, Bisset GS III, Siegel MJ, et al: Pediatric musculoskeletal MR imaging. Radiology *179*:345, 1991.
319. Bohndorf K, Benz-Bohm G, Gross-Engels W, et al: MRI of the knee region in leukemic children. I. Initial pattern in patients with untreated disease. Pediatr Radiol *20*:179, 1990.
320. Rosen BR, Fleming DM, Kushner DC, et al: Hematologic bone marrow disorders: Quantitative chemical shift MR imaging. Radiology *169*:799, 1988.
321. Smith SR, Williams CE, Davies JM, et al: Bone marrow disorders: Characterization with quantitative MR imaging. Radiology *172*:805, 1989.
322. Gerard EL, Ferry JA, Amrein PC, et al: Compositional changes in vertebral bone marrow during treatment for acute leukemia: Assessment with quantitative chemical shift imaging. Radiology *183*:39, 1992.
323. Mckinstry CS, Steiner RE, Young AT, et al: Bone marrow in leukemia and aplastic anemia: MR imaging before, during, and after treatment. Radiology *162*:701, 1987.
324. Islam A, Catovsky D, Galton D: Histologic study of bone marrow regeneration following chemotherapy for acute myeloid leukemia and chronic granulocytic leukemia in blast transformation. Br J Haematol *45*:535, 1980.
325. Schick F, Bongers H, Jung W-I, et al: Volume-selective proton MRS in vertebral bodies. Magn Reson Med *26*:207, 1992.
326. Jensen KE, Sorensen G, Thomsen C, et al: Magnetic resonance imaging of the bone marrow in patients with acute leukemia during and after chemotherapy. Changes in T1 relaxation. Acta Radiol (Diagn) *31*:361, 1990.
327. Hanna SL, Fletcher BD, Fairclough DL, et al: Magnetic resonance imaging of disseminate bone marrow disease in patients treated for malignancy. Skel Radiol *20*:79, 1991.
328. Pieters R, van Brenk AI, Veerman JP, et al: Bone marrow magnetic resonance studies in childhood leukemia. Evidence of osteonecrosis. Cancer *60*:2994, 1987.
329. van Zanten TEG, Golding RP, Van Amerongen AHMT, et al: Nuclear magnetic resonance imaging of bone marrow in childhood leukemia. Clin Radiol *39*:77, 1988.
330. Miller TP, Jones SE: Hodgkin's disease and non-Hodgkin's lymphoma. *In* JH Stein (Ed): Internal Medicine. 3rd Ed. Boston, Little, Brown and Company. 1990, p 1136.
331. Pond GD, Castellino RA, Horning S, et al: Non-Hodgkin lymphoma: Influence of lymphography, CT, and bone marrow biopsy on staging and management. Radiology *170*:159, 1989.
332. Franczyk J, Samuels T, Rubenstein J, et al: Skeletal lymphoma. J Can Assoc Radiol *40*:75, 1989.
333. Corres J, Morales A, Saban J, et al: Case report 674. Skel Radiol *20*:315, 1991.
334. Clayton F, Butler JJ, Ayala AG, et al: Non-Hodgkin's lymphoma in bone: Pathologic and radiologic features with clinical correlates. Cancer *60*:2494, 1987.
335. Giudici MAI, Eggli KD, Moser RP Jr, et al: Case report 730. Skel Radiol *21*:260, 1992.
336. Beatty PT, Björkengren AG, Moore SG, et al: Case report 764. Skel Radiol *21*:559, 1992.
337. Nghiem HV, Ellis BI, Haggar AM, et al: Juxta-articular large cell lymphoma. Skel Radiol *19*:353, 1990.
338. Gross SB, Robertson WW Jr, Lange BJ, et al: Primary Hodgkin's disease of bone. A report of two cases in adolescents and review of the literature. Clin Orthop *283*:276, 1992.
339. Klein MJ, Rudin BJ, Greenspan A, et al: Hodgkin disease presenting as a lesion in the wrist. A case report. J Bone Joint Surg [Am] *69*:1246, 1987.
340. Gaudin P, Juvin R, Rozand Y, et al: Skeletal involvement as the initial disease manifestation of Hodgkin's disease: A review of 6 cases. J Rheumatol *19*:146, 1992.
341. Manoli A II, Blaustein JC, Pedersen HE: Sternal Hodgkin's disease. Report of two cases. Clin Orthop *228*:20, 1988.
342. Sullivan WT, Solonick DM: Case report 414. Skel Radiol *16*:166, 1987.
343. Bloom RA, Peylan-Ramu N, Okon E: Case report 755. Skel Radiol *21*:474, 1992.
344. Nzeh DA: Importance of the jaw radiograph in diagnosis of Burkitt's lymphoma. Clinical Radiol *38*:519, 1987.
345. Berger RG: Mycosis fungoides with polyarthritis. Arthritis Rheum *31*:1335, 1988.
346. Berger RG, Knox SJ, Levy R, et al: Mycosis fungoides arthropathy. Ann Intern Med *114*:571, 1991.
347. Savin H, Zimmermann B III, Aaron RK, et al: Seronegative symmetric polyarthritis in Sezary syndrome. J Rheumatol *18*:464, 1991.
348. Dorfman HD, Siegel HL, Perry MC, et al: Non-Hodgkin's lymphoma of the synovium simulating rheumatoid arthritis. Arthritis Rheum *30*:155, 1987.
349. Mariette X, de Roqauncourt A, d'Agay M-F, et al: Monarthritis revealing non-Hodgkin's T cell lymphoma of the synovium. Arthritis Rheum *31*:571, 1988.
350. Seleznick MJ, Aguilar JL, Rayhack J, et al: Polyarthritis associated with cutaneous T cell lymphoma. J Rheumatol *16*:1379, 1989.
351. Malloy PC, Fishman EK, Magid D: Lymphoma of bone, muscle, and skin: CT findings. AJR *159*:805, 1992.
352. Pilepich MV, Carter BL: Muscle involvement in lymphoma patients. Radiology *134*:521, 1980.
353. Metzler JP, Fleckenstein JL, Vuitch F, et al: Skeletal muscle lymphoma: MRI evaluation. Magn Reson Imaging *10*:491, 1992.
354. Orzel JA, Sawaf NW, Richardson ML: Lymphoma of the skeleton: Scintigraphic evaluation. AJR *150*:1095, 1988.
355. Linden A, Zankovich R, Theissen P, et al: Malignant lymphoma: Bone marrow imaging versus biopsy. Radiology *173*:335, 1989.
356. Genez BM, Zirilli VL, Schlesinger AE, et al: Case report 487. Skel Radiol *17*:306, 1988.
357. Gückel F, Semmler W, Döhner H, et al: Kernspintomographische Darstellung von Knochenmarkinfiltrationen bei malignen Lymphomen. ROFO *150*:26, 1989.
358. Sundaram M, McLeod RA: MR imaging of tumor and tumorlike lesions of bone and soft tissue. AJR *155*:817, 1990.
359. Beltran J, Noto AM, Chakeres DW, et al: Tumors of the osseous spine: Staging with MR imaging versus CT. Radiology *162*:565, 1987.
360. Li MH, Holtš S, Larsson E-M: MR imaging of spinal lymphoma. Acta Radiol (Diagn) *33*:338, 1992.
361. Stiglbauer R, Augustin I, Kramer J, et al: MRI in the diagnosis of primary lymphoma of bone: Correlation with histopathology. J Comput Assist Tomogr *16*:248, 1992.
362. Moore SG, Sebag GH: Effect of trabecular bone on the appearance of marrow in gradient-echo imaging of the appendicular skeleton. Radiology *174*:855, 1990.
363. Erlemann R, Vassallo P, Bongartz G, et al: Musculoskeletal neoplasms: Fast low-angle shot MR imaging with and without Gd-DTPA. Radiology *176*:489, 1990.
364. Yufu Y, Nonaka S, Nobunaga M: Adult T cell leukemia-lymphoma mimicking rheumatic disease. Arthritis Rheum *30*:599, 1987.
365. Boumpas DT, Wheby MS, Jaffe ES, et al: Synovitis in angioimmunoblastic lymphadenopathy with dysproteinemia simulating rheumatoid arthritis. Arthritis Rheum *33*:578, 1990.
366. Castleman B, Ivers M, Menendez V: Localized mediastinal lymph node hyperplasia resembling lymphoma. Cancer *9*:822, 1956.
367. Keller AR, Hochholzer L, Castleman B: Hyaline-vascular and plasma-cell types of giant lymph node hyperplasia of the mediastinum and other locations. Cancer *29*:670, 1972.
368. Buckley JG, Sundaram M: Skeletal lymphoma in a patient with Castleman disease. AJR *157*:1035, 1991.
369. Boldt DH: Abnormalities of phagocytes, eosinophils, and basophils. *In* JH Stein (Ed): Internal Medicine. 3rd Ed. Boston, Little, Brown and Company. 1990, p 1115.
370. Huang T-Y, Yam LT, Li C-Y: Radiological features of systemic mast-cell disease. Br J Radiol *60*:765, 1987.
371. Travis WD, Li C-Y, Bergstralh EJ, et al: Systemic mast cell disease. Analysis of 58 cases and literature review. Medicine *67*:345, 1988.
372. Travis WD, Li C-Y, Yam LT, et al: Significance of systemic mast cell disease with associated hematologic disorders. Cancer *62*:965, 1988.
373. Roberts LJ II: Carcinoid syndrome and disorders of systemic mast-cell activation including systemic mastocytosis. Endocrinol Metab Clin North Am *17*:415, 1988.
374. Travis WD, Li C-Y, Bergstralh EJ: Solid and hematologic malignancies in 60 patients with systemic mast cell disease. Arch Pathol Lab Med *113*:365, 1989.
375. Schoenaers P, De Clerck LS, Timmermans U, et al: Systemic mastocytosis, an unusual cause of osteoporosis. Clin Rheumatol *6*:458, 1987.
376. Cook JV, Chandy J: Systemic mastocytosis affecting the skeletal system. J Bone Joint Surg [Br] *71*:534, 1989.
377. Grardel B, Hardouin P: Mastocytose et manifestations osseous. Rev Rhum Mal Osteoartic *59*:57, 1992.
378. Schweitzer ME, Irwin GAL: Case report 561. Skel Radiol *18*:411, 1989.
379. Alho A, Roald B B-H, Johnsen U, et al: A case of mastocytosis involving bone. Acta Orthop Scand *62*:485, 1991.
380. Meister HP, Rabben U: Case report 412. Skel Radiol *16*:158, 1987.
381. De Gennes C, Kuntz D, De Vernejoul MC: Bone mastocytosis. A report of nine cases with a bone histomorphometric study. Clin Orthop *279*:281, 1992.
382. Mason BA, Kressel BR, Cashdollar MR, et al: Periostitis associated with myelofibrosis. Cancer *43*:1568, 1979.
383. Nicholls MD, Concannon AJ, Biggs JC: Myelofibrosis associated with periostitis. Aust N Z J Med *12*:177, 1982.
384. Lagier R, Baud CA: Osteomyelosclerosis following polycythemia vera: Radiological-pathological correlation in a femur. Eur J Radiol *10*:15, 1990.
385. Pajus I, Amor B: Manifestations rhumatologiques associées aux syndromes myélodysplasiques et myéloprolifératifs. Rev Rhum Mal Osteoartic *59*:11, 1992.
386. Kaplan KR, Mitchell DG, Steiner RM, et al: Polycythemia vera and myelofibrosis: Correlation of MR imaging, clinical, and laboratory findings. Radiology *183*:329, 1992.
387. Brateman L: Chemical shift imaging: A review. AJR *146*:971, 1986.
388. Szumowski J, Eisen JK, Vinitski S, et al: Hybrid methods of chemical shift imaging. Magn Reson Med *9*:379, 1989.

389. Robinson SH: Hematopoiesis. *In* JH Stein (Ed): Internal Medicine. 3rd Ed. Boston, Little, Brown and Company, 1990, p 945.

390. Appelbaum FR: Bone marrow transplantation. *In* JH Stein (Ed): Internal Medicine. 3rd Ed. Boston, Little, Brown and Company, 1990, p 1002.

391. Patzik SB, Smith C, Kubicka RA, et al: Bone marrow transplantation: Clinical and radiologic aspects. RadioGraphics *11*:601, 1991.

392. Weisdorf DJ: Bone marrow transplantation for acute leukemia. Invest Radiol *22*:839, 1987.

393. Stevens SK, Moore SG, Amylon MD: Repopulation of marrow after transplantation: MR imaging with pathologic correlation. Radiology *175*:213, 1990.

394. Patrone S V-M, Resnik CS, Aisner SC, et al: Case report 761. Skel Radiol *21*:546, 1992.

395. Kook H, Hwang TJ, Kang HK, et al: Spinal intramedullary granulocytic sarcoma: Magnetic resonance imaging. Magn Res Imaging *11*:135, 1993.

396. Farrés MT, Dock W, Augustin I, et al: Radiologisches Erscheinungsbild des primären Knochenlymphoms. ROFO *158*:589, 1993.

397. Mulligan ME, Kransdorf MJ: Sequestra in primary lymphoma of bone: Prevalence and radiologic features. AJR *160*:1245, 1993.

398. Lombardi LJ, Cleri DJ, Present DA, et al: Systemic mastocytosis with pathologic fractures of distal long bones. Orthopedics *16*:320, 1993.

399. Mirowitz SA, Apicella P, Reinus WR, et al: MR imaging of bone marrow lesions: Relative conspicuousness on T1-weighted, fat-suppressed T2-weighted, and STIR images. AJR *162*:215, 1994.

400. Sullivan KM, Deeg HJ, Sanders JE, et al: Late complications after marrow transplantation. Semin Hematol *21*:53, 1984.

401. Deeg HJ, Sturb R, Thomas ED: Bone marrow transplantation: A review of delayed complications. Br J Hematol *57*:185, 1984.

402. Barrett A, Nicholls J, Gibson B: Late effects of total body irradiation. Radiother Oncol *9*:131, 1987.

403. Fletcher BD, Crom DB, Krance RA, et al: Radiation-induced bone abnormalities after bone marrow transplantation for childhood leukemia. Radiology *191*:231, 1994.

Bleeding Disorders

Donald Resnick, M.D.

Hemophilia is a term applied to a group of disorders characterized by an anomaly of blood coagulation due to a deficiency in a specific plasma clotting factor. This anomaly leads to easy bruising and prolonged and excessive bleeding. Of this group of disorders, two are associated most commonly with intraosseous and intra-articular bleeding: (1) classic hemophilia (hemophilia A), characterized by a functional deficiency of antihemophilic factor (AHF), factor VIII, and (2) Christmas disease (hemophilia B), marked by a functional deficiency of plasma thromboplastin component (PTC), factor IX. These two types of hemophilia are X-linked recessive disorders that are clinically manifested in men and carried by women.[1, 2, 112] Rarely, other disorders of blood coagulation may become manifest as bone and joint abnormalities. One such disorder is von Willebrand's disease, a rare familial disease of both men and women, apparently attributable to a dominant autosomal mutant gene in which both factor VIII and functional platelet abnormalities occur.

This chapter summarizes the clinical, radiologic, and pathologic features of skeletal involvement in the hemophilias. In addition, several other vascular disorders are discussed, including the Klippel-Trenaunay and Kasabach-Merritt syndromes, in which osteoarticular manifestations may simulate those of hemophilia.

HEMOPHILIA

Clinical Abnormalities

Classic hemophilia, related to a deficiency of AHF, occurs in approximately 1 in every 10,000 males in the United States. Christmas disease occurs about one tenth as often as classic hemophilia. Its laboratory features, which include the deficiency of PTC, represent the only major difference between the two forms of hemophilia. Although both forms are confined almost exclusively to male subjects, reports exist of significant clinical and radiographic abnormalities appearing in female patients.[112, 116, 174] Chromosomal abnormalities that have been detected in women with hemophilia include the XO syndrome, mosaicism, and partial deletion of an X chromosome; genetic factors responsible for this occurrence include testicular feminization syndrome, homozygosity for the hemophilia gene, autosomal transmission, and X-linked dominant transmission.[116]

The severity of the clinical manifestations in either form of hemophilia varies. In mild forms of disease, excessive bleeding may be apparent only during surgery. With moderate or severe forms, bleeding episodes may occur not only during operation but also spontaneously or after minor (or significant) trauma. Recurrent bleeding from the gastrointestinal or genitourinary tract can appear. Retroperitoneal hemorrhage may lead to significant abdominal pain and tenderness, and intraoral or retropharyngeal bleeding can compromise swallowing or respiration.[122] Rarely, subdural and intracerebral hemorrhages are evident.[123] The diagnosis is established by performing appropriate laboratory tests to detect defects in blood coagulation.

Hemarthrosis is a particularly characteristic abnormality in the hemophilias, which has been recognized for many years. Initially, joint changes in these disorders were attributed to atypical rheumatism until Volkmann in 1868 defined the role of hemorrhage in the pathogenesis of the articular findings.[3, 4] Hemarthrosis occurs in approximately 75 to 90 per cent of patients with hemophilia. It may begin in the early years of life and, in fact, young children and adolescents demonstrate more frequent episodes of joint bleeding than adults. It is not uncommon for the first episode of joint hemorrhage to occur between the ages of 2 and 3 years, and repeated hemorrhages are common between the ages of 8 and 13 years. Lower rates of occurrence of bleeding in older persons may be related to their being more careful because they comprehend more completely the nature of their disease.[5]

The joints altered most commonly are the knee, the elbow, the ankle, the hip, and the glenohumeral joint, in descending order of frequency. In general, articulations susceptible to stress and trauma are more likely to be sites of bleeding. Furthermore, joints such as the knee, whose stability depends on adjacent soft tissue structures rather than intrinsic factors, are particularly vulnerable. One episode of hemarthrosis predisposes the affected joint to another episode. Usually a single joint is involved in each episode, although polyarticular involvement occasionally is encountered. Eventually, multiple joints are affected in this disease. Joint involvement may be markedly asymmetric or even unilateral.

Clinical manifestations of hemophilic arthropathy can be divided into three types: acute, subacute, and chronic hemarthrosis.[1]

1. *Acute hemarthrosis.* Joint bleeding may occur rapidly, producing a tense, swollen, red, and tender articulation, which is painful and stiff. Associated muscle spasm leads to flexion of the extremity and restricted motion. Fever and leukocytosis are observed. Symptoms decrease quickly after administration of appropriate clotting factor.

2. *Subacute hemarthrosis.* This stage occurs subsequent to two or more acute hemarthroses. After these acute episodes, complete recovery of the joint is not evident. Periarticular swelling reflects the presence of thick soft tissues and boggy synovium. Joint motion is restricted, a finding that appears to best correlate with the degree of cartilaginous destruction,[158] and contractures become evident. Muscle atrophy is seen. Pain is not prominent.

3. *Chronic hemarthrosis.* After subacute hemarthrosis has been present for 6 months to 1 year, a chronic stage may develop. More severe and persistent contractures are found, particularly in the elbow and the knee. The final stage is a fibrotic, contracted, and destroyed joint.

Although it is convenient to divide the joint disease into these three stages, this division is not strongly defined, nor does it imply that all patients will develop severe articular abnormalities. Approximately 50 per cent of hemophilic patients, however, develop permanent changes in the peripheral joints, and only rarely do patients escape persistent deformity of any kind.[4] The usual outcome is chronic arthropathy of a few joints without significant abnormalities in the others.

Articular bleeding may be accompanied by hemorrhage into muscles, fascial planes, and bones.[117–119, 175] Soft tissue bleeding can lead to fixed joint deformities and soft tissue necrosis. Compartment syndromes may complicate intramuscular bleeding in the upper or lower extremities.[176] The most common of these in hemophilia are Volkmann's contractures related to massive hemorrhage into the volar muscles of the forearm.[6, 7, 117] Involvement of peripheral nerves in this disease generally is a consequence of intramuscular bleeding, although intraneural hemorrhage also has been reported.[177] Femoral neuropathy occasionally is observed in hemophilia and may be the result of hemorrhage into the iliopsoas muscle at the musculotendinous junction beneath the fascia iliaca, which compresses the femoral nerve between the iliopectineal ligament medially and the unyielding inguinal ligament superiorly.[8] Bleeding into the soleus or gastrocnemius muscle may lead to talipes equinus deformity. Common peroneal nerve entrapment in hemophilia also has been described.[124] Vascular compression from any soft tissue bleeding can produce gangrene.[5] Hemorrhage in and around the spinal cord can lead to neurologic abnormalities.[9–11, 120, 121] Subperiosteal and intraosseous bleeding can induce trabecular distortion and destruction, and large expansile lesions, particularly of the femur and ilium (hemophilic pseudotumors), may simulate neoplasm.

Pathologic Abnormalities

Characteristic pathologic abnormalities occur in hemophilia[5, 12–17, 125] (Table 63–1) (Fig. 63–1). After an acute episode of intra-articular bleeding, blackish fluid containing clots is apparent within the recesses of the articular cavity, embedded within the synovial membrane, or adherent to the joint capsule and periarticular tissues. In the interval before the second bleed, these hemorrhagic collections may disappear. With each recurring episode of bleeding, resorption of blood is less complete and more permanent findings are apparent, particularly in the synovial membrane.

Brownish discoloration of the synovial membrane is due to absorption of blood pigment. As a result of this absorption of hemosiderin, the synovial membrane demonstrates hypertrophy, hyperplasia, and increased vascularity. Hemosiderin appears as a fine particulate matter within the phagocytic lining cells and free or within macrophages in deeper synovial layers. Cellular infiltration with lymphocytes and plasma cells can be observed. Synovial villi become more numerous and enlarged, and the entire membrane thickens. The subsynovial tissue undergoes dense fibrous proliferation. A similar change also is apparent in the capsule, adjacent soft tissues, fasciae, ligaments, and muscles.

The altered synovial membrane appears as inflammatory tissue or pannus, which extends over the margins of the cartilage. Initially, the cartilage becomes discolored (gray-brown) and reveals focal areas of fibrillation, erosion, and

TABLE 63–1. Hemophilia:
Radiographic-Pathologic Correlation

Pathology	Radiology
Recurrent intra-articular hemorrhage with hemosiderin-laden hypertrophied synovial membrane	Radiodense joint effusions
Synovial inflammation and pannus formation; hyperemia	Osteoporosis; epiphyseal overgrowth; accelerated skeletal maturation
Cartilaginous erosion; subchondral trabecular resorption and collapse	Bony erosions and cysts
Cartilaginous denudation	Joint space narrowing
Bony proliferation	Sclerosis and osteophytosis
Soft tissue, subperiosteal, and intraosseous hemorrhage	Pseudotumors

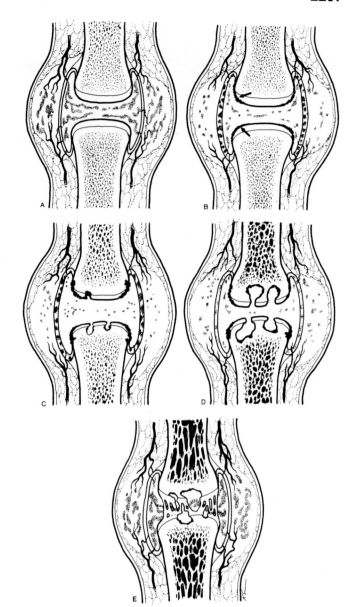

FIGURE 63–1. Hemophilia: Pathologic abnormalities—intra-articular findings.

A Acute episodes of bleeding lead to accumulation of blood in the articular cavity and periarticular soft tissues.

B After numerous bleeding episodes, absorption of blood is incomplete from the articular cavity and soft tissues. Brownish discoloration of the synovial membrane is associated with hypertrophy and hyperemia. Synovial inflammatory tissue or pannus appears at the margins of the articular cartilage (arrows).

C At a later stage, periarticular osteoporosis and focal areas of cartilage and osseous destruction become apparent. Cystic lesions are evident, which generally communicate with the joint cavity. Note areas of relatively normal cartilage and bone.

D Continued destruction of cartilage and bone leads to enlarging cystic lesions, surface irregularities, osteoporosis, and joint space narrowing.

E In late stages of the disease, fibrous adhesions extend across the articular space. New episodes of bleeding occur.

Illustration continued on following page

necrosis. Marginal cartilaginous erosion appears adjacent to synovial pannus, whereas more central defects may occur away from obvious synovial tissue. In either location, cartilaginous denudation may expose subchondral bone. Eventually, numerous small or large serrated erosions are scattered throughout the cartilaginous surface. In some of the defects, regenerated cartilage may be seen, whereas in others, discolored connective tissue is apparent.[18]

The subchondral bone becomes modified in several ways. Loss of the subchondral bone plate occurs, so that the calcified layer of cartilage rests on the cancellous bone.[5] Trabecular thinning and resorption lead to enlarging marrow spaces, which may appear cystic, and granulation tissue may extend from the bone into the overlying cartilage. Subchondral cysts also represent sites of intraosseous hemorrhage.[125] Osseous cystic lesions are particularly prominent in this disease. They frequently are multiple and of varying size and commonly are located beneath areas of abnormal cartilage, both marginally and centrally. Communication between cysts and articular cavity is common. These cysts contain loose, gelatinous tissue, collagenous fibrous tissue, brownish connective tissue, or hemorrhage.[5] Continued bone destruction leads to crevices and grooves within the osseous surface. Productive changes may appear, with sclerotic trabeculae and osteophytes.

Massive periosteal or intraosseous hemorrhage creates neoplastic-like lesions called hemophilic pseudotumors (Fig. 63–2). In subperiosteal locations, the periosteal membrane is lifted from the parent bone, and hemorrhage may extend into the adjacent soft tissues. Periosteal bone formation follows, creating expanded and irregular osseous contours. In intraosseous locations, large defects with geographic (relatively well-defined) bone destruction may be associated with distortion of traversing trabeculae.

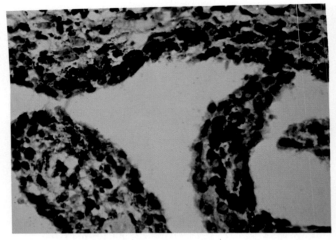

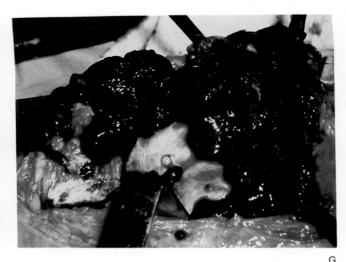

F   G

FIGURE 63–1 *Continued*

  F Synovial membrane abnormalities. Hemosiderin deposition and cellular proliferation are evident.

  G Synovial membrane and bony abnormalities. In the knee, discolored and proliferative synovial tissue is associated with widening of the intercondylar notch.

  (**F,** Courtesy of W. D. Arnold, M.D., and M. W. Hilgartner, M.D., New York, New York; **G,** From Arnold WD, Hilgartner MW: J Bone Joint Surg [Am] *59*:287, 1977.)

In the immature skeleton, chronic hyperemia of the epiphyseal cartilage can produce accelerated maturation and enlargement of epiphyses.

Radiographic Abnormalities

General Features. Distinctive radiologic findings accompany hemophilia.[5–7, 19–25, 101, 106] No uniformly accepted classification system exists, however.[1, 106, 178, 179] Suggested grading systems score a variety of radiographic abnormalities, including osteoporosis, soft tissue swelling, narrowing of the interosseous space, irregularity and erosion of bone, subchondral cystic lesions, incongruity of the joint surfaces, growth disturbances of bone, and deformities. The system of Arnold and Hilgartner[1] includes five stages (see following discussion), that of Pettersson and coworkers[106] emphasizes eight radiographic findings, and the system of Greene and coworkers[178] employs four radiographic alterations. The stages described by Arnold and Hilgartner are listed here (Fig. 63–3):

Stage I: Soft Tissue Swelling. After one or several episodes of intra-articular bleeding, soft tissue swelling be-

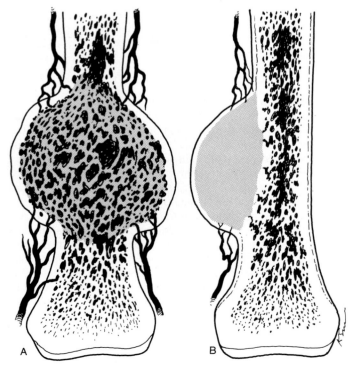

A   B

FIGURE 63–2. Hemophilia: Pathologic abnormalities—intraosseous **(A)** and subperiosteal **(B)** hemorrhage. These types of hemorrhage can lead to hemophilic pseudotumors, with destruction and deformity of bone.

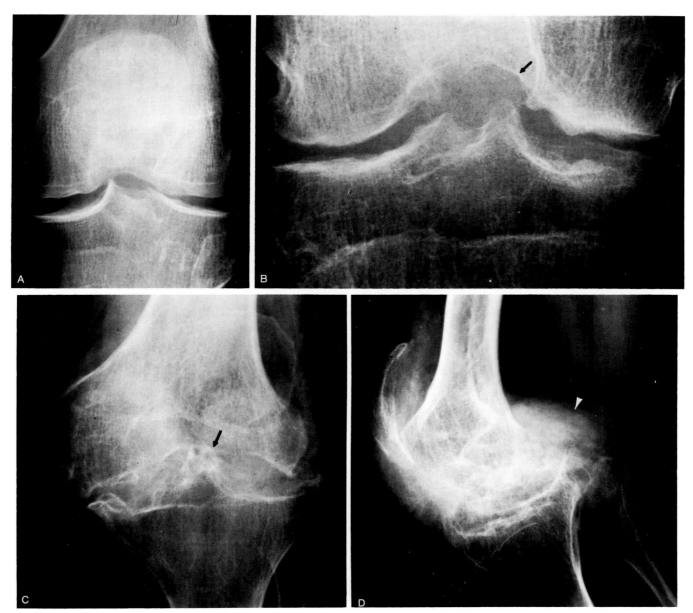

FIGURE 63–3. Hemophilia: Radiographic stages of disease.
  A Stage II. Major abnormalities are generalized osteoporosis and soft tissue swelling, although the latter feature is not well shown in this reproduction.
  B Stage IV. In this more advanced stage, abnormalities include osteoporosis, irregularity and erosion of subchondral bone, and mild cartilage destruction with joint space narrowing. Note the widening of the intercondylar notch of the femur (arrow) and bony eburnation.
  C, D Stage V. In this advanced stage, findings on frontal and lateral radiographs include osteoporosis, enlargement of the epiphyses, severe destruction of subchondral bone, subchondral cysts, and joint space narrowing. Observe the radiodense joint effusion (arrowhead) and widening of the intercondylar notch (arrow). The patella is grossly deformed.

comes evident. Typical signs of effusion are visualized. No bony or cartilaginous changes are seen.

Stage II: Osteoporosis. In this stage, periarticular osteoporosis is combined with soft tissue swelling. Epiphyseal lucency may be striking. In the immature skeleton, overgrowth of involved epiphyses becomes apparent.

Stage III: Osseous Lesions. Irregularity and erosion of bone are accompanied by subchondral cysts. The joint space usually is maintained, an important diagnostic clue that is not seen in many other arthropathies. Synovial effusions may appear relatively radiodense owing to the presence of hemosiderin deposition.

Stage IV: Cartilage Destruction. Joint space narrowing accompanies the bony abnormalities. This narrowing frequently is symmetric, involving the entire articulation. Occasionally, joint space diminution is asymmetric, localized to one aspect of the joint.

Stage V: Joint Disorganization. Severe cartilaginous and osseous abnormalities become apparent in this stage. These abnormalities include complete obliteration of the joint space, considerable bony erosion and irregularity, multiple cystic radiolucent lesions, secondary "degenerative" alterations with osteophytes and eburnation, severe epiphyseal overgrowth, and contractures.

The division of the radiographic changes of hemophilia into five stages does not imply that all cases follow this sequence of events. In some patients, articular involvement may never progress beyond the first or second stage; in other patients, despite appropriate medical or surgical therapy, severe arthropathy develops.[1, 26] Furthermore, radiographic abnormalities do not always develop in a systematic fashion. Although bone change usually precedes cartilaginous loss, this is not always the case. Joint space narrowing may appear before significant osseous findings become apparent. Joint contractures and muscular imbalance in response to soft tissue hemorrhage may antedate intra-articular findings. Finally, it has been recognized that radiologic alterations consistently underestimate the extent of joint damage.[125]

Distribution of Abnormalities. The knee, the ankle, and the elbow are the joints involved most frequently.[126, 127] No joint is exempt, however, although intra-articular bleeding distal to the elbows and the ankles is rare. Bilateral involvement is common, although the changes need not be symmetric.

Knee (Figs. 63–4 and 63–5). The knee is the joint affected most commonly in hemophilia.[111] Abnormalities occur at the femorotibial and patellofemoral joints. Dense joint effusions are common. Periarticular osteoporosis creates lucent epiphyses of both the distal end of the femur and the proximal part of the tibia. Irregularity of the articular surface of the femoral condyles, the tibial plateaus, and the posterior surface of the patella may become apparent. Multiple subchondral cysts are frequent.

Abnormalities of osseous shape have been emphasized in the diagnosis of hemophilia. Overgrowth of the distal femoral and proximal tibial epiphyses may result in osseous outlines that appear poorly fitted on the diaphyses, which are normal or diminished in size. The distal condylar surface may appear flattened. The intercondylar notch of the femur commonly is widened, a finding that has been attributed by some authors to hemorrhage about the cruciate ligaments. The patella may demonstrate an abnormal shape.

Squaring of the inferior pole of this bone was first described by Jordan in 1958[27] and later emphasized by other investigators.[28] This change has been detected in as many as 20 to 30 per cent of patients with hemophilia. It should be emphasized, however, that this squaring may be less evident than noted in these previous reports, that the patella can be of normal size and shape or long and thin, and that, when present, squaring of the patella is not specific for hemophilia, being a recognized manifestation of juvenile chronic arthritis. In fact, many of the distinctive alterations of the hemophilic knee are evident in patients with juvenile chronic arthritis. Differentiation between these two disorders on the basis of knee radiographs is very difficult.

One major complication resulting from knee damage in hemophilia is fixed flexion deformity and subluxation, particularly posterolateral displacement of the tibia on the femur.[29] Furthermore, flexion injury can result in patellar subluxation; the abnormally displaced patella occasionally may lock on the femoral condyles.[30, 128] Total joint replacement eventually may be required.[102, 103, 129–131, 162]

Ankle (Fig. 63–6). Ankle abnormalities also are common in this disease. The radiographic findings are similar to those in other involved joints, including soft tissue swelling, osteoporosis, marginal and central osseous erosions, and joint space narrowing. In the ankle, tibiotalar slanting may be observed, creating an angular joint surface.[180] This finding, which presumably is related to abnormal growth and premature fusion of the distal tibial physis, is not specific, being observed in epiphyseal dysplasias, juvenile chronic arthritis, and perhaps sickle cell anemia. Tibiotalar slanting, or tilt, also has been recorded in a variety of other diseases and as an artifact of radiographic technique.[132] Bony ankylosis of the subtalar joints likewise has been described in hemophilia.[5] Furthermore, osteonecrosis of the talus may be observed.[180] Ankle and foot deformities are not infrequent[24] and include plantar flexion of the ankle, inversion of the subtalar joints, and adduction of the forefoot. These deformities and others relate to intra-articular and intramuscular bleeding.

Elbow (Fig. 63–7). Radiodense effusion, osteoporosis, and cartilaginous and osseous destruction are evident in the elbow in hemophilia. The trochlear and radial notches of the ulna frequently are widened and the radial head may be enlarged.[4, 5, 100, 133]

Other Joints (Fig. 63–8). Typical hemophilic abnormalities can be apparent in other joints, including the hip,[110] the glenohumeral joint,[163, 181] and the small articulations of the hand[136, 182] and foot.[104] In the hip, unusual findings include severe bone resorption[134] and spontaneous dislocation.[135] In the shoulder, rotator cuff disruption has been reported to be a frequent finding.[181] In the hand and foot, predilection for the metacarpophalangeal, metatarsophalangeal, and subtalar joints exists.

Additional Abnormalities. Several other abnormalities may be associated with hemophilia.

Osteonecrosis (Fig. 63–9). Epiphyseal fragmentation and collapse may be apparent in hemophilia. These findings are most frequent in the hip (Fig. 63–9A) and ankle (see Fig. 63–6), although other locations may be affected (Fig. 63–9B). They appear to be related to intraosseous bleeding with subsequent collapse of bone or intracapsular bleeding with elevation of intra-articular pressure, vascular occlusion, and subsequent osteonecrosis. These changes are particularly

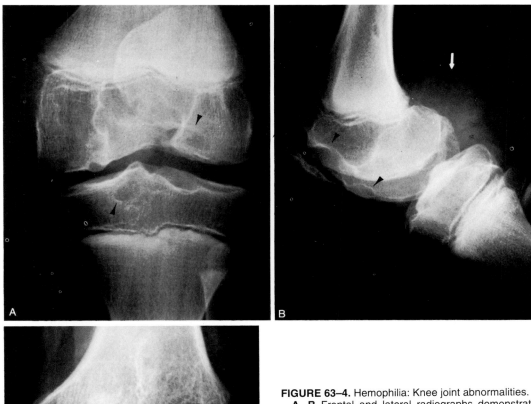

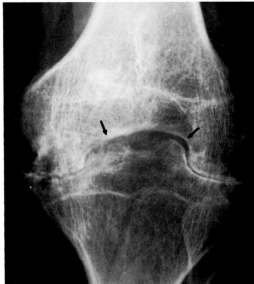

FIGURE 63–4. Hemophilia: Knee joint abnormalities.

A, B Frontal and lateral radiographs demonstrate characteristic findings of hemophilia. The bones are mildly osteoporotic and the epiphyses are enlarged. Note the well-defined or "etched" erosions of subchondral bone (arrowheads), the radiodense joint effusion (arrow), and the widened intercondylar notch of the femur.

C In a different patient, more extensive yet typical abnormalities are osteoporosis, enlargement and ballooning of the epiphyses, subchondral erosions and cysts, flattening of the distal femoral condyles, joint space obliteration, and striking enlargement of the intercondylar notch (arrows).

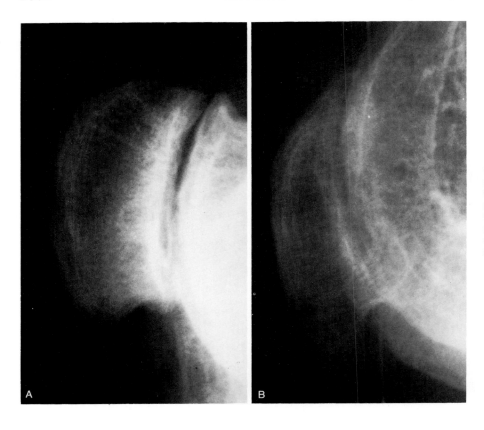

FIGURE 63–5. Hemophilia: Patellar abnormalities. Patellar size and shape are extremely variable in hemophilia. This bone may appear square (**A**) or elongated and thin (**B**). Abnormalities of the patellofemoral compartment are common in this disease. Osteoporosis, joint space narrowing, and osteophytes are evident.

common in the femoral head[5, 25, 31, 134, 183] and talus.[5, 31, 180] In the former location, resulting radiographic abnormalities resemble those of Legg-Calvé-Perthes disease.[184]

Ectopic Ossification (Fig. 63–10). Ossification may appear in periarticular soft tissues.[1, 32–34, 137] This complication most frequently is apparent in the lower one half of the body, particularly in the pelvis, at which site ossification extending from the lateral aspect of the ilium or ischium to the proximal end of the femur may be observed.[108] Other sites include the paraspinal regions, thigh, and knee.[137] Ossification may relate to traumatic tearing of the adjacent periosteum and intermuscular bleeding around the iliac, iliopsoas, and adductor muscles. Restricted joint motion can be observed, which may improve in rare instances in which the ectopic ossification has resolved spontaneously.[159]

Fractures. In hemophilia, fractures may occur spontaneously or after minor trauma.[35–37] This is not surprising in view of the presence of osteoporosis, joint contracture, and muscle imbalance in this disease. Patients with hemophilia and restricted knee motion frequently have supracondylar fractures.[1] Fracture healing in hemophilic patients proceeds normally,[107] although pseudotumors may develop at the site of fracture.[138]

Hemophilic Pseudotumor (Fig. 63–11). Hemophilic pseudotumor of bone and soft tissue first was described by Starker in 1918[38] in a patient with extensive destruction of the femur. Since that time, this complication has been noted with increasing frequency,[39–52] although it still remains a relatively uncommon manifestation of the disease, probably occurring in fewer than 2 per cent of cases. The bones that are implicated most frequently, in descending order of frequency, are the femur, the components of the osseous pelvis, the tibia, and the small bones of the hands. Rarely, more than one bone may contain a pseudotumor.[209] Pseudotumors may be intraosseous or subperiosteal or may occur within the soft tissues. It is probable that they arise from hemorrhage, a pathogenesis that is underscored by the many patients who relate an episode of trauma to the involved area. In some cases, hematomas within a muscle may dissect along the muscle bundles to reach the bone, producing considerable pressure deformity and subperiosteal elevation.

The radiographic appearance of a hemophilic pseudotumor is variable. Intraosseous lesions may be encountered. Medullary bone destruction may produce small or large central or eccentric radiolucent lesions that are fairly well demarcated. Trabeculae can extend across the lesions, and the surrounding bone frequently is sclerotic. Cortical violation and periosteal bone formation may reach considerable proportions. A large soft tissue mass may be encountered. Its characteristics and its relationship to adjacent structures can be well shown by ultrasonography, CT, or MR imaging.[109, 139–141, 188, 190–192, 210] Angiography documents the avascularity of the lesion.[141]

Mild, moderate, or massive bleeding may occur in subperiosteal locations. In the immature skeleton, the periosteum is lifted easily by the accumulation of blood. Cortical atrophy due to abnormal pressure, subperiosteal bone formation, and soft tissue extension are evident. Any bone may be involved, even those of the face,[142] although DePalma[5] has indicated that the fibula discloses this abnormality most frequently.

Tumors arising in the soft tissue enlarge slowly, develop a fibrous capsule, and distort the subjacent osseous tissue

Text continued on page 2307

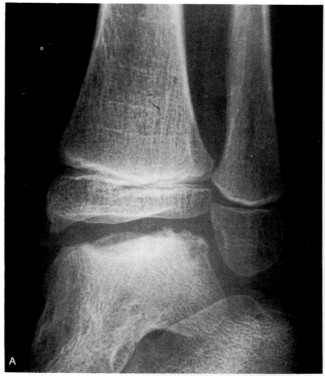

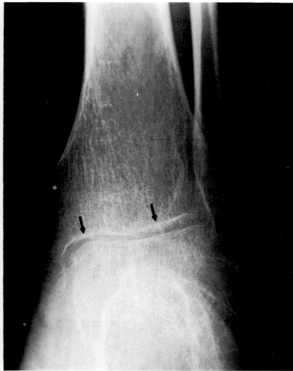

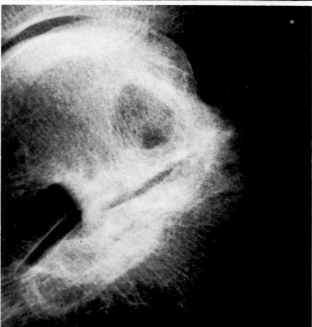

FIGURE 63–6. Hemophilia: Ankle and talocalcaneal joint abnormalities.

A Oblique radiograph in a child with hemophilia demonstrates flattening and erosion of the superior surface of the talus. These osseous abnormalities may be related to collapse of weakened subchondral bone or osteonecrosis. The joint space is relatively preserved. The bones are osteoporotic, and horizontal radiodense areas in the tibia represent growth recovery lines. Mild periostitis also is seen.

B In another patient, more extensive abnormalities in the ankle include osteoporosis and joint space narrowing. Note the tibiotalar slant with an angular joint surface (arrows).

C Severe posterior subtalar joint changes consist of joint space narrowing, sclerosis, cyst formation, and flattening of the bony surface.

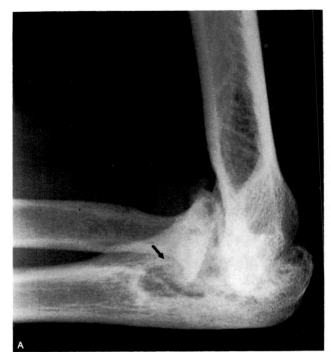

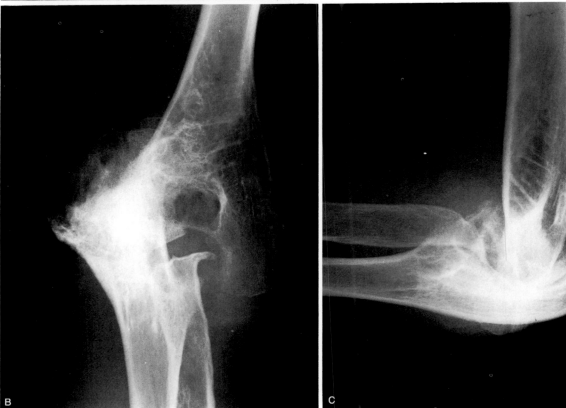

FIGURE 63–7. Hemophilia: Elbow joint abnormalities.

A Observe sclerosis, flattening, and deformity of the bones. The radial head is widened. Note the enlargement of the radial fossa (arrow).

B, C In a different patient, extensive destruction is evident. Osteoporosis, resorption, sclerosis, deformity, and a radiodense joint effusion are evident. The trochlear notch of the ulna is widened.

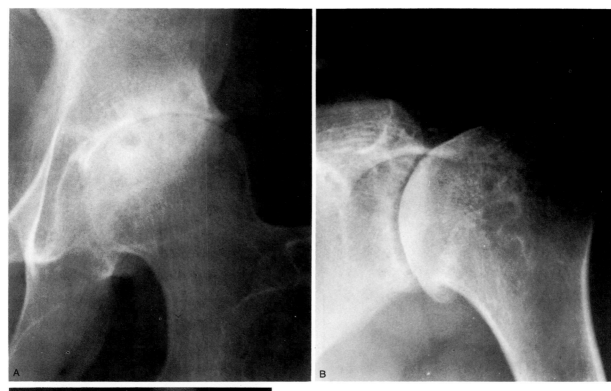

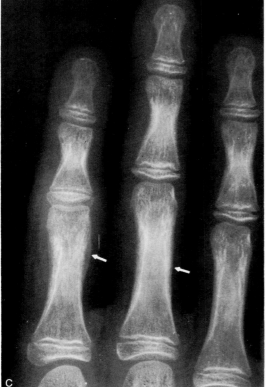

FIGURE 63–8. Hemophilia: Other articular abnormalities.
   A Hip: Symmetric loss of joint space, subchondral bone sclerosis, and cysts are seen.
   B Glenohumeral joint: Findings include joint space narrowing, sclerosis, and osteophytosis.
   C Hand: Soft tissue swelling and osteoporosis can be detected. Note periostitis of several phalanges (arrows).

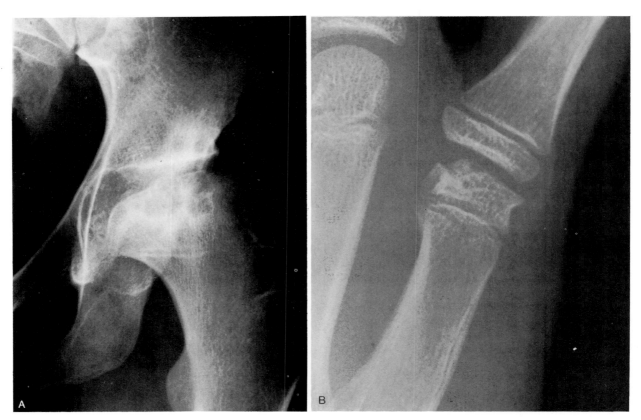

FIGURE 63–9. Hemophilia: Osteonecrosis.
  A Hip: Intra-articular bleeding can produce osteonecrosis of the femoral head. Findings include considerable flattening of the femoral head, subchondral cysts, mild joint space narrowing, and acetabular deformity.
  B Metacarpophalangeal joint: Observe collapse and irregularity of the metacarpal head.
  (**B,** Courtesy of M. Pathria, M.D., San Diego, California.)

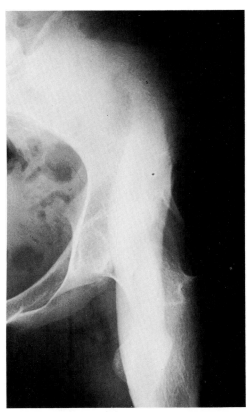

FIGURE 63–10. Hemophilia: Ectopic ossification. A large band of ossification extends from the lateral aspect of the ilium to the proximal portion of the femur. (Courtesy of M. Dalinka, M.D., Philadelphia, Pennsylvania.)

by pressure erosion. Soft tissue hemophilic pseudotumors are most common in the thigh and the gluteal region.[185] Infrequently, the soft tissue masses calcify.[186]

Although the radiographic characteristics of pseudotumors obviously depend on the initial site of hemorrhage (intramedullary, subperiosteal, soft tissue), eventually large and disorganized lesions may appear, which can lead to pathologic fracture. Secondary infection of these lesions is a rare but reported phenomenon; indeed, gas formation in a pseudotumor represents one radiographic characteristic of such infection, although gas within a hemophilic pseudotumor also may develop owing to its perforation into a viscus or on an iatrogenic basis related to attempted drainage.[187] Without treatment, the lesions progress slowly and eventually require radical surgery, often causing the patient's demise. With better recognition of this complication and its pathogenesis, definitive therapy (surgery, irradiation) can be instituted at an earlier stage.[105]

The differential diagnosis of hemophilic pseudotumors includes several other disorders. Initially, a subperiosteal hematoma in hemophilia produces periostitis that can simulate malignancy (Ewing's sarcoma, skeletal metastases) or infection. An intraosseous hematoma leading to osteolytic lesions of varying size simulates primary and secondary neoplasms, tumor-like lesions, and infection. In many patients, accurate diagnosis relies on knowledge of the patient's underlying disease. On rare occasions, diagnosis is not established adequately by the clinical and radiographic

features. In these cases, a biopsy followed by surgical extirpation may be necessary.

Other Articular Manifestations (Fig. 63–12). Chondrocalcinosis has been described in patients with hemophilia.[53, 143] Although this occurrence may be purely incidental, it is interesting to speculate that the presence of hemosiderin within a joint may alter the articular biomechanics and biochemistry, resulting in cartilage calcification. Septic arthritis occurring in patients with hemophilia also has been recorded.[54, 144–147] *Staphylococcus aureus* is the typical pathogen, and the knee is the most common site of involvement. The combination of hemophilia and septic arthritis may represent only a chance occurrence of two diseases, although intra-articular hemorrhagic fluid is an ideal culture medium for certain bacteria.[55] Furthermore, immunosuppression secondary to human immunodeficiency virus may play an important role in the pathogenesis of septic arthritis in patients with hemophilia.[189, 211] In hemophilia, joint contractures may complicate intra-articular destruction or soft tissue hemorrhage, with impingement on vessels and nerves.[117, 124]

Scintigraphy

The evaluation of patients with hemophilia using bone-seeking radionuclide agents has been advocated.[56, 57, 164, 165] Increased sensitivity of the isotopic examination over clinical and radiologic evaluation is not unexpected, particularly at sites of acute arthropathy. The radionuclide examination lacks specificity, however, and is less effective in evaluating joints with chronic arthropathy. Radioisotopic studies may be useful in assessing joint status during therapy. They also have been used to evaluate hemophilic pseudotumors.[49]

Computed Tomography

The major application of CT to the evaluation of patients with hemophilia is in assessing the extent of pseudotumors,[139–141] soft tissue hemorrhage,[118] or neurovascular compromise (Fig. 63–13). As hemophilic pseudotumors commonly arise in or extend to periosseous soft tissues, their excellent visualization by CT, a technique well known for its capabilities regarding soft tissue neoplasms, is not unexpected.[166, 191] CT is effective in establishing the diagnosis of extraosseous hemorrhage and in evaluating its extent and response to treatment.[118] Soft tissue ossification in hemophilia also is well shown with this technique.[137]

Magnetic Resonance Imaging

The remarkable ability of MR imaging to define soft tissue abnormalities and, specifically, hematomas[167, 168] indicates its promising potential in the evaluation of intra-articular and extra-articular hemorrhagic manifestations of hemophilia.[160, 169, 170] With regard to the intra-articular abnormalities of hemophilia, MR imaging has unique capabilities. It allows assessment of the extent of the process and provides information regarding its nature.[191, 193–195] Histologic abnormalities in hemophilic arthropathy are dependent on the stage of the disease: Initial episodes of bleeding lead to mild proliferation of synovial cells, acute perivascular inflammation, and synovial accumulation of iron from

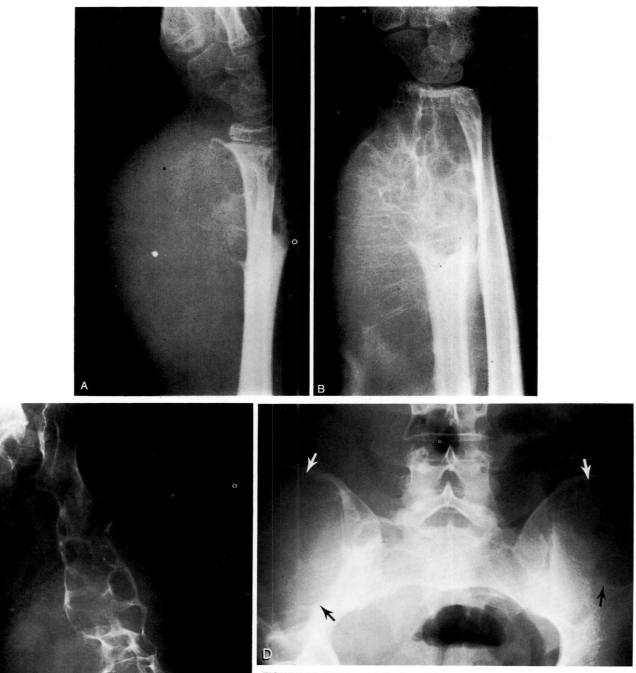

FIGURE 63–11. Hemophilia: Pseudotumors.

A, B Radiographs of the forearm obtained 7 years apart reveal a pseudotumor involving the distal portion of the radius. The initial radiograph **(A)** demonstrates an extensive soft tissue mass, scalloped erosion of the adjacent radius, and radiating trabeculae. The subsequent radiograph **(B)** reveals considerable new bone formation extending into the soft tissues with destruction and deformity of the underlying bone. (Courtesy of A. Brower, M.D., Norfolk, Virginia.)

C An example of the striking bone and soft tissue abnormalities that may accompany bleeding in hemophilia. The deformed femur has a "cystic" appearance and, in places, its contour has been obliterated completely. The hip also is abnormal.

D In this 30 year old man, bilateral pseudotumors of the ilia (arrows) are seen. (Courtesy of W. Murray, M.D., Boise, Idaho.)

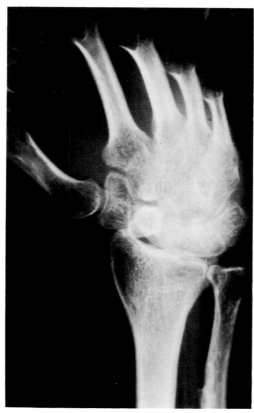

FIGURE 63–12. Hemophilia: Ischemic contracture. After extensive bleeding about the elbow, an ischemic contracture of the hand and wrist is evident.

nus composed of dense avascular, acellular fibrous tissue that adheres tightly to the cartilage; with chronicity, a fibrotic synovium develops.[196] In view of this varied and changing articular environment, the MR imaging features of hemophilic arthropathy are not expected to be uniform.

Most of the reported investigations of hemophilic arthropathy using MR imaging have focused on the knee, an appropriate choice owing to the frequency with which it is involved in this disease and to its large size, which more easily allows adequate MR imaging examination. Spin echo sequences, employed in most of these investigations, have revealed regions in the joint with low to intermediate signal intensity on T1- and T2-weighted images, with foci of increased signal intensity on T2-weighted images[193] (Figs. 63–14 and 63–15). Persistent low signal intensity in both types of images is consistent with the presence of synovial fibrosis or hemosiderin deposition, or both. The foci of high signal intensity on the T2-weighted images are consistent with areas of synovial inflammation or fluid. Owing to the changing signal characteristics of resolving hemorrhage, it may be difficult to distinguish between viscous joint fluid and fresh blood with MR imaging in this disease.[193] The role of intravenous administration of paramagnetic contrast agents such as those employing gadolinium in the differentiation among synovial inflammation, hemorrhage, and joint effusion in hemophilia has not yet been established.

The MR characteristics of hemosiderin deposition in this disease are similar to those in other disorders accompanied by recurrent episodes of intra-articular bleeding. Such processes include pigmented villonodular synovitis, neoplasms such as synovial hemangiomas, neuropathic osteoarthropathy, and chronic renal disease. Hemosiderin collections lead to low signal intensity on all spin echo sequences and, to a greater degree, on all gradient echo sequences. The deposits of hemosiderin within the synovial membrane are accentuated, in some sequences, by the presence of adjacent fluid and synovial inflammation of high signal intensity. Accu-

sequestered red blood cells; repeated hemarthroses produce villous hypertrophy and increased vascularity of the synovial membrane, the accumulation of hemosiderin in synovial and subsynovial macrophages, and an infiltrating pan-

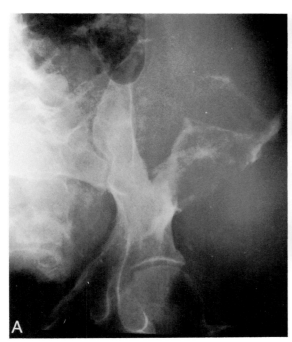

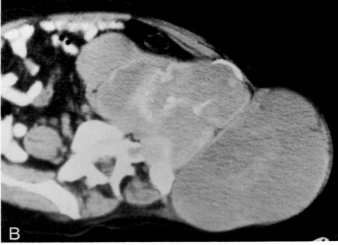

FIGURE 63–13. Hemophilia: Use of CT. Pseudotumor. In this 49 year old man with an enlarging mass of the buttock of 25 years' duration, routine radiography **(A)** and transaxial CT **(B)** reveal both the bone and soft tissue abnormalities. The extent of the process is better delineated with CT, which shows a lobulated mass of low attenuation with a partial rim of higher attenuation and residual and distorted trabeculae. (Courtesy of R. Cone, M.D., San Antonio, Texas.)

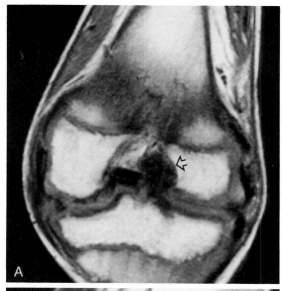

FIGURE 63–14. Hemophilia: Use of MR imaging. Knee arthropathy in a 10 year old boy.

A On a coronal T1-weighted (TR/TE, 800/25) spin echo MR image, an abnormal region of low signal intensity (arrow) is seen. Both menisci appear small and irregular.

B, C Sagittal proton density (TR/TE, 2000/30) **(B)** and T2-weighted (TR/TE, 2000/80) **(C)** spin echo MR images confirm the presence of a posterior lesion that demonstrates persistent low signal intensity (arrows). Additional areas of intermediate and low signal intensity are seen within the joint, extending into the suprapatellar recess (arrowheads) and deforming Hoffa's fat pad. The signal characteristics are those of synovial fibrosis or hemosiderin deposition, or both.

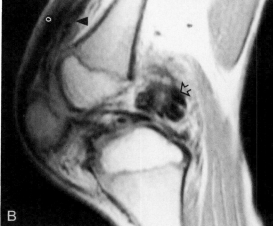

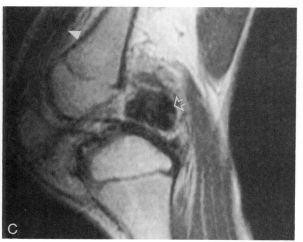

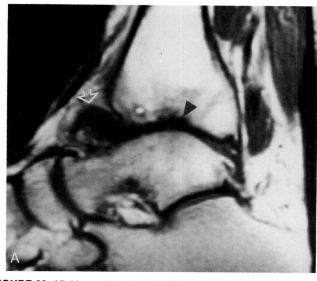

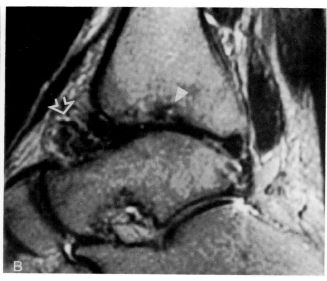

FIGURE 63–15. Hemophilia: Use of MR imaging. Ankle arthropathy in a 42 year old man.

A On a sagittal T1-weighted (TR/TE, 500/16) spin echo MR image, observe anterior extension of the joint (arrow). The intra-articular contents are of low signal intensity. Irregularity of the subchondral bone of the tibia is evident (arrowhead).

B On a sagittal T2-weighted (TR/TE, 2000/80) spin echo MR image, note persistent low signal intensity anteriorly with peripheral regions of higher signal intensity (arrow). Abnormal signal intensity also is seen in the tibia (arrowhead). The articular findings indicate synovial fibrosis or hemosiderin deposition (low signal intensity) and inflammation (high signal intensity).

rate differentiation among the many conditions that lead to hemosiderin accumulation is based primarily on clinical data.

As in other arthritic conditions, MR imaging may be used to assess the degree of cartilaginous and osseous destruction in hemophilia.[191, 193, 195] The optimal imaging sequence required for the accurate delineation of minor cartilaginous abnormalities is not yet clear (see Chapters 39 and 70), although regions of significant chondral thinning or denudation can be delineated with routine spin echo or gradient echo sequences. Subchondral cystic lesions, a prominent feature of hemophilic arthropathy, may be evaluated with MR imaging. The signal characteristics of these cysts, however, are dependent on the precise imaging sequence that is used and the contents of the lesions. Fluid, fibrotic material, hemorrhage or hemosiderin, in various combinations, may be present in the subchondral cysts.

Hemophilic pseudotumors also may be evaluated with MR imaging[190, 191] (Fig. 63–16), although the relative merits of this method compared with others, such as CT and ultrasonography, require further analysis. The signal behavior of these pseudotumors is complex, reflecting the effects of remote and recurrent bleeding and clot organization.[190] A peripheral margin of low signal intensity on T1- and T2-weighted spin echo MR sequences is consistent with the presence of fibrous tissue or hemosiderin, or both, in the wall of the pseudotumor. Less uniform, however, are the signal characteristics of the interior portions of the pseudotumor, which may reveal regions of either high or low signal intensity on one or both of these sequences. The full extent of the process and its relationship to bone and neurovascular structures are delineated with MR imaging (as well as with CT).

Pathogenesis of Hemophilic Arthropathy

Generally it is assumed that arthropathy in hemophilia results from intra- and periarticular hemorrhage, although most of the evidence for this arises from studies in animals.[58–62, 196] Experimental hemarthrosis leads to characteristic changes in articular tissues (Fig. 63–17).

In the synovial membrane, hypertrophy and inflammation, subsynovial fibrosis, and hemosiderin deposition are known responses to experimental hemarthrosis and resemble the findings of other articular disorders, particularly pigmented villonodular synovitis.[63] These same pathologic aberrations have been noted in hemophilia and posttraumatic hemarthrosis in humans.[64] The agent or agents in the blood causing synovial hypertrophy are not known.[1] Antigens in the red cell membrane may evoke autoimmune antibody formation, resulting in synoviocyte hypertrophy.

Cartilaginous abnormalities occurring after experimental hemarthrosis are less constant; some investigators have been unable to produce cartilaginous changes,[59] whereas others, employing more prolonged and extensive intra-articular bleeding, have noted cartilage fibrillation and degeneration.[65, 196] Some authors believe that after hemarthrosis, activated plasminogen degrades the chondromucoprotein in cartilage.[66] Investigators cite the presence of iron-containing bodies called siderosomes within the synovial lining and cartilage, which may release lysozymal enzymes and cause chondrocyte degeneration.[67, 68, 149] The levels of hydrolytic enzymes are increased in joint fluid and synovium in hemophilia.[1] A similar mechanism involving lysozymal degeneration of cartilage has been proposed in rheumatoid arthritis.[69] Additional factors that may contribute to cartilage damage in hemophilia are mechanical changes related to abnormal loading provoked by joint contractures and alterations occurring secondary to subchondral cystic lesions.[125]

The role of intra-articular iron deposits in the pathogenesis of hemophilic arthropathy is not clear.[1, 70] In this disease, iron is demonstrated in all layers of the synovium, both intracellularly and extracellularly; a similar distribution is apparent in hemochromatosis of exogenous origin. A potential role for iron in inhibition of pyrophosphatase enzymes, allowing accumulation of calcium pyrophosphate dihydrate crystals, has been suggested in the pathogenesis of chondrocalcinosis and arthropathy in hemochromatosis. Of interest in this regard is the report of cartilage calcification in patients with hemophilia.[53, 143] In addition, iron may alter the pH of synovial fluid[71] or the enzymatic activity of white blood cells.[72]

The osseous abnormalities in hemophilic joints may result from certain toxic and chemical effects on bone. In addition, elevation of intra-articular pressure (due to hemarthrosis) and intramarrow pressure (due to focal destruction of weight-bearing surfaces) may contribute to cystic defects[71, 148]; intraosseous bleeding accounting for the osseous cysts appears to be unlikely.[1, 58] Hyperemia may be responsible for epiphyseal overgrowth in hemophilia. Osteoporosis may relate to increased blood flow in capsular and epiphyseal blood vessels as well as to disuse and immobilization. Osteoporosis leads to mechanical weakening of the subchondral bone, which may contribute to osseous destruction and joint deformity.

Differential Diagnosis

Hemarthrosis is not confined to hemophilic arthropathy. It is frequent after trauma[197] (Fig. 63–18) and in other articular and nonarticular disorders, such as scurvy or myeloproliferative disease,[73] or after excessive administration of anticoagulant medication.[74, 150, 199] The radiographic findings associated with hemarthrosis are not specific, consisting mainly of soft tissue swelling, although after traumatic hemarthrosis, a distinctive fat-blood fluid level detectable on crosstable radiographs of the involved joint may be associated with obvious fracture.[75] In these conditions, permanent cartilaginous and osseous findings resembling those of hemophilia are not encountered.

Articular abnormalities of hemophilia most resemble changes of juvenile chronic arthritis (Table 63–2). This latter term has been applied to a variety of joint diseases occurring in children. One of these—juvenile-onset rheumatoid arthritis—may be associated with soft tissue swelling, periarticular osteoporosis, cartilage and osseous damage, and epiphyseal overgrowth, findings identical to those that are apparent in hemophilic arthropathy. It frequently is impossible to distinguish between these two disorders on the basis of radiographic abnormalities in a single joint. For example, osteoporosis, overgrowth of the distal femoral and proximal tibial epiphyses, osseous irregularity, numerous subchondral cysts, joint space narrowing, widening of the intercondylar notch, and squaring of the inferior pole of the patella may be observed in the knee in both hemophilia and

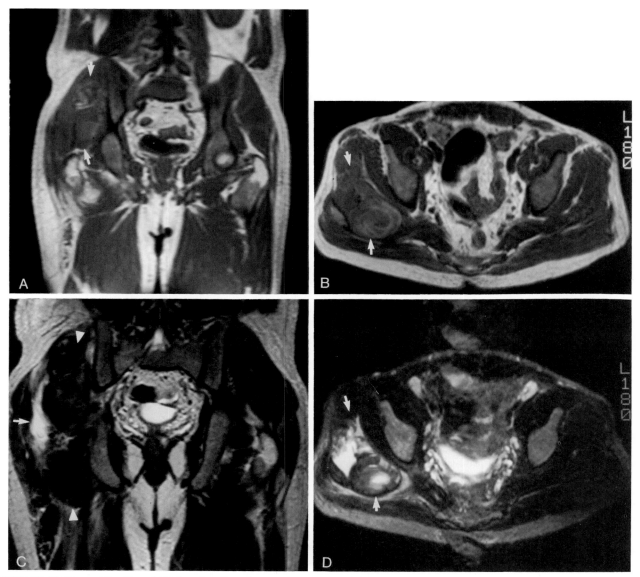

FIGURE 63–16. Hemophilia: Use of MR imaging. Pseudotumor in a 35 year old man.

A A T1-weighted (TR/TE, 600/10) spin echo MR image in the coronal plane reveals a large soft tissue mass (arrows), involving mainly the gluteus medius muscle. It is inhomogeneous in signal intensity, with some regions of the mass revealing signal intensity identical to that of muscle and other regions having greater signal intensity than muscle.

B A transaxial T1-weighted (TR/TE, 500/11) MR image confirms the presence of an intramuscular mass (arrows) with signal inhomogeneity.

C A coronal T2-weighted (TR/TE, 6000/102) fast spin echo MR image shows regions of low signal intensity, similar to that of muscle, and of very high signal intensity (arrow) in the mass. Note the full extent of the pseudotumor (between arrowheads).

D A transaxial T2-weighted (TR/TE, 8500/102) fast spin echo MR image, obtained with fat suppression technique (chemical presaturation), reveals the inhomogeneity of the signal intensity in the mass (arrows). Note its proximity to the ischium.

(Courtesy of M. Schweitzer, M.D., Philadelphia, Pennsylvania.)

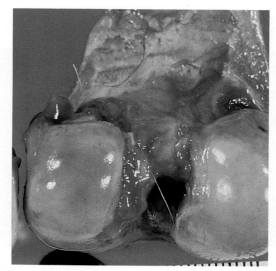

FIGURE 63–17. Experimental hemarthrosis. After continuous hemarthrosis of the knee in a dog, synovial and cartilaginous changes are evident. (Courtesy of F. R. Convery, M.D., San Diego, California.)

rheumatoid arthritis. Placing emphasis on any one of these radiographic manifestations as a useful finding in differentiating between these disorders frequently will lead to a mistaken diagnosis. Rather, it is the distribution of articular abnormalities in hemophilia and juvenile-onset rheumatoid arthritis (and other forms of juvenile chronic arthritis) that permits accurate radiographic diagnosis: In hemophilia, the knee, the ankle, and the elbow are altered most commonly; in juvenile-onset rheumatoid arthritis, the articulations of the hands and the wrists as well as the larger joints and spine may be affected.

In some joints, the findings of hemophilia may simulate those of pigmented villonodular synovitis (Fig. 63–19) or infection (Fig. 63–20). These latter disorders most characteristically are monoarticular, whereas joint involvement in hemophilia generally is polyarticular. Articular and skeletal alterations accompanying neuromuscular diseases, such as cerebral palsy, muscular dystrophy, and poliomyelitis, also may resemble those of hemophilia.[151] Such alterations include epiphyseal overgrowth, periarticular osteoporosis, soft tissue wasting, gracile bones, joint space narrowing, premature physeal closure, and tibiotalar slant. On rare oc-

FIGURE 63–18. Traumatic arthritis with hemarthrosis. After repetitive trauma to the knee, a sectional radiograph **(A)** and photograph **(B)** illustrate considerable degenerative alterations, consisting of joint space narrowing, osteophytes, cystic lesions, and bone sclerosis, as well as extensive hemarthrosis. The findings are reminiscent of those of hemophilia, neuropathic osteoarthropathy, and calcium pyrophosphate dihydrate crystal deposition disease.

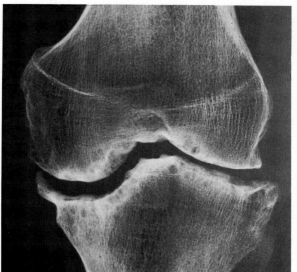

A

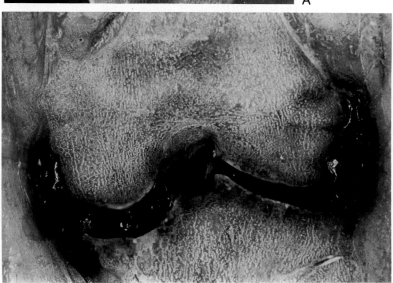

B

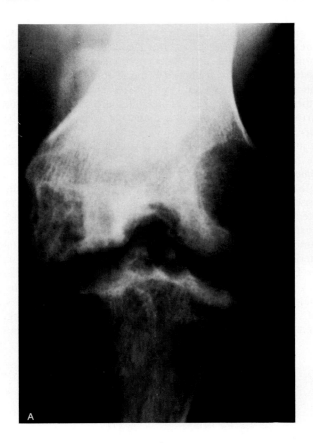

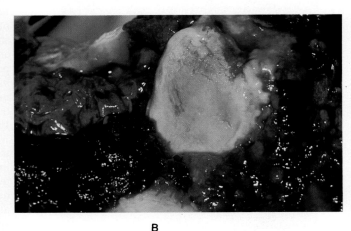

FIGURE 63–19. Pigmented villonodular synovitis.
A A radiograph of the knee outlines hemophilia-like changes, with osteoporosis, joint space narrowing, and subchondral bone irregularity and cyst formation. (Courtesy of H. Griffiths, M.D., Minneapolis, Minnesota.)
B A gross photograph of a knee involved with pigmented villonodular synovitis delineates the hypertrophied and pigmented synovium. (Courtesy of F. R. Convery, M.D., San Diego, California.)

casions, intra-articular bleeding in association with certain hemorrhagic diatheses may lead to an arthropathy identical to that of hemophilia.[171, 198, 200] Two of these diatheses are discussed subsequently. Additional disorders leading to intra-articular, intraosseous, or soft tissue hemorrhage include Glanzmann's thrombasthenia (rare autosomal recessive disorder with platelet abnormality)[113] (Fig. 63–21), congenital hereditary abnormalities of fibrinogen,[152, 153, 201] von Willebrand's disease, and thrombocytopenic purpura[114, 202] (Fig. 63–22) (Table 63–3).

TABLE 63–2. Hemophilia Versus Juvenile-Onset Rheumatoid Arthritis (JRA)

	Hemophilia	JRA
Common articular sites	Knee, ankle, elbow	Knee, ankle, wrist, hand
Soft tissue swelling	+	+
Osteoporosis	+	+
Joint space narrowing	±	±
Bony ankylosis	–	+
Epiphyseal overgrowth	+	+
Growth inhibition	–	+
Epiphyseal collapse or osteonecrosis	+	+
Periostitis	±	+
Pseudotumors	+	–
Spondylitis	–	+

BLEEDING DIATHESES AND HEMANGIOMAS

Background and General Features

Hemangiomas are vascular tumors, most frequently located in the skin, which appear in the early postnatal period.[76] Their occurrence in other tissues is well known, and they may arise within the synovial membrane, especially that of the knee.[203, 204] Synovial hemangiomas are discussed in detail elsewhere in this book (Chapter 84). Hemangiomas may be associated with unusual syndromes, some of which produce hematologic abnormality.

The association of varicose veins, soft tissue and bony hypertrophy, and cutaneous hemangiomas is known as the Klippel-Trenaunay syndrome, named after the two investigators who described this disorder in children and young adults in 1900.[77] An underlying vascular abnormality consisting of atresia and hypoplasia or obstruction of the deep venous system was noted in all cases. In 1918, Parke-Weber[78] demonstrated an arteriovenous fistula in this syndrome; when this feature is combined with the classic triad of findings, the term Parke-Weber syndrome commonly is employed. Additional variants have included cutaneous lymphangiomas, facial hemihypertrophy, cavernous hemangiomas of the colon, and varicosities of the pulmonary veins.[79, 80] Numerous other descriptions of the Klippel-Trenaunay syndrome also have emphasized the variability of its clinical and radiologic manifestations,[81–86, 154, 161, 172, 205, 206] which may include osseous abnormalities (syndactyly, polydactyly, clinodactyly, lobster-claw deformity, agenesis of phalanges, metatarsals, and metacarpals, hip or shoulder dislocation, pes equinovarus, scoliosis, and spina bifida)

TABLE 63–3. Heritable Disorders of Blood Coagulation

Disorder	Heredity	Hemorrhagic Tendency	Hemarthrosis
Classic hemophilia (factor VIII deficiency)	X-linked	Mild to severe	Common
Christmas disease (factor IX deficiency)	X-linked	Mild to severe	Common
Von Willebrand's disease (factor VIII deficiency, platelet abnormalities)	Autosomal dominant	Mild to severe	Uncommon
Plasma thromboplastin antecedent (PTA, factor IX) deficiency	Autosomal recessive	Mild	Rare
Hageman trait (deficiency of Hageman factor, factor XII)	Autosomal recessive	None to mild	Usually absent
Fletcher trait (deficiency of plasma prekallikrein)	Autosomal recessive	None	Absent
Fitzgerald trait (deficiency of high molecular weight kininogen)	Autosomal recessive	None	Absent
Parahemophilia (factor V deficiency)	Autosomal recessive	Moderate	Rare
Stuart factor deficiency (factor X deficiency)	Autosomal recessive	Severe	Variable
Factor VII deficiency	Autosomal recessive	Mild to moderate	Variable
Hereditary hypoprothrombinemia (prothrombin deficiency)	Autosomal recessive	Mild to severe	Variable
Congenital deficiency of fibrinogen	Autosomal recessive	Severe	Variable
Congenital dysfibrinogenemia (structural abnormality of fibrinogen)	Autosomal dominant	None to mild	Variable
Congenital deficiency of fibrin-stabilizing factor (factor XIII deficiency)	Unknown	Severe	Rare

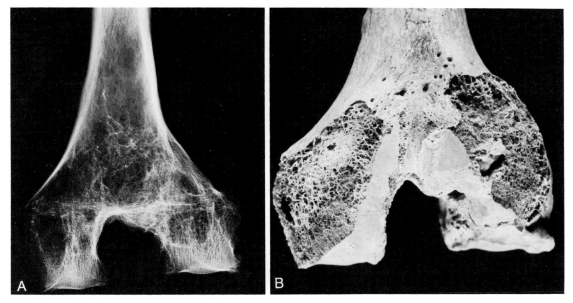

FIGURE 63–20. Septic arthritis. Femoral changes in the knee of a cadaver with chronic osteomyelitis and septic arthritis, consisting of osteopenia, flattening of the femoral condyles, and widening of the intercondylar notch, resemble those of hemophilia.

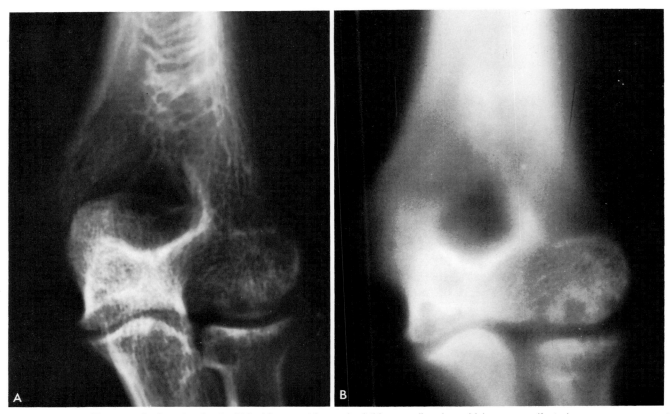

FIGURE 63–21. Glanzmann's thrombasthenia. This 19 year old man had this rare disorder, which was manifested as severe recurrent epistaxis. After suffering falls, he had developed hemarthroses of the knee and elbow. Continued elbow pain and locking led him to consult an orthopedic surgeon. A radiograph **(A)** and conventional tomogram **(B)** of the elbow reveal cystic changes in the humeral capitulum and trochlea and the radial head.

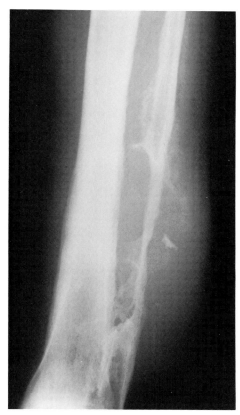

FIGURE 63–22. Thrombocytopenic purpura. A 29 year old man developed, over a period of 9 months, a mass in his leg. Eight years previously, a similar lesion had developed at this site, which, on biopsy, was interpreted as a hematoma. Laboratory evaluation indicated marked thrombocytopenia with prolonged bleeding time. A bone marrow aspirate showed good cellularity, normal granulocytic and erythroblastic morphology, presence of megakaryocytes, and no evidence of platelet formation. The frontal radiograph of the lower leg shows a large soft tissue mass above the ankle, containing bone fragments, with subjacent destruction of a long segment of the fibula. The margins of the lesion are well defined. Periosteal bone formation is evident in both the fibula and the tibia. At surgery, a large hematoma was found. (Courtesy of J. Vilar, M.D., Valencia, Spain.)

other than bony overgrowth.[87] The cause of the syndrome is not known, although it has been related to an intrauterine insult, perhaps during the embryologic period in which vascular differentiation and invasion of the limb bud are taking place.[155] An injury to the sympathetic ganglia or the intermediate lateral tract during intrauterine development also may be important. The association of the Klippel-Trenaunay syndrome and some of the phakomatoses, such as the Sturge-Weber syndrome, neurofibromatosis, and tuberous sclerosis, also has been reported.[154]

With regard to the clinical manifestations of this syndrome, both sexes are affected. The nevus usually is present at birth, and varices appear, sometimes at birth but typically in the first few years of life. Bony and soft tissue hypertrophy also is evident in early life but becomes more obvious during the adolescent growth spurt. Generally, only one lower limb is involved, although exceptions to this rule occur.[154] Reported cases have included combinations of upper and lower limb involvement and changes in all four limbs.[156, 157]

The natural history of the Klippel-Trenaunay syndrome is variable, although worsening of venous insufficiency is

the rule. The progressive nature of the condition commonly results in a shortened life span.

In 1940, Kasabach and Merritt[88] described the association of papillary hemangiomas and extensive purpura. Subsequent reports of hematologic abnormalities associated with the Kasabach-Merritt syndrome have included thrombocytopenia, deficiencies of factors V, VII, VIII, and IX, prothrombin depression, hypofibrinogenemia, and microangiopathic hemolytic anemia.[89, 90] A consumption coagulopathy due to intravascular coagulation within the hemangioma makes these patients (usually infants) susceptible to hemorrhage.[91, 207, 208] Subperiosteal[92] and intraosseous[92–94] hemangiomas have been described, most frequently in the flat bones. Occasionally, these hemangiomas can lead to fractures of the extremities.[94, 173] Surgical removal or embolization of the hemangioma leads to prompt correction of the coagulopathy.[207] Diagnostic methods used to study the hemangioma have included ultrasonography, CT, MR imaging, and scintigraphy.

Articular Abnormalities

Arthropathies are not reported commonly in either the Klippel-Trenaunay syndrome or the Kasabach-Merritt syndrome,[95] although in the latter condition, patients may suffer joint stiffness and "degenerative" changes.[96] Groh[97] has reported arthropathy of the knee resembling hemophilia in association with the Klippel-Trenaunay syndrome; a similar arthropathy in this same articulation can occur in the Kasabach-Merritt syndrome[98, 99] (Fig. 63–23).

The most likely explanation for the pathogenesis of the arthropathy resembling that accompanying hemophilia, which occurs in some patients with the Klippel-Trenaunay or Kasabach-Merritt syndrome, would involve recurrent episodes of intra-articular bleeding. This possible pathogenesis gains support from the appearance of this same arthropathy in patients with synovial hemangiomas without either of these syndromes.[99, 115] A generalized hemorrhagic tendency (Kasabach-Merritt syndrome) or localized abnormalities (synovial hemangiomas) would predispose the patient to intra-articular hemorrhage. The diagnosis of the precise cause for the radiographic findings is based on the appearance of calcified circular radiodense lesions (phleboliths) in soft tissue and periarticular locations in combination with abnormalities resembling those of hemophilia, including soft tissue swelling, osteoporosis, epiphyseal overgrowth, irregularities of subchondral bone, and widening of the intercondylar notch of the femur (Table 63–4).

SUMMARY

The skeletal abnormalities associated with hemophilia and other bleeding diatheses are characteristic. They result from hemorrhage in soft tissue, muscle, subperiosteal, in-

TABLE 63–4. Radiographic Features of Arthropathy Associated with Hemangiomas

Soft tissue swelling
Osteoporosis
Epiphyseal overgrowth
Subchondral bone erosions and cysts
Calcifications (phleboliths)

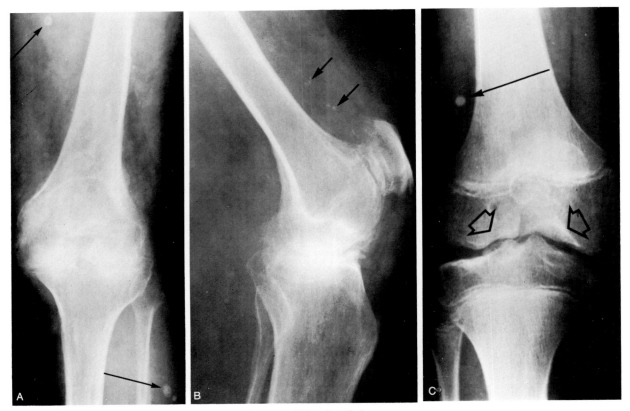

FIGURE 63–23. Arthropathy in association with hemangiomas and bleeding diatheses.

A, B A 45 year old man had pain in his left knee. He had had a vascular anomaly of the left leg since birth. Since the age of 15 years, he had experienced pain radiating from his left knee to his ankle. On physical examination, a vascular malformation of the left lower extremity was noted, extending from the buttock to the foot. Radiographs of the left knee reveal extensive osteoporosis, joint space narrowing, and sclerosis. The epiphyses appear enlarged in relation to the constricted diaphyses. Note the numerous phleboliths (arrows) in the soft tissues. **C** An 11 year old had recurrent bilateral knee pain and abdominal discomfort. At the age of 6 weeks, multiple hemangiomas of the lower extremities and abdomen were noted. Extensive clinical and laboratory evaluation confirmed the diagnosis of multiple giant hemangiomas and varicosities (Klippel-Trenaunay syndrome), Kasabach-Merritt syndrome, and a consumption coagulopathy. On this radiograph of the knee, a soft tissue phlebolith (arrow) is apparent. The distal femoral and proximal tibial epiphyses are enlarged, with irregularities of the subchondral bone and a widened intercondylar notch (open arrows).

(From Resnick D, Oliphant M: Radiology *114:* 323, 1975.)

traosseous, and intra-articular locations. In involved joints, typical findings are radiodense effusions, regional or periarticular osteoporosis, subchondral bony erosions and cysts, and joint space narrowing. Hyperemia may lead to epiphyseal overgrowth in a child affected by these disorders. Tumor-like lesions occasionally may be encountered owing to massive subperiosteal, osseous, or soft tissue hemorrhage with erosion and distortion of adjacent bone. Hemosiderin deposition in any of these disorders leads to characteristic findings with MR imaging. The differential diagnosis generally is not difficult when both clinical and imaging features are studied.

References

1. Arnold WD, Hilgartner MW: Hemophilic arthropathy. Current concepts of pathogenesis and management. J Bone Joint Surg [Am] *59:*287, 1977.
2. Schulman I, Smith CH: Coagulation disorders in infancy and childhood. Adv Pediatr *9:*231, 1957.
3. Key JA: Hemophilic arthritis. Ann Surg *95:*198, 1932.
4. Webb JB, Dixon AS: Haemophilia and haemophilic arthropathy. An historical review and a clinical study of 42 cases. Ann Rheum Dis *19:*143, 1960.
5. DePalma AF: Hemophilic arthropathy. Clin Orthop *52:*145, 1967.
6. Thomas HB: Some orthopaedic findings in ninety-eight cases of hemophilia. J Bone Joint Surg *18:*140, 1936.
7. Newcomer NB: The joint changes in hemophilia. Radiology *32:*573, 1939.
8. Goodfellow J, Fearn CB, Matthews JM: Iliacus haematoma. J Bone Joint Surg [Br] *49:*748, 1967.
9. Douglas AS, McAlpine SG: Neurological complications of haemophilia and Christmas disease. Scot Med J *1:*270, 1956.
10. Priest WM: Epidural haemorrhage due to haemophilia causing compression of the spinal cord. Lancet *2:*1289, 1935.
11. Cromwell LD, Kerber C, Ferry PC: Spinal cord compression and hematoma: An unusual complication in a hemophiliac infant. AJR *128:*847, 1977.
12. Mainardi CL, Levine PH, Werb Z, et al: Proliferative synovitis in hemophilia. Biochemical and morphologic observations. Arthritis Rheum *21:*137, 1978.
13. Hough AJ, Banfield WG, Sokoloff L: Cartilage in hemophilic arthropathy. Arch Pathol Lab Med *100:*91, 1976.
14. Handelsman JE, Lurie A: Pathological changes in the juvenile haemophilic knee. S Afr J Surg *13:*243, 1975.
15. Ghadially FN, Ailsby R, Yong NK: Ultrastructure of the haemophilic synovial membrane and electron-probe x-ray analysis of haemosiderin. J Pathol *120:*201, 1976.
16. Amouroux J, Adotti F: Lesions articulaires de l'hemophilie. Essai d'histogenese. Sem Hôp Paris *49:*955, 1973.
17. Rodnan GP, Brower TD, Hellstrom HR, et al: Postmortem examination of an elderly severe hemophiliac, with observations on the pathologic findings in hemophilic joint disease. Arthritis Rheum *2:*152, 1959.
18. Jaffe HL: Metabolic, Inflammatory and Degenerative Diseases of Bones and Joints. Philadelphia, Lea & Febiger, 1972, p 721.
19. Doub HP, Davidson EC: Roentgen ray examination of the joints of hemophiliacs. Radiology *6:*217, 1926.
20. Johnson JB, Davis TW, Bullock WH: Bone and joint changes in hemophilia. Radiology *63:*64, 1954.
21. Key JA: Hemophilic arthritis. Ann Surg *95:*198, 1932.

22. Gilchrist GS, Hagedorn AB, Stauffer RN: Severe degenerative joint disease. Mild and moderately severe hemophilia A. JAMA 238:2383, 1977.

23. Gilbert MS: Musculoskeletal manifestations of hemophilia. Mt Sinai J Med 44:339, 1977.

24. Zimbler S, McVerry B, Levine P: Hemophilic arthropathy of the foot and ankle. Orthop Clin North Am 7:985, 1976.

25. Moseley JE: Bone Changes in Hematologic Disorders. New York, Grune & Stratton, 1963, p 45.

26. Van Creveld S, Hoedemaeker PJ, Kingma JM, et al: Degeneration of joints in haemophiliacs under treatment by modern methods. J Bone Joint Surg [Br] 53:296, 1971.

27. Jordan HH: Hemophilic Arthropathies. Springfield, Ill, Charles C Thomas, 1958.

28. Gilbert M, Cockin J: An evaluation of the radiological changes in haemophilic arthropathy of the knee. In F Ala, KWE Denson (Eds): Proceedings of 7th Congress of the World Federation of Haemophilia. Amsterdam, Excerpta Medica, 1973, p 191.

29. Niemann KMW: Management of lower extremity contractures resulting from hemophilia. South Med J 67:437, 1974.

30. Ackroyd CE, Dinley RJ: The locked patella. An unusual complication of haemophilia. J Bone Joint Surg [Br] 58:511, 1976.

31. Boldero JL, Kemp HS: The early bone and joint changes in haemophilia and similar blood dyscrasias. Br J Radiol 39:172, 1966.

32. Hutcheson J: Peripelvic new bone formation in hemophilia. Report of three cases. Radiology 109:529, 1973.

33. Petersen J: A case of osseous change in a patient with hemophilia. Acta Radiol 28:323, 1947.

34. Samppinato F: Ossificazioni modellate nelle parti moli in soggetti emofilici. Rev Radiol 10:52, 1970.

35. Feil E, Bentley G, Rizza CR: Fracture management in patients with hemophilia. J Bone Joint Surg [Br] 56:643, 1974.

36. Ahlberg A, Nilsson IM: Fractures in haemophiliacs with special reference to complications and treatment. Acta Chir Scand 133:293, 1967.

37. Kemp HS, Matthews JM: The management of fractures in haemophilia and Christmas disease. J Bone Joint Surg [Br] 50:351, 1968.

38. Starker L: Knochensur durch ein hämophiles subperiostales hämatom. Mitt Grenzgeb Med Chir 31:381, 1918–1919.

39. Fraenkel GJ, Taylor KB, Richards WCD: Haemophilic blood cysts. Br J Surg 46:383, 1950.

40. Abell JM Jr, Bailey RW: Hemophilic pseudotumor. Two cases occurring in siblings. Arch Surg 81:569, 1960.

41. Chen YF: Bilateral hemophilic pseudotumors of calcaneus and cuboid treated by irradiation: Case report. J Bone Joint Surg [Am] 47:517, 1965.

42. Van Creveld S, Kingma MJ: Subperiosteal haemorrhage in hemophilia A and B. Acta Paediatr 50:291, 1961.

43. deValderrama JAF, Matthews JM: The haemophilic pseudotumor or haemophilic subperiosteal haematoma. J Bone Joint Surg [Br] 47:256, 1965.

44. Jones DM: Haemophilic blood cyst: Report of a case. J Bone Joint Surg [Br] 47:266, 1965.

45. Brant EE, Jordan HH: Radiologic aspects of hemophilic pseudotumors in bone. AJR 115:525, 1972.

46. Steel WM, Duthie RB, O'Connor BT: Haemophilic cysts: Report of five cases. J Bone Joint Surg [Br] 51:614, 1969.

47. Jensen PS, Putman CE: Hemophilic pseudotumor. Diagnosis, treatment and complications. Am J Dis Child 129:717, 1975.

48. Andes WA, Beltran G, Stuckey WJ: Pseudotumor in a patient with factor IX deficiency. South Med J 66:905, 1973.

49. Forbes CD, Moule B, Grant M, et al: Bilateral pseudotumors of the pelvis in a patient with Christmas disease. With notes on localization by radioactive scanning and ultrasonography. AJR 121:173, 1974.

50. Hilgartner MW, Arnold WD: Hemophilic pseudotumor treated with replacement therapy and radiation. Report of a case. J Bone Joint Surg [Am] 57:1145, 1975.

51. Ahlberg AKM: On the natural history of hemophilic pseudotumor. J Bone Joint Surg [Am] 57:1133, 1975.

52. Mulkey TF: Hemophilic pseudotumors of the mandible. J Oral Surg 35:561, 1977.

53. Jensen PS, Putman CE: Chondrocalcinosis and haemophilia. Clin Radiol 28:401, 1977.

54. Houghton GR: Septic arthritis of the hip in a hemophiliac. Report of a case. Clin Orthop 129:223, 1977.

55. Bulmer JH: Septic arthritis of the hip in adults. J Bone Joint Surg [Br] 48:289, 1958.

56. Cambouroglou G, Papathanassiou B, Koutolidis C, et al: Hemophilic arthropathy surveyed with whole-body gamma camera scintigraphy. Acta Orthop Scand 47:607, 1976.

57. Forbes CD, James W, Prentice CRM, et al: A comparison of thermography, radioisotope scanning and clinical assessment of the knee joints in hemophiliacs. Clin Radiol 26:41, 1975.

58. Swanton MC: Hemophilic arthropathy in dogs. Lab Invest 8:1269, 1959.

59. Wolf CR, Mankin HJ: The effect of experimental hemarthrosis on articular cartilage of rabbit knee joints. J Bone Joint Surg [Am] 47:1203, 1965.

60. Convery FR, Woo SL, Akeson WH, et al: Experimental hemarthrosis in the knee of the mature canine. Arthritis Rheum 19:59, 1976.

61. Ghadially FN, Lalonde JMA, Oryschak AF: Electron probe x-ray analysis of siderosomes in the rabbit haemarthrotic synovial membrane. Virchows Arch (Zellpathol) 22:135, 1976.

62. Roy S, Ghardially FN: Synovial membrane in experimentally produced chronic haemarthrosis. Ann Rheum Dis 28:402, 1969.

63. Young JM, Hudacek AG: Experimental production of pigmented villonodular synovitis in dogs. Am J Pathol 30:799, 1954.

64. Roy S, Ghadially FN: Ultrastructure of synovial membrane in human hemarthrosis. J Bone Joint Surg [Am] 49:1636, 1967.

65. Hoaglund FT: Experimental hemarthrosis. The response of canine knees to injections of autologous blood. J Bone Joint Surg [Am] 49:285, 1967.

66. Lack CH, Rogers HJ: Action of plasmin on cartilage. Nature 182:948, 1958.

67. Roy S: Ultrastructure of articular cartilage in experimental hemarthrosis. Arch Pathol 86:69, 1968.

68. Weissman G, Spilberg I: Breakdown of cartilage protein polysaccharide by lysosomes. Arthritis Rheum 11:162, 1968.

69. Barland P, Novikoff AB, Hamerman D, et al: Lysosomes in the synovial membrane in rheumatoid arthritis: A mechanism for cartilage erosion. Trans Assoc Am Physicians 77:239, 1964.

70. Muirden KD, Senator GB: Iron in the synovial membrane in rheumatoid arthritis and other joint diseases. Ann Rheum Dis 27:38, 1968.

71. Sokoloff L: Biochemical and physiological aspects of degenerative joint diseases with special reference to hemophilic arthropathy. Ann NY Acad Sci 240:285, 1975.

72. Oronsky AL, Perper RJ, Schroder HC: Phagocytic release and activation of human leukocyte procollagenase. Nature 246:417, 1973.

73. Harris BK, Ross HA: Hemarthrosis as the presenting manifestation of myeloproliferative disease. Arthritis Rheum 17:969, 1974.

74. Wild JH, Zvaifler NJ: Hemarthrosis associated with sodium warfarin therapy. Arthritis Rheum 19:98, 1976.

75. Kumar V: The shifting level in traumatic lipohaemarthrosis. Injury 3:13, 1971.

76. Stout AP, Lattes R: Tumors of the Soft Tissues. Atlas of Tumor Pathology, 2nd series, Fascicle 1. Washington DC, Armed Forces Institute of Pathology, 1967, p 67.

77. Klippel M, Trenaunay P: Du naevus variqueux osteo-hypertrophique. Arch Gen Med 185:641, 1900.

78. Weber FP: Hemangiectatic hypertrophy of limbs—congenital phlebacteriectasis and so-called congenital varicose veins. Br J Child Dis 15:13, 1918.

79. Belovic B, Nethercott J, Donsky HJ: An unusual variant of Klippel-Trenaunay-Weber syndrome. Can Med Assoc J 111:439, 1974.

80. Owens DW, Garcia E, Pierce RR, et al: Klippel-Trenaunay-Weber syndrome with pulmonary vein varicosity. Arch Dermatol 108:111, 1973.

81. Thomas ML, Macfie GB: Phlebography in the Klippel-Trenaunay syndrome. Acta Radiol (Diagn) 15:43, 1974.

82. Bourde C: Classification des syndromes de Klippel-Trénaunay et de Parkes-Weber d'après les données angiographiques. Ann Radiol 17:153, 1974.

83. Kontras SB: The Klippel-Trenaunay-Weber syndrome. Birth Defects 10:177, 1974.

84. Phillips GN, Gordon DH, Martin EC, et al: The Klippel-Trenaunay syndrome: Clinical and radiological aspects. Radiology 128:429, 1978.

85. Lindenauer SM: The Klippel-Trenaunay syndrome. Varicosity, hypertrophy and hemangioma with no arteriovenous fistula. Ann Surg 162:303, 1965.

86. Nöh, E, Steckenmesser R: Der angeborene Riesenwuchs, klinische and arteriographische Befunde an Hand und Arm beim Klippel-Trenaunay-Syndrom. Z Orthop 112:243, 1974.

87. D'Amico JA, Hoffman GC, Dyment PG: Klippel-Trénaunay syndrome associated with chronic disseminated intravascular coagulation and massive osteolysis. Cleve Clin Q 44:181, 1977.

88. Kasabach HH, Merritt KK: Capillary hemangioma with extensive purpura. Report of a case. Am J Dis Child 59:1063, 1940.

89. Inceman S, Tangün Y: Chronic defibrination syndrome due to a giant hemangioma associated with microangiopathic hemolytic anemia. Am J Med 46:997, 1969.

90. Rodriguez-Erdmann F: Bleeding due to increased intravascular blood coagulation. Hemorrhagic syndromes caused by consumption of blood-clotting factors (consumption-coagulopathies). N Engl J Med 273:1370, 1965.

91. McKay DG: Disseminated Intravascular Coagulation. An Intermediary Mechanism of Disease. New York, Hoeber, 1965.

92. Szilágyi G, Boga M, Rutkai P, et al: Complications of haemangiomatoses. Kasabach-Merritt syndrome in an adult. Haematologia (Budap) 7:69, 1973.

93. Hillman RS, Phillips LL: Clotting-fibrinolysis in a cavernous hemangioma. Am J Dis Child 113:649, 1967.

94. Lee JH Jr, Kirk RF: Pregnancy associated with giant hemangiomata, thrombocytopenia and fibrinogenopenia (Kasabach-Merritt syndrome). Report of a case. Obstet Gynecol 29:24, 1967.

95. Thompson LR, Umlauf HJ Jr: Hemangioma associated with thrombocytopenia: Report of two cases and review of the literature with emphasis on methods of therapy. Milit Med 129:652, 1964.

96. Rodriguez-Erdmann F, Button L, Murray JE, et al: Kasabach-Merritt syndrome: Coagulo-analytical observations. Am J Med Sci 261:9, 1971.

97. Groh P: "Blutergelenk" am Knie bei Morbus Klippel-Trenaunay. Arch Orthop Unfallchir 76:9, 1973.

98. Milikow E, Asch T: Hemangiomatosis, localized growth disturbance and intravascular coagulation disorder presenting with an unusual arthritis resembling hemophilia. Radiology 97:387, 1970.

99. Resnick D, Oliphant M: Hemophilia-like arthropathy of the knee associated

with cutaneous and synovial hemangiomas. Report of 3 cases and review of the literature. Radiology *114:*323, 1975.

100. Perri G: Widening of the radial notch of the ulna: A new articular change in haemophilia. Clin Radiol *29:*61, 1978.
101. Heylen W, Fabry G, Baert AL: Haemophilic arthropathy. J Belge Radiol *62:*41, 1979.
102. McCollough NC III, Enis JE, Lovitt J, et al: Synovectomy or total replacement of the knee in hemophilia. J Bone Joint Surg [Am] *61:*69, 1979.
103. Marmor L: Total knee replacement in hemophilia. Clin Orthop *125:*192, 1977.
104. Pavlov H, Goldman AB, Arnold WD: Haemophilic arthropathy in the joints of the hands and feet. Br J Radiol *52:*173, 1979.
105. Houghton GR, Duthie RB: Orthopedic problems in hemophilia. Clin Orthop *138:*197, 1979.
106. Pettersson H, Ahlberg Å, Nilsson IM: A radiologic classification of hemophilic arthropathy. Clin Orthop *149:*153, 1980.
107. Boardman KP, English P: Fractures and dislocations in hemophilia. Clin Orthop *148:*221, 1980.
108. Heim MD, Strauss S, Horoszowski H: Peripelvic new bone formation following straddle injuries in hemophiliac patients: Report of two cases. J Trauma *19:*846, 1979.
109. Guilford WB, Mintz PD, Blatt PM, et al: CT of hemophilic pseudotumors of the pelvis. AJR *135:*167, 1980.
110. Post M: Hemophilic arthropathy of the hip. Orthop Clin North Am *111:*65, 1980.
111. Handelsman JE: The knee joint in hemophilia. Orthop Clin North Am *10:*139, 1979.
112. Heller RM, Roloff JS, Kirchner SG, et al: Hemophilia and the female: Considerations for the radiologist. Radiology *133:*601, 1979.
113. Klofkorn RW, Lightsey AL: Hemarthrosis associated with Glanzmann's thrombasthenia. Arthritis Rheum *22:*1390, 1979.
114. Vilar J, Parra J, Monzo E: Case report 124. Skel Radiol *5:*197, 1980.
115. Thabe H: Das Synovialhämangiom des Kniegelenkes. Z Rheumatol *39:*95, 1980.
116. Burniat W, DeMartelaere N, Hariga C, et al: Two sisters with severe hemophilia A. Acta Paediatr Belg *34:*51, 1981.
117. Madigan RR, Hanna WT, Wallace SL: Acute compartment syndrome in hemophilia. A case report. J Bone Joint Surg [Am] *63:*1327, 1981.
118. Shirkhoda A, Mauro MA, Staab EV, et al: Soft tissue hemorrhage in hemophiliac patients. Computed tomography and ultrasound study. Radiology *147:*811, 1983.
119. Aronstam A, Browne RS, Wassef M, et al: The clinical features of early bleeding into the muscles of the lower limb in severe hemophiliacs. J Bone Joint Surg [Br] *65:*19, 1983.
120. Stanley P, McComb JG: Chronic spinal epidural hematoma in hemophilia A in a child. Pediatr Radiol *13:*241, 1983.
121. Roscoe MWA, Barrington TW: Acute spinal subdural hematoma. A case report and review of literature. Spine *9:*672, 1984.
122. Markowitz RI: Retropharyngeal bleeding in haemophilia. Br J Radiol *54:*521, 1981.
123. Iannaccone G, Pasquino AM: Calcifying splenic hematoma in a hemophilic newborn. Pediatr Radiol *10:*183, 1981.
124. Large DF, Ludlam CA, Macnicol MF: Common peroneal nerve entrapment in a hemophiliac. Clin Orthop *181:*165, 1983.
125. Speer DP: Early pathogenesis of hemophilic arthropathy. Evolution of the subchondral cyst. Clin Orthop *185:*250, 1984.
126. Brown IS, Toolis F, Prescott RJ: Haemophilic arthropathy: A ten year radiological and clinical study. Scott Med J *27:*279, 1982.
127. Soreff J, Blomback M: Arthropathy in children with severe hemophilia A. Acta Paediatr Scand *69:*667, 1980.
128. Leroux JL, Blotman F, Navarro M, et al: L'articulation fémoro-patellaire hémophilique. Rev Rhummal Osteoartic *49:*519, 1982.
129. Major M, Johnson P, Carrera G, et al: Arthrographic pseudoloosening of Marmor total knee in hemophilic arthropathy. Report of a case. Clin Orthop *160:*114, 1981.
130. Goldberg VM, Heiple KG, Ratnoff OD, et al: Total knee arthroplasty in classic hemophilia. J Bone Joint Surg [Am] *63:*695, 1981.
131. Small M, Steven MM, Freeman PA, et al: Total knee arthroplasty in haemophilic arthritis. J Bone Joint Surg [Br] *65:*163, 1983.
132. Griffiths H, Wandtke J: Tibiotalar tilt—a new slant. Skel Radiol *6:*193, 1981.
133. Benz HJ: Die Entwicklung der Epiphysen und Knochenkerne bei der hämophilen Arthropathie der Ellenbogens. ROFO *133:*305, 1980.
134. Longmaid HE III, Weissman BN: Resorptive hip arthropathy in hemophilia. J Can Assoc Radiol *33:*43, 1982.
135. Floman Y, Niska M: Dislocation of the hip joint complicating repeated hemarthrosis in hemophilia. J Pediatr Orthop *3:*99, 1983.
136. Heim M, Horoszowski H, Martinowitz U, et al: Haemophiliac hands—a three year follow-up study. Hand *14:*333, 1982.
137. Vaz W, Cockshott WP, Martin RF: Myositis ossificans in hemophilia. Skel Radiol *7:*27, 1981.
138. Wolff LJ, Lovrien EW: Management of fractures in hemophilia. Pediatrics *70:*431, 1982.
139. Pettersson H, Ahlberg A: Computed tomography in hemophilic pseudotumor. Acta Radiol (Diagn) *23:*453, 1982.
140. Coto H, Allen RC, Thomas E: CT scan diagnosis of hemophilic pseudotumor. Postgrad Med *70:*82, 1981.
141. Sundaram M, Wolverson MK, Joist JH, et al: Case report 133. Skel Radiol *6:*54, 1981.
142. Marquez JL, Vinageras E, Dorantes S, et al: Hemophilic pseudotumor of the inferior maxilla. Report of a case. Oral Surg *53:*347, 1982.
143. Leonello PP, Cleland LG, Norman JE: Acute pseudogout and chondrocalcinosis in a man with mild hemophilia. J Rheumatol *8:*841, 1981.
144. Rosner SM, Bhogal RS: Infectious arthritis in a hemophiliac. J Rheumatol *8:*519, 1981.
145. Wilkins RM, Wiedel JD: Septic arthritis of the knee in a hemophiliac. J Bone Joint Surg [Am] *65:*267, 1983.
146. Cobb WB: Septic polyarthritis in a hemophiliac. J Rheumatol *11:*87, 1984.
147. Hofmann A, Wyatt R, Bybee B: Septic arthritis of the knee in a 12-year-old hemophiliac. J Pediatr Orthop *4:*498, 1984.
148. Sancho FG: Experimental model of haemophilic arthropathy with high pressure haemarthrosis. Int Orthop (SICOT) *4:*57, 1980.
149. Mohr W, Kirkpatrick CJ, Kohler G: Arthropathie bei Hämophilie. Akt Rheumatol *7:*179, 1982.
150. Faux N, Manigand G: Hémarthroses spontanées de l'adolescent et de l'adulte, en dehors de l'hémophilie. Sem Hop Paris *58:*2367, 1982.
151. Richardson ML, Helms CA, Vogler JB III, et al: Skeletal changes in neuromuscular disorders mimicking juvenile rheumatoid arthritis and hemophilia. AJR *143:*893, 1984.
152. Lagier R, Bouvier CA, Van Strijthem N: Skeletal changes in congenital fibrinogen abnormalities. Skel Radiol *5:*233, 1980.
153. Zenny JC, Chevrot A, Sultan Y, et al: Lésions hémorragiques intra-osseuses des afibrinémies congénitales. J Radiol *62:*263, 1981.
154. You CK, Rees J, Gillis DA, et al: Klippel-Trenaunay syndrome: A review. Can J Surg *26:*399, 1983.
155. Woollard HH: The development of the principal arterial stems in the forelimbs of the pig. Contrib Embryol Carnegie Inst *14:*139, 1922.
156. Lal S, Sen SB, Narayanan PS: Klippel-Trenaunay syndrome involving the upper extremity. Indian J Med Sci *24:*430, 1970.
157. Lamar LM, Farber GA, O'Quinn SE: Klippel-Trenaunay-Weber syndrome. Arch Dermatol *91:*58, 1965.
158. Johnson RP, Babbitt DP: Five stages of joint disintegration compared with range of motion in hemophilia. Clin Orthop *201:*36, 1985.
159. Coblentz CL, Cockshott WP, Martin RF: Resolution of myositis ossificans in a hemophiliac. J Can Assoc Radiol *36:*161, 1985.
160. Pettersson H, Gilbert MS: Diagnostic Imaging in Hemophilia. Berlin, Springer-Verlag, 1985.
161. Servelle M: Klippel and Trénaunay's syndrome. 768 operated cases. Ann Surg *201:*365, 1985.
162. Lachiewicz PF, Inglis AE, Insall JN, et al: Total knee arthroplasty in hemophilia. J Bone Joint Surg [Am] *67:*1361, 1985.
163. Heim M, Horoszowski H, Martinowitz U: Hemophilic arthropathy resulting in a locked shoulder. Clin Orthop *202:*169, 1986.
164. Steven MM, Lewis D, Madhok R, et al: Radio-isotopic joint scans in haemophilic arthritis. Br J Rheumatol *24:*263, 1985.
165. Salimi Z, Vas W, Restrepo G: Joint scintigraphy using technetium-99m pyrophosphate in experimental hemarthrosis. J Nucl Med *27:*246, 1986.
166. Hermann G, Yeh H-C, Gilbert MS: Computed tomography and ultrasonography of the hemophilic pseudotumor and their use in surgical planning. Skel Radiol *15:*123, 1986.
167. Swenson SJ, Keller PL, Berquist TH, et al: Magnetic resonance imaging of hemorrhage. AJR *145:*921, 1985.
168. Unger EC, Glazer HS, Lee JKT, et al: MRI of extracranial hematomas: Preliminary observations. AJR *146:*403, 1986.
169. Cohen MD, McGuire W, Cory DA, et al: MR appearance of blood and blood products: An in vitro study. AJR *146:*1293, 1986.
170. Kulkarni MV, Drolshagen LF, Kaye JJ, et al: MR imaging of hemophiliac arthropathy. J Comput Assist Tomogr *10:*445, 1986.
171. Thakker S, McGehee W, Quismorio FP Jr: Arthropathy associated with factor XIII deficiency. Arthritis Rheum *29:*808, 1986.
172. Lewis BD, Doubilet PM, Heller VL, et al: Cutaneous and visceral hemangiomata in the Klippel-Trenaunay-Weber syndrome: Antenatal sonographic detection. AJR *147:*598, 1986.
173. Paley D, Evans DC: Angiomatous involvement of an extremity. A spectrum of syndromes. Clin Orthop *206:*215, 1986.
174. Nielsen FF, Christensen SE, de Carvalho A: Case report 475. Skel Radiol *17:*205, 1988.
175. Railton GT, Aronstam A: Early bleeding into upper limb muscles in severe haemophilia. Clinical features and treatment. J Bone Joint Surg [Br] *69:*100, 1987.
176. Nixon RG, Brindley GW: Hemophilia presenting as compartment syndrome in the arm following venipuncture. A case report and review of the literature. Clin Orthop *244:*176, 1989.
177. Katz SG, Nelson IW, Atkins RM, et al: Peripheral nerve lesions in hemophilia. J Bone Joint Surg [Am] *73:*1016, 1991.
178. Greene WB, Yankaskas BC, Guilford WB: Roentgenographic classifications of hemophilic arthropathy. J Bone Joint Surg [Am] *71:*237, 1989.
179. Hamel J, Pohlmann H, Schramm W: Radiological evaluation of chronic hemophilic arthropathy by the Pettersson score: Problems in correlation in adult patients. Skel Radiol *17:*32, 1988.
180. Gamble JG, Bellah J, Rinsky LA, et al: Arthropathy of the ankle in hemophilia. J Bone Joint Surg [Am] *73:*1008, 1991.

181. MacDonald PB, Locht RC, Lindsay D, et al: Haemophilic arthropathy of the shoulder. J Bone Joint Surg [Br] 72:470, 1990.
182. Hôgh J, Ludlam CA, Macnicol MF: Hemophilic arthropathy of the upper limb. Clin Orthop 218:225, 1987.
183. Paton RW, Evans DIK: Silent avascular necrosis of the femoral head in haemophilia. J Bone Joint Surg [Br] 70:737, 1988.
184. Pettersson H, Wingstrand H, Thambert C, et al: Legg-Calvé-Perthes disease in hemophilia: Incidence and etiologic considerations. J Pediatr Orthop 10:28, 1990.
185. Goldner BD: Osteolytic gluteal hematoma in hemophilia. AJR 151:833, 1988.
186. Hermann G, Gilbert M: Case report 471. Skel Radiol 17:152, 1988.
187. Ferenz CC, Tozzi JM: Sepsis due to an infected pseudocyst of hemophilia. A case report. Clin Orthop 244:254, 1989.
188. Liu SS, White WL, Johnson PC, et al: Hemophilic pseudotumor of the spinal canal. Case report. J Neurosurg 69:624, 1988.
189. Pappo AS, Buchanan GR, Johnson A: Septic arthritis in children with hemophilia. Am J Dis Child 143:1226, 1989.
190. Wilson DA, Prince JR: MR imaging of hemophilic pseudotumors. AJR 150:349, 1988.
191. Hermann G, Gilbert MS, Abdelwahab IF: Hemophilia: Evaluation of musculoskeletal involvement with CT, sonography, and MR imaging. AJR 158:119, 1992.
192. Wilson DJ, McLardy-Smith PD, Woodham CH, et al: Diagnostic ultrasound in haemophilia. J Bone Joint Surg [Br] 69:103, 1987.
193. Yulish BS, Lieberman JM, Strandjord SE, et al: Hemophilic arthropathy: Assessment with MR imaging. Radiology 164:759, 1987.
194. Armstrong SJ: Case report 661. Skel Radiol 20:369, 1991.
195. Pettersson H, Gillespy T, Kitchens C, et al: Magnetic resonance imaging in hemophilic arthropathy of the knee. Acta Radiol 28:621, 1987.
196. Madhok R, Bennett D, Sturrock RD, et al: Mechanisms of joint damage in an experimental model of hemophilic arthritis. Arthritis Rheum 31:1148, 1988.
197. Eiskjaer S, Larsen ST, Schmidt MB: The significance of hemarthrosis of the knee in children. Arch Orthop Trauma Surg 107:96, 1988.
198. Baker SR, Tartell J, Lawrence C, et al: Radiographic abnormalities in coagulation factor VII deficiency. J Can Assoc Radiol 38:64, 1987.
199. Riley SA, Spencer GE Jr: Destructive monarticular arthritis secondary to anticoagulant therapy. Clin Orthop 223:247, 1987.
200. Louthrenoo W, Abrahm J, Schumacher HR Jr: Hemarthrosis in patients with acquired factor VIII inhibitor. J Rheumatol 18:104, 1991.
201. Pellegrino M, Sacco M, Miglionico L, et al: Afibrinogenemia congenita: Descrizione di un caso con insolite lesioni ossee. Riv Ital Pediatr 17:115, 1991.
202. Moller DE, Goldstein K: Hemarthrosis and idiopathic thrombocytopenic purpora. J Rheumatol 14:382, 1987.
203. Lenchik L, Poznanski AK, Donaldson JS, et al: Case report 681. Skel Radiol 20:387, 1991.
204. Aalberg JR: Synovial hemangioma of the knee. A case report. Acta Orthop Scand 61:88, 1990.
205. Yousem DM, Scott WW Jr, Fishman EK: Case report 440. Skel Radiol 16:652, 1987.
206. McGrory BJ, Amadio PC, Dobyns JH, et al: Anomalies of the fingers and toes associated with Klippel-Trenaunay syndrome. J Bone Joint Surg [Am] 73:1537, 1991.
207. Larsen EC, Zinkham WH, Eggleston JC, et al: Kasabach-Merritt syndrome: Therapeutic considerations. Pediatrics 79:971, 1987.
208. Loh W Jr, Miller JH, Gomperts ED: Imaging with technetium 99m-labeled erythrocytes in evaluation of the Kasabach-Merritt syndrome. J Pediatr 113:856, 1988.
209. Shaw JA, Wilson SC: Multiple hemophilic bone cysts in the hand. J Hand Surg [Am] 18:262, 1993.
210. Iwata H, Oishi Y, Itoh A, et al: Surgical excision of hemophilic pseudotumor of the ilium. Clin Orthop 284:234, 1992.
211. Gregg-Smith SJ, Pattison RM, Dodd CAF, et al: Septic arthritis in haemophilia. J Bone Joint Surg [Br] 75:368, 1993.

SECTION
XIII
▼

Infectious Diseases

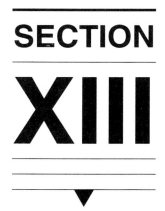

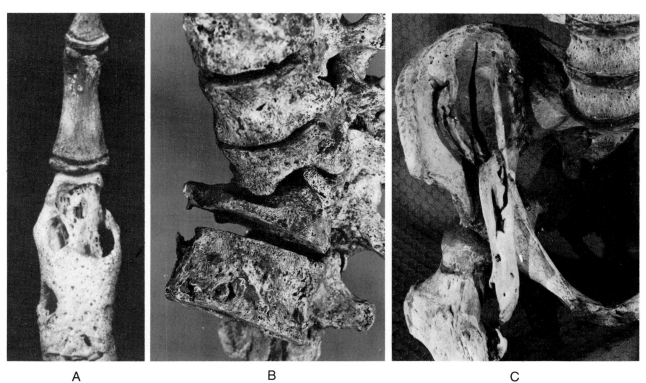

|A|B|C|

A Tuberculous dactylitis (spina ventosa): Note the expanded involucrum surrounding the remnant of the diseased phalanx with relative sparing of the epiphysis.

B Tuberculous spondylitis: In the midthoracic region, moderate to severe destruction of several adjacent vertebrae (with complete dissolution of one vertebral body and flattening of another) has resulted in kyphotic angulation.

C Tuberculous psoas abscess: The ossified right psoas abscess extends to the level of the lesser trochanter. (From Ortner DJ, Putschar WGJ: Identification of Pathological Conditions in Human Skeletal Remains. Washington, DC, Smithsonian Institution Press, 1981.)

64

Osteomyelitis, Septic Arthritis, and Soft Tissue Infection: Mechanisms and Situations

Donald Resnick, M.D., and Gen Niwayama, M.D.

Infection of bone and joint is a common and disturbing problem for children and adults alike, and it represents a diagnostic or therapeutic challenge to the pediatrician, internist, orthopedic surgeon, radiologist, and pathologist. Its manifestations are varied and depend on the site of involvement, the initiating event, the infecting organism, and the acute or chronic nature of the illness. Early diagnosis is imperative, as it allows prompt treatment, which can prevent many of the dreaded complications of the disease.

An adequate description of the imaging and pathologic features of bone and joint infection must address the problem from several aspects. Fundamental to this description is an analysis of the mechanisms by which the organisms reach the osseous and articular structures, the pathogenesis of the infective process itself, and any specific situations or circumstances that can influence the frequency and pattern of such contamination; this analysis is accomplished in the present chapter. Equally germane to the description of radiographic and pathologic abnormalities of skeletal infection is a discussion of the specific agents that are capable of infecting bones and joints and of the specific osseous and articular sites that can become contaminated. This chapter also discusses appendicular skeletal involvement, whereas axial skeletal involvement and specific causative agents of infection are addressed in Chapters 65 and 66.

TERMINOLOGY

Any discussion of bone and joint infection must make use of precise terms to describe the disease process. Definitions of these terms must be presented at the outset of the discussion so that the reader, in forging through the intricacies and complexities of the problem, does not become lost.

The term *osteomyelitis,* which was introduced by Nelaton[1] in 1844, implies an infection of bone and marrow. Osteomyelitis most commonly results from bacterial infections, although fungi, parasites, and viruses can infect the bone and the marrow. As used in this chapter, *infective (suppurative) osteitis* indicates contamination of the bone cortex. Infective osteitis can occur as an isolated phenomenon or, more frequently, as a concomitant to osteomyelitis. Radiographic and pathologic differentiation of osteitis and osteomyelitis can be extremely difficult; however, such differentiation is possible on many occasions, particularly with the use of CT and MR imaging, and can influence considerably the choice of an appropriate therapeutic regimen. Osteitis is not confined to infectious processes; inflammation of the cortex can be observed in numerous conditions, such as ankylosing spondylitis, psoriasis, and Reiter's syndrome, in which an infective cause has not been firmly established. *Infective (suppurative) periostitis* implies contamination of the periosteal cloak that surrounds the bone. In this situation, a subperiosteal accumulation of organisms frequently leads to infective osteitis and osteomyelitis, to interruption of periosteal blood supply to the cortex, producing necrosis, or to disruption of the periosteum and the accumulation of pus in the soft tissues. Routine radiography commonly is unable to delineate the precise extent of the infection (suppurative periostitis, osteitis, or osteomyelitis). Furthermore, periostitis can be noted in the absence of infection, being evident in neoplastic, metabolic, inflam-

matory, and traumatic disorders. *Soft tissue infection* indicates contamination of cutaneous, subcutaneous, muscular, fascial, tendinous, ligamentous, or bursal structures. This may be seen as an isolated condition, as a forerunner to infective periostitis, osteitis, or osteomyelitis, or as a complication of periosteal, osseous, marrow, or articular infection. Soft tissue infection can lead to inflammation of adjacent periosteal tissue (periostitis) without necessarily implying that the periosteum is contaminated. *Articular infection* implies a septic process of the joint itself. Septic arthritis can occur as an isolated condition that may soon spread to the neighboring bone or as a complication of adjacent osteomyelitis or soft tissue infection.

The clinical stages of osteomyelitis frequently are designated *acute, subacute,* and *chronic.*[575, 576] This does not imply that definitive divisions exist between one stage and another, nor does it signify that all cases of osteomyelitis progress through each of these phases. The relatively abrupt onset of clinical symptoms and signs during the initial stage of infection indicates clearly the acute osteomyelitic phase; if this acute phase passes without complete elimination of infection, subacute or chronic osteomyelitis can become apparent. The transition from acute to subacute and chronic osteomyelitis can indicate that therapeutic measures have been inadequate or inappropriate or that the organisms are especially resistant to accepted modes of therapy. Viable organisms can persist in small abscesses or fragments of necrotic bone, resisting all attempts at eradication of the septic process. At intervals of months or even years, the residual organisms can produce flare-ups of osteomyelitis. In contrast to those patients whose infections can be traced through each of the three clinical stages of osteomyelitis, other persons reveal chronic osteomyelitis at the initial time of evaluation,[2] having vague symptoms and signs on clinical examination and evidence of a long-standing process on radiographic evaluation.

Observations on large numbers of patients with infection underscore the difficulty in differentiating accurately among acute, subacute, and chronic osteomyelitis on the basis of clinical manifestations.[3] Some patients with apparently acute disease reveal historical evidence suggesting indolent infections; alternatively, patients with documented osteomyelitis for many years can appear with acute exacerbations characterized by fever, pain, tenderness, and warmth. This difficulty is compounded by histologic and imaging examinations that demonstrate the simultaneous occurrence of changes compatible with both acute and chronic disease. This evidence indicates that the physician should beware of applying the terms acute, subacute, and chronic osteomyelitis too rigorously.

Descriptive terms have been applied to certain radiographic and pathologic characteristics that are encountered during the course of osteomyelitis. A *sequestrum* represents a segment of necrotic bone that is separated from living bone by granulation tissue. Sequestra may reside in the marrow for protracted periods of time, harboring living organisms that have the capability of evoking an acute flare-up of the infection. An *involucrum* denotes a layer of living bone that has formed about the dead bone. It can surround and eventually merge with the parent bone, or it can become perforated by *tracts* through which pus may escape. An opening in the involucrum is termed a *cloaca;*

through it the granulation tissue and sequestra can be discharged. Tracts leading to the skin surface from the bone are termed *sinuses,* although they sometimes are described as *fistulae.* The latter term, however, is applied more rigidly to an abnormal passageway that exists between two internal organs or that extends between one internal organ and the surface of the body. A *bone abscess* (Brodie's abscess) is a sharply delineated focus of infection. It is of variable size, can occur at single or multiple locations, and represents a site of active infection. It is lined by granulation tissue and frequently is surrounded by eburnated bone. Occasionally, a sclerotic nonpurulent form of osteomyelitis exists, which is termed *Garré's sclerosing osteomyelitis.*[4] Although this term is applied carelessly to any form of osteomyelitis with severe osseous eburnation, it should be reserved for those cases in which intense proliferation of the periosteum leads to bony deposition and in which no necrosis or purulent exudate and little granulation tissue are present.[3] Sclerosing osteomyelitis of Garré is rare, typically results from *Staphylococcus aureus* infection, and is seen most commonly in the mandible.[5, 287]

OSTEOMYELITIS

Routes of Contamination

Osseous (and articular) structures can be contaminated by four principal routes.

1. Hematogenous spread of infection. Infection can reach the bone (or the joint) via the bloodstream. The vulnerability of any specific bone (or site within that bone) to infection is influenced by and dependent on the anatomy of the adjacent vascular tree.

2. Spread from a contiguous source of infection. Infection can extend into the bone (or the joint) from an adjacent contaminated site. Cutaneous, sinus, and dental infections are three important examples in which a primary extraskeletal infective focus subsequently can involve neighboring osseous and articular structures.

3. Direct implantation. In certain situations, there is direct implantation of infectious material into the bone (or the joint). Puncture and penetrating injuries represent important vehicles for this route of contamination.

4. Postoperative infection. In this age of aggressive orthopedic surgery, postoperative infection is becoming increasingly important. Although examples of this type of infection relate to direct implantation, spread from a contiguous septic focus, or hematogenous contamination of the bone (or the joint), infection occurring after surgery is so important that it deserves special emphasis.

In any particular person, the exact mechanism of the infection may not be clear. Furthermore, in some persons, more than one potential mechanism may be operational. Nonetheless, accurate interpretation of the imaging and pathologic characteristics of osteomyelitis (and septic arthritis) requires an awareness of the potential pathways by which organisms may reach the osseous and the articular structures.

Hematogenous Spread of Infection

Bacteremia

Fundamental to the development of hematogenous osteomyelitis is the presence of bacteria (or other types of organisms) in the blood stream. Bacteria usually enter the blood vessels (or the lymphatics and then the blood vessels) by direct extension from extravascular sites of infection, which include the genitourinary, gastrointestinal, biliary, and respiratory systems, the skin and soft tissue, and other structures. In some instances, no primary source of infection is identifiable. Surgical manipulation or instrumentation, particularly of sites that have a large indigenous bacterial flora, such as the teeth and colon, and the use of various intravascular devices constitute additional factors that predispose to bacteremia.[26–29, 328, 329] Although the presence of bacteria within the vascular system implies a risk for the subsequent development of distant infection, including osteomyelitis, such bacteremia often is transient and totally asymptomatic. In other instances, prominent clinical manifestations of the septicemia itself, including fever, chills, hypotension, coagulation abnormalities, cutaneous manifestations, and organ failure (lung, liver, kidney, heart), or manifestations of distant organ involvement become apparent.[330] Fatality rates are higher in cases of infection complicated by bacteremia than in localized infections alone.

It is not clear why certain species of bacteria, such as gram-positive and gram-negative cocci, are associated with metastatic complications, including osteomyelitis, whereas others, such as gram-negative bacilli, are not.[330] A single pathogenic organism usually is responsible for hematogenous osteomyelitis; polymicrobic hematogenous osteomyelitis is rare.[577] In the neonate or infant, *Staphylococcus aureus,* group B streptococcus, and *Escherichia coli* are the bone isolates recovered most frequently; in children over the age of 1 year, *Staphylococcus aureus, Streptococcus pyogenes,* and *Haemophilus influenzae* are responsible for most cases of hematogenous osteomyelitis; and in children older than 4 years, staphylococci are the major pathogens in this disease as the incidence of osteomyelitis related to *Haemophilus influenzae* decreases.[577] Gram-negative organisms assume importance as pathogens in bone and joint infections in adults and in intravenous drug abusers. A recent surgical procedure or concurrent soft tissue infection frequently is associated with staphylococcal septicemia and osteomyelitis[29]; disorders of the gastrointestinal and genitourinary tracts may initiate a gram-negative septicemia; and an acute or chronic respiratory infection is important in the pathogenesis of tuberculous, fungal, and pneumococcal osteomyelitis.[3] The ever-expanding list of organisms that are potential causes of hematogenous osteomyelitis underscores the need for careful microbiologic studies that identify the infecting agent precisely. Such identification is not uniformly rewarding. Blood cultures are positive in approximately 50 per cent of patients with acute hematogenous osteomyelitis and may obviate a bone biopsy,[327] although the isolation of organisms from the blood does not directly identify the cause of the osteomyelitis, nor does it exclude the possibility of a noninfectious cause of the osseous alterations. Furthermore, in some cases of presumed osteomyelitis, careful and repeated biopsy of bone fails to provide tissue from which bacteria or other organisms can be recovered, even though histologic features are interpreted as consistent with infection.[744]

General Clinical Features

The general clinical features of hematogenous osteomyelitis have been well outlined.[2, 3, 6–17, 326, 327] Traditionally, such osteomyelitis has been regarded as a disease of childhood (3 to 15 years of age),[18–20] although a rise in the frequency of hematogenous osteomyelitis in older patients has been noted.[3] Neonatal osteomyelitis also is well known.[13, 16, 21–25] Major clinical (and radiologic) differences exist in the presentation and course of hematogenous osteomyelitis in the child, the infant, and the adult. Childhood osteomyelitis can be associated with a sudden onset of high fever, a toxic state, and local signs of inflammation, although this presentation is certainly not uniform.[3] Indeed, as many as 50 per cent of children have vague complaints, including local pain of 1 to 3 months' duration with minimal if any temperature elevation.[577] In the infant, hematogenous osteomyelitis often leads to less dramatic findings, including pain, swelling, and an unwillingness to move the affected bones; in this age group, infected indwelling umbilical venous and arterial catheters can become the source of septicemia, resulting in osteomyelitis at multiple sites.[26–29, 334, 553, 578, 737] The adult form of hematogenous osteomyelitis may have a more insidious onset with a relatively longer period between the appearance of symptoms and signs and accurate diagnosis. In all age groups, the prior administration of antibiotics for treatment of the febrile state can attenuate or alter the clinical (and imaging) manifestations of the bone infection.[30] Most series indicate that in children, boys are affected more frequently than girls.[750] A similar male dominance is observed in adults. In infancy, boys and girls are affected with approximately equal frequency.

Single or multiple bones can be infected; involvement of multiple osseous sites appears to be particularly common in infants.[31, 334] In the younger age group, the long tubular bones of the extremities (femur, humerus, tibia) are especially vulnerable; in adults, hematogenous osteomyelitis is encountered more frequently in the axial skeleton. In infants, group B streptococcus typically involves a single bone, particularly the humerus.[15, 288, 289]

Vascular Anatomy

Overview. A distinct osseous circulation supplies the bone tissue and cells, the marrow, the perichondrium, the epiphyseal cartilage in the immature skeleton, and, in part, the articular cartilage.[32] The vascular supply of a tubular bone is derived from several points of arterial inflow, which become complicated sinusoidal networks within the bone (Fig. 64–1). Drainage is accomplished via venous channels that exit from multiple locations.

In tubular bones, one or two diaphyseal nutrient arteries pierce the cortex and divide into ascending and descending branches. As they extend to the ends of the bones, they branch repeatedly, becoming finer channels, and are joined by the terminals of metaphyseal and epiphyseal arteries. The metaphyseal arteries originate from neighboring systemic vessels, whereas the epiphyseal arteries arise from periarticular vascular arcades.

The arteries within the bone marrow form a series of cortical branches that connect with the fenestrated capillaries of the haversian systems. At the bony surface, the cortical capillaries form connections with overlying periosteal plexuses, which themselves are derived from the arteries of the neighboring muscles and soft tissues. The cortices of the tubular bones derive nutrition from both the periosteal and the medullary circulatory systems; the direction of blood flow in each of these systems and the specific contribution each makes in nourishing the cortex are controversial. Although it frequently is maintained that the periosteal vessels supply the outer one third of the cortex and that the medullary vessels supply the inner two thirds, the contribution of each may be age-dependent. Animal studies have shown the direction of arterial blood flow in the mature skeleton to be predominantly centrifugal and that of the venous drainage to be centripetal; in the immature animal, the contribution of the periosteal network is greater.[290] The exuberant anastomoses between the two systems allow blood to flow in either direction according to physiologic conditions.

The central arterioles drain into a thin-walled venous sinus, which subsequently unites with veins that retrace the course of the nutrient arteries, piercing the cortex at various points and joining larger and larger venous channels.

At the ends of the tubular bones, the nutrient arteries of the epiphysis form a series of intraosseous anastomoses with branches that pass into the subchondral regions. A series of end-arterial loops pierces the subchondral bone plate and, occasionally, the calcified zone of articular cartilage before turning to enter the venous sinusoid of the epiphysis.

The nature of the blood supply to the diaphysis, metaphysis, and epiphysis of tubular bones very much depends on the age of the patient (see discussion later in this chapter).[6, 32, 33] In the child, distinct epiphyseal and metaphyseal arteries can be distinguished on either side of the cartilaginous growth plate, and anastomoses between these vessels are either infrequent or absent. Furthermore, the periosteum of the bones of young patients is more vascular than that of adults; its vessels communicate more freely with those of the shaft and also give rise to many metaphyseal vessels.[32]

The blood supply also varies from one bone to another. Although the vascular anatomy of the tubular bones of the extremities has been emphasized in the preceding discussion, anastomosing periosteal and nutrient vessels also are fundamental to the blood supply of large, irregular bones such as those of the pelvis and scapula, whereas periosteal vessels supply compact and cancellous bone as well as marrow in the carpal and tarsal areas.

Joints receive blood vessels from periarterial plexuses that pierce the capsule to form a vascular plexus in the deeper part of the synovial membrane.[32] The blood vessels of the synovial membrane terminate at the articular margins as looped anastomoses (circulus articularis vasculosus). The epiphysis and the adjacent synovium share a common blood supply.[8, 34]

Vascular Patterns of the Tubular Bones. The radiologic and pathologic features of osteomyelitis differ in the child, the infant, and the adult, which is related in large part to peculiarities of the vascular anatomy of the tubular bones

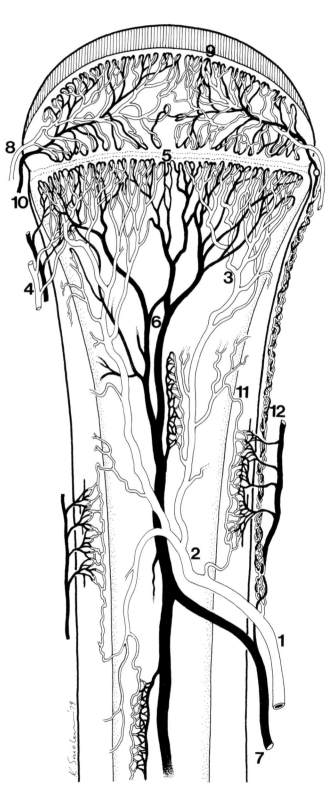

FIGURE 64–1. Normal osseous circulation to a growing tubular bone. Nutrient arteries (1) pierce the diaphyseal cortex and divide into descending and ascending (2) branches. These latter vessels continue to divide, becoming fine channels (3) as they approach the end of the bone. They are joined by metaphyseal vessels (4) and, in the subepiphyseal (growth) plate region, they form a series of end-arterial loops (5). The venous sinuses extend from the metaphyseal region toward the diaphysis, uniting with other venous structures (6) and eventually piercing the cortex as a large venous channel (7). At the ends of the bone, nutrient arteries of the epiphysis (8) branch into finer structures, passing into the subchondral region. At this site, arterial loops (9) again are evident, some of which pierce the sub-chondral bone plate before turning to enter the venous sinusoid and venous channels of the epiphysis (10). At the bony surface, cortical capillaries (11) form connections with overlying periosteal plexuses (12). Note that in the growing child, distinct epiphyseal and meta-physeal arteries can be distinguished on either side of the cartilaginous growth plate. Anastomoses between these vessels either do not occur or are infrequent.

in each of these three age groups (Figs. 64–2 and 64–3) (Table 64–1). Although the anatomic features outlined subsequently are not without exception, it is extremely instructive to consider each of the three vascular patterns separately, for these anatomic principles govern the radiographic and pathologic characteristics of the disease process.[6, 18]

Childhood Pattern. Between the ages of approximately 1 year and the time when the open cartilaginous growth plates fuse, a childhood vascular pattern can be recognized in the ends of the tubular bones (Fig. 64–2*A*). Apart from those vessels in a narrow fringe at the periphery of the cartilage, the capillaries on the metaphyseal side of the growth plate are the terminal ramification of a nutrient artery. It is here in the metaphysis that the vessels turn in acute loops to join large sinusoidal veins, which occupy the intramedullary portion of the metaphysis; and here the blood flow is slow and turbulent. The epiphyseal blood supply is distinct from that on the metaphyseal aspect of the plate, as the latter structure represents a barrier through which vessels do not pass. This anatomic characteristic, combined with additional features to be discussed later, explains the peculiar predilection of hematogenous osteomyelitis to affect metaphyses and equivalent locations in the child.[10]

Infantile Pattern. A fetal vascular arrangement may persist in some tubular bones up to the age of 1 year with local variations corresponding to the time of complete maturation of the epiphyseal bone nucleus (Fig. 64–2*B*). During fetal life, perichondral vessels progress toward the ends of the cartilaginous anlage, turning back when they reach the as yet unossified cartilaginous ends of the bone. In the terminal stages of intrauterine life and in the first 6 to 12 months following birth, when the growth cartilage is established but not yet limited by bone on its epiphyseal side, some vessels at the surface of the metaphysis penetrate the preexisting growth plate, ramifying in the epiphysis. After termination, they form large venous lakes not dissimilar to metaphyseal sinusoids. This arrangement affords a vascular connection between the metaphysis and epiphysis and explains the frequency of epiphyseal and articular infection in the infant.

Adult Pattern. With narrowing and closing of the physeal growth plate, metaphyseal vessels penetrate the dimin-

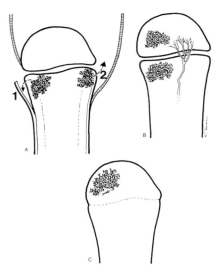

FIGURE 64–3. Sites of hematogenous osteomyelitis of a tubular bone in the child, the infant, and the adult.

A In the child, a metaphyseal focus is frequent. From this site, cortical penetration can result in a subperiosteal abscess in those locations in which the growth plate is extra-articular (1) or in a septic joint in those locations in which the growth plate is intra-articular (2).

B In the infant, a metaphyseal focus may be complicated by epiphyseal extension owing to the vascular anatomy in this age group.

C In the adult, a subchondral focus in an epiphysis is not unusual, owing to the vascular anatomy in this age group.

ishing cartilaginous structure progressively, reestablishing a vascular connection between the metaphysis and the epiphysis (Fig. 64–2*C*). Blood within the nutrient vessels then can reach the surface of the epiphysis through large anastomosing channels, and organisms within these vessels can gain quick access to the ends of bones and the adjacent articulations.

Hematogenous Osteomyelitis in the Child[2, 6, 18, 19, 35–49, 291, 331, 332] (Table 64–2)

Hematogenous osteomyelitis reaches the metaphysis by way of the nutrient vessels; with intravenous injection of bacteria, organisms localize in the vascular spaces in the metaphysis as early as 2 hours after inoculation.[40] In experimental situations using skeletally immature animals, such localization is accentuated by the presence of physeal injury.[579, 580] Metaphyseal location is related to (1) the peculiar anatomy of the vascular tree (Fig. 64–2 *A*), in which the last ramifications of the nutrient artery negotiate sharp turns just short of the growth plate, emptying into a system

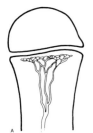 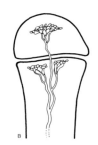 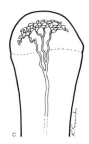

FIGURE 64–2. Normal vascular patterns of a tubular bone in the child, the infant, and the adult.

A In the child, the capillaries of the metaphysis turn sharply, without violating the open growth plate.

B In the infant, some metaphyseal vessels may penetrate or extend around the open growth plate, ramifying in the epiphysis.

C In the adult, with closure of the growth plate, a vascular connection between metaphysis and epiphysis can be recognized.

TABLE 64–1. Vascular Patterns of Tubular Bones

Pattern	Age	Characteristics
Infantile pattern	0–1 year*	Diaphyseal and metaphyseal vessels may perforate open growth plate
Childhood pattern	1–16 years†	Diaphyseal and metaphyseal vessels do not penetrate open growth plate
Adult pattern	>16 years	Diaphyseal and metaphyseal vessels penetrate closed growth plate

*Upper age limit depends on specific local anatomic variations in the appearance and growth of the ossification center.
†Upper age limit is related to the time at which the open growth plate closes.

TABLE 64–2. Hematogenous Osteomyelitis of Tubular Bones

	Infant	Child	Adult
Localization	Metaphyseal with epiphyseal extension	Metaphyseal	Epiphyseal
Involucrum	Common	Common	Not common
Sequestrum	Common	Common	Not common
Joint involvement	Common	Not common	Common
Soft tissue abscess	Common	Common	Not common
Pathologic fracture	Not common	Not common	Common*
Sinus tracts	Not common	Variable	Common

*In neglected cases.

of large sinusoidal veins; (2) the inability of vessels to penetrate the open physeal plate; (3) the slow rate of blood flow in this region; (4) a decrease in phagocytic ability of neighboring macrophages; or (5) secondary thrombosis of the nutrient artery. These factors create an ideal medium for the growth and multiplication of organisms (Figs. 64–3 to 64–5). The infection does not commonly localize in the epiphyseal, metaphyseal, or periosteal vessels, as these vessels do not possess a similar system of vascular loops proximal to the venous sinusoids[6]; however, reports of atypical localizations for the infectious process certainly exist. As an example, primary involvement of an epiphysis[333, 533, 581, 582] or secondary extension across the physis to an epiphysis[534] in hematogenous osteomyelitis is encountered. These patterns appear to predominate in the bones about the knee, especially the distal portion of the femur.

Inflammation in the adjacent bone of the metaphysis is characterized by vascular engorgement, edema, cellular response, and abscess formation.[35] The peripheral portion of one or more abscesses may be heavily infiltrated with viable polymorphonuclear leukocytes, but in the more central portion of the abscess cavity, necrotic leukocytes can be detected.[2] Extensive involvement of the metaphyseal veins leads to early edema. Transudates extend from the marrow to the adjacent cortex. A rise in intramedullary pressure, due to the presence of inflammatory and edematous tissue confined by the rigid cortical columns of bone, encourages infected fluid to enter the cortical bone and extend across it by way of the haversian and Volkmann's canals, especially in that area of the distal metaphysis in which the cortex is extremely thin.

Cortical porosity is produced, at least in part, by osteoclastosis, leading to enlargement of haversian canals and facilitating cortical penetration by the accumulating organisms. The inflammatory process soon reaches the outer surface of the cortex and abscesses develop, lifting the periosteum and disrupting the periosteal blood supply to the external cortical surface. Elevation of the periosteum is prominent in the immature skeleton because of its relatively loose attachment to the subjacent bone. The elevated periosteum lays down bone in the form of an involucrum that partially or completely surrounds the infected bone. Infec-

tion may penetrate the periosteal membrane, producing cloacae, and extend into the adjacent soft tissues, leading to single or multiple abscesses.

Cortical necrosis and sequestration subsequently can appear. Necrosis is facilitated by deprivation of blood supply to the inner portion of the cortex due to thrombosis of the metaphyseal vessels and by interruption of periosteal blood supply to the outer portion of the cortex as a result of lifting of the periosteum.

With treatment of the infection, with spontaneous escape of pus into the soft tissues, or with surgical decompression, a reparative response may supervene. Apposition of new bone on the walls of the widened haversian canals and cortical thickening can be seen. Osteoclastic activity at the junction of living and dead bone can produce resorption or fragmentation of the necrotic tissue. The marrow cavity becomes filled with granulation tissue, which later is replaced by fibrous elements. Further healing is characterized by transformation of abscesses into cystic cavities and replacement of scar tissue by either cellular or fatty marrow.[2]

Hematogenous osteomyelitis of the child is not confined to tubular bones.[10, 13, 41] Indeed, some evidence suggests that the frequency of involvement of tubular bones in such osteomyelitis is decreasing.[583] Infection in sites other than tubular bones may occur in 18 to 25 per cent of all cases of childhood osteomyelitis (Fig. 64–6).[43–45] In flat or irregular bones, such as the calcaneus,[584] the clavicle,[347] and the bones of the pelvis,[348] childhood osteomyelitis may show predilection for metaphyseal-equivalent osseous locations adjacent to an apophyseal cartilaginous plate and epiphyseal-equivalent locations adjacent to articular cartilage.[10] Preferential involvement of these sites as well as of metaphyseal-equivalent locations of long bones (e.g., adjacent to the apophyses of the tibial tuberosity and femoral trochanters) again is related to regional vascular anatomy, which, in these areas, is similar to that of the metaphyses of the tubular bones.[42] The radiographic and pathologic characteristics of osteomyelitis in metaphyseal- and epiphyseal-equivalent areas are similar to those in the long bones.[43, 44] Other reported sites of childhood osteomyelitis have included the talus[585] and the patella.[586–588]

Hematogenous Osteomyelitis in the Infant[6, 7, 14–16, 46, 47, 334, 335, 578] (Table 64–2)

Although there are fundamental similarities between the manifestations of hematogenous osteomyelitis in the infant and those in the child, certain differences also are apparent. In the infant, as some of the vessels in the metaphysis penetrate the growth plate, a suppurative process of the metaphysis may extend into the epiphysis (Figs. 64–3B and 64–7). Epiphyseal infection then can result in articular contamination and damage the cells on the epiphyseal side of the growth cartilage, leading to arrest or disorganization of growth and maturation. Articular involvement also is facilitated by the frequent localization of infantile osteomyelitis to ends of the bone in which the growth plate is intraarticular (e.g., hip), allowing direct contamination of the joint space from a metaphyseal septic focus[7] (see discussion later in this chapter).

Profuse involucrum formation also is characteristic of osteomyelitis in the infant; exuberant cloaks of bone may extend around the metaphysis and diaphysis of a tubular

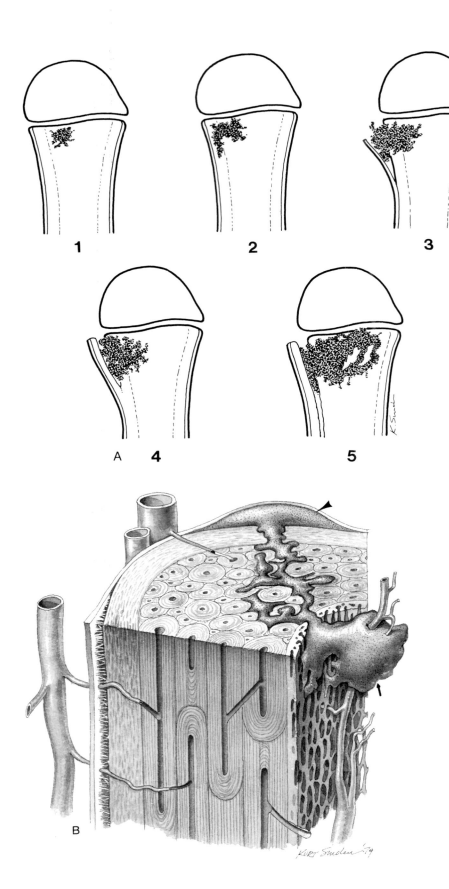

FIGURE 64–4. Hematogenous osteomyelitis of a tubular bone in the child.

A Sequential steps in the initiation and progression of infection. 1, A metaphyseal focus is common; 2, the infection spreads laterally, reaching and invading the cortical bone; 3, cortical penetration is associated with subperiosteal extension and elevation of the periosteal membrane; 4, subperiosteal bone formation leads to an involucrum or shell of new bone; 5, the involucrum may become massive with continued infection.

B A diagram of the manner in which an infectious process in the medullary canal (arrow) permeates the cortex and collects beneath the periosteal membrane (arrowhead).

Illustration continued on opposite page

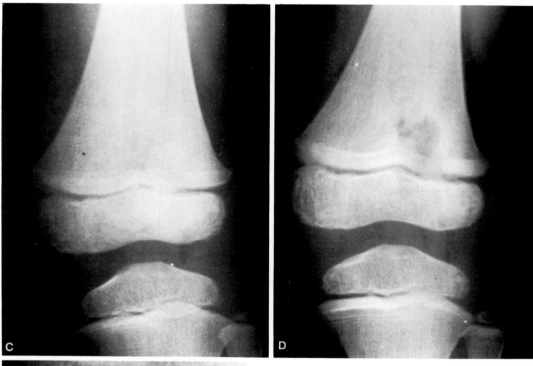

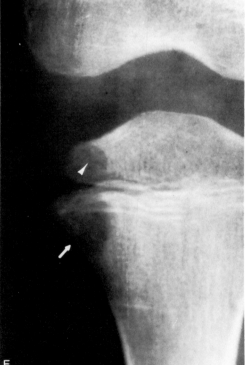

FIGURE 64–4 *Continued*

C, D In this child with pain and swelling of the knee, initial radiographs at the time of clinical presentation do not reveal osseous destruction. Two weeks later, a lytic metaphyseal focus in the femur readily is apparent. It extends to the growth cartilage (causative organism is Staphylococcus).

E Rarely, in the child, a metaphyseal infection (arrow) can violate the growth cartilage with epiphyseal involvement (arrowhead) (causative organism is Staphylococcus).

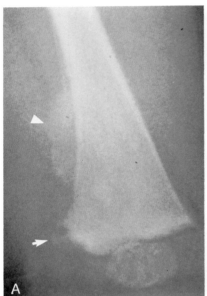
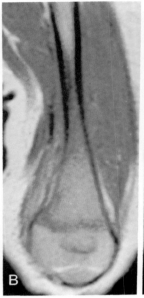
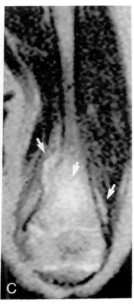

FIGURE 64–5. Hematogenous osteomyelitis of a tubular bone in the child.

A In this very young child, routine radiography shows subtle metaphyseal osteolysis with irregularity of the cortex (arrow) and prominent periosteal new bone (arrowhead)

B, C Coronal proton density (TR/TE, 1500/30) **(B)** and T2-weighted (TR/TE, 1500/100) **(C)** spin echo MR images show the extent of the infection. The intramedullary and subperiosteal involvement (arrows) is much more evident in **C,** owing to the high signal intensity of the process.

(Courtesy of R. Kerr, M.D., Los Angeles, California.)

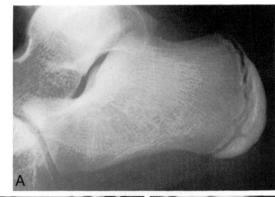

FIGURE 64–6. Hematogenous osteomyelitis of an irregular bone in the child.

A Routine radiograph in this 15 year old boy shows no obvious abnormalities.

B Sagittal T1-weighted (TR/TE, 800/20) spin echo MR image shows diffuse involvement of the calcaneus, with resultant low signal intensity of the marrow, and relative sparing of the apophysis.

C Transverse (plantar plane) T2-weighted (TR/TE, 1800/70) spin echo MR image reveals subtle increased signal intensity in the marrow of the calcaneus with subperiosteal extension of infection (arrows).

(Courtesy of C. Sebrechts, M.D., San Diego, California.)

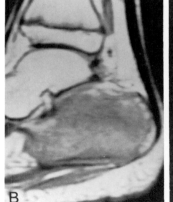
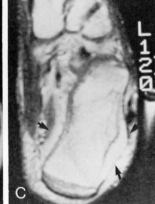

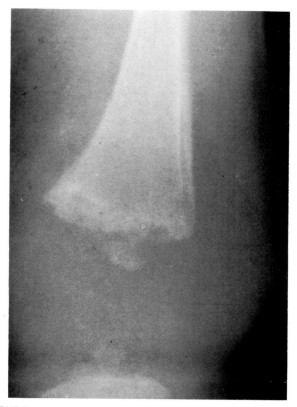

FIGURE 64–7. Hematogenous osteomyelitis of a tubular bone in the infant. In this infant with acute staphylococcal osteomyelitis, metaphyseal and epiphyseal involvement of the distal end of the femur is associated with periostitis and articular involvement.

bone, reflecting the ease with which the immature periosteum is lifted from the subjacent bone and the extreme richness of the periosteal vessels in infancy. The remarkable healing properties of osseous tissue in the first years of life are evidenced by the fact that the prominent involucrum commonly merges with cortex of the subjacent bone, eventually leaving little or no trace of previous osteomyelitis.

In addition to epiphyseal and joint involvement and massive involucrum formation, infantile osteomyelitis is associated with cortical sequestration and soft tissue alterations such as edema or abscess formation, which can lead to significant changes in the first days of the infection, prior to the appearance of osseous abnormalities.[9, 46] Apparently, in the younger age groups, infection more easily violates the adjacent periosteum, facilitating soft tissue contamination. Sinus tracts are relatively rare in infantile osteomyelitis.

Hematogenous Osteomyelitis in the Adult [6, 7, 18]
(Table 64–2)

Hematogenous osteomyelitis in the mature skeleton does not commonly localize in the tubular bones; hematogenous osteomyelitis of the spine, pelvis, and small bones is more common in the adult patient.[349] In cases in which involvement of tubular bones is evident, the free communication of the metaphyseal and epiphyseal vessels through the closed growth plate allows infection to localize in the subchondral (beneath the articular cartilage) regions of the bone (Figs. 64–3C and 64–8A). Joint contamination can complicate this epiphyseal location.

The fibrous and firm attachment of the periosteum to the cortex in the adult resists displacement and, therefore, subperiosteal abscess formation, extensive periostitis, and involucrum formation are relatively unusual in this age group. Furthermore, the intimacy of the periosteum and cortex in the adult ensures adequate cortical blood supply in most patients; extensive sequestration is not a common feature of adult-onset osteomyelitis. Rather, infection violates and disrupts the cortex itself, producing atrophy and osseous weakening, and predisposes the bone to pathologic fracture. Infection also may spread along the entire length of the tubular bone with involvement of large segments of the diaphysis (Fig. 64–8B,C); chronic osteomyelitis with sinus tracts is common.

Acute Hematogenous Osteomyelitis: Radiographic and Pathologic Abnormalities
(Table 64–3) (Fig. 64–9)

Radiographic evidence of significant osseous destruction in hematogenous pyogenic osteomyelitis is delayed for a period of days to weeks. It is the insensitivity of this technique in the early diagnosis of bone infection that has prompted the use of other methods such as scintigraphy and MR imaging for the prompt recognition of osteomyelitis (see discussion later in this chapter). Initial and subtle radiographic changes in the soft tissues may appear within 3 days of bacterial contamination of bone,[9, 554] however. Focal deep soft tissue swelling in the metaphyseal region of infants and children may be the first important radiographic sign. Such swelling, which is temporally related to the vascular changes and edema of the early osteomyelitic process, results in displacement of the lucent tissue planes from the underlying bone. In the neonate, this displacement

TABLE 64–3. Hematogenous Osteomyelitis: Radiographic-Pathologic Correlation

Pathologic Abnormality	Radiographic Abnormality
Vascular changes and edema of soft tissues	Soft tissue swelling with obliteration of tissue planes
Infection in medullary space with hyperemia, edema, abscess formation, and trabecular destruction	Osteoporosis, bone lysis
Infection in haversian and Volkmann's canals of cortex	Increasing lysis, cortical lucency
Subperiosteal abscess formation with lifting of the periosteum and bone formation	Periostitis, involucrum formation
Infectious penetration of periosteum with soft tissue abscess formation	Soft tissue swelling, mass formation, obliteration of tissue planes
Localized cortical and medullary abscesses	Single or multiple radiolucent cortical or medullary lesions with surrounding sclerosis
Deprivation of blood supply to cortex due to thrombosis of metaphyseal vessels and interruption of periosteal vessels, cortical necrosis	Sequestration
External migration of dead pieces of cortex with breakdown of skin and subcutaneous tissue	Sinus tracts

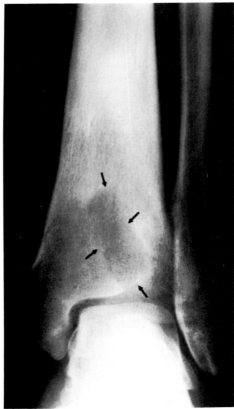

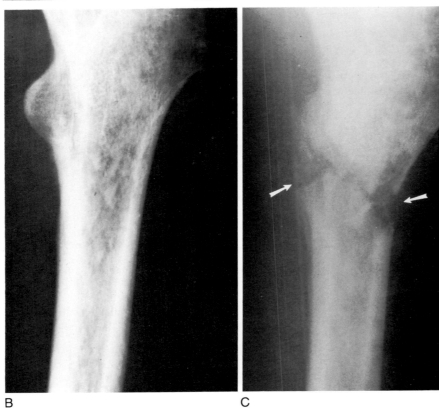

FIGURE 64–8. Hematogenous osteomyelitis of a tubular bone in the adult.

A An epiphyseal localization is not infrequent in this age group. Observe the lytic lesion (abscess) with surrounding sclerosis extending to the subchondral bone plate (arrows). Metaphyseal and diaphyseal sclerosis is evident. The elongated shape of the lesion is typical of infection (causative organism is Staphylococcus).

B, C This 20 year old man developed acute osteomyelitis after an aortic valve replacement. The initial film reveals mottled, poorly defined destruction of the metaphysis and diaphysis of the proximal end of the femur with endosteal erosion. Four weeks later, progressive lysis and sclerosis with a pathologic fracture (arrows) and soft tissue swelling are evident (causative organism is Staphylococcus).

A

B   C

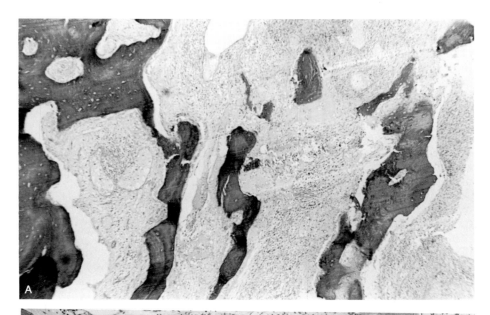

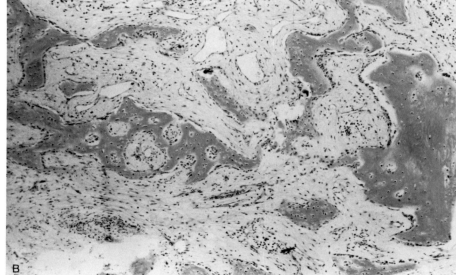

FIGURE 64–9. Hematogenous osteomyelitis: Histologic abnormalities.

A Acute osteomyelitis. Note necrosis of multiple bony trabeculae and an acute inflammatory cellular infiltration in the marrow spaces (100×).

B, C Chronic osteomyelitis. Low (100×) and high (250×) power photomicrographs reveal reactive bone formation in the vicinity of a chronic pyogenic inflammatory lesion. The normal hematopoietic marrow has been replaced by vascular connective tissue that contains lymphocytes and plasma cells. The newly formed woven bone is covered by large active osteoblasts.

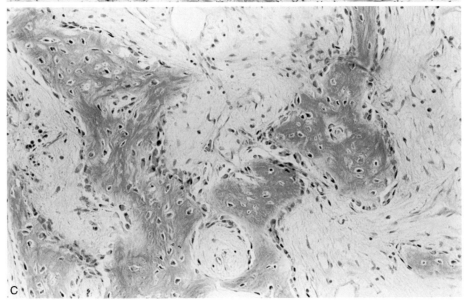

is difficult to detect because of the lack of subcutaneous fat and the presence of poorly defined fascial planes.[334] A few days after the appearance of the initial soft tissue changes, muscle swelling and obliteration of the soft tissue planes can be observed.[46, 48, 49] The deep muscles and soft tissues are affected first, followed later by involvement of the more superficial muscles and subcutaneous tissue.[9]

In pyogenic infection, radiographically evident bone destruction and periostitis can be delayed for 1 to 2 weeks after intraosseous lodgment of the organisms. At all early stages, the degree of bony involvement that is visible on the radiograph is considerably less than that which is evident on pathologic examination.[9] Eventually, large destructive lesions become evident on the radiograph. In the child, these lesions appear as enlarging, poorly defined lucent shadows of the metaphysis surrounded by varying amounts of eburnation; the lucent lesions extend to the growth plate and, on rare occasions, may violate it. In addition, destruction progresses horizontally, reaching the cortex, and periostitis follows.[751]

In the infant, the epiphyses are unossified or only partially ossified, so that radiographic recognition of epiphyseal destruction can be extremely difficult. Metaphyseal lucent lesions, periostitis, and a joint effusion are helpful radiographic clues. Arthrography is frequently of additional aid; joint aspiration allows documentation of the infection, and opacification of the joint can provide information regarding the integrity of the cartilaginous surface of the epiphysis. MR imaging also is able to provide similar information regarding the unossified cartilage.

In the adult, soft tissue alterations are more difficult to detect on radiographic examination. Epiphyseal, metaphyseal, and diaphyseal osseous destruction creates radiolucent areas of varying size, which are associated with mild periostitis. Cortical resorption can be identified as endosteal scalloping, intracortical lucent regions or tunneling,[336] and poorly defined subperiosteal bony defects or gaps.

Subacute and Chronic Hematogenous Osteomyelitis: Radiographic and Pathologic Abnormalities

Brodie's Abscess. Single or multiple radiolucent abscesses can be evident during subacute or chronic stages of osteomyelitis. These abscesses, which have been recognized in prehistoric paleopathologic remains,[337] initially were described in the tibial metaphyses by Brodie in 1832[50, 51] in a study of eight male patients between the ages of 13 and 34 years. Although this investigator did not have the advantages of radiographic and bacteriologic techniques, Brodie's detailed descriptive analysis has been honored by having his name applied to the pyogenic lesions. Further descriptions of Brodie's abscesses belong to Brickner,[52] Henderson and Simon,[53] Brailsford,[54] and, more recently, Harris and Kirkaldy-Willis.[55] These abscesses now are defined as circumscribed lesions showing predilection for (but not confinement to) the ends of tubular bones; they are found characteristically in subacute pyogenic osteomyelitis, usually of staphylococcal origin.

It has been suggested that bone abscesses develop when an infective organism has a reduced virulence or when the host demonstrates increased resistance to infection.[55] Brodie's abscesses are especially common in children, more typically boys. In this age group, they appear in the metaph-

ysis, particularly that of the distal or proximal portions of the tibia.[589] Less frequently, they occur in other tubular, flat, or irregular bones, including the vertebral bodies, and are diaphyseal in location.[2, 340] Rarely, they traverse the open growth plate,[342] affecting the epiphysis, although such extension does not commonly result in growth disturbance.[56] In young children and infants, Brodie's abscesses may occur in epiphyses and in the carpus and tarsus.[333, 338, 339, 341, 581, 582] Abscesses vary from less than 1 cm to over 4 cm in diameter. The wall of the abscess is lined by inflammatory granulation tissue that is surrounded by spongy bone eburnation (Fig. 64–10). The fluid in the abscess may be purulent or mucoid[2]; bacteriologic examination of the fluid may or may not reveal the infecting organisms.

Radiographs outline radiolucency with adjacent sclerosis (Fig. 64–11).[343, 590] This lucent region commonly is located in the metaphysis, where it may connect with the growth plate by a tortuous channel. Radiographic detection of this channel is important; identification of a metaphyseal defect connected to the growth plate by such a tract ensures the diagnosis of osteomyelitis. Furthermore, such channels usually indicate a pyogenic process and are uncommon in tuberculosis. Appropriate antibiotic treatment in children with metaphyseal abscesses may be accompanied by diminution in size and shaftward migration of the osteolytic focus.[534] In the diaphysis, the radiolucent abscess cavity can be located in central or subcortical areas of the spongiosa or in the cortex itself and may contain a central sequestrum.[57, 58, 281] In an epiphysis, a circular, well-defined osteolytic lesion is seen, which, in the immature skeleton, may border on the chondro-osseous junction or on the physis, where it may extend into the metaphysis. When an abscess

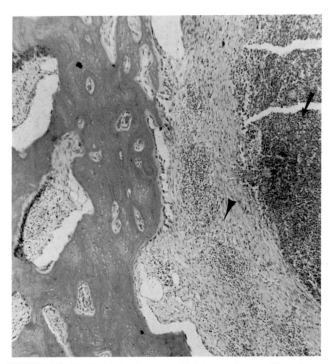

FIGURE 64–10. Brodie's abscess: Histologic abnormalities. On a low power (100×) photomicrograph, note the abscess mass consisting of cellular debris and neutrophils (arrow), a surrounding fibrotic reaction (arrowhead), and peripheral eburnated bone.

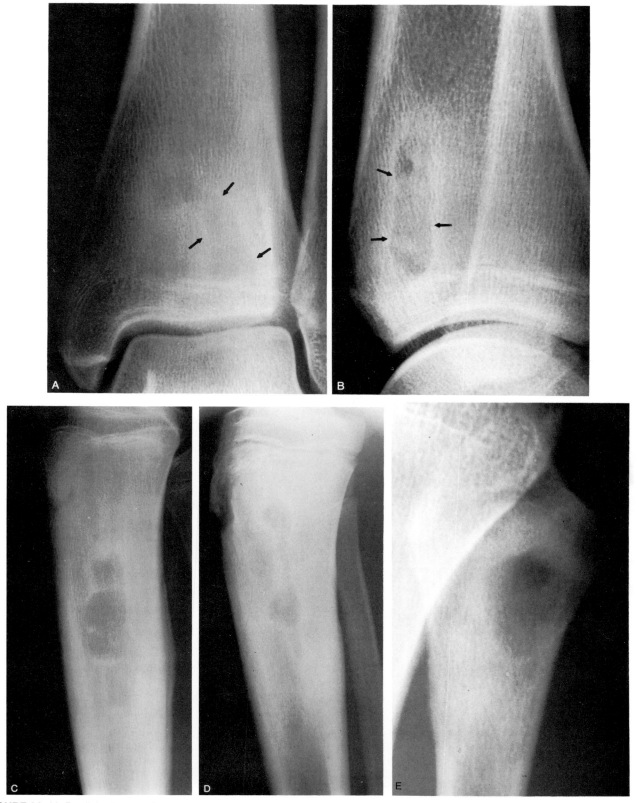

FIGURE 64–11. Brodie's abscess: Radiographic abnormalities.

A, B Anteroposterior and lateral radiographs outline a typical appearance of an abscess of the distal end of the tibia caused by staphylococci. Observe the elongated radiolucent lesion with surrounding sclerosis extending to the closing growth plate (arrows). The channel-like shape of the lesion is important in the accurate diagnosis of this condition.

C An example of an abscess of the proximal diaphysis of the tibia. Note its multiloculated appearance, surrounding sclerosis, and periosteal bone formation.

D In a different patient, a dumbbell-shaped lesion is evident. Note the channel-like characteristics of this abscess and surrounding bone eburnation of the tibia.

E This well-circumscribed abscess is located in the proximal end of the fibula. It too is contained within sclerotic bone.

is located in the cortex, its radiographic appearance, consisting of a lucent lesion with surrounding sclerosis and periostitis, simulates that of an osteoid osteoma or a stress fracture. A circular or elliptical radiolucent lesion without calcification that is smaller or larger than 2 cm is characteristic of a cortical abscess; a circular lucent area with or without calcification smaller than 2 cm is typical of an osteoid osteoma; and a linear lucent shadow without calcification is characteristic of a stress fracture. In any skeletal location, CT or MR imaging can be employed to better assess the extent of the abscess and any signs of its reactivation (Figs. 64–12 to 64–14).

Sequestration. During the course of hematogenous osteomyelitis, cortical sequestration can become evident. One or more areas of osseous necrosis commonly are situated in the medullary aspect of a tubular bone (sequestration is less prominent in flat bones), where they create radiodense bony

spicules (Figs. 64–15 and 64–16). The increased density is related primarily to the fact that a sequestrum does not possess a blood supply and does not participate in the hyperemia and resulting osteoporosis of the adjacent living bone. The sequestrum frequently is marginated sharply as it rests in a space surrounded by granulation tissue, and it varies in size from minute fragments to long necrotic segments. Sequestra may extrude through cortical breaks, extending into the adjacent soft tissues, where they eventually may be discharged through draining sinuses.[59] Conventional tomography[591] (Fig. 64–16) or CT scanning and sinus tract injections of contrast material are helpful procedures in documenting the presence and position of retained sequestra. MR imaging also may be employed (Fig. 64–17).

Sclerosing Osteomyelitis. In the subacute and chronic stages of osteomyelitis, considerable periosteal bone formation can surround the altered cortex, and an increased

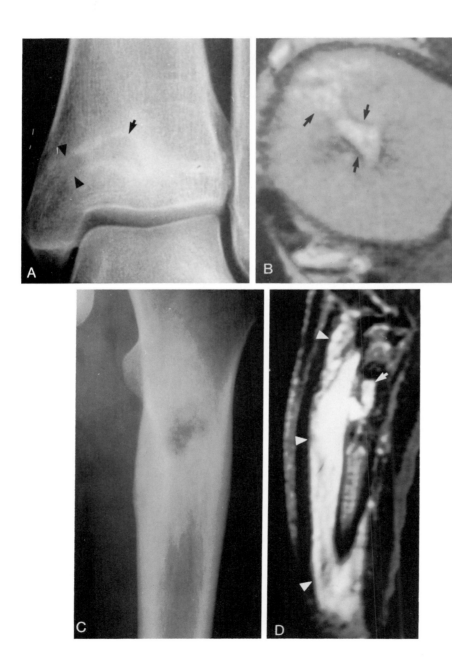

FIGURE 64–12. Brodie's abscess: MR imaging abnormalities.

A, B Tibial metaphyseal involvement in a 19 year old woman. The routine radiograph **(A)** shows a metaphyseal radiolucent lesion (arrow) with a medial channel (arrowhead). A transaxial T2-weighted (TR/TE, 2000/70) spin echo MR image **(B)** reveals the lesion consisting of a rim of low signal intensity (arrows) with central hyperintensity. (Courtesy of M. Mitchell, M.D., Halifax, Nova Scotia, Canada.)

C, D Femoral diaphyseal involvement in a 56 year old febrile man. The routine radiograph **(C)** shows an osteolytic focus, mature periostitis, and soft tissue fullness. A T2-weighted (TR/TE, 2000/70) spin echo MR image **(D)** reveals high signal intensity within the abscess (arrow), and a surrounding zone of low signal intensity. Note the disruption of the anterior cortex of the femur with extensive soft tissue involvement (arrowheads). (Courtesy of G. Greenway, M.D., Dallas, Texas.)

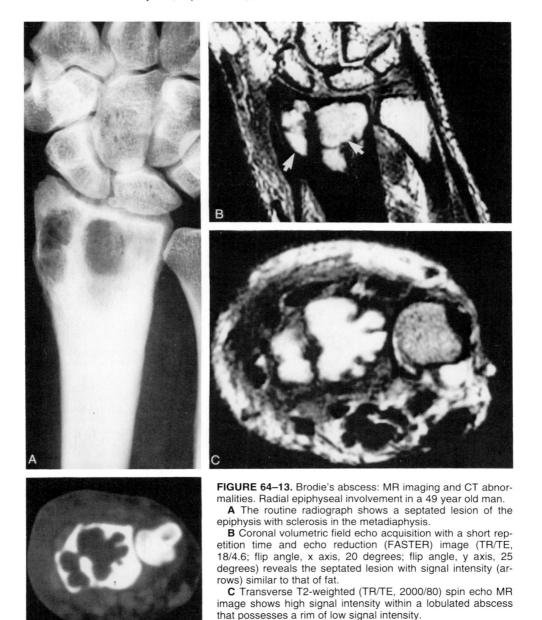

FIGURE 64–13. Brodie's abscess: MR imaging and CT abnormalities. Radial epiphyseal involvement in a 49 year old man.

A The routine radiograph shows a septated lesion of the epiphysis with sclerosis in the metadiaphysis.

B Coronal volumetric field echo acquisition with a short repetition time and echo reduction (FASTER) image (TR/TE, 18/4.6; flip angle, x axis, 20 degrees; flip angle, y axis, 25 degrees) reveals the septated lesion with signal intensity (arrows) similar to that of fat.

C Transverse T2-weighted (TR/TE, 2000/80) spin echo MR image shows high signal intensity within a lobulated abscess that possesses a rim of low signal intensity.

D Transverse CT scan reveals information regarding the size and shape of the lesion similar to that in **C**.

(**A, C, D,** Courtesy of S. Harms, M.D., and G. Greenway, M.D., Dallas, Texas; **B,** from Harms SE, et al, Radiology *173*:743, 1989).

FIGURE 64–14. Brodie's abscess: CT abnormalities. Patellar involvement in a 49 year old man. Routine radiography (**A**) and transaxial CT (**B**) reveal the osteolytic lesion of the patella. A sympathetic joint effusion was present.

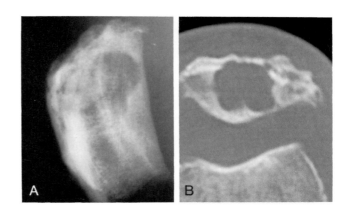

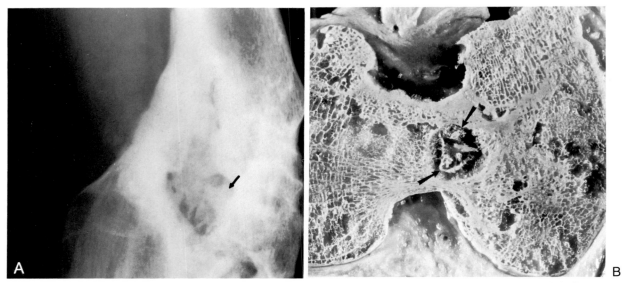

FIGURE 64–15. Chronic osteomyelitis: Sequestration. Routine radiography. A plain film **(A)** of the femur and a photograph **(B)** of a transverse section of the bone after amputation show necrotic bone (arrows) and deformity of the femur in a patient with long-standing draining osteomyelitis.

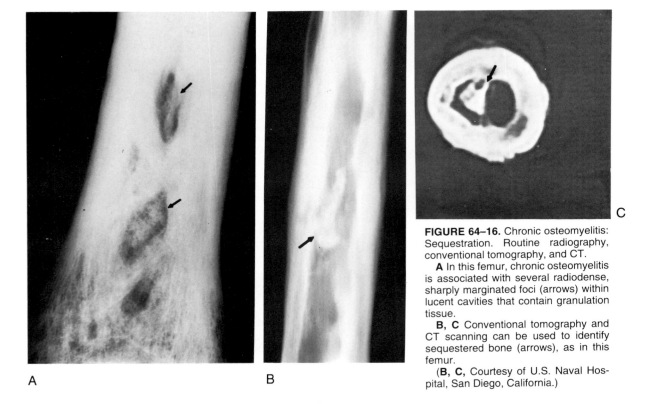

FIGURE 64–16. Chronic osteomyelitis: Sequestration. Routine radiography, conventional tomography, and CT.

A In this femur, chronic osteomyelitis is associated with several radiodense, sharply marginated foci (arrows) within lucent cavities that contain granulation tissue.

B, C Conventional tomography and CT scanning can be used to identify sequestered bone (arrows), as in this femur.

(B, C, Courtesy of U.S. Naval Hospital, San Diego, California.)

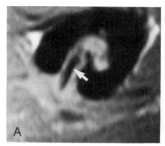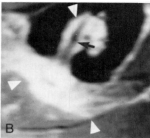

FIGURE 64–17. Chronic osteomyelitis: Sequestration. MR imaging. Humeral diaphyseal involvement in a 23 year old man with chronic pain and swelling. Transaxial T1-weighted (TR/TE, 886/15) **(A)** and gadolinium-enhanced T1-weighted (TR/TE, 886/15) **(B)** spin echo MR images reveal cortical thickening of the humerus, with perforation of the cortex. A sequestrum is evident (arrows). Note the medullary and soft tissue involvement, which is seen in **B** as regions of increased signal intensity (arrowheads).

number and size of spongy trabeculae can reappear in the affected marrow,[2] indicating a healing response and leading to considerable radiodensity and contour irregularity of the affected bone (Fig. 64–18). Cystic changes may occur within the sclerotic area, but sequestra are uncommon.[344] The mandible is the principal site of involvement,[592–595] although a similar histologic and radiologic process occurs in tubular bones, especially in the diaphysis.[345] The radiographic findings resemble those of osteoid osteoma, fibrous dysplasia, and Ewing's sarcoma.[346]

Spread from a Contiguous Source of Infection

General Clinical Features

Bone (and joint) contamination can result from spread from a contiguous source of infection. In most of the cases of osteomyelitis (and septic arthritis) arising from such a contiguous source, soft tissue infections are implicated (postoperative infection is discussed separately).[60] The contamination of bone from an adjacent soft tissue infection is particularly significant in the hands, the feet, the mandible (or maxilla), and the skull.[61–63] The importance of osteomyelitis of the mandible and maxilla in persons with poor dental hygiene (Fig. 64–19) and of the frontal portion of the skull and face in persons with chronic sinusitis is undeniable. Pott's puffy tumor refers to an indolent soft tissue swelling of the scalp that is due to subperiosteal infection or an osteomyelitis of the frontal bone resulting from frontal sinusitis.[350, 598, 599] Staphylococcus, *Streptococcus pneumoniae,* or *Haemophilus influenzae* commonly is implicated.[536] The occasional occurrence of osteomyelitis of the cervical spine after dental extraction is reported,[295] although it is not certain if the infection reaches the bone via tissue planes, lymphatics, or blood stream.

Soft tissue infections that lead to bone and joint contamination are frequent after trauma; animal and human bites[64–66] and puncture wounds[67–71] are especially troublesome in this regard. Diagnostic and therapeutic procedures such as venipuncture and catheterization can lead to secondary infec-

FIGURE 64–18. Chronic sclerosing osteomyelitis.

A Chronic osteomyelitis can be associated with considerable new bone formation. In this patient, a cortical abscess contains a sequestrum (arrow) and is surrounded by sclerosis (arrowheads). The appearance is reminiscent of that of an osteoid osteoma.

B A macerated coronal section of a femur in a patient with chronic osteomyelitis indicates the considerable osseous expansion and trabecular thickening that can accompany infection.

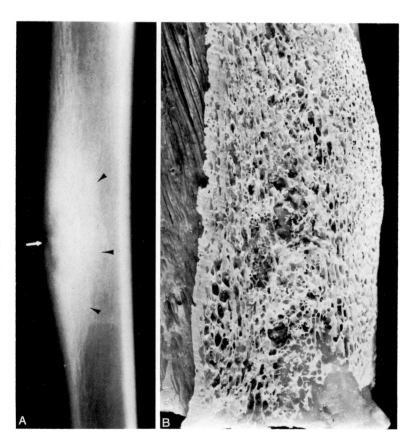

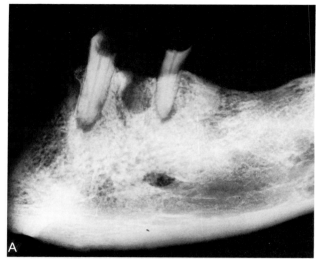

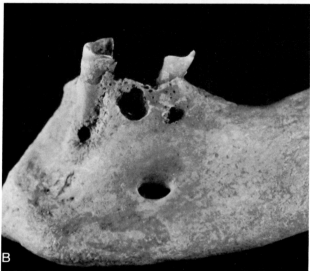

FIGURE 64–19. Osteomyelitis due to spread from a contiguous contaminated source: Mandible. Neglected dental infections can lead to osteomyelitis of the mandible (or the maxilla), which, as in this case, may be associated with considerable bone sclerosis. Note the radiolucent areas at the apex of the remaining teeth and the obvious caries.

tion of soft tissue and bone.[72, 73, 596] Irradiation, burns, and decubitus or pressure ulcers in paralyzed or immobilized patients are other important sources of soft tissue and osseous contamination.[597] Although the specific clinical manifestations vary with the site of soft tissue infection, local inflammatory symptoms and signs predominate, and gram-positive or gram-negative bacterial organisms usually are evident. Human and animal bites frequently are deep and extensive, allowing direct inoculation of osseous and articular structures; these are discussed later in this chapter.

General Radiographic and Pathologic Features
(Table 64–4)

Neglected soft tissue infections have a detrimental effect on neighboring osseous and articular structures. ''The destruction of bone that takes place might be compared with the erosive action of a turbulent stream of water upon a wall of rock''[74]; whereas the direction of contamination in hematogenous osteomyelitis is from the bone outward into the soft tissue, the direction of contamination in osteomyelitis resulting from adjacent sepsis is from the soft tissues inward into the bone (or joint) (Fig. 64–20). Thus, early evidence of soft tissue suppuration is the rule. Organisms within soft tissues disrupt fascial planes and form abscesses. They extend into the periosteum by initially invading its outer and more fibrous portion. Displacement of the periosteum is more frequent and marked in children because of its looser attachment. Resulting periosteal bone formation commonly is the initial radiographic manifestation of osteomyelitis. It must be noted, however, that after traumatic initiation of soft tissue infection, periostitis may appear early in response to injury and not reflect actual bone infection.[75] In addition, posttraumatic limitation of motion may produce osteoporosis with medullary radiolucent areas and intracortical tunneling (pseudoperiostitis), further simulating infection. New bone deposition can result also from stimulation of the periosteal membrane by adjacent infection.[76] Obviously, periostitis beneath suppurative soft tissues may not always indicate infective osteitis or osteomyelitis.

With further accumulation of pus, subperiosteal resorption of bone and cortical disruption ensue. The osseous response may be identical to that associated with soft tissue tumors.[77] As infection gains access to the spongiosa, it may spread in the marrow, producing lytic osseous defects on the radiograph (Fig. 64–21). Later radiographic and pathologic abnormalities (Fig. 64–22) are identical to those occurring in neglected hematogenous infections.

Specific Locations

Hand

Pathways of Spread of Infection. Three distinct routes are available to organisms that become lodged in the soft tissues of the hand; infection may disseminate via tendon sheaths, fascial planes, or lymphatics[78] (Figs. 64–23 and 64–24).

Tendon Sheaths. As noted previously (see Chapter 13), synovial sheaths surround the flexor tendons of each digit of the hand; they extend from the terminal phalanges in a proximal direction to the palm.[79] In the first and fifth digits, connection with the radial and ulnar bursae, two synovial sacs on the volar aspect of the wrist, frequently is apparent.

TABLE 64–4. Osteomyelitis due to Spread from a Contiguous Source of Infection: Radiographic-Pathologic Correlation

Pathologic Abnormality	Radiographic Abnormality
Soft tissue contamination and abscess formation	Soft tissue swelling, mass formation, obliteration of tissue planes
Infectious invasion of the periosteum with lifting of the membrane and bone formation	Periostitis
Subperiosteal abscess formation and cortical invasion	Cortical erosion
Infection in haversian and Volkmann's canals of cortex	Cortical lucency and destruction
Contamination and spread in marrow	Bone lysis

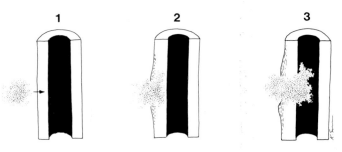

FIGURE 64–20. Osteomyelitis resulting from spread from a contiguous contaminated source. A diagrammatic representation of the sequential steps of osteomyelitis. **1,** Initially, a soft tissue focus of infection is apparent. Occasionally such a focus can irritate the underlying bone, producing periostitis without definite invasion of the cortex. **2,** The infection subsequently invades the cortex, spreading via haversian and Volkmann's canals. **3,** Finally, the medullary bone and marrow spaces are affected.

It is this communication that allows spread of infection from the first and fifth digits to the palm; such extension from the other digits is less constant (Fig. 64–25). Sequential contamination of the fifth finger, ulnar bursa, radial bursa, and first finger produces a typical horseshoe abscess.[80] The intimate relationship of the tendon sheaths to the volar aspect of the phalanges and proximal interphalangeal and metacarpophalangeal joints explains the occurrence of osteomyelitis and septic arthritis in cases of neglected tendon sheath infection.[81]

The extensor tendon sheaths extend in six compartments beneath the dorsal carpal ligament on the dorsum of the wrist (see Chapter 13). In this location, infection usually occurs in the subcutaneous or subaponeurotic space, whereas infective extensor tenosynovitis is less frequent. When present, such infection can contaminate the wrist[78] (Fig. 64–26).

Infective digital tenosynovitis can result from a puncture wound, particularly in a flexor crease of the finger, at which site skin and sheath are intimately related. Additional sources of infection are spread from the pulp space or dorsum of the hand or fingers.[82] A sheath infection may perforate into an adjacent bone or joint in the finger; the most characteristic site of such extension includes the proximal interphalangeal articulations and adjacent middle phalanx (Figs. 64–27 and 64–28). The metacarpophalangeal joints are altered less commonly. Infection within the volar sheaths of the first and fifth digits may spread quickly to the ulnar and radial bursae and from these latter areas into the wrist.[82] Such extensions more frequently involve the radial bursa. In the second, third, and fourth digits, the infective process can spill from the open proximal end of the sheath. Further extension along the lumbrical muscles can allow widespread contamination.

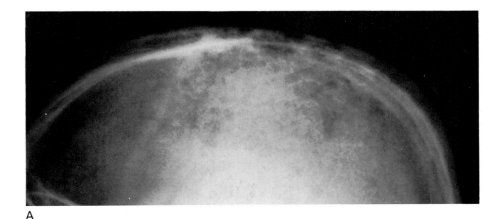

A

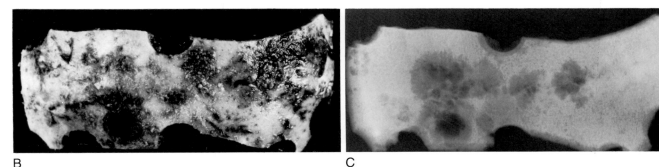

B   C

FIGURE 64–21. Osteomyelitis resulting from spread from a contiguous contaminated source. Skull. After a hair transplantation, this patient developed swelling of the scalp, local tenderness, and fever. The radiograph **(A)** of the skull demonstrates multiple osteolytic foci involving predominantly the outer table and diploic space. A photograph **(B)** and radiograph **(C)** of the resected cranial vault indicate the extent of the infectious process.

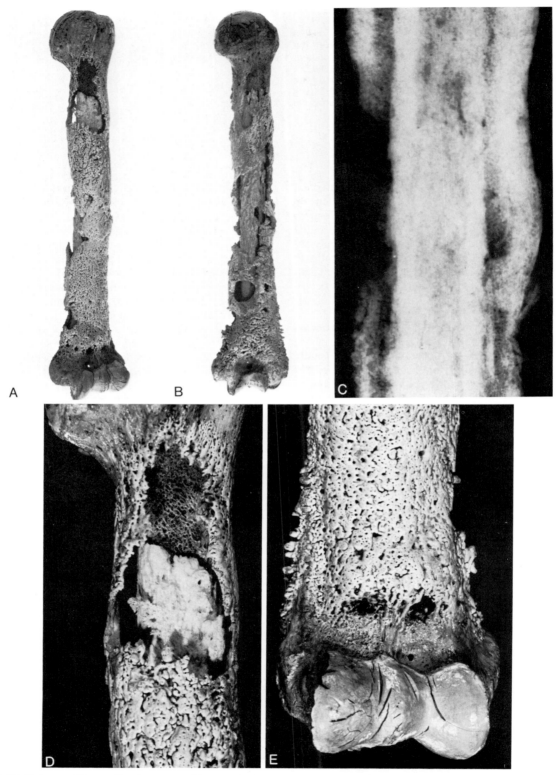

FIGURE 64–22. Osteomyelitis resulting from spread from a contiguous contaminated source. This 45 year old private in the Illinois Cavalry was wounded while charging the enemy on April 27, 1864. A musket ball penetrated the soft tissues of the arm near the elbow, flattening the bone but not entering it. The soldier continued to fight, carrying his weapon in the injured arm. Twelve days later, the ball was removed. Subsequently the limb rapidly became inflamed. Multiple soft tissue abscesses occurred over the ensuing 9 months, most treated by incision. Draining sinuses developed. Clinical deterioration occurred, necessitating an amputation at the level of the shoulder on November 10, 1865. The patient's condition improved and, although unable to continue in a military career, he became employed as a ward orderly.

The photographs and radiograph of the well-preserved macerated specimen reveal, in remarkable detail, the findings of chronic osteomyelitis. Note the extent of periosteal bone formation, creating layers of involucra. This bone is perforated by cloacae and, at the upper margin of the humerus **(A, D)**, a large sequestrum is seen.

(Courtesy of Armed Forces Institute of Pathology, Washington, D.C.)

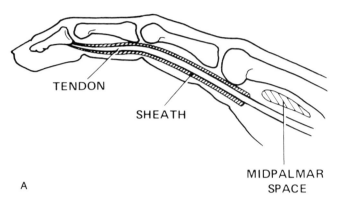

TENDON

SHEATH

MIDPALMAR SPACE

A

FIGURE 64–23. Spread of infection in the hand: Available anatomic pathways. Tendon sheaths.

A Digital tendon sheaths: The digital flexor tendon sheaths surround the tendon at its point of attachment to the terminal phalanx and extend proximally for a variable distance. In the second, third, and fourth fingers, they usually terminate just proximal to the metacarpophalangeal joint in close proximity to midpalmar space.

B Digital tendon sheaths: A digital tenogram outlines the tendon (T) within its sheath. Note the intimacy of the sheath to the proximal (arrow) and middle phalanges.

C Digital tendon sheaths: At the metacarpophalangeal joint, a sagittal section outlines the intimate relationship between the articulation and bones and the sheath. The tendon has been retracted (arrow) and is separated from the joint by a volar capsule (arrowhead). More distally, the sheath is adjacent to the proximal phalanx (open arrow).

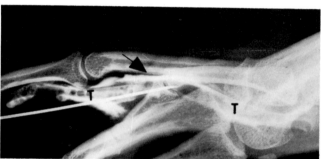

B

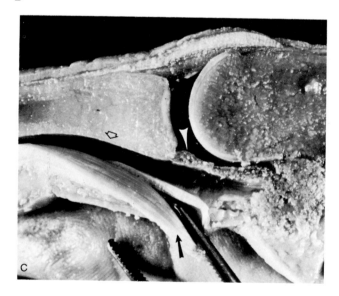

C

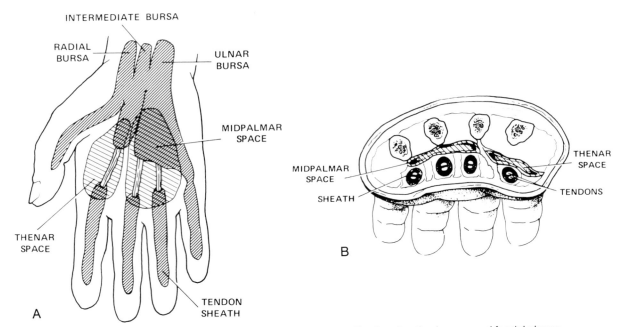

FIGURE 64–24. Spread of infection in the hand: Available anatomic pathways. Tendon sheaths, bursae, and fascial planes.
  A Drawing demonstrates the relationships of the tendon sheaths, bursae, and fascial planes (thenar space, midpalmar space).
  B Drawing of a section through the metacarpals outlines two spaces, the midpalmar and thenar spaces, separated by a septum and located above the digital flexor tendon sheaths. Note the close relationship between the sheath of the index finger and thenar space and between the sheaths of the third, fourth, and fifth fingers and midpalmar space.
  (**A, B,** From Resnick D: J Can Assoc Radiol *27*:21, 1976.)

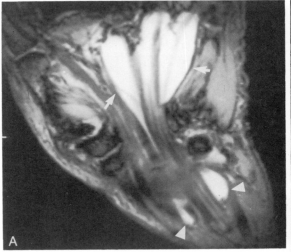

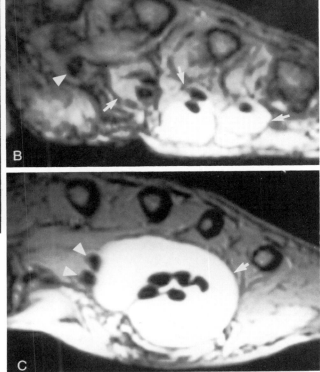

FIGURE 64–25. Spread of infection in the hand: Flexor tenosynovitis and ulnar bursitis. (No microorganisms recovered.)
  A Coronal multiplanar gradient recalled (MPGR) image (TR/TE, 350/20; flip angle, 30 degrees) shows fluid surrounding the flexor digitorum superficialis and flexor digitorum profundus tendons in the third, fourth, and fifth fingers (arrows) and in the ulnar bursa (arrowheads).
  B, C Transverse multiplanar gradient recalled (MPGR) images (TR/TE, 300/20; flip angle, 30 degrees) at the levels of the distal portion **(B)** and midportion **(C)** of the metacarpal bones show, in **B,** fluid in the tendon sheaths about the flexor digitorum superficialis and flexor digitorum profundus tendons in the third, fourth, and fifth fingers (arrows); in **C,** fluid in the ulnar bursa (arrow). Note that the flexor tendons and tendon sheath of the second finger are uninvolved (arrowheads).
  (Courtesy of G. Wesby, M.D., La Jolla, California.)

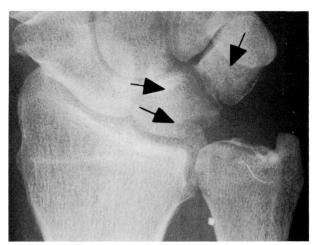

FIGURE 64–26. Spread of infection in the hand: Extensor tenosynovitis and osteomyelitis. A 50 year old man noted pain and swelling on the dorsum of the wrist for 3 weeks after trauma. At surgery, a staphylococcal tenosynovitis and osteomyelitis were confirmed. Lytic lesions and apposing cortical irregularities of the lunate and triquetrum (arrows) are apparent. Shrapnel from a previous injury is seen. (From Resnick D: J Can Assoc Radiol *27*:21, 1976.)

The diagnosis of tenosynovitis is accomplished from the four cardinal signs of Kanavel[81]: exquisite tenderness over the course of the sheath, semiflexed position of the finger, severe pain on extension of the finger, and symmetric swelling of the digit. On radiographs, diffuse soft tissue swelling

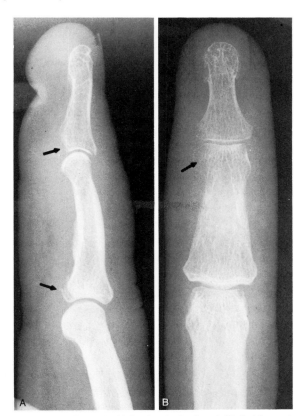

FIGURE 64–27. Spread of infection in the hand: Digital flexor tenosynovitis. This man had a chronic infection on the flexor surface of the finger. Observe the characteristic soft tissue swelling, especially on the volar aspect of the digit, and the resulting osteomyelitis of the phalanges (arrows). The distal interphalangeal joint became involved.

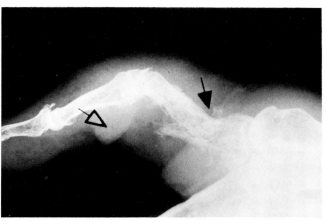

FIGURE 64–28. Spread of infection in the hand: Digital flexor tenosynovitis. After a neglected puncture wound, a 45 year old woman developed tenosynovitis and osteomyelitis. Note the soft tissue swelling, particularly along the volar surface of the proximal phalanx (open arrow), semiflexed position of the finger, and extensive permeative osseous destruction, with pathologic fracture (solid arrow) of the proximal phalanx. (From Resnick D: J Can Assoc Radiol *27*:21, 1976.)

is apparent. Osteoporosis and articular and osseous destruction, the latter commencing along the volar aspect of the bone, are evident.

Fascial Planes. Infections in the fascial planes of the hand are numerous but result in joint or bone alterations less frequently than those in the synovial sheaths. Although several fascial planes exist, two potential spaces dorsal to the volar sheaths and bursae are of particular importance.[81, 83] The midpalmar space extends in a triangular fashion along the ulnar aspect of the hand from the third metacarpal to the hypothenar eminence; the thenar space extends along the radial aspect of the hand from the third metacarpal bone to the thenar eminence (Fig. 64–24). The two are separated from each other by a firm septum. Through injection studies, Kanavel[81] demonstrated the frequent spread of fluid from the flexor tendon sheath of the index finger into the thenar space. Less frequently, communication between this space and the flexor tendon sheaths of the first and third digits was noted. Common communications between the flexor tendon sheaths of the third, fourth, and fifth digits and the midpalmar space were seen.

Infection in the midpalmar space may result from direct implantation during injury or by extension from suppurative sheaths. The proximity of the midpalmar space to the third, fourth, and fifth metacarpal bones may promote osteomyelitis in neglected infections[78, 81] (Fig. 64–29). Palmar swelling, semiflexion of the fingers, and bony destruction are the accompanying clinical and radiologic manifestations. Neglected infection of the thenar space, resulting from direct implantation or extension from adjacent flexor tendon sheaths (usually the second) or from the midpalmar space, also can lead to osteomyelitis of the metacarpal bones (Fig. 64–30). Extensive swelling along the radial aspect of the hand forces the thumb into abduction.[82] Web-space infections between the volar and dorsal skin may ascend through lumbrical muscle sheaths into the thenar and the midpalmar spaces.[80] The dorsal subaponeurotic and dorsal subcutaneous spaces are involved less frequently in hand infections, although lymphatic vessels at the latter site may pro-

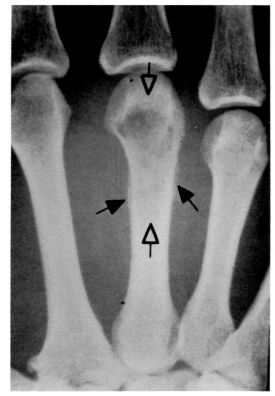

FIGURE 64–29. Spread of infection in the hand: Midpalmar space infection. Osteomyelitis of the third metacarpal bone has resulted from spread of infection from the midpalmar space. A large lytic lesion (open arrows) may be noted and periostitis is seen (solid arrows). (From Resnick D: J Can Assoc Radiol *27*:21, 1976.)

duce marked swelling and lymphedema in cases of palmar infections.[80]

Lymphatics. Lymphangitis may result from superficial injuries. Rapid extension can produce widespread swelling without clinical evidence of synovial sheath infection. In intense cases, complications, including tenosynovitis, septicemia, osteomyelitis, and septic arthritis, may be noted.[82]

Specific Entities

Felon. A felon results from infection in the terminal pulp space.[82–84] Bone involvement is not infrequent in neglected cases[85] because of the close proximity of the terminal phalanx (Fig. 64–31). In addition to osteomyelitis, soft tissue edema adjacent to the bone can produce relative ischemia and bone necrosis.[86] The tuft and diaphysis of the terminal phalanx are characteristically destroyed, with relative sparing of the phalangeal base.[85, 86] Sequestra may be evident. Furthermore, pyarthrosis of the distal interphalangeal joints and involvement of the flexor tendon sheaths occasionally are noted.[82]

Paronychia. Subcuticular abscesses of the nail fold are termed paronychia.[82, 84] On rare occasions, osseous destruction of a terminal phalanx may be evident[85] (Fig. 64–32).

Frequency of Osteomyelitis and Septic Arthritis After Hand Infections.

The reported frequency of bone and joint involvement during the course of hand infection has varied. Resnick[78] noted such involvement in 10 per cent of 78 patients, although in one third of the infected patients, the diagnosis of osteomyelitis and septic arthritis was not evident on radiographs and could be established only during

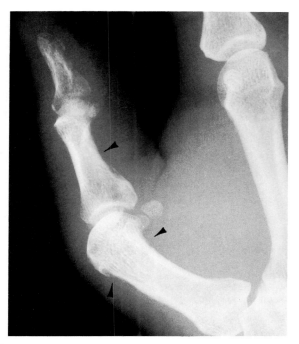

FIGURE 64–30. Spread of infection in the hand: Thenar space infection. The infection produced extensive soft tissue swelling, forcing the thumb into abduction. Two weeks later, osseous resorption and contamination of the metacarpal bone and proximal phalanx can be seen (arrowheads). The source of the infection, the soft tissues of the tip of the thumb, is evident on the film. (From Resnick D: J Can Assoc Radiol *27*:21, 1976.)

surgery (Fig. 64–33). Previous reports have indicated a much higher frequency of bone and joint involvement,[85] but with earlier diagnosis and current antibiotic and surgical therapy, obvious reduction of this dreaded complication has occurred. One study has indicated a 17 per cent prevalence of infective osteitis, tenosynovitis, or septic arthritis in an evaluation of 1400 cases of hand infection.[61]

The frequency of hand infection in drug addicts is noteworthy[78, 87]; infections commonly follow local injections with contaminated needles. Bilateral swelling of the dorsum of the hand in addicts, the puffy-hand syndrome (Fig. 64–34), however, can relate not to infection but to lymphedema resulting from lymphatic destruction and fibrosis of the subcutaneous tissues.[88, 89]

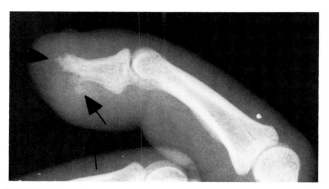

FIGURE 64–31. Spread of infection in the hand: Felon. An infection in the pulp space has produced considerable soft tissue swelling (open arrows). Extension into the tuft and diaphysis of the terminal phalanx is apparent (solid arrows). Shrapnel from a previous injury can be seen. (From Resnick D: J Can Assoc Radiol *27*:21, 1976.)

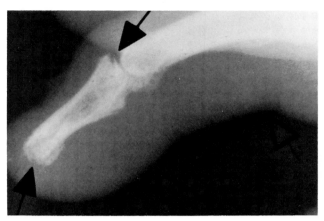

FIGURE 64–32. Spread of infection in the hand: Paronychia. Widespread infection of the pulp space, digital flexor tendon sheath, terminal tuft, and distal interphalangeal joint (solid arrows) resulted from an initial subcuticular abscess. Soft tissue swelling along the tendon sheath may be noted (open arrows). (From Resnick D: J Can Assoc Radiol *27*:21, 1976.)

Foot

Pathways of Spread of Infection. The plantar aspect of the foot is especially vulnerable to soft tissue infection. Foreign bodies, puncture wounds, or skin ulceration from weight-bearing can represent the portal of entry for various organisms. In a diabetic patient, soft tissue breakdown over certain pressure points (such as the metatarsal heads and calcaneus) leads to infection that is combined with vascular and neurologic abnormalities.[90–92]

There are three plantar muscle compartments—medial, intermediate, and lateral[93–96] (Fig. 64–35). These compartments are separated from each other by two intermuscular septa extending from the plantar fascia to the overlying osseous structures. The medial compartment contains the muscles to the great toe and the lateral compartment contains those to the fifth toe, with the intermediate compartment containing the remainder.

Cadaveric injection studies[97] have emphasized (1) that the intermediate compartment contains the greatest amount of potential space; when this compartment becomes filled, continued infusion of fluid will produce extravasation either into the medial compartment or more importantly along the flexor hallucis longus tendon into the lower leg; (2) that the lateral compartment has the least amount of potential space; extravasation from this area occurs into the dorsal compartment or plantar fat of the foot; and (3) that the medial compartment has a potential space somewhat greater than that of the lateral compartment and less than that of the intermediate compartment; extravasation from this area commonly occurs into the intermediate compartment.

These experimental observations can be applied to the evaluation of soft tissue infections in the plantar aspect of the foot. Initial contamination of skin and subcutaneous tissue at pressure points soon can lead to infective osteitis, osteomyelitis, and septic arthritis of adjacent bones and joints; this is especially frequent about the metatarsophalangeal joints, calcaneus, and terminal phalanges. Soft tissue dissemination of infection also can occur via the medial, lateral, or intermediate compartment; in these instances, osteomyelitis and septic arthritis can be seen to be remote from the initial site of soft tissue contamination. Furthermore, the intermediate compartment provides a pathway by which the infection can spread from the plantar aspect of the foot into the lower leg; neglected foot infections eventually may require amputations at levels above or below the knee.

The existence of these avenues within the soft tissues in the foot that allow dissemination of localized infection underscores the need for early diagnosis in the treatment of such infection, especially in a vulnerable person, such as

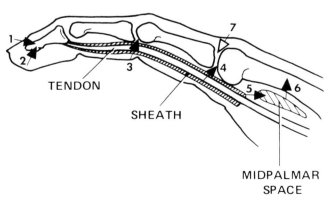

FIGURE 64–33. Spread of infection in the hand: Summary of pathways. A paronychia (1) rarely may invade the distal terminal phalanx. A felon (2) may produce destruction of the tuft and diaphysis of a distal phalanx. Suppurative tenosynovitis may spread to the proximal interphalangeal joint (3) and less frequently to the metacarpophalangeal joint (4). From the proximal end of the sheath of the third, fourth, and fifth digits, pus may reach the midpalmar space (5). Direct metacarpal invasion (6) then is possible. Puncture wounds of the metacarpophalangeal joint (7) are frequent during fist-fights (see text). (After Resnick D: J Can Assoc Radiol *27*:21, 1976.)

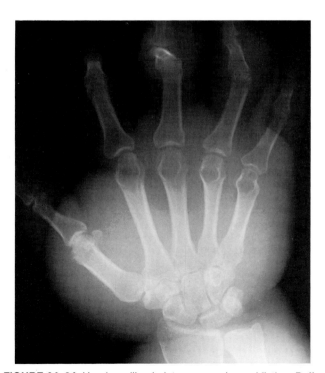

FIGURE 64–34. Hand swelling in intravenous drug addiction: Puffy-hand syndrome. Massive swelling of the hand in this 39 year old male drug addict is related to lymphatic obstruction. (Courtesy of M. Dalinka, M.D., Philadelphia, Pennsylvania.)

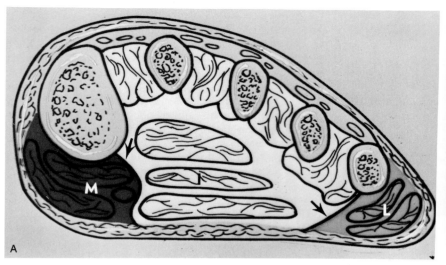
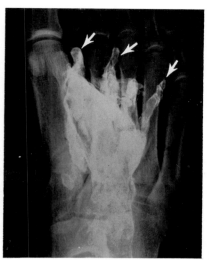

FIGURE 64–35. Spread of infection in the foot: Available anatomic pathways.

A, Plantar compartmental anatomy on cross section of the foot. Note the medial (M), intermediate (I), and lateral (L) compartments separated by two intermuscular septa (arrows).

B An injection into the intermediate plantar compartment reveals the extent of this space. Note the filling of the sheaths about the lumbrical muscles (arrows).

(From Feingold M, et al: Invest Radiol *12*:281, 1977.)

the patient with diabetes mellitus. Plain film radiography often is insensitive and inadequate in this regard, stimulating a search for other diagnostic techniques. Scintigraphy using a variety of radiopharmaceutical agents, CT, and MR imaging are three methods that provide information regarding the presence and the extent of soft tissue infection. With scintigraphy, problems arise in the differentiation of infection confined to soft tissue and that affecting adjacent bones or joints or both (see later discussion). With CT, the separation of suppuration, edema, and fibrosis in the soft tissue is difficult. MR imaging may represent the most sensitive and specific imaging technique, although diagnostic problems and pitfalls may be encountered (see later discussion).

Specific Entities

Puncture Wounds. Puncture wounds of the plantar aspect of the foot can lead to osteomyelitis and septic arthritis[67, 68, 70, 71, 292, 352, 600] (Fig. 64–36). These injuries are especially prominent in children who walk barefoot, exposing the unprotected foot to nails, glass, splinters, and other sharp objects. The infective organisms can vary,[353] but gram-negative agents such as *Pseudomonas aeruginosa* frequently are implicated[67, 68, 70, 98–100, 361]; this is not surprising, as these organisms usually are found in the soil and may be normal inhabitants of skin.[70] Typically, local pain and swelling appear within days after a puncture wound, although radiographs usually are normal at this time. After a delay of 1 to 3 weeks, the radiographs reveal typical abnormalities of osteomyelitis or septic arthritis. It has been suggested that *P. aeruginosa* has a propensity for infecting cartilage[67] with early evidence of cartilaginous destruction (articular or physeal growth cartilage) after intra-articular or metaphyseal introduction of organisms; infective chondritis due to Pseudomonas also can be noted in the sternoclavicular joints, intervertebral discs, and ear. Johanson[98] contended that Pseudomonas infections do not develop in puncture wounds in noncartilaginous areas of the foot.

Osteomyelitis of the os calcis is a recognized complication of repeated heel punctures in the neonate.[73, 355–358] The

mechanism of infection relates to the spread of soft tissue suppuration to the neighboring bone; subsequently, hematogenous dissemination with multifocal osteomyelitis may appear. Less commonly, direct intraosseous inoculation of

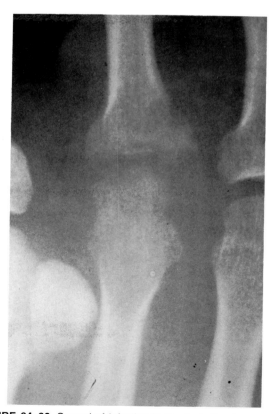

FIGURE 64–36. Spread of infection in the foot: Puncture wounds. After a puncture wound from a nail, this patient developed a plantar soft tissue infection that later led to osteomyelitis and septic arthritis. Observe osseous destruction of the metatarsal head and proximal phalanx, joint space narrowing, and soft tissue swelling.

organisms at the time of heel pad puncture leads to osteomyelitis. On radiographs, destruction of the plantar aspect of the bone is seen.

Wooden splinters and thorns can induce osseous and articular changes in the foot.[71] Areas of osteolysis, osteosclerosis, and periostitis may relate to secondary infection, simple irritation from the foreign body, or, perhaps, toxins within the thorns themselves.[325, 359, 360, 601] The clinical course characteristically is protracted, and the accurate diagnosis of the clinical and radiologic manifestations may be difficult, as the remote history of a puncture wound may seem insignificant to the patient and not be reported to the physician. CT or ultrasonography may be required to identify the splinter or thorn.[536]

Foot Infections in Diabetes Mellitus. Complete discussion of this common and complicated problem is beyond the scope of this book, and the interested reader should consult other sources.[91] Instead, an overview is presented.

Clinical, radiologic, and pathologic characteristics of osteomyelitis (and septic arthritis) complicating foot infections in diabetic patients are modified by the associated problems of these persons, including vascular insufficiency and neurologic deficit.[101, 362] Clinical differentiation between infection and gangrene can be difficult, although both processes may coexist in the same person. Systemic manifestations of sepsis are uncommon; local symptoms and signs dominate, including pain, swelling, erythema, and diminished peripheral pulses. Cellulitis and skin ulcerations are readily apparent.

The radiographic picture usually reveals significant soft tissue swelling and mottled osteolysis (Fig. 64–37). Osteosclerosis, fragmentation, and periostitis may be seen. Radiolucent areas within the soft tissues commonly are identified.[102] This finding can relate to the presence of air due to dissection around open wounds or after local débridement or to the presence of gas due to clostridial or nonclostridial infections. Although nonclostridial gas-producing infections can occur in nondiabetic as well as diabetic patients, the frequency is significantly higher in the latter persons. The responsible organisms may be either aerobic, such as *Escherichia coli, Aerobacter aerogenes, Klebsiella pneumoniae,* and non-hemolytic streptococci, or anaerobic, such as Bacteroides and anaerobic streptococci.[103–106] Cultures containing more than one organism, some of which are present in normal skin, are typical.[101]

In some diabetic patients with foot infections that are complicated by osteomyelitis and septic arthritis, pathologic fractures and subluxations are prominent. These findings can simulate those accompanying diabetic neuropathic osteoarthropathy, and differentiation of neurologic and infectious processes can be very difficult. In fact, both infection and neuropathic osteoarthropathy of the midfoot and forefoot frequently coexist in diabetic patients. The presence of poorly defined osseous contours is the most helpful radiologic clue to osteomyelitis. Additional techniques, including sinography,[363] scintigraphy,[362, 602] CT, and MR imaging,[603, 604] as discussed later in this chapter, may be required (Figs. 64–38 to 64–41).

Pelvis. Breakdown of soft tissue that occurs in debilitated persons who maintain a single position for long periods of time is referred to as a pressure sore, decubitus ulcer, or bedsore.[364, 597] It is seen most commonly in patients with spinal cord injury or other neurologic defects, although the complication is not confined to these persons, being evident in older patients with a variety of medical and surgical problems.[365] The cause of pressure sores is multifactorial, related both to extrinsic mechanical forces on the skin and soft tissue over a bone and to the intrinsic susceptibility to tissue breakdown, itself influenced by both systemic and local conditions.[365, 366] A relationship exists between the frequency of such sores and advancing age of the patients. Although other sites, such as the heels, may be affected, most pressure sores develop about the pelvis, especially near the sacrum, ischial tuberosities, trochanteric regions, and buttock.[367]

Local soft tissue infection and bacteremia commonly are associated with decubitus ulcers.[367] Typical organisms include *Staphylococcus aureus, Proteus mirabilis, Escherichia coli,* Bacteroides species, group A and other streptococci, Klebsiella, and *Pseudomonas aeruginosa.* The increased prevalence of certain of these organisms relates to the inevitable fecal contamination of the lesions (Bacteroides species) and the commonly associated nosocomial infections owing to long periods of hospitalization (Proteus species).[367] Although bacteremia implies an attendant risk for hematogenous spread of infection to distant bones and other tissues, osteomyelitis is observed most commonly in the innominate bones and proximal portions of the femora, areas subjacent to sites of skin breakdown, and is related to spread from a contiguous contaminated source. Superficial pressure sores extend through the dermis but not into the subcutaneous fat, whereas those penetrating the subcutaneous fat are referred to as deep pressure sores. Further extension into and through the deep fascia leads to osseous contamination with a sinus tract communicating with the skin or nearby joint.

The accurate diagnosis of osteomyelitis complicating pressure sores is difficult, owing to a number of other conditions that may become evident in the immobilized or paralyzed patient. Pressure-related changes in bone are not infrequent, leading to flattening and sclerosis of bony prominences, such as the femoral trochanters and ischial tuberosities.[364] Heterotopic ossification, a well-recognized accompaniment of neurologic injury, further complicates early diagnosis of osteomyelitis. Routine radiography is reported to be insensitive and nonspecific in the diagnosis of bone infection in patients with pressure sores,[364, 368, 565] related in part to the difficulty of differentiating changes caused by abnormal pressure from those of osteomyelitis, although this examination may disclose air within the soft tissues, allowing analysis of the size of the lesion. Sinography is indicated when there is clinical uncertainty about the extent of a pressure sore[364]; however, the examination is technically difficult when an appropriate catheter that will enter the wound cannot be found or when multiple soft tissue perforations are present. Fluoroscopic monitoring and spot-filming during the sinogram are mandatory in the accurate assessment of bone contamination. Additional diagnostic techniques, including radiographic magnification,[364] xeroradiography, ultrasonography, CT,[364, 369] MR imaging, and scintigraphy, sometimes are helpful, although precise diagnosis frequently requires histologic examination of the bone.[368] Cultures of material derived from bone biopsy are difficult to interpret owing to bacterial colonization or in-

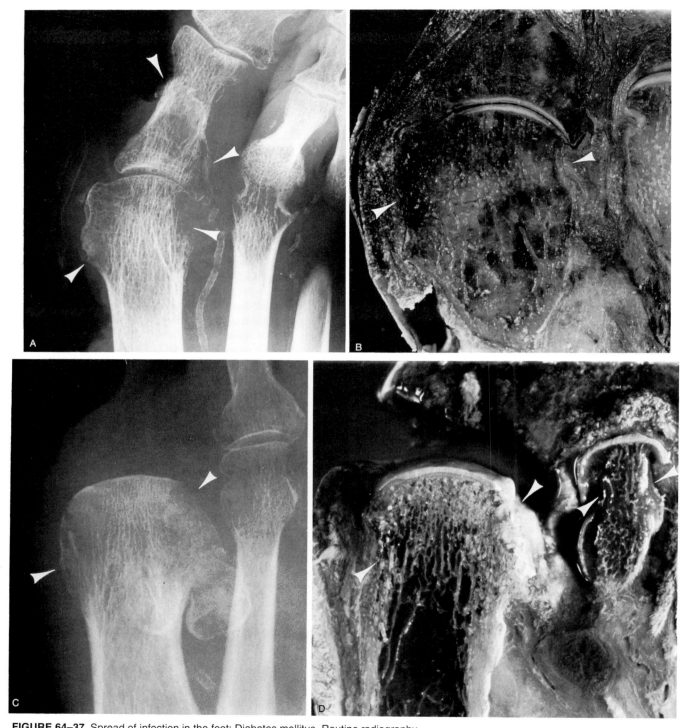

FIGURE 64–37. Spread of infection in the foot: Diabetes mellitus. Routine radiography.

  A, B Radiograph and transverse sectional photograph reveal a soft tissue infection about the first metatarsophalangeal joint with ulcerations and with erosion of bone (arrowheads). Observe vascular calcification and alterations at the second metatarsophalangeal joint.

  C, D In a different diabetic patient who had had the first toe amputated for infection, a radiograph and transverse sectional photograph illustrate contamination of the first and second metatarsal heads with osseous erosion (arrowheads).

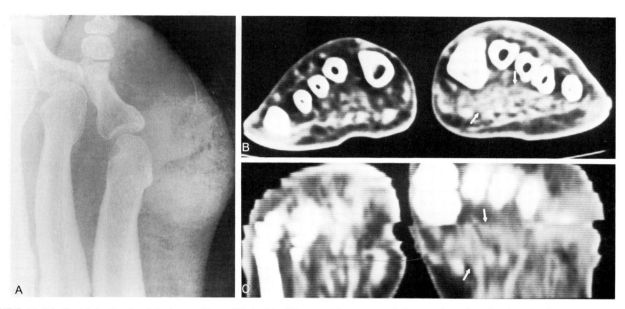

FIGURE 64–38. Foot infection in diabetes mellitus: CT. In this 55 year old man, a soft tissue ulceration developed adjacent to the lateral aspect of the fifth metatarsal head.

A The soft tissue prominence is apparent. Small radiolucent shadows within the soft tissue represent air attributable to the open wound. A bandage covers the area of ulceration. The bones and joints are normal.

B A coronal CT scan at the level of the proximal aspects of the metatarsal bones shows increased attenuation within the intermediate plantar compartment (arrows), which is more apparent when compared to the opposite (normal) side. The findings are compatible with the extension of infection although fibrosis and edema produce similar abnormalities. Edema in the dorsum of the foot also is seen.

C A transversely oriented reformation of the CT scan outlines the increased radiodensity (arrows) in the intermediate compartment. Compare with the opposite side.

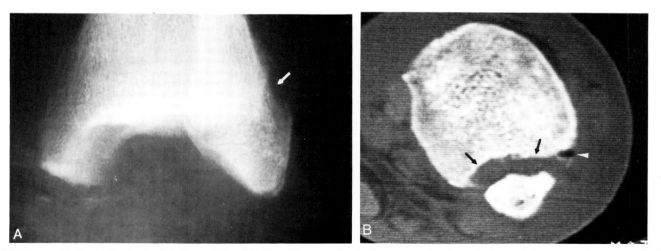

FIGURE 64–39. Foot infection in diabetes mellitus: CT. This 49 year old diabetic man required repeated amputations of portions of the foot for recurrent infections with osteomyelitis. Eventually the foot was disarticulated at the level of the ankle, but infection recurred.

A The plain film shows osteopenia and indistinctness and erosion of bone in the lateral aspect of the tibia and fibula (arrow). A soft tissue ulceration also is present.

B A transaxial CT scan at a level slightly above the ankle demonstrates soft tissue gas (arrowhead) and prominent erosion of the tibia (arrows).

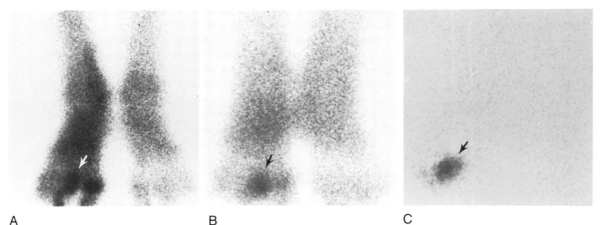

A   B   C

FIGURE 64–40. Foot infection in diabetes mellitus: Scintigraphy. A conventional frontal radiograph (not shown) revealed soft tissue swelling in the first and second toes of the foot.

A Frontal gamma camera image from a ^{99m}Tc-methylene diphosphonate bone scan reveals diffusely increased radioactivity in the infected foot related to hyperemia, with focal accentuation in the region of the second toe (arrow) and first metatarsophalangeal joint.

B Corresponding view from a ^{67}Ga-citrate scan demonstrates focal intense accumulation of the radiopharmaceutical agent in the vicinity of the infected second toe (arrow). The slight generalized accentuation of isotopic uptake in the involved foot reflects hyperemia.

C Frontal projection from an ^{111}In labeled leukocyte scan shows focal increased activity at the site of infection (arrow). All radionuclide agents have documented findings consistent with soft tissue and bone infection, but the abnormalities of the ^{111}In scan corresponded most accurately to the surgical findings.

(From Sartoris DJ, et al: Invest Radiol *20:*772, 1985.)

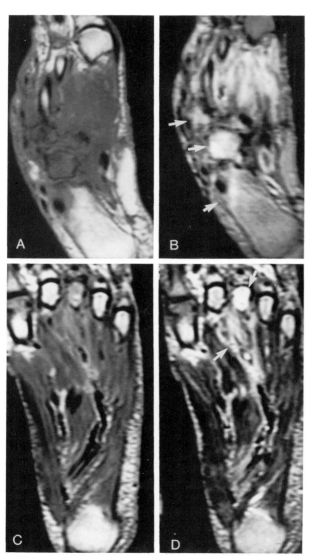

FIGURE 64–41. Foot infection in diabetes mellitus: MR imaging.

A, B Transverse T1-weighted (TR/TE, 700/12) **(A)** and T2-weighted (TR/TE, 2000/80) **(B)** spin echo MR images show the extent of soft tissue and bone involvement in the plantar aspect of the foot. The process is of low signal intensity in **A** and of high signal intensity in **B** and affects the fifth metatarsal base, cuboid bone, and calcaneus, better seen in **B** (arrows).

C, D In a different patient, proton density (TR/TE, 2000/30) **(C)** and T2-weighted (TR/TE, 2000/70) **(D)** spin echo MR images in the transverse plane show changes in signal intensity within areas of soft tissue and bone infection similar to those in **A** and **B**. Note the high signal intensity in the infected soft tissues and head of the third metatarsal bone in **D** (arrows).

fection of overlying pressure sores and should not be relied on unless histologic analysis of the tissue also is performed.[368]

Other Sites. Osteomyelitis of the clavicle and septic arthritis of the sternoclavicular joint have been associated with catheterization of the subclavian vein[72, 354, 370] as well as with Swan-Ganz catheterization.[371] The pathogenesis of the bone or joint involvement appears to relate to the spread of infection from a contiguous contaminated source, although seeding of the periosteum directly during the manipulation of the needle tip represents a second potential mechanism. The time interval from the insertion of the catheter to the onset of clinical and radiologic abnormalities varies regardless of whether the catheter is removed or left indwelling.[354] Osteomyelitis of the clavicle related to venous catheterization must be differentiated from nonseptic clavicular periostitis resulting from the trauma induced by the tip of the needle[372] and from hematogenous infection of the bone.[752]

Infection in a tubular bone of the lower or upper extremity is a rare complication of septic thrombophlebitis.[373] Extensive subperiosteal abscess formation is associated with minimal or late intramedullary contamination. It is possible that thrombophlebitis alters the intraosseous venous pressure, accentuating areas of sluggish blood flow and providing an environment well suited to osteomyelitis. Accurate diagnosis of this complication is difficult.

Direct Implantation

General Clinical Features

The direct route of contamination commonly is combined with spread from a contiguous source of infection. Thus, puncture wounds of the hand and the foot can lead to osteomyelitis (and septic arthritis) by contaminating adjacent soft tissues or directly inoculating the bone or joint (Fig. 64–42). This latter complication is especially prevalent in the foot, at which site nails, splinters, or glass can lead to deep puncture wounds, producing immediate bone (and joint) contamination; in the hand, at which site a human bite received during a fist-fight can directly injure osseous and articular structures; and in any site after animal bites.

General Radiographic Features

The features of bone (and joint) involvement after direct implantation of an infectious process are virtually identical to those occurring after spread of infection from a contiguous contaminated source. Commonly, osseous destruction and proliferation lead to focal areas of lysis, sclerosis, and periostitis. Soft tissue swelling is common, related not to infection but to edema resulting from the injury itself.

Specific Entities

Human Bites. The significance of this injury often is overlooked, and the delay that frequently occurs in the patient's seeking a physician's aid can result in serious sequelae.[107–111, 293, 374, 555, 605–607, 738] Although human bites occur in a variety of situations and are not infrequent in sex-related crimes and child abuse cases,[375] the most common cause of injury is a fist-blow to the mouth resulting in laceration of the dorsum of the metacarpophalangeal joint;

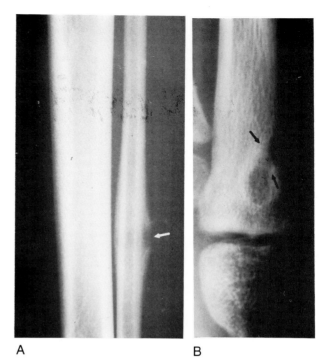

A   B

FIGURE 64–42. Infection due to direct implantation: Puncture wounds.

A Thorn granuloma. After a puncture wound with a thorn, a lytic lesion of the fibula became evident. Cultures repeatedly were negative. Note the considerable periostitis and the eccentric location with violation of the cortex (arrow), indicating an external source.

B After a puncture wound, an abscess of the distal end of the fibula due to staphylococci developed. Note the tract running from the cortex to the lesion (arrows), indicating the nature of the original injury.

(**A,** Courtesy of W. Pogue, M.D., San Diego, California.)

human bites also are frequent on the volar or dorsal aspect of the fingers. Joint infection is more common than bone infection in these cases. *Staphylococcus aureus* or Streptococcus species is the usual implicated organism. During a fist-fight, the flexed metacarpophalangeal joint striking the opponent's teeth has little protective superficial tissue; the third metacarpophalangeal joint is involved most frequently. As the hand is unclenched, the overlying tissue shifts and the organisms within the joint have no route of egress. The combination of *Bacillus fusiformis* and spirochetes does particularly well in this anaerobic setting; septic arthritis and osteomyelitis may be noted after a delay of days to weeks.[112] Tendon injuries also may occur.[605] The radiographic findings, which are particularly well shown on steep oblique and lateral radiographs,[537] include peculiar bony defects and fractures,[78] tooth fragments,[65] and osseous and articular destruction[78] (Fig. 64–43). Magnification radiography aids in early detection of these findings (Fig. 64–44).

Animal Bites. Superficial animal bites or scratches can inoculate local soft tissues, later leading to infection of underlying bones and joints, and deep animal bites can introduce organisms directly into both osseous and articular structures.[64, 66, 113–116, 293, 294] Dog bites account for approximately 90 per cent of these injuries and cat bites for about 10 per cent.[376] Miscellaneous other species, primarily ro-

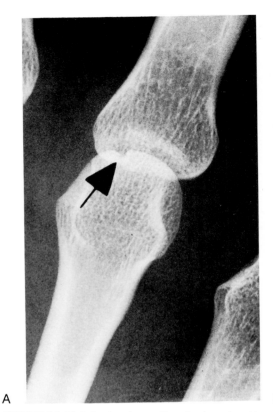
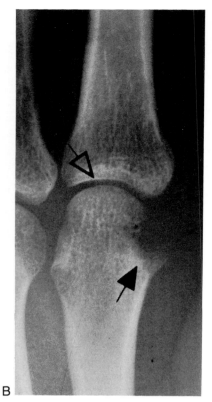
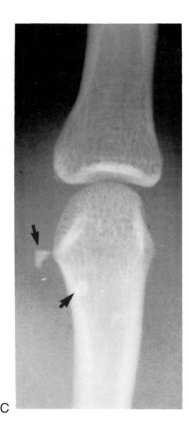

A B C

FIGURE 64–43. Infection due to direct implantation: Human bites.

A A small subchondral fracture of the metacarpal head (arrow) in this patient was produced by a fist-fight.

B Progressive destruction of the third metacarpal head (solid arrow) and a narrowed metacarpophalangeal joint (open arrow) resulted from infection after a fist-fight in which the fist struck the opponent's teeth. (From Resnick D: J Can Assoc Radiol *27*:21, 1976.)

C In this patient, small tooth fragments (arrows) can be seen. The joint space is normal.

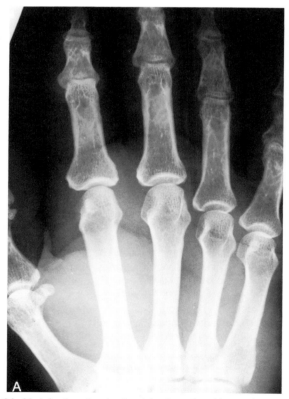
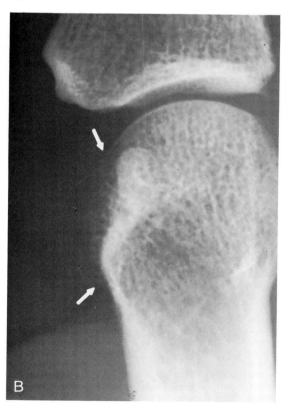

A B

FIGURE 64–44. Infection due to direct implantation: Human bites—magnification radiography. This 35 year old man developed pain and swelling over the second metacarpophalangeal joint after a fist-fight. *Staphylococcus aureus* was recovered from the joint fluid.

A The initial film, obtained 7 days after the fight, demonstrates soft tissue swelling about the second metacarpophalangeal joint. The interosseous space appears slightly narrowed.

B Direct radiographic magnification shows subchondral osteopenia and the interruption of the subchondral bone plate (between arrows), indicative of osseous infection.

dents and rabbits, infrequently are responsible. Approximately 5 per cent of dog bites and 20 to 50 per cent of cat bites become infected significantly.[376] The infecting organisms vary, but *Pasteurella multocida* commonly is implicated, especially in cat bites[376–379]; this latter organism is a normal isolate in the oral cavities of 12 to 54 per cent of dogs and 52 to 70 per cent of cats.[64, 117, 118] Other organisms include *Staphylococcus aureus, S. epidermidis,* and Bacteroides species.[293] It has been suggested that animal saliva, rather than the victim's skin flora, is the major source of the bacteria that are isolated from cultures of bite wounds.[376]

Clinical manifestations related to animal bites result not only from secondary infection but also from tissue crushing leading to areas of devitalization, especially with dog bites. A trained sentry dog can exert as much as 450 pounds per square inch, a force that is great enough to perforate sheet metal![376] Any anatomic site can be affected, although animal bites predominate in the hand, the arm, and the leg (Fig. 64–45). Inflammation with pain and swelling develops at the wound site in 1 to 3 days. Low-grade fever and lymphadenopathy also can be evident. In neglected cases, septicemia, infective synovitis, osteitis, osteomyelitis, and arthritis can develop.[66] These complications may not become apparent clinically until weeks or months after the

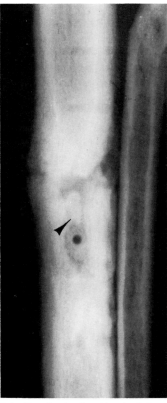

FIGURE 64–46. Infection due to direct implantation: Open fractures. This patient had a comminuted fracture of the tibia complicated by osteomyelitis. Operative intervention with application of a plate also was attempted, although the plate was removed because of continued drainage. Note a sequestrum in the tibia (arrowhead), fibrous union of the fracture, and the multiple osseous defects due to the removed screws.

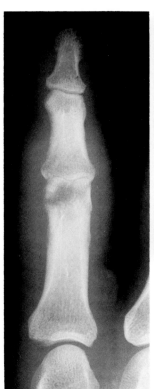
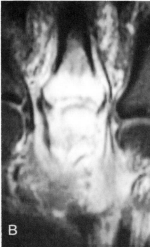

FIGURE 64–45. Infection due to direct implantation: Animal bites.
 A After a cat bite, this patient developed Pasteurella osteomyelitis and septic arthritis. Observe soft tissue swelling, osseous destruction of the proximal and middle phalanges, and joint space narrowing and flexion at the proximal interphalangeal joint.
 B In a different patient who developed Pasteurella osteomyelitis and septic arthritis after a cat bite, a coronal T1-weighted (TR/TE, 800/20) spin echo MR image obtained with fat saturation technique (ChemSat) and gadolinium enhancement shows high signal intensity in the third metacarpophalangeal joint and adjacent bone and soft tissues.

injury. Fractures also may be observed,[294] even in the cranium, at which site meningitis is a reported complication.[380]

Open Fractures and Dislocations. Whenever a fracture or dislocation is complicated by disruption of the overlying skin, direct inoculation of bones and joints can occur. This problem is especially relevant to injuries of the tibia; this is a superficially located bone, and extensive trauma at this site frequently is complicated by violation of the overlying soft tissues and skin. Despite the early administration of antibiotics, chronic osteomyelitis is frequent in this setting. Radiographic documentation of infection is not difficult; the poorly defined and irregular osseous destruction accompanying osteomyelitis rarely is confused with the manifestations of a nonsuppurative healing fracture (Fig. 64–46).

Postoperative Infection

Postoperative osteoarticular infections represent a problem of major concern, especially to the orthopedic surgeon and neurosurgeon. They may occur as a result of contamination of bones and joints from adjacent infected soft tissues, direct inoculation of osseous and articular tissue at the time of surgery, or, less frequently, hematogenous spread to an operative site from a distant location.[119, 120, 385, 386] Any surgical procedure can be complicated by osteomyelitis (and septic arthritis) (Fig. 64–47). Particularly troublesome are instances of infection occurring after internal fixation of fractures (Fig. 64–48), intervertebral disc surgery, median

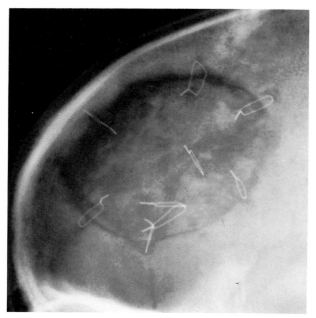

FIGURE 64–47. Postoperative infection: Craniotomy. An infection at a craniotomy site has resulted in considerable resorption of much of the osseous flap.

sternotomy, and various types of arthroplasty.[60, 121–123, 381–384] Clinically, considerable delay in diagnosis is not infrequent, as the signs of the infection are masked by the concomitant tissue injury or the suppressive effect of prophylactic agents, or the infecting organisms may be of limited pathogenicity. Any site can be affected, although the tibia and the femur are the most typical locations of infection after internal fixation of fractures, and the hip and the knee are the most typically infected sites after arthroplasty. One or more organisms may be implicated; *Staphylococcus aureus* is the most common pathogen.

Numerous radiographic techniques can be employed to evaluate postoperative infection. Routine radiography, conventional tomography, sinography, and arthrography all can be helpful; increasing osseous and cartilaginous destruction, periostitis, soft tissue swelling, and exaggerated lucency about cemented and noncemented metallic and polyethylene prostheses can be recognized (see Chapter 19).

One special type of postoperative infection relates to pin tracts. This complication particularly is troublesome after transcutaneous insertion of pins into bone, its reported frequency varying from almost zero to 4 per cent.[387, 392, 556] The causative organisms vary, but infections caused by gram-negative bacteria are common. The mechanisms of contamination also are variable; in some cases, the pins are inserted into bones that already are the site of osteomyelitis, whereas in others, osseous infection occurs at the time of or after pin insertion. Radiographs reveal progressive osteolysis about the metal or, after removal of the pin, a ring sequestrum (Fig. 64–49). In the latter instance the central circular radiolucent area created by the pin itself is surrounded by a ring of bone, which, in turn, is surrounded by an area of osteolysis.[392, 538] It is not clear whether loosening and separation of the osseous ring from the remainder of the bone precedes or follows the onset of sepsis.[392] Physical or thermal injury[393, 539] at the time of pin insertion produces a zone of osteosclerosis about the tract without a true sequestrum.[538] MR imaging also can be applied to the evaluation of pin tract infections (Figs. 64–50 and 64–51).

Rarely postoperative osteolysis is related not to infection, but to a reaction around a foreign body, such as a sponge[394] or Dacron or silicone material,[395] inserted at the time of surgery (see Chapter 19).

Complications

Severe Osteolysis

Although modern methods of diagnosis and treatment of infection usually ensure proper therapy before too long a

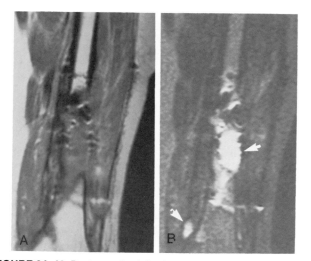

FIGURE 64–48. Postoperative infection: Internal fixation of fractures. A plate had been used in the treatment of a femoral shaft fracture but subsequent infection led to its removal. Coronal T1-weighted (TR/TE, 650/30) (**A**) and T2-weighted (TR/TE, 2000/200) (**B**) spin echo MR images show artifacts related to the removed metallic plate. The fracture site is evident. In **B**, the high signal intensity (arrows) in the soft tissues and the femoral diaphysis is consistent with active infection. (Courtesy of T. Mattsson, M.D., Riyadh, Saudi Arabia.)

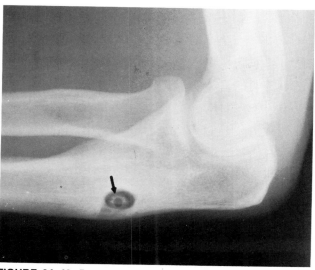

FIGURE 64–49. Postoperative infection: Pinhole ring sequestrum. Percutaneous pins were used to treat a fracture about the wrist in this 27 year old man. Purulent drainage occurred, requiring removal of the pins. Note the classic radiographic findings of a ring sequestrum (arrow).

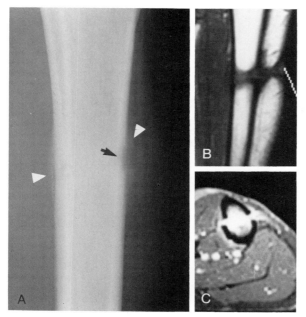

FIGURE 64–50. Postoperative infection: Pin tract. This 42 year old man developed drainage about one of the traction pins in the tibia used to treat a tibial plateau fracture. The pin was removed.

A Routine radiography shows an indistinct cortical hole (arrow) and periostitis (arrowheads).

B Coronal T1-weighted (TR/TE, 600/17) spin echo MR image reveals areas of low signal intensity in the tibia and soft tissue tract (marked with dotted line).

C Transaxial T1-weighted (TR/TE, 800/12) spin echo MR image obtained with fat saturation (ChemSat) after the intravenous injection of gadolinium contrast agent shows high signal intensity in the tibial marrow and soft tissues.

delay, this is not uniformly the case. Some persons with osteomyelitis do not receive early or adequate treatment, and in these patients, severe osteolysis may ensue.[124, 125] Large foci of destruction eventually can lead to disappearance of long segments of tubular or flat bones. Although institution of proper chemotherapeutic agents may reverse some of the deleterious effects of the infection, bizarre

deformity consisting of osteosclerosis and osteolysis may require courageous reconstructive procedures.[282]

Epiphyseal Growth Disturbance

In the infant, infection that has spread to the epiphysis of a tubular bone can produce significant damage.[126–128] Injury to the cartilage cells on the epiphyseal side of the growth plate is irreparable,[129] and subsequent growth disturbances are to be expected.[396] Even with severe epiphyseal disintegration, however, some regeneration of the epiphysis can occur after eradication of the infection (Fig. 64–52).[130, 131, 299, 566] Unfortunately, it is difficult to predict accurately the occurrence and extent of epiphyseal recovery after injury.[128] Thus, in all infants, the documentation of osteomyelitis with epiphyseal involvement must be accomplished at an early stage, so that prompt therapy is instituted and later complications, such as shortening of the limb and secondary degenerative arthritis, are avoided.

Neoplasm

Epidermoid carcinoma arising in a focus of chronic osteomyelitis is not uncommon[101] and may be evident in at least 0.5 per cent of patients with long-term draining infections of bone.[132, 540] Men are affected more frequently than women.[541] The latent period between the onset of osteomyelitis and the appearance of neoplasm is variable, although a time span of 20 to 30 years is typical. Neoplasm most frequently arises adjacent to the femur and the tibia, being evident clinically as pain, increasing drainage, onset of a foul odor from the sinus tract, a mass, and lymphadenopathy; and radiographically as progressive destruction of bone (Fig. 64–53).[397, 608]

An epidermoid carcinoma can develop at any site along the sinus tract, although it commonly is quite deep; the epithelial lining of the tract undergoes repeated degeneration because of the presence of pus within the sinus tract.[2] It is in this setting that malignant degeneration occurs. The prognosis is guarded, as distant metastasis is not infrequent, particularly in instances of poorly differentiated tumors.[608]

Although epithelial carcinoma is the most common neoplasm that is encountered in osteomyelitis,[132–138] fibro-

FIGURE 64–51. Postoperative infection: Pin tract. This 37 year old man developed pain and swelling about the left femur near the site of a previously removed femoral pin that had been used for halo-femoral traction prior to spinal manipulation. The opposite femur was affected similarly. Staphylococcus was the causative organism.

A A coronal T1-weighted (TR/TE, 900/20) spin echo MR image shows abnormal signal intensity in the marrow of the femur.

B On a transaxial T2-weighted (TR/TE, 2000/80) spin echo MR image, gross distortion of the soft tissues is evident. Note the infection, which is characterized by high signal intensity in the femur and adjacent soft tissues, particularly posteriorly.

(Courtesy of G. Greenway, M.D., Dallas, Texas.)

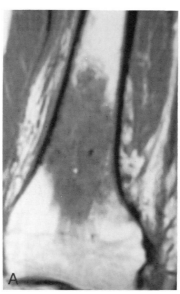

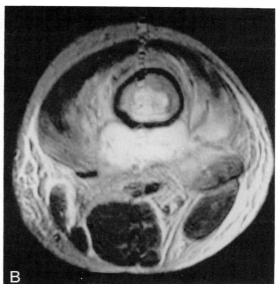

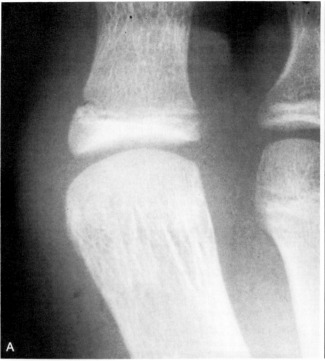

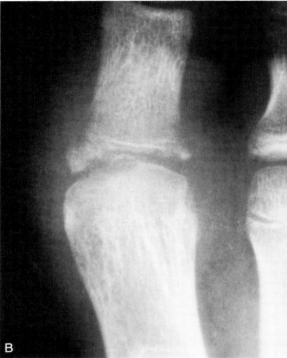

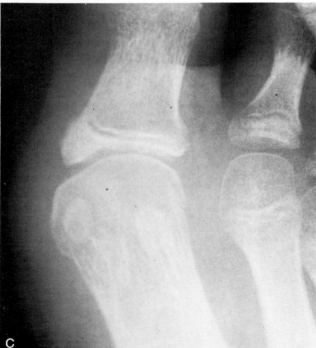

FIGURE 64–52. Complications of osteomyelitis: Epiphyseal destruction. This 11 year old boy developed osteomyelitis and septic arthritis of the first metatarsophalangeal joint.

A An initial film reveals metaphyseal irregularity, soft tissue swelling, and a radiodense epiphysis of the proximal phalanx.

B One week later, the epiphysis has fragmented and largely disappeared, and osteolysis of both the metatarsal bone and the phalanx can be noted. Joint space narrowing is seen.

C Four weeks later, reconstitution of the epiphysis is seen.

(Courtesy of T. Goergen, M.D., Escondido, California.)

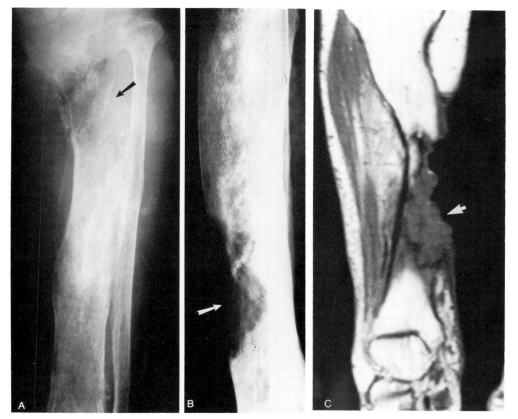

FIGURE 64–53. Complications of osteomyelitis: Neoplasm.

A Epidermoid carcinoma. This 63 year old man with chronic draining osteomyelitis developed a mass in the proximal portion of the tibia about a sinus tract. Superimposed on the radiographic changes of chronic infection of the tibia is a lytic lesion of the proximal aspect of the bone (arrow), which represented an epidermoid carcinoma invading the osseous tissue.

B Histiocytic lymphoma. In this patient with chronic osteomyelitis of the tibia, the area of osseous destruction (arrow) was related to a lymphoma.

C Epidermoid carcinoma. The tumor (arrow) is of low signal intensity and is invading the tibia, as shown in this coronal T1-weighted (TR/TE, 500/15) spin echo MR image.

(**C,** Courtesy of M. Schweitzer, M.D., Philadelphia, Pennsylvania.)

sarcoma,[133, 139, 140] angiosarcoma,[133] rhabdomyosarcoma,[133] histiocytic lymphoma, adenocarcinoma,[141] basal cell carcinoma,[142] and plasmacytoma,[143, 398, 609] also have been noted.[101] At times, the tissue consists of proliferative fibrous or granulation tissue and has been termed granulation tissue sarcoma.[144] Surgical manipulation at a site of osteomyelitis in an infant has been associated with the subsequent appearance of an osteochondroma.[399]

Amyloidosis

Secondary amyloidosis can complicate chronic osteomyelitis.[101] This complication has become less frequent, a fact that is attributable to improvement in the chemotherapy of infection. In studies of 105 cases of secondary amyloidosis, only five were associated with chronic osteomyelitis.[145–147]

Modifications and Difficulties in Diagnosis

Antibiotic Modified Osteomyelitis

The previous discussion has concerned itself with the radiologic and pathologic findings of untreated osteomyelitis. In the modern era of sophisticated chemotherapeutic techniques, the infective process often is interrupted at a relatively early stage. If therapy is adequate, complete healing of the osseous abnormalities can occur, although clinical improvement initially is not paralleled by radiographic improvement. During the early healing phase of osteomyelitis, bone resorption continues as damaged osseous tissue is removed. Thus, radiographically evident increased destruction can occur at a time when the clinical picture is improving. Knowledge of this phenomenon ensures that the clinician, alarmed at worsening radiographs, does not modify beneficial therapeutic regimens. Obviously, the patient, not the radiograph, must be treated. Soon the image, too, will reveal evidence of osseous reconstitution, and the benefits of therapy become equally obvious to both the clinician and the radiologist.

Inappropriate or inadequate chemotherapy can mask the clinical and radiographic manifestations of osteomyelitis for a period of time.[30] Most typically, acute lesions are obscured and the osteomyelitic process appears in a subacute or chronic form.

"Active" and "Inactive" Chronic Osteomyelitis

Although the radiographic features of chronic osteomyelitis are well established, differentiation of active and inactive chronic osteomyelitis by imaging techniques can be extremely difficult (Table 64–5). The extensive osteolytic and osteosclerotic changes of a chronic osteomyelitic proc-

TABLE 64–5. Radiographic Signs of Activity in Chronic Osteomyelitis

Change from previous radiograph
Poorly defined areas of osteolysis
Thin, linear periostitis
Sequestration

ess that is dormant can obscure the changes of reactivation for a period of time. Other diagnostic methods, such as magnification radiography, MR imaging, or radionuclide examination using technetium and gallium pharmaceuticals, can be helpful in this setting (see discussion later in this chapter). Certain indications on the radiograph may aid in the differentiation of active and inactive chronic osteomyelitis, however. In cases of active infection, comparison with earlier available radiographs can detect a changing pattern or image that is characterized by new areas of destruction. Periostitis that is thin and linear in quality and separated from the subjacent bone suggests activity. Furthermore, poorly defined or fluffy periosteal excrescences extending into the adjacent soft tissues also suggest active infection (Fig. 64–54). Finally, the documentation of sequestration on routine radiography, on conventional tomography or CT scanning, or with MR imaging implies activity, as necrotic osseous fragments commonly harbor viable organisms.[610]

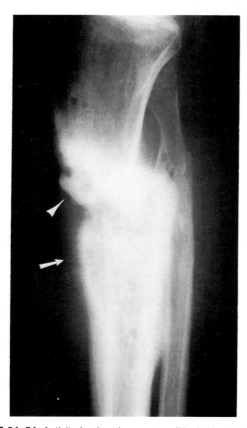

FIGURE 64–54. Activity in chronic osteomyelitis. In this patient with chronic osteomyelitis, the presence of poorly defined destruction, fluffy periostitis (arrow), and a sequestrum (arrowhead) indicates activity.

Differential Diagnosis

General Features

The combination of clinical and imaging characteristics in osteomyelitis usually ensures correct diagnosis. Occasionally, aggressive bone destruction combined with periostitis and soft tissue swelling simulates the changes in malignant neoplasms, especially Ewing's sarcoma or osteosarcoma in the child, histiocytic lymphoma in the young adult, and skeletal metastasis in the older person. In aggressive neoplastic disorders and in infection, the pattern of osseous destruction is of motheaten appearance or permeative nature: The area of abnormality is not clearly separated or marginated from the adjacent normal bone; rather, the marginal characteristics of the lesion(s) are poorly defined and the zone of transition from normal to abnormal bone extends over a relatively long distance. With very aggressive behavior, the lesion(s) may merge imperceptibly with the surrounding bony tissue.

Periostitis

The nature of the periosteal proliferation accompanying osteomyelitis is varied. In some patients, single or multiple osseous shells appear about the parent bone and later merge with it. This "onion-skinning" is not specific for osteomyelitis, as it also may be evident in malignant neoplasm, such as Ewing's sarcoma. A triangular area (Codman's triangle) of periostitis similar to that in osteosarcoma may be evident in osteomyelitis. In cases of osteomyelitis in which a single thick layer of periosteal bone is seen, the changes are reminiscent of eosinophilic granuloma or traumatic periostitis.

Osteolytic Foci

The identification in a child of a metaphyseal radiolucent lesion abutting on the growth plate or connecting with it by a channel certainly suggests the presence of an abscess. In these instances, the lucent focus is surrounded by sclerotic bone and may be accompanied by periostitis. Although osteosarcoma typically is metaphyseal in location and Ewing's sarcoma may be metaphyseal, the osteolytic foci in these tumors are more poorly marginated, and with osteosarcoma considerable neoplastic bone production may be evident. In an adult, osteolytic foci within an infected epiphysis can simulate the appearance of a giant cell tumor, clear cell chondrosarcoma, osteonecrosis, fibrous dysplasia, intraosseous ganglion, or subchondral cyst. In a child, epiphyseal infection with abscess formation leads to radiographic features similar to those of chondroblastoma, enchondroma, or eosinophilic granuloma.

Cortical lucent lesions can indicate an abscess, osteoid osteoma, or stress fracture. The nature of the lesion and the surrounding bony eburnation generally allows differentiation among these conditions (see earlier discussion).

Osteosclerosis

In some cases of osteomyelitis, exuberant bone formation produces widespread sclerosis. This may be of uniform quality or combined with mottled radiolucent shadows. The resulting radiographic picture can simulate malignant bone tumors (such as osteosarcoma, Ewing's sarcoma, histiocytic lymphoma, and chondrosarcoma), osteonecrosis, fibrous dysplasia, or Paget's disease. If the abnormal area does not extend down to the subchondral bone of an epiphysis in a tubular bone, the diagnosis of Paget's disease generally can be eliminated. The absence of large lytic areas, cortical disruption, soft tissue masses, and visible tumor matrix militates against the diagnosis of sarcomas.

Sequestration

Radiodense foci representing sequestra are reliable indicators of infection. Their occasional appearance in tumors (e.g., fibrosarcoma) does not significantly diminish the diagnostic nature of the finding.[591]

Soft Tissue Masses and Swelling

Soft tissue prominence is a common finding in infectious and neoplastic conditions. In general, tumors are associated with circumscribed soft tissue masses that displace surrounding soft tissue planes and frequently contain visible tumor matrix. Infections lead to infiltration and obscuring of soft tissue planes. This differentiation is not uniformly reliable.

Soft tissue infections or neoplasms can infiltrate subjacent osseous tissue. The pattern of cortical and medullary destruction and associated periostitis accompanying the process usually is not specific enough to allow a single diagnosis.

SEPTIC ARTHRITIS

Articular Manifestations of Infection

As is discussed in Chapter 31, septic arthritis is but one of several processes that can cause or perpetuate articular disease in patients with infection. An infectious agent may trigger a sterile synovitis at a site distant from the primary infective focus, as the joint reacts to its presence in the form of an inflammatory, hypersensitivity, or immune-mediated response.[400] Classic examples of reactive arthritis include acute rheumatic fever occurring as a complication of streptococcal throat infection, Reiter's syndrome, intestinal bypass surgery, and hepatitis.[403] Although the mechanism leading to reactive arthritis is not clear and probably depends on the specific underlying disease, experimental evidence supports the role of nonviable bacterial components in the development of acute and chronic arthritis.[400] When injected systemically or in the joints of laboratory animals, certain bacterial wall antigens, such as peptidoglycan, cause arthritis.[401, 402] An immune-mediated or hypersensitivity reaction to a cell wall component that persists within a joint or in the circulation could explain the occurrence of sterile synovitis in patients with various bacterial and nonbacterial infections, including gonococcal infection. In the latter disorder, failure to recover *Neisseria gonorrhoeae* from the skin, joint, and blood of patients with disseminated disease is well known and further supports the role of nonviable bacterial components.[400]

Clinical characteristics common to reactive arthritides include a symptom-free interval (generally 2 to 3 weeks) between the inciting infection and the rheumatic reaction; a self-limited course in which cartilage or bone destruction is rare; a characteristic clinical presentation that includes acute migratory polyarthritis, especially of large joints, such as

the knees and ankles, fever, and an elevated erythrocyte sedimentation rate; a tendency in some patients toward involvement of the heart; and a negative serologic test for rheumatoid factor.[404] Inciting infections commonly reach the body through one of three portals of entry: the oronasopharynx and respiratory tract, the urogenital tract, and the intestinal tract.[404] The infections themselves may be entirely asymptomatic, the major clinical manifestations relating to the reaction of distant organs and sites to the infecting agent.

The existence of reactive arthritis in patients with infection underscores the importance of joint aspiration and attempts at isolation of the causative organisms in all cases of suspected septic arthritis. Such attempts are not uniformly successful; the reported frequency of negative cultures of synovial fluid in patients with "septic" arthritis is as high as 75 per cent, and the success of the procedure is related, in part, to the patient's age and the specific infection that is present.[405] For example, in disseminated gonococcal infection, cultures of synovial fluid as well as blood may be negative in as many as 75 to 80 per cent of cases,[406, 407] again lending support to the presence of joint reaction rather than infection in many of these cases. Furthermore, successful recovery of an infecting organism depends on inoculation of the specimen into the proper culture medium and examination of a gram-stained smear.[408] In some cases, such as those with granulomatous synovitis related to tuberculosis or fungal disease, biopsy and culture of the synovial membrane may be required.

Even when infection of the musculoskeletal system has been well documented, the cause of an accompanying inflamed joint may relate not to a septic arthritis but to a sympathetic joint effusion. Sterile synovial reaction to osteomyelitis in an adjacent bone[409, 410] or to nearby septic arthritis[411] or septic bursitis[542] has been recorded, although in the first situation, the vascular continuity that exists between the epiphysis and the synovial membrane can explain the occurrence of septic arthritis in cases of osteomyelitis even when the synovial fluid is sterile.[8]

Routes of Contamination

The potential routes of contamination of joints can be divided into the same categories as were used in the previous discussion of osteomyelitis (Figs. 64–55 and 64–56).

1. Hematogenous spread of infection. Hematogenous seeding of the synovial membrane is due to either direct transport of organisms within the synovial vessels or spread from an adjacent epiphyseal focus of osteomyelitis by means of vascular continuity between the epiphysis and the synovial membrane.[8]

2. Spread from a contiguous source of infection. A joint may become contaminated by intra-articular extension of osteomyelitis from an epiphyseal or metaphyseal focus, or of neighboring suppurative soft tissue processes.

3. Direct implantation. Inoculation of a joint can occur during aspiration or arthrography or after a penetrating wound.

4. Postoperative infection. An intra-articular suppurative process can occur after arthroscopy or any other type of joint surgery.

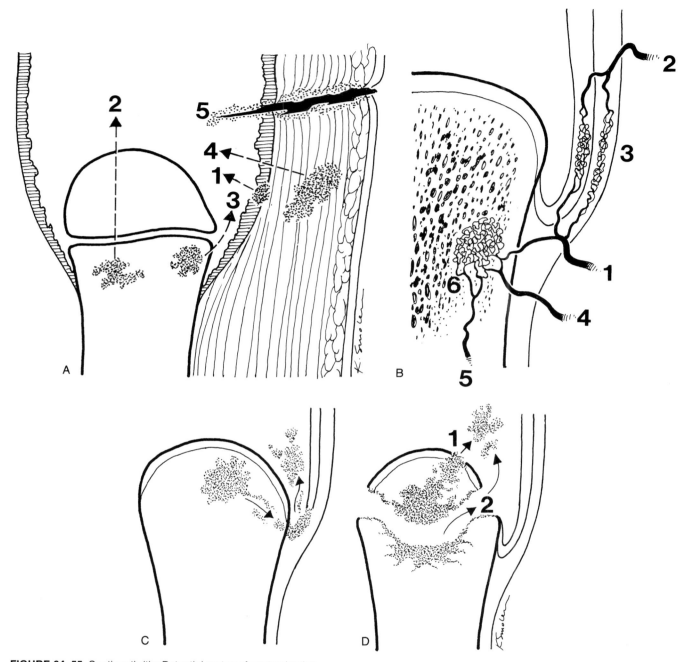

FIGURE 64–55. Septic arthritis: Potential routes of contamination.

  A Hematogenous spread of infection to a joint can result from direct lodgment of organisms in the synovial membrane (1) or, as illustrated in **B,** direct vascular continuity between an infected epiphysis and the synovial membrane. Spread into the joint from a contiguous source can occur from a metaphyseal focus that extends into the epiphysis and from there into the joint (2); from a metaphyseal focus with extension into the joint when the growth plate is intra-articular (3); or from a contiguous soft tissue infection (4). Direct implantation after a penetrating wound (5) also can lead to septic arthritis.

  B, C Hematogenous spread of infection to a joint can occur owing to vascular continuity between the epiphysis and synovial membrane. In **B** the vessels shown include arterioles (1), venules (2), and capillaries (3) of the capsule, periosteal vessels (4), the nutrient artery (5), and metaphyseal-epiphyseal anastomoses (6). In this fashion, the synovial membrane may become infected from an osseous focus before the joint fluid is contaminated. In **C,** this sequence of events is diagrammed.

  D Spread from a contiguous osseous surface can result from penetration of the cartilage (1) or pathologic fracture with articular contamination (2). In this situation, synovial fluid may become infected before the synovial membrane.

Hematogenous Spread of Infection

Pathogenesis

Hematogenous spread of infection to a joint indicates that organisms are transported within the vasculature of the synovial membrane directly from a distant infected source or indirectly from an adjacent bone infection.[557] In either case, infection of the synovial membrane precedes contamination of the synovial fluid.[8, 300] Thus, initial arthrocentesis may suggest bland inflammation of the joint. Lodgment of organisms (bacteria) in the synovial membrane has been documented experimentally after their intravenous injection; similar studies have indicated that living bacteria obtain access to synovial fluid more readily than to spinal fluid, aqueous humor, or urine.[148]

The reaction of the synovial tissue to the contained organisms varies according to the local and general resistance of the patient and the number, type, and virulence of the infecting agents. Thus, in some cases of infective arthritis, a limited and locally confined reaction of the synovial membrane is encountered; in other cases, severe tissue inflammation is seen. Although the precise pathogenesis of subsequent injury to intra-articular structures is not known, the appearance of fibrin deposition in septic arthritis may be important in this regard.[149] Fibrin deposits adherent to articular cartilage could interfere with proper cartilaginous nutrition from the adjacent synovial fluid and also could impede the release of metabolic products from the cartilage.[148] Fibrin possibly could attract leukocytes chemotactically; these cells phagocytize fibrin, and degranulation of the leukocytes and release of enzymes into the synovial fluid may accentuate the intra-articular inflammatory process.[148] If this mechanism indeed is operational, the elimination of fibrin clots through surgical drainage may afford some control over the extent of joint destruction.

As collagenase appears to be important in the pathogenesis of cartilage destruction in rheumatoid arthritis, this substance also may be important in the chondrolysis of infective arthritis.[150] Enzymatic release by the lysosomes in the leukocytes probably is important in cartilaginous injury in septic arthritis.[148] The possibility that additional abnormalities in this process also result from an autoimmune response to damaged cartilage has been suggested.[151] The extent of articular destruction accompanying infective arthritis, whatever its pathogenesis, is influenced by the defense mechanisms of the host. Elderly patients, patients with serious chronic illnesses, patients who are receiving immunosuppressive therapy, and those with preexisting joint diseases have an increased frequency of articular infection.[152, 153]

The reader also should refer to Chapter 23 for further details regarding enzymatic destruction of cartilage in septic arthritis.

General Clinical Features

Septic arthritis affects men and women of all ages, although it predominates in the young.[154–156, 296, 611, 612] Monoarticular involvement is the major pattern of presentation, especially in the younger age groups, although polyarticular localization occurs in approximately 20 per cent of cases,[613, 745] particularly in patients with rheumatoid arthritis. The specific site(s) of infection depend on the age of the patient, the organism, and the existence of an underlying disease or problem. The knee, particularly in children, infants, and adults,[152, 153, 612] and the hip, especially in children and infants,[157–160, 614] frequently are affected. With pyogenic infection, an acute onset with fever and chills is typical, although a prodromal phase of several days' duration with malaise, arthralgia, and low grade fever can be encountered.[161, 615] Pain, tenderness, redness, heat, and soft tissue swelling of the involved joint are common. Leukocytosis and positive blood and joint cultures are important laboratory parameters of pyogenic arthritis. The bacteria most commonly implicated are *Staphylococcus aureus*[408]; others include alpha- and beta-hemolytic streptococci, pneumococci, Haemophilus, Pseudomonas, gonococcus, *Escherichia coli,* and Serratia. Mycobacterial and fungal agents also may be implicated.

Haemophilus influenzae represents an important and common cause of septic arthritis in children less than 5 years of age.[612] In neonates and in infants less than 6 months old, *Haemophilus influenzae* articular infection is reported to be uncommon, however. Infectious arthritis in neonates is caused by the bacteria frequently associated with sepsis: staphylococci, group B streptococci, and Enterobacteriaceae.[616] In older children, gram-positive cocci (staphylococci and streptococci) predominate as the cause of joint infections. In adults, a similar pattern is seen, although septic arthritis related to gram-negative bacilli, anaerobes, and multiple microorganisms appears to be increasing in frequency.[616] In elderly patients with septic arthritis, *Staphylococcus aureus* and streptococci are implicated most frequently.[611] In patients with polyarticular involvement, an increased association with pneumococcal, group G streptococcal, and *Haemophilus influenzae* microorganisms has been noted.[613]

In addition to age, other factors may predispose to articular infection with specific pathogens.[616] Examples include *Staphylococcus aureus, Pseudomonas aeruginosa,* and *Serratia marcescens* infections in the parenteral drug abusers; opportunistic pathogens such as *Staphylococcus epidermidis* causing joint sepsis as a complication of catheter-associated bacteremia; and anaerobic bacterial infections of joints as a complication of traumatic injuries and elective musculoskeletal surgery.

Radiographic-Pathologic Correlation (Table 64–6)

In response to bacterial infection, the synovial membrane becomes edematous, swollen, and hypertrophied.[2, 162, 163] In-

TABLE 64–6. Septic Arthritis: Radiographic-Pathologic Correlation

Pathologic Abnormality	Radiographic Abnormality
Edema and hypertrophy of synovial membrane with fluid production	Joint effusion, soft tissue swelling
Hyperemia	Osteoporosis
Inflammatory pannus with chondral destruction	Joint space loss
Pannus destruction of bone	Marginal and central osseous erosion
Fibrous or bony ankylosis	Bony ankylosis

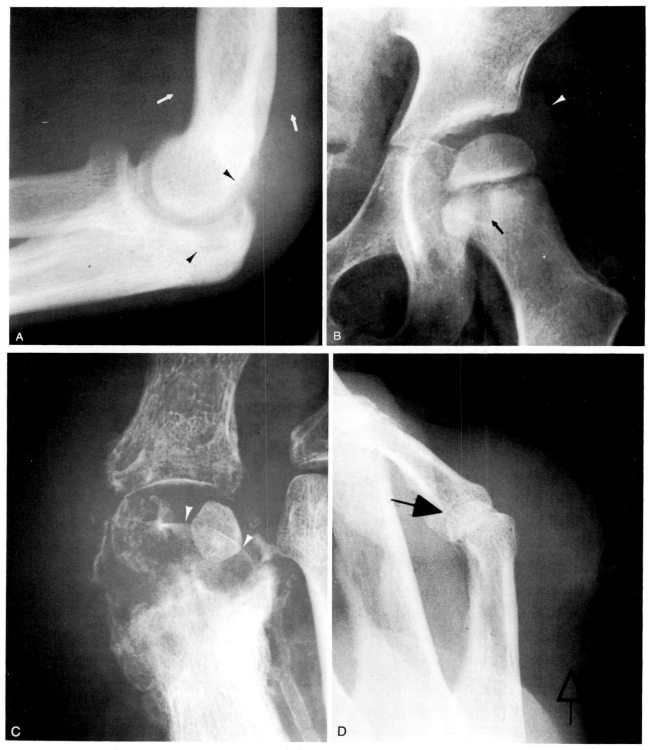

FIGURE 64–56. Septic arthritis: Potential routes of contamination.

A Hematogenous spread of infection. Septic arthritis in this patient was related to implantation of organisms into the synovial membrane. An effusion with elevation of the fat pads (arrows) was evident long before osseous involvement occurred (arrowheads).

B Spread from a contiguous metaphyseal focus in a child. In the hip, the growth plate is an intra-articular structure. Thus, an osteomyelitic focus in the metaphysis (arrow) can lead to joint contamination, with widening of the articular space and soft tissue swelling (arrowhead).

C Spread from a contiguous epiphyseal focus in an adult. Osteomyelitis of the first metatarsal bone in this diabetic patient preceded the occurrence of joint infection. Note the collapse of the articular surface with depression of the subchondral bone (arrowheads), allowing contamination of the joint contents.

D Spread from a contiguous soft tissue infection. An infection in soft tissue (open arrows) after an injury led to contamination of the proximal interphalangeal joint of the fifth finger with bony erosion and joint space narrowing (solid arrow).

Illustration continued on opposite page

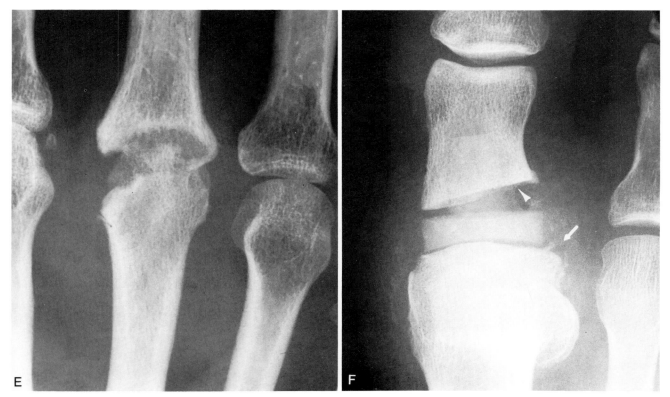

FIGURE 64–56 *Continued*

E Direct implantation of organisms in a metacarpophalangeal joint after a fist-fight in which the opponent's tooth penetrated the articulation. Observe soft tissue swelling, joint space narrowing, and poorly defined destruction of bone.

F Postoperative infection. After the placement of a phalangeal prosthesis for degenerative joint disease, infection developed that required the removal of the prosthesis. Note soft tissue swelling and mild osseous erosion and fragmentation (arrow). Resorption of a small part of the phalangeal surface also is evident (arrowhead).

creased amounts of synovial fluid are produced; the fluid may be thin and cloudy, contain large numbers of leukocytes, and reveal a lowered sugar level and elevated protein count. After a few days, frank pus accumulates in the articular cavity and destruction of cartilage begins[35] (Fig.

64–57). The early site of cartilaginous change varies. Prominent abnormality may appear at the margins or central portions of joints, accompanied by growth of the inflamed synovium across the surface of the cartilage or between cartilage and bone. Even or uneven cartilaginous erosion

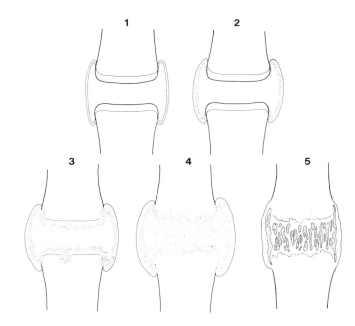

FIGURE 64–57. Septic arthritis: Pathologic abnormalities. 1, Normal synovial joint; 2, an edematous swollen and hypertrophic synovial membrane becomes evident; 3, 4, accumulating inflammatory pannus leads to chondral destruction and to marginal and central osseous erosions; 5, bony ankylosis eventually can result.

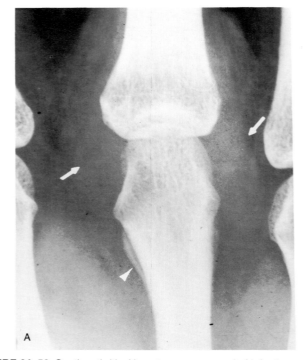 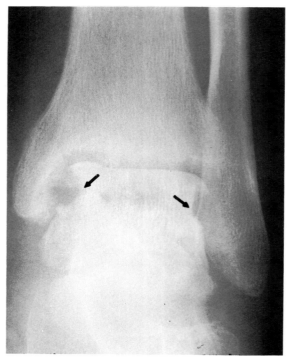

FIGURE 64–58. Septic arthritis: Hematogenous spread of infection.
A Metacarpophalangeal joint. A low KV radiograph of an infected metacarpophalangeal joint demonstrates soft tissue edema (arrows), osteoporosis, and periostitis (arrowhead).
B Ankle. A radiograph reveals joint space narrowing and osseous erosions, which predominate at the margins of the talus (arrows).
(**A,** Courtesy of J. Weston, M.D., Lower Hutt, New Zealand.)

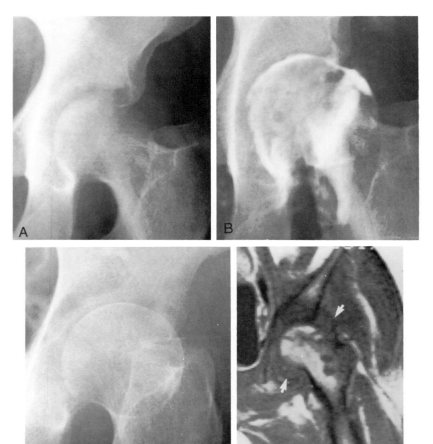

FIGURE 64–59. Septic arthritis: Hematogenous spread of infection.

A, B Hip. The routine radiograph **(A)** shows osteopenia, loss of the subchondral bone plate in the femoral head, and mild joint space loss. Arthrography **(B)** confirms cartilage loss and irregularity of the contrast material consistent with synovial proliferation.

C, D Hip. The routine radiograph **(C)** reveals osteopenia and joint space loss. A coronal T1-weighted (TR/TE, 500/20) spin echo MR image **(D)** shows low signal intensity in portions of the marrow in the acetabulum and proximal femur, a joint effusion (arrows), and possible osteonecrosis in the femoral head.

(**C, D,** Courtesy of R. Stiles, M.D., Atlanta, Georgia.)

(from superficially located pannus) and disruption or separation (from subchondral pannus) can develop. With further accumulation of hypertrophied synovium and fluid, the capsule becomes distended, surrounding soft tissue edema is evident, and osseous abnormalities ensue. Superficial marginal and central bony erosions may progress to extensive destruction of large segments of the articular surface. Fibrous or bony ankylosis eventually can occur.

Radiographic abnormalities parallel the pathologic changes in pyogenic arthritis[164, 558] (Figs. 64–58 and 64–59). Radiographically evident soft tissue swelling accompanies synovial hypertrophy. Interosseous space narrowing, which frequently is diffuse, reflects damage and disruption of the chondral surface. Osseous erosions at the edges of the joint, related to the effects of diseased synovium on bone, lead to marginal defects that are similar in appearance and location to those of rheumatoid arthritis. They predominate at the unprotected osseous surfaces that do not possess cartilaginous coats at the periphery of the joint. Subchondral extension of pannus destroys the bone plate and adjacent trabeculae, leading to poorly defined gaps in the subchondral "white" line on the radiograph. Further destruction of bone becomes evident and, in late stages, bony ankylosis of the joint may be seen.

These pathologic and radiographic abnormalities are modified in accordance with the infecting organism. Rapid destruction of bone and cartilage is characteristic of bacterial arthritis, whereas in tuberculosis and fungal diseases, articular changes occur more slowly. In tuberculosis, marginal osseous erosions with preservation of joint space and periarticular osteoporosis can be prominent. Pathologically, in this disease, subchondral extension of pannus, masslike intra-articular protrusion of granulation tissue, and fibrous ankylosis, rather than bony ankylosis, can be evident.[2]

In all varieties of septic arthritis, involvement of adjacent osseous structures produces typical features of osteomyelitis. Poorly defined motheaten bony destruction and periostitis are seen. In some instances of pyogenic arthritis, calcification in and around the joint is observed.[165, 166] These deposits are more common in those patients with severe and lengthy illness, occur after a period of 4 to 12 weeks, and probably are related to dystrophic calcification in association with rupture of the joint capsule and extension of the infection into the adjacent soft tissue. They have been produced in experimental joint infections.[167, 168] In humans, soft tissue calcification may be responsible for residual pain owing to local mechanical factors.

Rarely, gas formation within a joint can complicate septic arthritis due to *Escherichia coli, Serratia (Enterobacter) liquefaciens,* streptococci, and *Clostridium perfringens*[169–174, 414–416] (Fig. 64–60). Gas formation can occur from infection by obligate anaerobes (Bacteroides, Clostridium, Fusobacterium, and Peptococcus) or by facultative organisms capable of growth in either aerobic or anaerobic environments (Enterobacteriaceae such as *Escherichia coli* and Serratia).[416] Much more frequently, the appearance of radiolucent collections in an infected joint indicates that a prior arthrocentesis has been performed or that an open wound exists with communication between the joint and the skin surface.

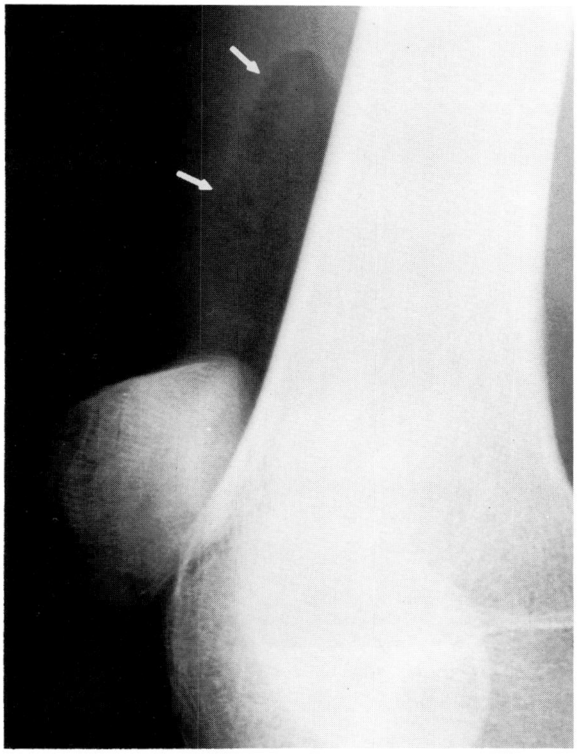

Spread from a Contiguous Source of Infection

Pathogenesis

In certain age groups, osteomyelitis can be complicated by contamination of the adjacent articulation. In the infant the presence of vascular communication between metaphyseal and epiphyseal segments of tubular bones allows organisms within nutrient vessels to localize in the epiphysis and subsequently extend into the joint. This may occur via the common vascular pathways of the epiphysis and synovial membrane (hematogenous spread of infection) or as a result of transchondral extension directly into the articular cavity (spread from a contiguous source). In the latter situation, radiographic evidence of osteomyelitis generally precedes that of articular infection. In the adult, vascular connections between the epiphysis and metaphysis are reestablished as the growth plate closes. Hematogenous osteomyelitis thus can affect the epiphysis in this age group. Once again, subsequent joint contamination can occur via hematogenous pathways or through disruption of the chondral surface.

A second situation in which septic arthritis can occur as a result of contamination from a contiguous source is related to adjacent soft tissue infection or, more rarely, nearby visceral infection (e.g., vesicoacetabular or enteroacetabular fistulae)[175, 297, 417–420, 617] (Figs. 64–61 and 64–62). In these instances, the organisms first are evident in periarticular locations and only later penetrate the capsule to enter the synovial membrane and articular cavity. Predisposing factors include pelvic trauma, surgical manipulation, and diverticulitis.

FIGURE 64–60. Septic arthritis: Intra-articular gas formation. *Escherichia coli* pyogenic arthritis rarely can lead to intra-articular "bubbly" collections of gas (arrows). Much more frequently, radiolucent collections within the joint relate to air introduced during arthrocentesis or by means of a tract that communicates with the skin.

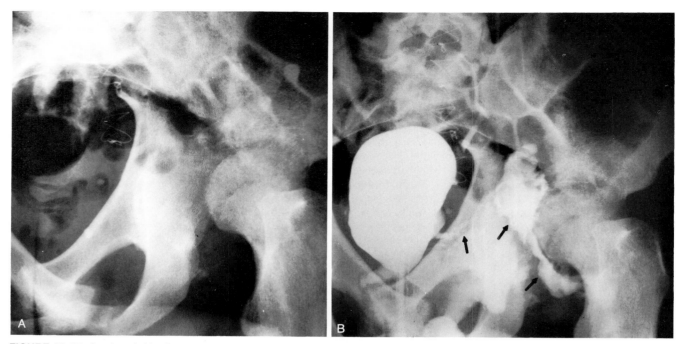

FIGURE 64–61. Septic arthritis: Contamination from a contiguous source of infection. During an automobile accident, this patient sustained pelvic trauma resulting in fractures and injury to the bladder.

A Radiograph reveals, in addition to the obvious comminuted fractures of the pelvis, a poorly defined osteoporotic femoral head.

B Cystogram after an intravenous pyelogram demonstrates communication between the bladder and the hip, with accumulation of contrast material in the joint (arrows).

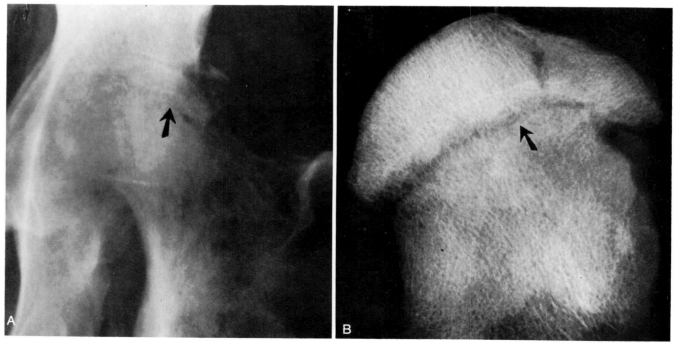

FIGURE 64–62. Septic arthritis: Contamination from a contiguous source of infection. This 43 year old man with rheumatoid arthritis had undergone a laparotomy and bowel resection with a colostomy for sigmoid diverticulitis. A tract developed between the bowel, left hip, and skin, which was related to *Escherichia coli* infection.

A Radiograph of the hip outlines the narrowed joint space and bony destruction. A radiolucent line can be seen in the femoral head (arrow).

B After a modified Girdlestone procedure, a radiograph of the removed femoral head allows identification of the osseous destruction and fracture line (arrow).

(From Resnick D: Radiology *114*:581, 1975.)

A third situation in which joint infection develops as a result of extension from a surrounding suppurative process occurs in those locations in which the growth plate has an intra-articular location; the most important such sites are the hip and the glenohumeral joint.[421] Because of this anatomic arrangement, osteomyelitis localized to the metaphysis can enter the joint by extending laterally without violating the growth plate. With penetration of the thin metaphyseal cortex, organisms can extend directly into the synovium or the articular cavity. Another mechanism by which a metaphyseal infection can reach a joint relates to cortical violation and subsequent contamination of an extra-articular tendon that along its course becomes located within the joint; as an example of this, a metaphyseal infection of the proximal portion of the humerus spreading through the adjacent cortex can contaminate the glenohumeral joint by extending along the tendon of the long head of the biceps brachii muscle.[618]

Radiographic-Pathologic Correlation

Generally, radiographic evidence exists that the infective process originates outside the articulation. This evidence may include soft tissue deficit, swelling, or gas formation; osteomyelitis with typical epiphyseal or metaphyseal destruction; and diverticulitis or cystitis with fistulization, detected on appropriate contrast examination. In certain situations, however, joint effusion and cartilaginous and subchondral osseous destruction are the first radiographic clues to infection; radiographic abnormalities in the adjacent structures may be subtle or absent entirely. In the infant in whom the epiphysis is unossified or only partially ossified, detection of primary osteomyelitis can be extremely difficult, and an enlarging effusion, displacement or subluxation of the ossified epiphyseal nucleus, or blurring of the subchondral white line in the opposite bone (e.g., acetabulum) may be the first evidence of sepsis. In the adult with diabetes mellitus, joint space narrowing or marginal and central osseous erosion of the metatarsophalangeal or interphalangeal joint may alert the physician to a clinically unsuspected septic arthritis.

Once the articulation has been violated, the radiographic and pathologic abnormalities of the infection are virtually identical to those associated with hematogenously derived suppurative joint disease. Soft tissue swelling, diffuse loss of joint space, poorly defined marginal and central osseous defects, periostitis, fragmentation, and calcification can be observed. In some cases, fistulography or sinography with retrograde injection of contrast material will opacify the joint, providing definite evidence of communication of the joint and overlying skin surfaces or viscera. CT and MR imaging also can be used for this purpose.

Specific Entities

Septic Arthritis of the Hip in Infancy and Childhood. Although additional mechanisms of hip infection in infants and children can include hematogenous seeding of the synovium and direct implantation following needle puncture when drawing blood from the femoral vessels,[176–178] the spread of infection into the hip from a metaphyseal (or epiphyseal) focus is well known, common, and of such importance that it deserves special emphasis.[159, 179–185]

Neonatal septic arthritis was first documented by Smith in 1874.[186] The hip is the joint affected most frequently,

and *Staphylococcus aureus* is the organism most commonly implicated. In this age group, infection can reach the hip by spreading from a metaphyseal focus of osteomyelitis either directly into the joint (the growth plate is intra-articular) or to the epiphysis by way of vascular channels that cross the growth plate, and, from there, into the articulation. Clinically, infants with septic arthritis of the hip may reveal irritability, loss of appetite, and fever.[413] Local symptoms and signs may be absent or minimal, complicating accurate diagnosis, although swelling in the thigh and a hip held in flexion, abduction, and external rotation are helpful clues.[187, 614] Initial radiographs of the hip frequently are unremarkable. Soft tissue or capsular swelling[188] and a positive obturator sign[189] are not readily apparent on neonatal radiographs, although the findings, when present, may be more reliable in this age group than in adults[190, 298] (Fig. 64–63). With accumulation of intra-articular fluid, pathologic subluxation or dislocation of the femoral head can occur,[191, 413] although the lack of ossification in most of the proximal capital femoral epiphysis makes this sign difficult to apply (Fig. 64–64). Helpful, however, is radiographically detectable osteomyelitis of the femoral metaphysis manifested as osteolysis, osteosclerosis, or periostitis.

The radiographic findings of hip infection in infants can simulate those accompanying other conditions. Displacement of the femoral head or metaphysis occurs in infants with developmental dysplasia of the hip, neurologic deficits, and traumatic epiphyseal separations. Thus, aspiration of the joint is mandatory in firmly establishing the diagnosis of septic arthritis as well as in providing guidelines for adequate therapy. Appropriate antibiotic administration combined with repeated aspiration or surgical drainage, or both, applied at an early stage of the septic process will diminish the likelihood of subsequent destruction of the cartilaginous femoral head and acetabulum. Only as the child develops and ossification of the immature skeleton proceeds will the degree of residual deformity become apparent (Fig. 64–65). Such deformities may include coxa magna, complete dissolution of the femoral head and neck with the lesser trochanter articulating with the acetabulum, or persistent dislocation of the femoral head or femoral shaft.[185, 324, 422, 619]

Septic arthritis of the hip also is frequent in the child, although the overall frequency of this problem and its devastating effects on local cartilage and bone are less prominent in children than in neonates. Furthermore, in the child, septic arthritis of the hip resulting from contamination by an adjacent focus of osteomyelitis is not so common as in the infant; the vascular channels that extend across the growth plate from metaphysis to epiphysis in the infant largely have become obliterated, and the increased cortical thickness of the child's metaphysis over that in the neonate may provide increased resistance to intra-articular spread from a metaphyseal infection.[22] A childhood hip infection may be associated with the acute onset of fever, pain, swelling, and limping, as well as with dramatic leukocytosis. On radiographs, accumulation of intra-articular fluid may produce soft tissue swelling, capsular distention, and subtle lateral displacement of the ossified epiphysis (Fig. 64–66). Recognition of this last finding is facilitated by comparison radiographs of the opposite hip. Concentric loss of joint space, subchondral osseous defects, and lytic foci of the femoral metaphysis can be evident.[192] Although the radio-

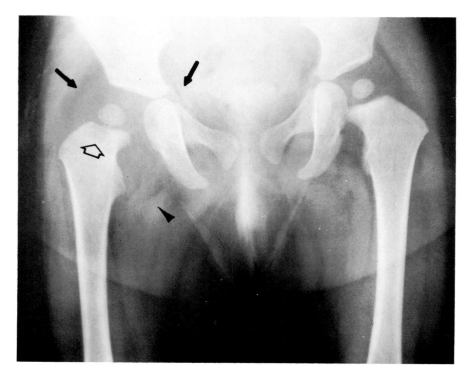

FIGURE 64–63. Septic arthritis of the hip: Infancy. This infant developed septic arthritis of the right hip and osteomyelitis. Note displacement of the "capsular" and obturator fat planes (solid arrows), obliteration of the iliopsoas fat plane (arrowhead), and a metaphyseal focus of infection (open arrow). The femoral head is displaced laterally and is enlarged slightly. The soft tissue findings indicative of intra-articular fluid may be more helpful in diagnosis in this age group than in adults. (Courtesy of J. Weston, M.D., Lower Hutt, New Zealand.)

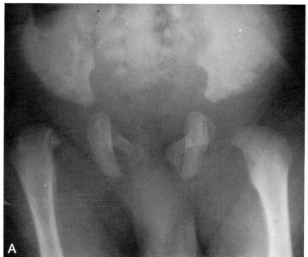

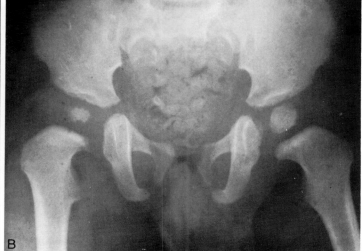

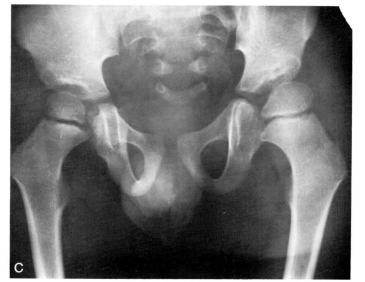

FIGURE 64–64. Septic arthritis of the hip: A 21 day old infant developed bilateral septic arthritis of the hips.

A The right hip is subluxated laterally and periosteal reaction is evident along the proximal portion of the femur. The left hip shows minimal lateral displacement.

B At 13 months of age, both hips are well located in the acetabulum. The left acetabulum is shallow, and the left epiphyseal ossification center is larger.

C At 3½ years of age, the right femoral head is small, and coxa magna is present on the left side. The shallow left acetabulum again is seen.

(Reproduced with permission from Freiberger RH, et al: Hip disease of infancy and childhood. In RD Moseley Jr et al (Eds): Current Problems in Radiology. Copyright 1973 by Year Book Medical Publishers, Inc, Chicago.)

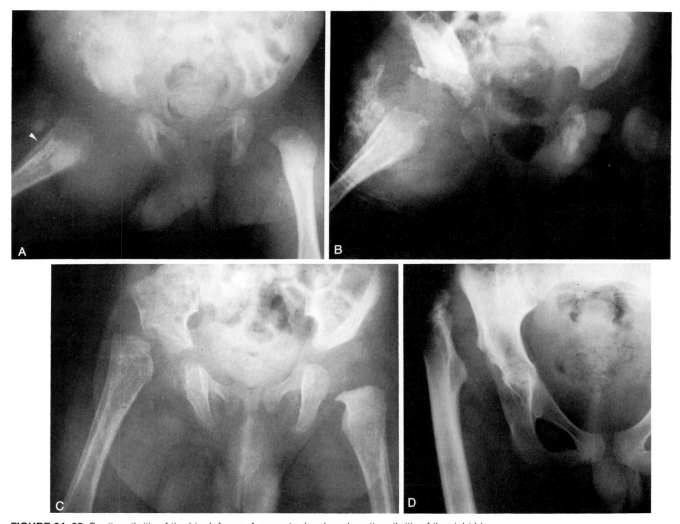

FIGURE 64–65. Septic arthritis of the hip: Infancy. A neonate developed septic arthritis of the right hip.
 A An initial radiograph reveals soft tissue swelling and periosteal reaction along the femur (arrowhead).
 B Two weeks later, extensive periosteal reaction and soft tissue ossification are evident.
 C At 2 months of age, superior subluxation of the femur is seen.
 D At age 13 years, the ossification centers of the greater and lesser trochanters are apparent. Femoral dislocation, acetabular shallowness, and absence of epiphyseal ossification are evident.
 (Reproduced with permission from Freiberger RH, et al: Hip disease of infancy and childhood. *In* RD Moseley Jr et al (Eds): Current Problems in Radiology. Copyright 1973 by Year Book Medical Publishers, Inc, Chicago.)

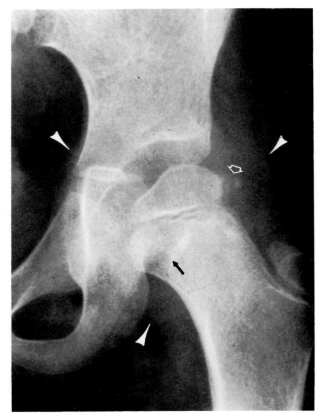

FIGURE 64–66. Septic arthritis of the hip: Childhood. Septic arthritis complicated metaphyseal osteomyelitis in this child. Observe osseous destruction (solid arrow), soft tissue swelling with displacement of fat planes (arrowheads), widening of the joint space due to lateral subluxation of the femoral head, and periarticular calcification or ossification (open arrow).

graphs eventually are quite diagnostic of infection, initial abnormalities may be mistaken for those associated with juvenile chronic arthritis or Legg-Calvé-Perthes disease.[185] Joint aspiration is mandatory for definite diagnosis and appropriate treatment. The prognosis of septic arthritis of the hip for a child is far better than that for an infant, although growth disturbances (coxa vara or coxa valga, leg shortening or overgrowth),[193] fibrous or bony intra-articular ankylosis, and osteonecrosis of the femoral head[194, 195] can be observed.

Osteonecrosis of the femoral head occurring after metaphyseal or epiphyseal infection in the child (or infant) is a very important complication of the disease (Figs. 64–67 and 64–68). In the hip, the vascular circle formed by the ascending branches of the circumflex femoral vessels is intimate with the capsular attachment. In the setting of proximal femoral osteomyelitis, these branches can become obliterated primarily by two mechanisms: septic thrombosis and compression by a sterile sympathetic effusion with a rise in intra-articular pressure.[195–197] In either case, aseptic ischemic necrosis may accompany the septic process of the neighboring bone, although the osteonecrotic epiphysis subsequently may become contaminated by the adjacent suppurative focus. Osteonecrosis of the epiphysis usually is not recognized until 6 to 8 weeks after the onset of infection. The epiphysis can reveal a generalized increase in radiodensity, followed by fragmentation and, less commonly, col-

lapse. Persistent clinical and radiologic deformity can occur after healing of the osteomyelitis and septic arthritis.

Direct Implantation

Direct inoculation of organisms into a joint can occur in many different clinical situations. Arthrocentesis accomplished for evaluation of synovial contents or used for arthrography can introduce gram-positive or gram-negative bacteria.[198] Similarly, penetrating injury, such as occurs in a fist-fight (see earlier discussion) or from a bullet, knife, nail, or other sharp object, can lead to septic arthritis. In these instances, articular abnormalities become evident in a variable period of time (which is determined by the type and virulence of the infective organism), with soft tissue swelling, joint space widening or narrowing, and osseous erosion.

Postoperative Infection

As outlined previously, articular surgery in the form of arthroscopy, arthrotomy, arthrodesis, arthroplasty, or other procedure can be complicated by joint infection in the postoperative period. This complication is rare after arthroscopy[620] but may occur in 1 to 10 per cent of patients undergoing more extensive procedures, the frequency being related to many factors, including the type and length of surgery and the presence of an underlying disorder, such as rheumatoid arthritis, osteoarthritis, ankylosing spondylitis, and systemic lupus erythematosus. Infections occurring soon after such procedures usually are related to direct inoculation of the joint during the operation or to intra-articular spread from an adjacent contaminated focus (e.g., soft tissue abscess). Joint infection occurring long after surgery frequently is associated with obvious preceding sepsis elsewhere in the body and may relate to hematogenous spread to the joint from this distant process.[199–202, 385, 386, 621] The reported frequency of this latter phenomenon after total hip arthroplasty is approximately 0.3 per cent.[202, 203]

Radiographic evaluation of postoperative joint infection may be complicated by the presence of metallic implants and radiopaque or radiolucent cement. Increased radiolucency at the interfaces between the metallic or polyethylene component and cement and between cement and bone can indicate a suppurative process, although similar abnormalities are encountered in asymptomatic patients and in those with loose, noninfected prostheses. Additional evidence of endosteal erosion and of lysis and sclerosis of the medullary bone is strongly indicative of infection. Arthrography can be especially helpful in this situation; the puncture allows aspiration of intra-articular contents for laboratory evaluation, and the injected contrast material may dissect between the cement and osseous surface, fill abscess cavities, or reveal synovial irregularity and lymphatic vessels. Similar radiographic and arthrographic findings can be used in the assessment of noncemented prostheses (see Chapter 19).

Complications

Several potential complications of septic arthritis, such as epiphyseal destruction and osteonecrosis, have been discussed previously. Several others deserve emphasis.

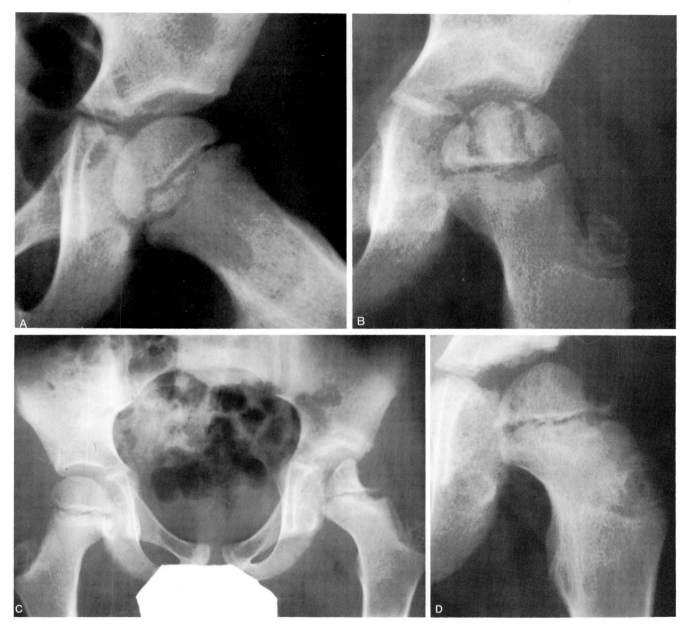

FIGURE 64–67. Septic arthritis of the hip: Childhood. A 4½ year old boy developed suppurative arthritis of the left hip.

A An initial radiograph was normal except for soft tissue swelling.

B One month later, after incision and drainage as well as antibiotic therapy, lateral subluxation of the femoral head indicates reaccumulation of fluid. The fissuring and increased density of the head reflect osteonecrosis.

C Ten months later, lateral subluxation persists, and the lateral half of the epiphyseal ossification center has been resorbed.

D Three months later, some reconstitution of the femoral head has taken place.

(Reproduced with permission from Freiberger RH, et al: Hip disease in infancy and childhood. *In* RD Moseley Jr et al (Eds): Current Problems in Radiology. Copyright 1973 by Year Book Medical Publishers, Inc, Chicago.)

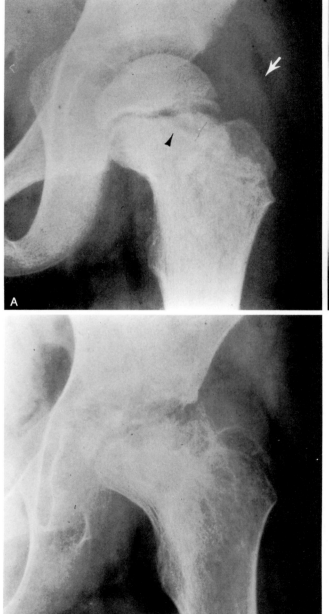

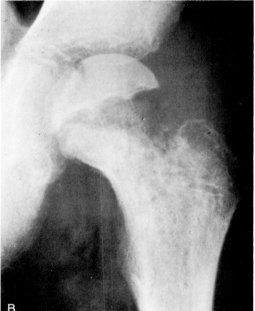

FIGURE 64–68. Septic arthritis of the hip: Childhood. The complication of osteonecrosis in a child with septic arthritis of the hip is well demonstrated in this patient.

A The initial radiograph outlines metaphyseal destruction (arrowhead), soft tissue swelling (arrow), and subtle lateral displacement of the femoral head.

B Subsequently, progressive osteomyelitis and septic arthritis have produced increased intra-articular fluid and osteonecrosis of the femoral head manifested as increased radiodensity.

C Eventually, disintegration of the femoral head occurred.

Synovial Cysts

The frequency of synovial cyst formation in septic arthritis appears to be low, judging by the paucity of available literature on the subject. Occasionally, sepsis in a joint may become evident as distention and contamination of a communicating cyst.[543, 567] Rarely, synovial rupture of the cyst with or without sinus tract formation can be observed.[204, 205, 283, 423–425] In patients with rheumatoid arthritis, sinus tracts about superficial joints can result from superimposed articular infection[206] (see Chapter 25).

Soft Tissue and Tendon Injury

Septic arthritis can result in disruption of adjacent capsular, tendinous, and soft tissue structures. This complication has been well documented in the glenohumeral joint,[426] at which site arthrography may indicate intra-articular synovial inflammation, tears of the rotator cuff, and soft tissue abscess formation[207, 208, 622] (see Chapter 13). Similar phenomena are to be expected at other locations.

Osteomyelitis

Radiographic and pathologic evidence of osteomyelitis commonly is associated with septic arthritis. Bony abnormalities can antedate and be the source of the suppurative joint process or can indicate the contamination of adjacent bony surfaces from a primary joint infection.

Intra-articular Bony Ankylosis

Partial or complete osseous fusion may represent the residual findings of septic arthritis. This complication is not frequent, especially when effective chemotherapy is instituted at an early stage. Bone ankylosis, however, occasionally is encountered after pyogenic processes (Figs. 64–69 and 64–70) and, rarely, after tuberculosis.

Degenerative Joint Disease

Significant destruction of articular cartilage from joint sepsis can lead to incongruity of apposing articular surfaces and, later, to changes of secondary degenerative joint disease. The resulting radiographic findings consisting of joint space narrowing, sclerosis, and osteophytosis may be difficult to differentiate from primary degenerative joint disease, although concentric loss of interosseous space and bony erosions are helpful indicators of preexisting articular disease.

Other Complications

Numerous other complications may occur after septic arthritis. These include epiphyseal displacement (not only of the proximal femoral capital epiphysis but also of the proximal humeral epiphysis[623]), widening of the joint space with subluxation or dislocation (e.g., drooping shoulder[624]),[696] overgrowth of epiphyses and apophyses (e.g., patella[625]), soft tissue and muscle abscesses (particularly in the hip and glenohumeral and sternoclavicular joints[626, 627, 746]), and resorption of sesamoid bones (in the hands and feet[628]).

Modifications and Difficulties in Diagnosis

Antibiotic Modified Septic Arthritis

Inadequate or inappropriate administration of antibiotics can modify articular infection. Clinical manifestations can be masked, appearing relatively late in the course of the disease, and radiographic changes may be less dramatic,

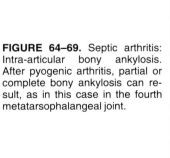

FIGURE 64–69. Septic arthritis: Intra-articular bony ankylosis. After pyogenic arthritis, partial or complete bony ankylosis can result, as in this case in the fourth metatarsophalangeal joint.

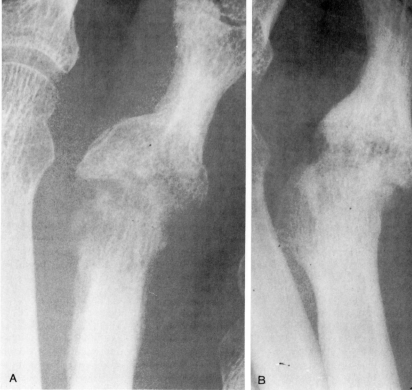

A

B

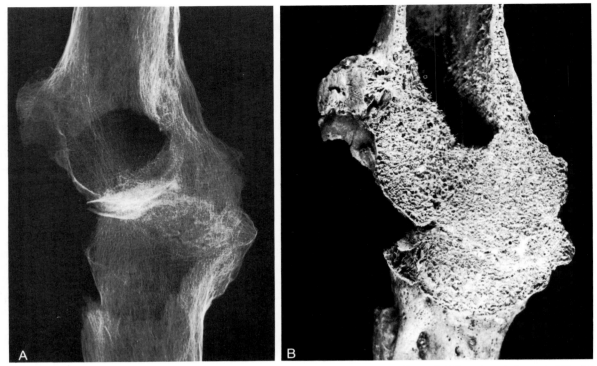

FIGURE 64–70. Septic arthritis (presumed diagnosis): Intra-articular bony ankylosis. A radiograph **(A)** and a photograph **(B)** of a sagittal section reveal solid bone fusion between femur and tibia. The protuberance on the anterior surface of the femur probably represents the patella.

less extensive, and much delayed. Furthermore, radiographic improvement after control of the infection lags behind the amelioration of clinical signs.

Pre-existing Articular Abnormality

When infection is superimposed on a previous articular disorder such as rheumatoid arthritis, calcium pyrophosphate dihydrate crystal deposition disease (see Chapter 44), or osteoarthritis, the clinical and radiographic abnormalities can be hidden or changed by the underlying disease process. In the septic rheumatoid joint, for example, the findings of soft tissue swelling, joint space narrowing, and osseous destruction related to the suppurative process are difficult to differentiate from those of rheumatoid arthritis[200, 427] (see Chapter 25). In this clinical situation, progressive effusion and rapid acceleration of joint destruction should be viewed cautiously as the findings may indicate that worsening clinical manifestations are related not to the rheumatoid process itself but rather to a superimposed infection. Furthermore, polyarticular involvement may characterize septic arthritis superimposed on rheumatoid arthritis or other joint diseases.

Differential Diagnosis

General Features

Any destructive monoarticular process should be regarded as infection until proved otherwise. Although numerous disorders such as pigmented villonodular synovitis, idiopathic synovial osteochondromatosis, juvenile chronic arthritis, and even adult-onset rheumatoid arthritis can be associated with monoarticular changes, infection must be considered the prime diagnostic possibility until appropriate aspiration and culture document its absence. This is particularly true when the joint process is associated with loss of interosseous space, poorly defined or "fuzzy" osseous margins, and a sizeable effusion. In patients with pyogenic infection, the articular destruction can be very rapid, with complete loss of joint space and large destructive osseous foci appearing within a period of 1 to 3 weeks; in patients with tuberculosis or fungal disease, the articular abnormalities appear more slowly and may be associated with extensive periarticular osteoporosis. Diagnostic difficulty arises when the septic process involves more than one joint or when septic arthritis appears during the course of another articular disorder.

Of all the radiographic features of infection, it is the poorly defined nature of the bony destruction that is most characteristic. Osseous erosions or cysts in gout, rheumatoid arthritis, seronegative spondyloarthropathies, osteoarthritis, pigmented villonodular synovitis, idiopathic synovial osteochondromatosis, hemophilia, and calcium pyrophosphate dihydrate crystal deposition disease are more sharply marginated. Furthermore, concentric loss of interosseous space is typical in infection. A similar pattern of joint space loss accompanies rheumatoid arthritis, the seronegative spondyloarthropathies, calcium pyrophosphate dihydrate crystal deposition disease, chondrolysis, and chondral atrophy, but focal diminution of the articular space, as noted in osteoarthritis, and relative preservation of articular space, as seen in gout, pigmented villonodular synovitis, idiopathic synovial osteochondromatosis, and hemophilia, are rare in pyogenic infection (although late loss of joint space can be encountered in tuberculosis and fungal disorders).

Osseous erosions at the marginal areas of synovial joints are frequent in processes associated with significant synovial inflammation, such as sepsis, rheumatoid arthritis, and the seronegative spondyloarthropathies. They also may be observed in gout and, less commonly, in pigmented villonodular synovitis and idiopathic synovial osteochondromatosis. Centrally located erosions and cysts are seen in many disorders, including septic arthritis. Similarly, periarticular osteoporosis can be encountered in rheumatoid arthritis, Reiter's syndrome, juvenile chronic arthritis, hemophilia, and nonpyogenic suppurative processes, such as tuberculosis or fungal disease.

Intra-articular bony ankylosis can represent the end stage of septic arthritis, the seronegative spondyloarthropathies, and, in some locations, rheumatoid arthritis and juvenile chronic arthritis.

Specific Joint Involvement

Any articulation can be the site of an infectious process. The joint selection is influenced by the age of the patient and the specific clinical situation. In children and infants, the joints of the appendicular skeleton, especially the knee and the hip, commonly are affected in hematogenous infections; in children and adults, the joints of the axial skeleton, particularly the sacroiliac joint and those in the spine, not uncommonly are involved. These patterns of distribution frequently are modified when infection relates to a nonhematogenous process; any joint can be affected after soft tissue suppuration, penetrating injury, or surgery. Furthermore, joint selection in septic arthritis is influenced by other factors. In the intravenous drug abuser, the sacroiliac, sternoclavicular, and acromioclavicular joint and the spine are common sites of involvement. In the person with rheumatoid arthritis, any joint affected by the primary disease process represents a potential site of infection. In the diabetic patient with infection, joints of the foot commonly are altered. Because of this variability, the distribution of infectious processes overlaps that of other disorders.

SOFT TISSUE INFECTION

Routes of Contamination

Infection of soft tissue structures commonly results from direct contamination after trauma. Any process that disrupts the skin surface potentially can lead to secondary infection, particularly in the person with a debilitating illness (e.g., diabetes mellitus) (Fig. 64–71) or one who is being treated with immunosuppressive agents; furthermore, nonpenetrating trauma can lead to soft tissue infection, although the exact mechanism for this complication is not entirely clear. Hematogenous spread is less important as a mechanism in soft tissue contamination than it is in osteomyelitis and septic arthritis.

Radiographic-Pathologic Correlation

Swelling with obliteration of adjacent tissue planes is characteristic of soft tissue infection. Radiolucent streaks within the contaminated area can relate to collections of air derived from the adjacent skin surface or gas formation by various bacteria[169–174, 210–212] (Fig. 64–72) (see Chapter 66). Erosion of bone due to pressure from an adjacent soft tissue mass is much more frequent when the mass is neoplastic

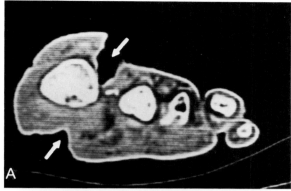

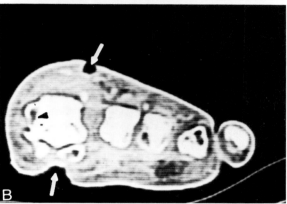

FIGURE 64–71. Soft tissue infection: Diabetes mellitus. This patient had a plantar infection confined to the medial compartment.

A Coronal CT scan at the level of the base of the first proximal phalanx reveals plantar and dorsal cutaneous ulcerations (arrows).

B Approximately 1.5 cm proximal to **A**, skin ulcerations (arrows) and soft tissue abnormalities in the medial plantar compartment and dorsal aspect of the foot are seen. Osteomyelitis involves the first metatarsal head (arrowhead) and lateral sesamoid of the flexor hallucis brevis.

(From Sartoris DJ, et al: Invest Radiol 20:772, 1985.)

rather than infectious in origin (Fig. 64–73). When osseous abnormalities appear after soft tissue contamination, infective periostitis, osteitis, or osteomyelitis usually is present (Fig. 64–74). Occasionally, periostitis of the underlying bone may represent irritation rather than true suppuration (Fig. 64–75).

A well-defined soft tissue mass is less typical of infection than of neoplasm. The edema of an infectious process usually leads to infiltration of surrounding soft tissues rather than displacement, but radiographic differentiation between infiltration and displacement of tissue planes can be exceedingly difficult. Furthermore, reaction of the soft tissue to an adjacent infection can produce pseudoneoplastic masses, which are difficult to differentiate from tumors on clinical, radiographic, and pathologic examination.[213, 214]

Complications

Although there are several complications of soft tissue infection, the most important in terms of the musculoskeletal structures is contamination of underlying osseous and articular tissues. This complication has been amply discussed earlier in this chapter.

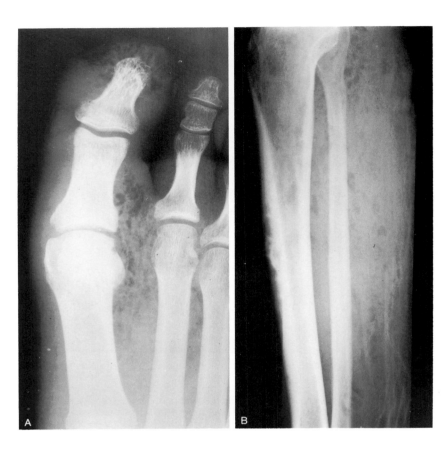

FIGURE 64–72. Soft tissue infection: Gas formation. Two examples of *Escherichia coli* infection in diabetes mellitus. Note the "bubbly" radiolucent collections in the foot and lower leg.

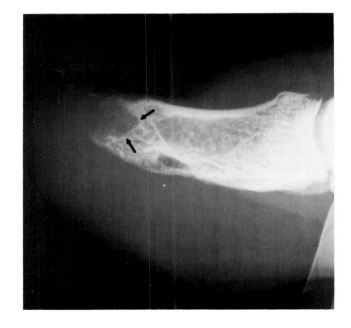

FIGURE 64–73. Soft tissue infection: Osseous erosion. This 55 year old woman developed a chronic bacterial infection of the great toe, which was associated with osseous involvement. Note the erosion of the terminal tuft (arrows). Most frequently such abnormalities reflect contamination of the underlying bone rather than pressure erosion.

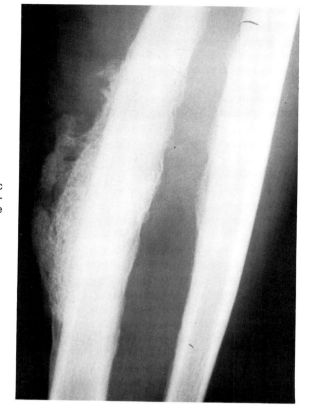

FIGURE 64–74. Soft tissue infection: Infective periostitis and osteitis. A chronic soft tissue ulceration and bacterial infection of the forearm have led to contamination of the underlying periosteum and cortex, with exuberant new bone formation. The marrow does not appear to be involved.

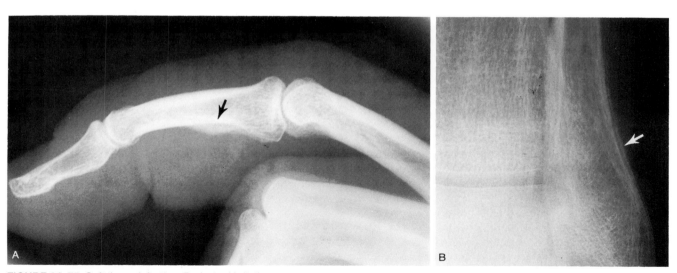

FIGURE 64–75. Soft tissue infection: Periosteal irritation.
   A Chronic infective tenosynovitis has produced irritation of the underlying phalangeal bone with periostitis (arrow). Note the soft tissue swelling and semiflexion of the digit.
   B Chronic soft tissue ulceration and infection have led to noninfective periostitis of the underlying fibula (arrow).

Specific Entities

Septic Subcutaneous Bursitis

Numerous subcutaneous bursae are found in the human body.[215, 301] Afflictions of these structures have led to such well-known terms as housemaid's knee (prepatellar bursitis), miner's elbow (olecranon bursitis), and weaver's bottom (ischial bursitis). In addition, bursal swelling often is apparent in rheumatoid arthritis and gout, as well as after trauma.

Septic bursitis is less well recognized. In most cases, bursal infection localizes to the olecranon and the prepatellar and, less frequently, the subdeltoid regions.[216–220, 301, 302, 323, 568, 629–632] Other sites of infection include the infrapatellar bursae,[633] the trochanteric bursae,[642] the subgluteal bursa,[642] the retrocalcaneal and superficial tendo Achillis bursae,[642] and the iliopsoas bursa.[634] At most sites, septic bursitis is more common in men (Fig. 64–76). Prepatellar septic bursitis is especially frequent in children.[428] A history of recent injury, occupational trauma, or puncture (e.g., steroid administration) frequently, although not invariably, is present. Other reported predisposing factors are diabetes mellitus, alcoholism, an immunocompromised state,[629] eczema, psoriasis, and rheumatoid and gouty arthritis.[632] Clinically detectable skin breakage and bacteriologically evident isolates of Staphylococcus aureus[431, 631] in the absence of bacteremia suggest that direct penetration by skin pathogens accounts for many cases of bursal infection. Other agents that are

implicated less typically are Streptococcus pneumoniae,[216] other streptococci,[430] Staphylococcus epidermidis,[408] gram-negative bacilli,[408] Serratia marcescens,[429] Mycobacterium marinum,[217] and Sporothrix schenckii.[22, 220, 222] Septic subcutaneous bursitis due to hematogenous spread is very rare[219, 221] although it is reported,[629] particularly in deeply situated bursae. This fact may be related to a blood supply that is less exuberant than that of the intra-articular synovial membrane, although the laboratory findings of infected bursal fluid are similar to those of septic joint fluid.[219] In some cases, the bursal reaction to infection is less intense than that of the joint.[286]

Clinical manifestations include painful swelling localized to the involved bursa, subcutaneous edema, a normal range of joint motion, and fever in approximately 40 per cent of cases.[408] As nonseptic bursitis rarely is associated with fever, this finding is an important clue to the correct diagnosis. Cellulitis commonly is present.[631] Routine radiography, bursography,[630, 634] CT,[634] and MR imaging[629] can be used to define the extent of the soft tissue infection.

Septic bursitis usually is not associated with infectious arthritis.[322] Erosion and proliferation of subjacent bone (e.g., ulna, patella, humerus) indicate complicating infective periostitis, osteitis, and osteomyelitis.[633] The radiographic and clinical findings (redness, warmth, tenderness, soft tissue swelling) may be misinterpreted as those of gout or rheumatoid arthritis. As these latter conditions can coexist with infection,[223] appropriate clinical and laboratory tests

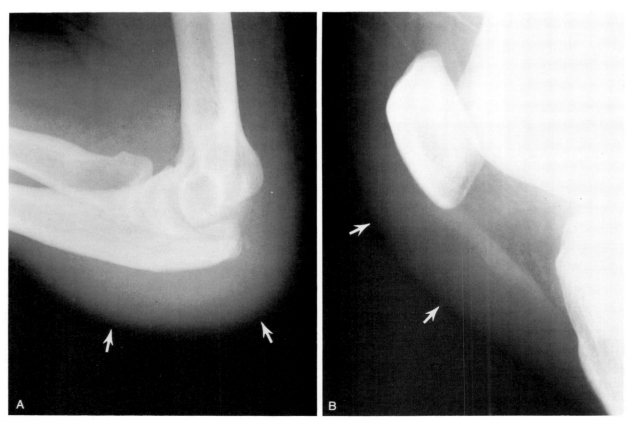

FIGURE 64–76. Septic bursitis.
  A Olecranon bursitis. Note olecranon swelling (arrows) and soft tissue edema due to Staphylococcus aureus. Previous surgery and trauma are the causes of the adjacent bony abnormalities.
  B Prepatellar bursitis. This 28 year old carpenter who had worked on his knees for prolonged periods of time developed tender swelling in front of the knee (arrows). Inflammatory fluid that was culture positive for Staphylococcus aureus was recovered from the bursa.

should be undertaken to exclude their presence. Because a sympathetic sterile effusion of a neighboring joint can be associated with septic bursitis,[302, 432] the detection of joint fluid by imaging techniques does not necessarily imply that a septic arthritis is present.

Septic Periarticular Bursitis

Infection of bursae that are located about articulations (e.g., popliteal) usually is related to extension of an infective process within the joint. Rarely, primary infection of a synovial cyst can occur, although the neighboring joints soon are contaminated.

Septic Tenosynovitis

Inflammation of the synovial lining of tendon sheaths is a common finding in various rheumatologic conditions, especially rheumatoid arthritis. Septic processes originating from a distant or local focus or occurring after trauma also can lead to tenosynovitis.[642] Various bacteria, mycobacteria, fungi, viruses, or protozoa may be implicated.[224–227, 301, 321] Soft tissue swelling and surface resorption and erosion of underlying bony structures may be evident (Fig. 64–77). Appropriate microbiologic studies confirm the infective nature of the lesion. Osteomyelitis of adjacent sesamoid bones sometimes can be identified.[303] Routine radiography, CT, MR imaging, and ultrasonography are appropriate diagnostic methods applied to the assessment of suppurative tenosynovitis.[635]

Granulomatous tenosynovitis may occur in sarcoidosis or after exposure to beryllium, or it may result from puncture wounds (i.e., blackthorn, stingray)[304, 305, 601] (Fig. 64–78).

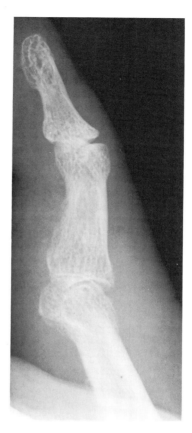

FIGURE 64–78. Tenosynovitis: Stingray injury. A 64 year old man was stung by a stingray while diving. A soft tissue puncture wound on the dorsum of the fifth finger was extremely painful and, over the next 6 weeks, was associated with stiffness of the entire digit. A radiograph shows considerable soft tissue swelling on both the dorsal and the volar aspects of the finger. Surgery documented chronic inflammation and fibrosis of the tendons and sheath with no growth of organisms.

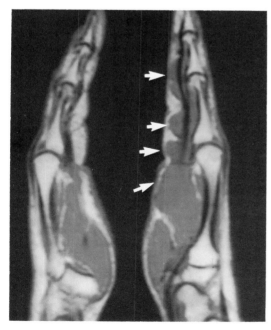

FIGURE 64–77. Infective tenosynovitis: Flexor tendons of finger. Atypical mycobacterial infection in farmer. A sagittal T1-weighted (TR/TE, 600/20) spin echo MR image shows lobulated fluid collections (arrows) of low signal intensity extending along the course of the flexor digitorum superficialis and flexor digitorum profundus tendons of the index finger of one hand. Compare with the opposite (normal) hand.

Lymphadenitis

Lymphadenitis, usually with an accompanying cellulitis, can complicate streptococcal or staphylococcal infections. Although many sites can be involved, acute epitrochlear lymphadenitis about the elbow can produce clinical and radiologic findings that simulate osteomyelitis.[228] Nodular or diffuse soft tissue swelling and underlying periostitis can be encountered.

Cellulitis

Cellulitis represents an acute inflammatory process of the deeper subcutaneous tissue, affecting male and female patients of all ages. Drug addicts are particularly susceptible to this condition. It can involve the upper or lower extremities, thorax, abdomen, neck, or head, including the orbital region. Clinical findings include pain or tenderness, redness, swelling, warmth, and mild to moderate fever.[433, 434] Cellulitis results generally from a streptococcal or, less commonly, a staphylococcal infection, although diverse organisms, including *Haemophilus influenzae*,[435] *Streptococcus pneumoniae*,[436] *Neisseria meningitidis*,[437] and Cryptococcus,[438] may be responsible.[434, 439] Radiographic findings are nonspecific and usually are confined to the soft tissues, although septicemia and osteomyelitis are recognized complications.

Necrotizing Fasciitis

Necrotizing fasciitis represents a rare type of soft tissue infection that is accompanied by widespread fascial necrosis in the absence of muscular and cutaneous infection.[636] It is a serious condition associated with systemic toxicity and, if untreated, death. Predisposing factors include trauma, cutaneous lesions, intravenous drug abuse, surgical wounds, and thermal injury.[637] Although identified most commonly in the extremities, necrotizing fasciitis also may be encountered in the neck, face, perineum, genitalia, and trunk.[636, 638, 639] A variety of bacteria, particularly streptococci and staphylococci, are responsible for most cases.[640] Routine radiography may reveal evidence of soft tissue gas,[641] although the clinical findings consisting of fever, pain, swelling, and bullae usually allow accurate diagnosis.[636]

Infectious Myositis

Inflammation of muscle may occur in a variety of infectious disorders caused by viruses, bacteria, protozoa, and parasites. In some instances, as in viral myositis, the precise mechanism leading to muscle inflammation is not clear, whereas in others, direct involvement of the muscle by the infectious agent is implicated. A summary of some of these processes is included here, but the interested reader should consult other sources[440, 441] for a more detailed description.

Myalgia is a common finding in certain viral diseases and generally is of short duration. Some viruses, including members of the influenza, coxsackie, echo, herpes, and hepatitis groups, can lead to an inflammatory myopathy of longer duration. Epidemic pleurodynia (Bornholm's disease) usually is related to coxsackievirus infection, and positive virologic cultures from the inflamed intercostal muscles have been obtained.[440, 442] Of interest is the isolation from skeletal muscles of the coxsackieviral particles in patients with polymyositis, dermatomyositis, and necrotizing myopathy.[441]

Pyogenic myositis (pyomyositis) is a well-recognized and serious infection affecting children and young adults in tropical regions (tropical pyomyositis) and, less frequently, in other locations.[443–451] The prevalence of the disorder in East Africa is underscored by the fact that it represents the cause of approximately 4 per cent of surgical admissions to hospitals.[446] Children and young adults are affected, but in the United States, the vast majority of cases occur in children.[451] Although the disease, as described classically, occurs in otherwise healthy persons, it also is seen in malnourished and immunodeficient patients, including those with acquired immunodeficiency syndrome (AIDS).[645, 649, 650] It has been reported as a complication of other muscle diseases (such as dermatomyositis) as well.[651] The initial clinical findings are pain and tenderness of the muscle, and hard, "woody" induration of the overlying skin; subsequently, fluctuance occurs with swelling of the regional lymph nodes.[441] Musculature in the lower extremity, especially in the thigh and buttocks, is affected more frequently than that in the upper extremity or trunk.[441, 648, 652] Abscesses isolated to centrally located musculature such as the psoas muscle may be encountered, however[654] (Fig. 64–79). Although involvement of a single muscle group is typical, two or three muscles occasionally are affected.[450, 646] Fever, mal-

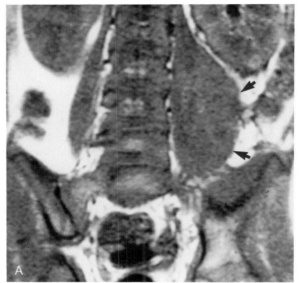

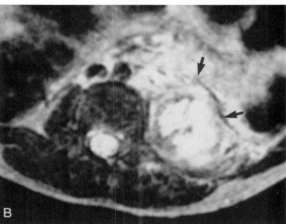

FIGURE 64–79. Infectious myositis: Psoas muscle. *Staphylococcus aureus* infection in a 6 year old otherwise healthy child.

A Coronal T1-weighted (TR/TE, 500/11) spin echo MR image shows enlargement of the left psoas muscle (arrows). Its signal intensity is similar to that of normal muscle.

B A transaxial T2-weighted (TR/TE, 2000/80) spin echo MR image reveals an enlarged left psoas muscle (arrows) of inhomogeneous but mainly high signal intensity. At surgery, chronic inflammatory tissue and fat necrosis without abscess formation or pus were found.

(Courtesy of G. Greenway, M.D., Dallas, Texas.)

aise, muscle spasm and contracture, leukocytosis, and eosinophilia (in the tropics) are additional manifestations of the disease. Levels of the serum enzymes that reflect muscle damage generally are not elevated.

Pyomyositis is related to *Staphylococcus aureus* infection in about 90 per cent of cases (streptococci account for most of the remaining cases),[739, 740] and staphylococcal septicemia with metastatic seeding of bacteria to vital organs may be present.[441] In the tropics, the lack of footwear may predispose to minor trauma and insect bites, and resulting skin infections may go untreated; pyoderma in the feet is evident in more than 50 per cent of such patients who develop pyomyositis.[450, 451] As skeletal muscle generally is highly resistant to metastatic infections,[441] the pathogenesis of staphylococcal localization in muscle with the development of abscesses is not clear, although it is suggested that an

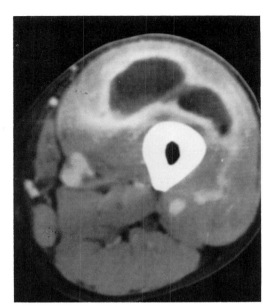

FIGURE 64–80. Infective myositis: Quadriceps femoris muscles. *Staphylococcus aureus* infection in an adult patient with the acquired immunodeficiency syndrome. A transaxial contrast enhanced CT scan reveals a lobulated abscess with enhancement of its wall.

initial muscular insult is required to allow such localization. Proposed causes of this insult have included trauma, nutritional deficiency, parasitic or viral infections, and leptospirosis.[451, 452]

Accurate diagnosis of this condition outside of the tropics is difficult as its clinical abnormalities resemble those of more common disorders; prolonged periods of hospitalization, reflecting this diagnostic difficulty, are characteristic.[451] The hard, ''woody,'' tumor-like quality of the affected muscle has led to the incorrect diagnosis of sarcoma.[450] Accurate analysis requires aspiration of the infected area with culture of the recovered material. As plain film radiography provides little information regarding the proper diagnosis or the ideal site of tissue aspiration, attention has been directed toward other imaging techniques.

Sonographically guided percutaneous drainage may be helpful in the diagnosis and management of the condition.[449, 453, 454, 644] CT[451, 454–456, 463, 643, 646, 647] and MR imaging[643, 645, 646, 653, 753] may further delineate the location and extent of the disease process, and CT has been used to monitor aspiration attempts. The CT findings of pyogenic myositis (Fig. 64–80) include enlargement of the muscle(s), effacement of the intramuscular and intermuscular fat planes, fluid or gas collections within involved musculature, enhancement of inflamed areas after intravenous administration of contrast material, and bone involvement.[647] Abscesses may be identified.[646] MR imaging findings (Fig. 64–81) include muscle enlargement, abscesses characterized by a peripheral rim of increased signal intensity on T1-weighted spin echo MR images and a central region, representing fluid, of intense signal on T2-weighted spin echo MR images and by peripheral enhancement after intravenous administration of gadolinium-based contrast medium, and associated abnormalities of subcutaneous edema in some cases.[645] Radionuclide studies with gallium[453, 454, 457–459] or indium[646] are helpful in defining additional nearby or distant abscesses. Surgical procedures including myotomy and abscess drainage, when combined with antimicrobial therapy, usually ensure complete resolution.

Clostridial myonecrosis, or gas gangrene, is a rare disease resulting from the presence of *Clostridium perfringens*[440] or *C. septicum*[460, 461] (see Chapter 66). Gas within the soft tissues and muscles is an important diagnostic sign (Fig. 64–82), although other organisms can produce a similar finding.[462, 464] Toxoplasmosis, trichinosis, schistosomiasis, cysticercosis, and sarcosporidiasis are parasitic causes of myositis.[440]

SPECIFIC SITUATIONS

A variety of situations and systemic disorders are associated with an increased frequency of bone, joint, and soft tissue infection. Examples, such as sickle cell anemia, diabetes mellitus, rheumatoid arthritis, crystal-induced arthropathy, myeloproliferative disorders, systemic lupus erythematosus, endogenous and exogenous hypercortisolism, and

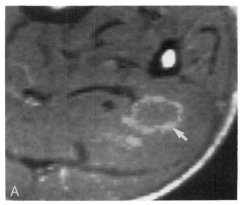
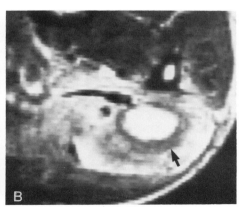

FIGURE 64–81. Infective myositis: Soleus muscle. *Staphylococcus aureus* infection in a 34 year old patient with the acquired immunodeficiency syndrome.
 A On a transaxial T1-weighted (TR/TE, 500/30) spin echo MR image, a rim of increased signal intensity (arrow) is evident.
 B With T2 weighting (TR/TE, 2000/90), a similar transaxial image shows a central area of marked hyperintensity surrounded by a hypointense band (arrow) which itself is surrounded by a more diffuse region of hyperintensity. The MR imaging findings are those of an abscess.
 (From Fleckenstein JL, et al: Radiology *179*:653, 1991.)

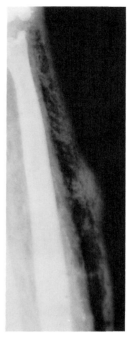

FIGURE 64–82. Myonecrosis related to *Clostridium perfringens* infection. Observe diffuse intramuscular and soft tissue gas in the forearm. (Courtesy of B. Howard, M.D., Charlotte, North Carolina.)

hypo- and agammaglobulinemia, are discussed elsewhere in the book. A few additional situations that predispose to musculoskeletal infection are noted here.

Chronic Granulomatous Disease

This heterogeneous disorder is a hereditary condition, usually transmitted as an X-linked recessive trait, which occurs in male children,[247–250, 280] although a similar syndrome has been identified in female and male children without a family history of disease.[251] The syndrome is characterized by purulent granulomatous and eczematoid skin lesions, granulomatous lymphadenitis with suppuration, hepatosplenomegaly, recurrent and persistent pneumonias, and chronic osteomyelitis (25 to 35 per cent); it frequently is fatal (40 per cent). In its classic form, chronic granulomatous disease is manifested as infections early in life, sometimes within the first week but usually during the first year.[465] A fatal outcome before adolescence is common. Variants of the disease, in which infections begin or become more prominent in adolescents or adults or are confined to one organ system, such as the skin, are described.[466, 657] Virtually every organ or tissue is vulnerable to infection in this disorder. Histologically, granulomas composed primarily of plasma cells, lymphocytes, macrophages, and multinucleated giant cells, with or without central caseation, are seen. Small or large abscesses also may be evident. A defect has been noted in the ability of the polymorphonuclear leukocytes and monocytes to destroy certain pathogenetic organisms adequately.[250, 252, 253] Thus, although the leukocytes can phagocytize bacteria normally, they are incapable of killing them, especially certain strains of relatively low virulence, such as *Staphylococcus epidermidis, Staphylococcus aureus,* species of Enterobacteriaceae, *Serratia marcescens,* and certain fungi (Aspergillus

strains, *Candida albicans, Torulopsis glabrata, Hansenula polymorpha,* and Mucor)[465, 655, 656, 658] (Fig. 64–83). Affected children demonstrate a normal spectrum of immunoglobulins, a normal ability to develop and express a hypersensitivity response, and normal complement and complement component levels.[254, 255] Investigations suggest that enzyme deficiencies, abnormal elicited membrane potential changes, abnormal acidification of the phagocytic vacuole, and deficiencies of an electron transport cascade are important in the pathogenesis of the disorder.[467, 657]

Certain clinical and radiologic peculiarities characterize the osteomyelitis of chronic granulomatous disease of childhood.[256, 659]

1. The disease lacks the usual early clinical signs and symptoms of osteomyelitis, so that initial radiographs frequently reveal considerable bony involvement.

2. The causative organisms usually are of low virulence.

3. The most frequent site of involvement is the small bones of the hands and feet. Involvement of the chest wall and spine also is common.

4. Osteomyelitis may result either from contamination related to an adjacent focus of infection, especially in the thoracic region, or from hematogenous dissemination.

5. The radiographic abnormalities are characterized by extensive osseous destruction with minimal reactive sclerosis. Sequestrum formation is unusual.

6. The osteomyelitis may develop in new areas despite continuous therapy.

7. The osteomyelitis eventually responds to long-term antibiotic therapy, so that operative intervention rarely is necessary.

The radiographic features related to the osteomyelitis of chronic granulomatous disease are not diagnostic. The pre-

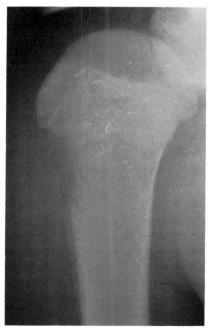

FIGURE 64–83. Chronic granulomatous disease: Aspergillus osteomyelitis. Humeral involvement in a 15 year old boy. Note metaphyseal destruction and periostitis. (From Heinrich SD, et al: J Bone Joint Surg [Am] *73*:456, 1991.)

dilection for the small bones of the hands and feet, the presence of extensive osteolysis, and the absence of significant bony sclerosis are helpful clues, although similar abnormalities can accompany tuberculous dactylitis. The changes also may simulate those of primary hypogammaglobulinemia and other immunodeficiency states.[257] In chronic granulomatous disease, the progression of the osseous alterations with the development of new areas of involvement, even during continuous antibiotic therapy, reflects the immunologic incompetence of the patient, although the eventual appearance of complete healing suggests that the immunologic mechanisms ultimately are capable of destroying the relatively indolent organisms that are causing the osteomyelitis.[256]

Chronic Recurrent Multifocal Osteomyelitis (CRMO)

CRMO, which also is discussed in Chapter 93, is a variety of subacute and chronic osteomyelitis of unknown cause that occurs in childhood and that frequently reveals multiple and symmetric alterations.[258–261, 306, 468–474, 544–546, 569, 570, 660–675] It also has been referred to as condensing osteitis of the clavicle in childhood, chronic symmetric plasma cell osteomyelitis, chronic sclerosing osteomyelitis, multifocal chronic osteomyelitis, SAPHO (*s*ynovitis, *a*cne, *p*ustulosis, *h*yperostosis, *o*steitis) syndrome, cleidometaphyseal osteomyelitis, plasma cell osteomyelitis, and primary chronic osteomyelitis. The usual age of onset of the disease is 5 to 10 years, although infants and adults also may be affected. Pain, tenderness, and swelling are common initial clinical manifestations. The metaphyses of the bones of the lower extremity and the medial ends of the clavicles particularly are vulnerable (Figs. 64–84 and 64–85), although other osseous sites, including those in the face, the spine and pelvis, and the upper extremity (Fig. 64–86), can be altered.[754] Indeed, virtually any skeletal site, including irregular and small bones such as the sternum, ribs, and carpal and tarsal bones, may be involved.[661] Osteolysis with intense sclerosis may be noted. In certain locations, such as the clavicle, the bone may become massive and a diagnosis of fibrous dysplasia, Paget's disease, or sarcoma is suggested.[468, 660, 673] In fact, the dominant radiographic feature at any skeletal site is bone sclerosis (Fig. 64–87) which, in some locations, is combined with periostitis that may be exuberant.[671] This feature is similar or identical to that described in cases of sclerosing osteomyelitis of Garré. The radiographic abnormalities in the spine resemble those of idiopathic hemispherical sclerosis (see Chapter 40), those about the symphysis pubis resemble the changes of osteitis pubis, and those in the ilium simulate the changes of osteitis condensans ilii. Destructive lesions of bone also are encountered, however, which can lead to a variety of complications including vertebra plana.[667, 672] Rarely, soft tissue calcification in the form of tumoral calcinosis occurs in patients with CRMO.[747]

Laboratory analysis generally is nonspecific, and cultures of the blood or of the bone following biopsy may be nonrewarding.[662] Occasionally organisms, including pneumococci, are recovered. There is no evidence of reduced cellular or humoral immunity. Histologic evaluation is reported to be relatively specific, characterized by the predominance of plasma cells in the center of the osteolytic foci.[258, 262] Other reports, however, indicate that plasma cell accumulation is not always present[306] and that early osteomyelitic foci are associated with the accumulation of poly-

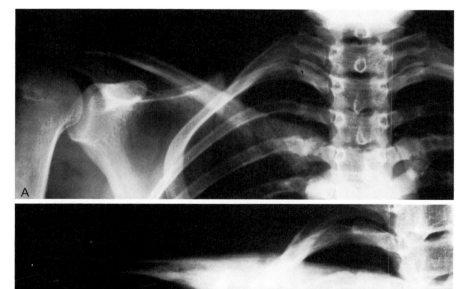

FIGURE 64–84. Chronic recurrent multifocal osteomyelitis: Clavicle. A 16 year old girl developed pain and progressive enlargement of the medial portion of the right clavicle over a 6 month period. She had no fever or erythema. Radiographs obtained 8 months apart reveal a process that is associated initially with permeative bone destruction and subsequently with massive enlargement of the clavicle. Biopsy and histologic evaluation indicated only chronic osteitis. Cultures were negative. (Courtesy of G. Greenway, M.D., Dallas, Texas.)

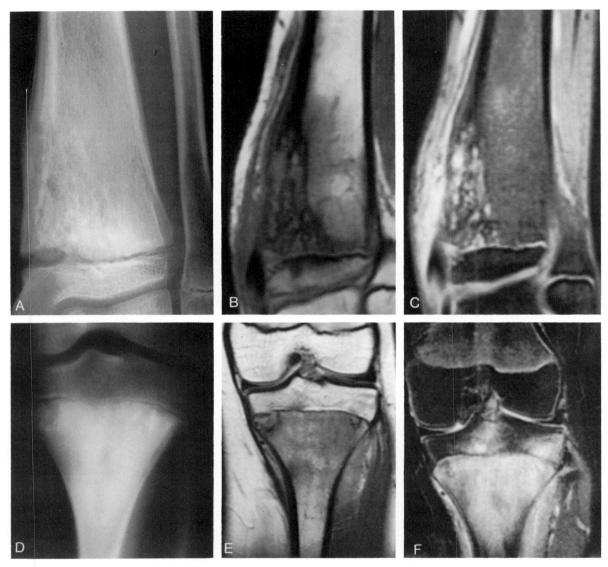

FIGURE 64–85. Chronic recurrent multifocal osteomyelitis: Tibia.

A–C In this 12 year old boy, progressive pain developed in the lower extremity. Subsequent biopsy of the tibia revealed material that on histologic analysis showed chronic inflammation. Cultures were negative. The routine radiograph **(A)** shows a combination of osteolysis and osteosclerosis in the distal tibial metaphysis, with irregularity of the physis and extensive periostitis. A coronal T1-weighted (TR/TE, 700/12) spin echo MR image **(B)** shows predominantly low signal intensity in the involved bone marrow, periosteal new bone, and soft tissue edema. A multiplanar gradient recalled (MPGR) image (TR/TE, 600/15; flip angle, 30 degrees) **(C)** shows regions of high signal intensity in the bone, beneath the periosteal membrane, and in the soft tissues. (Courtesy of R. Taketa, M.D., Long Beach, California.)

D–F In this 11 year old girl with lower extremity pain, a conventional tomogram **(D)** shows metaphyseal irregularity and diffuse sclerosis in the tibia. A coronal proton density (TR/TE, 2100/18) spin echo MR image **(E)** reveals predominantly low signal intensity in the metaphyseal marrow and soft tissues. A coronal short tau inversion recovery (STIR) image (TR/TE, 2000/27; inversion time, 160 msec) **(F)** shows high signal intensity in the metaphysis and epiphysis of the tibia and in the soft tissues. No biopsy was done.

(Courtesy of M. Gallagher, M.D., Billings, Montana.)

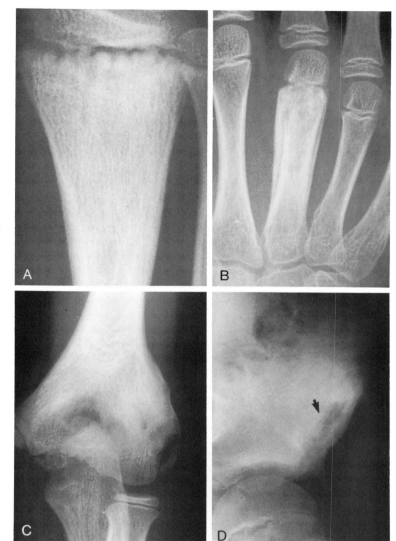

FIGURE 64–86. Chronic recurrent multifocal osteomyelitis: Upper extremity and pelvis.

A Radius. In this 12 year old boy, note metaphyseal sclerosis and physeal irregularity. The distal end of the tibia also was involved.

B Metacarpal bone. In this 10 year old girl, observe osteolysis, osteosclerosis, and periostitis in the third metacarpal bone. The epiphysis is unaffected.

C, D Humerus and ilium. Radiographs in this 12 year old boy reveal increased density in the lateral metaphyseal region of the distal humerus **(C)** and osteolysis and osteosclerosis (arrow) in the ilium **(D)**.

(**A,** Courtesy of S. Cassell, M.D., Eugene, Oregon.)

morphonuclear leukocytes, whereas chronic lesions are accompanied by lymphocyte and histiocyte infiltration.[307] Although the long-term prognosis is good, the condition may run a protracted course with resultant skeletal deformities.[667]

The peculiar features of this variety of osteomyelitis in-

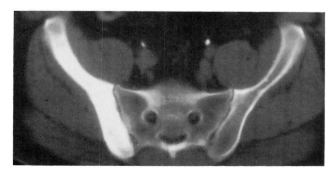

FIGURE 64–87. Chronic recurrent multifocal osteomyelitis: Pelvis. Transaxial CT scan shows diffuse sclerosis of the ilium. Note that the sacrum is unaffected. (Courtesy of M. Pathria, M.D., San Diego, California.)

clude a protracted clinical course with exacerbations and remissions, a striking degree of symmetric bone involvement (not an invariable pattern[663]), a predilection for the metaphyseal regions of the lower extremity (especially in the tibia and femur), common involvement of the clavicle, difficulty in implicating specific organisms from blood or bone, and histologic evidence of plasma cells. The radiographic features may simulate those of other types of osteomyelitis, chronic granulomatous disease of childhood, infantile cortical hyperostosis, vitamin D-resistant rickets, or bone infarction.

Of considerable interest, selective hyperostosis of the clavicle, as noted in this condition, also may be seen in two additional disorders. Osteitis condensans (condensing osteitis) of the medial end of the bone has been reported, especially in young women[284] (see Chapter 58). Sternoclavicular hyperostosis of unknown cause with painful swelling of the sternum, clavicles, and upper ribs also has been described.[285] Men and women are both affected, and the usual age of onset is in the fifth and sixth decades of life. In some of the patients, unilateral or bilateral subclavian vein occlusion can be seen. Hyperostotic spongiosa trabeculae are noted on histologic examination, but microorganisms are not recovered. This syndrome, termed sternocostoclavicular hyperostosis, is discussed further in Chapter 93.

The relationship of CRMO to these other conditions is not clear. That all three involve the clavicle may represent only a coincidence, but several features suggest otherwise. A peculiar pustular lesion in the hands and feet, pustulosis palmaris et plantaris, is observed both in sternoclavicular hyperostosis and CRMO, perhaps indicating a strong association between skin disease and alterations of the sternoclavicular region[475]; psoriasis, which also affects this area, is characterized in some cases by pustular cutaneous lesions that are difficult to distinguish from pustulosis palmaris et plantaris.[668] Long-term radiographic studies firmly linking CRMO of the young with sternocostoclavicular hyperostosis of the aged have not been undertaken. Pustular skin disease, lesions of tubular bones, and sclerotic changes in the manubrium sterni and spine of young and elderly women also have been described,[476] and histologic analysis of the manubrial lesion in some of these patients has documented plasma cell infiltration. The authors have seen plasma cells within sclerotic bone in persons with condensing osteitis of the clavicle, and, furthermore, plasma cell dyscrasia in the form of the POEMS syndrome (see Chapter 60) is accompanied by distinctive bone proliferation in both the axial and the appendicular skeleton. All of these observations support a firm link between plasma cell infiltration and new bone formation. As such cells are known to elaborate an osteoclast-activating factor, it is attractive to suggest that they may produce an osteoclast-deactivating or osteoblast-promoting factor as well.

In recent years, the designation SAPHO syndrome has been used to describe a group of disorders, including CRMO, that have in common (although not invariably) pustular skin lesions and bone proliferation, especially of the anterior chest wall.[674, 748] The SAPHO syndrome is discussed in Chapter 93.

Osteomyelitis and Septic Arthritis in Intravenous Drug Abusers

An increased frequency of infectious disease has been noted in intravenous drug abusers.[263, 264, 308, 309, 676, 677, 680, 681]

The mechanisms for this association are not entirely known. Although it appears that leukocyte function is altered in these persons, this possibility has not been established firmly. In laboratory analyses, morphine has inhibited migration of polymorphonuclear leukocytes in animals[265] and has reduced phagocytic power of neutrophils in humans[266]; however, other experiments have indicated little effect of narcotics on bacterial destruction by polymorphonuclear leukocytes.[267] Use of contaminated narcotics or needles, colonization of the skin during previous hospitalizations, and alterations of the bacterial flora by pretreatment with antibiotics are three other potential mechanisms that may explain an increased frequency of infection in intravenous drug abusers.[277, 278]

Hematogenous osteomyelitis and septic arthritis in drug users are characterized by unusual localization and organisms. Although staphylococcal infection may be seen, Pseudomonas,[268–272, 477] Klebsiella,[272] and Serratia[273, 274] commonly are implicated. Other organisms include Enterobacter, Streptococcus, Candida, and Mycobacterium.[478] Furthermore, the axial skeleton frequently is affected, especially the spine, the sacroiliac joint, and the sternoclavicular joints, with less common involvement of the manubriosternal joint,[559] the acromioclavicular joint, the hip, the pubic symphysis,[479] the ribs, and the ischial tuberosities[268–276] (Figs. 64–88 and 64–89). Alteration of the bones in the appendicular skeleton is less typical. Although the precise cause of axial skeletal involvement in intravenous drug abusers is not clear, the insertion of contaminated needles directly into the jugular vein may lead to adjacent inflammation in the prevertebral and thoracic soft tissues, accounting for osteomyelitis and septic arthritis in the cervical spine and sternoclavicular joints.[679]

The occurrence of systemic candidiasis in heroin addicts deserves emphasis. Contamination of the lemon used to dissolve the ''brown'' heroin by strains of Candida albicans previously colonizing the oropharynx and skin in heroin addicts probably is the source of the infection.[682] Musculoskeletal sites of involvement include, foremost, the costochondral joints and, less commonly, the spine, sacroiliac joints, knees, and wrists.[682–684] (see also Chapter 66). Such involvement occurs in approximately one third of

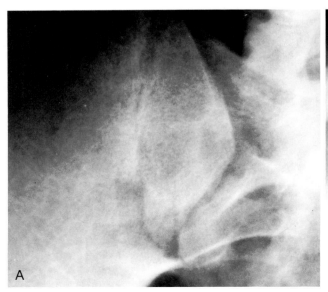

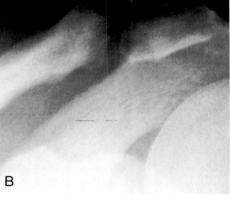

FIGURE 64–88. Hematogenous osteomyelitis and septic arthritis in the intravenous drug abuser. Common sites of involvement are the sacroiliac joint **(A)**, the sternoclavicular and acromioclavicular **(B)** joints, and the spine. Atypical organisms frequently are recovered.

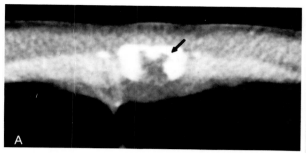

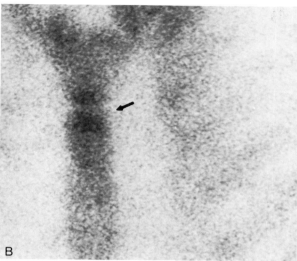

FIGURE 64–89. Hematogenous osteomyelitis and septic arthritis in the intravenous drug abuser. This 56 year old man developed pain and swelling over the manubriosternal joint. Radiographs revealed bone irregularity at this site.
A Transaxial CT scan at the level of the manubriosternal joint shows bone destruction (arrow) and minimal soft tissue prominence.
B Bone scan documents increased accumulation of the radiopharmaceutical agent in the manubriosternal region (arrow). Pseudomonas organisms were recovered.

heroin addicts with systemic candidiasis, either as an isolated phenomenon or, more typically, subsequent to cutaneous or ocular lesions, or both.[682] A hard, slightly tender mass occurs at the affected costochondral junction, which may resolve spontaneously or lead to fistulization. Routine radiography may be normal, but scintigraphy using bone tracers or gallium generally is diagnostic[682] (Fig. 64–90). An inflammatory infiltrate in soft tissue, cartilage, bone, and muscle may be evident on histologic examination. A similar costochondral lesion in heroin addicts can result from bacterial infections, including tuberculosis.

Additional musculoskeletal manifestations in intravenous drug abusers include lymphedema, thrombophlebitis, subcutaneous fat necrosis, atrophy and calcification, pyomyositis (Fig. 64–91), myonecrosis, tenosynovitis, and chemical inflammation of the synovium due to direct intra-articular

administration of the drug.[478, 480, 481, 678] Furthermore, introduction of bacteria directly into the periosteum of the bones (radius, ulna) in the nondominant arm during injection of the drug may lead to osteomyelitis with extensive periostitis.[560]

Osteomyelitis and Septic Arthritis in Lymphedema

A report has appeared of two elderly patients with lymphedema who developed beta-hemolytic streptococcal infection of the knee.[279] In these persons, synovitis persisted for months despite the presence of adequate levels of antibiotics in the synovial fluid. Because lymphatic vessels normally drain synovial fluid from the joint, their obstruction may have interrupted normal egress of the intra-articular organisms and aided in retrograde passage of microorganisms from the site of cellulitis into the joint. Other reports have confirmed the occurrence of septic arthritis in patients with primary hereditary lymphedema (Milroy's disease)[685] and lymphedema resulting from mastectomy for carcinoma of the breast.[686]

OTHER DIAGNOSTIC TECHNIQUES

Magnification Radiography

Optical and radiographic magnification techniques can be helpful in evaluating patients with infectious disorders.[571] The early alterations of osteomyelitis, infective osteitis or periostitis, and septic arthritis may be apparent readily on magnification studies when conventional radiographs are equivocal or negative. The detection of small osteolytic foci in osteomyelitis, minor disruption of the subchondral bone plate in infectious arthritis, and slight periosteal proliferation in infective osteitis, periostitis, or osteomyelitis may be possible with this technique (Fig. 64–92). The authors have used magnification techniques routinely with good success in the evaluation of the feet of diabetic patients and in the differentiation of active versus inactive chronic osteomyelitis (Fig. 64–93). Magnification radiography may show definite bony disruption, indicating

FIGURE 64–90. Systemic candidiasis with costochondral involvement in the intravenous drug abuser. In this heroin addict, a ⁶⁷Ga scan reveals uptake of the radiopharmaceutical agent at the fourth left costochondral junction. (From Miro JM, et al: Arthritis Rheum *31:*793, 1988.)

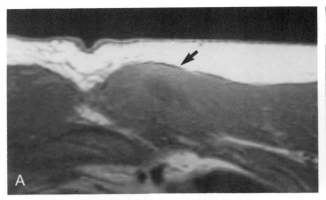
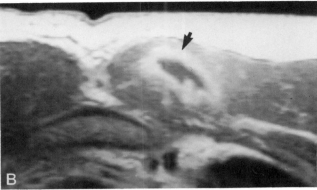

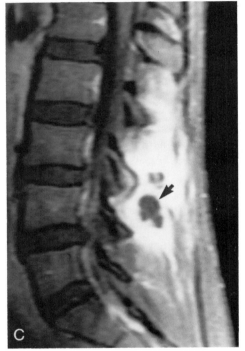

FIGURE 64–91. Pyomyositis in the intravenous drug abuser.

A, B In a 36 year old man, a transaxial T1-weighted (TR/TE, 600/20) spin echo MR image **(A)** shows a mass (arrow) anterior to the sternum in the pectoralis major muscle. The central portion of the mass has signal intensity slightly lower than that of muscle, and its appearance is consistent with fluid in an abscess. A similar T1-weighted image (TR/TE, 700/12) after the intravenous injection of gadolinium contrast agent **(B)** shows enhancement of signal intensity (arrow) in the wall of the abscess.

C In a 38 year old woman, a sagittal T1-weighted (TR/TE, 700/12) fat suppressed (ChemSat), gadolinium-enhanced MR image shows considerable inflammation in the posterior soft tissues of the lumbar spine. Fluid collections (arrow) of low signal intensity are seen within abscess cavities.

infection, in the diabetic person in whom osseous structures are obscured on routine radiography by the presence of soft tissue gas or calcification. In chronic osteomyelitis, the documentation of poorly defined periosteal bone formation with magnification techniques implies existence of active chronic osteomyelitis at a time when the changes may be obscured on conventional radiographs by the subperiosteal alterations of the chronic infection itself.

Conventional Tomography

The major role of conventional tomography in infectious disorders is the detection of sequestra in a patient with chronic osteomyelitis, as these pieces of necrotic bone can be obscured by the surrounding osseous abnormalities on routine radiography. With conventional tomography, they become readily apparent, surrounded by radiolucent granulation tissue (Fig. 64–94). Because the presence of pieces of sequestered bone suggests activity of the infectious process, their detection is important to the orthopedic surgeon and guides the choice of therapy. Occasionally, conven-

tional tomographic examination outlines definite destruction of the subchondral bone plate, indicating the likely presence of septic arthritis rather than simple osteoporosis (which usually produces a thin but otherwise intact plate).

Computed Tomography

The primary applications of CT to the evaluation of infections of the musculoskeletal system are the delineation of the osseous and soft tissue extent of the disease process, especially in areas of complex anatomy such as the vertebral column,[246, 319, 482–487, 572] and the monitoring of percutaneous aspiration and biopsy procedures, particularly of the spine, retroperitoneal tissues, and sacroiliac joints[488, 489] (see Chapter 65).

With regard to the specificity of CT abnormalities in osteomyelitis, many of the findings are shared by primary and secondary malignant neoplasms affecting the skeleton. An increased attenuation value in the medullary canal, destruction of cortical bone, new bone formation, and a soft tissue mass are abnormalities common to both infectious

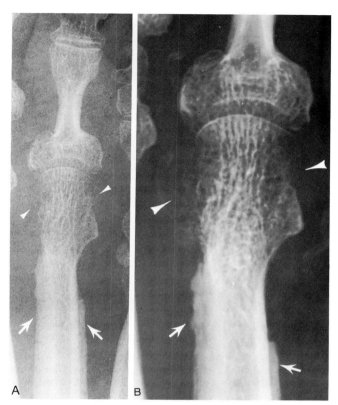

FIGURE 64–92. Osteomyelitis and septic arthritis: Magnification radiography. Although the radiographic changes of infection, including periostitis (arrows) and osseous destruction (arrowheads), are apparent on the routine radiograph **(A)**, they are more obvious with magnification techniques **(B)**.

and neoplastic disorders. With CT, the detection of gas within the medullary canal is an infrequent but reliable diagnostic sign of osteomyelitis that may not be evident on plain film radiography[490, 547, 687, 688] (Fig. 64–95). It is analogous to the presence of gas within soft tissue abscesses.[491] Fat-fluid levels within the medullary canal (Fig. 64–96) or in the adjacent joint also are reported in osteomyelitis and septic arthritis and may relate to necrosis of fat in the bone marrow with release of free fatty globules.[492, 687] These globules can be trapped within the bone or, in the presence of cortical perforation, within the articular cavity. Although relatively specific for osteomyelitis, a similar abnormality (fluid levels) has been observed in patients with tumors and tumor-like lesions such as giant cell tumors, chondroblastomas, and aneurysmal or unicameral bone cysts.[493, 494]

Defining the proximal extent of an infection in a tubular bone is possible with CT owing to the increased attenuation values that are characteristic of the inflammatory reaction of the bone marrow. This finding, however, also is evident in tumorous replacement of the bone, myelofibrosis, and fractures. Furthermore, in certain locations such as the fibula, especially in younger children, the thin size of the marrow space does not allow accurate assessment of the attenuation coefficient.[487]

CT evaluation in patients with subacute or chronic osteomyelitis may reveal cortical sequestration, cloacae, and bone and soft tissue abscesses (Figs. 64–97 and 64–98).[487, 495, 548, 689, 742] This information is important to an orthopedic surgeon who is contemplating operative intervention in a patient with chronic active osteomyelitis.[489]

Joint effusions in cases of septic arthritis of the hip (or other articulation) may be detected by CT when routine radiographs are normal.[561, 688] Furthermore, CT allows the detection of intra-articular fragments complicating septic arthritis (see Fig. 64–105).

Localization of foreign bodies in the soft tissues may be difficult with standard imaging techniques, depending on the nature of the embedded material. Although metallic fragments are well shown on plain film radiography, particles of wood or glass within the soft tissues commonly escape detection. CT has been used successfully in this clinical situation.[496, 497]

Sinography

Opacification of a sinus tract can produce important information that influences the choice of therapy.[310, 320] A small catheter can be placed securely within a cutaneous opening or a Foley catheter can be placed against the opening with the balloon inflated and pressed tightly against the skin to prevent or diminish leakage. Retrograde injection of contrast material will define the course and extent of the sinus tract and its possible communication with an underlying bone or joint (Fig. 64–99). Sinography may be combined with CT for better delineation of the sinus tracts.[690] Although septicemia has been recorded after sinography,[311] this indeed is a rare occurrence.

Arthrography

The principal reason for performing a joint puncture in the clinical setting of infection is to obtain fluid for bacte-

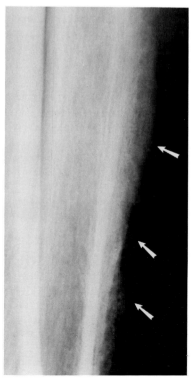

FIGURE 64–93. Active versus inactive chronic osteomyelitis: Magnification radiography. The poorly defined bone proliferation (arrows) in the lateral aspect of the fibula documents the presence of active chronic osteomyelitis.

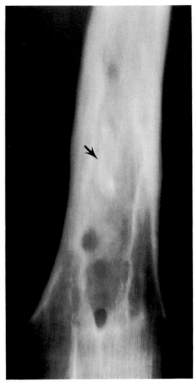

FIGURE 64–94. Chronic osteomyelitis: Conventional tomography. A frontal tomogram of the femur shows a large osteolytic region containing smaller areas of osteolysis and a sequestrum (arrow).

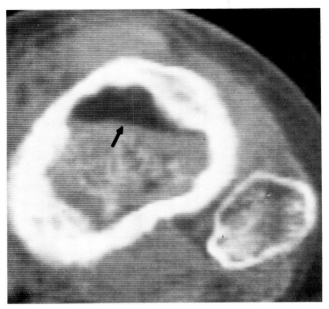

FIGURE 64–96. Acute osteomyelitis: CT. In a 42 year old woman with osteomyelitis of the tibia caused by *Escherichia coli,* a transaxial CT scan at the level of the proximal portion of the tibia shows a fat-fluid level (arrow) in the medullary cavity and osseous erosion and reaction. Aspiration of the intramedullary contents documented purulent material and a small amount of fat; organisms subsequently were recovered from the aspirate. (From Rafii M, et al: Radiology *153*:493, 1984.)

riologic examination.[691] Following removal of the joint contents, however, contrast opacification of the joint will outline the extent of the synovial inflammation and the presence of capsular, tendinous, and soft tissue injury (Fig. 64–100). This is especially helpful in those joints such as the hip and the glenohumeral joint that are relatively inaccessible to direct clinical examination because of their deep location.[312] In performing this procedure, the arthrographer should first attempt to recover some joint fluid by moving

the needle about the joint. If this fails, nonbacteriostatic saline solution should be injected and then aspirated and sent to the laboratory. These techniques should be employed prior to the injection of contrast material, although the precise effect of contrast agents on the growth of bacteria is debated. Some in vitro experiments have indicated that contrast medium inhibits bacterial growth[498, 499] whereas others have not.[500, 501] The conflicting data are related, in part, to the influence of the size of the bacterial inoculum, the specific contrast material that is studied, and the solution in which the bacteria are recovered (e.g., urine, synovial fluid).[502, 503] Lidocaine has been found to have a significant antibacterial effect.[504] Because of all of these variables, the author prefers to obtain a joint sample before injecting the contrast agent.

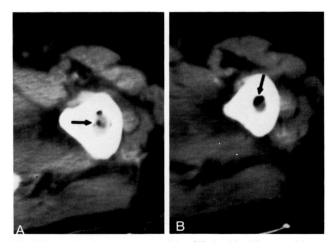

FIGURE 64–95. Acute osteomyelitis: CT. In this 54 year old man with Enterobacter osteomyelitis of the hip and the femur, two transaxial CT scans at the level of the proximal portion of the femur reveal intramedullary gas collections (arrows). (Courtesy of V. Vint, M.D., San Diego, California.)

Ultrasonography

As discussed in Chapter 81, ultrasonography represents a useful technique for the detection of effusions in the hip in children with transient synovitis, septic arthritis, and Legg-Calvé-Perthes disease. The absence of joint fluid in this joint on sonographic examination excludes the diagnosis of septic arthritis, although it does not eliminate the possibility of osteomyelitis.[692] Furthermore, sonography can be used to monitor aspiration of the effusion. Ultrasonography also can be employed in the detection of joint fluid in adults with septic arthritis of the hip[693] and, in a similar fashion, can be used to assess the presence and extent of infected fluid in superficially located joints, synovial cysts, bursae, and tendon sheaths, both in children and in adults. The role of ultrasonography in the clinical setting of osteomyelitis is

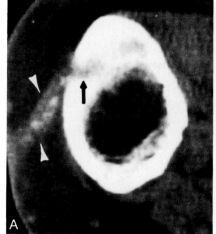
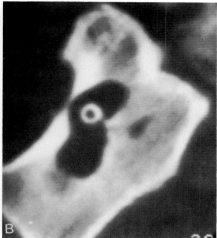

FIGURE 64–97. Chronic osteomyelitis: CT.

A On this transaxial scan, osteomyelitis has resulted in erosion of the anterior cortex of the tibia (arrow) and a sinus tract (arrowheads). (From Wing VW, et al: Radiology *154*:171, 1985.)

B In a second patient, transverse CT reveals bone destruction and a sequestrum in the calcaneus that have resulted from a pin tract infection.

more limited, although this technique allows detection of periosseous abscesses and fluid collections.[694, 695]

Radionuclide Examination

Although the use of scintigraphy in the evaluation of musculoskeletal infections is discussed elsewhere (see Chapter 15), a few comments are appropriate here. The role of this examination in the evaluation of bone,[229–237, 331, 505–507, 697–701] joint,[238–240, 702, 703] and soft tissue[239, 240] infectious processes is firmly established.

The most widely used radionuclide agents for bone imaging are ^{99m}Tc-methylene diphosphonate (Tc-MDP) and hydroxymethylene diphosphonate (Tc-HMDP). Over the course of several hours after their intravenous administration, half or more of the injected radionuclide accumulates in bone with the remainder being excreted in the urine.[705] The reported sensitivities of bone scintigraphy for the detection of osteomyelitis have varied from 32 to 100 per cent; recent technical improvements such as high resolution cameras, powerful computer systems, digital processing methods, and single photon emission computed tomography (SPECT) have led to improved diagnostic sensitivity.[705] Such sensitivity may be lower in children and neonates than

in adults and when osteomyelitis occurs in a complicated clinical setting or in elderly patients. The examination lacks specificity in any age group, however.[705]

Technetium phosphate bone scans become abnormal within hours to days of the onset of bone infection and days to weeks before the disease becomes manifest on conventional radiographs. The scintigraphic abnormality initially may be evident as a photodeficient area (''cold'' spot),[508, 509, 749] a finding that is related to fulminant infection with thrombosis or vascular compression, but, within a few days, increased accumulation of the radioisotope (''hot''

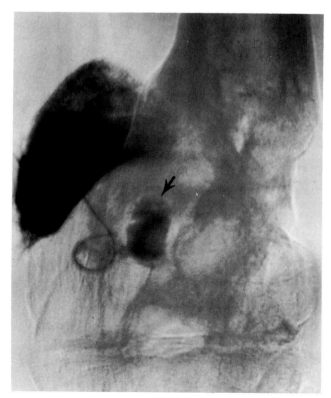

FIGURE 64–99. Chronic osteomyelitis: Sinography. Subtraction film obtained during retrograde opacification of a sinus tract confirms the communication with an abscess in the distal portion of the femur (arrow).

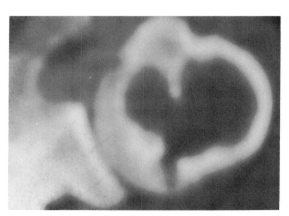

FIGURE 64–98. Subacute osteomyelitis: CT. Note the abscess in the proximal portion of the humerus, shown on a transaxial CT image. Its internal ridges are highly specific for a Brodie's abscess.

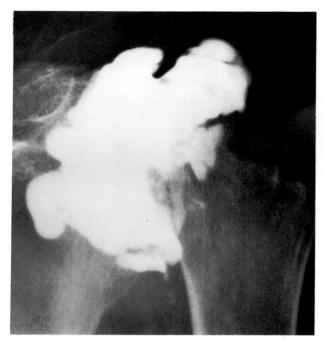

FIGURE 64–100. Septic arthritis: Arthrography. Arthrography of an infected glenohumeral joint reveals the degree of synovial irregularity and the presence of outpockets or diverticula.

spot) is typical (Fig. 64–101). The bone scan also can be used to follow the infected patient and the response to treatment, although several weeks may be required before the scan returns to an entirely normal appearance, and the correlation between clinical and scintigraphic improvement is not uniformly good.[505] Occasional difficulty in interpreting the bone scan in younger patients arises from an inability to differentiate between normal and abnormal activity in the metaphyseal region (Fig. 64–102).[315, 316, 549] Although use of higher resolution gamma cameras and magnification techniques may diminish this difficulty,[510] using gallium scans in this situation, even though these are associated with less radionuclide accumulation, may allow more accurate interpretation of the metaphyseal activity.

Gallium-67 is produced by cyclotron and, therefore, is a relatively expensive scintigraphic agent. After intravenous administration of ⁶⁷Ga-citrate, rapid binding to serum proteins, particularly transferrin, occurs, as well as cellular uptake in the blood, especially by leukocytes.[705] In the normal situation, prominent activity is seen in the liver and spleen and some uptake in the bone itself. In addition, gallium accumulates in the hematopoietic marrow, salivary and lacrimal glands, breasts, and external genitalia.[705] In the abnormal situation, ⁶⁷Ga-citrate imaging is a useful technique for the detection of inflammation. The accumulation of gallium in inflamed areas is believed to be related to the exudation of in vivo labeled serum proteins and the accumulation of in vivo labeled leukocytes, primarily neutrophils.[241, 242] Leukocytes are rich in lactoferrin, and gallium, which accumulates in leukocytes, is bound primarily to lactoferrin. Thus leukocytic uptake of gallium may explain, at least in part, augmented activity at sites of skeletal infection on gallium scans. Similar accumulation of gallium in patients without circulating leukocytes indicates that other factors also are important, however.[313] It has been suggested that lactoferrin binding may be a second important mechanism explaining gallium accumulation in inflammatory foci.[511] The lactoferrin contained in leukocytes is excreted at sites of inflammation, and the discharged lactoferrin may adhere to receptor sites in tissue macrophages. It also is possible that infective organisms themselves may take up gallium, perhaps owing to siderophore production by the microorganisms.

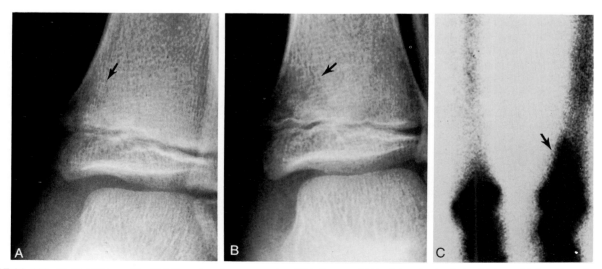

FIGURE 64–101. Acute osteomyelitis: Scintigraphy—bone scanning. This 6 year old black boy had a 6 day history of left ankle pain after an injury. He was febrile, with a warm, red, swollen and tender lower leg.

  A The initial radiograph reveals soft tissue swelling and mild focal osteopenia (arrow).

  B Three days later, a repeat radiograph shows progression of the osteolysis (arrow).

  C A technetium phosphate bone scan documents increased accumulation of the radiopharmaceutical agent in the distal portion of the tibia (arrow). Compare to the opposite (normal) side. Surgical irrigation and débridement were accomplished, and *Staphylococcus aureus,* coagulase-positive, was recovered.

  (Courtesy of G. Greenway, M.D., Dallas, Texas.)

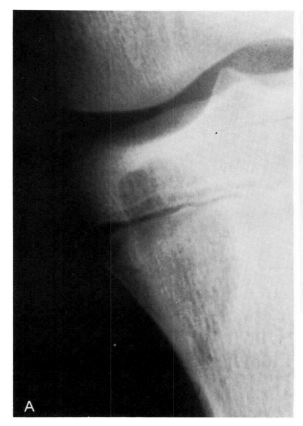

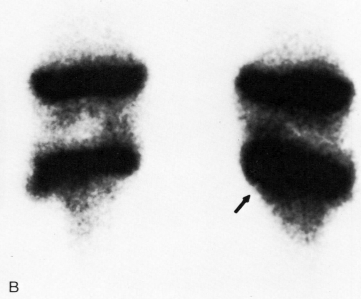

FIGURE 64–102. Subacute osteomyelitis: Scintigraphy—bone scanning. A 12 year old girl had left knee pain of approximately 3 months' duration.

A Radiograph shows a large osteolytic lesion in the metaphyseal region of the tibia, which is extending across the physis to involve the epiphysis.

B Technetium phosphate bone scan demonstrates increased accumulation of the radiopharmaceutical agent in the proximal portion of the tibia (arrow). At surgery, an abscess (related to *Staphylococcus aureus*) was found.

The rationale for the use of gallium as an adjunct to technetium phosphates in evaluating inflammatory lesions of bone is based on several considerations.[317, 318] As technetium accumulation is related to the integrity of the vascular tree, increased intramedullary pressure accompanying osteomyelitis can partially prevent augmented blood flow and prevent significant accumulation of the radionuclide.[314] Gallium, being less dependent on the vascular flow, might still localize at the site of infection. Thus, in the presence of a clinical suspicion of bone or joint infection and a negative bone scan, a gallium study could be useful. Unfortunately, as gallium accumulation occurs also with soft tissue infection, differentiation of cellulitis and osteomyelitis usually is not possible with this agent, although use of good image quality may allow some differentiation of bone, joint, and soft tissue uptake (Fig. 64–103).[317, 573]

A gallium scan can be obtained in conjunction with a technetium scan in the same patient, and the information that is obtained may be even more useful than that of either examination alone (Table 64–7).[562] After administration of technetium agents, scans can be obtained within a few hours, documenting the presence of an inflammatory process; optimal scanning with gallium, on the other hand, may necessitate a delay of 10 to 24 hours. Gallium scans may reveal abnormal accumulation in patients with active osteomyelitis when technetium scans reveal decreased activity ("cold" lesions) or perhaps normal activity (transition period between "cold" and "hot" lesions). Furthermore, gallium accumulation appears to correlate more closely with activity in cases of osteomyelitis than does technetium uptake,[563] and it may be superior in determining the response of acute osteomyelitis and chronic osteomyelitis to various therapeutic regimens. Increased accumulation of gallium in sites of cellulitis can be helpful in establishing the presence of soft tissue infection; initial technetium accumulation also occurs in cases of cellulitis, but its activity diminishes rapidly, thus affording a mechanism for differentiating between cellulitis and osteomyelitis, as the latter situation is associated with persistent increased radionuclide accumulation.[243, 244] This differentiation may not be possible in the first few days of infection.[514] Initial abnormal technetium activity also persists in patients with septic arthritis.[233]

TABLE 64–7. Radionuclide Evaluation of Osseous and Soft Tissue Infection

Agent	Cellulitis	Acute Osteomyelitis	Chronic Osteomyelitis
Technetium phosphates	Early scans show increased uptake; later scans are normal	Early and late scans show increased uptake (scans in early acute osteomyelitis may reveal "cold" spots)	Scans may remain positive even in inactive disease
Gallium	Increased uptake	Increased uptake	Increased uptake in areas of active disease

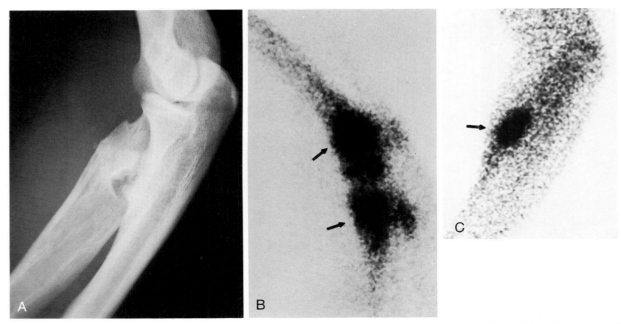

FIGURE 64–103. Soft tissue infection: Scintigraphy—gallium imaging. This 37 year old man, with a history of chronic inactive osteomyelitis of the proximal portion of the radius, developed a staphylococcal soft tissue infection.
A Radiograph shows soft tissue swelling and osseous deformity of the proximal portion of the radius and ulna.
B Technetium phosphate bone scan reveals accentuated uptake of the radiopharmaceutical agent (arrows) in the humerus, radius, and ulna about the elbow.
C Gallium scan indicates abnormality of soft tissue alone (arrow).
(Courtesy of V. Vint, M.D., San Diego, California.)

It should be remembered that gallium is a bone scanning agent, accumulating in regions of increased bone remodeling that occur in osteomyelitis. Therefore, its accumulation in osseous sites that also are positive on technetium phos-

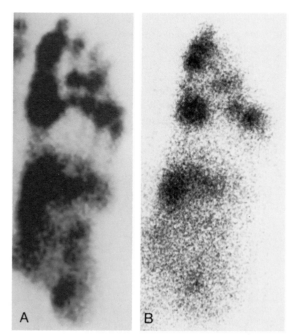

FIGURE 64–104. Alcoholic neuropathic osteoarthropathy without infection: Scintigraphy—gallium imaging. A bone scan (**A**) and gallium scan (**B**) are shown. The periarticular uptake of gallium in **B** reflects its bone scanning characteristics. This uptake, which is not out of proportion to that of technetium diphosphonate in A, has occurred at sites of neuropathic osteoarthropathy.

phate scans is not unexpected, and such accumulation by itself does not increase the specificity of the radionuclide examination (Fig. 64–104). Rather, when *both* technetium phosphate and gallium scanning are employed, it becomes important to compare the degree and extent of radionuclide uptake on the two examinations.[743] Disparate distribution of uptake or increased intensity of uptake on the gallium study is an important sign of osteomyelitis.[706] As many of the advantages of gallium imaging in cases of osteomyelitis, however, are provided by indium leukocyte imaging, which appears to be a superior technique in such cases (see later discussion), gallium rarely is used as a radiopharmaceutical agent for the diagnosis of osteomyelitis when indium-111 labeled leukocytes are available.[706]

The changing patterns of scintigraphic activity on initial and subsequent images after injection of bone-seeking radiopharmaceutical agents underscore the inaccuracy in interpretation that may occur during the analysis of single phase bone images alone. Although a definitely negative delayed bone image appears to be quite specific in excluding infection,[512] a positive finding during the delayed static phase of the examination lacks specificity for infection, being observed in a variety of other conditions as well. Furthermore, as noted earlier, the differentiation of cellulitis, osteomyelitis, and even septic arthritis may be difficult or impossible on the basis of alterations in this phase of the study. These problems have stimulated considerable interest in "three-phase" examinations in patients with musculoskeletal infection: Serial images are obtained during the first minute after the bolus injection of the technetium compound (angiographic phase); a postinjection image then is obtained at the end of the first minute or several minutes (blood pool phase); and additional images are obtained 2 or

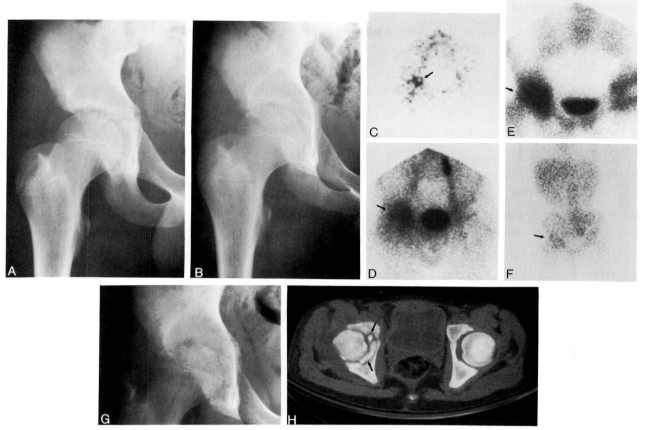

FIGURE 64–105. Septic arthritis: Scintigraphy—"three phase" bone scanning. A 12 year old boy developed severe pain in the hip. He initially was given a "flu" shot, but the pain continued. On physical examination, the hip was held in external rotation and was tender to palpation. An aspiration of its contents revealed several milliliters of thick, purulent material which, on Gram stain, was found to contain gram-positive cocci. Culture of the material led to the recovery of *Staphylococcus aureus*.

A, B Radiographs obtained 6 days apart show progressive joint space narrowing and osteopenia.

C–E A three-phase technetium phosphate study documents increased flow (arrow) in the angiographic phase **(C)**, diffuse hyperemia about the hip (arrow) in the blood pool stage **(D)**, and increased uptake of the radiopharmaceutical agent (arrow) in the delayed image **(E)**. The findings indicate septic arthritis.

F Gallium scan also is abnormal, with increased scintigraphic activity about the hip (arrow).

G Radiograph obtained 3 weeks after **A** documents significant erosion in the acetabulum and femoral head.

H Transaxial CT scan at the level of the femoral head shows sequestered bone (arrows) in the joint space. At surgery, fragments of cartilage and bone were discovered in the joint.

(Courtesy of G. Greenway, M.D., Dallas, Texas.)

3 hours later (delayed phase).[513] Although radionuclide angiography and blood pool imaging do not increase the sensitivity in detecting osteomyelitis, they do increase the specificity of scintigraphy for patients without osteomyelitis.[513] If increased accumulation of the radionuclide within the bone is observed in all three phases of the examination, the diagnosis of osteomyelitis is highly likely. Conversely, if such an increase is present only on the delayed image, an alternative diagnosis should be considered. Soft tissue infections are characterized by delayed images that either are normal or reveal minimally increased tracer accumulation within the bone, presumably because of regional hyperemia; by blood pool images that reveal diffuse hyperemia; and by radionuclide angiograms that show soft tissue hyperemia.[513] Septic arthritis usually is accompanied by increased uptake of the radiopharmaceutical agent in juxtaarticular bone in the delayed images, moderate and diffuse blood pool hyperemia, and, on the radionuclide angiogram,

increased flow to the joint space (Fig. 64–105).[513] Direct visualization of the synovium during the blood pool phase in this condition also has been observed.[518] In general, joint aspiration or arthrography prior to the bone scan does not interfere significantly with the scintigraphic diagnosis of septic arthritis.[552] Transient photopenia of the femoral head, however, has been reported when bone scintigraphy is performed within 30 minutes of the completion of an arthrogram of the hip, perhaps related to a venous tamponade resulting from the elevation of intra-articular pressure that accompanies joint distention.[704]

Although not without technical problems or diagnostic dilemmas, three-phase bone scintigraphy has been used successfully by a number of investigators in a variety of clinical situations.[515–517] The study has been applied with some success to the preoperative[516] and postoperative[517] evaluation of the feet in patients with diabetes mellitus, although in these persons the differentiation of neuropathic osteoarthropathy and osteomyelitis may not be possible.[516] The addition of a fourth phase to the scintigraphic examination, representing a static image obtained 24 hours after the injection of the bone-seeking radiopharmaceutical agent, may help in this differentiation.[550] Advantages of the 24-hour image relate to continued accumulation of the technetium phosphate radionuclide in the abnormal woven bone that is present about foci of infection (or neoplasm).[706] The sensitivity of both the three-phase and four-phase bone scans is decreased in neonatal osteomyelitis, in which regions of decreased accumulation of the radionuclide are encountered. In some cases, such regions may reflect the presence of a subperiosteal abscess that disrupts the important periosteal vessels that normally supply a large portion of the blood to bone in neonates.[697] The usefulness of the 24-hour delayed static image in the differentiation of osteomyelitis and soft tissue infection without adjacent osteomyelitis, particularly when a ratio of bone uptake at 24 hours and that at 4 hours is employed, has been emphasized.[712]

Bone marrow imaging with technetium sulfur-colloid has been used experimentally to evaluate osteomyelitis.[236] Decrease in accumulation of the radioactive agent that is observed in osteomyelitis but not in septic arthritis may reflect obstruction to blood flow in small arteries supplying the bone and bone marrow and influx of inflammatory cells into the affected area. A similar pattern of decreased activity, presumably related to bone infarction,[245] can be noted after technetium sulfur-colloid injection in patients with sickle cell anemia.

The accumulation of leukocytes at sites of abscess formation has led, in recent years, to attempts to isolate and label autologous leukocytes with radioactive tracers.[506] Of the potential agents that have been studied, indium-111, with a half-life of 67 hours, appears to be the most suitable, providing reasonable images as early as 4 to 6 hours after injection of the labeled leukocytes. The method, which requires removal of 50 ml of the patient's blood and leukocyte separation, isolation, and incubation, requires technical expertise and is somewhat time-consuming.[519–521] The success of ^{111}In leukocyte labeling in the identification of septic foci requires the migration of the leukocytes to the site of infection. Although it has been demonstrated that separation and labeling do not affect leukocyte function,[519, 521] the technique is better applied to acute infections associated with vigorous leukocyte infiltration, as opposed to chronic infections in which such migration may be insufficient.[519, 522–524, 551] Antibiotic administration does not appear to influence the sensitivity of detection. In general, ^{111}In labeled leukocyte scintigraphy is less sensitive in detecting bone infections than soft tissue infections (see Fig. 64–40) and leads to difficulty in differentiating osteomyelitis and septic arthritis.[524] It can demonstrate soft tissue extension from an area of bone infection.[524, 574] In the evaluation of a painful arthroplasty, abnormal accumulation of the labeled leukocytes usually indicates infection.[710]

Positive leukocyte images are encountered in musculoskeletal conditions other than infection. Rheumatoid arthritis and other synovial inflammatory disorders[525] can lead to findings simulating those of septic arthritis. Primary or secondary tumors in the soft tissues or bone can produce positive leukocyte images similar to those accompanying infection.[564] Iatrogenic osseous changes (sites of marrow aspiration and bone graft donor sites) and soft tissue ab-

normalities (hematomas, contusions, and thrombophlebitis) also can lead to scintigraphic alterations that resemble those of infection.[524] Although some reports have indicated that ^{111}In labeled leukocyte imaging can be used effectively in the diagnosis of infections complicating healing fractures (in which case radionuclide uptake is more prominent and prolonged than in noninfected healing fractures[708]), difficulties in the interpretation of the examination are encountered.[701] Similar difficulties arise in the assessment of infection in traumatized periarticular bone sites.[709] Furthermore, although the hallmark of a positive indium study for infection is an abnormal region of increased activity, regions of decreased activity at sites of infection also are seen, particularly in the spine, where indium uptake in hematopoietic bone marrow may be greater than that in the infected site.[705] These observations have led to some caution in the acceptance of the technique and to comparison studies using ^{111}In, ^{99m}Tc phosphate compounds, and [67]Ga. Compared to bone imaging with ^{99m}Tc compounds, ^{111}In scintigraphy has increased sensitivity in the detection of early osteomyelitis, but preparation of the labeled leukocytes is more time-consuming and the technique requires delayed imaging.[526] Although combined scans with both of these agents have been employed,[527, 711] [111]In leukocyte imaging, when performed within 24 hours of the bone scan, may yield artifacts unless meticulous technical guidelines are followed.[528] Such guidelines also must be followed when radionuclide bone imaging, bone marrow imaging, and leukocyte imaging are used together in an individual patient.[711] Compared to ^{67}Ga imaging, leukocyte scanning is preferable in infections of short duration, but, in cases of more prolonged sepsis, the latter technique may be falsely negative.[519] In such instances, gallium studies also should be employed. Despite its lack of specificity, ^{67}Ga imaging appears preferable in low grade infections,[519] although attempts to label with ^{111}In an increased number of lymphocytes, as opposed to polymorphonuclear leukocytes, have resulted in more successful identification of sites of low grade musculoskeletal sepsis.[529] Furthermore, the administration of ^{111}In labeled human nonspecific polyclonal immunoglobulin G also may prove useful in the assessment of musculoskeletal infections.[707] An advantage of this method over ^{67}Ga imaging is the absence of gastrointestinal or bone uptake that often interferes with interpretation; its advantages over ^{111}In leukocyte imaging include simple preparation procedure (without the need for phlebotomy or laborious labeling methods), avoidance of significant radiation exposure to labeled cells, reduction of radiation exposure to the patient, and the absence of a potentially confusing amount of uptake in the bone marrow.[705] Additional newer radionuclide imaging strategies for the diagnosis of musculoskeletal infections are discussed in Chapter 15.

Magnetic Resonance Imaging

After preliminary studies indicated the diagnostic potential of MR imaging in the assessment of osteomyelitis in both extraspinal and spinal sites,[530–532] a great deal of attention was directed to this topic. Many of the earlier investigations relied on the results of spin echo MR imaging alone and modifications in the signal intensity of marrow fat that occurred in hematogenous osteomyelitis or that related to spread from a contiguous contaminated source (particularly the soft tissues).[713–717] The signal intensity of normal bone marrow is variable, being influenced by the percentage of hematopoietic and fatty elements present. The normal orderly conversion of hematopoietic to fatty marrow that occurs during the first two decades of life, which results in an adult distribution by the age of approximately 25 years, has been described in detail elsewhere (see Chapters 10, 59, 65, and 85).[718, 719] This adult distribution, consisting of hematopoietic marrow confined mainly to the bones of the axial skeleton and proximal metaphyses of the femora and humeri and of fatty marrow in the bones of the appendicular skeleton and, to a lesser extent, regions of the axial skeleton, results in a "canvas" of variable signal intensity on which the finding of osteomyelitis is "painted." A canvas consisting of yellow marrow is of high signal intensity on

T1-weighted spin echo MR images and of somewhat lesser signal intensity on T2-weighted spin echo MR images; a canvas consisting of red marrow is of low signal intensity on both T1- and T2-weighted spin echo MR images. As described in these earlier publications,[713, 714, 716] the process of acute osteomyelitis typically appears as an area of low signal intensity on T1-weighted spin echo MR images and high signal intensity on T2-weighted spin echo MR images, its conspicuity being influenced by the hematopoietic or fatty nature of the adjacent marrow (Fig. 64–106). The process of subacute and chronic osteomyelitis has a more variable MR imaging appearance, although in cases of chronic active infection, similar characteristics of signal intensity are observed[715, 716] (Fig. 64–107). Additional MR imaging abnormalities in either acute or chronic osteomy-

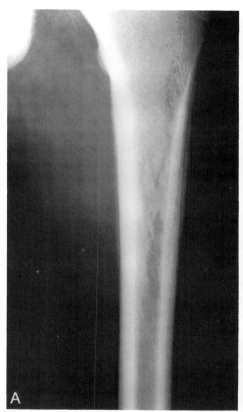

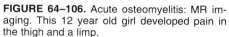

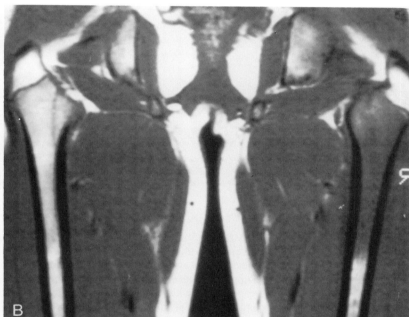

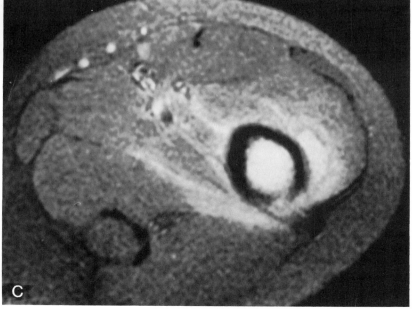

FIGURE 64–106. Acute osteomyelitis: MR imaging. This 12 year old girl developed pain in the thigh and a limp.

A The routine radiograph reveals poorly defined osteolysis in the femoral diaphysis with periostitis.

B Coronal T1-weighted (TR/TE, 650/20) spin echo MR image shows a long segment of abnormal bone marrow manifested as a region of low signal intensity.

C Transaxial T2-weighted (TR/TE, 2000/80) spin echo MR image shows that the infection, demonstrating high signal intensity, has extended from the marrow through the posterior cortex into the soft tissues. Documentation of the extent of the soft tissue infection, which requires its differentiation from edema, is difficult.

(Courtesy of G. Greenway, M.D., Dallas, Texas.)

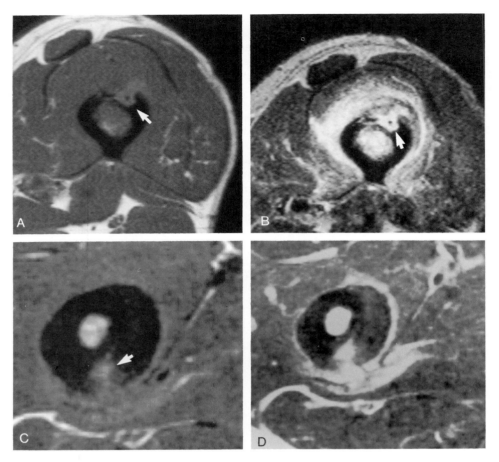

FIGURE 64–107. Subacute and chronic osteomyelitis: MR imaging.

A, B Osteomyelitis of the femur is well displayed on transaxial T1-weighted (TR/TE, 730/20) **(A)** and T2-weighted (TR/TE, 1800/80) **(B)** spin echo MR images. In **A,** note a cortical abscess (arrow) containing a sequestrum and abnormal marrow of low signal intensity. The soft tissue extension of infection is poorly seen. In **B,** the cortical abscess (arrow) again is identified. Infection in the marrow, cortex, and soft tissues is of high signal intensity. (Courtesy of M. Schweitzer, M.D., Philadelphia, Pennsylvania.)

C, D In a different patient with chronic active osteomyelitis of the femur, a transaxial T1-weighted (TR/TE, 500/40) spin echo MR image **(C)** shows diffuse cortical thickening, a cortical abscess (arrow), and soft tissue abnormalities. With T2 weighting (TR/TE, 2000/60) **(D),** the infectious process, including that in the marrow, is of high signal intensity. Note the soft tissue extension of the infection. (Courtesy of J. Robins, M.D., San Diego, California.)

elitis include cortical erosion or perforation, periosteal bone formation, and soft tissue involvement and, in chronic osteomyelitis, abscesses, bone sequestration, and sinus tracts.

Simultaneously with or subsequent to these initial investigations, several studies were reported in which MR imaging was used to investigate experimentally produced infections of the musculoskeletal system.[720–722] Results of these studies indicated an increased sensitivity and accuracy of MR imaging in the detection of soft tissue infection and equal sensitivity and accuracy of MR imaging in the detection of osteomyelitis when compared with three phase bone scintigraphy[720]; a slightly better overall accuracy of MR imaging when compared with contrast material–enhanced CT in the detection of either osteomyelitis or soft tissue abscesses[721]; and increased sensitivity of MR imaging when compared with CT in the detection of infective periostitis.[722]

In both clinical and experimental situations, modifications of MR imaging technique affect the sensitivity of this method in the detection of musculoskeletal infection as well as the manner in which such infection is displayed. With short tau inversion recovery (STIR) imaging, osteomyelitis and soft tissue infection appear as areas of markedly increased signal intensity that have been reported to be more conspicuous than on routine spin echo MR images[723, 724] (Fig. 64–108). T1- and T2-weighted contrasts are additive with STIR imaging; the combination of fat suppression and the additive effects of tissue brightening with this technique leads to the very high signal intensity of infectious (as well as neoplastic) lesions.[724] As STIR sequences are very sensitive to changes in water content, as occurs in peri-infectious (as well as peritumoral) edema, they may lead to an overestimation of the size of the lesion, however.[724, 725]

In experimental[726, 727] and clinical[728–731] situations, gadolinium-enhanced MR imaging has been used to study musculoskeletal infections. After intravenous administration of gadolinium contrast agent, areas of vascularized inflammatory tissue reveal enhancement of signal intensity, but nonvascularized abscess collections show either no enhancement or enhancement at the margin of the lesion.[728] The rim of enhancement of signal intensity about abscesses relates to a peripheral, cellular inflammatory zone, and the central nonenhancing region indicates necrotic tissue.[727] Brodie's abscesses, which typically appear as well-defined intraosseous regions of low signal intensity on T1-weighted spin echo MR images and of high signal intensity on T2-weighted spin echo MR images, with a rim of low signal intensity due to sclerotic bone, may be better delineated with gadolinium-enhanced MR imaging.[728] Such enhanced imaging can be used to demonstrate effectively areas of disease activity in patients with chronic osteomyelitis and the location and course of sinus tracts.[728] Sequestra appear as regions of low to intermediate signal intensity on both T1- and T2-weighted images and do not show enhancement of signal intensity after intravenous administration of gadolinium-based contrast agent. The inflamed synovial membrane in cases of septic arthritis, as in rheumatoid arthritis, will enhance after the intravenous injection of gadolinium agent.

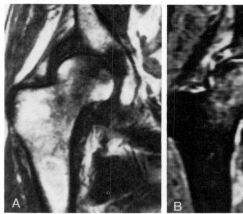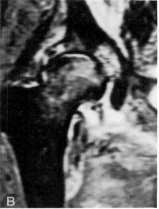

FIGURE 64–108. Septic arthritis and osteomyelitis: MR imaging.

A Coronal T1-weighted (TR/TE, 350/20) spin echo MR image displays the infectious process in this 75 year old woman as areas of low signal intensity in the proximal end of the right femur and adjacent acetabulum. A joint effusion of low signal intensity is evident.

B Coronal short tau inversion recovery (STIR) image (TR/TE, 2700/30; inversion time, 160 msec) better delineates the bone and soft tissue abnormalities, which are of high signal intensity. Although extremely sensitive in the documentation of inflammation, STIR imaging can lead to an overestimation of the extent of the process.

(Courtesy of M. Pathria, M.D., and D. Bates, M.D., San Diego, California.)

Reported data related to the use of gadolinium-enhanced MR imaging indicate clearly the increase in signal intensity that occurs in areas of active infection, whether they be in the bone or in the soft tissues. Although this might be interpreted as a distinct advantage in the diagnosis of such infection, this is not always the case. When osteomyelitis is present in regions of fatty marrow, enhancement of the signal intensity of the lesion may decrease its conspicuity on T1-weighted spin echo MR images owing to the high signal intensity of the adjacent marrow. The combination of gadolinium enhancement and fat suppression techniques may overcome this diagnostic difficulty (Fig. 64–109). Several fat suppression methods are available, some of which rely on chemical shift imaging that allows the selection of the correct transmission frequency so that fat preferentially can first be excited and then suppressed.[732] When used alone, fat suppression techniques may lead to decreased conspicuity of osteomyelitis; with suppression of fat signal on T1-weighted spin echo MR images, an infective lesion in the marrow, with its low signal intensity, may no longer be separated clearly from the surrounding fatty marrow. Similar fat suppression combined with heavily T2-weighted images (e.g., fast spin echo MR images) may display the site of osteomyelitis adequately, however. Use of a paramagnetic contrast agent (i.e., gadolinium based) in combination with the fat suppression technique improves the contrast between pathologic lesions, including infection, and normal structures, particularly those containing fat (e.g., marrow, soft tissues).[732]

When comparison is made between two popular methods of fat suppression, STIR and chemical presaturation (ChemSat) imaging, advantages and disadvantages of each can be identified.[732] The advantages of STIR imaging are that it can markedly suppress the signal from fat at several field strengths, requires no additional heating over normal inversion recovery, leads to fewer problems with an inho-

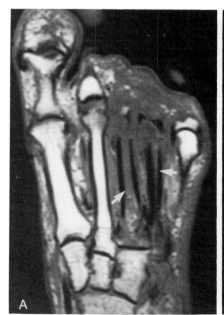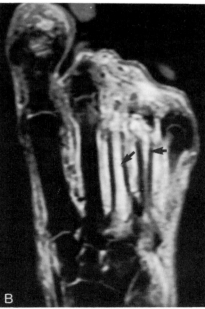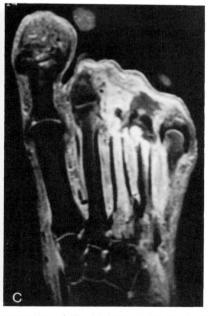

FIGURE 64–109. Diabetic foot infection: MR imaging. This 63 year old man had required amputation of the third toe at the level of the metatarsophalangeal joint for control of infection. He later developed clinical manifestations of recurrent infection.

A Transverse T1-weighted (TR/TE, 700/15) spin echo MR image shows abnormally low signal intensity in the third and fourth metatarsal bones (arrows) and in the adjacent soft tissues. The head of the second metatarsal bone also appears to be involved.

B Transverse short tau inversion recovery (STIR) image (TR/TE, 1800/25; inversion time, 160 msec) reveals high signal intensity in these metatarsal bones (arrows) and soft tissues.

C Transverse T1-weighted (TR/TE, 900/13) fat suppressed (ChemSat) image obtained in conjunction with intravenous administration of gadolinium contrast agent gives information similar to that in **B**. A third and fourth ray resection confirmed the presence of osteomyelitis.

mogeneous magnetic field, and allows the operator to lengthen the echo time and obtain cumulation contrast effects from T1 recovery and T2 decay; the disadvantages of STIR imaging include longer duration (repetition times may be as long as 2000 msec), relative incompatibility with other MR techniques, suppression of signals from tissues with similar T1 values (e.g., resolving hematoma and paramagnetically enhanced tissues), and for a given repetition time, fewer imaging slices than with conventional spin echo MR imaging techniques. The advantages of ChemSat include its application to many other MR imaging techniques, fat specificity, and compatibility with gadolinium-enhanced MR imaging. Its disadvantages include image degradation related to inhomogeneities in the magnetic field, reliance on high field strength magnets, and an increase in time due to the application of the fat-selective saturation radiofrequency pulse and dephasing gradient.

The appearance of musculoskeletal infections in sequences using gadolinium enhancement and fat suppression is similar to that obtained with gadolinium enhancement alone, although in some instances the former combination leads to increased conspicuity of the disease process. For example, by enhancing the signal intensity of a focus of osteomyelitis using gadolinium-based agent and depressing the signal intensity of the adjacent marrow using fat suppression, the disease process is displayed vividly. Enhancement of signal intensity about abscesses in bone and soft tissue and at the margins of sinus tracts also is well seen.

Although numerous reviews of the subject have emphasized the sensitivity of MR imaging in the diagnosis of musculoskeletal infections,[733, 734] it is this very sensitivity that can lead to diagnostic problems, particularly in defining the extent of the process.[735] Several specific problem areas can be defined:

1. In *acute osteomyelitis,* differentiation of soft tissue extension of infection and soft tissue edema. This diagnostic problem is not unique to MR imaging (e.g., it occurs as well with CT) nor to infection. (e.g., tumor). Both soft tissue infection and soft tissue edema lead to similar characteristics with MR imaging, including high signal intensity on T2-weighted spin echo and STIR imaging in muscles and fascial planes. Localized soft tissue abscesses, however, more typically produce a mass effect, focal disruption of fascial planes, and peripheral or rim enhancement after the intravenous administration of gadolinium contrast agent.

2. In *septic arthritis,* differentiation of secondary osteomyelitis and bone marrow edema; or in *acute osteomyelitis affecting epiphyses,* differentiation of secondary septic arthritis and sympathetic effusions. The occurrence of marrow edema in subarticular bone about septic joints produces, on spin echo and STIR sequences, changes in signal intensity identical to those of secondary osteomyelitis. Although it is suggested that high signal intensity of the marrow on both types of sequences is more suggestive of infection than edema,[735] more supportive data are required. The presence of bone marrow changes isolated to one side of the infected joint, of marginal erosions of bone, and of periosteal reaction is more consistent with osteomyelitis than with edema. The occurrence of sympathetic effusions (Fig. 64–110) in cases of acute epiphyseal osteomyelitis (particularly involving the proximal femoral epiphysis in infants and children) is well recognized (see earlier discussion). The intravenous administration of gadolinium contrast agent, allowing delineation of the degree and extent of

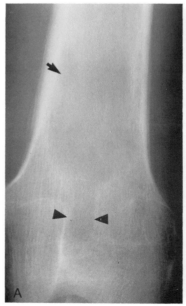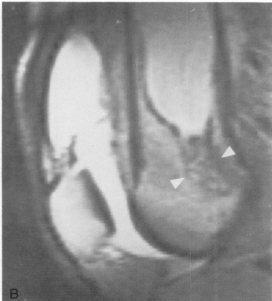

FIGURE 64–110. Osteomyelitis with sympathetic joint effusion: MR imaging. This 23 year old man developed osteomyelitis after a fracture of the femur at the age of 13 years. He has had a 4 month history of thigh pain. Although arthrocentesis of the knee revealed noninfected fluid, surgery confirmed a femoral abscess related to *Staphylococcus aureus* infection.

A On the routine radiograph, observe an abscess of the femoral diaphysis (arrow) with a distal tract (arrowheads) extending into the metaphysis. The latter finding is diagnostic of infection.

B Sagittal T2-weighted (TR/TE, 2000/120) spin echo MR image reveals high signal intensity in the diaphyseal abscess and joint, consistent with fluid. Note the low signal intensity in the tract (arrowheads).

(Courtesy of G. Greenway, M.D., Dallas, Texas.)

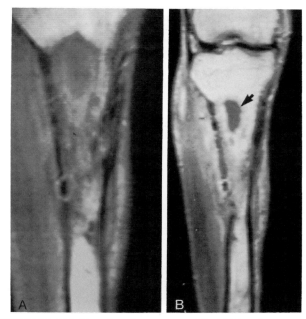

FIGURE 64–111. Chronic active osteomyelitis: MR imaging.
A Coronal T1-weighted (TR/TE, 600/30) spin echo MR image of the lower leg shows low signal intensity in the marrow of the proximal end of the tibia. Artifact related to a previously removed metal plate is seen.
B Coronal T1-weighted (TR/TE, 600/30) spin echo MR image obtained after the intravenous injection of gadolinium contrast agent reveals enhancement of signal intensity in the actively infected marrow and fluid of low signal intensity in an abscess (arrow).
(Courtesy of T. Mattsson, M.D., Riyadh, Saudia Arabia.)

synovial proliferation, may prove helpful in differentiating between sterile and infective effusions, although diagnostic arthrocentesis usually is required.

3. In *chronic osteomyelitis,* differentiation of active and inactive disease. This differentiation can be difficult, not just with MR imaging but with other imaging techniques as well. MR imaging findings more compatible with inactive chronic osteomyelitis are the absence of sequestra and the presence of normal marrow fat in involved regions. MR imaging findings more compatible with active chronic osteomyelitis are the presence of sequestra, periosteal elevation with bone formation and subperiosteal fluid, and areas of high signal intensity in the involved marrow on T2-weighted spin echo and STIR images and on gadolinium-enhanced images (Fig. 64–111). None of these findings, however, is diagnostic of active or inactive chronic osteomyelitis.

4. In *soft tissue infections,* differentiation of infective periostitis, osteitis, or osteomyelitis and bone marrow edema. This problem, which has its greatest clinical importance in the assessment of the foot in diabetic patients (see later discussion), is encountered with routine radiography, CT, scintigraphy, and MR imaging. With the last of these techniques, areas of high signal intensity in the marrow adjacent to sites of soft tissue infection on standard T2-weighted spin echo, gadolinium-enhanced T1-weighted spin echo, and STIR images are not diagnostic of bone contamination. The more diffuse the intraosseous abnormalities, the more likely it is that secondary osteomyelitis is present. Additional MR imaging findings supporting the diagnosis of osteomyelitis are cortical erosion or violation

and extensive periosteal bone formation. The absence of marrow abnormalities in cases of soft tissue infection generally eliminates the possibility of osteomyelitis (Fig. 64–112).

The assessment of infection in the feet of diabetic patients provides unique challenges. Although reported data indicate the value of scintigraphic methods, particularly ^{111}In leukocyte imaging with or without bone scintigraphy in this assessment,[602, 736] the day-to-day clinical experience of many physicians suggests otherwise. A normal bone scan virtually excludes the presence of osteomyelitis, but this is relatively uncommon in diabetic patients whose routine radiographs of the feet reveal changes of soft tissue infection, neuropathic osteoarthropathy, or both.[736] The hyperemia associated with either process can lead to positive results with three-phase bone scintigraphy.[604] Although ^{67}Ga-citrate scintigraphy may increase the specificity for diagnosing osteomyelitis, uptake of this agent in neuropathic osteoarthropathic sites is encountered (see Fig. 64–104). Decreased blood flow and possible impaired leukocyte responsiveness limit the sensitivity achievable with ^{111}In leukocyte scintigraphy in diabetic foot infections, although specificity may be increased.[736] Reports indicate that the finding of definite increased uptake on leukocyte scans has a high positive predictive value but a somewhat lower sensitivity in the diagnosis of osteomyelitis complicating soft tissue infection, whereas absence of increased leukocyte uptake in or near bone makes the diagnosis of osteomyelitis very unlikely.[736] When increased leukocyte uptake is subtle or cannot be localized exclusively to soft tissue, other imaging techniques may be necessary.[736]

It is not surprising, therefore, that MR imaging has been applied to the analysis of infections in the feet of diabetic patients.[603, 604] Although high signal intensity in the bone marrow on T2-weighted spin echo and STIR images and on T1-weighted spin echo MR images (with or without fat saturation) after the intravenous administration of gadolin-

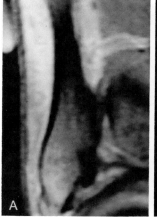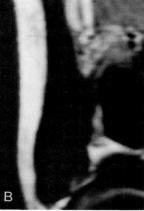

FIGURE 64–112. Cellulitis: MR imaging.
A Coronal gadolinum-enhanced, fat suppressed T1-weighted (TR/TE, 517/12) spin echo MR image shows high signal intensity in the inflamed soft tissues but no marrow abnormalities in the adjacent fibula.
B Coronal STIR MR image (TR/TE, 2100/35; inversion time, 160 msec) demonstrates similar findings.
(Courtesy of M. Pathria, M.D., and D. Bates, M.D., San Diego, California.)

TABLE 64–8. MR Imaging Signal Intensity Characteristics of Normal and Abnormal Bone Marrow

Marrow Type	T1-Weighted Spin Echo Images	T2-Weighted Spin Echo Images	Gadolinium-Enhanced T1-Weighted Spin Echo Images	Gadolinium-Enhanced Fat Suppressed T1-Weighted Spin Echo Images
Normal red marrow	Low	Variable	Variable*	Variable
Normal yellow marrow	High	Intermediate	High	Low
Osteomyelitis	Low	High	High	High

*Marrow may enhance in children.

ium contrast agent is compatible with the diagnosis of osteomyelitis, it is not a specific finding (Fig. 64–113). Some investigators indicate that neuropathic osteoarthropathy in the absence of coexistent infection is accompanied by persistent low signal intensity in the bone marrow on T2-weighted spin echo MR images,[603] although this is not a constant finding. Furthermore, sympathetic joint effusions in the feet of diabetic patients produce MR imaging findings that are very similar to those of septic arthritis, and differentiation of soft tissue edema and soft tissue infection with MR imaging in this clinical setting is a problem.

The specificity of the MR imaging findings in cases of osteomyelitis at any skeletal site is limited. Other processes associated with marrow infiltration, such as tumors, myelofibrosis, and Gaucher's disease, produce similar alterations. Bone marrow ischemia and edema also can lead to problems in differential diagnosis. It becomes mandatory to review carefully all clinical and other imaging data prior to performing the MR imaging examination in patients with suspected musculoskeletal infection and to select thoughtfully the most appropriate MR imaging sequences to be performed. To again use the analogy of the creation of a painting, the selection of the specific MR imaging sequence or technique must be accomplished with the idea of providing the most vivid contrast between the canvas (i.e., the bone marrow, joint, or soft tissues) and the paint (i.e., the disease process such as osteomyelitis, septic arthritis, or soft tissue infection) with skillful strokes of the brush (i.e., the MR imaging sequence or technique). In cases of active

osteomyelitis, the choice of MR imaging technique is based on providing high contrast between the signal intensity characteristics of the infection and those of the bone marrow (Table 64–8). Some guidelines for this choice in instances of osteomyelitis, septic arthritis, and soft tissue infections are provided in Table 64–9.

SUMMARY

A thorough understanding of regional anatomy is fundamental to the accurate interpretation of clinical, radiologic, and pathologic characteristics of infections of bone, joint, and soft tissue. In most persons with such infections, a specific mechanism of contamination can be recognized; infection may be derived from hematogenous seeding, spread from a contiguous source, direct implantation, or operative contamination. The radiographic findings of osteomyelitis (including abscess, involucrum, sequestration), septic arthritis (including joint space loss, marginal and

TABLE 64–9. Some Useful MR Imaging Protocols in Assessment of Musculoskeletal Infections

Condition	Suggested Protocols
Osteomyelitis in red marrow	T2-weighted spin echo T1-weighted spin echo with gadolinium contrast enhancement STIR
Osteomyelitis in yellow marrow	T1-weighted spin echo T1-weighted spin echo with gadolinium contrast enhancement and fat suppression STIR
Septic arthritis	T1-weighted spin echo with gadolinium contrast enhancement with or without fat suppression
Soft tissue infection	T1-weighted spin echo with gadolinium contrast enhancement with or without fat suppression

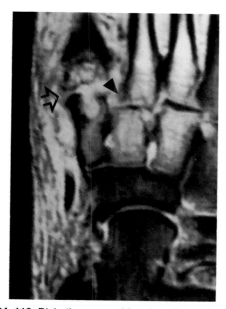

FIGURE 64–113. Diabetic neuropathic osteoarthropathy and osteomyelitis: MR imaging. A transverse short tau inversion recovery (STIR) image (TR/TE, 1800/20; inversion time, 125 msec) shows high signal intensity in the marrow of the second and third metatarsal bones, in the intermediate and lateral cuneiforms, and in the soft tissues. Note the neuropathic changes about the first tarsometatarsal joint (arrow) and a Lisfranc pattern of subluxation (arrowhead). Differentiating sites of osteomyelitis and of neuropathic disease with marrow edema in such cases is difficult.

central osseous erosions), and soft tissue suppuration (including swelling, radiolucent streaks, and periostitis) generally are delayed for a variable period after the clinical onset of infection. Other diagnostic techniques, including scintigraphy and MR imaging, allow accurate diagnosis at an earlier stage of the process.

References

1. Nelaton A: Elements de pathologie chirurgicale. Paris, Germer-Bailliere, 1844–1859.
2. Jaffe HL: Metabolic, Degenerative, and Inflammatory Diseases of Bones and Joints. Philadelphia, Lea & Febiger, 1972.
3. Waldvogel FA, Medoff G, Swartz MN: Osteomyelitis: A review of clinical features, therapeutic considerations and unusual aspects. Part I. N Engl J Med 282:198, 1970.
4. Garré C.: Über besondere Formen und Folgezustande der akuten infektiosen Osteomyelitis. Bruns Beitr Klin Chir 10:241, 1893.
5. Thoma, KH, Goldman HM: Oral Pathology. 5th Ed. St Louis, CV Mosby Co, 1960, p 719.
6. Trueta J: Studies of the Development and Decay of the Human Frame. Philadelphia, WB Saunders Co, 1968, p 254.
7. Kahn DS, Pritzker KPH: The pathophysiology of bone infection. Clin Orthop 96:12, 1973.
8. Atcheson SG, Ward JR: Acute hematogenous osteomyelitis progressing to septic synovitis and eventual pyarthrosis. Arthritis Rheum 21:968, 1978.
9. Capitanio MA, Kirkpatrick JA: Early roentgen observations in acute osteomyelitis. AJR 108:488, 1970.
10. Nixon GW: Hematogenous osteomyelitis of metaphyseal-equivalent locations. AJR 130:123, 1978.
11. Lindberg L, Lidgren L: Bone and joint infections. Int Orthp (SICOT) 1:191, 1977.
12. Ferguson AB Jr: Osteomyelitis in children. Clin Orthop 96:51, 1973.
13. Mollan RAB, Piggot J: Acute osteomyelitis in children. J Bone Joint Surg [Br] 59:2, 1977.
14. Troger J, Eibner D, Otte G, et al: Diagnose und Differential-diagnose der akuten hämatogen Osteomyelitis des Sauglings. Radiologe 19:99, 1979.
15. Edwards MS, Baker CJ, Wagner ML, et al: An etiologic shift in infantile osteomyelitis: The emergence of the group B streptococcus. J Pediatr 93:578, 1978.
16. Brill PW, Winchester P, Krauss AN, et al: Osteomyelitis in a neonatal intensive care unit. Radiology 131:83, 1979.
17. Butt WP: The radiology of infection. Clin Orthop 96:20, 1973.
18. Trueta J: The three types of acute hematogenous osteomyelitis. A clinical and vascular study. J Bone Joint Surg [Br] 41:671, 1959.
19. Winters JL, Cahen I: Acute hematogenous osteomyelitis: A review of sixty-six cases. J Bone Joint Surg [Am] 42:691, 1960.
20. Shandling B: Acute hematogenous osteomyelitis: A review of 300 cases treated during 1952–1959. S Afr Med J 34:520, 1960.
21. Weissberg ED, Smith AL, Smith DH: Clinical features of neonatal osteomyelitis. Pediatrics 53:505, 1974.
22. Green WT: Osteomyelitis in infancy. JAMA 105:1835, 1935.
23. Ogden JA, Lister G: The pathology of neonatal osteomyelitis. Pediatrics 55:474, 1975.
24. Dich VQ, Nelson JD, Haltalin KC: Osteomyelitis in infants and children. A review of 163 cases. Am J Dis Child 129:1273, 1975.
25. Clarke AM: Neonatal osteomyelitis: A disease different from osteomyelitis of older children. Med J Aust 1:237, 1958.
26. Lim MQ, Gresham EL, Franklin EA Jr, et al: Osteomyelitis as a complication of umbilical artery catheterization. Am J Dis Child 131:142, 1977.
27. Krauss AN, Albert RF, Kannan MM: Contamination of umbilical catheters in the newborn infant. J Pediatr 77:965, 1970.
28. Simmons PB, Harris LE, Bianco AJ Jr: Complications of exchange transfusion. Report of two cases of septic arthritis and osteomyelitis. Mayo Clin Proc 48:190, 1973.
29. Cohen LS, Fekety FR Jr, Cluff LE: Studies of the epidemiology of staphylococcal infection. VI. Infections in the surgical patient. Ann Surg 159:321, 1964.
30. Davis LA: Antibiotic modified osteomyelitis. AJR 103:608, 1968.
31. Blanche DW: Osteomyelitis in infants. J Bone Joint Surg [Am] 34:71, 1952.
32. Warwick R, Williams PL (Eds): Gray's Anatomy. 35th British Ed. Philadelphia, WB Saunders Co, 1973, pp 220, 406.
33. Crock HV: The Blood Supply of the Lower Limb Bones in Man. London, E & S Livingstone Ltd, 1967, p 29.
34. Gardner E: Blood and nerve supply of joints. Stanford Med Bull 11:203, 1953.
35. Tachdjian MO: Pediatric Orthopedics. Philadelphia, WB Saunders Co, 1972, p 352.
36. Trueta J: Acute hematogenous osteomyelitis: Its pathology and treatment. Bull Hosp Joint Dis 14:5, 1953.
37. Trueta J: Acute hematogenous osteomyelitis: Its pathology and treatment. Bull NY Acad Med 35:25, 1959.
38. Trueta J: The normal vascular anatomy of the human femoral head during growth. J Bone Joint Surg [Br] 39:358, 1957.
39. Hobo T: Zur Pathogenese der akuten haematogenen Osteomyelitis mit Berucksichtigung der Vitalfarbungslehre. Acta Sch Med Univ Kioto 4:1, 1921.
40. Koch J: Untersuchungen über die Lokalisation der Bakterien: Das Verhalten des Knochenmarkes und die Veranderungen der Knochen, insbesondere der Epiphysen bei Infektionskrankheiten. Z Hyg Infektionskr 69:436, 1911.
41. Morrey BF, Bianco AJ, Rhodes KH: Hematogenous osteomyelitis at uncommon sites in children. Mayo Clin Proc 53:707, 1978.
42. Brookes M: The Blood Supply of Bone. London, Butterworths, 1971.
43. Wilensky AO: Osteomyelitis: Its Pathogenesis, Symptomatology and Treatment. New York, Macmillan Co, 1934, p 114.
44. Green M, Nyhan WL Jr, Fousek MD: Acute hematogenous osteomyelitis. Pediatrics 17:368, 1956.
45. Gilmour WN: Acute haematogenous osteomyelitis. J Bone Joint Surg [Br] 44:841, 1962.
46. Moyson FR, Brombart JC, Wittek FR: Ostéomyélite de l'enfant. Signes radiologiques précoces. J Belge Radiol 55:645, 1972.
47. Bretagne M-C, Jolly A, Mouton J-N, et al: Mémoires originaux. Ostéomyélite pseudo-sarcomateuse de l'enfant. J Radiol Electrol Med Nucl 58:1, 1977.
48. Jorup S, Kjellberg SR: Early diagnosis of acute septic osteomyelitis, periostitis and arthritis, and its importance in treatment. Acta Radiol 30:316, 1948.
49. Griffin PP: Bone and joint infections in children. Pediatr Clin North Am 14:533, 1967.
50. Brodie BC: An account of some cases of chronic abscess of the tibia. Trans Med Chir Soc 17:238, 1832.
51. Brodie BC: Pathological and Surgical Observations on the Diseases of the Joint. 4th Ed. London, Longman, 1836, p 298.
52. Brickner WM: The treatment of chronic bone abscesses by simple evacuation through a small drill hole. Its application in non-sterile abscesses. J Bone Joint Surg 5:492, 1923.
53. Henderson MS, Simon ME: Brodie's abscess. Arch Surg 9:504, 1924.
54. Brailsford JF: Brodie's abscess and its differential diagnosis. Br Med J 2:119, 1938.
55. Harris NH, Kirkaldy-Willis WH: Primary subacute pyogenic osteomyelitis. J Bone Joint Surg [Br] 47:526, 1965.
56. Kandel SN, Mankin HJ: Pyogenic abscess of the long bones in children. Clin Orthop 96:108, 1973.
57. Gledhill RB: Subacute osteomyelitis in children. Clin Orthop 96:57, 1973.
58. Cabanela ME, Sim FH, Beabout JW, et al: Osteomyelitis appearing as neoplasms. A diagnostic problem. Arch Surg 109:68, 1974.
59. Weston WT: Case report 44. Skel Radiol 2:125, 1977.
60. Waldvogel FA, Medoff G, Swartz MN: Osteomyelitis: A review of clinical features, therapeutic considerations and unusual aspects. Part 2. N Engl J Med 282:260, 1970.
61. VanNiekerk JP de V: Hand infections: Management and results based on a new classification: A study of more than 1000 cases. S Afr Med J 40:316, 1966.
62. Kinnman JEG, Lee HS: Chronic osteomyelitis of the mandible: Clinical study of thirteen cases. Oral Surg 25:6, 1968.
63. Blumenfeld RJ, Skolnik EM: Intracranial complications of sinus disease. Trans Am Acad Ophthalmol Otolaryngol 70:899, 1966.
64. Francis DP, Holmes MA, Brandon G: Pasteurella multocida infections after domestic animal bites and scratches. JAMA 233:42, 1975.
65. Hooper G: Tooth fragment in a metacarpophalangeal joint. Hand 10:215, 1978.
66. Lavine LS, Isenberg HD, Rubins W, et al: Unusual osteomyelitis following superficial dog bites. Clin Orthop 98:251, 1974.
67. Chusid MJ, Jacobs WM, Sty JR: Pseudomonas arthritis following puncture wounds of the foot. J Pediatr 94:429, 1979.
68. Miller EH, Semian DW: Gram-negative osteomyelitis following puncture wounds of the foot. J Bone Joint Surg [Am] 57:535, 1975.
69. Tscherne H, Trentz O: Gelenkinfektionen nach perforierenden Wunden, Punktionen und Injektioner. Langenbecks Arch Chir 334:521, 1973.
70. Brand RA, Black H: Pseudomonas osteomyelitis following puncture wounds in children. J Bone Joint Surg [Am] 56:1637, 1974.
71. Swischuk LE, Jorgenson F, Jorgenson A, et al: Wooden splinter induced "pseudotumors" and "osteomyelitis-like lesions" of bone and soft tissue. AJR 122:176, 1974.
72. Manny J, Haruzi I, Yosipovitch Z: Osteomyelitis of the clavicle following subclavian vein catheterization. Arch Surg 106:342, 1973.
73. Lilien LD, Harris VJ, Ramamurthy RS, et al: Neonatal osteomyelitis of the calcaneus: Complication of heel puncture. J Pediatr 88:478, 1976.
74. Koch SL: Osteomyelitis of the bones of the hand. Surg Gynecol Obstet 64:1, 1937.
75. Whitehouse WM, Smith WS: Osteomyelitis of the feet. Semin Roentgenol 5:367, 1970.
76. Suydam MJ, Mikity VG: Cellulitis with underlying inflammatory periostitis of the mandible. AJR 106:133, 1969.
77. Martel W, Abell MR: Radiologic evaluation of soft tissue tumors. A retrospective study. Cancer 32:352, 1973.
78. Resnick D: Osteomyelitis and septic arthritis complicating hand injuries and infections: Pathogenesis of roentgenographic abnormalities. J Can Assoc Radiol 27:21, 1976.
79. Resnick D: The roentgenographic anatomy of the tendon sheaths of the hand and wrist: Tenography. AJR 124:44, 1975.
80. Lampe EW: Surgical anatomy of the hand with special reference to infections and trauma. Clin Symp 21:66, 1969.
81. Kanavel A: Infections of the Hand. A Guide to the Surgical Treatment of Acute

and Chronic Suppurative Processes in the Fingers, Hand, and Forearm. 7th Ed. Philadelphia, Lea & Febiger, 1939.

82. Boyes JH: Bunnell's Surgery of the Hand. 5th Ed. Philadelphia, JB Lippincott, 1970.
83. Flynn JE: Clinical and anatomical investigations of deep fascial space infections of the hand. Am J Surg 55:467, 1942.
84. Carter SJ, Mersheimer WL: Infections of the hand. Orthop Clin North Am 1:455, 1970.
85. Robins RHC: Infections of the hand. A review based on 1000 consecutive cases. J Bone Joint Surg [Br] 34:567, 1952.
86. Macey HB: Paronychia and bone felon. Am J Surg 50:553, 1940.
87. Daniel DM: The acutely swollen hand in the drug user. Arch Surg 107:548, 1973.
88. Neviaser RJ, Butterfield WC, Wiehe DR: The puffy hand of drug addiction. A study of the pathogenesis. J Bone Joint Surg [Am] 54:629, 1972.
89. Whitaker LA, Graham WP III: Management of hand infections in the narcotic addict. Plast Reconstr Surg 52:384, 1973.
90. Ellenberg M: Diabetic foot. NY State J Med 73:2778, 1973.
91. Levin M, O'Neal LW: The Diabetic Foot. St Louis, CV Mosby, 1973.
92. Meade JW, Mueller CB: Major infections of the foot. Med Times 96:154, 1968.
93. Godinsky M: A study of the fascial spaces of the foot and their bearing on infections. Surg Gynecol Obstet 49:737, 1929.
94. Kamel R, Sakla FB: Anatomical compartments of the sole of the human foot. Anat Rec 140:57, 1961.
95. Martin BF: Observations on the muscles and tendons of the medial aspect of the sole of the foot. J Anat 98:437, 1964.
96. Rao VR, Kini MG: Infections of the foot—an anatomical and experimental study of the fascial spaces and tendon sheaths with clinical correlations of certain types of infections of the foot. Indian Med Res Memoirs 37:1, 1957.
97. Feingold ML, Resnick D, Niwayama G, Garetto L: The plantar compartments of the foot: A roentgen approach. I. Experimental observations. Invest Radiol 12:281, 1977.
98. Johanson PH: Pseudomonas infections of the foot following puncture wounds. JAMA 204:262, 1968.
99. Hagler DJ: Pseudomonas osteomyelitis: Puncture wounds of the feet. Pediatrics 48:672, 1971.
100. Minnefor AB, Olson MI, Carver DH: Pseudomonas osteomyelitis following puncture wounds of the foot. Pediatrics 47:598, 1971.
101. Waldvogel FA, Medoff G, Swartz MN: Osteomyelitis: A review of clinical features, therapeutic considerations and unusual aspects. Part 3. N Engl J Med 282:316, 1970.
102. Lipscomb H, Dobson HL, Greene JA: Infection in the diabetic. South Med J 52:16, 1959.
103. Spring M, Kahn S: Nonclostridial gas infection in the diabetic. Review of the literature and report of three cases. Arch Intern Med 88:373, 1951.
104. Wills MR, Reece MW: Non-clostridial infections in diabetes mellitus. Br Med J 2:566, 1960.
105. Warren S, LeCompte PM, Legg MA: The Pathology of Diabetes Mellitus. 4th Ed. Philadelphia, Lea & Febiger, 1966, p 167.
106. Deutsch SD: Non-clostridial gas infection of a fracture in a diabetic. A case report. J Bone Joint Surg [Am] 57:1009, 1975.
107. Boyce FF: Human bites. An analysis of 90 (chiefly delayed and late) cases from Charity Hospital of Louisiana at New Orleans. South Med J 35:631, 1942.
108. Farmer CB, Mann RJ: Human bite infections of the hand. South Med J 59:515, 1966.
109. Lowry TM: Infected human bites. Analysis of treatment and results in twenty-eight cases. Surg Clin North Am 21:565, 1941.
110. Miller H, Winfield JM: Human bites of the hand. Surg Gynecol Obstet 74:153, 1942.
111. Chuinard RG, D'Ambrosia R: Human bite infections of the hand. J Bone Joint Surg [Am] 59:416, 1977.
112. Mason ML, Koch SL: Human bite infections of the hand with a study of the routes of extension of infection from the dorsum of the hand. Surg Gynecol Obstet 51:591, 1930.
113. Tindall JP, Harrison CM: Pasteurella multocida infections following animal injuries, especially cat bites. Arch Dermatol 105:412, 1972.
114. Lee MLH, Buhr AJ: Dog bites and local infection with Pasteurella septica. Br Med J 1:169, 1960.
115. Hubbert WT, Rosen MN: Pasteurella multocida infection due to animal bite. Am J Public Health 60:1103, 1970.
116. Carithers HA: Mammalian bites of children: A problem in accident prevention. Am J Dis Child 95:150, 1958.
117. Smith JE: Studies on Pasteurella septica. The occurrence in the nose and tonsils of dogs. J Comp Pathol 65:239, 1955.
118. Owen CR, Buker EO, Bell JF, et al: Pasteurella multocida in animals' mouths. Rocky Mountain Med J 65:45, 1968.
119. Stevens DB: Postoperative orthopaedic infections. A study of etiological mechanisms. J Bone Joint Surg [Am] 46:96, 1964.
120. Harris WH: Sinking prostheses. Surg Gynecol Obstet 123:1297, 1966.
121. Petty W, Bryan RS, Coventry MB, et al: Infection after total knee arthroplasty. Orthop Clin North Am 6:1005, 1975.
122. Kaushal SP, Galante JO, McKenna R, et al: Complication following total knee replacement. Clin Orthop 121:181, 1976.
123. Patterson FP, Brown CS: Complications of total hip replacement arthroplasty. Orthop Clin North Am 4:503, 1973.

124. Bryson AF, Mandell BB: Primary closure after operative treatment of gross chronic osteomyelitis. Lancet 1:1179, 1964.
125. Griffiths JC: Defects in long bones from severe neglected osteitis. J Bone Joint Surg [Br] 50:813, 1968.
126. Potter CMC: Osteomyelitis in the new-born. J Bone Joint Surg [Br] 36:578, 1954.
127. Smith T: On the acute arthritis of infants. St Bartholomew's Hosp Rep 10:189, 1874.
128. Roberts PH: Disturbed epiphyseal growth at the knee after osteomyelitis in infancy. J Bone Joint Surg [Br] 52:692, 1970.
129. Trueta J, Amato VP: The vascular contributions to osteogenesis. III. Changes in the growth cartilage caused by experimentally induced ischaemia. J Bone Joint Surg [Br] 42:571, 1960.
130. Hall R McK: Regeneration of the lower femoral epiphysis. J Bone Joint Surg [Br] 36:116, 1954.
131. Lloyd-Roberts GC: Suppurative arthritis of infancy. Some observations upon prognosis and management. J Bone Joint Surg [Br] 42:706, 1960.
132. Sedlin ED, Fleming JL: Epidermoid carcinoma arising in chronic osteomyelitic foci. J Bone Joint Surg [Am] 45:827, 1963.
133. Johnston RM, Miles JS: Sarcomas arising from chronic osteomyelitic sinuses. A report of two cases. J Bone Joint Surg [Am] 55:162, 1973.
134. Dränert K, Rüter A, Burri C, et al: Fistelmalignome bei chronischer Osteomyelitis. Arch Orthop Unfallchir 84:199, 1976.
135. Henderson MS, Swart HA: Chronic osteomyelitis associated with malignancy. J Bone Joint Surg 18:56, 1936.
136. Fitzgerald RH, Brewer NS, Dahlin DC: Squamous-cell carcinoma complicating chronic osteomyelitis. J Bone Joint Surg [Am] 58:1146, 1976.
137. Bereston ES, Ney C: Squamous cell carcinoma arising in a chronic osteomyelitic sinus tract with metastasis. Arch Surg 43:257, 1941.
138. Lidgren L: Neoplasia in chronic fistulating osteitis. Acta Orthop Scand 44:152, 1973.
139. Waugh W: Fibrosarcoma occurring in chronic bone sinus. J Bone Joint Surg [Br] 34:642, 1952.
140. Akbarnia BA, Wirth CR, Colman N: Fibrosarcoma arising from chronic osteomyelitis. Case report and review of the literature. J Bone Joint Surg [Am] 58:123, 1976.
141. Buxton SD: Malignant change in sinuses resulting from osteomyelitis. Med Press 232:45, 1954.
142. Dal Monte A: Neoplasie in processi osteomielitici. Chir Organi Mov 38:252, 1953.
143. Heilmann D: Plasmozytom auf dem Boden einer chronischen Osteomyelitis bei gleichzeitiger Ostitis deformans Paget. München Med Wochenschr 99:1586, 1957.
144. Cruickshank AH, McConnell EM, Miller DG: Malignancy in scars, chronic ulcers, and sinuses. J Clin Pathol 16:573, 1963.
145. Dahlin DC: Secondary amyloidosis. Ann Intern Med 31:105, 1949.
146. Briggs GW: Amyloidosis. Ann Intern Med 55:943, 1961.
147. Cohen AS: Amyloidosis. N Engl J Med 277:522, 1967.
148. Curtiss PH Jr: The pathophysiology of joint infections. Clin Orthop 96:129, 1973.
149. Barnhart MI, Riddle JM, Bluhm GB, et al: Fibrin promotion and lysis in arthritic joints. Ann Rheum Dis 26:206, 1967.
150. Harris ED, Cohen GL, Krane SM: Synovial collagenase: Its presence in culture from joint disease of diverse etiology. Arthritis Rheum 12:92, 1969.
151. Bobechko WP, Mandell L: Immunology of cartilage in septic arthritis. Clin Orthop 108:84, 1975.
152. Goldenberg DL, Cohen AS: Acute infectious arthritis. A review of patients with nongonococcal joint infections (with emphasis on therapy and prognosis). Am J Med 60:369, 1976.
153. Kauffman CA, Watanakunakorn C, Phair JP: Pneumococcal arthritis. J Rheumatol 3:409, 1976.
154. Paterson DC: Acute suppurative arthritis in infancy and childhood. J Bone Joint Surg [Br] 52:474, 1970.
155. Borella L, Goobar JE, Summitt RL, et al: Septic arthritis in childhood. J Pediatr 62:742, 1963.
156. Gillespie R: Septic arthritis of childhood. Clin Orthop 96:152, 1973.
157. Cole WG, Elliott BG, Jensen F: The management of septic arthritis in childhood. Aust NZ J Surg 45:178, 1975.
158. Newman JH: Review of septic arthritis throughout the antibiotic era. Ann Rheum Dis 35:198, 1976.
159. Hallel T, Salvati EA: Septic arthritis of the hip in infancy: End result study. Clin Orthop 132:115, 1978.
160. Samilson RL, Bersani FA, Watkins MB: Acute suppurative arthritis in infants and children: The importance of early diagnosis and surgical drainage. Pediatrics 21:798, 1958.
161. Ward J, Cohen AS, Bauer W: The diagnosis and therapy of acute suppurative arthritis. Arthritis Rheum 3:522, 1960.
162. Guiraudon C: Problèmes diagnostiques posés à l'histologiste par les monoarthrites infectieuses. Rev Rhum Mal Osteoartic 39:787, 1972.
163. Phemister DB: Changes in the articular surfaces in tuberculosis and in pyogenic infections of joints. AJR 12:1, 1924.
164. Butt WP: Radiology of the infected joint. Clin Orthop 96:136, 1973.
165. Shawker TH, Dennis JM: Periarticular calcifications in pyogenic arthritis. AJR 113:650, 1971.
166. Kluge RM, Schmidt MC, Barth WF: Pneumococcal arthritis and joint calcification (Abstr). Arthritis Rheum 14:394, 1971.

167. Bardenheimer JA, Morgan HC, Stamp WG: Treatment and sequelae of experimentally produced septic arthritis. Surg Gynecol Obstet 122:249, 1966.
168. Clark RL, Cuttino JT Jr, Anderle SK, et al: Radiologic analysis of arthritis in rats after systemic injection of streptococcal cell walls. Arthritis Rheum 22:25, 1979.
169. Miller JM, Engle RL Jr: Metastatic suppurative arthritis with subcutaneous emphysema caused by *Escherichia coli*. Am J Med 10:241, 1951.
170. McNae J: An unusual case of *Clostridium welchii* infection. J Bone Joint Surg [Br] 48:512, 1966.
171. Torg JS, Lammot TR III: Septic arthritis of the knee due to *Clostridium welchii*. Report of two cases. J Bone Joint Surg [Am] 50:1233, 1968.
172. Bliznak J, Ramsey J: Emphysematous septic arthritis due to *Escherichia coli*. J Bone Joint Surg [Am] 58:138, 1976.
173. Ziment I, Davis A, Finegold SM: Joint infection by anaerobic bacteria: A case report and review of the literature. Arthritis Rheum 12:627, 1969.
174. Meredith HC, Rittenberg GM: Pneumoarthropathy: An unusual radiographic sign of gram negative septic arthritis. Radiology 128:642, 1978.
175. Morganstern S, Seery W, Borshuk S, et al: Septic arthritis secondary to vesico-acetabular fistula: a case report. J Urol 116:116, 1976.
176. Chacha PB: Suppurative arthritis of the hip joints in infancy. A persistent diagnostic problem and possible complication of femoral venipuncture. J Bone Joint Surg [Am] 53:538, 1971.
177. Asnes RS, Arendar GM: Septic arthritis of the hip: A complication of femoral venipuncture. Pediatrics 38:837, 1966.
178. Samilson RL, Bersani FA, Watkins MB: Acute suppurative arthritis in infants and children. The importance of early diagnoses and surgical drainage. Pediatrics 21:798, 1958.
179. Morrey BF, Bianco AJ, Rhodes KH: Suppurative arthritis of the hip in children. J Bone Joint Surg [Am] 58:388, 1976.
180. Glassberg GB, Ozonoff MB: Arthrographic findings in septic arthritis of the hip in infants. Radiology 128:151, 1978.
181. Eyre-Brook AL: Septic arthritis of the hip and osteomyelitis of the upper end of the femur in infants. J Bone Joint Surg [Br] 42:11, 1960.
182. Obletz BE: Suppurative arthritis of the hip joint in infants. Clin Orthop 22:27, 1962.
183. Obletz BE: Acute suppurative arthritis of the hip in the neonatal period. J Bone Joint Surg [Am] 42:23, 1960.
184. Stetson JW, DePonte RJ, Southwick WO: Acute septic arthritis of the hip in children. Clin Orthop 56:105, 1968.
185. Kaye JJ: Bacterial infections of the hips in infancy and childhood. Curr Probl Radiol 3:17, 1973.
186. Smith T: On the acute arthritis of infants. St Bartholomew's Hosp Rep 10:189, 1874.
187. Howard PJ: Sepsis in normal and premature infants with localization in the hip joint. Pediatrics 20:279, 1957.
188. White H: Roentgen findings of acute infectious disease of the hip in infants and children. Clin Orthop 22:34, 1962.
189. Hefke HW, Turner VC: The obturator sign as the earliest roentgenographic sign in the diagnosis of septic arthritis and tuberculosis of the hip. J Bone Joint Surg 24:857, 1942.
190. Guerra J, Armbuster T, Resnick D, et al: The adult hip: An anatomic study. Part II. The soft tissue landmarks. Radiology 128:11, 1978.
191. Chont LK: Roentgen sign of early suppurative arthritis of the hip in infancy. Radiology 38:708, 1942.
192. Phemister DB: Changes in the articular surfaces in tuberculosis and in pyogenic infections of joints. AJR 12:1, 1924.
193. Siffert RS: The effect of juxta-epiphyseal pyogenic infection on epiphyseal growth. Clin Orthop 10:131, 1957.
194. McWhorter GL: Operation on the neck of the femur following acute symptoms in a case of osteochondritis deformans juvenilis coxae (Perthes' disease). Surg Gynecol Obstet 38:632, 1924.
195. Kemp HBS, Lloyd-Roberts GC: Avascular necrosis of the capital epiphysis following osteomyelitis of the proximal femoral metaphysis. J Bone Joint Surg [Br] 56:688, 1974.
196. Tachdjian MO, Grana L: Response of the hip joint to increased intraarticular hydrostatic pressure. Clin Orthop 61:199, 1968.
197. Kemp HBS: Perthes' disease. An experimental and clinical study. Ann R Coll Surg 52:18, 1973.
198. Goldenberg DL, Brandt KD, Cathcart ES, et al: Acute arthritis caused by gram-negative bacilli: A clinical characterization. Medicine 53:197, 1974.
199. Burton DS, Schurman DJ: Hematogenous infection in bilateral total hip arthroplasty. J Bone Joint Surg [Am] 57:1004, 1975.
200. Cruess RL, Bickel WS, von Kessler KLC: Infections in total hips secondary to a primary source elsewhere. Clin Orthop 106:99, 1975.
201. Mallory TH: Sepsis in total hip replacement following pneumococcal pneumonia. J Bone Joint Surg [Am] 55:1753, 1973.
202. Ahlberg A, Carlsson AS, Lindberg L: Hematogenous infection in total joint replacement. Clin Orthop 137:69, 1978.
203. Carlsson AS, Lidgren L, Lindberg L: Prophylactic antibiotics against early and late, deep infections after total hip replacements. Acta Orthop Scand 48:405, 1977.
204. Good CJ, Jones MA: Posterior rupture of the knee joint in septic arthritis: Case report. Br J Surg 61:553, 1974.
205. Stewart IM, Swinson DR, Hardinge K: Pyogenic arthritis presenting as a ruptured popliteal cyst. Ann Rheum Dis 38:181, 1979.
206. Shapiro RF, Resnick D, Castles JJ, et al: Fistulization of rheumatoid joints: A spectrum of identifiable syndromes. Ann Rheum Dis 34:489, 1975.
207. Master R, Weisman MH, Armbuster TG, et al: Septic arthritis of the glenohumeral joint. Arthritis Rheum 20:1500, 1977.
208. Armbuster T, Slivka J, Resnick D, et al: Extra-articular manifestations of septic arthritis of the glenohumeral joint. AJR 129:667, 1977.
209. Resnick D: Pyarthrosis complicating rheumatoid arthritis: Report of 5 patients and a review of the literature. Radiology 114:581, 1975.
210. Altemeier WA: Diagnosis, classification and general management of gas-producing infection, particularly those produced by *Clostridium perfringens*. In IW Brown Jr, BG Cox (Eds): Proceedings of the Third International Conference on Hyperbaric Medicine. Duke University, Durham, North Carolina, 1965. Washington DC National Academy of Sciences-National Research Council, 1966, p 481.
211. Bornstein DL, Weinberg AN, Swartz MN, et al: Anaerobic infections—review of current experience. Medicine 43:207, 1964.
212. Fee NF, Dobranski A, Bisla RS: Gas gangrene complicating open forearm fractures. Report of five cases. J Bone Joint Surg [Am] 59:135, 1977.
213. Angervall L, Stener B, Stener I, et al: Pseudomalignant osseous tumor of soft tissue. J Bone Joint Surg [Br] 51:654, 1969.
214. Fu FH, Scranton PE Jr: Pseudosarcomatous proliferation of soft tissue secondary to localized infection. Orthopedics 1:474, 1978.
215. Bywaters EGL: The bursae of the body. Ann Rheum Dis 24:215, 1965.
216. Marchildon A, Slonim RR, Brown HE Jr, et al: Primary septic bursitis. J Fla Med Assoc 50:139, 1963.
217. Winter FE, Runyon EH: Prepatellar bursitis caused by *Mycobacterium marinum*: Case report, classification, and review of the literature. J Bone Joint Surg [Am] 47:375, 1965.
218. Ho G Jr, Tice AD, Kaplan SR: Septic bursitis in the prepatellar and olecranon bursae. An analysis of 25 cases. Ann Intern Med 89:21, 1978.
219. Canoso JJ, Sheckman PR: Septic subcutaneous bursitis. Report of sixteen cases. J Rheumatol 6:96, 1979.
220. Thompson GR, Manshady BM, Weiss JJ: Septic bursitis. JAMA 240:2280, 1978.
221. Garcia-Kutzbach A, Masi AT: Acute infectious agent arthritis (IAA): A detailed comparison of proved gonococcal and other blood-borne bacterial arthritis. J Rheumatol 1:93, 1974.
222. Levinsky WJ: Sporotrichial arthritis. Report of a case mimicking gout. Arch Intern Med 129:118, 1972.
223. McConville JH, Pototsky RS, Calia FM, et al: Septic and crystalline joint disease: A simultaneous occurrence. JAMA 231:841, 1975.
224. Stratton CW, Phelps DB, Reller LB: Tuberculoid tenosynovitis and carpal tunnel syndrome caused by *Mycobacterium szulgai*. Am J Med 65:349, 1978.
225. Danzig LA, Fierer J: Coccidioidomycosis of the extensor tenosynovium of the wrist. A case report. Clin Orthop 129:245, 1977.
226. Iverson RE, Vistnes LM: Coccidioidomycosis tenosynovitis in the hand. J Bone Joint Surg [Am] 55:413, 1973.
227. Vass M, Kulmann L, Csoka, R, et al: Polytenosynovitis caused by *Toxoplasma gondii*. J Bone Joint Surg [Br] 59:229, 1977.
228. Currarino G: Acute epitrochlear lymphadenitis. Pediatr Radiol 6:160, 1977.
229. Letts RM, Sutherland JB: Technetium bone scanning as an aid in the diagnosis of atypical acute osteomyelitis in children. Surg Gynecol Obstet 140:899, 1975.
230. Handmaker H, Leonards R: The bone scan in inflammatory osseous disease. Semin Nucl Med 6:95, 1976.
231. Teates CD, Williamson BRJ: "Hot and cold" bone lesion in acute osteomyelitis. AJR 129:517, 1977.
232. Garnett ES, Cockshott WP, Jacobs J: Classical acute osteomyelitis with a negative bone scan. Br J Radiol 50:757, 1977.
233. Majd M: Radionuclide imaging in early detection of childhood osteomyelitis and its differentiation from cellulitis and bone infarction. Ann Radiol 20:9, 1977.
234. Treves S, Khettry J, Broker FH, et al: Osteomyelitis: Early scintigraphic detection in children. Pediatrics 57:173, 1976.
235. Kolyvas E, Rosenthall, L, Ahronheim GA, et al: Serial 67Ga-citrate imaging during treatment of acute osteomyelitis in childhood. Clin Nucl Med 3:461, 1978.
236. Feigin DS, Strauss HW, James AE Jr: The bone marrow scan in experimental osteomyelitis. Skel Radiol 1:103, 1976.
237. Smith PW, Petersen RJ, Ferlic RM: Gallium scan in sternal osteomyelitis. AJR 132:840, 1979.
238. Lisbona R, Rosenthall L: Observations on the sequential use of 99mTc-phosphate complex and 67Ga imaging in osteomyelitis, cellulitis and septic arthritis. Radiology 123:123, 1977.
239. Atcheson SG, Coleman RE, Ward JR: Septic arthritis mimicking cellulitis: Distinction using radionuclide bone imaging. Clin Nucl Med 4:79, 1979.
240. Lisbona R, Rosenthall L: Radionuclide imaging of septic joints and their differentiation from periarticular osteomyelitis and cellulitis in pediatrics. Clin Nucl Med 2:337, 1977.
241. Hayes RL, Nelson B, Swartzendruber DC, et al: Studies of the intra-cellular deposition of 67Ga (Abstr). J Nucl Med 12:364, 1971.
242. Swartzendruber DC, Nelson B, Hayes RL: Gallium-67 localization in lysosomal-like granules of leukemic and nonleukemic murine tissues. J Natl Cancer Inst 46:941, 1971.
243. Gilday DL, Paul DJ: The differentiation of osteomyelitis and cellulitis in chil-

dren using a combined blood pool and bone scan (Abstr). J Nucl Med *15*:494, 1974.

244. Gilday DL, Paul DJ, Paterson J: Diagnosis of osteomyelitis in children by combined blood pool and bone imaging. Radiology *117*:331, 1975.

245. Alavi A, Bond JP, Kuhl DE, et al: Scan detection of bone marrow infarcts in sickle cell disorders. J Nucl Med *15*:1003, 1974.

246. Kuhn JP, Berger PE: Computed tomographic diagnosis of osteomyelitis. Radiology *130*:503, 1979.

247. Good RA, Quie PG, Windhorst DB, et al: Fatal (chronic) granulomatous disease of childhood: A hereditary defect of leukocyte function. Semin Hematol *5*:215, 1968.

248. Berendes H, Bridges RA, Good RA: A fatal granulomatosis of childhood. The clinical studies of a new syndrome. Minn Med *40*:309, 1957.

249. Landing BH, Shirkey HS: A syndrome of recurrent infection and infiltration of viscera by pigmented lipid histiocytes. Pediatrics *20*:431, 1957.

250. Holmes B, Quie PG, Windhorst DB, et al: Fatal granulomatous disease of childhood: An inborn abnormality of phagocytic function. Lancet *1*:1225, 1966.

251. Quie PG, Kaplan EL, Page AR, et al: Defective polymorphonuclear-leukocyte function and chronic granulomatous disease in two female children. N Engl J Med *278*:976, 1968.

252. Holmes B, Page AR, Windhorst DB, et al: The metabolic pattern and phagocytic function of leukocytes from children with chronic granulomatous disease. Ann NY Acad Sci *155*:888, 1968.

253. Quie PG, White JG, Holmes B, et al: In vitro bactericidal capacity of human polymorphonuclear leukocytes: Diminished activity in chronic granulomatous disease of childhood. J Clin Invest *46*:668, 1967.

254. Bridges RA, Berendes H, Good RA: A fatal granulomatous disease of childhood. Am J Dis Child *97*:387, 1959.

255. Carson MJ, Chadwick DL, Brubaker CA, et al: Thirteen boys with progressive septic granulomatosis. Pediatrics *35*:405, 1965.

256. Wolfson JJ, Kane WJ, Laxdal SD, et al: Bone findings in chronic granulomatous disease of childhood. A genetic abnormality of leukocyte function. J Bone Joint Surg [Am] *51*:1573, 1969.

257. Renton P, Webster ADB: Case report 70. Skel Radiol *3*:131, 1978.

258. Giedion A, Holthusen W, Masel LF, et al: Subacute and chronic symmetrical osteomyelitis. Ann Radiol *15*:329, 1972.

259. Probst FP: Chronic multifocal cleido-metaphyseal osteomyelitis of childhood. Report of a case. Acta Radiol (Diagn) *17*:531, 1976.

260. Gustavson K-H, Wilbrand HF: Chronic symmetric osteomyelitis. Report of a case. Acta Radiol *15*:551, 1974.

261. Willert H-G, Enderle A: Multifocale, symmetrische, chronische Osteomyelitis. Acta Orthop Unfallchir *89*:109, 1977.

262. Exner GU: Die plasmacelluläre Osteomyelitis. Langenbecks Arch Chir *326*:165, 1970.

263. Louria DB, Hensle T, Rose J: The major medical complications of heroin addiction. Ann Intern Med *67*:1, 1967.

264. Cherubin CE: The medical sequelae of narcotic addiction. Ann Intern Med *67*:23, 1967.

265. Krueger H, Eddy NB, Sumwalt M: The Pharmacology of the Opium Alkaloids. Part I. Washington, DC, Government Printing Office, 1941, p 426.

266. Arkin A: The influence of strychnine, caffeine, chloral, antipyrin, cholesterol, and lactic acid on phagocytosis. J Infect Dis *13*:408, 1913.

267. Nickerson DS, Williams RC, Boxmeyer M, et al: Increased opsonic capacity of serum in chronic heroin addiction. Ann Intern Med *72*:671, 1970.

268. Goldwin RH, Chow AW, Edwards JE Jr, et al: Sternoarticular septic arthritis in heroin users. N Engl J Med *289*:616, 1973.

269. Salahuddin NI, Madhavan T, Fisher EJ, et al: Pseudomonas osteomyelitis. Radiologic features. Radiology *109*:41, 1973.

270. Gifford DB, Patzakis M, Ivler D, et al: Septic arthritis due to pseudomonas in heroin addicts. J Bone Joint Surg [Am] *57*:631, 1975.

271. Wiesseman GJ, Wood VE, Kroll LL: Pseudomonas vertebral osteomyelitis in heroin addicts. Report of five cases. J Bone Joint Surg [Am] *55*:1416, 1973.

272. Kido D, Bryan D, Halpern M: Hematogenous osteomyelitis in drug addicts. AJR *118*:356, 1973.

273. Ross GN, Baraff LJ, Quismorio FP: Serratia arthritis in heroin users. J Bone Joint Surg [Am] *57*:1158, 1975.

274. Donovan TL, Chapman MW, Harrington KD, et al: Serratia arthritis. Report of seven cases. J Bone Joint Surg [Am] *58*:1009, 1976.

275. Holzman RS, Bishko F: Osteomyelitis in heroin addicts. Ann Intern Med *75*:693, 1971.

276. Lewis R, Gorbach S, Altner P: Spinal pseudomonas chondro-osteomyelitis in heroin users. N Engl J Med *286*:1303, 1972.

277. Tuazon CU, Sheagren JN: Increased rate of carriage of *Staphylococcus aureus* among narcotic addicts. J Infect Dis *129*:725, 1974.

278. Tuazon CU, Hill R, Sheagren JN: Microbiologic study of street heroin and injection paraphernalia. J Infect Dis *129*:327, 1974.

279. Scott JE, Harrison DH: Septic arthritis in association with primary lymphoedema. Acta Orthop Scand *47*:676, 1976.

280. Kirkpatrick JA, Capitanio MA, Pereira RM: Immunologic abnormalities: Roentgen observations. Radiol Clin North Am *10*:245, 1972.

281. Miller WB, Murphy WA, Gilula LA: Brodie abscess: Reappraisal. Radiology *132*:15, 1979.

282. Fowles JV, Lehoux J, Zlitni M, et al: Tibial defect due to acute haematogenous osteomyelitis. Treatment and results in twenty-one children. J Bone Joint Surg [Br] *61*:77, 1979.

283. Terho P, Viikari J, Makela P, et al: Ruptured bilateral synovial cysts in presumed gonococcal arthritis. Sex Trans Dis *4*:100, 1977.

284. Brower AC, Sweet DE, Keats TE: Condensing osteitis of the clavicle: A new entity. AJR *121*:17, 1974.

285. Kohler H, Uehlinger E, Kutzner J, et al: Sternocostoclavicular hyperostosis: Painful swelling of the sternum, clavicles, and upper ribs. Ann Intern Med *87*:192, 1977.

286. Canoso JJ, Yood RA: Reaction of superficial bursae in response to specific disease stimuli. Arthritis Rheum *22*:1361, 1979.

287. Rabe WC, Angelillo JC, Leipert DW: Chronic sclerosing osteomyelitis: Treatment considerations in an atypical case. Oral Surg *49*:117, 1980.

288. Memon IA, Jacobs NM, Yeh TF, et al: Group B streptococcal osteomyelitis and septic arthritis. Its occurrence in infants less than 2 months old. Am J Dis Child *133*:921, 1979.

289. Chilton SJ, Aftimos SF, White PR: Diffuse skeletal involvement of streptococcal osteomyelitis in a neonate. Radiology *134*:390, 1980.

290. Trias A, Fery A: Cortical circulation of long bones. J Bone Joint Surg [Am] *61*:1052, 1979.

291. Petersen S, Knudsen FU, Andersen EA, et al: Acute haematogenous osteomyelitis and septic arthritis in childhood. A 10-year review and follow-up. Acta Orthop Scand *51*:451, 1980.

292. Green NE, Bruno J III: Pseudomonas infections of the foot after puncture wounds. South Med J *73*:146, 1980.

293. Peeples E, Boswick JA Jr, Scott FA: Wounds of the hand contaminated by human or animal saliva. J Trauma *20*:383, 1980.

294. Pinckney LE, Kennedy LA: Fractures of the infant skull caused by animal bites. AJR *135*:197, 1980.

295. Pinckney LE, Currarino G, Highgenboten CL: Osteomyelitis of the cervical spine following dental extraction. Radiology *135*:335, 1980.

296. Sharp JT, Lidsky MD, Duffy J, et al: Infectious arthritis. Arch Intern Med *139*:1125, 1979.

297. Cooke CP III, Levinsohn EM, Baker BE: Septic hip in pelvic fractures with urologic injury. Clin Orthop *147*:253, 1980.

298. Hayden CK Jr, Swischuk LE: Paraarticular soft-tissue changes in infections and trauma of the lower extremity in children. AJR *134*:307, 1980.

299. Wood BP: The vanishing epiphyseal ossification center: A sequel to septic arthritis of childhood. Radiology *134*:387, 1980.

300. Wofsy D: Culture negative septic arthritis and bacterial endocarditis. Diagnosis by synovial biopsy. Arthritis Rheum *23*:605, 1980.

301. Bywaters EGL: Lesions of bursae, tendons, and tendon sheaths. Clinics Rheum Dis *5*:883, 1979.

302. Ho G Jr, Tice AD: Comparison of nonseptic and septic bursitis. Arch Intern Med *139*:1269, 1979.

303. Brock JG, Meredith HC: Case report 102. Skel Radiol *4*:236, 1979.

304. Nicholl EDV, Foster EA: Granulomatous tenosynovitis due to beryllium. J Bone Joint Surg [Am] *42*:1087, 1966.

305. Kelly JJ: Blackthorn inflammation. J Bone Joint Surg [Br] *48*:474, 1966.

306. Solheim LF, Paus B, Liverud K, et al: Chronic recurrent multifocal osteomyelitis. Acta Orthop Scand *51*:37, 1980.

307. Bjorkstén B: Histopathological aspects of chronic recurrent multifocal osteomyelitis. J Bone Joint Surg [Br] *62*:376, 1980.

308. Yarchoan R, Davies SF, Fried J, et al: Isolated *Candida parapsilos* arthritis in a heroin addict. J Rheumatol *6*:447, 1979.

309. Roca RP, Yoshikawa TT: Primary skeletal infections in heroin users. Clin Orthop *144*:238, 1979.

310. Metges PJ, Silici R, Kleitz C, et al: La fistulographie. A propos de 126 éxamens. J Radiol *61*:57, 1980.

311. Halpern AA, Hasson N, Javier M: Septicemia following sinogram. Clin Orthop *145*:187, 1979.

312. Gelberman RH, Menon J, Austerlitz MS, et al: Pyogenic arthritis of the shoulder in adults. J Bone Joint Surg [Am] *62*:550, 1980.

313. Hofer P: Gallium: Mechanisms. J Nucl Med *21*:282, 1980.

314. Hofer P: Gallium and infection. J Nucl Med *21*:484, 1980.

315. Gilday DL: Problems in the scintigraphic detection of osteomyelitis. Radiology *135*:791, 1980.

316. Sullivan DC, Rosenfield NS, Ogden J, et al: Problems in the scintigraphic detection of osteomyelitis in children. Radiology *135*:731, 1980.

317. Handmaker H: Acute hematogenous osteomyelitis: Has the bone scan betrayed us? Radiology *135*:787, 1980.

318. Murray IPC: Bone scanning in the child and young adult. Skel Radiol *5*:65, 1980.

319. Ralls PW, Boswell W, Henderson R, et al: CT of inflammatory disease of the psoas muscle. AJR *134*:767, 1980.

320. Sequeira FW, Smith WL: Seldinger sinography. Radiology *137*:238, 1980.

321. Atdjian M, Granda JL, Ingberg HO, et al: Systemic sporotrichosis polytenosynovitis with median and ulnar nerve entrapment. JAMA *243*:1841, 1980.

322. Viggiano DA, Garrett JC, Clayton ML: Septic arthritis presenting as olecranon bursitis in patients with rheumatoid arthritis. J Bone Joint Surg [Am] *62*:1011, 1980.

323. Ahbel DE, Alexander AH, Kleine ML, et al: Prothecal olecranon bursitis. J Bone Joint Surg [Am] *62*:835, 1980.

324. Dias L, Tachdjian MO, Schroeder KE: Premature closure of the triradiate cartilage. J Bone Joint Surg [Br] *62*:46, 1980.

325. Carandell M, Roig D, Benasco C: Plant thorn synovitis. J Rheumatol *7*:567, 1980.

326. Weinstein AJ: Osteomyelitis—microbiologic, clinical and therapeutic considerations. Primary Care 8:557, 1981.

327. Waldvogel FA, Vasey H: Osteomyelitis: The past decade. N Engl J Med 303:360, 1980.

328. Collins R, Braun PA, Zinner SH, et al: Risk of local and systemic infection with polyethylene intravenous catheters: A prospective study of 213 catheterizations. N Engl J Med 279:340, 1968.

329. Goldmann DA, Maki DG: Infection control in total parenteral nutrition. JAMA 223:1360, 1973.

330. McCabe WR, Treadwell TL, DeMaria A Jr: Pathophysiology of bacteremia. Am J Med 75:7, 1983.

331. Nade S: Acute haematogenous osteomyelitis in infancy and childhood. J Bone Joint Surg [Br] 65:109, 1983.

332. O'Brien T, McManus F, MacAuley PH, et al: Acute haematogenous osteomyelitis. J Bone Joint Surg [Br] 64:450, 1982.

333. Green NE, Beauchamp RD, Griffin PP: Primary subacute epiphyseal osteomyelitis. J Bone Joint Surg [Am] 63:107, 1981.

334. Mok PM, Reilly BJ, Ash JM: Osteomyelitis in the neonate. Clinical aspects and the role of radiography and scintigraphy in diagnosis and management. Radiology 145:677, 1982.

335. Ekengren K, Bergdahl S, Eriksson M: Neonatal osteomyelitis. Radiographic findings and prognosis in relation to site of involvement. Acta Radiol (Diagn) 23:305, 1982.

336. Rosen RA, Morehouse HT, Karp HJ, et al: Intracortical fissuring in osteomyelitis. Radiology 141:17, 1981.

337. Lagier R, Baud C-A, Kramar C: Brodie's abscess in a tibia dating from the neolithic period. Virchows Arch (Pathol Anat) 401:153, 1983.

338. Kozlowski K: Brodie's abscess in the first decade of life. Report of eleven cases. Pediatr Radiol 10:33, 1980.

339. Skevis XA: Primary subacute osteomyelitis of the talus. J Bone Joint Surg [Br] 66:101, 1984.

340. Laurent F, Diard F, Calabet A, et al: Les osteomyelites circonscrites non tuberculeuses de l'enfant. Apropos de 31 cas. J Radiol 65:545, 1984.

341. Lindenbaum S, Alexander H: Infections simulating bone tumors. A review of subacute osteomyelitis. Clin Orthop 184:193, 1984.

342. Bogoch E, Thompson G, Salter RB: Foci of chronic circumscribed osteomyelitis (Brodie's abscess) that traverse the epiphyseal plate. J Pediatr Orthop 4:162, 1984.

343. Bonakdar-pour A, Gaines VD: The radiology of osteomyelitis. Orthop Clin North Am 14:21, 1983.

344. Mollan RAB, Craig BF, Biggart JD: Chronic sclerosing osteomyelitis. An unusual case. J Bone Joint Surg [Br] 66:583, 1984.

345. Collert S, Isacson J: Chronic sclerosing osteomyelitis (Garré). Clin Orthop 164:136, 1982.

346. Blockey NJ: Chronic osteomyelitis. An unusual variant. J Bone Joint Surg [Br] 65:120, 1983.

347. Leeson M, Weiner DS, Klein L: Osteomyelitis of the clavicle in children. Orthopedics 5:428, 1982.

348. Highland TR, Lamont RL: Osteomyelitis of the pelvis in children. J Bone Joint Surg [Am] 65:230, 1983.

349. Hedstrom SA, Lidgren L: Acute hematogenous pelvic osteomyelitis in athletes. Am J Sports Med 10:44, 1982.

350. Mosher HP: Osteomyelitis of the frontal bone. JAMA 107:942, 1936.

351. Tudor RB, Carson JP, Pulliam MW, et al: Pott's puffy tumor, frontal sinusitis, frontal bone osteomyelitis, and epidural abscess secondary to a wrestling injury. Am J Sports Med 9:390, 1981.

352. Jacobs RF, Adelman L, Sack CM, et al: Management of Pseudomonas osteochondritis complicating puncture wounds of the foot. Pediatrics 69:432, 1982.

353. Congeni BL, Weiner DS, Izsak E: Expanded spectrum of organisms causing osteomyelitis after puncture wounds. Orthopedics 4:531, 1981.

354. Lindsey RW, Leach JA: Sternoclavicular osteomyelitis and pyoarthrosis as a complication of subclavian vein catheterization. Orthopedics 7:1017, 1984.

355. Leftridge CA: Osteomyelitis of the calcaneus secondary to heel pad puncture: A case report. JAMA 69:507, 1977.

356. Canale ST, Manugian AH: Neonatal osteomyelitis of the os calcis. A complication of repeated heel punctures. Clin Orthop 156:178, 1981.

357. Nelson DL, Hable KA, Matsen JM: Proteus mirabilis osteomyelitis in two neonates following heel puncture. Am J Dis Child 125:109, 1973.

358. Goldberg I, Shauer L, Klier I, et al: Neonatal osteomyelitis of the calcaneus following a heel pad puncture: A case report. Clin Orthop 158:195, 1981.

359. Cahill N, King JD: Palm thorn synovitis. J Pediatr Orthop 4:175, 1984.

360. Southgate GW, Murray RO: Case report 190. Skel Radiol 8:79, 1982.

361. De SD, McAllister TA: Pseudomonas osteomyelitis following puncture wounds of the foot in children. Injury 12:334, 1981.

362. Mendelson EB, Fisher MR, Deschler TW, et al: Osteomyelitis in the diabetic foot: A difficult diagnostic challenge. RadioGraphics 3:248, 1983.

363. Goldman F, Manzi J, Carver A, et al: Sinography in the diagnosis of foot infections. J Am Podiatry Assoc 71:497, 1981.

364. Hendrix RW, Calenoff L, Lederman RB, et al: Radiology of pressure sores. Radiology 138:351, 1981.

365. Versluyen M: Pressure sores in elderly patients. The epidemiology related to hip operations. J Bone Joint Surg [Br] 67:10, 1985.

366. Barton AA, Barton M: The Management and Prevention of Pressure Sores. London, Faber and Faber, 1981.

367. Bryan CS, Dew CE, Reynolds KL: Bacteremia associated with decubitus ulcers. Arch Intern Med 143:2093, 1983.

368. Sugarman B, Hawes S, Musher DM, et al: Osteomyelitis beneath pressure sores. Arch Intern Med 143:683, 1983.

369. Firooznia H, Rafii M, Golimbu C, et al: Computed tomography of pressure sores, pelvic abscess, and osteomyelitis in patients with spinal cord injury. Arch Phys Med Rehabil 63:545, 1982.

370. Lee YH, Kerstein MD: Osteomyelitis and septic arthritis: Complication of subclavian catheterization. N Engl J Med 285:1179, 1971.

371. Hunter D, Moran JF, Venezio FR: Osteomyelitis of the clavicle after Swan-Ganz catheterization. Arch Intern Med 143:153, 1983.

372. Friedman AP, Velcek FT, Haller JO, et al: Clavicular periostitis: An unusual complication of percutaneous subclavian venous catheterization. Radiology 148:692, 1983.

373. Jupiter JB, Ehrlich MG, Novelline RA, et al: The association of septic thrombophlebitis with subperiosteal abscesses in children. J Pediatr 101:690, 1982.

374. Resnick D: Hand pain and swelling after the fight. J Musculoskel Med 1:61, 1984.

375. Vale GL, Noguchi TT: Anatomical distribution of human bite marks in a series of 67 cases. J Forensic Sci 28:61, 1983.

376. Marcy SM: Infections due to dog and cat bites. Pediatr Infect Dis 1:351, 1982.

377. Arons MS, Polayes IM: Pasteurella multocida—the major cause of hand infections following domestic animal bites. J Hand Surg 7:47, 1982.

378. Jarvis WR, Banko S, Snyder E, et al: Pasteurella multocida osteomyelitis following dog bites. Am J Dis Child 135:625, 1981.

379. Pechter EA, Miller TA: Severe osteomyelitis of the wrist following a cat bite. Hand 15:242, 1983.

380. Belardi FG, Pascoe JM, Beegle ED: Pasteurella multocida meningitis in an infant following occipital dog bite. J Fam Pract 14:778, 1982.

381. Culliford AT, Cunningham JN, Zeff RH, et al: Sternal and costochondral infections following open-heart surgery. A review of 2,594 cases. J Thorac Cardiovasc Surg 72:714, 1976.

382. Wray TM, Bryant RE, Killen DA: Sternal osteomyelitis and costochondritis after median sternotomy. J Thorac Cardiovasc Surg 66:227, 1973.

383. Grmoljez PF, Barner HH, Willman VL, et al: Major complications of median sternotomy. Am J Surg 130:679, 1975.

384. Goodman LR, Kay HR, Teplick SK, et al: Complications of median sternotomy: Computed tomographic evaluation. AJR 141:225, 1983.

385. Glynn MK, Sheehan JM: An analysis of the causes of deep infection after hip and knee arthroplasties. Clin Orthop 178:202, 1983.

386. Ainscow DA, Denham RA: The risk of haematogenous infection in total joint replacements. J Bone Joint Surg [Br] 66:580, 1984.

387. Anderson LD, Hutchins WC, Wright PE, et al: Fractures of the tibia and fibula treated by casts and transfixing pins. Clin Orthop 105:179, 1974.

388. Fellander M: Treatment of fractures and pseudoarthroses of the long bones by Hoffman's transfixation method (osteotaxis). Acta Orthop Scand 33:132, 1963.

389. Horwitz T: Surgical treatment of chronic osteomyelitis complicating fractures. A study of 50 patients. Clin Orthop 96:118, 1973.

390. Siris IE: External pin transfixion of fractures. An analysis of eighty cases. Ann Surg 120:911, 1944.

391. Lawyer RB Jr, Lubbers LM: Use of the Hoffman apparatus in the treatment of unstable tibial fractures. J Bone Joint Surg [Am] 62:1264, 1980.

392. Green SA, Ripley MJ: Chronic osteomyelitis in pin tracks. J Bone Joint Surg [Am] 66:1092, 1984.

393. Matthews LS, Green CA, Goldstein SA: The thermal effects of skeletal fixation—pin insertion in bone. J Bone Joint Surg [Am] 66:1077, 1984.

394. Sexton CC, Lawson JP, Yesner R: Case report 174. Skel Radiol 7:211, 1981.

395. Vives P, de Lestang M, Dorde T, et al: Réaction ostéolytique tardive massive autour de fils trans-osséux. Rev Chir Orthop 66:395, 1980.

396. Langenskiold A: Growth disturbance after osteomyelitis of femoral condyles in infants. Acta Orthop Scand 55:1, 1984.

397. Greenspan A, Norman A, Steiner G: Case report 146. Skel Radiol 6:149, 1981.

398. Parsons SW, Downey T: Solitary myeloma in chronic osteomyelitis presenting as a lower femoral fracture. Injury 16:17, 1984.

399. Van Winkle GN, Mazur JM: Iatrogenic exostosis in a patient treated for osteomyelitis. J Pediatr Orthop 3:610, 1983.

400. Goldenberg DL: "Postinfectious" arthritis. New look at an old concept with particular attention to disseminated gonococcal infection. Am J Med 74:925, 1983.

401. Cromartie WJ, Craddock JG, Schwab MH, et al: Arthritis in rats after systemic injection of streptococcal cells or cell walls. J Exp Med 146:1585, 1977.

402. Hadler NM, Granovetter DA: Phlogistic properties of bacterial debris. Semin Arthritis Rheum 8:1, 1978.

403. Keat A: Reiter's syndrome and reactive arthritis in perspective. N Engl J Med 309:1606, 1983.

404. Olhagen B: Diagnosis and treatment of reactive arthritis. IM 4:69, 1983.

405. Nelson JD, Koontz WC: Septic arthritis in infants and children: A review of 117 cases. Pediatrics 38:966, 1966.

406. Brandt KD, Cathcart ES, Cohen AS: Gonococcal arthritis. Clinical features correlated with blood, synovial fluid and genitourinary cultures. Arthritis Rheum 17:503, 1974.

407. Rice PA, Goldenberg DL: Clinical manifestations of disseminated infection caused by Neisseria gonorrhoeae are linked to differences in bactericidal reactivity of infecting strains. Ann Intern Med 96:175, 1981.

408. Ho G Jr, Toder JS, Zimmermann B III: An overview of septic arthritis and septic bursitis. Orthopedics 7:1571, 1984.

409. Platt PN, Griffiths ID: Pyogenic osteomyelitis presenting as an acute sterile arthropathy. Ann Rheum Dis 43:607, 1984.

410. Le Goff P, Fauchier CH, Pennec Y, et al: Subacute monoarthritis of the knee as the presentation of hematogenic chronic osteomyelitis in the adult. Two cases. Rev Rhum Mal Osteoartic *49:*185, 1982.

411. Baker SB, Robinson DR: Sympathetic joint effusion in septic arthritis. JAMA *240:*1989, 1978.

412. Peltola H, Vahvanen V: Acute purulent arthritis in children. Scand J Infect Dis *15:*75, 1983.

413. Nade S: Acute septic arthritis in infancy and childhood. J Bone Joint Surg [Br] *65:*234, 1983.

414. Lever AML, Owen T, Forsey J: Pneumoarthropathy in septic arthritis caused by *Streptococcus milleri.* Br Med J *285:*24, 1982.

415. Lowery CE, Stern PJ: Septic dislocation of the hip with extension of emphysema. Clin Orthop *178:*241, 1983.

416. Anderson RB, Dorwart BB: Pneumarthrosis in a shoulder infected with *Serratia liquefaciens:* Case report and literature review. Arthritis Rheum *26:*1166, 1983.

417. Levitin B, Rubin LA, Rubenstein JD: Occult retroperitoneal abscess presenting as septic arthritis of the hip. J Rheumatol *9:*904, 1982.

418. Cotler HB, Meadowcroft JA, Smink RD: Enteric fistula as a complication of a pelvic fracture. J Bone Joint Surg [Am] *65:*854, 1983.

419. Kumar JM, Jowett RL: Fistula between the hip and the caecum. J Bone Joint Surg [Br] *66:*603, 1984.

420. McCrea ES, Wagner E: Femoral osteomyelitis secondary to diverticulitis. J Can Assoc Radiol *32:*181, 1981.

421. Schmidt D, Mubarak S, Gelberman R: Septic shoulders in children. J Pediatr Orthop *1:*67, 1981.

422. Hunka L, Said SE, MacKenzie DA, et al: Classification and surgical management of the severe sequelae of septic hips in children. Clin Orthop *171:*30, 1982.

423. Richards AJ: Ruptured popliteal cyst and pyogenic arthritis. Br Med J *282:*1120, 1981.

424. Hall S, Wong C, Littlejohn GO: Popliteal cyst rupture in septic arthritis. Med J Aust *2:*385, 1982.

425. Shuckett R, Fam AG: Pseudothrombophlebitis syndrome in pyogenic arthritis. Can Med Assoc J *128:*294, 1983.

426. Gordon EJ, Hutchful GA: Pyarthrosis simulating ruptured rotator cuff syndrome. South Med J *75:*759, 1982.

427. Kraft SM, Panush RS, Longley S: Unrecognized staphylococcal pyarthrosis with rheumatoid arthritis. Semin Arthritis Rheum *14:*196, 1985.

428. Paisley JW: Septic bursitis in childhood. J Pediatr Orthop *2:*57, 1982.

429. Kahl LE, Rodnan GP: Olecranon bursitis and bacteremia due to *Serratia marcescens.* J Rheumatol *11:*402, 1984.

430. Borbas E, Genti G, Balint G: Septic prepatellar bursitis due to erysipelas. Arthritis Rheum *24:*1213, 1981.

431. Ho G Jr, Su EY: Antibiotic therapy of septic bursitis. Its implication in the treatment of septic arthritis. Arthritis Rheum *24:*905, 1981.

432. Sebaldt RJ, Tenenbaum J: Sympathetic synovial effusion associated with septic prepatellar bursitis: Synovial fluid analysis with therapeutic implications. J Rheumatol *11:*555, 1984.

433. Schirger A, Martin WJ, Spittle JA Jr: Acute lymphangitis and cellulitis. Minn Med *48:*191, 1965.

434. Ginsberg MB: Cellulitis: Analysis of 101 cases and review of the literature. South Med J *74:*530, 1981.

435. Rapkin RH, Bautista G: *Hemophilus influenzae* cellulitis. Am J Dis Child *124:*540, 1972.

436. Lewis RJ, Richmond AS, McGrory JP: *Diplococcus pneumoniae* cellulitis in drug addicts. JAMA *232:*54, 1975.

437. Ploy-Song-Sang Y, Winkle RA, Phair JP: *Neisseria meningitidis* cellulitis. South Med J *65:*1243, 1972.

438. Gauder JP: Cryptococcal cellulitis. JAMA *237:*672, 1977.

439. Fleisher G, Ludwig S, Campos J: Cellulitis: Bacterial etiology, clinical features and laboratory findings. J Pediatr *97:*591, 1980.

440. Bradley WA: Inflammatory diseases of muscle. *In* WN Kelley, ED Harris Jr, S Ruddy, et al (Eds): Textbook of Rheumatology. 2nd Ed. Philadelphia, WB Saunders Co, 1985, p 1225.

441. Kagen LJ: Less common causes of myositis. Clin Rheum Dis *10:*175, 1984.

442. Lepine P, Desse G, Sautter V: Biopsies musculaires avec éxamen histologique et isolement du virus coxsackie chez l'homme atteint de myalgie épidemique (maladie de Bornholm). Bull Acad Nat Med *136:*66, 1952.

443. Horn CV, Masters S: Pyomyositis tropicans in Uganda. E Afr Med J *45:*463, 1968.

444. Levin MJ, Gardner P, Waldvogel FA: "Tropical" pyomyositis. N Engl J Med *284:*196, 1971.

445. Altrocchi PH: Spontaneous bacterial myositis. JAMA *217:*819, 1971.

446. Goldberg JS, London WL, Nagel DM: Tropical pyomyositis: A case report and review. Pediatrics *63:*298, 1979.

447. Grose C: Staphylococcal pyomyositis in South Texas. J Pediatr *93:*457, 1978.

448. Jordan GW, Bauer R, Wong GA, et al: Staphylococcal myositis in a compromised host. West J Med *124:*140, 1976.

449. Kallen P, Nies KN, Louie JS, et al: Tropical polymyositis. Arthritis Rheum *25:*107, 1982.

450. Brown JD, Wheeler B: Pyomyositis. Report of 18 cases in Hawaii. Arch Intern Med *144:*1749, 1984.

451. Schlech WF III, Moulton P, Kaiser AB: Pyomyositis: Tropical disease in a temperate climate. Am J Med *71:*900, 1981.

452. Taylor JF, Fluck D, Fluck D: Tropical myositis: Ultrastructural studies. J Clin Pathol *29:*1081, 1976.

453. Datz EL, Lewis SE, Conrad MR, et al: Pyomyositis diagnosed by radionuclide imaging and ultrasonography. South Med J *73:*649, 1980.

454. Yousefzadeh DK, Schumann EM, Mulligan GM, et al: The role of imaging modalities in diagnosis and management of pyomyositis. Skel Radiol *8:*285, 1982.

455. Chaitow J, Martin HC, Knight P, et al: Pyomyositis tropicans: A diagnostic dilemma. Med J Aust *2:*512, 1980.

456. McLoughlin MJ: CT and percutaneous fine-needle aspiration biopsy in tropical myositis. AJR *134:*167, 1980.

457. Hirano T, Spinivasan G, Janakiraman N, et al: Gallium-67 citrate scintigraphy in pyomyositis. J Pediatr *97:*596, 1980.

458. Rao BR, Gerber FH, Greaney RB, et al: Gallium-67 citrate imaging of pyomyositis. J Nucl Med *22:*836, 1981.

459. Lamki L, Willis RB: Radionuclide findings of pyomyositis. Clin Nucl Med *7:*465, 1982.

460. Lee AB, Waffle CM, Trebbin WM, et al: Clostridial myonecrosis. Origin from an obturator hernia in a dialysis patient. JAMA *246:*1232, 1981.

461. Kizer KW, Ogle LC: Occult clostridial myonecrosis. Ann Emerg Med *10:*307, 1981.

462. Ramirez H Jr, Brown JD, Evans JW Jr: Case report 225. Skel Radiol *9:*223, 1983.

463. Kvernebo K, Stiris G, Haaland M: CT in idiopathic pyogenic myositis of the iliopsoas muscle. A report of 2 cases. Eur J Radiol *3:*1, 1983.

464. Bessman AN, Wagner W: Nonclostridial gas gangrene: Report of 48 cases and review of the literature. JAMA *233:*958, 1975.

465. Tauber AI, Borregaard N, Simons E, et al: Chronic granulomatous disease: A syndrome of phagocyte oxidase deficiencies. Medicine *62:*286, 1983.

466. Perry HB, Boulanger M, Pennoyer D: Chronic granulomatous disease in an adult with recurrent abscesses. Arch Surg *115:*200, 1980.

467. Buescher ES, Seligmann BE, Nath J, et al: Recent advances in chronic granulomatous disease. Ann Intern Med *99:*657, 1983.

468. Appell RG, Oppermann HC, Becker W, et al: Condensing osteitis of the clavicle in childhood: A rare sclerotic bone lesion. Review of literature and report of seven patients. Pediatr Radiol *13:*301, 1983.

469. Exner GU: Plasmacellular osteomyelitis in children. Clinical and radiological features. Follow-up. Z Kinderchir *31:*262, 1980.

470. Murray SD, Kehl DK: Chronic recurrent multifocal osteomyelitis. A case report. J Bone Joint Surg [Am] *66:*1110, 1984.

471. Probst FP: Chronisch rekurrierende multifokale Osteomyelitis (CRMO). Radiologe *24:*24, 1984.

472. Kozlowski K, Hochberger O: Rare forms of chronic osteomyelitis (multifocal recurrent periostitis and chronic symmetric osteomyelitis—report of 3 cases). Australas Radiol *28:*152, 1984.

473. Speer DP: Chronic multifocal symmetrical osteomyelitis. Am J Dis Child *138:*340, 1984.

474. Jani L, Remagan W: Primary chronic osteomyelitis. Int Orthop (SICOT) *7:*79, 1983.

475. Nilsson BE, Uden A: Skeletal lesions in palmar-plantar pustulosis. Acta Orthop Scand *55:*366, 1984.

476. Jurik AG, Graudal H, de Carvalho A: Sclerotic changes of the manubrium sterni. Skel Radiol *13:*195, 1985.

477. Miskew DEW, Lorenz MA, Pearson RL, et al: *Pseudomonas aeruginosa* bone and joint infection in drug abusers. J Bone Joint Surg [Am] *65:*829, 1983.

478. Firooznia H, Golimbu C, Rafii M, et al: Radiology of musculoskeletal complications of drug addiction. Semin Roentgenol *18:*198, 1983.

479. Sequeira W, Jones E, Siegel ME, et al: Pyogenic infections of the pubic symphysis. Ann Intern Med *96:*604, 1982.

480. Dhaliwal AS, Garnes AL: Tenosynovitis in drug addicts. J Hand Surg *7:*626, 1982.

481. Kiburz D: Intra-articular drug abuse. J Bone Joint Surg [AM] *66:*1469, 1984.

482. Jeffrey RB, Callen PW, Federle MP: Computed tomography of psoas abscesses. J Comput Assist Tomogr *4:*639, 1980.

483. Firooznia H, Rafii M, Golimbu C, et al: Computerized tomography of pelvic osteomyelitis in patients with spinal cord injuries. Clin Orthop *181:*126, 1983.

484. Firooznia H, Rafii M, Golimbu C, et al: Computerized tomography in diagnosis of pelvic abscess in spinal-cord-injured patients. Comput Radiol *7:*335, 1983.

485. Wechsler RJ, Schilling JF: CT of the gluteal region. AJR *144:*185, 1985.

486. Morgan GJ Jr, Schlegelmilch JG, Spiegel PK: Early diagnosis of septic arthritis of the sacroiliac joint by use of computed tomography. J Rheumatol *8:*979, 1981.

487. Azouz EM: Computed tomography in bone and joint infections. J Can Assoc Radiol *32:*102, 1981.

488. Mueller PR, Ferrucci JT Jr, Wittenberg J, et al: Iliopsoas abscess: Treatment by CT-guided percutaneous catheter drainage. AJR *142:*359, 1984.

489. Seltzer SE: Value of computed tomography in planning medical and surgical treatment of chronic osteomyelitis. J Comput Assist Tomogr *8:*482, 1984.

490. Ram PC, Martinez S, Korobkin M, et al: CT detection of intraosseous gas: A new sign of osteomyelitis. AJR *137:*721, 1981.

491. Callen PW: Computed tomographic evaluation of abdominal and pelvic abscesses. Radiology *131:*171, 1979.

492. Rafii M, Firooznia H, Golimbu C, et al: Hematogenous osteomyelitis with fat-fluid level shown by CT. Radiology *153:*493, 1984.

493. Hertzanu Y, Mendelsohn DB, Gottschalk F: Aneurysmal bone cyst of the calcaneus. Radiology *151:*51, 1984.

494. Hahn PF, Rosenthal DI, Ehrlich MG: Case report 286. Skel Radiol *12:*214, 1984.

495. Wing VW, Jeffrey RB Jr, Federle MP, et al: Chronic osteomyelitis examined by CT. Radiology 154:171, 1985.
496. Rhoades CE, Soye I, Levine E, et al: Detection of a wooden foreign body in the hand using computed tomography—case report. J Hand Surg 7:306, 1982.
497. Bauer AR Jr, Yutani D: Computed tomographic localization of wooden foreign bodies in children's extremities. Arch Surg 118:1084, 1983.
498. Narins DJ, Chase RM: The effect of Hypaque upon urine cultures. J Urol 105:433, 1971.
499. Kuhns LR, Baublis JV, Gragory J, et al: In vitro effect of cystographic contrast media on urinary tract pathogens. Invest Radiol 7:112, 1972.
500. Melson GL, McDaniel RC, Southern PM, et al: In vitro effects of iodinated arthrographic contrast media on bacterial growth. Radiology 112:593, 1974.
501. Johansen JG, Clausen OG: Antibacterial effects of metrizoate and metrizamide on bacterial growth in vitro. Acta Radiol (Diagn) 18:269, 1977.
502. Kim KS, Lachman R: In vitro effects of iodinated contrast media on the growth of staphylococci. Invest Radiol 17:305, 1982.
503. Dawson P, Becker A, Holton JM: The effect of contrast media on the growth of bacteria. Br J Radiol 56:809, 1983.
504. Dory MA, Wautelet MJ: Arthroscopy in septic arthritis. Lidocaine- and iodine-containing contrast material are bacteriostatic. Arthritis Rheum 28:198, 1985.
505. Scoles PV, Hilty MD, Sfakianakis GN: Bone scan patterns in acute osteomyelitis. Clin Orthop 153:210, 1980.
506. Merkel KD, Fitzgerald RH Jr, Brown ML: Scintigraphic evaluation in muscoloskeletal sepsis. Orthop Clin North Am 15:401, 1984.
507. Sullivan JA, Vasileff T, Leonard JC: An evaluation of nuclear scanning in orthopaedic infections. J Pediatr Orthop 1:73, 1981.
508. Barron BJ, Dhekne RD: Cold osteomyelitis. Radionuclide bone scan findings. Clin Nucl Med 9:392, 1984.
509. Murray IPC: Photopenia in skeletal scintigraphy of suspected bone and joint infection. Clin Nucl Med 7:13, 1982.
510. Bressler EL, Conway JJ, Weiss SC: Neonatal osteomyelitis examined by bone scintigraphy. Radiology 152:685, 1984.
511. Tsan M-F: Mechanism of gallium-67 accumulation in inflammatory lesions. J Nucl Med 26:88, 1985.
512. Fihn SD, Larson EB, Nelp WB, et al: Should single-phase radionuclide bone imaging be used in suspected osteomyelitis? J Nucl Med 25:1080, 1984.
513. Maurer AH, Chen DCP, Camargo EE, et al: Utility of three-phase skeletal scintigraphy in suspected osteomyelitis: Concise communication. J Nucl Med 22:941, 1981.
514. Norris SH, Watt I: Radionuclide uptake during the evolution of experimental acute osteomyelitis. Br J Radiol 54:207, 1981.
515. Wellman HN, Siddiqui A, Mail JT, et al: Choice of radiotracer in the study of bone and joint infection in children. Ann Radiol 26:411, 1983.
516. Park H-M, Wheat LJ, Siddiqui AR, et al: Scintigraphic evaluation of diabetic osteomyelitis: Concise communication. J Nucl Med 23:569, 1982.
517. Gonzalez AC, Macon PF, Sankey RR, et al: Amputation stumps studied by bone scanning. Work in progress. Radiology 151:225, 1984.
518. Yon JW Jr, Spicer KM, Gordon L: Synovial visualization during Tc-99m MDP bone scanning in septic arthritis of the knee. Clin Nucl Med 8:249, 1983.
519. Sfakianakis GN, Al-Sheikh W, Heal A, et al: Comparisons of scintigraphy with In-111 leukocytes and Ga-67 in the diagnosis of occult sepsis. J Nucl Med 23:618, 1982.
520. McAfee JG, Subramanian G, Gagne G: Technique of leukocyte harvesting and labeling: Problems and perspective. Semin Nucl Med 14:83, 1984.
521. Thakur ML, Coleman RE, Welch MJ: Indium-111-labeled leukocytes for the localization of abscesses: Preparation, analysis, tissue distribution, and comparison with gallium-67 citrate in dogs. J Lab Clin Med 89:217, 1977.
522. McDougall IR, Baumert JE, Lantieri RL: Evaluation of ¹¹¹In leukocyte whole body scanning. AJR 133:849, 1979.
523. Seabold JE, Wilson DG, Lieberman LM, et al: Unsuspected extra-abdominal sites of infection—scintigraphic detection with indium-111-labeled leukocytes. Radiology 151:213, 1984.
524. McAfee JG, Samin A: In-111 labeled leukocytes: A review of problems in image interpretation. Radiology 155:221, 1985.
525. Segal AW, Arnot RN, Thakur ML, et al: Indium-111-labeled leukocytes in localisation of abscesses. Lancet 2:1056, 1976.
526. Raptopoulos V, Doherty PW, Goss TP, et al: Acute osteomyelitis: Advantages of white cell scans in early detection. AJR 139:1077, 1982.
527. Goss TP, Monahan JJ: Indium-111 white blood cell scan. Orthop Rev 10:91, 1981.
528. Fernandez-Ulloa M, Hughes JA, Krugh KB, et al: Bone imaging in infections: Artifacts from spectral overlap between a Tc-99m tracer and In-111 leukocytes. J Nucl Med 24:589, 1983.
529. Merkel KD, Brown ML, Dewanjee MK, et al: Comparison of indium-labeled-leukocyte imaging with sequential technetium-gallium scanning in the diagnosis of low-grade musculoskeletal sepsis. J Bone Joint Surg [Am] 67:465, 1985.
530. Fletcher BD, Scoles PV, Nelson AD: Osteomyelitis in children: Detection by magnetic resonance. Work in progress.
531. Aguila LA, Piraino DW, Modic MT, et al: The intranuclear cleft of the intervertebral disk: Magnetic resonance imaging. Radiology 155:155, 1985.
532. Baker HL, Berquist TH, Kispert DB, et al: Magnetic resonance imaging in a routine clinical setting. Mayo Clin Proc 60:75, 1985.
533. Rosenbaum DM, Blumhagen JD: Acute epiphyseal osteomyelitis in children. Radiology 156:89, 1985.
534. Ross ERS, Cole WG: Treatment of subacute osteomyelitis in childhood. J Bone Joint Surg [Br] 67:443, 1985.
535. Kozlowski K, Anderson RJ, Hochberger O, et al: Tumorous osteomyelitis. Report of two cases. Pediatr Radiol 14:404, 1984.
536. Klein B, McGahan JP: Thorn synovitis: CT diagnosis. J Comput Assist Tomogr 9:1135, 1985.
537. Resnick D, Pineda CJ, Weisman MH, et al: Osteomyelitis and septic arthritis of the hand following human bites. Skel Radiol 14:263, 1985.
538. Nguyen VD, London J, Cone RO III: Ring sequestrum: Radiographic characteristics of skeletal pin-tract osteomyelitis. Radiology 158:129, 1986.
539. Eriksson RA, Albrektsson T, Magnusson B: Assessment of bone viability after heat trauma. A histological, histochemical and vital microscopic study in the rabbit. Scand J Plast Reconstr Surg 18:261, 1984.
540. Lifeso RM, Bull CA: Squamous cell carcinoma of the extremities. Cancer 55:2862, 1985.
541. Sankaran-Kutty M, Corea JR, Ali MS, et al: Squamous cell carcinoma in chronic osteomyelitis. Report of a case and review of the literature. Clin Orthop 198:264, 1985.
542. Strickland RW, Raskin RJ, Welton RC: Sympathetic synovial effusions associated with septic arthritis and bursitis. Arthritis Rheum 28:941, 1985.
543. Batlle-Gualda E, Pascual-Gomez E: Septic arthritis of the knee presenting as an abscess in the thigh. J Rheumatol 12:650, 1985.
544. Kozlowski K, Beluffi G, Feltham C, et al: Multifocal, chronic osteomyelitis of unknown etiology. A further report. ROFO 142:440, 1985.
545. Cyrlak D, Pais MJ: Chronic recurrent multifocal osteomyelitis. Skel Radiol 15:32, 1986.
546. Zahran MH, Kaufmann HJ: Case report 336. Skel Radiol 14:296, 1985.
547. Azouz EM, Raymond J: Case report 316. Skel Radiol 13:327, 1985.
548. Hernandez RJ: Visualization of small sequestra by computerized tomography. Report of 6 cases. Pediatr Radiol 15:238, 1985.
549. Park H-M, Rothschild PA, Kernek CB: Scintigraphic evaluation of extremity pain in children: Its efficacy and pitfalls. AJR 145:1079, 1985.
550. Alazraki N, Dries D, Datz F, et al: Value of a 24-hour image (four-phase bone scan) in assessing osteomyelitis in patients with peripheral vascular disease. J Nucl Med 26:711, 1985.
551. Al-Sheikh W, Sfakianakis GN, Mnaymneh W, et al: Subacute and chronic bone infections: Diagnosis using In-111, Ga-67 and Tc-99m MDP bone scintigraphy, and radiography. Radiology 155:501, 1985.
552. Traughber PD, Manaster BJ, Murphy K, et al: Negative bone scans of joints after aspiration or arthrography: Experimental studies. AJR 146:87, 1986.
553. Seibert JJ, McCarthy RE, Alexander JE, et al: Acquired bone dysplasia secondary to catheter-related complications in the neonate. Pediatr Radiol 16:43, 1986.
554. Bar-Ziv J, Barki Y, Maroko A, et al: Rib osteomyelitis in children. Early radiologic and ultrasonic findings. Pediatr Radiol 15:315, 1985.
555. Dreyfuss UY, Singer M: Human bites of the hand: A study of one hundred six patients. J Hand Surg [Am] 10:884, 1985.
556. Stewart MC, Little RE, Highland TR: Osteomyelitis of the ilium secondary to external pelvic fixation. J Trauma 26:284, 1986.
557. Alderson M, Speers D, Emslie K, et al: Acute hematogenous osteomyelitis and septic arthritis—a single disease. An hypothesis based upon the presence of transphyseal blood vessels. J Bone Joint Surg [Br] 68:268, 1986.
558. Bjorkengren A, Resnick D, Sartoris DJ: Radiographic changes in pyogenic arthritis. IM 7:119, 1986.
559. López-Longo FJ, Monteagudo I, Vaquero FJ, et al: Primary septic arthritis of the manubriosternal joint in a heroin user. Clin Orthop 202:230, 1986.
560. Taylor CR, Lawson JP: Periostitis and osteomyelitis in chronic drug addicts. Skel Radiol 15:209, 1986.
561. Lopez M, Sauerbrei E: Septic arthritis of the hip joint: Sonographic and CT findings. J Can Assoc Radiol 36:322, 1985.
562. Lewin JS, Rosenfield NS, Hoffer PB, et al: Acute osteomyelitis in children: Combined Tc-99m and Ga-67 imaging. Radiology 158:795, 1986.
563. Tumeh SS, Aliabadi P, Weissman BN, et al: Chronic osteomyelitis: Bone and gallium scan patterns associated with active disease. Radiology 158:685, 1986.
564. Fortner A, Datz FL, Taylor A Jr, et al: Uptake of ¹¹¹In-labeled leukocytes by tumor. AJR 146:621, 1986.
565. Thornhill-Joynes M, Gonzales F, Stewart CA, et al: Osteomyelitis associated with pressure ulcers. Arch Phys Med Rehabil 67:314, 1986.
566. Singson RD, Berdon WE, Feldman F, et al: "Missing" femoral condyle: An unusual sequela to neonatal osteomyelitis and septic arthritis. Radiology 161:359, 1986.
567. Buehler M, Bird CB: Posterior leg sepsis associated with pyogenic arthritis of the knee. A report of two cases. Clin Orthop 209:172, 1986.
568. Ho G Jr, Mikolich DJ: Bacterial infection of superficial subcutaneous bursae. Clinics Rheum Dis 12:437, 1986.
569. Wiener MD, Newbold RG, Merten DF: Chronic recurrent multifocal osteomyelitis (case report). AJR 146:87, 1986.
570. Jurik AG, Moller BN: Inflammatory hyperostosis and sclerosis of the clavicle. Skel Radiol 15:284, 1986.
571. Lee SM, Lee RGL, Wilinsky J, et al: Magnification radiography in osteomyelitis. Skel Radiol 15:625, 1986.
572. Stark P, Jaramillo D: CT of the sternum. AJR 142:72, 1986.
573. Borman TR, Johnson RA, Sherman FC: Gallium scintigraphy for diagnosis of septic arthritis and osteomyelitis in children. J Pediatr Orthop 6:317, 1986.
574. Mauer AH, Millmond SH, Knight LC, et al: Infection in diabetic osteoarthropathy: Use of indium-labeled leukocytes for diagnosis. Radiology 161:221, 1986.
575. Waldvogel FA: Acute osteomyelitis. In D Schlossberg (Ed): Orthopedic Infection. New York, Springer-Verlag, 1988, p 1.

576. Braun TI, Lorber B: Chronic osteomyelitis. In D Schlossberg (Ed): Orthopedic Infection. New York, Springer-Verlag, 1988, p 9.

577. Mader JT: Osteomyelitis. In JH Stein (Ed): Internal Medicine. 3rd Ed. Boston, Little Brown, and Company, 1990, p 1310.

578. Knudsen CJM, Hoffman EB: Neonatal osteomyelitis. J Bone Joint Surg [Br] 72:846, 1990.

579. Whalen JL, Fitzgerald RH, Morrissy RT: A histological study of acute hematogenous osteomyelitis following physeal injuries in rabbits. J Bone Joint Surg [Am] 70:1383, 1988.

580. Morrissy RT, Haynes DW: Acute hematogenous osteomyelitis: A model with trauma as an etiology. J Pediatr Orthop 9:447, 1989.

581. Sørensen TS, Hedeboe J, Christensen ER: Primary epiphyseal osteomyelitis in children. Report of three cases and review of the literature. J Bone Joint Surg [Br] 70:818, 1988.

582. Azouz EM, Greenspan A, Marton D: CT evaluation of primary epiphyseal bone abscesses. Skel Radiol 22:17, 1993.

583. Craigen MAC, Watters J, Hackett JS: The changing epidemiology of osteomyelitis in children. J Bone Joint Surg [Br] 74:541, 1992.

584. Wang EHM, Simpson S, Bennet GC: Osteomyelitis of the calcaneum. J Bone Joint Surg [Br] 74:906, 1992.

585. Grattan-Smith JD, Wagner ML, Barnes DA: Osteomyelitis of the talus: An unusual cause of limping in childhood. AJR 156:785, 1991.

586. Papavasiliou VA, Sferopoulos NK: Ostéomyélite hématogène aiguë de la rotule. Rev Chir Orthop 75:128, 1989.

587. Roy DR, Greene WB, Gamble JG: Osteomyelitis of the patella in children. J Pediatr Orthop 11:364, 1991.

588. Alexander JE, Seibert JJ, Aronson J: Dorsal defect of the patella and infection. Pediatr Radiol 30:325, 1987.

589. Stephens MM, MacAuley P: Brodie's abscess. A long-term review. Clin Orthop 234:211, 1988.

590. Jones NS, Anderson DJ, Stiles PJ: Osteomyelitis in a general hospital. A five-year study showing an increase in subacute osteomyelitis. J Bone Joint Surg [Br] 69:779, 1987.

591. Helms CA, Jeffrey RB, Wing VW: Computed tomography and plain film appearance of a bony sequestrum: Significance and differential diagnosis. Skel Radiol 16:117, 1987.

592. Wood RE, Nortje CJ, Grotepass F, et al: Periostitis ossificans versus Garré's osteomyelitis. Part I. What did Garré really say? Oral Surg 65:773, 1988.

593. Nortje CJ, Wood RE, Grotepass F, et al: Periostitis ossificans versus Garré's osteomyelitis. Part II. Radiographic analysis of 93 cases in the jaws. Oral Surg 66:249, 1988.

594. Van Merkesteyn JPR, Groot RH, Bras J, et al: Diffuse sclerosing osteomyelitis of the mandible: A new concept of its etiology. Oral Surg 70:414, 1990.

595. Van Merkesteyn JPR, Groot RH, Bras J, et al: Diffuse sclerosing osteomyelitis of the mandible: Clinical, radiographic and histologic findings in twenty-seven patients. J Oral Maxillofac Surg 46:825, 1988.

596. Buckley SL, Alexander AH, Barrack RL: Scapular osteomyelitis. An unusual complication following subacromial corticosteroid injection. Orthop Rev 18:321, 1989.

597. Borgström PS, Ekberg O, Lasson Å: Radiography of pressure ulcers. Acta Radiol 29:581, 1988.

598. Belli AM, Dow CJ, Monro P: Radiographic appearance of frontal osteomyelitis in two patients with extradural abscess. Br J Radiol 60:1026, 1987.

599. Feder HM Jr, Cates KL, Cementina AM: Pott puffy tumor: A serious occult infection. Pediatrics 79:625, 1987.

600. Siegel IM: Identification of non-metallic foreign bodies in soft tissue: Eikenella corrodens metatarsal osteomyelitis due to a retained toothpick. A case report. J Bone Joint Surg [Am] 74:1408, 1992.

601. Olenginski TP, Bush DC, Harrington TM: Plant thorn synovitis: An uncommon cause of monoarthritis. Semin Arthritis Rheum 21:40, 1991.

602. Schauwecker DS, Park HM, Burt RW, et al: Combined bone scintigraphy and indium-111 leukocyte scans in neuropathic foot disease. J Nucl Med 29:1651, 1988.

603. Beltran J, Campanini DS, Knight C, et al: The diabetic foot: Magnetic resonance imaging evaluation. Skel Radiol 19:37, 1990.

604. Yuh WTC, Corson JD, Baraniewski HM: Osteomyelitis of the foot in diabetic patients: Evaluation with plain film, 99mTc-MDP bone scintigraphy, and MR imaging. AJR 152:795, 1989.

605. Patzakis MJ, Wilkins J, Bassett RL: Surgical findings in clenched-fist injuries. Clin Orthop 220:237, 1987.

606. Lindsey D, Christopher M, Hollenbach J, et al: Natural course of the human bite wound: Incidence of infection and complications in 434 bites and 803 lacerations in the same group of patients. J Trauma 27:45, 1987.

607. Phair IC, Quinton DN: Clenched fist human bite injuries. J Hand Surg [Br] 14:86, 1989.

608. Lifeso RM, Rooney RJ, El-shaker M: Post-traumatic squamous-cell carcinoma. J Bone Joint Surg [Am] 72:12, 1990.

609. Roger DJ, Bono JV, Singh JK: Plasmacytoma arising from a focus of chronic osteomyelitis. A case report. J Bone Joint Surg [Am] 74:619, 1992.

610. Tumeh SS, Aliabadi P, Weissman BN, et al: Disease activity in osteomyelitis: Role of radiography. Radiology 165:781, 1987.

611. Vincent GM, Amirault JD: Septic arthritis in the elderly. Clin Orthop 251:241, 1990.

612. Barton LL, Dunkle LM, Habib FH: Septic arthritis in childhood. A 13-year review. Am J Dis Child 141:898, 1987.

613. Epstein JH, Zimmermann B III, Ho G Jr: Polyarticular septic arthritis. J Rheumatol 13:1105, 1986.

614. Bennett OM, Namnyak SS: Acute septic arthritis of the hip joint in infancy and childhood. Clin Orthop 281:123, 1992.

615. O'Meara PM, Bartal E: Septic arthritis: Process, etiology, treatment outcome. A literature review. Orthopedics 11:623, 1988.

616. Parker RH: Acute infectious arthritis. In D Schlossberg (Ed): Orthopedic Infection. New York, Springer-Verlag, 1988, p 69.

617. Magen AB, Moser RP Jr, Woomert CA, et al: Septic arthritis of the hip: A complication of a rectal tear associated with pelvic fractures. AJR 157:817, 1991.

618. Danielsson LG, Gupta RP: Four cases of purulent arthritis of the shoulder secondary to hematogenous osteomyelitis. Acta Orthop Scand 60:591, 1989.

619. Betz RR, Cooperman DR, Wopperer JM, et al: Late sequelae of septic arthritis of the hip in infancy and childhood. J Pediatr Orthop 10:365, 1990.

620. Armstrong RW, Bolding F, Joseph R: Septic arthritis following arthroscopy: Clinical syndromes and analysis of risk factors. J Arthrosc Rel Surg 8:213, 1992.

621. Northmore-Ball MD, Requesens-Gruber JG, Ferreira CEV: Sequential haematogenous infection of bilateral cementless total hip replacements. J Bone Joint Surg [Br] 75:22, 1993.

622. Leslie BM, Harris JM III, Driscoll D: Septic arthritis of the shoulder in adults. J Bone Joint Surg [Am] 71:1516, 1989.

623. Rankin KC, Rycken JM: Bilateral dislocation of the proximal humeral epiphyses in septic arthritis: A case report. J Bone Joint Surg [Br] 75:329, 1993.

624. Resnik CS: Septic arthritis: A rare cause of drooping shoulder. Skel Radiol 21:307, 1992.

625. Dirschl DR, Henderson RC: Patellar overgrowth after infection of the knee. A case report. J Bone Joint Surg [Am] 73:940, 1991.

626. Wohlgethan JR, Newberg AH, Reed JI: The risk of abscess from sternoclavicular septic arthritis. J Rheumatol 15:1302, 1988.

627. Van Linthoudt D, Velan F, Ott H: Abscess formation in sternoclavicular joint septic arthritis. J Rheumatol 16:413, 1989.

628. Conway WF, Hayes CW, Murphy WA: Case report 568. Skel Radiol 18:483, 1989.

629. Chartash EK, Good PK, Gould ES, et al: Septic subdeltoid bursitis. Semin Arthritis Rheum 22:25, 1992.

630. Co DL, Baer AN: Staphylococcal infection of the subacromial/subdeltoid bursa. J Rheumatol 17:849, 1990.

631. Raddatz DA, Hoffman GS, Franck WA: Septic bursitis: Presentation, treatment and prognosis. J Rheumatol 14:1160, 1987.

632. Smith DL, McAfee JM: Staphylococcal bacteremia complicating septic prepatellar bursitis. J Rheumatol 14:634, 1987.

633. Walters P, Kasser J: Infection of the infrapatellar bursa. A report of two cases. J Bone Joint Surg [Am] 72:1095, 1990.

634. Manueddu CA, Hoogewoud HM, Balague F, et al: Infective iliopsoas bursitis. A case report. Int Orthop (SICOT) 15:135, 1991.

635. Jeffrey RB, Laing FC, Schecter WP, et al: Acute suppurative tenosynovitis of the hand: Diagnosis with US. Radiology 162:741, 1987.

636. Wilkerson R, Paull W, Coville FV: Necrotizing fasciitis. Review of the literature and case report. Clin Orthop 216:187, 1987.

637. Freeman HP, Oluwole SF, Ganepola GAP, et al: Necrotizing fasciitis. Am J Surg 142:377, 1981.

638. Bahlmann JCM, Fourie IJ, Arndt TCH: Fournier's gangrene: Necrotizing fasciitis of the male genitalia. Br J Urol 55:85, 1983.

639. Schecter W, Meyer A, Schecter G, et al: Necrotizing fasciitis of the upper extremity. J Hand Surg [Am] 7:15, 1982.

640. Giuliano A, Lewis F, Hadley K, et al: Bacteriology of necrotizing fasciitis. Am J Surg 134:52, 1977.

641. Fischer JR, Conway MJ, Takeshita RT, et al: Necrotizing fasciitis: Importance of roentgenographic studies for soft-tissue gas. JAMA 241:803, 1979.

642. LaCour EG, Schmid FR: Infection of bursae and tendons. In D Schlossberg (Ed): Orthopedic Infection. New York, Springer-Verlag, 1988, p 92.

643. Audran M, Masson C, Bregeon CH, et al: Pyomyositis. Study of five cases. Rev Rhum [Eng] 60:49, 1993.

644. Belli L, Reggiori A, Cocozza E, et al: Ultrasound in tropical myositis. Skel Radiol 21:107, 1992.

645. Fleckenstein JL, Burns DK, Murphy FK, et al: Differential diagnosis of bacterial myositis in AIDS: Evaluation with MR imaging. Radiology 179:653, 1991.

646. Applegate GR, Cohen AJ: Pyomyositis: Early detection utilizing multiple imaging modalities. Magn Reson Imaging 9:187, 1991.

647. Tumeh SS, Butler GJ, Maguire JH, et al: Pyogenic myositis: CT evaluation. J Comput Assist Tomogr 12:1002, 1988.

648. Andrew JG, Czyz WM: Pyomyositis presenting as septic arthritis. A report of 2 cases. Acta Orthop Scand 59:587, 1988.

649. Watts RA, Hoffbrand BI, Paton DF, et al: Pyomyositis associated with human immunodeficiency virus infection. Br Med J 294:1524, 1987.

650. Widrow CA, Kellie SM, Saltzman BR, et al: Pyomyositis in patients with the human immunodeficiency virus: An unusual form of disseminated bacterial infection. Am J Med 91:129, 1991.

651. Soriano ER, Barcan L, Clara L, et al: Streptococcus pyomyositis occurring in a patient with dermatomyositis in a country with temperate climate. J Rheumatol 19:1305, 1990.

652. Hall RL, Callaghan JJ, Moloney E, et al: Pyomyositis in a temperate climate. Presentation, diagnosis, and treatment. J Bone Joint Surg [Am] 72:1240, 1990.

653. Yuh WTC, Schreiber AE, Montgomery WJ, et al: Magnetic resonance imaging of pyomyositis. Skel Radiol 17:190, 1988.
654. Malhotra R, Singh KD, Bhan S, et al: Primary pyogenic abscess of the psoas muscle. J Bone Joint Surg [Am] 74:278, 1992.
655. Heinrich SD, Finney T, Craver R, et al: Aspergillus osteomyelitis in patients who have chronic granulomatous disease. Case report. J Bone Joint Surg [Am] 73:456, 1991.
656. Kawashima A, Kuhlman JE, Fishman EK, et al: Pulmonary Aspergillus chest wall involvement in chronic granulomatous disease: CT and MRI findings. Skel Radiol 20:487, 1991.
657. Schapiro BL, Newburger PE, Klemper MS, et al: Chronic granulomatous disease presenting in a 69-year-old man. N Engl J Med 325:1786, 1991.
658. Gill PJ, Goddard E, Beatty DW, et al: Chronic granulomatous disease presenting with osteomyelitis: Favorable response to treatment with interferon-γ. J Pediatr Orthop 12:398, 1992.
659. Sponseller PD, Malech HL, McCarthy EF Jr, et al: Skeletal involvement in children who have chronic granulomatous disease. J Bone Joint Surg [Am] 73:37, 1991.
660. Jurik AG, Møller BN: Chronic sclerosing osteomyelitis of the clavicle. A manifestation of chronic recurrent multifocal osteomyelitis. Arch Orthop Trauma Surg 106:144, 1987.
661. Jurik AG, Helmig O, Ternowitz T, et al: Chronic recurrent multifocal osteomyelitis: A follow-up study. J Pediatr Orthop 8:49, 1988.
662. Pelkonen P, Ryöppy S, Jääskeläinen J, et al: Chronic osteomyelitislike disease with negative bacterial cultures. Am J Dis Child 142:1167, 1988.
663. Manson D, Wilmot DM, Laxer RM: Physeal involvement in chronic recurrent multifocal osteomyelitis. Pediatr Radiol 20:76, 1989.
664. Jurik AG, Møller SH, Mosekilde L: Chronic sclerosing osteomyelitis of the iliac bone. Etiological possibilities. Skel Radiol 17:114, 1988.
665. Ezra E, Khermosh O, Assia A, et al: Primary subacute osteomyelitis of the axial and appendicular skeleton. J Pediatr Orthop 1:148, 1993.
666. Foy MA: Primary subacute osteomyelitis of the ilium. Clin Orthop 248:254, 1989.
667. Brown T, Wilkinson RH: Chronic recurrent multifocal osteomyelitis. Radiology 166:493, 1988.
668. Laxer RM, Shore AD, Manson D, et al: Chronic recurrent multifocal osteomyelitis and psoriasis—a report of a new association and review of related disorders. Semin Arthritis Rheum 17:260, 1988.
669. Van Howe RS, Starshak RJ, Chusid MJ: Chronic, recurrent multifocal osteomyelitis. Case report and review of the literature. Clin Pediatr 28:54, 1989.
670. Mortensson W, Edeburn G, Fries M, et al: Chronic recurrent multifocal osteomyelitis in children. A roentgenologic and scintigraphic investigation. Acta Radiol 29:565, 1988.
671. Starinsky R: Multifocal chronic osteomyelitis with exuberant periosteal formation. Pediatr Radiol 21:455, 1991.
672. Yu L, Kasser JR, O'Rourke E, et al: Chronic recurrent multifocal osteomyelitis. Association with vertebra plana. J Bone Joint Surg [Am] 71:105, 1989.
673. Rosenberg ZS, Shankman S, Klein M, et al: Chronic recurrent multifocal osteomyelitis. AJR 151:142, 1988.
674. Kahn M-F, Chamot A-M: SAPHO syndrome. Rheum Dis Clin North Am 18:225, 1992.
675. Huaux J-P, Esselinckx W, Rombouts J-J, et al: Pustulotic arthroosteitis and chronic recurrent multifocal osteomyelitis in children. Report of three cases. J Rheumatol 15:95, 1988.
676. Guyot DR, Manoli A II, Kling GA: Pyogenic sacroiliitis in IV drug abusers. AJR 149:1209, 1987.
677. Lopez-Longo F-J, Ménard H-A, Carreño L, et al: Primary septic arthritis in heroin users: Early diagnosis by radioisotopic imaging and geographic variations in the causative agents. J Rheumatol 14:991, 1987.
678. Miknowski E, Schechter GP, Nashel DJ: Acute monocytic arthritis in a patient with a long history of heroin abuse. Arthritis Rheum 30:356, 1987.
679. Endress C, Guyot DR, Fata J, et al: Cervical osteomyelitis due to IV heroin use: Radiographic findings in 14 patients. AJR 155:333, 1990.
680. Brancós MA, Peris P, Miró JM, et al: Septic arthritis in heroin addicts. Semin Arthritis Rheum 21:81, 1991.
681. Lohr KM: Rheumatic manifestations of diseases associated with substance abuse. Semin Arthritis Rheum 17:90, 1987.
682. Miro JM, Brancos R, Abello R, et al: Costochondral involvement in systemic candidiasis in heroin addicts: Clinical, scintigraphic, and histologic features in 26 patients. Arthritis Rheum 31:793, 1988.
683. Rowe IF, Wright ED, Higgens CS, et al: Intervertebral infection due to Candida albicans in an intravenous heroin abuser. Ann Rheum Dis 47:522, 1988.
684. Podzamczer D, Nolla JM, Juanola X, et al: Candidal osteomyelitis and septic arthritis in heroin abusers. J Rheumatol 16:256, 1989.
685. Albornoz MA, Myers AR: Recurrent septic arthritis and Milroy's disease. J Rheumatol 15:1726, 1988.
686. Chaudhuri K, Lonergan D, Portek I, et al: Septic arthritis of the shoulder after mastectomy and radiotherapy for breast carcinoma. J Bone Joint Surg [Br] 75:318, 1993.
687. Greiner K, Vorbrüggen W: High resolution CT in the diagnosis of osteomyelitis. Medicamundi 33:87, 1988.
688. Resnik CS, Ammann AM, Walsh JW: Chronic septic arthritis of the adult hip: Computed tomographic features. Skel Radiol 16:513, 1987.
689. Ochsner PE, Sokhegyi A, Petralli C: Der Wert der Computertomographie bei der Abklärung der chronischen Osteomyelitis. Z Orthop 128:313, 1990.
690. Égund N, Pettersson H: Computed tomographic sinography in orthopedic radiology. Skel Radiol 17:96, 1988.
691. Goldman AB: Arthrography for rheumatic disease. When, why, and for whom. Rheum Dis Clin North Am 17:505, 1991.
692. Zawin JK, Hoffer FA, Rand FF, et al: Joint effusion in children with an irritable hip: US diagnosis and aspiration. Radiology 187:459, 1993.
693. Wingstrand H, Egund N, Forsberg L: Sonography and joint pressure in synovitis of the adult hip. J Bone Joint Surg [Br] 69:254, 1987.
694. Abiri MM, Kirpekar M, Ablow RC: Osteomyelitis: Detection with US. Radiology 172:509, 1989.
695. Howard CB, Einhorn M, Dagan R, et al: Ultrasound in diagnosis and management of acute haematogenous osteomyelitis in children. J Bone Joint Surg [Br] 75:79, 1993.
696. Walker JL, Rang M: Radial head dislocation following septic arthritis of the elbow. Orthopedics 16:314, 1993.
697. Allwright SJ, Miller JH, Gilsanz V: Subperiosteal abscess in children: Scintigraphic appearance. Radiology 179:725, 1991.
698. Palestro CJ, Roumanas P, Swyer AJ, et al: Diagnosis of musculoskeletal infection using combined In-111 labeled leukocyte and Tc-99m SC marrow imaging. Clin Nucl Med 17:269, 1992.
699. Seabold JE, Nepola JV, Conrad GR, et al: Detection of osteomyelitis at fracture nonunion sites: Comparison of two scintigraphic methods. AJR 152:1021, 1989.
700. Schauwecker DS: Osteomyelitis: Diagnosis with In-111-labeled leukocytes. Radiology 171:141, 1989.
701. Kim EE, Pjura GA, Lowry PA, et al: Osteomyelitis complicating fracture: Pitfalls of 111In leukocyte scintigraphy. AJR 148:927, 1987.
702. Hansen ES, Hjortdal VE, Noer I, et al: Three-phase [99mTc] diphosphonate scintimetry in septic and nonseptic arthritis of the immature knee: An experimental investigation in dogs. J Orthop Res 7:543, 1989.
703. Zalutsky MR, De Sousa M, Venkatesan P, et al: Evaluation of indium-111 chloride as a radiopharmaceutical for joint imaging in a rabbit model of arthritis. Invest Radiol 22:733, 1987.
704. Mandell GA, Harcke HT, Bowen JR, et al: Transient photopenia of the femoral head following arthrography. Clin Nucl Med 14:397, 1989.
705. Wegener WA, Alavi A: Diagnostic imaging of musculoskeletal infection. Roentgenography; gallium, indium-labeled white blood cell, gammaglobulin bone scintigraphy; and MRI. Orthop Clin North Am 22:401, 1991.
706. Schauwecker DS: The scintigraphic diagnosis of osteomyelitis. AJR 158:9, 1992.
707. Oyen WJG, van Horn JR, Claessens RAMJ, et al: Diagnosis of bone, joint, and joint prosthesis infections with In-111-labeled nonspecific human immunoglobulin G scintigraphy. Radiology 182:195, 1992.
708. Van Nostrand D, Abreu SH, Callaghan JJ, et al: In-111-labeled white blood cell uptake in noninfected closed fracture in humans: Prospective study. Radiology 167:495, 1988.
709. Seabold JE, Ferlic RJ, Marsh JL, et al: Periarticular bone sites associated with traumatic injury: False-positive findings with In-111-labeled white blood cell and Tc-99m MDP imaging. Radiology 186:845, 1993.
710. Ouzounian TJ, Thompson L, Grogan TJ, et al: Evaluation of musculoskeletal sepsis with indium-111 white blood cell imaging. Clin Orthop 221:304, 1987.
711. Seabold JE, Nepola JV, Marsh JL, et al: Postoperative bone marrow alterations: Potential pitfalls in the diagnosis of osteomyelitis with In-111-labeled leukocyte scintigraphy. Radiology 180:741, 1991.
712. Israel O, Gips S, Jerushalmi J, et al: Osteomyelitis and soft-tissue infection: Differential diagnosis with 24 hour/4 hour ratio of Tc-99m MDP uptake. Radiology 163:725, 1987.
713. Beltran J, Noto AM, McGhee RB, et al: Infections of the musculoskeletal system: High-field-strength MR imaging. Radiology 164:449, 1987.
714. Tang JSH, Gold RH, Bassett LW, et al: Musculoskeletal infection of the extremities: Evaluation with MR imaging. Radiology 166:205, 1988.
715. Mason MD, Zlatkin MB, Esterhai JL, et al: Chronic complicated osteomyelitis of the lower extremity: Evaluation with MR imaging. Radiology 173:355, 1989.
716. Cohen MD, Cory DA, Kleiman M, et al: Magnetic resonance differentiation of acute and chronic osteomyelitis in children. Clin Radiol 41:53, 1990.
717. Williamson MR, Quenzer RW, Rosenberg RD, et al: Osteomyelitis: Sensitivity of 0.064 T MRI, three-phase bone scanning and indium scanning with biopsy proof. Magn Reson Imaging 9:945, 1991.
718. Vogler JB III, Murphy WA: Bone marrow imaging. Radiology 168:679, 1988.
719. Moore SG, Bisset GS III, Siegel MJ, et al: Pediatric musculoskeletal MR imaging. Radiology 179:345, 1991.
720. Beltran J, McGhee RB, Shaffer PB, et al: Experimental infections of the musculoskeletal system: Evaluation with MR imaging and Tc-99m MDP and Ga-67 scintigraphy. Radiology 167:167, 1988.
721. Chandnani VP, Beltran J, Morris CS, et al: Acute experimental osteomyelitis and abscesses: Detection with MR imaging versus CT. Radiology 174:233, 1990.
722. Spaeth HJ, Chandnani VP, Beltran J, et al: Magnetic resonance imaging detection of early experimental periostitis. Invest Radiol 26:304, 1991.
723. Unger E, Moldofsky P, Gatenby R, et al: Diagnosis of osteomyelitis by MR imaging. AJR 150:605, 1988.
724. Jones KM, Unger EC, Granstrom P, et al: Bone marrow imaging using STIR at 0.5 and 1.5 T. Magn Reson Imaging 10:169, 1992.
725. Shuman WP, Patten RM, Baron RL, et al: Comparison of STIR and spin-echo imaging at 1.5 T in 45 suspected extremity tumors: Lesion conspicuity and extent. Radiology 179:247, 1991.

726. Paajanen H, Brasch RC, Schmiedl U, et al: Magnetic resonance imaging of local soft tissue inflammation using gadolinium-DTPA. Acta Radiol 28:79, 1987.

727. Paajanen H, Grodd W, Revel D, et al: Gadolinium-DTPA enhanced MR imaging of intramuscular abscesses. Magn Reson Imaging 5:109, 1987.

728. Dangman BC, Hoffer FA, Rand FF, et al: Osteomyelitis in children: Gadolinium-enhanced MR imaging. Radiology 182:743, 1992.

729. Donovan Post MJ, Sze G, Quencer RM, et al: Gadolinium-enhanced MR in spinal infection. J Comput Assist Tomogr 14:721, 1990.

730. de Roos A, van Persijn van Meerten EL, Bloem JL, et al: MRI of tuberculous spondylitis. AJR 146:79, 1986.

731. Beltran J, Chandnani V, McGhee RA Jr, et al: Gadopentetate dimeglumine-enhanced MR imaging of the musculoskeletal system. AJR 156:457, 1991.

732. Tien RD: Fat-suppression MR imaging in neuroradiology: Techniques and clinical application. AJR 158:369, 1992.

733. Gold RH, Hawkins RA, Katz RD: Bacterial osteomyelitis: Findings on plain radiography, CT, MR, and scintigraphy. AJR 157:365, 1991.

734. Tehranzadeh J, Wang F, Mesqarzadeh M: Magnetic resonance imaging of osteomyelitis. CRC Crit Rev Diagn Imaging 33:495, 1992.

735. Erdman WA, Tamburro F, Jayson HT, et al: Osteomyelitis: Characteristics and pitfalls of diagnosis with MR imaging. Radiology 180:533, 1991.

736. Jacobson AF, Harley JD, Lipsky BA, et al: Diagnosis of osteomyelitis in the presence of soft-tissue infection and radiologic evidence of osseous abnormalities: Value of leukocyte imaging. AJR 157:807, 1991.

737. Frederiksen B, Christiansen P, Knudsen FU: Acute osteomyelitis and septic arthritis in the neonate, risk factors and outcome. Eur J Pediatr 152:577, 1993.

738. Gonzalez MH, Papierski P, Hall RF Jr: Osteomyelitis of the hand after a human bite. J Hand Surg [Am] 18:520, 1993.

739. Flory P, Brocq O, Euller-Ziegler L, et al: Pyomyositis: Cervical localization. J Rheumatol 20:1411, 1993.

740. Fam AG, Rubenstein J, Saibel F: Pyomyositis: Early detection and treatment. J Rheumatol 20:521, 1993.

741. Carr AJ, Cole WG, Roberton DM, et al: Chronic multifocal osteomyelitis. J Bone Joint Surg [Br] 75:582, 1993.

742. Bonfiglio M: Case report 791. Skel Radiol 22:367, 1993.

743. Sorsdahl OA, Goodhart GL, Williams HT, et al: Quantitative bone gallium scintigraphy in osteomyelitis. Skel Radiol 22:239, 1993.

744. Howard CB, Einhorn M, Dagan R, et al: Fine-needle bone biopsy to diagnose osteomyelitis. J Bone Joint Surg [Br] 76:311, 1994.

745. Dubost J-J, Fis I, Denis P, et al: Polyarticular septic arthritis. Medicine 72:296, 1993.

746. Chen W-S, Wan Y-L, Lui C-C, et al: Extrapleural abscess secondary to infection of the sternoclavicular joint. Report of two cases. J Bone Joint Surg [Am] 75:1835, 1993.

747. Majeed SA: Chronic recurrent multifocal osteomyelitis associated with tumoral calcinosis. J Bone Joint Surg [Br] 76:325, 1994.

748. Kasperczyk A, Freyschmidt J: Pustulotic arthroosteitis: Spectrum of bone lesions with palmoplantar pustulosis. Radiology 191:207, 1994.

749. Tuson CE, Hoffman EB, Mann MD: Isotope bone scanning for acute osteomyelitis and septic arthritis in children. J Bone Joint Surg [Br] 76:306, 1994.

750. Lauschke FHM, Frey C: Hematogenous osteomyelitis in infants and children in the Northwestern Region of Namibia. J Bone Joint Surg [Am] 76:502, 1994.

751. Chew FS, Schulze ES, Mattia AR: Osteomyelitis. AJR 162:942, 1994.

752. Gerscovich EO, Greenspan A: Osteomyelitis of the clavicle: Clinical, radiologic, and bacteriologic findings in ten patients. Skeletal Radiol 23:205, 1994.

753. De Boeck H, Noppen L, Desprechins B: Pyomyositis of the adductor muscles mimicking an infection of the hip. J Bone Joint Surg [Am] 76:747, 1994.

754. Stewart A, Carneiro R, Pollock L, et al: Case report 834. Skeletal Radiol 23:225, 1994.

Osteomyelitis, Septic Arthritis, and Soft Tissue Infection: Axial Skeleton

Donald Resnick, M.D., and Gen Niwayama, M.D.

The distribution of osteomyelitis and septic arthritis is influenced dramatically by the age of the patient, the specific causative organism, and the presence or absence of any underlying disorder or situation. In the child and the infant, frequent involvement of the bones and the joints of the appendicular skeleton is evident, whereas in the adult, localization of infection to the osseous and articular structures of the vertebral column is common. Pyogenic organisms can affect axial or extra-axial sites and commonly are implicated in hematogenous osteomyelitis of the tubular bones in children and infants. Tuberculous organisms also can localize in appendicular or axial skeletal sites, although the occurrence of tuberculous spondylitis is especially well known. In specific circumstances, infection also may show predilection for certain musculoskeletal locations. Examples of such predilection include osteomyelitis and septic arthritis of the spine and the sacroiliac and sternoclavicular joints in the drug addict, of the foot in the diabetic patient, of the diaphyses of tubular bones in persons with sickle cell anemia, and of altered articular sites in various patients with arthritides.

Chapter 64 has described in detail the mechanism and the pathogenesis of bone and joint infection in various age groups and situations and has emphasized alterations of the appendicular skeleton. This chapter delineates the radiographic and pathologic characteristics of infection in important axial skeletal locations, especially the spine and the sacroiliac joint.

SPINAL INFECTIONS

Routes of Contamination

Hematogenous Spread of Infection. Organisms may reach the vertebrae in several fashions.[1, 2, 188] Hematogenous spread via arterial and venous routes (Batson's paravertebral venous system) can result in lodgment of organisms in the bone marrow of the vertebrae.[3–8] The basic arrangement of the nutrient vessels is similar in the cervical, the thoracic, and the lumbar spine; a vertebral, intercostal, or a lumbar artery lying closely apposed to the vertebral body supplies minute vessels to the nearby bone, which penetrate the cortex and ramify within the marrow.[9] In addition, at each intervertebral foramen, a posterior spinal branch enters the vertebral canal and divides into an ascending and a descending branch, which anastomose with similar branches from the segments above and below and from the other side, creating an arterial network on the dorsal or posterior surface of each vertebral body.[9] Three or four nutrient arteries are derived from this network and enter the vertebral body through a large dorsal, centrally placed nutrient foramen.

The venous drainage of the vertebral body is treelike in configuration. Minute tributaries drain from the peripheral portion of the vertebral body to its center, the blood being collected by a large valveless venous channel that emerges

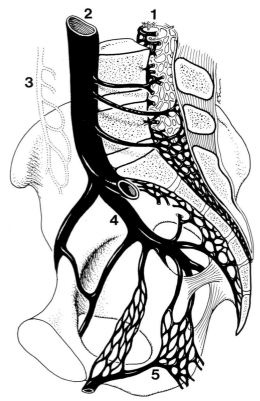

FIGURE 65–1. Anatomic considerations: Batson's paravertebral venous system. This valveless, plexiform set of veins lies outside the thoracoabdominal cavity, anastomosing with the cavitary veins at each segmental level. Thus, communication exists between the pelvic and vertebral venous system, femoral and iliac veins, inferior vena cava and superior vena cava, and other important venous structures. 1, Paravertebral venous plexus; 2, inferior vena cava; 3, inferior mesenteric vein; 4, internal iliac vein; 5, pelvic plexus. (After Vider M, et al: Cancer 40:67, 1977.)

from the central dorsal nutrient foramen and drains into an extensive loose plexus lining the vertebral canal.[9] The branching tributaries of the vertebral body are connected by channels that perforate the cortex and enter veins lying on the lateral and anterior surfaces of the vertebrae. This represents the paraspinal and spinal venous plexus of Batson (Fig. 65–1). Within the vertebral body, the ramification of blood vessels at the subchondral superior and inferior limits is reminiscent of the vascular arrangement in the childhood metaphysis and adulthood epiphysis of tubular bones.

The intraosseous venous anatomy is well depicted on the transaxial sections afforded by CT scanning (Fig. 65–2). In this plane, a treelike configuration is seen. The trunk of the tree is the major sagittally oriented posterior channel, which leads to the anterior internal plexus, and the branches of the tree are the radially coursing, generally smaller tunnels, which variably open onto the anterior and lateral surfaces of the vertebral body. Often, the two most prominent of the latter are symmetrically arranged and appear to divide the vertebral body into three nearly equal parts, resulting in a Y configuration. This CT appearance usually is differentiated easily from an abnormal configuration that may accompany traumatic, neoplastic, and infectious processes of the vertebral body (Fig. 65–3).

This vascular arrangement allows two direct routes for the hematogenous spread of infection: via the nutrient arter-

ies and via the paravertebral venous system. Although the contribution of each system to cases of spinal osteomyelitis is a matter of debate, it is attractive to implicate the valveless venous plexus, whose direction and extent of flow are influenced dramatically by changes in abdominal pressure, in the frequent spread of infection (and neoplasm) to the spine from pelvic sources.[10] Urinary tract infections or surgery,[11–17] rectosigmoid disease and enteric fistulae,[18, 19] and septic abortion or postpartum infection[20] are well recognized pelvic precursors of vertebral osteomyelitis (Fig. 65–4). Although experimental evidence can be found documenting the spread of malignant disease from the pelvic veins into the vertebral bodies through the paravertebral plexus,[21] the evidence is less decisive in cases of infectious diseases,[22, 23] suggesting to some investigators[9] that the role of Batson's plexus in the dissemination of infectious disease has been greatly exaggerated. In addition, the common localization of early foci of osteomyelitis in the subchondral region of the vertebral body, an area richly supplied by nutrient arterioles,[112, 169, 170] emphasizes that arterial rather than venous pathways may be more important in hematogenous osteomyelitis of the spine. This concept is further underscored by the distribution of infection along the route of the ascending and descending nutrient branches of the posterior spinal arteries, the presence of prodromal findings consistent with septicemia in cases of vertebral osteomyelitis, and the absence of pathologic documentation of a spreading extradural thrombophlebitis in these cases.[9] Thus, in many examples of pelvic and extrapelvic infection complicated by spinal contamination, the arterial hematogenous route may be the real pathway of sepsis.

The role of hematogenous spread of infection directly into the intervertebral disc has stimulated great interest. It has been suggested that in children and adolescents below the age of 19 or 20 years, vascular channels perforate the vertebral endplate,[24] allowing organisms in the blood stream to have direct access to the intervertebral disc.[25] This concept has led to the popular terms of "discitis,"[26] spondylarthritis,[26–28] intervertebral disc space infection[29–31] or inflammation,[32, 33] benign osteomyelitis of the spine, nonspecific spondylitis,[34, 35] and pyogenic vertebral osteomyelitis[36] that are applied to such infection.[37] A similar occurrence in adults[38, 113] has been attributed to a persistent discal blood supply[39] or to a supply that has been reinstated by vascular invasion of degenerating discal tissue. Because of the great interest in "discitis" that has been sparked by a most heated debate, this condition is discussed separately later in this chapter.

Spread from a Contiguous Source of Infection. Vertebral or intervertebral discal infection can result from contamination by an adjacent soft tissue suppurative focus[40] (Fig. 65–5). This mechanism is not common, as many paravertebral abscesses dissect away from the spine along normal and abnormal soft tissue planes.[114] Even in those cases in which bone or cartilage involvement follows soft tissue infection, it is extremely difficult to eliminate the possibility that osteomyelitis or discal infection does not result from hematogenous or lymphatic seeding. Tuberculous and fungal infection, however, can extend from the spine to the neighboring tissue, dissect along the subligamentous areas for a considerable distance, and then reenter the vertebral body or intervertebral disc. Furthermore, examples of osteomyelitis and infective discitis as a complication of co-

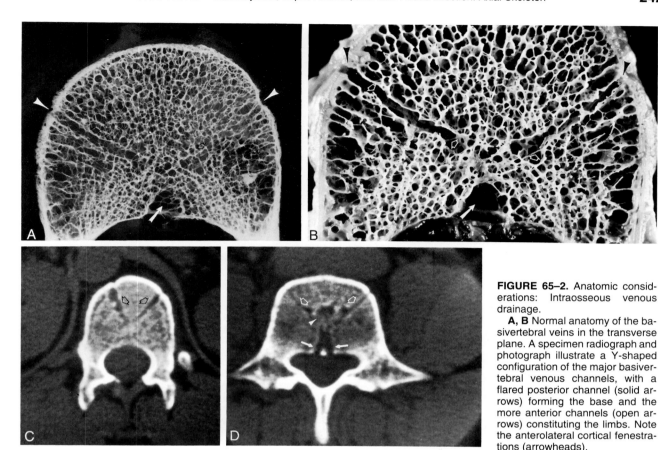

FIGURE 65–2. Anatomic considerations: Intraosseous venous drainage.

A, B Normal anatomy of the basivertebral veins in the transverse plane. A specimen radiograph and photograph illustrate a Y-shaped configuration of the major basivertebral venous channels, with a flared posterior channel (solid arrows) forming the base and the more anterior channels (open arrows) constituting the limbs. Note the anterolateral cortical fenestrations (arrowheads).

C On the transaxial CT scan of a normal thoracic vertebra, a V-shaped configuration of the anterior channels is observed (open arrows).

D In a similar image of a lumbar vertebra, a Y-shaped configuration composed of paired posterior channels (solid arrows) and anterior channels (open arrows) is observed. A prominent central confluence of vessels (arrowhead) is evident.

lonic,[171] hypopharyngeal,[115] and esophageal[116, 189] perforation or instrumentation, fistulous communication with a pelvic abscess,[40] and arteritis (due to Salmonella infection)[117] have been reported. Dental extractions[121] may be associated with cervical osteomyelitis. In all of these examples, however, the role of bacteremia with subsequent hematogenous seeding of the spine must be considered. In cases of osteomyelitis and discal infection resulting from contamination by a contiguous suppurative focus, soft tissue abnormalities are followed by sequential invasion of the periosteum, cortex, and marrow of the vertebrae or of the ligaments and anulus fibrosus and nucleus pulposus of the intervertebral disc.

A specific entity that may be related to this mechanism of infection is Grisel's syndrome,[118] in which spontaneous atlantoaxial subluxation accompanies inflammation of neighboring soft tissues mainly in children (Fig. 65–6).[119, 120, 190, 191] Proposed causes of this phenomenon have included muscle spasm, ligamentous laxity, and synovial effusion; the direct continuity of the periodontoidal venous plexus and the suboccipital epidural sinuses with the pharyngovertebral veins[122] suggests the existence of a hematogenous route for the transport of peripharyngeal septic exudates to the upper cervical spine structures. Predisposing events in cases of Grisel's syndrome include rhinopharyngitis, tonsillitis and tonsillectomy, alveolar periostitis, acute rheumatic fever, tuberculous adenitis, and syphylitic pharyngeal ulceration.[190] Clinical manifestations, which vary in their time of onset after the predisposing event, include neck pain, stiffness, and torticollis. Imaging studies reveal rotational abnormalities between the atlas and the axis, anterior atlantoaxial subluxation, and, in some cases, compromise of the spinal cord.

Direct Implantation. Organisms can be implanted directly into the intervertebral disc (and far less commonly the vertebra) during attempted punctures of the spinal canal, intervertebral disc, paravertebral and peridural tissues, or aorta[41, 123] or in penetrating injuries. Usually the intervertebral disc is the initial site of infection, especially in cases of misguided puncture, and the vertebra becomes contaminated as a secondary event. After inadvertent administration of a paravertebral anesthetic into the intervertebral disc, discal narrowing occasionally can represent not an infection but, perhaps, a chemical destruction of tissue.[42] Similarly, injection of chymopapain (chemical diskectomy) or iodinated contrast material (discography) may lead to noninfectious destruction of the intervertebral disc, although disc space infections can complicate these procedures.[124, 192, 193] Spinal infections occurring after percutaneous diskectomy also are recognized.[194, 195] (Fig. 65–7).

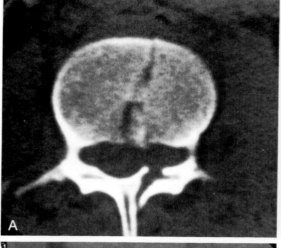

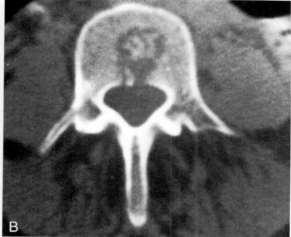

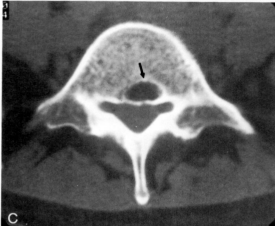

FIGURE 65–3. Pathologic changes simulating normal venous anatomy.

A Sagittal fracture of lumbar vertebral body. The transaxial CT appearance resembles the normal Y configuration of the venous channels minus one limb. Observe minimal displacement of bone, irregular, poorly defined margins of the fracture line, and an off-midline position of an apparent normal posterior septum, representing a displaced bone fragment encroaching on the spinal canal. A fracture of the posterior portion of the vertebra also is present.

B Metastasis of malignant melanoma to lumbar vertebral body. A large, poorly defined osteolytic lesion with bone sequestration is seen in this transaxial CT image.

C Cartilaginous (Schmorl's) node in lumbar vertebral body. A transaxial CT scan demonstrates an oval osseous defect (arrow) that was continuous with the intervertebral disc.

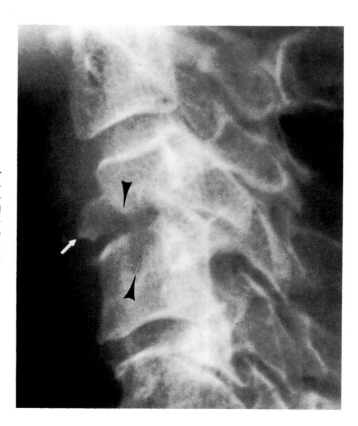

FIGURE 65–4. Spinal infection: Hematogenous spread. This 54 year old diabetic man developed emphysematous pyelonephritis and cystitis with septicemia and progressive neck pain (causative microorganism is *Escherichia coli*). Note the destructive foci in the third and fourth cervical vertebrae (arrowheads) and loss in height of the intervening interverteral disc space. The anteriorly located ledge of bone (arrow) may represent a preexisting osteophyte that now is infected. Soft tissue swelling also is evident along the anterior aspect of the spine.

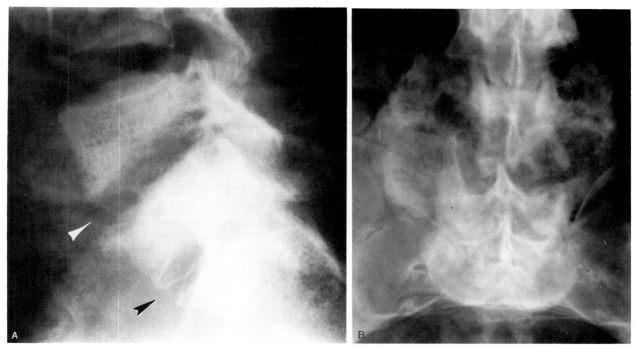

FIGURE 65–5. Spinal infection: Spread from a contiguous contaminated source.

A This 30 year old man developed a buttock abscess complicated by peripelvic abscess formation and osteomyelitis (causative microorganisms were mixed gram-positive and gram-negative bacteria). A radiograph reveals considerable destruction of the fourth and fifth lumbar vertebral bodies and, possibly, the superior surface of the sacrum with involvement of two intervening disc spaces (arrowheads).

B In this 38 year old paraplegic man, extensive decubitus ulcers in the lower back were associated with a soft tissue infection that eventually contaminated the lumbar spine. Note the prominent destruction of the fourth and fifth lumbar vertebrae, accompanied by new bone formation. The sacroiliac joints are narrowed or ankylosed as a result of cartilage atrophy.

FIGURE 65–6. Grisel's syndrome. This 11 year old boy developed a head tilt after an ear infection.

A The scout view from a CT study reveals the deviation of the head to the left side.

B A transaxial CT scan at the level of the atlas shows that it is rotated about the odontoid process with the right side of the atlas located anterior to the left side.

C A transaxial T1-weighted (TR/TE, 300/15) spin echo MR image obtained after the intravenous injection of gadolinium contrast agent reveals a similar position of the atlas, which is rotated with respect to the axis. The adjacent soft tissues show some degree of hyperintensity, reflecting gadolinium enhancement. The rotational abnormality resolved slowly over a period of months.

(Courtesy of S. Wall, M.D., San Francisco, California.)

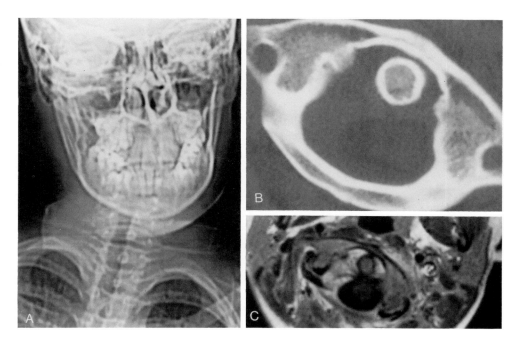

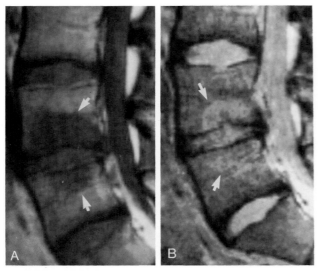

FIGURE 65–7. Spinal infection: Direct implantation. Percutaneous diskectomy. This 26 year old man developed an infection at the L4-L5 spinal level with progressive back pain that began several weeks after percutaneous diskectomy. Subsequent surgery confirmed the presence of pus in the intervertebral disc. Sagittal T1-(TR/TE, 450/20) **(A)** and proton density (TR/TE, 2200/45) **(B)** weighted MR images reveal abnormalities consistent with infection. In **A**, abnormal regions of low signal intensity (arrows) are evident in the L4 and L5 vertebral bodies. In **B**, the signal intensity in these intraosseous regions (arrows) is slightly greater than that of the adjacent bone marrow. Note the loss of the normal intranuclear cleft in the L4-L5 intervertebral disc.

Postoperative Infection. The more frequent and aggressive spinal operations that currently are undertaken have led to an increase in postoperative infection of the spinal column. Laminectomy, diskectomy, instrumentation, and fusion can each be complicated by osteomyelitis or discal infection[43-46, 196, 197] (Fig. 65–8). Staphylococcus species generally are implicated,[125, 126, 186] although the failure to recover organisms in some patients, particularly those undergoing discal surgery, has suggested that trauma or vascular disturbance without infection may produce similar abnormalities.[126-128] The localization of osseous or articular contamination depends on the precipitating surgical event; infection may involve the vertebral body, the posterior osseous elements, the intervertebral disc, or even the spinal canal in any region of the vertebral column. In some cases of diskectomy, infection of an intervertebral disc at a nonsurgical level may occur, perhaps related to hematogenous seeding.[197]

Clinical Abnormalities

The clinical abnormalities of spinal infection depend on the site and extent of involvement and on the specific organisms that are implicated. Most of the following observations concern pyogenic infections of the spine.[1, 2, 47–58, 103]

With increasing interest in and the development of more sophisticated diagnostic techniques, the reported frequency of osteomyelitis and disc space infection (together these will be termed infective spondylitis) has risen dramatically. Initially infective spondylitis was thought to represent less than 1 per cent of all cases of osteomyelitis[59]; now it appears that 2 to 4 per cent is a more accurate estimation.[2, 6, 47, 60] This frequency rises rapidly in patients with pelvic infection and in those who are debilitated or who have other predisposing factors. Men are affected more commonly than women with ratios ranging between 1.5 to 1 and 3 to 1. The highest frequency of septic spondylitis occurs in the fifth and sixth decades of life, although infants, children, and elderly persons also are affected.[53, 55, 61–63, 198] The lumbar spine is the most typical site of involvement, followed by the thoracic spine, with sacral and cervical abnormalities

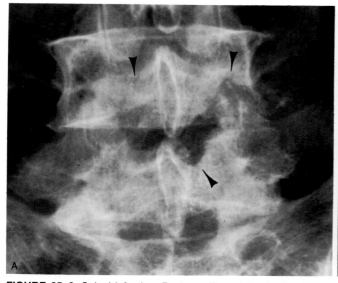
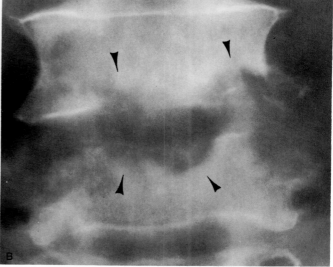

FIGURE 65–8. Spinal infection: Postoperative contamination. This 71 year old man developed the onset of back and gluteal pain after a recent laminectomy. A subsequent biopsy demonstrated necrotic osseous and fibrous tissue with acute and chronic inflammatory cellular infiltration.

A An anteroposterior radiograph delineates destruction of apposing margins of the fourth and fifth lumbar vertebrae (arrowheads) with narrowing of the intervening disc space.

B Frontal tomography confirms the extent of the vertebral destruction with surrounding sclerosis (arrowheads).

about equal in frequency.[64] The usual location of infection in the vertebra is the vertebral body.[2, 54] Alterations in the posterior osseous elements, including the apophyseal joints, and in unusual sites such as the occiput, atlas, and odontoid process certainly are encountered, however.[2, 65–68, 199–204, 212]

A history of recent primary infection (urinary tract, respiratory tract, or skin infection), instrumentation (catheterization, cystoscopy), or diagnostic or surgical procedure (myelography, discography; bowel, urinary, or back operation) is common.[47] The most frequently encountered (55 to 90 per cent) pyogenic organism is *Staphylococcus aureus,* although other gram-positive (Streptococcus, pneumococcus) and, less typically, gram-negative (*Escherichia coli,* Pseudomonas, Klebsiella, and Salmonella) agents may be implicated. Associations of particular bacterial pathogens with vertebral osteomyelitis include Pseudomonas infection in the intravenous drug abuser, streptococcal infection in patients with endocarditis, *Streptococcus bovis* infection in patients with colonic polyposis, *Haemophilus aphrophilus* infection after meningitis, and *Nocardia asteroides* infection in patients with pulmonary involvement.[188] Brucella infection of the spine may be encountered in international travelers, abattoir workers, farmers, veterinarians, and laboratory personnel.[188] Nonpyogenic organisms accounting for infective spondylitis include tuberculous and syphilis organisms and various fungi.[1]

Clinical manifestations vary with the virulence of the organisms and the nature of the host resistance. General findings include fever, malaise, anorexia, and weight loss. Back pain is a common initial local manifestation and may be intermittent or constant, exacerbated by motion and throbbing at rest. It may have a radicular distribution. Spinal tenderness and rigidity also may be observed. With accompanying soft tissue abscess formation, hip contracture can occur (psoas muscle irritation).[2] Paraplegia, which can be reversible with appropriate antibiotic therapy, is evident in fewer than 1 per cent of cases.[47] This complication is most frequent in cervical infections and in patients with underlying diseases such as diabetes mellitus and rheumatoid arthritis.[129]

The erythrocyte sedimentation rate is elevated almost universally. Evaluation of the peripheral blood can reveal a normal or elevated leukocyte count. Appropriate culture of the blood can identify the causative organism in some cases, although more drastic methods, such as needle biopsy or aspiration, may be necessary.

Clinical diagnosis may be especially difficult in four situations[47, 188]: After surgical removal of a herniated intervertebral disc, the postoperative manifestations may mask the symptoms and signs of infection; in young children, absence of local manifestations can be misleading; lack of sensation in paraplegic or quadriplegic patients may prevent early diagnosis; and, in the intravenous drug abuser, extraspinal abnormalities may overshadow the vertebral alterations.

Radiographic-Pathologic Correlation

Early Abnormalities. Hematogenous spread of infection frequently leads to a focus in the anterior subchondral regions of the vertebral body adjacent to the intervertebral disc (Fig. 65–9).[130, 131] Extension to the ventral surface of the vertebra can be associated with infection of the adjacent longitudinal ligaments[1] but more typically, discal perforation soon ensues. At this stage, radiographs may be entirely normal. Soon (1 to 3 weeks), however, a decrease in height of the intervertebral disc is accompanied by loss of normal definition of the subchondral bone plate and enlarging destructive foci within the neighboring vertebral body (Fig. 65–10). The combination of rapid loss of intervertebral disc height and adjacent lysis of bone is most suggestive of an infectious process. With further spread of infection, progressive destruction of the vertebral body and the intervertebral disc becomes evident, and the process soon contaminates the adjacent vertebra.[50] Such involvement of two contiguous vertebral bodies almost uniformly is associated with transdiscal infection and rarely is the result of multicentric involvement.[47] In a series of 150 patients with infective spondylitis, approximately two thirds had infection limited to the disc space and two vertebral bodies, 23 per cent had changes at more than one level, and in less than 1 per cent the changes were isolated to a single intervertebral disc and a single vertebral body.[50]

It has been suggested that vertebral osteomyelitis in infants may have an unusual radiographic appearance in which progressive dissolution of involved vertebral bodies

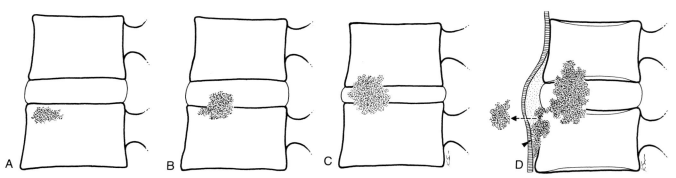

FIGURE 65–9. Spinal infection: Sequential stages.
  A An anterior subchondral focus in the vertebral body is typical.
  B Infection then may perforate the vertebral surface, reaching the intervertebral disc space.
  C With further spread of infection, contamination of the adjacent vertebral body and narrowing of the intervertebral disc space are recognizable.
  D With continued dissemination, infection may spread in a subligamentous fashion, eroding the anterior surface of the vertebral body (arrowhead), or perforating the anterior ligamentous structures (arrow).

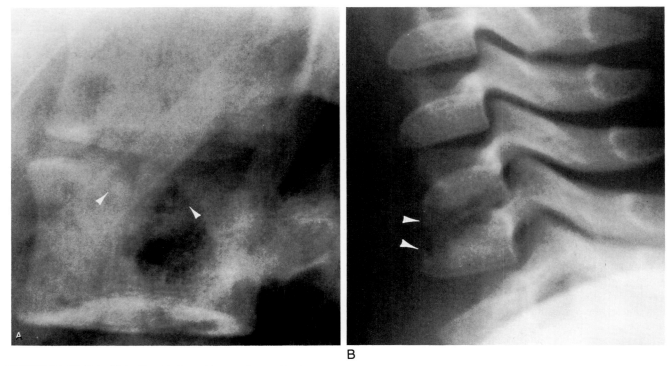

B

FIGURE 65–10. Spinal infection: Early and later radiographic abnormalities.

A Observe loss of definition of the superior aspect of a lumbar vertebral body (arrowheads) with narrowing of the adjacent intervertebral disc space. This appearance (in a middle-aged man with pyogenic infection) conforms to the stage in Figure 65–9**B**.

B In this young child, a staphylococcal infection has led to destruction of two adjacent vertebral bodies (arrowheads) and narrowing of the intervening intervertebral disc. A soft tissue mass was apparent. This appearance corresponds to the stage in Figure 65–9**D**.

occurs in the absence of loss of discal height.[132] Years later, resultant kyphotic deformity resembles that in congenital kyphosis. Furthermore, in adults with underlying disorders such as diffuse idiopathic skeletal hyperostosis that lead to bony bridging of vertebral bodies, the disc space may be maintained in cases of infective spondylitis.[205]

Later Abnormalities. After a variable period (10 to 12 weeks), regenerative changes appear in the bone with sclerosis or eburnation[50] (Fig. 65–11). The osteosclerotic response is variable in severity and has been used in the past as a helpful sign in differentiating pyogenic from tuberculous infection.[69] Although such sclerosis is indeed common in pyogenic (nontuberculous) spondylitis,[54] it also may be evident in tuberculosis, particularly in black patients.[70, 71] Furthermore, some persons with pyogenic spinal infection do not reveal significant eburnation, particularly when symptoms and signs have not been of long duration, so that using the presence or absence of bony sclerosis as a foolproof way of differentiating tuberculous and nontuberculous spondylitis can lead to an erroneous diagnosis. More helpful in this differentiation is a combination of findings that strongly indicates tuberculous spondylitis, including the presence of a slowly progressive vertebral process with preservation of intervertebral discs, subligamentous spread of infection with erosion of anterior vertebral margins, large and calcified soft tissue abscesses, and the absence of severe bony eburnation (Fig. 65–12).

Soft tissue extension of infection can be observed in

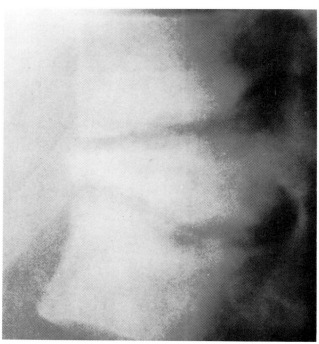

FIGURE 65–11. Spinal infection: Later radiographic abnormalities. Involvement of several vertebrae is evident. Note the destruction and collapse of bone with reactive sclerosis and narrowing of two intervertebral disc spaces. Observe the poorly defined or "fuzzy" discovertebral junctions (pyogenic infection).

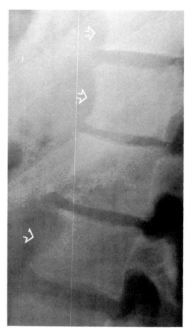

FIGURE 65–12. Spinal infection: Tuberculosis. Subligamentous spread. Note erosion of the anterior surface (arrows) of multiple vertebral bodies. (Courtesy of A. Nemcek, M.D., Chicago, Illinois.)

approximately 20 per cent of cases of pyogenic spondylitis.[47] In the lumbar spine, such extension can lead to obliteration or displacement of the psoas margin; in the thoracic spine, a paraspinal mass can be encountered; and in the cervical spine, retropharyngeal swelling can lead to displacement and obliteration of adjacent prevertebral fat planes[25, 50, 54] (Fig. 65–13).

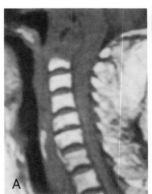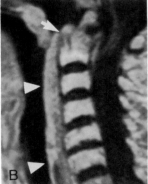

FIGURE 65–13. Spinal infection: Soft tissue extension. This 72 year old woman developed a staphylococcal infection of the upper cervical spine, presumably spread hematogenously.

A Sagittal T1-weighted (TR/TE, 500/10) spin echo MR image reveals replacement of the axis, particularly the odontoid process, with tissue of low signal intensity. Prominent prevertebral soft tissues are evident.

B After the intravenous injection of gadolinium contrast agent, an identical T1-weighted (TR/TE, 500/10) spin echo MR image shows enhancement of signal intensity in the abnormal intraosseous (arrow), prevertebral (arrowheads), and intraspinal infected tissue. A pathologic fracture of the odontoid process and posterior displacement of the atlas and odontoid process are present. Note that because of the increased signal intensity of the abnormal marrow in the axis, its differentiation from normal marrow is more difficult than in **A.**

(Courtesy of M. Schweitzer, M.D., Philadelphia, Pennsylvania.)

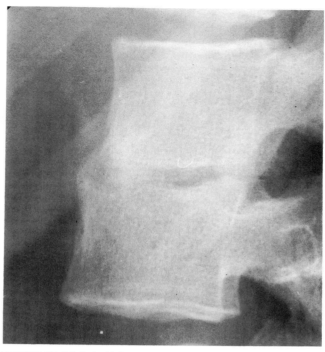

FIGURE 65–14. Spinal infection: Bony fusion. After a pyogenic infection, partial (or complete) bony ankylosis can result. Such bony fusion also can accompany trauma or congenital disorders, although the lack of hypoplasia of the vertebral bodies suggests that the process did not occur prior to the cessation of growth.

With early and proper treatment, reconstitution can result, with production of a radiodense (ivory) vertebra, a relatively intact or ankylosed intervertebral disc, and surrounding osteophytosis[50, 72–74] (Fig. 65–14). Without such treatment, complete bony lysis and collapse, discal obliteration, deviation and deformity of the vertebral column (Fig. 65–15), and massive soft tissue abscesses, which ascend or descend along the spine, extending here and there into the bone or disc (migrating osteomyelitis),[1] can appear.

Special Types of Spinal Infection

Intervertebral Disc Infection ("Discitis"). Most infections of the intervertebral disc occur as an extension of vertebral osteomyelitis or direct inoculation during diagnostic or surgical procedures. In children, however, a hematogenous route to the disc still exists, which may persist until the age of 20 or 30 years[24, 75] and, according to some investigators, may be found even in the elderly.[39] Thus, certainly in children, hematogenous contamination of the discal tissue is possible.[28–37, 76–79] Although organisms are not always isolated in cases of childhood discitis, a bacterial cause is proposed most frequently; however, some investigators believe the condition is a noninfectious inflammatory or traumatic disorder. Clinical symptoms and signs may become evident between 1 and 16 years of age, and a preexisting infectious condition (upper respiratory tract, urinary tract, or ear infection) usually is apparent. Manifestations generally are mild. Back pain, abdominal pain, hip irritability, and altered gait may be evident.[206] Low grade fever, irritability, malaise, elevation of the erythrocyte sedimentation rate, and, on occasion, leukocytosis are noted in many cases. When positive, blood or bone biopsy culture

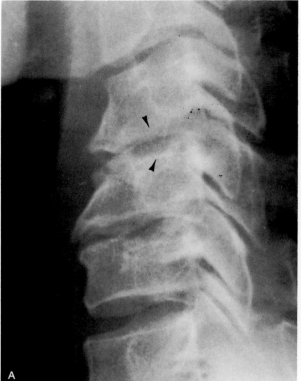

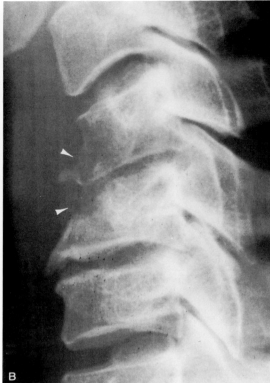

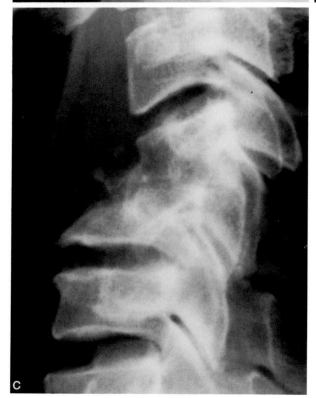

FIGURE 65–15. Spinal infection: Residual deformity. A 41 year old man developed Klebsiella spondylitis in the cervical region.

A Initial radiograph reveals minimal bony indistinctness and destruction (arrowheads) at the C4-C5 level. Considerable degenerative disease of the intervertebral discs has resulted in disc space narrowing and osteophytes at multiple sites.

B Three weeks later, note the collapse and fragmentation of the superior aspect of the fifth cervical vertebral body and lysis of the inferior aspect of the fourth cervical vertebral body (arrowheads). Soft tissue swelling is evident.

C Two weeks after **B,** angulation and subluxation are apparent. Soft tissue swelling again is seen.

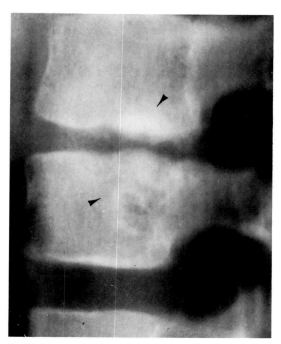

FIGURE 65–16. Intervertebral disc infection: Discitis. This 6 year old girl developed symptoms and signs consistent with spinal infection. Bacteriologic studies were not helpful. Observe the narrowing of the intervertebral disc between the second and third lumbar vertebral bodies with osseous lucency and sclerosis (arrowheads). The appearance is consistent with infection. (Courtesy of L. Lurie, M.D., Chula Vista, California.)

most typically reveals *Staphylococcus aureus.* Negative culture results are reported in 50 to 90 per cent of cases.

Radiologic abnormalities of discitis in children commonly are delayed (several weeks), although scintigraphy may reveal increased accumulation of bone-seeking pharmaceuticals at a relatively early stage.[133, 134] Radiographic changes are most frequent in the lumbar spine, followed, in descending order of frequency, by the thoracic and cervical segments. Intervertebral disc space narrowing later is accompanied by erosion of the subchondral bone plate and osseous eburnation (Figs. 65–16 and 65–17). Antibiotic therapy usually is administered on an empirical basis, and reconstitution of the intervertebral disc, although not complete, commonly results. Rarely, psoas abscesses may develop,[135] a finding that is well shown with CT or MR imaging.[136] Other reported late manifestations are partial or complete interbody fusion, osteophytosis, spondylolisthesis, kyphosis, scoliosis, and vertebra magnum or wedging.[206–208] Intraspinal extension of an inflammatory mass is unusual,[136] and neurologic findings are rare.

MR imaging in cases of childhood discitis reveals findings similar to those in adults with infective spondylitis (see later discussion).[209–211] High signal intensity in the intervertebral disc and adjacent portions of the vertebral bodies on T2-weighted spin echo MR images or on gadolinium-enhanced images is characteristic (Fig. 65–18). Posterior discal displacement and paraspinal masses also may be evident.

The occurrence of hematogenous spread of infection to the adult intervertebral disc also has been proposed.[80, 113] Kemp and associates[38] described 13 men and two women between the ages of 17 and 72 years who revealed findings compatible with isolated discal infection, related primarily to staphylococci. They interpreted the radiographic manifestations, which included early decrease in the vertical height of the affected intervertebral disc and subsequent sclerosis of the neighboring bone and irregularity of the vertebral plate, as indicative of discal infection with noninfectious reactive osseous response, an interpretation that

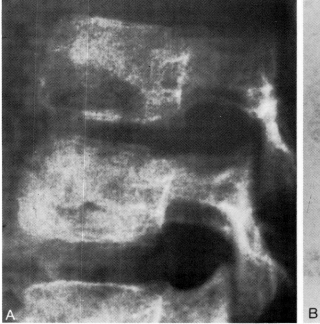
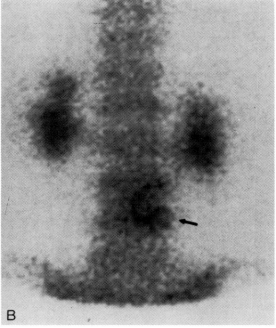

FIGURE 65–17. Intervertebral disc infection: Discitis. A lateral radiograph **(A)** shows subtle narrowing of the disc space between the third and the fourth lumbar vertebral bodies, which, on bone scan **(B)**, is associated with increased accumulation of the radionuclide (arrow). (Courtesy of T. Goergen, M.D., San Diego, California.)

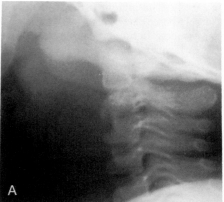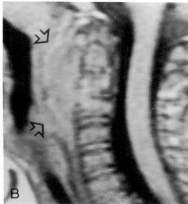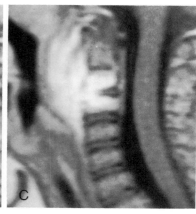

FIGURE 65–18. Intervertebral disc infection: Discitis.

   A The routine lateral radiograph in this 1 year old child reveals destruction of the third and fourth cervical vertebral bodies and a prominent anterior soft tissue mass.

   B This sagittal T1-weighted (TR/TE, 600/20) MR image reveals a soft tissue mass (arrows) of signal intensity similar to that of muscle. The osseous and discal involvement is not well shown in this image.

   C After intravenous administration of gadolinium contrast agent, an identical image (TR/TE, 600/20) shows dramatic hyperintensity of the infective process in the vertebral bodies, anterior portion of the C3-C4 intervertebral disc, and anterior soft tissues.

   (Courtesy of K. Kortman, M.D., San Diego, California.)

was strengthened by the lack of evidence of osteomyelitis on pathologic examination. Histologic changes included inflammatory granulation tissue within the affected disc, deposition of new bone or osteoid on existing trabeculae of the vertebral body, and fibroblastic tissues within the intertrabecular spaces. The outcome of discitis in these patients was variable. In some, attempted repair was associated with circumferential formation of bone across the anulus; intervertebral disc fusion was not evident. Partial or complete paraplegia was observed in some of these patients.

Although the pathologic observations in this report are consistent with noninfectious bone response, it is not possible to state with certainty that some foci of infection were not present in the vertebrae. The difficulty of obtaining adequate biopsy samples and of isolating organisms from the bone successfully in documented cases of osteomyelitis is well known. Furthermore, radiologic findings in the cases reported by Kemp and coworkers and by others[113] are similar or identical to those in vertebral osteomyelitis. Although the concept of hematogenous infection isolated to the intervertebral disc of the adult due to persistent normal or abnormal vascular channels is indeed intriguing, further documentation of this entity is required before its existence truly is established.

Other Diagnostic Techniques

As at other sites of infection, a variety of diagnostic techniques in addition to routine radiography can be employed in cases of infective spondylitis. These include conventional tomography, myelography, scintigraphy, CT, and MR imaging. The role of *radionuclide studies* in establishing the presence of spinal infection at a stage when radiographs are entirely normal is well documented. Technetium and gallium radiopharmaceutical agents can be used in this regard[37, 47, 58, 76, 107, 108, 137–139, 213, 214]; gallium may have a special role in the diagnosis of discitis.[81, 139] The value of ^{111}In-labeled leukocytes in the early diagnosis of spinal infections is not clear.[172, 183] The abnormal technetium scan

may be characterized by augmented uptake in two adjacent vertebral bodies or a more diffuse pattern, reflecting reactive hyperemia[47]; with gallium, paravertebral uptake of the isotope leads to a butterfly appearance.[138] The application of single photon emission computed tomography (SPECT) has increased further the sensitivity of bone scanning in the diagnosis of infective spondylitis.

CT also can be used in the investigation of patients with infective spondylitis.[106, 136, 140–146, 173, 174, 184] The examination, which can be performed with or without subarachnoid injection of contrast material, allows definition of the extent of osseous and discal destruction and of paravertebral and intraspinal involvement (Fig. 65–19). The intravenous injection of contrast material aids in the separation of abnormal and normal soft tissues. Gas may be identified in the infected soft tissues[140] or, rarely, in the intervertebral disc itself.

Hypodensity of the intervertebral disc on CT has been reported as a reliable indicator of infection,[147, 175] and a similar decrease in attenuation numbers (Hounsfield units) has been identified in infected bone and soft tissue.[143] The precise cause of the decreased radiodensity is not clear but appears to be related to the edema and inflammatory exudate present within the granulation tissue. During the healing process, a decrease in the size of soft tissue abscesses and an increase in attenuation numbers are expected.

CT criteria have been proposed that aid in the differential diagnosis of infections and neoplastic diseases of the spine.[215] The most reliable criteria for pyogenic infection are complete prevertebral soft tissue involvement, diffuse motheaten or permeative bone destruction, gas formation within both bone and soft tissue, and a process centering on the intervertebral disc. Nonpyogenic, or granulomatous, infection is associated with geographic or motheaten bone destruction and marginal bone sclerosis. CT criteria for skeletal metastasis include posterior osseous element involvement, osteolytic and osteoblastic response, and focal or absent prevertebral swelling or mass formation. Such criteria are helpful but not without exceptions; diagnostic

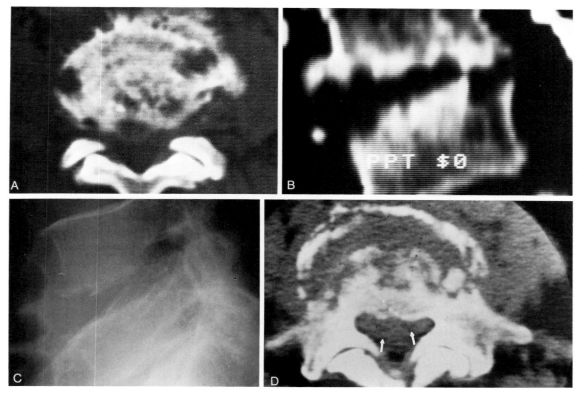

FIGURE 65–19. Spinal infection: Role of CT.

A, B In this 72 year old man with a 2 month history of weight loss, malaise, and back pain, involvement of the lumbar spine by *Staphylococcal aureus* infection is well shown on a transaxial CT scan with sagittal reformation. Findings include osseous and discal destruction with a soft tissue mass that obliterated the right psoas muscle.

C, D In a 70 year old man with spinal infection caused by the same microorganisms, a plain film documents loss of height of the intervertebral disc between the fourth and fifth lumbar vertebral bodies with bone erosion. The transaxial CT scan at this level documents the extent of spinal destruction with a soft tissue mass in paraspinal and intraspinal locations (arrows). This mass explained the patient's prominent neurologic manifestations.

errors can best be avoided when the CT findings are correlated with other imaging studies, including plain films.

CT can be helpful during attempts to aspirate fluid or tissue from sites of vertebral infection. It also can be used in guiding correct placement of percutaneous catheters for paravertebral soft tissue drainage.[148]

Even the early studies employing *MR imaging* in cases of spinal infection emphasized its diagnostic sensitivity, its ability to allow delineation of the extent of vertebral and paravertebral involvement, and its usefulness in gauging the response of the disease process to therapy.[149–152, 176–178, 187] Subsequent investigations have confirmed the many advantages of this imaging method when applied to the assessment of spinal infection, whether pyogenic or nonpyogenic, whether it is extradural, intradural extramedullary, or intramedullary. The vast majority of spinal infections involve one or more of the extradural structures, including the vertebral bodies, intervertebral discs, posterior osseous elements, epidural space, and paraspinal soft tissues. Indeed, as indicated previously, infective spondylitis of hematogenous origin typically localizes in the vertebral body of adults and in the vertebral body or intervertebral disc of children. Alterations in morphology and signal intensity of these two structures are fundamental to detection of infective spondylitis using MR imaging.

As described in detail elsewhere in this book, a gradual conversion of red to yellow marrow occurs during growth and development. At birth, virtually the entire fetal marrow space is hematopoietic in nature; subsequently, during the first two decades of life, conversion of hematopoietic to fatty marrow takes place, beginning in the appendicular skeleton and then extending to portions of the axial skeleton, such that by the age of approximately 25 years, an adult pattern is achieved.[216] At this time, red marrow is located primarily in the vertebrae, ribs, sternum, skull, and innominate bones and, to a lesser extent, the proximal metaphyses of the femora and humeri. With regard to the spine, foci of fatty marrow may be present in the vertebral bodies, although hematopoietic marrow usually predominates. The specific distribution patterns of red and yellow marrow in the vertebral bodies, as delineated by MR imaging, have been summarized by Ricci and coworkers[217]: linear areas of fatty marrow along the basivertebral veins; bandlike and triangular areas of fatty marrow in the peripheral portions of the vertebral bodies; and multiple small or large areas of fatty marrow scattered throughout the vertebral bodies. In general, with increasing age of the person, the foci of fatty marrow (as depicted by MR imaging) become more numerous and prominent, although individual variations in this distribution are encountered (Fig. 65–20).

The MR imaging characteristics of infective spondylitis will be influenced by the specific nature and extent of

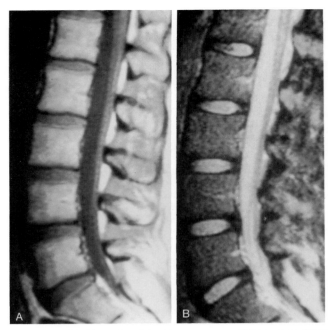

FIGURE 65–20. Normal vertebral bone marrow: MR imaging. Adult pattern.

A On a sagittal T1-weighted (TR/TE, 800/20) spin echo MR image, most of the vertebral bone marrow has signal intensity indicative of fat.

B With multiplanar gradient recalled (MPGR) imaging (TR/TE, 400/15; flip angle, 15 degrees), low signal intensity of the bone marrow is evident.

(Courtesy of L. L. Baker, M.D., La Jolla, California.)

the process and the precise imaging protocols that are used.[218-224] Furthermore, the age of the patient (child versus adult) will affect these characteristics owing to the changing constituency of the bone marrow (i.e., red versus yellow marrow). In instances of acute pyogenic osteomyelitis, an inflammatory reponse occurs, leading to an increase in extracellular fluid in the marrow of the vertebral body. Typically, in affected regions, signal intensity decreases on T1-weighted spin echo MR images and increases on T2-weighted spin echo images (Fig. 65–21). The conspicuity of the bone marrow infection on these MR images depends on the extent of red and yellow marrow in the vertebral body. For example, in children, adolescents, or young adults, the low signal intensity of the infective process seen on T1-weighted images may be less obvious as the adjacent bone marrow is predominantly hematopoietic in nature; in the elderly, however, in whom much of the vertebral marrow is fatty, this region of low signal intensity on such images becomes more apparent. The conspicuity of the infective process in the bone marrow on T2-weighted spin echo MR images also is variable; sufficient T2-weighting provided by repetition times of 2000 msec or longer and echo times of 100 to 120 msec is important in the differentiation of the inflammatory process and the marrow fat.[220]

Classically, in adults with pyogenic spondylitis, the process extends quickly from one vertebral body to an adjacent one through the intervertebral disc (Fig. 65–22). With MR imaging, irregularity of the vertebral endplates and narrowing of the intervertebral disc may be evident. On T2-weighted spin echo MR sequences, the infected disc reveals increased signal intensity with absence of the normal nu-

clear cleft (normal anatomic structure that on T2-weighted images appears as an area of signal void in the center of the lumbar discs in subjects 30 years of age or older).[218] The high signal intensity of the intervertebral disc in cases of pyogenic spondylitis is a very important diagnostic sign that is not evident in degenerative processes of the disc. Additional MR imaging findings of pyogenic spondylitis are less frequent but include epidural and paraspinal extension, vertebral collapse, and spinal deformity.

Modifications in imaging protocol can be used to accentuate the MR imaging findings in pyogenic spondylitis. Intravenous administration of gadolinium contrast agent in such cases has several advantages: enhancement of signal intensity in the vertebral body and intervertebral disc increases the conspicuity of the infectious process; epidural extension of infection, which may lead to minor abnormalities on standard MR imaging examinations, is seen to better advantage; sites of enhancement in the vertebral body, intervertebral disc, or paraspinal tissues, corresponding to regions of active infection, are better identified, leading to increased accuracy of percutaneous biopsy procedures; and the response of the infection to antibiotic therapy can be ascertained.[225] The infected marrow usually enhances diffusely after administration of gadolinium (Fig. 65–23). In some instances, this may produce a decrease rather than an increase in the contrast between normal and infected vertebral bodies[226] (Fig. 65–24). The combination of contrast-enhancement and fat suppression in cases of pyogenic spondylitis may eliminate this problem. Increased conspicuity of the enhancing infective foci relates to the suppressed signal intensity in the background fatty marrow. The use of fat suppression without intravenous administration of gadolinium agent, however, is not recommended in pyogenic spondylitis; on T1-weighted spin echo MR images, the suppressed signal intensity of the fatty marrow may become identical to that of infected marrow. Vertebral marrow involvement in cases of infection (or tumor) also may be demonstrated effectively by employing short tau (inversion time) inversion recovery (STIR) sequences.[227, 228] T1- and T2-weighted contrasts are additive on STIR images, and infective (and neoplastic) lesions in the vertebral bone marrow are of high signal intensity; in addition, they are made more obvious by fat suppression of the normal marrow. Limitations of STIR imaging include sensitivity to artifacts, especially motion artifacts, which produce problems in the assessment of the spinal cord and canal, and overestimation of the size of the lesion.[227]

The MR imaging characteristics of infective spondylitis also depend on the nature of the process (e.g., granulomatous versus pyogenic)[219] and the mechanism of vertebral contamination. In tuberculous and brucellar spondylitis (see Chapter 66), intraosseous abscesses, meningeal involvement, subligamentous spread, and paraspinal extension may be evident[218, 219] (Fig. 65–25). Spinal infections resulting from spread from neighboring tissues or organs or from direct implantation also can be studied with MR imaging, and the full extent of the infection can be determined.[218]

With regard to the differential diagnosis of the MR imaging features of vertebral osteomyelitis, other processes may produce similar abnormalities. Certain of the changes in signal intensity that occur in the vertebral bodies in association with degenerative disc disease simulate those of infective spondylitis (see Chapter 40), although high signal

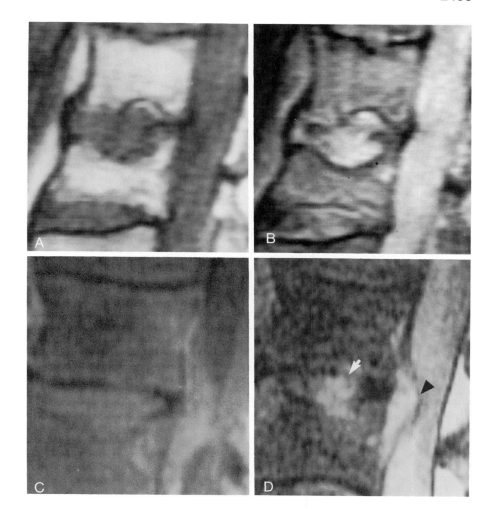

FIGURE 65–21. Spinal infection: MR imaging. Pyogenic spondylitis.

A, B Sagittal T1-weighted (TR/TE, 600/25) **(A)** and T2-weighted (TR/TE, 2000/60) **(B)** spin echo MR images reveal characteristic findings of infective spondylitis. Abnormal morphology of the endplates of the first and second lumbar vertebral bodies and of the L1-L2 intervertebral disc is evident in both images. In **B**, note the increased signal intensity in the infected disc.

C, D Sagittal proton density (TR/TE, 1000/20) **(C)** and T2-weighted (TR/TE, 1000/80) **(D)** spin echo MR images reveal abnormalities similar to those in **A** and **B**. In **D**, note the high signal intensity in the involved disc (arrow) and anterior epidural space (arrowhead).

(**A, B,** Courtesy of D. Belovich, M.D., Mechanicsburg, Pennsylvania.)

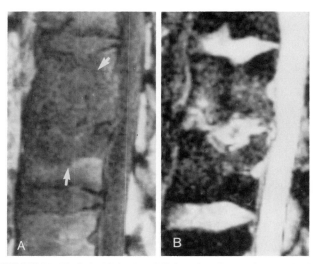

FIGURE 65–22. Spinal infection: MR imaging. Pyogenic spondylitis. This 20 year old man developed infective spondylitis after a percutaneous lumbar sympathetic block.

A Sagittal T1-weighted (TR/TE, 600/20) spin echo MR image shows regions of abnormally low signal intensity (arrows) in the second and third lumbar vertebral bodies. The signal intensity of the L2-L3 intervertebral disc also is abnormal.

B Sagittal multiplanar gradient recalled (MPGR) image (TR/TE, 500/17; flip angle, 30 degrees) reveals altered morphology at the L2-L3 spinal levels.

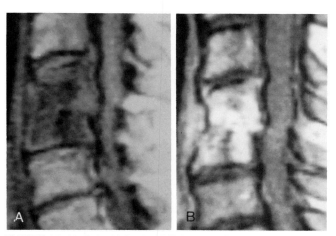

FIGURE 65–23. Spinal infection: MR imaging. Pyogenic spondylitis.

A In this 61 year old man, a sagittal T1-weighted (TR/TE, 300/20) spin echo MR image shows abnormally low signal intensity in the marrow of the fourth and fifth cervical vertebral bodies with narrowing of the intervening disc.

B A gadolinium-enhanced sagittal T1-weighted (TR/TE, 300/20) image reveals hyperintensity in the infected vertebral bodies and intervertebral disc. Similar hyperintensity is seen in the prevertebral soft tissues.

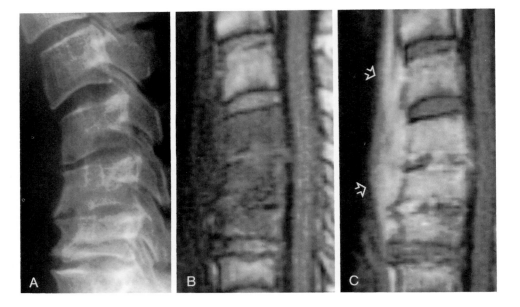

FIGURE 65–24. Spinal infection: MR imaging. Pyogenic spondylitis. This 40 year old man developed infective spondylitis after multilevel cervical discography.

A Routine radiography shows narrowing of the intervertebral discs at the C4-C5 and the C5-C6 levels. Prevertebral soft tissue swelling also was evident.

B Sagittal T1-weighted (TR/TE, 500/12) spin echo MR image reveals low signal intensity of the marrow of the fourth, fifth, and sixth cervical vertebral bodies.

C After intravenous administration of gadolinium contrast agent, a sagittal T1-weighted (TR/TE, 500/12) spin echo MR image shows hyperintensity in the prevertebral soft tissues (arrows). In comparison with the findings in **B,** the marrow involvement is less apparent.

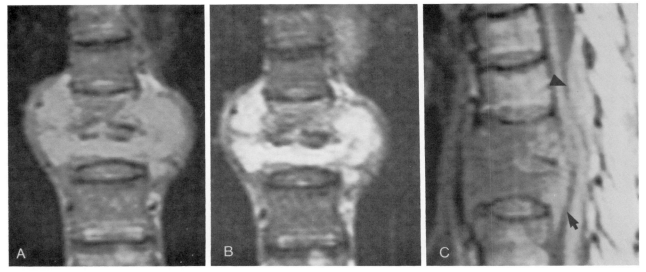

FIGURE 65–25. Spinal infection: MR imaging. Tuberculosis.

A, B Coronal proton density (TR/TE, 1800/50) **(A)** and T2-weighted (TR/TE, 1800/100) **(B)** spin echo MR images reveal spinal and paraspinal involvement in the midthoracic region. The infectious process is of higher signal intensity in **B.**

C Sagittal T1-weighted (TR/TE, 450/30) spin echo MR image in the same patient reveals tuberculous involvement of contiguous vertebral bodies with extension anteriorly. Also note anterior (arrow) and posterior (arrowhead) extradural disease.

(Courtesy of T. Mattsson, M.D., Riyadh, Saudi Arabia.)

intensity in the degenerating intervertebral disc on T2-weighted spin echo MR images is not characteristic. Also, enhancement of discal signal intensity after intravenous administration of gadolinium contrast agent is not typical of disc degeneration. MR imaging findings that are more typical of vertebral neoplasms than of vertebral infections are a normal appearing intervertebral disc, better defined vertebral endplates, pediculate involvement, changes isolated to a single vertebral body, and displacement or focal obliteration of fat planes in the adjacent soft tissues (as compared with diffuse obliteration of these planes in infection).[221] Diagnostic difficulties arise, however, in cases of (1) spinal neoplasm affecting consecutive vertebral bodies and intervertebral discs (e.g., lymphoma, plasma cell myeloma, and chordoma), (2) coexistent infection and neoplasm, (3) bizarre infections (e.g., echinococcosis), and (4) infection in which the vertebral endplates or discs are not altered.[218, 224]

Hematogenous spread of pyogenic microorganisms rarely may cause an epidural abscess in the absence of detectable bone or disc disease.[218, 229–232] *Staphylococcus aureus* is the most common cause of localized epidural infection, and the risk of such infection is increased in patients with chronic illness, underlying immunosuppression, or a history of intravenous drug abuse.[231] The thoracic spine is involved most frequently (approximately 50 per cent of cases), followed by the lumbar (35 per cent) and cervical (15 per cent) spine.[232] Spinal epidural abscesses usually can be detected on routine spin echo MR images. On T1-weighted images, an extradural mass isointense with the vertebral marrow, compressing the spinal cord or thecal sac, is seen; homogeneously increased signal intensity within the mass is apparent on T2-weighted images and, occasionally, the epidural mass is completely silhouetted by the high signal of the cerebrospinal fluid.[218, 231] Subsequent to the intravenous administration of gadolinium contrast agent, there may be homogeneous or peripheral enhancement of the epidural infection[244]; contrast-enhanced images aid in the differentiation of a necrotic liquid abscess from phlegmonous granulation tissue with embedded microabscesses.[231] The demonstration of an abscess that can be drained has clinical importance. The differentiation of an epidural abscess from other epidural masses, such as tumor and hematoma, generally can be accomplished when a combination of unenhanced and enhanced MR images is employed, although in some instances such differentiation is very difficult.

Intradural extramedullary infections (i.e., infectious leptomeningitis) can be caused by bacterial, fungal, viral, and parasitic organisms. Transmission of infection can occur either by the hematogenous route or by direct spread from infective spondylitis, cranial meningitis, or parenchymal brain or spinal cord infections.[218] MR imaging features of infectious leptomeningitis include loss of the normal spinal cord–cerebrospinal fluid interface on T1-weighted images; increased signal intensity of the infected meninges on T2-weighted images that may be obscured by the high signal intensity of the cerebrospinal fluid; and linear, nodular, or diffuse enhancement of the infected tissue on images obtained after the administration of gadolinium contrast agent. These MR imaging findings are virtually indistinguishable from those of leptomeningeal tumor spread.[218]

Intramedullary (i.e., spinal cord) infection generally results from hematogenous transmission, although extension of disease from vertebral osteomyelitis or brain and meningeal infections also may lead to spinal cord involvement. Bacterial, fungal, parasitic, or viral organisms may be responsible for such infection. With regard to bacterial infections, pyogenic or granulomatous (e.g., tuberculous) myelitis may be encountered. The MR imaging features in cases of intramedullary infection are not well documented, although nodular or diffuse swelling of the spinal cord and enhancement after administration of gadolinium contrast agent are reported.[233]

Postoperative infection of the intervertebral disc can be evaluated with MR imaging, although some overlap in MR findings occurs in postoperative patients who have discitis and those who are asymptomatic.[234, 235] On standard MR images, the most important findings of discitis are decreased signal intensity within the disc and adjacent marrow of the vertebral body on T1-weighted images and increased signal intensity in the disc (often with obliteration of the intranuclear cleft) and in the vertebral marrow on T2-weighted images. Unfortunately, some postoperative patients without discitis have similar findings, and some patients with postoperative discitis have only a portion of these findings.[234] Intravenous administration of gadolinium-based contrast agent may be useful in diagnosing postoperative disc infection more accurately. Enhancing lesions in the vertebral bone marrow on either side of the disc space, enhancement of the intervertebral disc itself, and enhancement in the posterior portion of the anulus fibrosus are among the MR imaging findings of discitis. This diagnosis is more certain when the entire triad of abnormalities is encountered.[234]

Differential Diagnosis

The radiographic hallmark of infective spondylitis is intervertebral disc space narrowing, frequently accompanied by lysis or sclerosis of adjacent vertebrae (Table 65–1). A similar radiographic pattern can be encountered in various articular disorders, such as rheumatoid arthritis, the seronegative spondyloarthropathies, calcium pyrophosphate dihydrate crystal deposition disease, alkaptonuria, and neuropathic osteoarthropathy, but in each of these disorders, clinical and additional radiographic features usually ensure accurate differential diagnosis.[82] Sarcoidosis occasionally can be associated with disc space narrowing and bone eburnation at one or more levels of the spine.

Diminution of intervertebral disc height and bony sclerosis are associated with cartilaginous node formation (Schmorl's node), which accompanies many disease processes, including traumatic, articular, and metabolic disorders.[83–85] In general, the poor definition of the subchondral bone plate is less in cases of cartilaginous nodes than in those of infection; the latter condition is characterized by "fuzzy" spiculated osseous contours. Furthermore, conventional tomography or CT scanning may define lucent intraosseous discal fragments accurately in patients with cartilaginous nodes, although an intraosseous abscess can create similar lucency. Widespread cartilaginous nodes are detected in Scheuermann's disease (juvenile kyphosis), creating an appearance that should not be confused with that of infection.

Intervertebral (osteo)chondrosis also produces intervertebral disc space narrowing and reactive sclerosis of the

TABLE 65–1. Differential Diagnosis of Some Disorders Producing Discal Narrowing

Disorder	Discovertebral Margin	Sclerosis	Vacuum Phenomena	Osteophytosis	Other Findings
Infection	Poorly defiend	Variable[1]	Rare[2]	Absent	Vertebral lysis, soft tissue mass
Intervertebral osteochondrosis	Well defined	Prominent	Present	Variable	Cartilaginous nodes
Rheumatoid arthritis	Poorly or well defined with ''erosions''	Variable	Absent	Absent or mild	Apophyseal joint abnormalities, subluxation
Calcium pyrophosphate dihydrate crystal deposition disease	Poorly or well defined	Prominent	Variable	Variable	Fragmentation, subluxation
Neuropathic osteoarthropathy	Well defined	Prominent	Variable	Prominent	Fragmentation, subluxation, disorganization
Trauma	Well defined	Prominent	Variable	Variable	Fracture, soft tissue mass
Sarcoidosis	Poorly or well defined	Variable, may be prominent	Absent	Absent	Soft tissue mass

[1]Usually evident in pyogenic infections and in tuberculosis in the black patient.

[2]Vacuum phenomena initially may be evident when intervertebral osteochondrosis also is present or, rarely, when a gas-forming microorganism is responsible for the infection.

neighboring bone (see Chapter 40). The resulting radiographic picture can resemble that of infective spondylitis. In intervertebral (osteo)chondrosis, the vertebral endplates usually are smooth and well defined, although focal defects can represent sites of intravertebral discal displacement (cartilaginous nodes). Of particular diagnostic significance is the presence of one or more radiolucent collections overlying the intervertebral disc in intervertebral (osteo)chondrosis (Fig. 65–26). These vacuum phenomena represent gaseous collections (nitrogen) within the nucleus pulposus and are a reliable sign of discal degeneration. They are exceedingly rare in cases of discal infection, and their detection makes the diagnosis of infection very unlikely. Occasionally, however, infection that is initiated in a site of previously existing discal degeneration can be associated with a vacuum phenomenon. Usually, in these cases, the dissemination of infection throughout the intervertebral disc leads to disappearance of the gaseous collections (Fig. 65–27). Additionally, in rare occasions, infections with gas-forming bacteria may lead to a vacuum phenomenon–like appearance.[102]

Idiopathic hemispherical (segmental) sclerosis (Fig. 65–28) leads to a well-defined radiodense area in a vertebral body that borders on an intervertebral disc (see Chapter 40). The adjacent intervertebral disc and vertebral body usually are normal. Involvement of the lumbar spine is characteristic.

In general, primary or metastatic tumor in the spine does not lead to significant loss of intervertebral disc space; the combination of widespread lysis or sclerosis of a vertebral body and an intact adjacent intervertebral disc is much more characteristic of tumor than of infection. Certain neoplasms such as plasma cell myeloma, chordoma, and even skeletal metastasis can extend across or around the intervertebral disc to involve the neighboring vertebra, however. Furthermore, neoplastic disruption of the subchondral bone can produce osseous weakening, allowing intraosseous discal displacement.[86] In these latter cases, some degree of disc space narrowing may accompany the bony destruction, producing a radiographic picture that simulates that of infection.

In patients with infective spondylitis involving primarily the posterior elements, bony destruction and production can simulate the findings of tumor. This is especially true when significant pediculate involvement is present.

Paraspinal masses occur in infective spondylitis and traumatic and neoplastic disorders. Infection is likely if such masses contain gas. Intervertebral disc space ossification leading to bridging of vertebral bodies is encountered as a sequela of infective spondylitis. It also may be seen in congenital disorders and after surgery or trauma.

The accurate radiographic differentiation of pyogenic infective spondylitis from granulomatous infections (tuberculosis and fungal disorders) can be difficult. Rapid loss of intervertebral disc height, extensive sclerosis, and the absence of calcified paraspinal masses are findings that are more typical of pyogenic infection, although one or more of these signs can be encountered in some cases of tuberculous or fungal spondylitis (Fig. 65–29).

SACROILIAC JOINT INFECTIONS

Routes of Contamination

The sacroiliac joint may become infected by the hematogenous route, by contamination from a contiguous suppurative focus, by direct implantation, or after surgery (Fig. 65–30). In many instances, the exact mechanism leading to infective arthritis at this site is not clear.[87–91]

Although a hematogenous route appears likely in cases of septic sacroiliac joint disease occurring in the clinical setting of preexisting infection in a distant site (e.g., skin, pharynx) or in intravenous drug addicts, in most patients it is not certain whether the primary focus is in the adjacent osseous structures or in the joint itself.[87] The subchondral circulation of the ilium is slow, resembling the situation in the metaphysis of long bones in children. Thus, hematogenous implantation at this site is to be expected; the ilium is the most frequently infected flat bone of the body.[92, 93] From this location, extension of infection into the sacroiliac or hip joint can occur. Similarly, the association of sacroiliac joint infection with suppurative conditions of the pelvis or

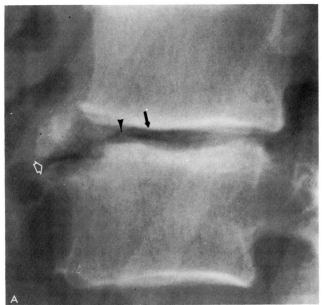

FIGURE 65–26. Intervertebral osteochondrosis.

A With degeneration of the intervertebral disc, narrowing of the discal space and reactive bone formation can be seen. Note the well-defined appearance of the eburnated bone (solid arrow) and the presence of a vacuum phenomenon (arrowhead). The lucent zone can be traced anteriorly beneath a separated vertebral ossicle (open arrow), confirming that a limbus vertebra is related to anterolateral displacement of discal material.

B, C In this patient with back pain, an initial radiograph **(B)** reveals obvious intervertebral osteochondrosis at the L4-L5 vertebral level (arrow), characterized by disc space narrowing, a vacuum phenomenon, and well-defined sclerotic vertebral margins. The changes at the L3-L4 vertebral level (arrowhead) are more difficult to interpret. The vertebral bodies are irregular, and a vacuum phenomenon is not definite. On a second radiograph exposed during back extension **(C),** vacuum phenomena now are apparent at both vertebral levels, indicating that infection is highly unlikely. A subsequent gallium scan (not shown) failed to reveal augmented spinal activity and provided further documentation that infection is not present.

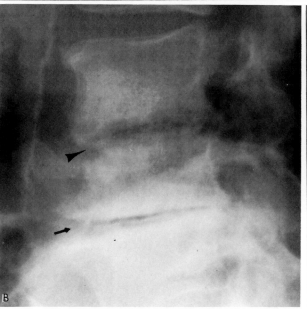

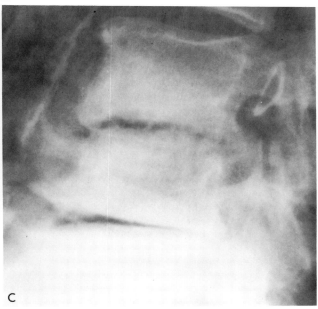

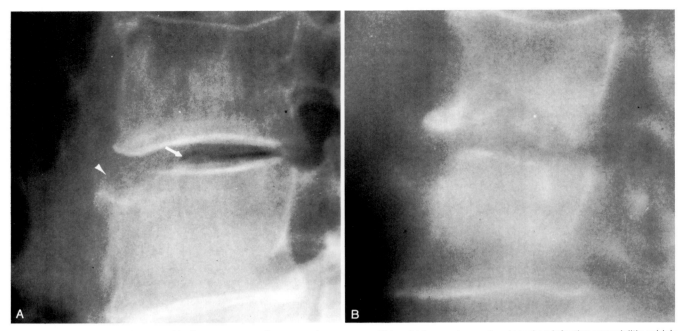

FIGURE 65–27. Spinal infection with disappearance of vacuum phenomenon. This middle-aged man developed an infective spondylitis, which on histologic and laboratory examination was found to be related to brucellosis.

A An initial radiograph outlines intervertebral disc space narrowing, erosion of the anterosuperior aspect of the vertebral body (arrowhead), bony proliferation, and a vacuum phenomenon (arrow). Although the appearance is reminiscent of that in intervertebral (osteo)chondrosis with cartilaginous node formation, the poorly defined nature of the destruction is more consistent with infection.

B Two weeks later, a midline lateral tomogram reveals the progressive nature of the osseous destruction and the disappearance of the vacuum phenomenon. At this time, the classic radiographic features of an infection are evident. The rapidity with which the abnormalities progressed in this case is consistent with brucellosis.

(Courtesy of J. Usselman, M.D., and V. Vint, M.D., LaJolla, California.)

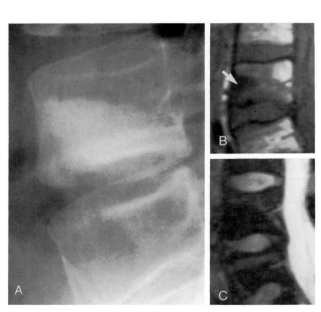

FIGURE 65–28. Idiopathic hemispheric (segmental) sclerosis. In this 50 year old woman, an initial radiograph **(A)** shows well-defined sclerosis involving the inferior portion of the fourth lumbar vertebral body and extending to a normal L4-L5 intervertebral disc. A sagittal T1-weighted (TR/TE, 600/20) MR image **(B)** reveals low signal intensity in the corresponding portion of the vertebral body (arrow). With multiplanar gradient recalled (MPGR) imaging (TR/TE, 500/25; flip angle, 25 degrees) **(C)**, the abnormal vertebral region is not well shown. The L4-L5 intervertebral disc appears normal.

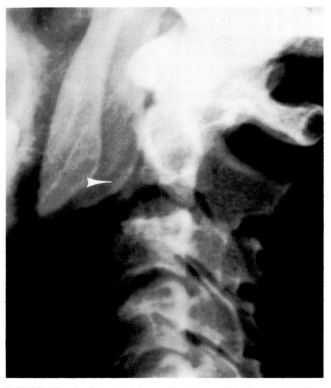

FIGURE 65–29. Spinal infection due to coccidioidomycosis. This man, living in Arizona, developed progressive neck pain. A lytic lesion of the second cervical vertebral body (arrowhead) with soft tissue swelling is evident. The absence of sclerosis and the preservation of adjacent intervertebral disc height are not uncommon in fungal or tuberculous spondylitis.

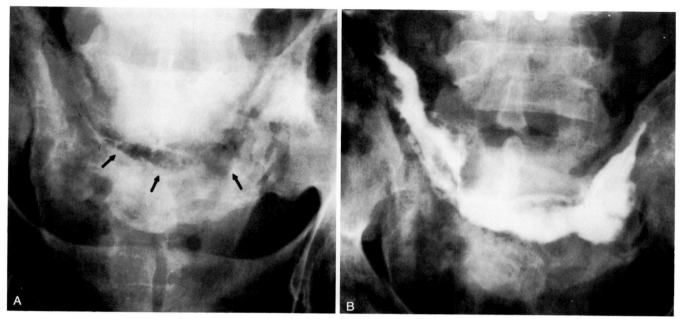

FIGURE 65–30. Sacroiliac joint and sacral infection: Spread from a contiguous contaminated source. This 28 year old paralyzed man developed soft tissue infection with a sinus tract leading to the sacrum and sacroiliac joint.
A Note irregular channel-like destruction of the sacrum (arrows), with articular space widening and poorly defined bone about the left sacroiliac joint. The fifth lumbar vertebra also is affected.
B Sinogram confirms the communication of the tract with the sacrum and sacroiliac joint.

previous pelvic surgical procedures may indicate the importance of hematogenous spread via the paravertebral venous system of Batson, although, once again, the initial site of contamination (osseous or synovial) is difficult to document. The observation of a destructive process in both the iliac and the sacral aspects of the joint in the early phases of infection suggests that direct hematogenous intra-articular contamination may be incriminated in many patients.[87]

Contamination of the sacroiliac joint or neighboring bone can occur from an adjacent infection. Pelvic abscesses can disrupt the anterior articular capsule or the periosteum and cortex of the ilium or sacrum.[114, 153] Thus, vaginal, uterine, ovarian, bladder, and intestinal processes can lead to iliac or sacral osteomyelitis and sacroiliac joint suppuration by contiguous contamination (as well as by hematogenous spread via Batson's plexus).[94, 95] Trauma can aggravate this situation by disrupting viscera, soft tissue, and osseous and articular structures. Pressure sores related to prolonged immobilization are not infrequent in the sacral region and can lead to subsequent articular and osseous infection (Fig. 65–30). Abscesses following intragluteal injection of medication can lead to osteomyelitis and sacroiliac joint septic arthritis. Even infective conditions of the spine subsequently can spread beneath the spinal ligaments into the pelvis and sacroiliac articulations.[96]

Direct implantation of organisms following diagnostic or surgical procedures represents another, although uncommon, source of sacroiliac joint infection. Needle aspiration of the joint or closed or open biopsy of the adjacent bone can be complicated by infection.

Clinical Abnormalities

Pyogenic infection of the sacroiliac joint can lead to severe clinical manifestations, especially in children and adolescents.[104, 154–158, 179, 236] Unilateral alterations predominate, although cases of bilateral sacroiliac joint involvement in infection are described.[157] Fever, local pain and tenderness, and a limp can be evident. Radiation of pain to the buttock, in a sciatic distribution, and even to the abdomen can be recorded. Widespread discomfort is not infrequent, perhaps reflecting the proclivity of suppurative sacroiliac joint disease to spread beyond the confines of the joint. The discharged purulent material may follow the iliac fossa, track along the tendon of the iliopsoas muscle to the hip and toward the thigh, follow the tendons of the short external rotators to the buttock, ascend into the lumbar region or along the crest of the ilium, or penetrate the pelvic floor to be discharged through the vagina or rectum.[87] Delay in accurate diagnosis in cases of septic sacroiliitis is frequent, increasing the frequency of such extra-articular contamination.

Elevation of the erythrocyte sedimentation rate and leukocytosis are common but variable laboratory features. The identification of the causative organisms from blood culture or joint aspiration can be difficult.[105] Staphylococci, streptococci, pneumococci, Proteus, Klebsiella, Pseudomonas, Brucella, mycobacteria, and fungi can be implicated. Gram-negative bacterial agents are especially common in pyogenic arthritis of the sacroiliac joint in intravenous drug abusers.

Radiographic-Pathologic Correlation

In almost all cases of sacroiliac joint infection, a unilateral distribution is encountered. In pyogenic arthritis, radiographic findings generally occur in 2 or 3 weeks, characterized by blurring and indistinctness of the subchondral osseous line and narrowing or widening of the interosseous space. Although these two alterations frequently coexist,

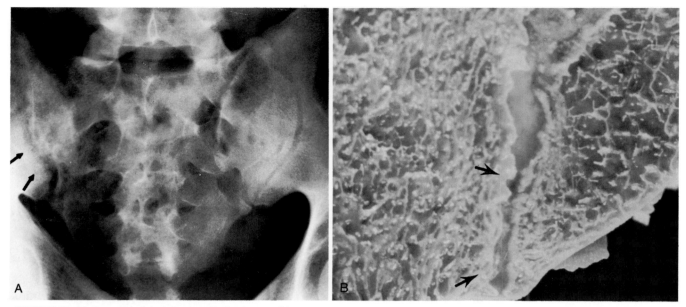

FIGURE 65–31. Sacroiliac joint infection: Early abnormalities.
  A A 35 year old male heroin addict developed Pseudomonas osteomyelitis and septic arthritis. The radiograph reveals the changes in the right sacroiliac joint, consisting of subchondral osseous erosion, poorly defined articular margins, and widening of the joint space (arrows).
  B In the coronal section of an infected sacroiliac joint in a cadaver, observe the erosions, which predominate in the ilium (arrows).

their time of appearance is dictated by the initial site of contamination: If osteomyelitis precedes septic arthritis, bony abnormalities may antedate articular changes; if the joint is affected initially, cartilaginous and osseous alterations may coexist. In both situations, the most extensive findings commonly are evident about the inferoanterior aspect of the joint. Progressive changes are accompanied by erosions, which usually are predominant in the lower ilium (Fig. 65–31). Surrounding condensation of bone is variable in frequency and degree, and it is influenced by the type and virulence of the infecting microorganisms. With treatment, intra-articular osseous fusion may be encountered,[238] ultimately leading to complete bridging of the interosseous space and disappearance of bone eburnation (Fig. 65–32).

Other Diagnostic Techniques

Conventional tomography and radionuclide examination are two important diagnostic methods that can be employed in patients with suspected sacroiliac joint infection. Tomograms may detect early erosive alterations when initial radiographs are normal; scintigraphy, using technetium phosphate or gallium agents, or both, may outline increased accumulation of radionuclide at a time when findings on routine radiographs and conventional tomograms are unimpressive.[87, 90, 159–161, 180, 237] Abnormal unilateral uptake of isotope in the sacroiliac joint indicates infection until proved otherwise.[111] Scintigraphic improvement mirrors the clinical features of resolution.

Although CT has been advocated as a technique that is valuable in the early diagnosis of septic sacroiliitis (Fig. 65–33), revealing cartilaginous and bony destruction,[162] as well as intraosseous gas,[163] it is better applied to the detection of soft tissue extension of the infection[163–167, 181] (Figs.

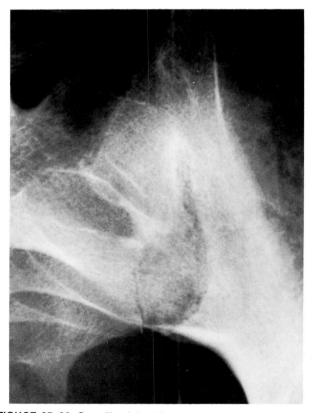

FIGURE 65–32. Sacroiliac joint infection: Later abnormalities. This 28 year heroin addict had severe back pain. Pseudomonas was cultured from a bone biopsy specimen. Note the articular space narrowing and osseous sclerosis about the left sacroiliac joint, especially in the ilium. Osseous fusion ultimately can result from pyogenic septic arthritis.

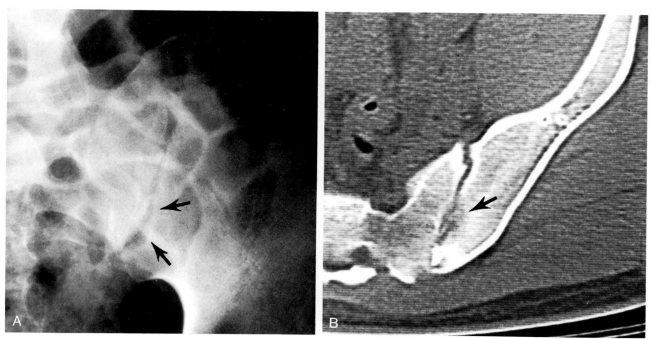

FIGURE 65–33. Sacroiliac joint infection: CT scanning. An infected left sacroiliac joint in this 32 year old man has led to subtle radiographic abnormalities **(A)** consisting of osteopenia and superficial erosion of bone (arrows). A transaxial CT scan **(B)** at the level of the lower part of the articulation shows the bone destruction to better advantage (arrow).

65–34 and 65–35) and as an aid to aspiration and biopsy techniques. The latter procedures can be difficult without CT guidance.[168] Although a report has indicated that, experimentally, the administration of a perfluorocarbon macro-

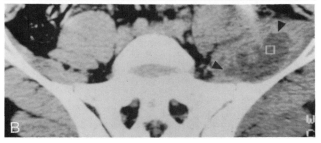

FIGURE 65–34. Sacroiliac joint infection: CT scanning. In this 20 year old intravenous drug abuser, CT scans with bone **(A)** and soft tissue **(B)** windows show involvement of the left sacroiliac joint (arrow) and an abscess (arrowheads) in the iliacus muscle. (Courtesy of J. Hodler, M.D., Zurich, Switzerland.)

phage-labeling contrast agent, perfluoroctylbromide, may increase the specificity of CT for infection,[182] further investigation in this area is required.

The precise value of MR imaging in the assessment of septic sacroiliitis is not clear (Figs. 65–36 to 65–38). Reported findings are those of marrow edema in the sacrum and ilium, irregularity of the subchondral bone on either side of the joint space, joint fluid, muscle edema, and fluid-filled channels, sinus tracts, and fistulae.[239, 240] Intravenous administration of gadolinium contrast agent may be used to accentuate the MR imaging abnormalities and can be employed to delineate adjacent soft tissue involvement.[247]

Differential Diagnosis

It is the unilateral nature of infective sacroiliac joint disease that is its most useful diagnostic feature. Bilateral symmetric or asymmetric articular changes are characteristic of ankylosing spondylitis, psoriasis, Reiter's syndrome, osteitis condensans ilii, and hyperparathyroidism (Fig. 65–39). Unilateral changes can be encountered in rheumatoid arthritis, gout, Reiter's syndrome, and psoriasis. They also may appear on the paralyzed side in hemiplegic patients (due to chondral atrophy) and on the contralateral side in patients with osteoarthritis of the hip. Unilateral sacroiliac joint disease characterized by blurring or poor definition of subchondral bone and loss of joint space is virtually diagnostic of infection.

INFECTION AT OTHER AXIAL SITES

Infection can involve almost any additional site in the axial skeleton. As elsewhere, infection can result from hematogenous spread, spread from a contiguous source, and direct or postsurgical contamination. In the intravenous

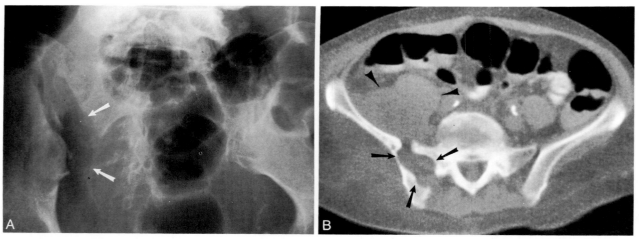

FIGURE 65–35. Sacroiliac joint infection: CT scanning. Although the plain film shows the destruction of ilium and sacrum (arrows) that accompanies this infection, a transaxial CT scan further documents this destruction (arrows) and reveals a large soft tissue mass (arrow-heads).

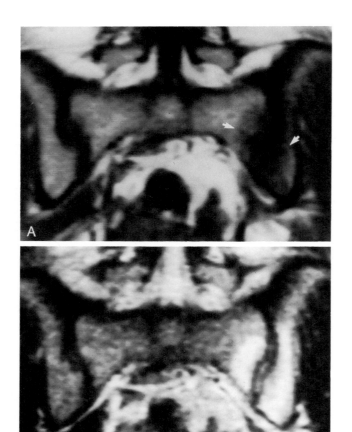

FIGURE 65–36. Sacroiliac joint infection: MR imaging. In this 15 year old patient with hematogenous spread of infection to the left sacroiliac joint, routine radiographs (not shown) were normal.

A Coronal T1-weighted (TR/TE, 600/20) MR image reveals low signal intensity in the marrow (arrows) about the left sacroiliac joint.

B Coronal T2-weighted (TR/TE, 2000/70) MR image shows high signal intensity in the infected marrow.

(Courtesy of H.S. Kang, M.D., Seoul, Korea.)

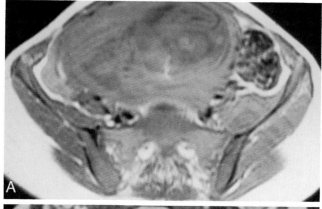
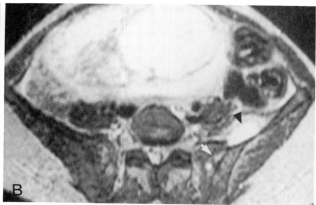
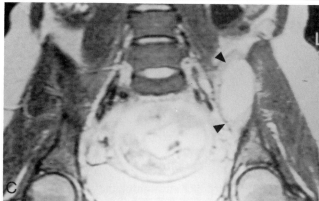

FIGURE 65–37. Sacroiliac joint infection: MR imaging. This 19 year old pregnant woman developed septic arthritis of the left sacroiliac joint.

A, B Transaxial T1-weighted (TR/TE, 800/20) **(A)** and T2-weighted (TR/TE, 3000/70) **(B)** spin echo MR images document the pregnancy and the septic arthritis of the left sacroiliac joint. In **B,** observe the high signal intensity about the infected joint (arrow) and within the anterior tissues (arrowhead).

C The coronal T2-weighted (TR/TE, 2000/70) spin echo MR image reveals the extent of the soft tissue involvement (arrowheads). This pattern of soft tissue extension, including fluid collections posterior to the iliopsoas muscle, is very typical of sacroiliac joint infections.

FIGURE 65–38. Sacroiliac joint infection: MR imaging. This 48 year old woman developed a staphylococcal infection of the left sacroiliac joint.

A Transaxial T1-weighted (TR/TE, 650/11) spin echo MR image does not show well the infectious process in the sacrum and ilium owing to the similar signal intensity characteristics of the inflammatory response and the hematopoietic bone marrow. The soft tissue extension of infection also is not very evident.

B Transaxial T2-weighted (TR/TE, 6000/102) fast spin echo MR image (echo train, 4) reveals high signal intensity in the sacrum and ilium as well as in the anterior and posterior soft tissues and musculature (arrows).

C Transaxial T1-weighted (TR/TE, 500/11) spin echo MR image obtained with fat saturation technique (ChemSat) after the intravenous injection of gadolinium contrast agent reveals the inflammatory reaction with high signal intensity in the bone and about anterior and posterior abscesses. Note the low signal intensity of the fluid in the joint and in the soft tissues and musculature.

(Courtesy of M. Schweitzer, M.D., Philadelphia, Pennsylvania.)

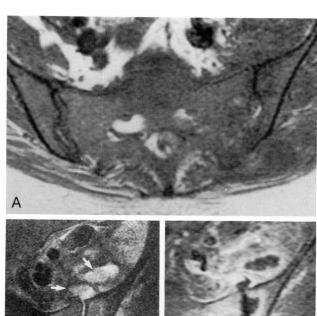
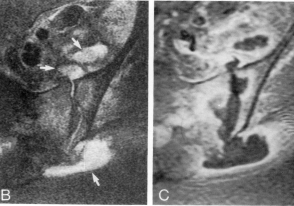

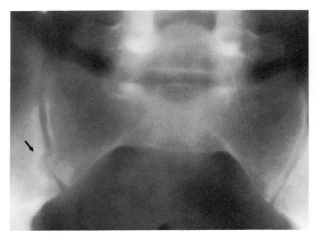

FIGURE 65–39. Reiter's syndrome simulating infection. Conventional tomography indicates an iliac erosion with surrounding sclerosis on the right side (arrow) and superficial osseous irregularity about the left sacroiliac joint. Although the sacroiliac joint alterations are asymmetric, the fact that they appear to be bilateral militates against the diagnosis of infection.

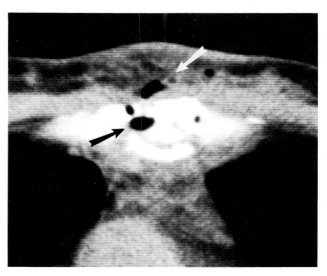

FIGURE 65–41. Sternal infection. This 47 year old man developed group B streptococcal septicemia resulting in infections in the hip, spine, and sternum. In a transaxial image, CT shows a destroyed sternum and an anterior soft tissue mass, both containing gas (arrows), and mediastinal adenopathy. Mediastinitis was confirmed at surgery.

drug abuser, osteomyelitis and septic arthritis of the sternoclavicular and acromioclavicular joints in addition to the spine and sacroiliac joint can be evident[97] (Fig. 65–40). After urologic procedures, osteomyelitis of the symphysis pubis may be difficult to differentiate from osteitis pubis. Infection of the sternum and manubriosternal joint can result from direct hematogenous inoculation (Fig. 65–41) or secondary contamination due to local injury, surgery, or diagnostic or therapeutic procedure (subclavian vein catheterization).[98–101, 109, 185] In all cases, typical clinical and radiologic features of osteomyelitis and septic arthritis usually are apparent, allowing differentiation from other conditions.[110] In some sites, such as the sternoclavicular joint, abscess formation and inflammation in nearby tissues are common, and these complications are well studied by CT or MR imaging[241–243, 245, 246] (Fig. 65–41).

SUMMARY

The routes of contamination of the spine, the sacroiliac joint, and other axial skeletal sites are identical to those of the appendicular skeleton. In the spine, early loss of intervertebral disc space is characteristic of pyogenic infection and is associated with lysis and sclerosis of neighboring bone. These findings can simulate those of other disorders, such as rheumatoid arthritis, intervertebral (osteo)chondrosis, and conditions complicated by cartilaginous node formation. Sacroiliac joint infection typically is unilateral in distribution, a feature that allows differentiation from many other articular processes. Additional locations in the axial skeleton not uncommonly are infected in intravenous drug abusers and in patients after trauma, surgery, or diagnostic or therapeutic procedures.

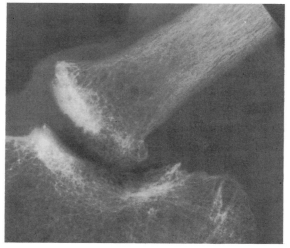

FIGURE 65–40. Sternoclavicular joint infection. A coronal section through an infected sternoclavicular articulation reveals osseous destruction and reactive eburnation of both the clavicle and the sternum.

References

1. Schmorl G, Junghanns H: The Human Spine in Health and Disease. Translated by EF Besemann. 2nd Ed. New York, Grune & Stratton, 1971, p 307.
2. Hodgson AR: Infectious disease of the spine. *In* RH Rothman, FA Simeone (Eds): The Spine. Philadelphia, WB Saunders Co, 1975, p 567.
3. Batson OV: The function of the vertebral veins and their role in the spread of metastases. Ann Surg *112:*138, 1940.
4. Batson OV: The vertebral vein system. AJR *78:*195, 1957.
5. Harris RS, Jones DM: The arterial supply to the adult cervical vertebral bodies. J Bone Joint Surg [Br] *38:*922, 1956.
6. Wilensky AO: Osteomyelitis of the vertebrae. Ann Surg *89:*561, 1929.
7. Willis TA: Nutrient arteries of the vertebral bodies. J Bone Joint Surg [Am] *31:*538, 1949.
8. Ferguson WR: Some observations on the circulation in foetal and infant spines. J Bone Joint Surg [Am] *32:*640, 1950.
9. Wiley AM, Trueta J: The vascular anatomy of the spine and its relationship to pyogenic vertebral osteomyelitis. J Bone Joint Surg [Br] *41:*796, 1959.
10. Carson HW: Acute osteomyelitis of the spine. Br J Surg *18:*400, 1930.
11. Turner P: Acute infective osteomyelitis of the spine. Br J Surg *26:*71, 1938.
12. Henriques CQ: Osteomyelitis as a complication in urology with special reference to the paravertebral venous plexus. Br J Surg *46:*19, 1958.
13. Henson SW Jr, Coventry MB: Osteomyelitis of the vertebrae as a result of infection of the urinary tract. Surg Gynecol Obstet *102:*207, 1956.
14. Leigh TF, Kelly RP, Weens HS: Spinal osteomyelitis associated with urinary tract infections. Radiology *65:*334, 1955.

15. Liming RW, Youngs FJ: Metastatic vertebral osteomyelitis following prostatic surgery. Radiology 67:92, 1956.
16. De Feo E: Osteomyelitis of the spine following prostatic surgery. Radiology 62:396, 1954.
17. Alderman EJ, Duff J: Osteomyelitis of cervical vertebrae as a complication of urinary tract disease. JAMA 148:283, 1952.
18. O'Leary JM, Lipscomb PR, Dixon CF: Enteric fistula associated with osteomyelitis of the hip and spinal column. Ann Surg 140:897, 1954.
19. Lame EL: Vertebral osteomyelitis following operation on the urinary tract or sigmoid. AJR 75:938, 1956.
20. Sherman M, Schneider GT: Vertebral osteomyelitis complicating postabortal and postpartum infection. South Med J 48:333, 1955.
21. Coman DR, deLong RP: The role of the vertebral venous system in the metastasis of cancer to the spinal column. Cancer 4:610, 1951.
22. Collis JL: The aetiology of cerebral abscess as a complication of thoracic disease. J Thorac Surg 13:445, 1944.
23. Barrington FJF, Wright HD: Bacteriaemia following operations on the urethra. J Pathol Bacteriol 33:871, 1930.
24. Coventry MB, Ghormley RK, Kernohan JW: The intervertebral disc: Its microscopic anatomy and pathology. J Bone Joint Surg [Am] 27:105, 1945.
25. Stauffer RN: Pyogenic vertebral osteomyelitis. Orthop Clin North Am 6:1015, 1975.
26. Alexander CJ: The aetiology of juvenile spondylarthritis (discitis). Clin Radiol 21:178, 1970.
27. Moes CAF: Spondylarthritis in childhood. AJR 91:578, 1964.
28. Saenger EL: Spondylarthritis in children. AJR 64:20, 1950.
29. Boston HC Jr, Bianco AJ Jr, Rhodes KH: Disc space infections in children. Orthop Clin North Am 6:953, 1975.
30. Lascari AD, Graham MH, MacQueen JC: Intervertebral disk infection in children. J Pediatr 70:751, 1967.
31. Milone FP, Bianco AJ Jr, Ivins JC: Infections of the intervertebral disk in children. JAMA 181:1029, 1962.
32. Spiegel PG, Kengla KW, Isaacson AS, et al: Intervertebral disc-space inflammation in children. J Bone Joint Surg [Am] 54:284, 1972.
33. Smith RF, Taylor TKF: Inflammatory lesions of intervertebral discs in children. J Bone Joint Surg [Am] 49:1508, 1967.
34. Dupont A, Andersen H: Nonspecific spondylitis in childhood. Acta Paediatr 45:361, 1956.
35. Jamison RC, Heimlich EM, Miethke JC, et al: Non-specific spondylitis of infants and children. Radiology 77:355, 1961.
36. Bonfiglio M, Lange TA, Kim YM: Pyogenic vertebral osteomyelitis. Disk space infections. Clin Orthop 96:234, 1973.
37. Wenger DR, Bobechko WP, Gilday DL: The spectrum of intervertebral disc-space infection in children. J Bone Joint Surg [Am] 60:100, 1978.
38. Kemp HBS, Jackson JW, Jeremiah JD, et al: Pyogenic infections occurring primarily in intervertebral discs. J Bone Joint Surg [Br] 55:698, 1973.
39. Smith NR: The intervertebral discs. Br J Surg 18:358, 1931.
40. Gordon EJ: Infection of disc space secondary to fistula from pelvic abscess. South Med J 70:114, 1977.
41. Buetti VC, Lüdi H: Spondylitis nach Paravertebralanästhesie. Helv Chir Acta 25:261, 1958.
42. Rohr H: Die angeborenen knöcherenen Fehlbildungen in der Occipito-Cervikal-Gegend und ihre Behandlung. Zbl Neurochir 16:276, 1956.
43. McLaurin RL: Spinal suppuration. Clin Neurosurg 14:314, 1966.
44. Keon-Cohen BT: Epidural abscess simulating disc hernia. J Bone Joint Surg [Br] 50:128, 1968.
45. Sullivan CR, Bickel WH, Svien HJ: Infection of the vertebral interspaces after operations on intervertebral disks. JAMA 166:1973, 1958.
46. Stern WE, Balch RE: Surgical aspects of nonspecific inflammatory and suppurative disease of the vertebral column. Am J Surg 112:314, 1966.
47. Goldman AB, Freiberger RH: Localized infectious and neuropathic diseases. Semin Roentgenol 14:19, 1979.
48. Ross PM, Fleming JL: Vertebral body osteomyelitis. Spectrum and natural history. A retrospective analysis of 37 cases. Clin Orthop 118:190, 1976.
49. Musher DM, Thorsteinsson SB, Minuth JN, et al: Vertebral osteomyelitis. Still a diagnostic pitfall. Arch Intern Med 136:105, 1976.
50. Malawski SK: Pyogenic infection of the spine. Int Orthop (SICOT) 1:125, 1977.
51. Collert S: Osteomyelitis of the spine. Acta Orthop Scand 48:283, 1977.
52. Chari PR: Haematogenous pyogenic osteomyelitis of the spine: A study of 17 cases. Aust N Z J Surg 42:381, 1973.
53. Bolivar R, Kohl S, Pickering LK: Vertebral osteomyelitis in children: Report of four cases. Pediatrics 62:549, 1978.
54. Griffiths HED, Jones DM: Pyogenic infection of the spine. A review of twenty-eight cases. J Bone Joint Surg [Br] 53:383, 1971.
55. Berant M, Shrem M: Vertebral osteomyelitis in a young infant. Clin Pediatr 13:677, 1974.
56. Fredrickson B, Yuan H, Olans R: Management and outcome of pyogenic vertebral osteomyelitis. Clin Orthop 131:160, 1978.
57. Wedge JH, Oryschak AF, Robertson DE, et al: Atypical manifestations of spinal infections. Clin Orthop 123:155, 1977.
58. Partio E, Hatanpaa S, Rokkanen P: Pyogenic spondylitis. Acta Orthop Scand 49:165, 1978.
59. Hahn O: In Wilensky AO: Osteomyelitis of the vertebrae. Ann Surg 89:561, 1929.
60. Kulowski J: Pyogenic osteomyelitis of the spine. An analysis and discussion of 102 cases. J Bone Joint Surg 18:343, 1936.
61. Bremner AE, Neligan GA: Benign form of acute osteitis of the spine in young children. Br Med J 1:856, 1953.
62. Finch PG: Staphylococcal osteomyelitis of the spine in a baby aged three weeks. Lancet 2:134, 1947.
63. Epremian BE, Perez LA: Imaging strategy in osteomyelitis. Clin Nucl Med 2:218, 1977.
64. Garcia A Jr, Grantham SA: Haematogenous pyogenic vertebral osteomyelitis. J Bone Joint Surg [Am] 42:429, 1960.
65. Shehadi WH: Primary pyogenic osteomyelitis of the articular processes of the vertebra. J Bone Joint Surg 21:969, 1939.
66. Leach RE, Goldstein H, Younger D: Osteomyelitis of the odontoid process. J Bone Joint Surg [Am] 49:369, 1967.
67. Selvaggi G: Wirbelsäulenosteomyelitis. Zentr Org Ges Chir 63:622, 1933.
68. Chinaglia A: Die akute Osteomyelitis der Wirbelsäule. Zentr Org Ges Chir 83:342, 1937.
69. Richards AJ: Non-tuberculous pyogenic osteomyelitis of the spine. J Can Assoc Radiol 11:45, 1960.
70. Allen EH, Cosgrove D, Millard FJC: The radiological changes in infections of the spine and their diagnostic value. Clin Radiol 29:31, 1978.
71. Jacobs P: Osteo-articular tuberculosis in coloured immigrants: A radiological study. Clin Radiol 15:59, 1964.
72. Waisbren BA: Pyogenic osteomyelitis and arthritis of the spine treated with combinations of antibiotics and gamma globulin. J Bone Joint Surg [Am] 42:414, 1960.
73. Dini P: Le spondiliti infettiose. Arch Putti Chir Organi Mov 16:117, 1962.
74. Weber R: Considérations sur l'ostéomyélite vértébrale. Rev Chir Orthop 51:273, 1965.
75. Mineiro JD: Coluna vertebral humana: Alguns aspectos da sua estrutura e vascularizacao. Lisboa, Dissertacao de Doutoramento, 1965.
76. Fischer GW, Popich GA, Sullivan DE, et al: Diskitis: A prospective diagnostic analysis. Pediatrics 62:543, 1978.
77. Rocco HD, Eyring EJ: Intervertebral disk infections in children. Am J Dis Child 123:448, 1972.
78. Doyle JR: Narrowing of the intervertebral disc space in children. J Bone Joint Surg 42:1191, 1960.
79. Mathews SS, Wiltse LL, Karbelnig MJ: A destructive lesion involving the intervertebral disc in children. Clin Orthop 9:162, 1957.
80. Ghormley RK, Bickel WH, Dickson DD: A study of acute infectious lesions of the intervertebral disks. South Med J 33:347, 1940.
81. Norris S, Ehrlich MG, Keim DE, et al: Early diagnosis of disk-space infection using Gallium-67. J Nucl Med 19:384, 1978.
82. Patton JT: Differential diagnosis of inflammatory spondylitis. Skel Radiol 1:77, 1976.
83. Resnick D, Niwayama G: Intravertebral disk herniations: Cartilaginous (Schmorl's) nodes. Radiology 126:57, 1978.
84. Williams JL, Moller GA, O'Rourke TL: Pseudoinfections of the intervertebral disk and adjacent vertebrae. AJR 103:611, 1968.
85. Sauser R, Goldman AB, Kaye JJ: Discogenic vertebral sclerosis. J Can Assoc Radiol 29:44, 1978.
86. Resnick D, Niwayama G: Intervertebral disc abnormalities associated with vertebral metastasis: Observations in patients and cadavers with prostate cancer. Invest Radiol 13:182, 1978.
87. Coy JT III, Wolf CR, Brower TD, et al: Pyogenic arthritis of the sacro-iliac joint. Long term follow-up. J Bone Joint Surg [Am] 58:845, 1976.
88. Avila L Jr: Primary pyogenic infection of the sacroiliac articulation. A new approach to the joint. Report of 7 cases. J Bone Joint Surg 23:922, 1941.
89. L'Episcopo JB: Suppurative arthritis of the sacroiliac joint. Ann Surg 104:289, 1936.
90. Ailsby RL, Staheli LT: Pyogenic infections of the sacroiliac joint in children. Radioisotope bone scanning as a diagnostic tool. Clin Orthop 100:96, 1974.
91. Delbarre F, Rondier J, Delrieu F, et al: Pyogenic infection of the sacro-iliac joint. Report of thirteen cases. J Bone Joint Surg [Am] 57:819, 1975.
92. Young F: Acute osteomyelitis of the ilium. Surg Gynecol Obstet 58:986, 1934.
93. Morgan A, Yates AK: The diagnosis of acute osteomyelitis of the pelvis. Postgrad Med J 42:74, 1966.
94. Ghahremani GG: Osteomyelitis of the ilium in patients with Crohn's disease. AJR 118:364, 1973.
95. Goldstein MJ, Nasr K, Singer HC, et al: Osteomyelitis complicating regional enteritis. Gut 10:264, 1969.
96. Oppenheimer A: Paravertebral abscesses associated with Strumpell-Marie disease. J Bone Joint Surg 25:90, 1943.
97. Goldin RH, Chow A, Edwards JE Jr, et al: Sternoarticular septic arthritis in heroin users. N Engl J Med 289:616, 1973.
98. Biesecker GL, Aaron BL, Mullen JT: Primary sternal osteomyelitis. Chest 63:236, 1973.
99. Wray TM, Bryant RE, Killen DA: Sternal osteomyelitis and costochondritis after median sternotomy. J Thorac Cardiovasc Surg 65:227, 1973.
100. Lee HY, Kerstein MD: Osteomyelitis and septic arthritis, a complication of subclavian venous catheterization. N Engl J Med 285:1179, 1971.
101. Glushakow AS, Carlson D, DePalma AF: Pyarthrosis of the manubriosternal joint. Clin Orthop 114:214, 1976.
102. Pate D, Katz A: Clostridia discitis: A case report. Arthritis Rheum 22:1039, 1979.

103. Digby JM, Kersley JB: Pyogenic nontuberculous spinal infection. An analysis of thirty cases. J Bone Joint Surg [Br] 61:47, 1979.

104. Beaupre A, Carroll N: The three syndromes of iliac osteomyelitis in children. J Bone Joint Surg [Br] 61:1087, 1979.

105. Miskew DB, Block RA, Witt PF: Aspiration of infected sacro-iliac joints. J Bone Joint Surg [Am] 61:1071, 1979.

106. Ralls PW, Boswell W, Henderson R, et al: CT of inflammatory disease of the psoas muscle. AJR 134:767, 1980.

107. Murray IPC: Bone scanning in the child and young adult. Skel Radiol 5:65, 1980.

108. Norris S, Ehrlich MG, McKusick K: Early diagnosis of disk space infection with ^{67}Ga in an experimental model. Clin Orthop 144:293, 1979.

109. Mittapalli MR: Value of bone scan in primary sternal osteomyelitis. South Med J 72:1603, 1979.

110. Borgmeier PJ, Kalovidouris AE: Septic arthritis of the sternomanubrial joint due to *Pseudomonas pseudomallei*. Arthritis Rheum 23:1057, 1980.

111. Gordon G, Kabins SA: Pyogenic sacroiliitis. Am J Med 69:50, 1980.

112. Crock HV, Goldwasser M: Anatomic studies of the circulation in the region of the vertebral end-plate in adult greyhound dogs. Spine 9:702, 1984.

113. McCain GA, Harth M, Bell DA, et al: Septic discitis. J Rheumatol 8:100, 1981.

114. Simons GW, Sty JR, Starshak RJ: Retroperitoneal and retrofascial abscesses. J Bone Joint Surg [Am] 65:1041, 1983.

115. Lloyd TV, Johnson JC: Infectious cervical spondylitis following traumatic endotracheal intubation. Spine 5:478, 1980.

116. Mattingly WT, Dillon ML, Todd EP: Cervical osteomyelitis after esophageal perforation. South Med J 75:626, 1982.

117. Baird RA, Anderson NJ, Bloch JH: Salmonella vertebral osteomyelitis: A complication of salmonella aortitis. Orthopedics 4:1127, 1981.

118. Grisel P: Enucleation de l'atlas et torticolis naso-pharyngien. Presse Med 38:50, 1930.

119. Sullivan AW: Subluxation of the atlanto-axial joint: Sequel to inflammatory processes of the neck. J Pediatr 35:451, 1949.

120. Hess JH, Bronstein IP, Abelson SM: Atlanto-axial dislocations unassociated with trauma and secondary to inflammatory foci in the neck. Am J Dis Child 49:1137, 1935.

121. Pinckney LE, Currarino G, Higgenboten CL: Osteomyelitis of the cervical spine following dental extraction. Radiology 135:335, 1980.

122. Parke WW, Rothman RH, Brown MD: The pharyngovertebral veins: An anatomical rationale for Grisel's syndrome. J Bone Joint Surg [Am] 66:568, 1984.

123. Hadden WA, Swanson AJG: Spinal infection caused by acupuncture mimicking a prolapsed intervertebral disc. A case report. J Bone Joint Surg [Am] 64:624, 1982.

124. Deeb ZL, Schimel S, Daffner RH, et al: Intervertebral disk-space infection after chymopapain injection. AJR 144:671, 1985.

125. Rawlings CE III, Wilkins RH, Gallis HA, et al: Postoperative intervertebral disc space infection. Neurosurgery 13:371, 1983.

126. Lindholm TS, Pylkkanen P: Discitis following removal of intervertebral disc. Spine 7:618, 1982.

127. Puranen J, Makela J, Lahde S: Postoperative intervertebral discitis. Acta Orthop Scand 55:461, 1984.

128. Seifert V, Stolke D, Vogelsang H: Die postoperative discitis intervertebralis lumbalis. Akt Neurol 10:161, 1983.

129. Eismont FJ, Bohlman HH, Soni PL, et al: Pyogenic and fungal vertebral osteomyelitis with paralysis. J Bone Joint Surg [Am] 65:19, 1983.

130. Byrd SE, Biggers SL, Locke GE: The radiographic evaluation of infections of the spine. J Nat Med Assoc 75:969, 1983.

131. Devereaux MD, Hazelton RA: Pyogenic spinal osteomyelitis—its clinical and radiological presentation. J Rheumatol 10:491, 1983.

132. Eismont FJ, Bohlman HH, Soni PL, et al: Vertebral osteomyelitis in infants. J Bone Joint Surg [Br] 64:32, 1982.

133. O'Brien TM, McManus F: Discitis—the irritable back of childhood. Irish J Med Sci 152:404, 1983.

134. Scoles PV, Quinn TP: Intervertebral discitis in children and adolescents. Clin Orthop 162:31, 1982.

135. Short DJ, Webley M, Hadfield J: Septic discitis presenting as a psoas abscess. J R Soc Med 76:1066, 1983.

136. Sartoris DJ, Moskowitz PS, Kaufman RA, et al: Childhood diskitis: Computed tomographic findings. Radiology 149:701, 1983.

137. Gaucher A, Columb JN, Pourel J, et al: What can one expect from bone scanning in the investigation of infectious spondylodiscitis and septic arthritis? Rev Rhum Mal Osteoartic 49:171, 1982.

138. Haase D, Martin R, Marrie T: Radionuclide imaging in pyogenic vertebral osteomyelitis. Clin Nucl Med 5:533, 1980.

139. Bruschwein DA, Brown ML, McLeod RA: Gallium scintigraphy in the evaluation of disk-space infections: Concise communication. J Nucl Med 21:925, 1980.

140. Jeffrey RB, Callen PW, Federle MP: Computed tomography of psoas abscesses. J Comput Assist Tomogr 4:639, 1980.

141. Price AC, Allen JH, Eggers FM, et al: Intervertebral disk-space infection: CT changes. Work in progress. Radiology 149:725, 1983.

142. Brant-Zawadzki M, Burke VD, Jeffrey RB: CT in the evaluation of spine infection. Spine 8:358, 1983.

143. Kattapuram SV, Phillips WC, Boyd R: CT in pyogenic osteomyelitis of the spine. AJR 140:1199, 1983.

144. Hermann G, Mendelson DS, Cohen BA, et al: Role of computed tomography in the diagnosis of infectious spondylitis. J Comput Assist Tomogr 7:961, 1983.

145. Golimbu C, Firooznia H, Rafii M: CT of osteomyelitis of the spine. AJR 142:159, 1984.

146. Nino-Murcia M, Wechsler RJ, Brennan RE: Computed tomography of the iliopsoas muscle. Skel Radiol 10:107, 1983.

147. Larde D, Mathieu D, Frija J, et al: Vertebral osteomyelitis: Disk hypodensity on CT. AJR 139:963, 1982.

148. Mueller PR, Ferrucci JT Jr, Wittenberg J, et al: Iliopsoas abscess: Treatment by CT-guided percutaneous catheter drainage. AJR 142:359, 1984.

149. Baker HL Jr, Berquist TH, Kispert DB, et al: Magnetic resonance imaging in a routine clinical setting. Mayo Clin Proc 60:75, 1985.

150. Modic MT, Weinstein MA, Pavlicek W, et al: Magnetic resonance imaging of the cervical spine: Technical and clinical observations. AJR 141:1129, 1983.

151. Han JS, Benson JE, Yoon YS: Magnetic resonance imaging in the spinal column and craniovertebral junction. Radiol Clin North Am 22:805, 1984.

152. Aguila LA, Piraino DW, Modic MT, et al: The intranuclear cleft of the intervertebral disk: Magnetic resonance imaging. Radiology 155:155, 1985.

153. Faerber EN, Leonidas JC, Leape LL: Retroperitoneal iliac abscess with periostitis. AJR 136:828, 1981.

154. Iczkovitz JM, Leek JC, Robbins DL: Pyogenic sacroiliitis. J Rheumatol 8:157, 1981.

155. Lewkonia RM, Kinsella TD: Pyogenic sacroiliitis. Diagnosis and significance. J Rheumatol 8:153, 1981.

156. Roubergue A, Beauvais P: Arthrites aigues sacro-iliaques à pyogénes de l'enfant. Ann Pediatr 30:81, 1983.

157. Oka M, Mottonen T: Septic sacroiliitis. J Rheumatol 10:475, 1983.

158. Jajic IS, Furst Z, Kralj K, et al: Septic sacroiliitis. An analysis of 14 patients. Acta Orthop Scand 54:210, 1983.

159. Gupta S, Herrera N, Chen C: Scintigraphic demonstration of pyogenic sacroiliitis. Clin Nucl Med 7:295, 1982.

160. Kumar R, Balachandran S: Unilateral septic sacro-iliitis. Importance of the anterior view of the bone scan. Clin Nucl Med 8:413, 1983.

161. Horgan JG, Walker M, Watt I: Scintigraphy in the diagnosis and management of septic sacro-iliitis. Clin Radiol 34:337, 1983.

162. Morgan GJ Jr, Schlegelmich JG, Spiegel PK: Early diagnosis of septic arthritis of the sacroiliac joint by use of computed tomography. J Rheumatol 8:979, 1981.

163. Rosenberg D, Baskies AM, Deckers PJ, et al: Pyogenic sacroiliitis. An absolute indication for computerized tomographic scanning. Clin Orthop 184:128, 1984.

164. Firooznia H, Rafii M, Golimbu C, et al: Computed tomography of pelvic osteomyelitis in patients with spinal cord injuries. Clin Orthop 181:126, 1983.

165. Firooznia H, Rafii M, Golimbu C, et al: Computerized tomography in diagnosis of pelvic abscess in spinal-cord-injured patients. Comput Radiol 7:335, 1983.

166. Wechsler RJ, Schilling JF: CT of the gluteal region. AJR 144:185, 1985.

167. Simons GW, Sty JR, Starshak RR: Iliacus abscess. Clin Orthop 183:61, 1984.

168. Vinceneux PH, Lasserre PP, Grossin M: Technique of percutaneous trocar puncture biopsy of the sacroiliac joint for the bacteriological and histological diagnosis of sacroiliitis. Rev Rhum Mal Osteoartic 49:180, 1982.

169. Ratcliffe JF: Anatomic basis for the pathogenesis and radiologic features of vertebral osteomyelitis and its differentiation from childhood discitis. A microarteriographic investigation. Acta Radiol (Diagn) 26:137, 1985.

170. Whalen JL, Parke WW, Mazur JM, et al: The intrinsic vasculature of developing vertebral end plates and its nutritive significance to the intervertebral discs. J Pediatr Orthop 5:403, 1985.

171. Romanick PC, Smith TK, Kopaniky DR, et al: Infection about the spine associated with low-velocity-missile injury to the abdomen. J Bone Joint Surg [Am] 67:1195, 1985.

172. Fernandez-Ulloa M, Vasavada PJ, Hanslits ML, et al: Diagnosis of vertebral osteomyelitis: Clinical radiological and scintigraphic features. Orthopedics 8:1141, 1985.

173. Heuck F, Weiske R: Informationswert der Röntgen-Computer-Tomographie für den Nachweis und die Kontrolle der Spondylitis. Radiologe 25:307, 1985.

174. Raininko RK, Aho AJ, Laine MO: Computed tomography in spondylitis. CT versus other radiographic methods. Acta Orthop Scand 56:372, 1985.

175. Lahde S, Puranen J: Disk-space hypodensity in CT: The first radiological sign of postoperative diskitis. Eur J Radiol 5:190, 1985.

176. Modic MT, Feiglin DH, Piraino DW, et al: Vertebral osteomyelitis: Assessment using MR. Radiology 157:157, 1985.

177. Weinreb JC, Cohen JM, Maravilla KR: Iliopsoas muscles: MR study of normal anatomy and disease. Radiology 156:435, 1985.

178. Wall SD, Fisher MR, Amparo EG, et al: Magnetic resonance imaging in the evaluation of abscesses. AJR 144:1217, 1985.

179. Shanahan MDG, Ackroyd CE: Pyogenic infection of the sacro-iliac joint. A report of 11 cases. J Bone Joint Surg [Br] 67:605, 1985.

180. Hernandez RJ, Conway JJ, Poznanski AK, et al: The role of computed tomography and radionuclide scintigraphy in the localization of osteomyelitis in flat bones. J Pediatr Orthop 5:151, 1985.

181. Rafii M, Firooznia H, Golimbu C: Computed tomography of septic joints. CT 9:51, 1985.

182. Sartoris DJ, Guerra J Jr, Mattrey RF, et al: Perfluoroctylbromide as a contrast agent for computed tomographic imaging of septic and aseptic arthritis. Invest Radiol 21:49, 1986.

183. Georgi P, Kaps HP, Sinn HJ: Leukozytenszintigraphie bei entzündlichen Prozessen der Wirbelsäule. Radiologe 25:324, 1985.

184. Williams MP: Non-tuberculous psoas abscess. Clin Radiol 37:253, 1986.

185. Watanakunakorn C: *Serratia marcescens* osteomyelitis of the clavicle and ster-

noclavicular arthritis complicating infected indwelling subclavian vein catheter. Am J Med *80:*753, 1986.

186. Fernand R, Lee CK: Postlaminectomy disc space infection. A review of the literature and a report of three cases. Clin Orthop *209:*215, 1986.

187. Lee JKT, Glazer HS: Psoas muscle disorders: MR imaging. Radiology *160:*683, 1986.

188. Piercy EA, Smith JW: Vertebral osteomyelitis. *In* D Schlossberg (Ed): Orthopedic Infection. New York, Springer-Verlag, 1988, p 21.

189. Barr RJ, Hannon DG, Adair IV, et al: Cervical osteomyelitis after rigid oesophagoscopy: Brief report. J Bone Joint Surg [Br] *70:*147, 1988.

190. Wetzel FT, La Rocca H: Grisel's syndrome. A review. Clin Orthop *240:*141, 1989.

191. Mathern GW, Batzdorf U: Grisel's syndrome. Cervical spine clinical, pathologic, and neurologic manifestations. Clin Orthop *244:*131, 1989.

192. Fraser RD, Osti OL, Vernon-Roberts B: Discitis after discography. J Bone Joint Surg [Br] *69:*26, 1987.

193. Osti OL, Fraser RD, Vernon-Roberts B: Discitis after discography. The role of prophylactic antibiotics. J Bone Joint Surg [Br] *72:*271, 1990.

194. Blankstein A, Rubinstein E, Ezra E, et al: Disc space infection and vertebral osteomyelitis as a complication of percutaneous lateral discectomy. Clin Orthop *225:*234, 1987.

195. Dendrinos GK, Polyzoides JA: Spondylodiscitis after percutaneous discectomy. Acta Orthop Scand *63:*219, 1992.

196. Bircher MD, Tasker T, Crawshaw C, et al: Discitis following lumbar surgery. Spine *13:*98, 1988.

197. Nielsen VAH, Iversen E, Ahlgren P: Postoperative discitis. Radiology of progress and healing. Acta Radiol *31:*559, 1990.

198. Cahill DW, Love LC, Rechtine GR: Pyogenic osteomyelitis of the spine in the elderly. J Neurosurg *74:*878, 1991.

199. Chevalier X, Marty M, Larget-Piet B: *Klebsiella pneumoniae* septic arthritis of a lumbar facet joint. J Rheumatol *19:*1817, 1992.

200. Peris P, Brancós MA, Gratacós J, et al: Septic arthritis of spinal apophyseal joint. Report of two cases and review of the literature. Spine *17:*1514, 1992.

201. Ehara S, Khurana JS, Kattapuram SV: Pyogenic vertebral osteomyelitis of the posterior elements. Skel Radiol *18:*175, 1989.

202. Roberts WA: Pyogenic vertebral osteomyelitis of a lumbar facet joint with associated epidural abscess. A case report with review of the literature. Spine *13:*948, 1988.

203. Halpin DS, Gibson RD: Septic arthritis of a lumbar facet joint. J Bone Joint Surg [Br] *69:*457, 1987.

204. Rousselin B, Gires F, Vallée C, et al: Case report 627. Skel Radiol *19:*453, 1990.

205. Fontaine S, Dumas J-M, Brassard R, et al: Pyogenic spondylodiscitis without disc space collapse. J Can Assoc Radiol *38:*129, 1987.

206. Crawford AH, Kucharzyk DW, Ruda R, et al: Diskitis in children. Clin Orthop *266:*70, 1991.

207. Jansen BRH, Hart W, Schreuder O: Discitis in childhood. 12–35-year follow-up of 35 patients. Acta Orthop Scand *64:*33, 1993.

208. Wynne AT, Southgate GW: Discitis causing spondylolisthesis. A case report. Spine *11:*970, 1986.

209. Szalay EA, Green NE, Heller RM, et al: Magnetic resonance imaging in the diagnosis of childhood discitis. J Pediatr Orthop *7:*164, 1987.

210. Gabriel KR, Crawford AH: Magnetic resonance imaging in a child who had clinical signs of discitis. Report of a case. J Bone Joint Surg [Am] *70:*938, 1988.

211. Heller RM, Szalay EA, Green NE, et al: Disc space infection in children: Magnetic resonance imaging. Radiol Clin North Am *26:*207, 1988.

212. Zigler JE, Bohlman HH, Robinson RA, et al: Pyogenic osteomyelitis of the occiput, the atlas, and the axis. J Bone Joint Surg [Am] *69:*1069, 1987.

213. Swanson D, Blecker I, Gahbauer H, et al: Diagnosis of discitis by SPECT technetium-99m MDP scintigram. A case report. Clin Nucl Med *12:*210, 1987.

214. Nolla-Solé JM, Mateo-Soria L, Rozadilla-Sacanell A, et al: Role of technetium-99m diphosphonate and gallium-67 citrate bone scanning in the early diagnosis of infectious spondylodiscitis. A comparative study. Ann Rheum Dis *51:*665, 1992.

215. Van Lom KJ, Kellerhouse LE, Pathria MN, et al: Infection versus tumor in the spine: Criteria for distinction with CT. Radiology *166:*851, 1988.

216. Vogler JB III, Murphy WA: Bone marrow imaging. Radiology *168:*679, 1988.

217. Ricci C, Cova M, Kang YS, et al: Normal age-related patterns of cellular and fatty bone marrow distribution in the axial skeleton: MR imaging study. Radiology *177:*83, 1990.

218. Sharif HS: Role of MR imaging in the management of spinal infections. AJR *158:*1333, 1992.

219. Sharif HS, Clark DC, Aabed MY, et al: Granulomatous spinal infections: MR imaging. Radiology *177:*101, 1990.

220. Post MJD, Bowen BC, Sze G: Magnetic resonance imaging of spinal infection. Rheum Dis Clin North Am *17:*107, 1991.

221. An HS, Vaccaro AR, Dolinskas CA, et al: Differentiation between spinal tumors and infections with magnetic resonance imaging. Spine *16:*334, 1991.

222. Kramer J, Schratter M, Pongracz N, et al: Spondylitis: Erscheinungsbild und Verlaufsbeurteilung mittels Magnetresonanztomographie. ROFO *153:*131, 1990.

223. Post MJD, Quencer RM, Montalvo BM, et al: Spinal infection: Evaluation with MR imaging and intraoperative US. Radiology *169:*765, 1988.

224. Michael AS, Mikhael MA: Spinal osteomyelitis: Unusual findings on magnetic resonance imaging. Comput Med Imaging Graph *12:*329, 1988.

225. Post MJD, Sze G, Quencer RM, et al: Gadolinium-enhanced MR in spinal infection. J Comput Assist Tomogr *14:*721, 1990.

226. Saini S, Modic MT, Hamm B, et al: Advances in contrast-enhanced MR imaging. AJR *156:*235, 1991.

227. Jones KM, Unger EC, Granstrom P, et al: Bone marrow imaging using STIR at 0.5 and 1.5T. Magn Reson Imaging *10:*169, 1992.

228. Stimac GK, Porter BA, Olson DO, et al: Gadolinium-DTPA–enhanced MR imaging of spinal neoplasms: Preliminary investigation and comparison with enhanced-spin echo and STIR sequences. AJNR *150:*605, 1988.

229. Angtuaco EJ, McConnell JR, Chadduck WM, et al: MR imaging of spinal epidural sepsis. AJNR *8:*879, 1987.

230. Angtuaco EJC, McConnell JR, Chadduck WM, et al: MR imaging of spinal epidural sepsis. AJR *149:*1249, 1987.

231. Sandhu FS, Dillon WP: Spinal epidural abscess: Evaluation with contrast-enhanced MR imaging. AJR *158:*405, 1992.

232. Kricun R, Shoemaker EI, Chovanes GI, et al: Epidural abscess of the cervical spine: MR findings in five cases. AJR *158:*1145, 1992.

233. Gero B, Sze G, Sharif H: MR imaging of intradural inflammatory diseases of the spine. AJNR *12:*1009, 1991.

234. Boden SD, Davis DO, Dina TS, et al: Postoperative diskitis: Distinguishing early MR imaging findings from normal postoperative disk space changes. Radiology *184:*765, 1992.

235. Ross JS: Magnetic resonance assessment of the postoperative spine. Degenerative disc disease. Radiol Clin North Am *29:*793, 1991.

236. Vyskocil JJ, McIlroy MA, Brennan TA, et al: Pyogenic infection of the sacroiliac joint: Case reports and review of the literature. Medicine *70:*188, 1991.

237. Reilly JP, Gross RH, Emans JB, et al: Disorders of the sacro-iliac joint in children. J Bone Joint Surg [Am] *70:*31, 1988.

238. Haanpää M, Hannonen P, Kaira P, et al: Clinical sequelae and sacroiliac joint changes by computed tomography after recovery from septic sacroiliitis. Clin Rheumatol *8:*197, 1989.

239. Wilbur AC, Langer BG, Spigos DG: Diagnosis of sacroiliac joint infection in pregnancy by magnetic resonance imaging. Magn Reson Imaging *6:*341, 1988.

240. Klein MA, Winalski CS, Wax MR, et al: MR imaging of septic sacroiliitis. J Comput Assist Tomogr *15:*126, 1991.

241. Van Linthoudt D, Velan F, Ott H: Abscess formation in sternoclavicular joint septic arthritis. J Rheumatol *16:*413, 1989.

242. Wohlgethan JR, Newberg AH, Reed JI: The risk of abscess from sternoclavicular septic arthritis. J Rheumatol *15:*1302, 1988.

243. Pollack MS: Staphylococcal mediastinitis due to sternoclavicular pyarthrosis: CT appearance. J Comput Assist Tomogr *14:*924, 1990.

244. Numaguchi Y, Rigamonti D, Rothman MI, et al: Spinal epidural abscess: Evaluation with gadolinium-enhanced MR imaging. RadioGraphics *13:*545, 1993.

245. Chen W-S, Wan Y-L, Lui C-C, et al: Extrapleural abscess secondary to infection of the sternoclavicular joint. Report of two cases. J Bone Joint Surg [Am] *75:*1835, 1993.

246. Covelli M, Lapadula G, Pipitone N, et al: Isolated sternoclavicular joint arthritis in heroin addicts and/or HIV positive patients: Three cases. Clin Rheumatol *12:*422, 1993.

247. Sandrasegaran K, Saifuddin A, Coral A, et al: Magnetic resonance imaging of septic sacroiliitis. Skeletal Radiol *23:*289, 1994.

66

Osteomyelitis, Septic Arthritis, and Soft Tissue Infection: Organisms

Donald Resnick, M.D., and Gen Niwayama, M.D.

Bacterial Infection
  Gram-Positive Cocci
    Staphylococcal Infection
    Streptococcal Infection
  Gram-Negative Cocci
    Meningococcal Infection
    Gonococcal Infection
  Enteric Gram-Negative Bacilli
    Coliform Bacterial Infection
    Proteus *Infection*
    Pseudomonas *Infection*
    Klebsiella *Infection*
    Salmonella *Infection*
    Shigella *Infection*
    Yersinia *Infection*
    Serratia *Infection*
    Campylobacter *Infection*
    Citrobacter *Infection*
    Kingella (Moraxella) *Infection*
  Other Gram-Negative Bacilli
    Haemophilus *Infection*
    Brucella *Infection*
    Aeromonas *Infection*
    Pasteurella *Infection*
  Other Bacteria
    Corynebacterium *(Diphtheroid) Infection*
    Clostridial Infection
    Bacteroides *and Related Anaerobic Infection*
  Mycobacteria
    Tuberculous Infection
    BCG Vaccination-Induced Infection
    Atypical Mycobacterial Infection
    Leprosy (Hansen's Disease, Mycobacterium leprae
      Infection)
  Spirochetes and Related Organisms
    Syphilis
    Yaws
    Bejel
    Tropical Ulcer
    Leptospirosis
    Rat Bite Fever
    Lyme Disease
Fungal and Higher Bacterial Infection
  Actinomycosis
    General Features
    Musculoskeletal Abnormalities
  Nocardiosis

Cryptococcosis (Torulosis)
  General Features
  Musculoskeletal Abnormalities
North American Blastomycosis
  General Features
  Musculoskeletal Abnormalities
South American Blastomycosis (Paracoccidioidomycosis)
Coccidioidomycosis
  General Features
  Musculoskeletal Abnormalities
Histoplasmosis
  General Features
  Musculoskeletal Abnormalities
Sporotrichosis
  General Features
  Musculoskeletal Abnormalities
Candidiasis (Moniliasis)
  General Features
  Musculoskeletal Abnormalities
Mucormycosis
Aspergillosis
Maduromycosis (Mycetoma)
Other Mycoses
Viral Infection
  Rubella Infection (German Measles)
    Postnatal Rubella
    Intrauterine Rubella
  Cytomegalic Inclusion Disease
  Varicella (Chickenpox)
  Varicella and Herpes Zoster
  Herpes Simplex
  Mumps
  Variola (Smallpox)
  Vaccinia
  Infectious Mononucleosis and Epstein-Barr Virus Infection
  Human Immunodeficiency Virus Infection
    Rheumatologic Disorders
    Infectious Disorders
    Bacillary Angiomatosis
    Miscellaneous Abnormalities
  Other Viral or Viral-like Diseases
Rickettsial Infection
Mycoplasma Infection
Protozoan Infection
  Toxoplasmosis
  Leishmaniasis
  Amebiasis

The discussions of mechanisms, situations, and sites of musculoskeletal infection given in Chapters 64 and 65 leave one major area still to be covered. To correct this deficiency, consideration is directed now toward the specific microorganisms themselves. Although the skeleton can react in only a limited number of ways, certain characteristics of its response to a particular infectious agent may differ, at least subtly, from the changes that are encountered in the presence of a different agent. Thus, certain organisms produce rapid and destructive osseous or articular disease, whereas others are associated with a more indolent process. Furthermore, some agents show predilection for certain anatomic regions of the skeleton, whereas other agents produce changes at different sites. What follows is a survey of some of the organisms that can infect the musculoskeletal system, with emphasis given to a few of the more important disorders.

BACTERIAL INFECTION

Gram-Positive Cocci

Staphylococcal Infection

The two major pathogens are *Staphylococcus aureus* (coagulase positive) and *Staphylococcus epidermidis* (coagulase negative). Staphylococci are responsible for the majority of cases of acute osteomyelitis[1] and nongonococcal infectious arthritis.[561, 562, 569] Estimates of the frequency of one or another strain of staphylococcus (*S. aureus* is most typical) in pyogenic osteomyelitis can reach 80 to 90 per cent. Staphylococcal osteomyelitis is primarily a disease of children under the age of 12 or 13 years, particularly boys. In cases of hematogenous spread of infection to bone, a history of a septic process at a distant site, such as the skin, the respiratory tract, or the genitourinary system,[2] and of local trauma is frequent; thus, the disease occurs in children after a minor injury or in teenage athletes engaged in contact sports. Localization of the infection to the metaphysis of tubular bones of children is typical, although virtually any extra-axial or axial skeletal site may be affected. Brodie's abscesses may be seen[924] (Fig. 66–1). Staphylococci (*S. aureus* and *S. epidermidis*) are responsible also for many of the deep infections that occur after bone or joint surgery[3-5]; the foot infections in diabetic patients; cases of osteomyelitis and septic arthritis seen in hemodialysis patients with infected shunts, in intravenous drug addicts, and in patients with rheumatoid arthritis; and the osseous, articular, and soft tissue suppurative processes that follow penetrating or open wounds. *Staphylococcus aureus* is impli-

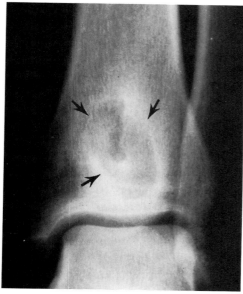

FIGURE 66–1. Staphylococcal osteomyelitis. A well-defined lucent lesion surrounded by a sclerotic margin at the end of the tubular bone (arrows) is typical of a Brodie's abscess.

cated in most cases of pyomyositis (Fig. 66–2) (see Chapter 64).

The clinical and radiologic features of musculoskeletal infections due to staphylococci are discussed in Chapters 64 and 65.

Streptococcal Infection

Streptococci are gram-positive cocci that can be classified on the basis of the type of hemolysis that they produce on sheep blood agar plates. Many of the organisms, especially beta-hemolytic streptococci, can cause osteomyelitis. These latter microorganisms can be further divided into groups A, B, C, D, G, and other groups. In infants, hemolytic streptococcal agents were a frequent cause of osteomyelitis prior to 1940[6] and have been recognized as an important etiologic factor in neonatal or infantile osteomyelitis.[7-11, 520, 529, 530, 948] The clinical manifestations of streptococcal bone infection may be mild even in the presence of significant radiologic alterations, a feature that is evident in other types of infantile osteomyelitis as well. Typically, the disease is discovered in the first few weeks of life.[10] Infection of a single bone is most frequent, and predilection for humeral involvement has been noted by some investigators. Indeed, it has been postulated that involvement of the humerus, particularly its proximal portion, is related to shoulder trauma of the fetus occurring during delivery.[948] Lytic lesions with mild or absent sclerosis and periostitis can be seen. After recovery of the organism from the blood or elsewhere, antibiotic therapy usually leads to rapid healing.

The joints may be infected by streptococcal organisms either by extension from a neighboring site of osteomyelitis or cellulitis or directly,[12] although the prevalence of such articular infection appears to be declining. Residual joint damage is infrequent if appropriate antibiotic treatment is instituted without significant delay.

Anaerobic streptococci can contaminate soft tissue wounds and fractures, producing a crepitant myositis that resembles clostridial gas gangrene. Osteomyelitis and septic

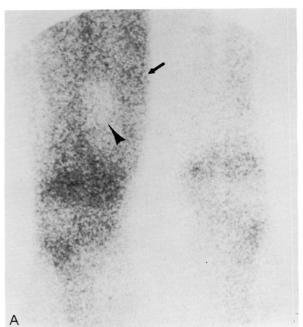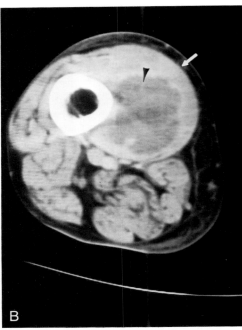

FIGURE 66–2. Staphylococcal pyomyositis. A 51 year old man, with a recent abscess in the back, developed pain and swelling in the knee. Although the initial attempt at aspiration was unrewarding, the pain increased and the mass became erythematous. The radionuclide study **(A)** reveals a diffuse increase in the accumulation of the bone-seeking radiopharmaceutical agent in the soft tissue of the thigh (arrow). A central area of focal photopenia is evident (arrowhead). A transaxial CT scan **(B)** at the level of the mass (arrow) demonstrates its location in the vastus medialis muscle. A rim or rind of increased radiodensity is accompanied by an irregular central zone with decreased attenuation values (arrowhead). Infiltration of the subcutaneous fat adjacent to the mass is present. Needle aspiration and incisional drainage were accomplished. At the time of surgery, a 3 × 5 × 8 cm abscess containing necrotic material was identified. *Staphylococcus aureus* was recovered from the abscess. Subsequently this patient was found to also have diabetes mellitus and subacute bacterial endocarditis. (Courtesy of G. Greenway, M.D., Dallas, Texas.)

arthritis due to streptococcal infection can follow human bites.[13]

With regard to specific groups of streptococci, an increasing number of isolated reports in recent years suggest that almost any variety of the microorganisms can cause bone or joint infection. Group A beta-hemolytic streptococcus *(Streptococcus pyogenes)* is a frequent cause of bacterial infection in children, although skin, pharyngeal, and upper respiratory tract involvement predominates. Myositis related to *S. pyogenes* resembles clostridial myonecrosis.[949] Osteomyelitis and septic arthritis are infrequent. Serious group B streptococcal infections are particularly characteristic in neonates, postpartal women or those who have undergone gynecologic surgery, and aged patients with an underlying disorder, such as chronic renal failure, malignancy, cirrhosis, and diabetes mellitus.[950] Osteomyelitis and suppurative arthritis can occur as a localized infection or as a manifestation of generalized septicemia.[570–572, 913, 951, 952] Single or multiple joint involvement and contamination of prosthetic components characterize the articular manifestations.

Group C streptococci, especially *Streptococcus equisimilis,* have been associated with osteomyelitis and septic arthritis.[573, 574, 953] Group F streptococci are rare causes of musculoskeletal infection.[954] Group G streptococci, which along with group C microorganisms normally inhabit the skin, upper respiratory and gastrointestinal tracts, and vagina, can cause serious infection, especially endocarditis and septicemia. Suppurative arthritis, bursitis, spondylitis, and tenosynovitis are described.[575–578, 875, 914, 955, 956]

Other streptococci, including enterococci (e.g., *S. faecalis*),[579, 957] peptostreptococci (i.e., *Peptococcus*),[958, 959]

Streptococcus milleri,[960–962] and the viridans group of microorganisms,[580–582] rarely can lead to musculoskeletal infections.

Pneumococcal Infection. Formerly termed *Diplococcus pneumoniae,* the pneumococcus now is referred to as *Streptococcus pneumoniae,* as it shares many characteristics with streptococci. Pulmonary infections and those of the upper respiratory tract predominate. Pneumococcal arthritis is not frequent.[14–16, 963] One report of 12 patients with this disease emphasized the prominence of underlying conditions (alcoholism, hypogammaglobulinemia), preexisting joint alterations (rheumatoid arthritis, osteoarthritis), and coexistent pneumococcal infection (meningitis, endocarditis).[17] Children[583] or adults[584] may be affected, and the knee appears to be the site involved most commonly. Soft tissue swelling, joint space narrowing, osseous erosions, periostitis, and periarticular calcification are encountered.[18] Antibiotic therapy usually produces a favorable response with return of normal joint function.

Pneumococcal osteomyelitis is rare and generally is confined to periarticular bone or the spine (Fig. 66–3). Sickle cell anemia may be an underlying problem.[583]

Gram-Negative Cocci

Meningococcal Infection

Meningococcal infection, related to the presence of *Neisseria meningitidis,* occurs almost exclusively in persons who have no measurable antimeningococcal antibody. It varies remarkably in its severity, appearing as a benign and asymptomatic illness in some persons and as a fulminant

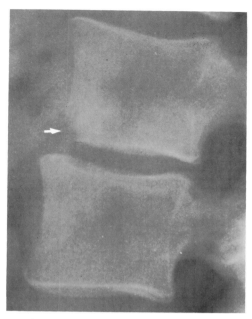

FIGURE 66–3. Pneumococcal osteomyelitis. Observe erosion of the anteroinferior corner (arrow) of a lumbar vertebral body with narrowing of the adjacent intervertebral disc.

and fatal disorder in others. Septicemia may lead to contamination of many sites, but the microorganisms commonly lodge in the central nervous system, skin, adrenal glands, and serosal surfaces.

Meningococcemia leads to the rapid development of fever, shaking chills, skin eruption, petechiae, myalgias, and a variety of neurologic manifestations. In fulminant cases (Waterhouse-Friderichsen syndrome), hypotension, confusion, tachypnea, and peripheral cyanosis develop, and disseminated intravascular coagulation with a consumptive coagulopathy, evident in some patients, produces diffuse bleeding from mucosal surfaces and the skin. Disseminated intravascular coagulation is associated with occlusion of small blood vessels and subsequent necrosis in the skin, brain, kidneys, adrenal glands, and other tissues. If the patient survives, brain damage and gangrene (requiring limb amputation) may be evident.[585, 964, 965] In children, months or years after recovery from the acute illness, characteristic skeletal abnormalities have been described[586–589, 876, 966, 967] in which the localized premature fusion of part of several physes is seen, usually in a bilateral and relatively symmetric distribution (Fig. 66–4). Commonly, it is the central aspect of the physes that is affected, and a cupped or cone-shaped metaphysis results. Subsequently, epiphyseal disintegration and bowing and angular deformities appear, especially in the legs, leading to limb shortening.

Although the cause is not known precisely, a vascular insult is the most likely candidate for the metaphyseal alterations.[586, 966] Predilection for the central portion of the physis, although not present uniformly, is consistent with vascular compromise of the most vulnerable portion of the epiphysis, the center of the germinal plate nearest the physis. Evidence of necrosis at other sites, including the fingertips, toes, skin, scalp, and nasal and auricular cartilage, supports this concept, as does the occurrence of osteolysis and periostitis, consistent with bone infarction, in the

tubular bones of adults after meningococcal septicemia and disseminated intravascular coagulation.[590] Bone infection is not a likely cause.

Meningococcal arthritis is not a common condition.[19–22, 521] Three forms are recognized: an acute transient polyarthritis associated with marked pain and tenderness occurring simultaneously with a petechial rash, and perhaps related to intra-articular hemorrhage or reactive arthritis; a purulent arthritis involving one or more joints, often the knee, occurring after the fifth day of illness; and arthritis occurring after serum therapy, a variety that is not seen currently.[23, 24] The frequency of purulent arthritis in cases of meningococcal infection is 5 to 10 per cent.[22] It may arise during septicemia[591] or as the infection is being controlled with chemotherapy.[25] Rapid resolution of the joint disease is typical, although occasionally a protracted course with radiologic evidence of cartilaginous and osseous destruction is evident.[26, 27] Tenosynovitis related to meningococcal infection also is encountered.[877, 878, 968]

Gonococcal Infection

Clinical Abnormalities. The frequency of gonococcal arthritis is rising. Although the reasons for this rise are not entirely clear, evidence suggests that there has been an increasing resistance of the gonococcus to antibiotics over the last few decades. The role of changing sexual mores in the resurgence of gonococcal arthritis in recent years is controversial.

Gonorrhea is produced by the microorganism *Neisseria gonorrhoeae,* which infects the mucous membranes of the urethra, cervix, rectum, and pharynx. The disease is transmitted almost exclusively through sexual contact with persons who have asymptomatic or ignored symptomatic infection. Although gonorrhea is more frequent in women than in men, the disease may become evident in homosexual men. It also is encountered during pregnancy and after gonococcal vulvovaginitis in children and in the neonate.[23, 28–36] It is clear that as an infant passes through the birth canal, any of its orifices may act as a portal of entry for the gonococcus; susceptible sites include the conjunctiva and the anogenital, oropharyngeal, and umbilical orifices.[34]

Only a minority of gonococcal infections eventually disseminate.[593] Gonococcemia leads to skin rash, fever, and arthritis,[1248] the last occurring in approximately 75 per cent of disseminated cases. The articular disease may have an insidious onset with fleeting arthralgias or a sudden onset with fever and red, hot, swollen, and tender joint(s). Polyarticular findings are frequent, although the infection tends to localize in one or two joints.[592, 971] The affected articulations, in decreasing order of frequency, are the knee, the ankle, the wrist, and the joints of the shoulder, foot, and spine (Fig. 66–5). The joints of the lower extremity are involved more commonly than those of the upper extremity in most series, although some reports indicate predominant involvement of the upper extremities, especially the wrists.[593] In approximately 50 to 70 per cent of cases, acute asymmetric tenosynovitis or periarthritis, particularly in the dorsal aspect of the fingers, hand, or wrist, or in the ankle, is evident.[593, 594] This represents a characteristic and early manifestation of the disease. Other clinical manifestations include skin rash[37] and, rarely, suppurative myositis.[38]

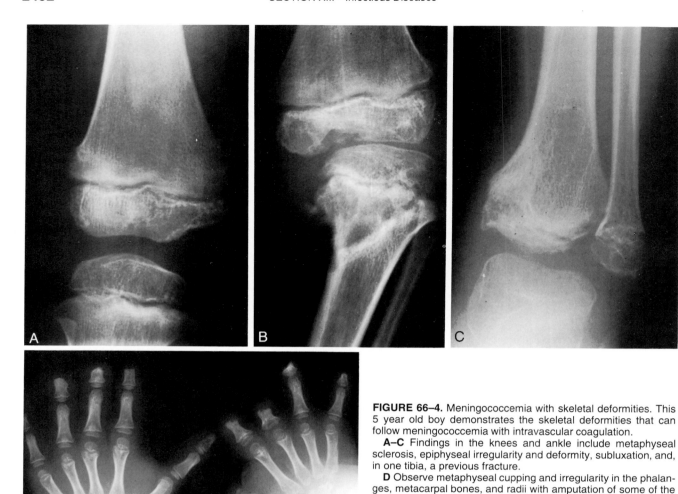

FIGURE 66–4. Meningococcemia with skeletal deformities. This 5 year old boy demonstrates the skeletal deformities that can follow meningococcemia with intravascular coagulation.

A–C Findings in the knees and ankle include metaphyseal sclerosis, epiphyseal irregularity and deformity, subluxation, and, in one tibia, a previous fracture.

D Observe metaphyseal cupping and irregularity in the phalanges, metacarpal bones, and radii with amputation of some of the digits. (Courtesy of M. Dalinka, M.D., Philadelphia, Pennsylvania.)

Several stages of this articular disease have been recognized.[35] In patients with a positive blood culture or typical skin rash, clinical findings appear earlier in the disease course than in patients with positive joint culture without organisms recoverable from the blood. Dissemination of the microorganisms from the primary site of infection via the blood stream leads to a typical and frequently toxic syndrome consisting of fever, chills, skin lesions, and polyarthritis. During this stage of the illness (1 to 3 days) aspiration of joint contents frequently is unrewarding, and polyarthritis is evanescent. By the fourth to sixth day, articular manifestations dominate the clinical picture and involve one or a few joints that commonly contain fluid from which the microorganisms can be cultured.[35, 39]

Pathologic Abnormalities. A reliable diagnosis of gonococcal arthritis depends on recovery of the bacteria from the blood, the synovial tissue, the synovial fluid, the genitourinary tract, or the skin. This is accomplished in 50 to 60 per cent of suspected cases. The synovial fluid is an exudate that can be frankly purulent or straw-colored. The appearance of the synovial membrane is typical of that of pyogenic articular processes.[40] Initially, infiltration of the membrane with polymorphonuclear leukocytes, lympho-

cytes, and plasma cells is identified. With progression, the synovial lining may be destroyed and the inner surface of the articular capsule is covered with granulation tissue containing polymorphonuclear leukocytes, macrophages, and plasma cells.[1] The articular cartilage and subchondral bone may become involved in later stages of joint infection[595] or in early stages when hematogenous implantation has produced a primary osteomyelitis.[36, 41, 42, 969]

Radiologic Abnormalities. When antibiotic treatment is instituted at an early stage, the only significant radiographic features are soft tissue swelling and osteoporosis. If appropriate treatment is delayed, more prominent radiographic findings are encountered, including joint space narrowing, marginal and central osseous erosions, lytic destruction of adjacent metaphyses and epiphyses, and periostitis (Fig. 66–5). Healing can be associated with intra-articular osseous fusion. These features are identical to those accompanying other pyogenic infections. The appearance of abnormalities at multiple joints and tenosynovitis are helpful clues to a specific diagnosis of gonococcal infection.[43, 970]

Pathogenesis. The pathogenesis of the various inflammatory lesions in disseminated gonococcemia is controversial. Numerous theories have been proposed to explain the

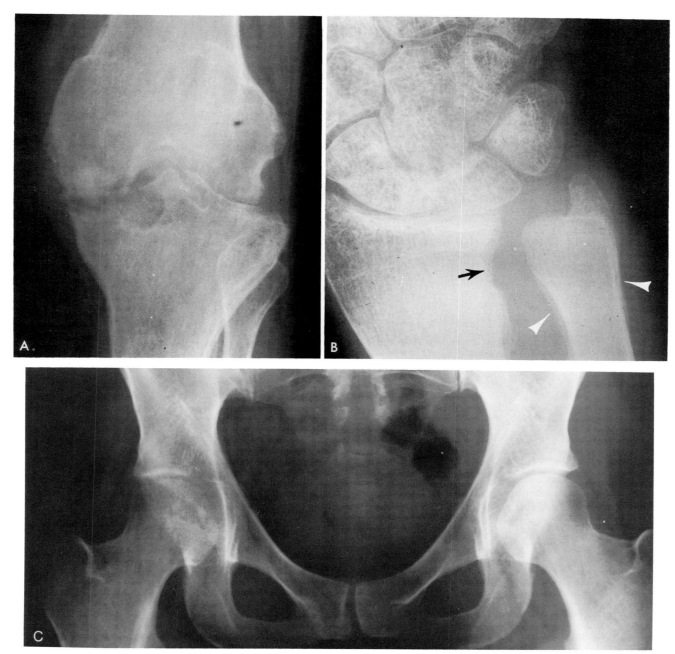

FIGURE 66–5. Gonococcal arthritis.

A Knee. Observe joint space loss, poorly defined marginal and central osseous erosions, and soft tissue swelling. The lack of osteoporosis is impressive. Bone proliferation is evident along the distal medial portion of the femur.

B Inferior radioulnar joint. Note massive soft tissue swelling about the distal end of the ulna, scalloped osseous erosions (arrow), and periostitis (arrowheads). Carpal osteoporosis is seen.

C In this patient, gonococcal arthritis of the right hip has led to periarticular osteoporosis and joint space loss. The findings simulate those of transient osteoporosis of the hip.

cutaneous and articular manifestations of the disease. Although attempts at demonstrating *Neisseria gonorrhoeae* by culture and smear of the skin lesions rarely are successful,[44] identification of typical organisms through the use of immunofluorescent staining techniques of the involved cutaneous tissue[45] supports one current explanation of the skin lesions, which is that they represent embolization of gonococcal organisms to cutaneous vessels.[46] Circulating immune complexes have been detected in the migratory polyarthralgic phase of gonococcal arthritis.[47] Other evidence supporting[48, 49, 531] and refuting[46] the role of immune complexes and gonococcal antigen in the pathogenesis of disseminated gonococcal disease is available.[879] Some investigators[596] have summarized what they consider to be mounting evidence that a sterile or ''reactive'' arthritis is a prominent feature of such disseminated disease: The articular manifestations commonly resemble serum sickness or an immune complex disorder rather than a purulent arthritis; *Neisseria gonorrhoeae* frequently is absent in joint effusions; gonococcal arthritis uncommonly leads to joint destruction; gonococcal osteomyelitis is rare; circulating immune complexes are evident in some patients with disseminated gonococcal infection; and reactive arthritis may accompany other infectious diseases (see Chapters 31 and 64). At this writing, the exact mechanism by which gonococcal organisms or their products affect skin and joint is not known.

Differential Diagnosis. The accurate differentiation of gonococcal joint disease and that related to other pyogenic organisms on the basis of radiographic findings usually is not possible; this differentiation depends on the interpretation of the radiographic abnormalities in light of the clinical findings. Furthermore, differentiating the radiographic features of gonococcal pyarthrosis and Reiter's syndrome can be extremely difficult; clinical differentiation is complicated by the presence of skin rash, urethral discharge, and articular abnormalities in both conditions. Gonococcal arthritis and Reiter's syndrome both produce soft tissue swelling, osteoporosis, joint space narrowing, osseous erosion, and periostitis in one or more joints, particularly in the lower extremity. Involvement of the joints of the foot, the calcaneus, the spine, and the sacroiliac articulation; the presence of poorly defined periosteal proliferation about the involved joints; and the absence of fuzzy or frayed central osseous margins are helpful in accurately diagnosing Reiter's syndrome.

Enteric Gram-Negative Bacilli

Although the terminology related to this group of bacteria is not constant, two major families of microorganisms are identified: Enterobacteriaceae and Pseudomonadaceae. In the former family, genus types include Escherichia, Klebsiella, Proteus, Enterobacter, Serratia, Morganella, Providencia, Citrobacter, Shigella, Salmonella, Hafnia, Yersinia, Edwardsiella, Arizona, and Erwinia. Related groups of bacteria, frequently classified as enteric gram-negative rods, include the Bacteroides family (Bacteroides, Fusobacterium, Leptotrichia), Vibrio group (Vibrio, Campylobacter), and nonfermenter group (Moraxella, Achromobacter, Acinetobacter, Bordetella, and others). Some of the more important of these infective agents that are responsible for musculoskeletal disease are discussed here. In general,

these gram-negative bacilli are responsible for as many as 25 per cent of skeletal infections.

Coliform Bacterial Infection

The coliform bacteria are gram-negative bacilli that normally inhabit the human intestinal tract. The best-known organisms in this group are *Escherichia coli* and *Enterobacter (Aerobacter) aerogenes.* Articular and osseous infections with these agents (and the other gram-negative bacilli that are discussed subsequently) are rare except in the intravenous drug abuser, the person with preexisting joint disease, and the patient with a chronic debilitating disorder.[50, 597] The usual mechanism of articular infection is hematogenous, although direct inoculation after a diagnostic or therapeutic procedure or injury can be implicated in some patients. Monoarticular involvement, especially of the knee, generally is associated with a poor therapeutic response. No specific radiographic features are evident, although emphysematous septic arthritis has been noted in patients with *E. coli* infection.[51, 52]

Proteus Infection

Proteus mirabilis infection of a joint rarely is observed.[50] The clinical situation is similar to that which is evident with coliform bacterial infection. Urinary tract abnormalities may coexist. Monoarticular involvement of the knee or another joint is typical. Osteomyelitis related to this microorganism also is rare.[598]

Pseudomonas Infection

Serious infection with pseudomonas is associated almost invariably with diminished resistance of the host or damage to local tissues (Fig. 66–6). Premature infants, children with congenital anomalies, intravenous drug abusers, patients with myeloproliferative disorders or those receiving immunosuppressive agents, and geriatric patients with debilitating diseases are persons who may develop osteomyelitis or septic arthritis due to *Pseudomonas aeruginosa.*[50, 53–56, 599] Hematogenous spread of infection is common in intravenous drug abusers; Pseudomonas infection commonly localizes in the axial skeleton, affecting the spine and the sacroiliac, sternoclavicular, and acromioclavicular joints.[972] The peculiar proclivity of intravenous drug abusers to develop Pseudomonas osteomyelitis and septic arthritis and the common localization of such disease within the central skeleton are interesting but unexplained observations.

Pseudomonas contamination of bone and joint can result also from spread of infection in an adjacent focus or from direct inoculation.[973] Pseudomonas osteomyelitis is a recognized complication of puncture wounds,[57–60, 532] although Proteus, *E. coli,* and other agents also may be implicated in this clinical situation.[59] Other types of trauma and surgery can lead to Pseudomonas involvement of osseous and articular structures. No specific radiographic features characterize skeletal involvement with this organism.

Meliodosis, related to *Pseudomonas pseudomallei,* rarely involves the musculoskeletal system. During the conflict in Vietnam, cases of meliodosis increased in frequency, presumably related to exposure of soldiers to wet rice fields. In this environment, the organism was introduced into the body by inhalation or through the skin. Although respiratory symptoms and signs predominate, musculoskeletal in-

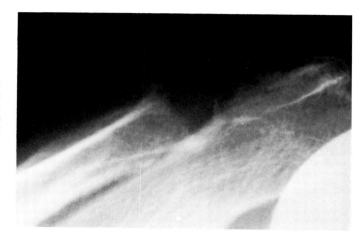

FIGURE 66–6. Pseudomonas osteomyelitis and septic arthritis. In this intravenous drug abuser, osteomyelitis of the distal end of the clavicle and septic arthritis of the acromioclavicular joint with osseous destruction and periostitis were related to Pseudomonas infection. Infection with this organism and in this location is not infrequent in the intravenous drug abuser.

volvement, particularly infective spondylitis and septic arthritis, is reported.[1264]

Klebsiella Infection

Rarely, *Klebsiella pneumoniae* results in osteomyelitis and septic arthritis in a host with diminished resistance.[50] Adults or children[600] are affected (Fig. 66–7). Emphysematous septic arthritis may be seen.[974]

Salmonella Infection

A variety of Salmonella organisms cause human disease, with great variation in the spectrum and severity of such disease. Bacteremia is a constant feature of infection by some of these organisms, such as *S. typhi,* and a common feature of others, such as *S. choleraesuis*. Bacteremia predominates in the very young and the aged and in persons with underlying disorders such as malignancy and cirrhosis. In the presence of Salmonella bacteremia, localized infec-

tions can develop at distant sites and are particularly characteristic in areas of preexisting abnormalities, including congenital cysts, calculous gallbladders, bone infarction (see later discussion), and vascular aneurysms. With regard to the last abnormality, Salmonella organisms, especially *S. choleraesuis* and *S. typhimurium,* invade the lamina intima of diseased and atherosclerotic abdominal aortas, penetrating their walls and leading to mycotic aneurysms. Subsequently, infections of the retroperitoneal tissues, psoas musculature, and lumbar spine may develop.[605]

Salmonella typhi produces a systemic infection, typhoid fever. Before the advent of antibiotics, bone infection was encountered in approximately 1 per cent of patients with typhoid fever[61]; more recently, such cases indeed have become rare.[62–68, 601] Involvement can occur in extraspinal or spinal locations. In the latter site, the radiographic picture resembles that in tuberculosis.[602] The similarity is accentuated by histologic findings revealing an inflammatory process with or without caseating necrosis.[63, 67]

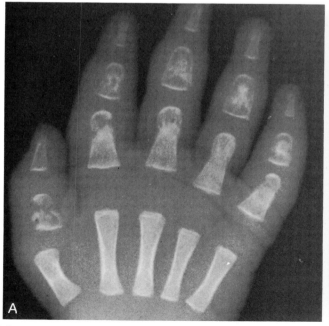
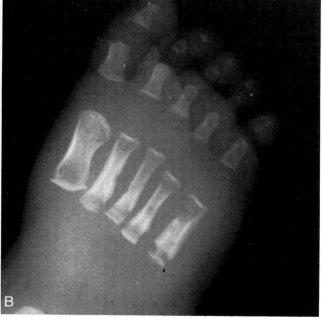

FIGURE 66–7. Klebsiella osteomyelitis. In this 6 day old infant, Klebsiella septicemia was associated with toxic shock and osteomyelitis with involvement of multiple bones in the hands and feet. Observe soft tissue swelling and osteolytic lesions, especially in the phalanges of the hand and metatarsals of the foot. (From Diard F, et al: Australas Radiol 27:39, 1983.)

Other Salmonella organisms can involve bone and joint.[69, 70, 533, 975–979] Salmonella arthritis is not common, predominates in infants and young children, may occur in persons harboring the human immunodeficiency virus, and may be the initial or major manifestation of infection.[603] It usually is monoarticular, most frequently affecting the knee, the glenohumeral joint, and the hip.[23] Swelling, pain, tenderness, and limitation of articular motion may be evident.[69]

An association exists between Salmonella infection and sickle cell anemia or other hemoglobinopathies,[71–73] as well as leukemia, lymphoma, bartonellosis, cirrhosis of the liver, and systemic lupus erythematosus.[67] In patients with sickle cell disease, infection with *S. choleraesuis, S. paratyphi,* or *S. typhimurium* is most typical.[74] The basis for the unusual propensity of these persons to develop Salmonella infection is not known. It has been postulated that multiple bowel infarcts allow the organisms to leave the colon and enter the blood stream, and that Salmonella organisms are well suited for survival in areas of medullary bone infarction.[74] In fact, Salmonella osteomyelitis frequently originates in the medullary cavity of a tubular bone, although epiphyses and other osseous structures occasionally can be affected.[75] Salmonella spondylitis is reported to be rare, however.[1, 604, 978] In tubular bones, Salmonella infection may be characterized by a symmetric distribution, a combination of lysis and sclerosis, and periostitis, findings that are difficult to differentiate from infarction alone. In addition to suppurative arthritis and osteomyelitis, a nonbacterial polyarthritis (reactive arthritis) may be observed 1 to 2 weeks after infection with *S. typhimurium.*[76, 77] Its clinical manifestations resemble those of rheumatic fever.[23] A relationship between this variety of postinfectious polyarthritis and Reiter's syndrome, spondylitis, and the presence of HLA-B27 antigen has been noted.[23, 78]

A Salmonella subspecies, *Salmonella arizonae (Arizona hinshawii)* bacillus, also is capable of producing osteomyelitis and septic arthritis, especially in association with immunosuppression and sickle cell disease.[96–98, 606] As snakes constitute the main reservoir of *S. arizonae,* patients ingesting uncooked snake flesh, most often as a folk remedy for joint pain, may develop septic arthritis related to this organism.[980]

Shigella Infection

Two to 3 weeks after an episode of acute bacillary dysentery, a noninfectious polyarthritis showing predilection for the knees, the elbows, the wrists, or the fingers can be evident, which simulates rheumatic fever and which may be associated with Reiter's syndrome and the presence of HLA-B27 antigen.[23, 78]

Yersinia Infection

Two types of bone or joint affliction can occur in association with infection caused by *Yersinia enterocolitica.* A nonsuppurative, self-limited polyarthritis, especially of the knees and the ankles, can appear approximately 3 weeks after the onset of the illness.[23, 79, 80, 607] This articular manifestation may be complicated by sacroiliitis and the presence of the HLA-B27 antigen. The second type of affliction relates to the presence of *Y. enterocolitica* septicemia, particularly in patients with underlying abnormalities (hemoglobinopathies, leukemia, diabetes mellitus, alcoholism).

Septic arthritis or osteomyelitis may appear in this setting.[81–84] Tenosynovitis also has been described after a puncture wound.[981]

Serratia Infection

Serratia marcescens can cause infection of the musculoskeletal system, especially in persons with underlying disorders such as diabetes mellitus, systemic lupus erythematosus, neutrophil dysfunction syndromes, and rheumatoid arthritis or after trauma, placement of intravenous, arterial, or urinary catheters, ischemic necrosis of bone, or intravenous drug abuse.[50, 109–113, 536, 608–610, 982] The usual pathway for articular and osseous infection with this organism is the blood stream. Radiographic features of septic arthritis include soft tissue swelling, osteoporosis, and osseous destruction, and these are entirely nonspecific. Similarly, involvement of the bone leads to radiographic changes common to many types of osteomyelitis at one or more sites.

Campylobacter Infection

Campylobacter infections are increasing in frequency and vary considerably in severity. *Campylobacter fetus jejuni* is a common cause of inflammatory diarrhea, whereas other subspecies, including *C. fetus (Vibrio fetus),* can produce more serious disease as a result of the presence of septicemia, endocarditis, thrombophlebitis, meningitis, and lung abscesses in normal and compromised hosts. Osteomyelitis and septic arthritis are described in this clinical setting.[611, 983]

Citrobacter Infection

Although *Citrobacter diversus* is considered an unusual opportunistic microorganism, it can be associated with significant clinical disease, especially in the compromised host.[612] Septic arthritis related to infection by this organism has been reported.[613]

Kingella (Moraxella) Infection

Kingella and Moraxella are closely related organisms that occur as part of the normal oropharyngeal flora and, rarely, lead to clinical infection, especially in infants, children, and elderly persons. Reported manifestations of hematogenous dissemination of infection include abscesses in the brain and soft tissue, endocarditis, osteomyelitis, and septic arthritis.[614–618, 984, 985] The knee is affected most commonly.

Other Gram-Negative Bacilli

Haemophilus Infection

Acute septic arthritis due to *Haemophilus influenzae* has been recorded.[85–93, 522, 534, 637, 925, 926] It is more frequent in children, particularly between the ages of 7 months and 4 years, than in adults[925] (Fig. 66–8). In fact, this microorganism appears to be the leading cause of pyarthrosis in children in the first 2 years of life. In adult patients, *H. influenzae* accounts for 1 or 2 per cent of cases of septic arthritis, and alcoholism, diabetes mellitus, the acquired immunodeficiency syndrome, the nephrotic syndrome, or agammaglobulinemia may be present.[90, 94, 620, 986, 987] Hematogenous spread is the usual mechanism of joint infection. Single or, less commonly, multiple joints may be affected,

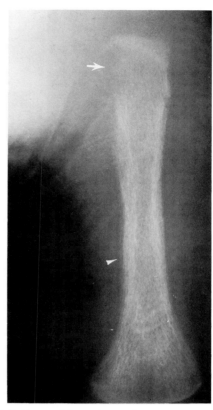

FIGURE 66–8. Haemophilus osteomyelitis and septic arthritis. This infant developed osteomyelitis of the proximal metaphysis and diaphysis of the humerus with glenohumeral joint involvement due to Haemophilus infection. Observe metaphyseal erosion (arrow), permeative bone destruction, and periostitis (arrowhead).

with the knee and the ankle being the most frequent sites of involvement. Less frequently, localization in joints of the hand and the foot is apparent; a case of infection of the first metatarsophalangeal joint resembling gout has been noted.[93] Vertebral osteomyelitis caused by this organism also has been reported.[95, 988] A relationship of Haemophilus pyarthrosis and trauma has been suggested; in this regard, it is of interest that the majority of cases have affected the right side of the body (the dominant side?). Haemophilus tenosynovitis also has been described.[535, 563]

Other Haemophilus species that can produce septic arthritis include *H. parainfluenzae* and *H. aphrophilus*.[619, 638, 989]

Brucella Infection

Brucellosis (undulant fever) can result from human infection with one of a variety of organisms, including *Brucella abortus, B. melitensis,* and *B. suis.*[99, 100] *B. canis* also can cause human infection.[1265] The disease, which is endemic in Saudi Arabia, South America, Spain, Italy, and in the Midwest region of the United States, is transmitted to humans from lower animals such as the goat, the cow, and the hog through the ingestion of milk or milk products containing viable bacteria or through contact of skin with infected tissues or secretions. The disease is transmitted very rarely from one human to another. The invading organisms localize in tissues of the reticuloendothelial system, such as the liver, the spleen, the lymph nodes, and the bone marrow. After an incubation period, which varies

from 7 to 21 days (or longer), fever, headaches, weakness, sweats, myalgia, and arthralgia become apparent.

Involvement of joints, bones, and bursae is relatively uncommon, although an inflammatory process in any one of these sites in a farmer or meathandler should arouse suspicion of brucellosis.[101] The inability to recover the causative organisms in many cases of brucellosis with articular involvement has raised the possibility that such involvement may be reactive rather than representing a true septic arthritis.[631] The arthritis usually is monoarticular or pauciarticular, with the hip and knee being involved most frequently.[23, 990–993] Sacroiliac joint abnormalities also are common.[621–624, 927, 991, 994, 997] Such involvement may be unilateral or, less commonly, bilateral.[998, 999] Sternoclavicular joint involvement has received increasing attention.[994, 995, 1249] Alterations of bursae may be especially characteristic, with common inflammation in the prepatellar region.[101, 102] Other bursae, including that of the subdeltoid area, also may be involved.[103]

Osteomyelitis of long, short, or flat bones may be encountered; it frequently is chronic, and the osseous tissues may be invaded secondarily by staphylococci.[101, 625–628, 880, 996] Brucellar spondylitis, which appears to be the most common form of musculoskeletal disease, typically affects the lumbar spine and is associated with an acute clinical onset and rapid progression of radiologic findings (Fig. 66–9).[629, 999–1004] Other regions of the spine and multiple sites may be involved.[630, 881] Abnormalities include destruction of vertebrae and intervertebral discs, sclerosis, paravertebral abscess formation, and healing with intraosseous fusion and osteophytosis.[74, 101, 104–106] A large parrot-beak–like osteophyte has been reported as a characteristic feature of spinal brucellosis.[999] These radiographic abnormalities resemble those in other types of pyogenic or tuberculous spondylitis. Osteoporosis, large soft tissue abscesses, and paraspinal calcification may be somewhat less common in brucellosis than in tuberculosis.[107, 881] Other findings that are reported to be more characteristic of brucellosis than of tuberculosis are less disc space loss and more commonly evident bone ankylosis between affected vertebral bodies.[1004] A peripherally located intradiscal gas collection also may be characteristic of brucellosis.[1003] As in tuberculous spondylitis, MR imaging may be used to further evaluate brucellar spondylitis (Fig. 66–10).[1265]

The diagnosis of brucellosis frequently is difficult to establish.[23] Culture of the organisms from a joint or bursa provides an absolute diagnosis; a rising serum agglutination titer in conjunction with developing spinal or extraspinal clinical and radiographic findings allows a confident diagnosis. Skin tests are of little diagnostic value. Histologic examination of the synovial membrane shows granulomatous tissue, cellular infiltration with large or small mononuclear cells, and granuloma formation.[108] A granulomatous osteomyelitis may be evident on bone biopsy (Fig. 66–9).

Aeromonas Infection

Aeromonas hydrophila is an aerobic gram-negative rod found in fresh water, tap water, swimming pools, and soil, as well as in stools from some persons. Although rarely a pathogen, it can cause infection in patients with neoplasm or chronic liver disease.[114, 115] A history of exposure to water in a pool or lake, especially when combined with trauma,

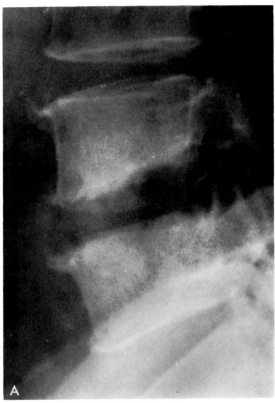

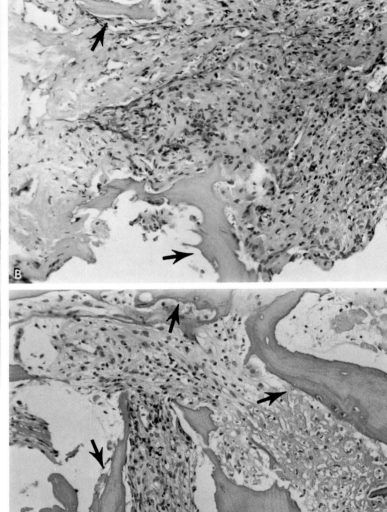

FIGURE 66–9. Brucellar spondylitis.

A Lumbar spine involvement is characterized by irregular destruction of the osseous surfaces of two adjacent vertebrae with reactive sclerosis. Note the parrot beak–like osteophytes.

B A photomicrograph (50×) in a different patient with brucellar spondylitis reveals necrotic osseous trabeculae (arrows) surrounded by active chronic inflammatory cells (predominantly lymphocytes and polymorphonuclear leukocytes), cellular debris, and fibroblastic cells with stromal fibrosis.

C In another photomicrograph (50×), osseous trabeculae show complete or incomplete necrosis (arrows). The intervening stroma reveals active chronic inflammation with polymorphonuclear leukocytes, lymphocytes, cellular debris, fibrinous exudate, and fibrosis.

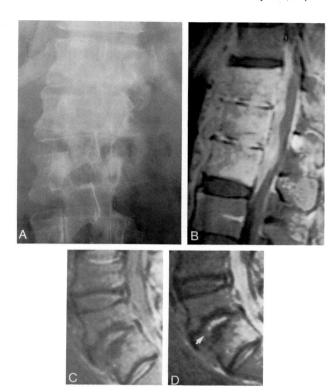

FIGURE 66–10. Brucellar spondylitis.

A, B In this 47 year old man with back pain, a routine frontal radiograph **(A)** shows involvement of the twelth thoracic and first and second lumbar vertebrae. Findings include disc space loss at two levels (T12-L1; L1-L2) with osteophyte formation. A sagittal T1-weighted (TR/TE, 600/20) spin echo MR image obtained with chemical presaturation of fat (ChemSat) and after intravenous administration of a gadolinium contrast agent **(B)** reveals high signal intensity in the affected vertebral bodies and intervertebral discs, as well as in the anterior soft tissues and intraspinal regions.

C, D In a 66 year old man, sagittal proton density (TR/TE, 1700/50) **(C)** and T2-weighted (TR/TE, 1700/100) **(D)** spin echo MR images show involvement of the fourth and fifth lumbar vertebral bodies and intervening disc. Note the high signal intensity in the infected disc (arrow) in **D.**

(C, D, Courtesy of T. Mattsson, M.D., Riyadh, Saudi Arabia.)

is characteristic.[1005] Manifestations include septicemia, soft tissue and muscle infection, meningitis, osteomyelitis, and septic arthritis.[632–634] Necrotizing lesions can lead to gas formation. After initiation of septic arthritis resulting from hematogenous spread of infection, the patients respond poorly to therapy.

Pasteurella Infection

Typical pathogens in animals, pasteurellae can produce human infections, including cutaneous abscesses, septicemia, endocarditis, osteomyelitis, and septic arthritis. *Pasteurella multocida* and, more rarely, *P. haemolytica, P. pneumotropica,* and *P. ureae,* are the species implicated most commonly in human disease.

Pasteurella multocida frequently is isolated from both wild and domestic animals, especially cats, dogs, swine, and rats, explaining the association of human infections with animal exposure, bites, or scratches.[882, 1006] Contact with animals, however, is not a uniform feature in such infections. Cutaneous and subcutaneous abscesses, cellulitis, and lymphangitis are local and regional manifestations

of Pasteurella infection and can be followed by septicemia and involvement of distant sites. Localization of infection in the knee is common, although any joint, especially those with preexisting disease or with prosthetic components, can be affected.[635] Bone and joint contamination in the hand or foot commonly is related to direct inoculation of organisms or spread of infection from involved soft tissues owing to the injury (animal bite or scratch) itself (see Chapter 64). Osteolysis, periostitis, and soft tissue swelling are observed (Fig. 66–11).[636]

Other Bacteria

Corynebacterium (Diphtheroid) Infection

Diphtheroid bacteria belong to the genus Corynebacterium and are part of the normal flora of the skin, mucous membranes, and gastrointestinal tract.[116] Although these bacteria are identified in 1 to 30 per cent of all blood cultures[117] and in 3 per cent of surgical specimens obtained at total hip arthroplasty,[118] usually they are regarded as contaminants. Rarely, diphtheroid bacteria can cause septic arthritis or osteomyelitis.[116, 119, 120, 639] In these circumstances, a preexisting condition or disease usually is evident, or previous surgery has been accomplished.

Clostridial Infection

Gas Gangrene. Wounds that are contaminated by gas gangrene may contain a mixture of clostridial organisms, including *Clostridium tetani, C. perfringens, C. septicum,* and *C. novyi.* These organisms are anaerobic and are capable of producing extensive tissue destruction with gas for-

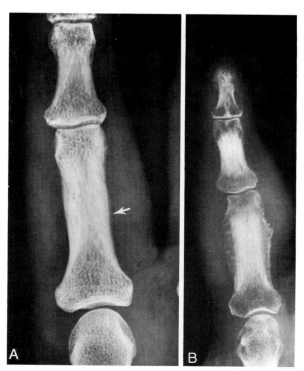

FIGURE 66–11. Pasteurella osteomyelitis: Phalanges of the hand. In **A,** soft tissue swelling and minimal periostitis (arrow) are seen. In **B,** more dramatic alterations are apparent. (From Lequesne M, et al: Rev Rheum Mal Osteoartic *48:*163, 1981.)

mation at the site of invasion. Soft tissue contamination with gas gangrene develops in devitalized tissues in which arterial blood supply has been compromised. War wounds, vehicular trauma, surgery, burns, decubitus ulcers, and septic abortions are some predisposing factors.[640] Nontraumatic gas gangrene can occur at sites adjacent or distant to a visceral lesion,[640, 641, 1007] particularly a gastrointestinal malignancy. Three patterns are recognized in this situation: visceral anaerobic cellulitis, in which a local infection is accompanied by septicemia; visceral anaerobic cellulitis, with contiguous spread to adjacent muscles (i.e., to the iliopsoas muscle or muscles of the abdominal wall); and metastatic myonecrosis, in which organisms deposit in distant muscles subsequent to septicemia.[1007] Edema, necrotizing myositis, vascular thrombosis, cellular infiltration, and interstitial gas bubbles are evident at infected sites.

Clinical manifestations of clostridial myonecrosis may become evident within 6 to 8 hours of injury and include severe pain and an edematous, pulseless, and gangrenous limb. Crepitation with detection of gas in the soft tissue is apparent in the later stages of the disease. Systemic manifestations include prostration, a normal or slightly elevated temperature, anorexia, and, ultimately, circulatory collapse, coma, and death.[537]

Clinical manifestations of clostridial cellulitis are less striking. This condition relates to infection of skin and subcutaneous tissue with subsequent necrosis. The underlying skeletal muscle is not affected. Local pain and crepitus can be detected, but systemic manifestations are absent or mild.

On radiographs, radiolucent collections may appear within the subcutaneous or muscular tissues (Fig. 66–12). In the former location, they produce linear or netlike lucent areas that can extend both proximally and distally. Gas in the muscular tissues may produce circular collections of varying size. It should be emphasized, however, that soft tissue gas is not specific for clostridial infections, being evident in some cases related to infections with *E. coli*, other coliform bacteria, streptococci, and Bacteroides species. Nonbacterial mechanisms responsible for gas in the soft tissues include visceral rupture (lung and pleura, esophagus, pharynx), skin lacerations and open fractures, explosive-type injuries, cutaneous ulcerations, and chemical exposures (hydrogen peroxide, magnesium).[642, 883]

Arthritis. *Clostridium perfringens* (or rarely *C. bifermentans*) can be introduced into a joint by contamination from a penetrating injury or, rarely, by hematogenous spread from its normal site of residence in the gastrointestinal tract.[121–126, 643] *C. septicum* also has been implicated as a cause of septic arthritis.[915] Diabetes mellitus, rheumatoid arthritis, thermal burns, and plasma cell myeloma have been present in some patients with clostridial infection.[1008, 1009] Monoarticular disease, particularly of the knee, is typical, although polyarticular involvement has been described.[1008] Synovial edema and inflammation and cartilaginous destruction can be evident, perhaps related to the effect of the highly toxic enzymes produced by these bacteria.[125, 127] In addition to joint space narrowing and osseous defects, radiographs may delineate gas in the adjacent soft tissues or articulation itself. Although the diagnosis of septic arthritis usually is readily apparent, noninfectious or reactive arthritis also has been associated with clostridial infections at distant sites.[1010]

Clostridial organisms rarely may cause infective spondylitis,[916, 1011] which may be associated with intradiscal gas.

Bacteroides and Related Anaerobic Infection

In comparison to clostridia, which are spore-forming obligate anaerobic bacteria, Bacteroides, Fusobacterium, Propionibacterium, Leptotrichia, Lactobacillus, Peptococcus, Peptostreptococcus, Veillonella, and several strains of Eikenella represent some of the non-spore-forming obligate anaerobes. Many of these organisms exist as part of the normal microflora on the skin and adjacent mucous membranes, including those in the lower intestinal tract, vagina,

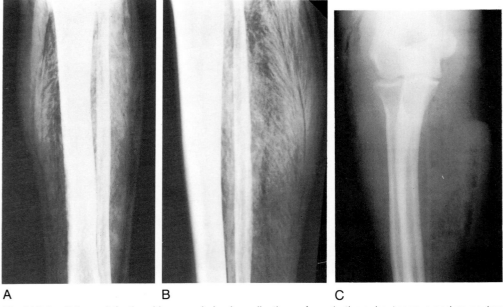

A   B   C

FIGURE 66–12. Clostridial soft tissue infection. Linear and circular collections of gas in the subcutaneous and muscular tissues reflect the presence of clostridial myositis and cellulitis.

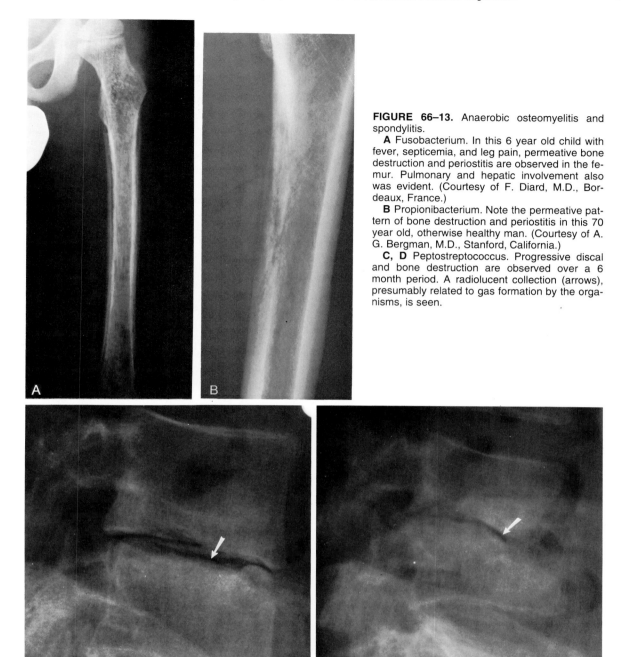

FIGURE 66–13. Anaerobic osteomyelitis and spondylitis.

A Fusobacterium. In this 6 year old child with fever, septicemia, and leg pain, permeative bone destruction and periostitis are observed in the femur. Pulmonary and hepatic involvement also was evident. (Courtesy of F. Diard, M.D., Bordeaux, France.)

B Propionibacterium. Note the permeative pattern of bone destruction and periostitis in this 70 year old, otherwise healthy man. (Courtesy of A. G. Bergman, M.D., Stanford, California.)

C, D Peptostreptococcus. Progressive discal and bone destruction are observed over a 6 month period. A radiolucent collection (arrows), presumably related to gas formation by the organisms, is seen.

urethra, and gingiva. Clinically evident infections result when breaks in the mucosa or skin allow the microflora to become displaced into deeper tissues and to reach the blood stream, and generally they relate to the presence of more than one type of anaerobe. Characteristics of such infections include localization to a site normally inhabited by anaerobic bacteria, traumatic disruption of the skin or mucous membrane, and a history of diabetes mellitus, other chronic debilitating diseases, recent surgical procedures, aspiration of mouth contents, or a human or animal bite.

With regard to the musculoskeletal system, crepitant cellulitis, necrotizing fasciitis, and myonecrosis are typical expressions of anaerobic infections related primarily to contamination of contiguous tissue. Septic arthritis, infective spondylitis, and osteomyelitis[644–649, 1012–1015] are rare and may

be manifestations of hematogenous dissemination (Fig. 66–13). Gas formation in the soft tissues or, rarely, the articular cavity or intervertebral disc aids in precise radiographic diagnosis.

The relationship of Propionibacterium infection, pustulosis palmaris et plantaris, and sternocostoclavicular hyperostosis is discussed in Chapter 93.

Mycobacteria

Tuberculous Infection

Frequency and Pattern. The frequency of tuberculosis has changed dramatically since the advent of appropriate chemotherapy for this disease.[128, 523] Even when pulmonary tuberculosis was a common and largely uncontrolled disorder, musculoskeletal involvement was not very frequent, occurring in approximately 10 cases per 10,000 subjects.[1, 129, 130] In the 1940s and 1950s, osseous involvement occurred in approximately 3 to 5 per cent of tuberculous patients, although in persons with extrapulmonary tuberculosis, the frequency of skeletal abnormalities was approximately 30 per cent.[1] These statistics varied with the country (as well as with the racial population) under consideration, the prevalence of the disease being greater in impoverished, undernourished, and overcrowded areas. Currently, the frequency of tuberculosis in general, and of skeletal tuberculosis in particular, has diminished, although the use of modern therapeutic techniques, including BCG vaccination, has produced examples of iatrogenic infection (see discussion later in this chapter).

Furthermore, the pattern of osteoarticular tuberculosis has changed over the years.[23] Initially, the disease usually was encountered in children and young adults; currently, patients of all ages are affected. Persons with underlying disorders, those receiving corticosteroid medication, alcoholic patients, intravenous drug abusers, persons who harbor the human immunodeficiency virus, and immigrants are not infrequent hosts for this disease.[131–133, 650–652, 928] In the past, two modes of infection were recognized: inhalation and ingestion.[134] The latter mechanism was more common for the bovine tubercle bacillus, *Mycobacterium bovis,* and was responsible for approximately 20 per cent of all cases of bone and joint tuberculosis, especially in children.[135, 652] This mechanism of infection largely has been eradicated, although *Mycobacterium tuberculosis* remains an important source of the musculoskeletal alterations. Although such alterations are considered to result from hematogenous infection secondary to tuberculosis at a distant site, rarely no primary lesion can be found.[136]

Tuberculous spondylitis is the most typical form of the disease, the spine being involved in more than 25 per cent (and probably more than 50 per cent) of cases of skeletal tuberculosis. In recent years, however, articular changes in extraspinal sites, such as the hip, the knee, the wrist, and the elbow, have been more prominent.[134, 651] Tuberculous dactylitis, multiple sites of involvement, and tendon sheath abnormalities also are encountered commonly.

Clinical Abnormalities. Skeletal tuberculosis can affect persons of all ages, although it is rare in the first year of life. No significant predilection for either sex is seen. The vertebral column, the hip, and the knee are the most frequent sites of involvement. The joints of the lower extremity are affected more commonly than are those of the upper extremity.

The presenting symptoms and signs of the disease vary considerably.[1, 134] Tuberculous arthritis can lead to pain, swelling, weakness, muscle wasting, a draining sinus, and other manifestations, which may be present for 1 to 2 years prior to diagnosis. A history of local trauma may be obtained in 30 to 50 per cent of cases. Tuberculous spondylitis is first manifested clinically with the insidious onset of back pain, stiffness, local tenderness, and possibly fever. Neurologic abnormalities also may be apparent. In fact, paralysis is encountered as a result of spinal cord compression from abscesses, granulation tissue or bone fragments, arachnoiditis, ischemia of the cord resulting from endarteritis, or intramedullary granulomas. The mortality rate for tubercu-

lous spondylitis, reported previously as 26 to 30 per cent,[1] has decreased in recent years but still is relatively high. This form of tuberculosis is associated most clearly with pulmonary disease. Tuberculous dactylitis usually appears as painless swelling of the hand or the foot. Tuberculous tenosynovitis and bursitis can produce soft tissue swelling and tenderness in the ulnar or radial bursa, the fingers, and the toes.[137]

A positive skin test for tuberculosis is of little help in the diagnosis of this disease, although a negative skin test usually (but not invariably) excludes the diagnosis. A negative chest radiograph in the adult patient does not exclude the possibility of skeletal tuberculosis. In a child, such a radiograph makes tuberculosis an unlikely cause of bony abnormalities. The disorder is confirmed by the demonstration of the tubercle bacilli in smear or culture; this may require aspiration of joint contents or biopsy of the synovial membrane in cases of tuberculous arthritis and closed or open biopsy of bone in cases of tuberculous osteomyelitis.[23, 138, 1266]

Pathogenesis. It generally is accepted that skeletal involvement in tuberculosis occurs mainly by the hematogenous route. The localization to metaphyseal segments of long bones is noted in this disease as in hematogenously derived pyogenic osteomyelitis, perhaps related to tuberculous infarcts from emboli within the nutrient vessels[181] or to an obliterative endarteritis.[182]

Hematogenous seeding of the skeleton may arise from a primary infection of the lung, particularly in children, or, at a later date, from a quiescent primary site or an extraosseous focus. With healing of the primary complex, there is a tendency toward resolution of skeletal foci, most healing without residua.[77] Occasionally, reactivation of bone and joint tuberculosis is evident. This phenomenon may occur after decreased local resistance (e.g., trauma, debilitation)[183] and is especially frequent in the hip.[134]

The frequency of associated visceral disease in patients with skeletal tuberculosis varies with the age of the patient and the method of tissue analysis (clinical, surgical, radiographic, pathologic).[177] Pulmonary involvement may be evident in 50 per cent of cases, is more frequent in children, and on radiographs may appear either active or inactive; urogenital lesions may coexist with skeletal involvement in 20 to 45 per cent of cases.[182–186]

General Pathologic Considerations. Although the specific response to tuberculosis is influenced by the anatomic structure of the skeletal part that is affected, some general characteristics can be noted.[1] The typical response of the tissue is the formation of tubercles that are sharply demarcated from the surrounding tissue (Fig. 66–14). Around a central zone are clusters of epithelioid cells with elongated vesicular nuclei. In the central part of the tubercle are multinucleated giant cells, whereas at the periphery of the tubercle is a mantle of lymphocytes.

Central caseating necrosis is characteristic of these tubercles, incited by the tuberculin produced by the bacilli.[1] During the progression of necrosis, the epithelioid cells degenerate and become grouped into an amorphous mass. Peripheral growth of the tubercle relates to the influx of new mononuclear cells, which mature into the epithelioid cells, a process that continues so long as neighboring viable tubercle bacilli are present. A prominent role of degenerating bacilli in tubercle formation also is probable.

Healing of lesions is associated with the production of

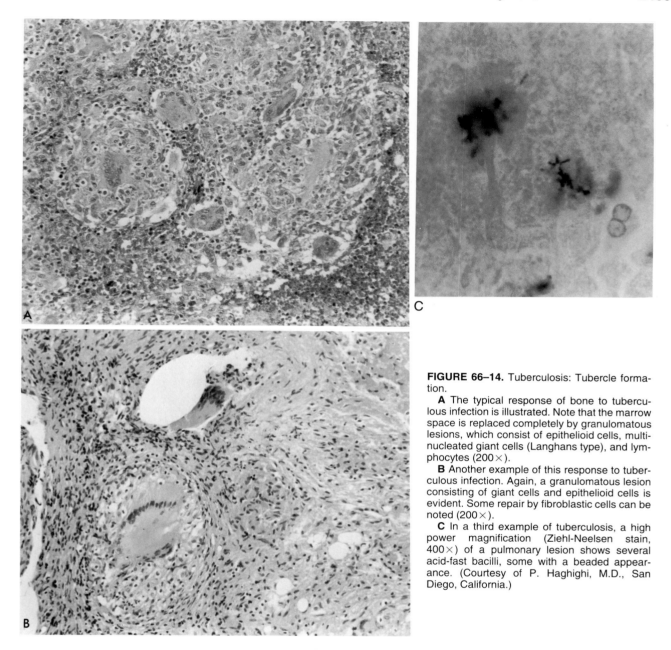

FIGURE 66–14. Tuberculosis: Tubercle formation.

A The typical response of bone to tuberculous infection is illustrated. Note that the marrow space is replaced completely by granulomatous lesions, which consist of epithelioid cells, multinucleated giant cells (Langhans type), and lymphocytes (200×).

B Another example of this response to tuberculous infection. Again, a granulomatous lesion consisting of giant cells and epithelioid cells is evident. Some repair by fibroblastic cells can be noted (200×).

C In a third example of tuberculosis, a high power magnification (Ziehl-Neelsen stain, 400×) of a pulmonary lesion shows several acid-fast bacilli, some with a beaded appearance. (Courtesy of P. Haghighi, M.D., San Diego, California.)

hyaline fibrous nodules. Encapsulation of large caseous foci may lead ultimately to tubercle replacement with a connective tissue scar. Calcification and ossification of caseating lesions also may be encountered.

It should be emphasized that granulomatous disease, including that of the bone marrow, is a nonspecific response to a persistent antigenic stimulus and has been identified in a wide range of illnesses (Table 66–1).[653] This has led to attempts to subdivide granulomas according to specific histologic aberrations. A proliferative or epithelioid granuloma (with or without giant cells or areas of caseation) is characteristic of tuberculosis, sarcoidosis, lymphoma, and infectious mononucleosis; suppurative granulomas may be seen in a variety of infections, including lymphogranuloma venereum, brucellosis, tularemia, and cat-scratch disease.[653] Such attempts at classification are difficult and, sometimes, inaccurate. Rather, it is suggested that the most accurate diagnosis of the nature of marrow granulomatous disease requires evaluation of the tissue derived from a second biopsy after specific therapy has been instituted; a decrease in size or disappearance of the granuloma is indicative of the appropriateness of the therapeutic regimen.[653]

Tuberculous Spondylitis

History. Tuberculous spondylitis is a disease of antiquity, having been described in a mummy from the time of 3000 BCE[139, 515] and in the writings of Hippocrates (450 BCE).[140] The first full account of the disease belongs to Pott in 1779.[141]

Frequency and Distribution. Currently it is estimated that the vertebral column is affected in 25 to 60 per cent of cases of skeletal tuberculosis.[1, 142] The first lumbar vertebra is affected most commonly and the frequency of involvement decreases equally on proceeding in either direction from this level.[142] The disease is relatively infrequent in the cervical and sacral segments of the vertebral column, although tuberculous infection of the upper cervical

TABLE 66–1. Diseases Associated with Bone Marrow Granuloma

Infectious Diseases
  Bacterial Infections and Exposures
    Mycobacterial diseases
      Tuberculosis
      BCG vaccination
      Leprosy
    Brucellosis
    Tularemia
    Glanders
  Fungal Infections (Disseminated)
    Histoplasmosis
    Cryptococcosis
    Paracoccidioidomycosis
    Saccharomyces cerevisiae infection
  Viral Infections
    Infectious mononucleosis
    Cytomegalovirus infection
    Viral hepatitis
  Parasitic Infections
    Toxoplasmosis
    Leishmaniasis
  Other
    Rocky Mountain spotted fever
    Q-fever
    Mycoplasma pneumoniae infection

Malignant Diseases
  Hodgkin's disease
  Non-Hodgkin's lymphoma
  Metastatic carcinoma
  Acute lymphocytic leukemia

Drugs
  Chlorpropamide
  Phenylbutazone (oxyphenbutazone)
  Allopurinol
  Procainamide
  Ibuprofen
  Phenytoin

Autoimmune or Allergic Diseases
  Rheumatoid arthritis (Felty's syndrome)
  Systemic lupus erythematosus
  Primary biliary cirrhosis
  Farmer's lung

Miscellaneous
  Syndrome of marrow and lymph node granuloma, uveitis, and
    reversible renal failure
  Berylliosis
  Sarcoidosis

(From Bodem CR, et al: Medicine 62:372, 1983. ©1983, The Williams & Wilkins Co, Baltimore.)

Forssman[146] noted that 82 per cent of early spinal tuberculosis began in the anterior portion of the vertebral body and only 18 per cent originated in the posterior portion.

Men are affected slightly more frequently than women. Tuberculous spondylitis can occur in children or in adults.

Cause and Pathogenesis. Tuberculous spondylitis is generally accepted to result from hematogenous spread of infection. A debate has existed whether the primary vascular pathway is supplied by the arterial route or the paravertebral venous plexus of Batson. It is Hodgson's belief that the latter vascular system is more important in the dissemination of tuberculosis to the spine,[142] a belief that is founded on several observations: the unusual predilection for spinal tuberculosis to involve the thoracolumbar junction; the higher frequency of spinal involvement in tuberculosis than in pyogenic osteomyelitis, in which the arterial tree appears important in vertebral contamination; the failure to produce spinal tuberculosis experimentally by injecting the bacilli locally into the vertebrae or into the left ventricle of the heart[147]; the similarity in the distribution of spinal tuberculosis and pyogenic infectious spondylitis after urologic procedures, in which Batson's plexus may be an important pathway[148]; and the production of tuberculous spinal lesions by injecting the bacilli into the abdominal or pelvic organs. Although these findings implicate the venous plexus in the spread of tuberculosis to the vertebral column, they are not incontrovertible, and a final judgment must await additional experimental or anatomic studies.

Radiographic-Pathologic Correlation. The radiographic

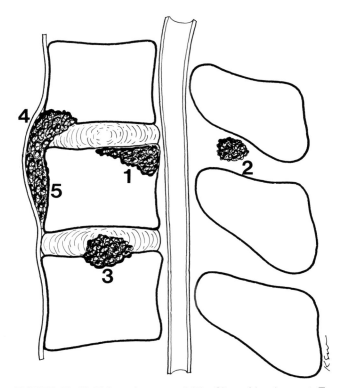

FIGURE 66–15. Tuberculous spondylitis: Sites of involvement. Tuberculous lesions can localize in the vertebral body (1) or, more rarely, the posterior osseous or ligamentous structures (2). Extension to the intervertebral disc (3) or prevertebral tissues (4) is not infrequent. Subligamentous spread (5) can lead to erosion of the anterior vertebral surface.

spine[1016–1018, 1250] and lumbosacral junction[1019] has received recent attention, and involvement of the sacroiliac joint[1020] is not rare. Although solitary lesions are not uncommon,[655] especially in the cervical spine, more than one vertebra typically is affected, and it is not unusual for as many as five or ten to be altered.[1] Involved vertebrae can be located in one segment of the spine, suggesting that the disease began in a single focus and spread to neighboring vertebrae by violating the intervertebral disc. Separate foci of tuberculosis can be detected in 1 to 4 per cent of cases, however.[143] With regard to its location within the vertebra, the vertebral body is involved more commonly than the posterior elements, although these latter structures may be affected initially or predominantly in some persons[144, 145, 1021, 1022] (Fig. 66–15), leading to neurologic compromise or spinal instability. In the vertebral body, an anterior predilection is striking. In a radiographic study, Westermark and

and pathologic features of tuberculous spondylitis have been described exhaustively.[1, 47, 134, 142, 143, 149–154, 654, 1023, 1024]

Discovertebral Lesion. In most cases, tuberculous spondylitis begins as an infectious focus in the anterior aspect of the vertebral body adjacent to the subchondral bone plate (Fig. 66–16). Enlargement and caseation of the lesion lead to an identifiable radiographic abnormality in approximately 2 to 5 months.[155] During this time, infection may spread to the adjacent intervertebral discs. This may occur if the bacilli extend beneath the anterior longitudinal ligament or posterior longitudinal ligament to violate the peripheral discal tissue (Fig. 66–17); if the organisms penetrate the subchondral bone plate and overlying cartilaginous endplate to enter the intervertebral disc; or if an intraosseous lesion weakens the vertebral body to such a degree that it produces a discal displacement (cartilaginous node), contamination of invading discal tissue, and subsequent spread through the defect into the intervertebral disc. Any or all of these events can lead to decrease in height of the disc space. The combination of vertebral body and discal destruction in tuberculosis is similar to that occurring in pyogenic spondylitis, although the tuberculous process usually is not rapidly progressive. Only rarely does vertebral body tuberculosis extend into the pedicles, laminae, or transverse or spinous processes.

Once infection has reached the intervertebral disc, the loose structure of the nucleus pulposus allows its further dissemination. Extension into neighboring vertebral bodies and intervertebral discs subsequently may become evident, and eventually long segments of the spine can be affected.

Paraspinal Extension. Extension of tuberculosis from vertebral and discal sites to the adjacent ligaments and soft tissues is frequent. This extension usually occurs anterolaterally; rarely, it is observed posteriorly in the peridural space (Fig. 66–18).[539] Once infection has been established in the paraspinal tissues, it may remain localized or extend for a considerable distance. With enlargement, the paravertebral abscesses can strip the periosteal coverings of the vertebral bodies, rendering them avascular and producing osteonecrosis.[142] Subligamentous extension of a tuberculous abscess can allow osseous and discal invasion at distant sites (Fig. 66–19). The osseous changes may be subtle, including mild contour irregularity (gouge defects) and sparing of the intervertebral discs.

Burrowing abscesses can extend for extraordinary distances before perforating an internal viscus or the body surface. The direction and extent of burrowing are influenced by the site of spinal infection, the anatomy of the adjacent soft tissues, and the effect of gravity. In the lumbar region, pus collecting beneath the fascia of the psoas muscle produces a psoas abscess, which can extend into the groin and the thigh. Among the organs and tissues that have been penetrated by paravertebral abscesses are the esophagus, bronchus, lung, mediastinum, liver, kidney, intestine, urinary bladder, rectum, vagina, and aorta; the organ involved most frequently is the lung.[156, 157, 656] Other body structures that have been violated by burrowing abscesses of tuberculosis are the abdominal wall, thigh, buttocks, and back.

Abscess formation in tuberculosis can produce soft tissue swelling on radiographs that appears out of proportion to the degree of osseous and discal destruction (Fig. 66–18). Rarely, such abscesses develop in the absence of bone and cartilage abnormalities.[657] The swelling commonly is bilat-

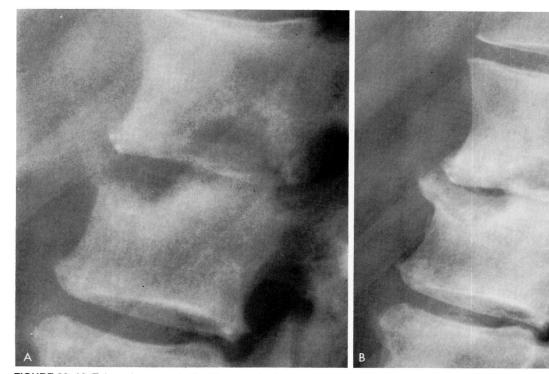

FIGURE 66–16. Tuberculous spondylitis: Discovertebral lesion.
 A The initial radiograph reveals subchondral destruction of two vertebral bodies with mild surrounding eburnation and loss of intervertebral disc height. The appearance is identical to that in pyogenic spondylitis.
 B Several months later, osseous response is evident. Note the increased sclerosis. Osteophytosis and improved definition of the osseous margins can be seen.

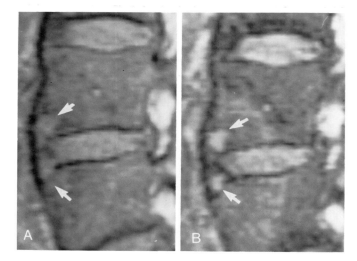

FIGURE 66–17. Tuberculous spondylitis: Discovertebral lesion. In a 55 year old man who had had low back pain for 2 months, sagittal proton density (TR/TE, 2000/30) **(A)** and T2-weighted (TR/TE, 2000/70) **(B)** spin echo MR images show tuberculous changes at the L3-L4 spinal level. Note anterior lesions of the vertebral bodies (arrows) with bowing of the adjacent anterior longitudinal ligament and contamination of the anterior portion of the L3-L4 intervertebral disc. The lesions are of higher signal intensity in **B**. (Courtesy of P. VanderStoep, M.D., St. Cloud, Minnesota.)

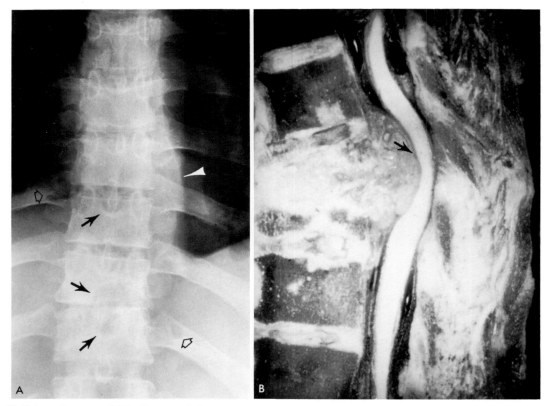

FIGURE 66–18. Tuberculous spondylitis: Paraspinal abscess.

A Tuberculous spondylitis, resulting in vertebral and discal destruction (solid arrows), has been complicated by paraspinal swelling (arrowhead). Rib involvement also is seen (open arrows).

B Tuberculous spondylitis, producing vertebral and discal destruction, is associated with posterior extension, causing encroachment on the spinal cord (arrow). (Courtesy of The Arthritis Foundation.)

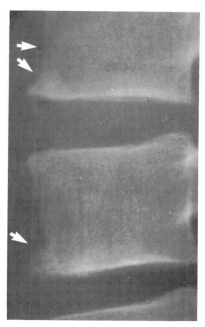

FIGURE 66–19. Tuberculous spondylitis: Subligamentous extension. The findings, although subtle, include erosion of the anterior surface of the vertebral bodies (arrows). (Courtesy of C. Resnik, M.D., Baltimore, Maryland.)

eral and fusiform, associated with scalloping of the anterior and lateral aspects of the vertebral bodies. Psoas abscesses usually are easy to identify and may contain calcification (Fig. 66–20). Nontuberculous psoas abscesses rarely calcify. Tuberculous abscesses of the psoas muscle calcify in two distinct patterns: faint amorphous deposits, which may become quite dense with progressive healing; and teardrop-shaped calcification.[152] In either situation, the calcification appears in the paraspinal area between L1 and L5. In rare instances, diminution or disappearance of such calcification may be observed on serial radiographs.[1025]

Although psoas abscess formation can complicate 5 per cent of cases of tuberculous spondylitis, abscesses also may appear in nontuberculous conditions. Examples include inflammatory intestinal disorders (diverticulitis, appendicitis, Crohn's disease, perinephric abscess), postpartum or postoperative infections, bowel neoplasm with necrosis, and trauma with secondary infection.[152, 158–160] Implicated organisms in these cases include staphylococcus and gram-negative agents.

Other diagnostic methods, including ultrasonography, CT, and MR imaging, can provide important information in patients with psoas or paraspinal abscesses.[658–664,929,932,1026–1031] The first of these techniques is sensitive in this clinical situation but is limited by the presence of adjacent intestinal gas, overlying dressings, and surgical appliances.[658] CT is even more sensitive in the detection of these abscesses and is less affected by gaseous collections in the intestinal tract; accurate interpretation of the CT scans requires the examiner's familiarity with regional anatomy.[664] Transaxial images generally are sufficient, although the use of reformatted displays and intravenous contrast agents occasionally is required. CT findings indicative of abscess include an abnormal mass of low attenuation number, displacement of surrounding structures, obliteration of normal fascial

planes, a "rind" sign (consisting of a rim of increased tissue attenuation that enhances after intravenous administration of contrast material), and abnormal gaseous collections.[658] Intraspinal extension of the process also may be apparent. None of these findings is specific for infection, as hematomas and tumors produce similar alterations; none distinguishes between tuberculous and nontuberculous abscesses, although calcification is more frequent in tuberculosis.

With regard to MR imaging of tuberculous spondylitis, this technique in common with CT provides an accurate display of paraspinal and intraspinal extension of disease as well as of the extent of bone and disc involvement (Figs. 66–21 and 66–22). Furthermore, sagittal images in addition to transaxial images may be obtained so that long segments of the spine may be evaluated.[1029] MR imaging provides more information in these cases than does routine radiography, and some of the features (such as posterior vertebral body and pediculate involvement and focal soft tissue masses) resemble those of neoplasm.[1031] Although one report has indicated the presence of high signal intensity in diseased areas on T1-weighted spin echo MR images,[1030] low signal intensity on such images and high signal intensity on T2-weighted images are more typical (Figs. 66–23 and 66–24).[1031] These MR imaging findings are similar to those of pyogenic spondylitis, although preservation of discal morphology and normal discal signal intensity, posterior element involvement, large and sometimes calcified paraspinal masses, and subligamentous spread of infection are more characteristic of tuberculosis.[1031] Also, involvement of several segments of the spine and of several contiguous vertebral bodies and focal, rather than diffuse, involvement of bone suggest the diagnosis of tuberculosis. The MR imaging findings (as well as the routine radiographic findings) of tuberculous and brucellar spondylitis are similar, however.[1032]

Posterior Element Lesions. Occasionally, the posterior elements may be the initial spinal site of tuberculosis (Fig. 66–25). In these instances, radiographic findings include pediculate or laminal destruction, erosion of the posterior cortex of the vertebral body and adjacent ribs, a large paraspinal mass, and relative sparing of the intervertebral discs.[47, 145, 538, 665, 666, 1021, 1022] Single or multiple levels may be affected. With involvement of the pedicles, paraplegia is frequent owing to granulomatous extension into the spinal canal. During the reparative phase, the pedicles may be reconstituted. Differential diagnosis of tuberculous spondylitis of the posterior elements includes other infections and neoplasms.

Solitary Vertebral Involvement. Rarely, tuberculosis leads to isolated involvement of a single vertebral body.[47, 1251] In adults, osseous destruction will resemble that which is evident in tumors or with cartilaginous node formation (Fig. 66–26).[538, 667] In children or adults, vertebra plana can appear, simulating the appearance of eosinophilic granuloma (Fig. 66–27).

Vertebra Within a Vertebra. The appearance of growth recovery lines within single or multiple vertebrae in patients with tuberculosis has been noted by O'Brien.[161] These are analogous to those lines within bones of the appendicular skeleton that accompany chronic illnesses in children.

Kyphosis. Collapse of partially destroyed vertebral bodies during the course of tuberculous spondylitis can lead to

Text continued on page 2472

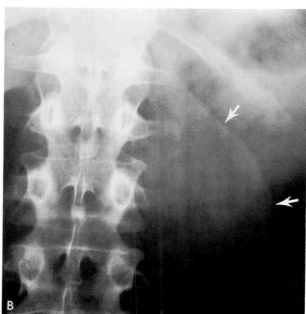

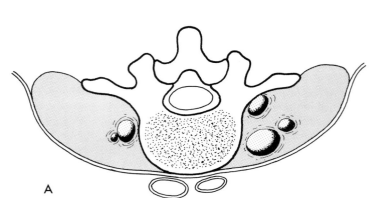

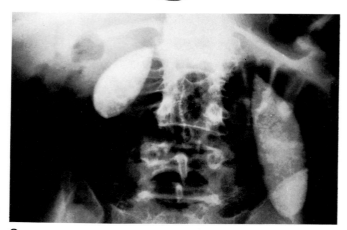

FIGURE 66–20. Tuberculous spondylitis: Psoas abscess.

A The typical appearance of bilateral and fusiform psoas abscesses is illustrated in a cross-sectional drawing through a lumbar vertebral body.

B A large left noncalcified psoas abscess (arrows) can be seen.

C Diffusely calcified psoas abscesses are noted in association with spinal abnormalities.

FIGURE 66–21. Tuberculous spondylitis: Paraspinal and intraspinal extension—MR imaging.

A, B In this patient, a coronal proton density (TR/TE, 2800/19) spin echo MR image **(A)** shows paraspinal extension of disease, more evident on the right side (arrows), originating from a discovertebral lesion (arrowhead). A coronal T2-weighted (TR/TE, 1800/80) spin echo image **(B)** confirms psoas extension (arrows). (Courtesy of R. Kerr, M.D., Los Angeles, California.)

C, D In a different patient, a sagittal T1-weighted (TR/TE, 767/20) spin echo MR image **(C)** demonstrates both anterior (arrow) and posterior (arrowhead) extension of disease. A coronal T1-weighted (TR/TE, 767/20) spin echo image **(D)** reveals more prominent extension on the left side (arrows) with displacement of the kidney. Note regions of low signal intensity (arrowheads) in the abscess, consistent with fluid. (Courtesy of T. Broderick, M.D., Orange, California.)

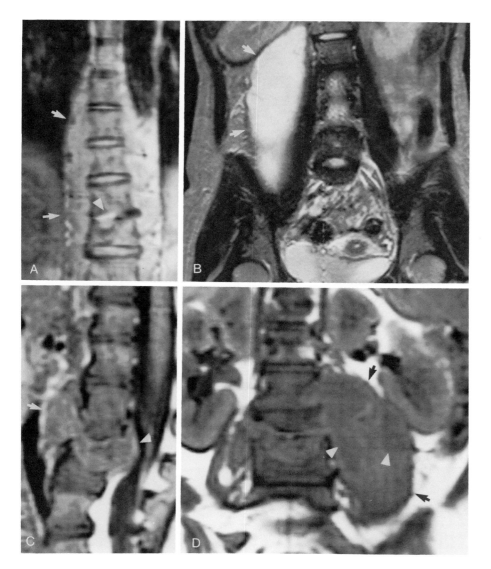

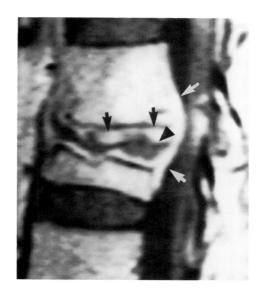

FIGURE 66–22. Tuberculous spondylitis: Intraspinal extension—MR imaging. A sagittal T1-weighted (TR/TE, 700/20) spin echo MR image after the intravenous administration of a gadolinium-based contrast agent reveals enhancement of signal intensity (arrows) in the discovertebral region and anterior epidural space. Note low signal intensity centrally (arrowhead). The findings are consistent with an abscess. (Courtesy of H. S. Kang, M.D., Seoul, Korea.)

FIGURE 66–23. Tuberculous spondylitis: Discovertebral lesion—MR imaging. In a 40 year old woman, a sagittal proton density (TR/TE, 3000/18) spin echo MR image **(A)** shows discovertebral destruction and posterior extension (arrow) of the infection. With T2 weighting (TR/TE, 3000/90) **(B),** the discovertebral and anterior epidural (arrow) foci of infection show higher signal intensity. Note subligamentous extension (arrowheads) of infection as well. (Courtesy of J. Hodler, M.D., Zurich, Switzerland.)

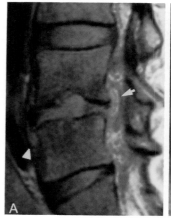
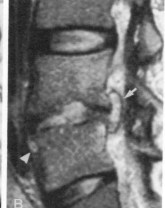

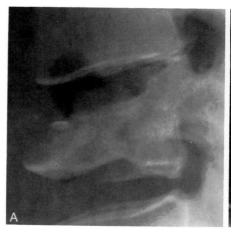
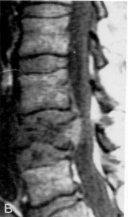
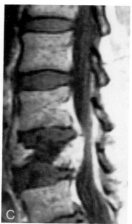

FIGURE 66–24. Tuberculous spondylitis: Vertebral lesion—MR imaging.

A The routine radiograph shows fracture and collapse of the fourth lumbar vertebral body with minimal discal changes.

B, C Sagittal T1-weighted (TR/TE, 550/20) spin echo MR images obtained prior to **(B)** and after **(C)** intravenous administration of a gadolinium contrast agent reveal the extent of the process. In **B,** the signal intensity in the involved vertebral body is decreased. In **C,** it is increased.

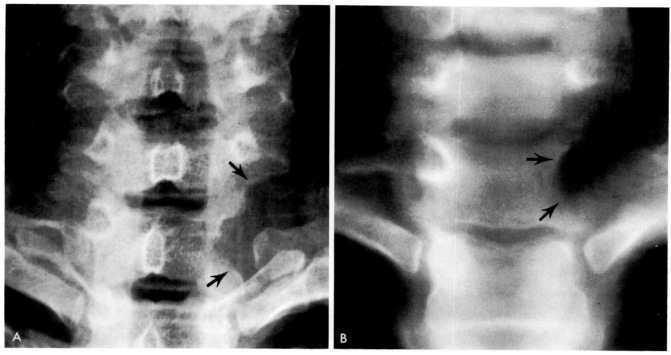

FIGURE 66–25. Tuberculous spondylitis: Posterior element lesions.
A Observe destruction of the left pedicle and lateral mass of the seventh cervical vertebra (arrows).
B The abnormalities are better delineated on anteroposterior conventional tomography (arrows).

FIGURE 66–26. Tuberculous spondylitis: Solitary vertebral involvement.
A collapsed vertebral body (arrow) represents the site of tuberculous involvement in this adult patient.

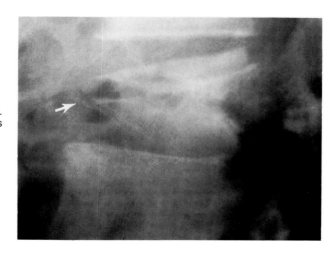

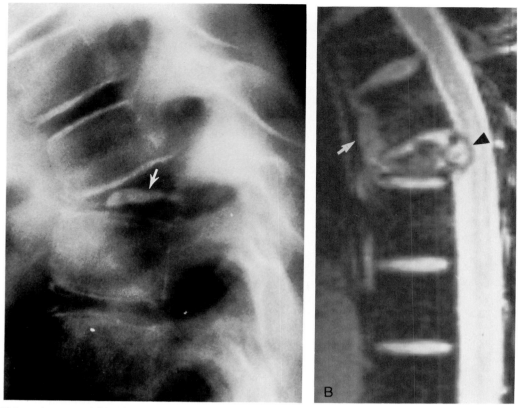

FIGURE 66–27. Tuberculous spondylitis: Vertebra plana and kyphosis.
  A In this child, a wafer-like remnant of the infected vertebral body can be seen (arrow). Abnormal kyphosis is present. The adjacent vertebrae appear normal. (Courtesy of A. D'Abreu, M.D., Porto Alegre, Brazil.)
  B In a different patient, a sagittal multiplanar gradient recalled (MPGR) image (TR/TE, 425/12; flip angle, 20 degrees) shows vertebral plana and anterior (arrow) and posterior (arrowhead) extension of disease.

severe deformities. Typically, an angulated posterior projection appears at the site of maximum spinal involvement, leading to tuberculous kyphosis or gibbus deformity.[1033] The degree of angulation varies with the site and extent of vertebral disease; angulation is more acute in the thoracic spine than in the cervical or lumbar region, and it is more severe when only one or two vertebrae are affected.[1] Despite the striking nature of the deformity, the diameter of the spinal canal may not be altered significantly. Radiography indicates destroyed and, rarely, extruded[1034] vertebral

bodies in the area of angulation (Fig. 66–28) and, in some cases of thoracic kyphosis, a remarkable increase in height of the vertebral bodies in the lordotic lumbar area.[143] Such "long" vertebrae are found only in those cases in which the growth of the vertebral bodies had not ceased at the time the disease affected the thoracic spine; they also are observed in other conditions associated with spinal deformity. A variety of operative techniques have been advocated in the treatment of tuberculous kyphosis.[162]

Scoliosis. Although not so frequent as kyphosis, lateral

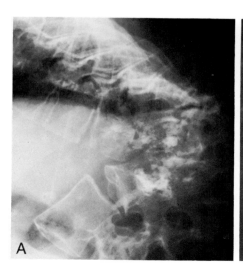
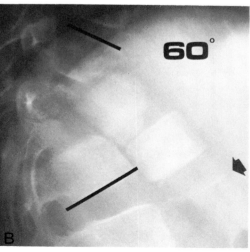

FIGURE 66–28. Tuberculous spondylitis: Kyphosis.
  A Severe thoracolumbar kyphosis, associated with calcification and an increased superoinferior dimension of a lumbar vertebral body, is evident. (Courtesy of T. Yochum, D.C., Denver, Colorado.)
  B In this patient, the vertebral bodies of T11 and T12 are seen in front of the first lumbar vertebral body. An arrow marks the superior endplate of L1. Using the horizontal lines, a kyphotic angle of 60 degrees is present. (From Louw JA, et al: Spine *12*:942, 1987.)

deviation of the spine can occur in tuberculous spondylitis.[142, 163] This accompanies asymmetric or unilateral destruction of vertebral bodies and intervertebral discs and is virtually confined to the lower thoracic and lumbar vertebrae.

Bony Ankylosis of Vertebral Bodies. Healing in tuberculous spondylitis can be associated with osseous fusion of vertebral bodies. This manifestation, which also is evident in congenital block vertebrae and after trauma or other infectious diseases, leads to partial or complete obliteration of the intervening intervertebral disc. Not uncommonly, four to eight vertebrae are coalesced into a large osseous mass, particularly in areas of angular spinal deformity.

Ivory Vertebrae. Increased radiodensity of the vertebral body in tuberculosis can lead to an ivory vertebra.[164] This phenomenon usually is evident in the lumbar region in association with healing of the disease. At surgery, the involved vertebrae are hard; histologic examination reveals revascularization and reossification, apparently indicating a healing response to osteonecrosis.[142]

Atlantoaxial Destruction. Tuberculosis involving the upper cervical spine is a rare but important manifestation of the disease, occurring in fewer than 2 per cent of cases of tuberculous spondylitis.[655, 668–673, 885, 1016–1018] Clinical manifestations include pain and decreased range of motion in the neck, dysphagia, and weakness in one or more extremities. Quadriparesis may be observed in as many as 40 per cent of patients with cervical tuberculosis in general.[674] Radiographic abnormalities include occipitoatlantoaxial subluxation, bone erosion, and a prevertebral soft tissue mass (Figs. 66–29 and 66–30). They may simulate the findings of trauma, accounting for a delay in accurate diagnosis. Furthermore, identical abnormalities are seen in occasional cases of fungal infection.

Extraosseous, Extradural Granuloma. In rare circumstances, tuberculosis leads to an extradural granulomatous lesion in the absence of bone involvement.[666, 675, 886] This manifestation is more common in men than in women, in the dorsal epidural space, and in the thoracic segment (and should be distinguished from a similar finding that is observed more frequently in tuberculous patients with osseous and discal destruction). Clinically, compressive radiculomyelopathy is evident. On pathologic examination, a thick granulomatous membrane ensheathing and compressing the spinal cord or cauda equina is found.[666]

Intramedullary Spinal Cord Involvement. Intramedullary involvement of the spinal cord in tuberculosis is very rare.[1035] Although young adults typically are affected, children and elderly patients also may be involved.[1036] Lesions more frequently are solitary than multiple, although addi-

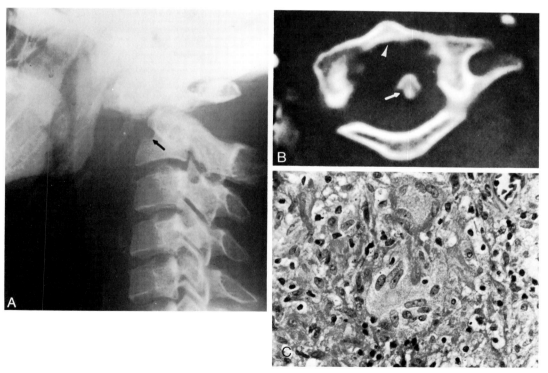

FIGURE 66–29. Tuberculous spondylitis: Atlantoaxial destruction. This 36 year old man had a 2 month history of increasing intermittent neck pain and a 1 month history of generalized weakness of all extremities with numbness in the fingers of both hands. He also had dysphagia. The patient denied previous trauma to the neck. A chest radiograph was normal but the tuberculin skin test was strongly positive.

A A lateral radiograph of the cervical spine documents a large anterior soft tissue mass displacing the pharynx. Atlantoaxial subluxation is seen, the odontoid process is poorly visualized, and an erosion of the anterior portion of the axis is present (arrow).

B A transaxial CT scan at the level of the atlas confirms the presence of atlantoaxial subluxation. Note the increased space between the anterior arch of the atlas (arrowhead) and the odontoid process (arrow). Observe that the latter is displaced laterally, indicating rotation between the two bones. Osseous erosion of both the odontoid process and the atlas is evident.

C Histologic evaluation of material obtained from the soft tissue mass shows granulomatous inflammatory changes consisting of multinucleated giant cells, epithelioid histiocytes, and chronic inflammatory cells (lymphocytes and plasma cells) (hematoxylin and eosin stain, 160×). *Mycobacterium tuberculosis* was cultured from the soft tissue mass and bone.

(From Dowd CF, et al: Skel Radiol *15:*65, 1986.)

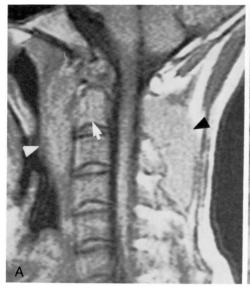
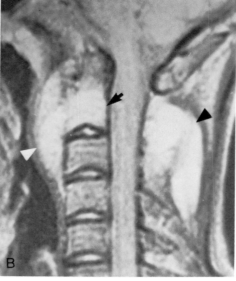

FIGURE 66–30. Tuberculous spondylitis: Atlantoaxial destruction. In a 23 year old man, sagittal T1-weighted (TR/TE, 450/30) **(A)** and more T2-weighted (TR/TE, 1800/50) **(B)** spin echo MR images reveal tuberculous involvement of the upper cervical spine. Findings include abnormalities of the axis (arrows) with anterior and posterior extension of the process (arrowheads). (Courtesy of T. Mattsson, M.D., Riyadh, Saudia Arabia.)

tional lesions of the spinal cord or brain, or both, may be encountered.[1252] Accurate diagnosis is accomplished with MR imaging (see Chapter 65), particularly when a patient has typical clinical manifestations and evidence of active tuberculosis at other sites.

Differential Diagnosis. The differential diagnosis of tuberculous spondylitis includes a wide variety of other infectious disorders of the spine. Differentiation of tuberculous and pyogenic vertebral osteomyelitis can be extremely difficult. Clinical data that favor a diagnosis of tuberculosis are an insidious onset of symptoms, a typical tuberculous pulmonary infiltrate, the late onset of paraplegia after back pain of many months' duration, and a normal erythrocyte sedimentation rate.[47] Radiographic features favoring tuberculosis are involvement of one or more segments of the spine, a delay in destruction of intervertebral discs, a large and calcified paravertebral mass, and absence of sclerosis. None of the radiographic findings is pathognomonic of tuberculosis. Furthermore, reactive bony eburnation, which is common in pyogenic osteomyelitis, also is encountered in tuberculosis, particularly in the black race.[153]

Tuberculous spondylitis may simulate tumor. Intervertebral disc space destruction is more characteristic of infectious lesions of the spine, although it occasionally is evident in neoplastic disorders. Scalloping of the anterior surface of the vertebral bodies, evident in tuberculosis with subligamentous spread, also can be seen with paravertebral lymphadenopathy due to metastasis, myeloma, or lymphoma. Sarcoidosis can produce multifocal lesions of vertebrae and intervertebral discs with paraspinal masses, findings identical to those of tuberculosis.

Tuberculous Osteomyelitis

Frequency and Distribution. Tuberculous osteomyelitis can remain localized to bone or involve adjacent joints. In general, tuberculosis confined to bone is relatively infrequent; occasionally, however, a tuberculous focus in one or more osseous structures is not associated with tuberculous arthritis. Virtually any bone can be affected, including the pelvis, the phalanges and metacarpals (tuberculous dactylitis), the long bones, the ribs, the sternum, the scapula, the skull (Fig. 66–31), the patella, and the carpal and tarsal regions.[133, 134, 165–169, 542, 543, 564, 676–687, 1037–1048, 1275]

In the long tubular bones, tuberculosis usually originates in one of the epiphyses and soon spreads into the neighboring joint (Fig. 66–32). In fact, tuberculous osteomyelitis originating in the shaft of a long bone represents fewer than 1 per cent of all cases of the disease,[1, 688, 689, 1040, 1042] although in Chinese patients, the frequency is somewhat greater.[170] Pathologic fractures also are rare.[1038] Metaphyseal foci in the child occasionally can violate the growth plate (Fig. 66–32).[677] This feature deserves emphasis, as pyogenic infections arising in the metaphyseal segment of a child's tubular bone generally do not extend across the physis. The detection of transphyseal spread of infection favors a granulomatous infectious process.

Although tuberculous osteomyelitis almost is uniformly related to hematogenous dissemination, on rare occasions it can result from the spread of adjacent infectious foci. Traveling abscesses and fistulae represent examples of this latter mechanism. In addition, tuberculous involvement of the skin, which may result from accidental injury or be related to such procedures as ear piercing and ritual circumcision when performed by carriers of the disease, can lead to osteomyelitis of adjacent bones.[690] Other examples of this mechanism of infection are rib involvement due to extra-

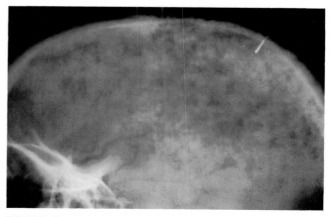

FIGURE 66–31. Tuberculous osteomyelitis: Skull. Observe widespread osteolysis of the cranial vault. (Courtesy of B. Howard, M.D., Charlotte, North Carolina.)

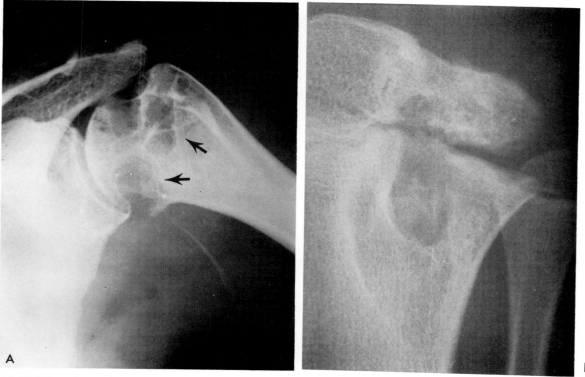

FIGURE 66–32. Tuberculous osteomyelitis: Tubular bones.
   A In this patient, an initial epiphyseal lesion (arrows) subsequently involved the glenohumeral joint. The lesions are well circumscribed, and the glenoid and acromion also are affected.
   B Transphyseal spread of a metaphyseal lesion into the epiphysis is evident in this 6 year old child.

pleural abscesses[683] and osseous contamination occurring secondary to bursal or tendon sheath disease (see later discussion).

Radiographic-Pathologic Correlation. The pathologic process is initiated by tubercle formation in the marrow with secondary infection of the trabeculae[1] (Fig. 66–33). These trabeculae are resorbed as the focus of infection enlarges and as tuberculous granulation tissue insinuates itself between the bands of spongy trabecular bone. Caseous necrosis may be prominent or limited. In the latter situation, circumscribed lytic lesions of bone may be evident, termed cystic tuberculosis (see later discussion). With caseation and liquefaction, an abscess cavity is created containing pus and small granules of bone—"bone sand."[1] About the abscess are zones of marrow-containing granulation tissue, connective tissue with cellular elements (lymphocytes, polymorphonuclear leukocytes), and sclerotic trabeculae.

On radiographs, foci of osteolysis are accompanied by varying amounts of eburnation and periostitis. Sequestrum formation can be encountered as a spicule of increased radiodensity within the zone of destruction.[1046, 1047] Intracortical lesions rarely are encountered (Fig. 66–34). The initial radiographic appearance in tuberculous osteomyelitis is similar to that in other types of osteomyelitis and even in nonaggressive or aggressive neoplasm.[1039–1041] Differentiation of tuberculous from pyogenic infection on the basis of increased osteoporosis and decreased eburnation is not feasible in most cases.

Special Types of Tuberculous Osteomyelitis

Cystic Tuberculosis. A rare variety of tuberculosis is associated with disseminated lesions of the axial and the extra-axial skeleton.[165] This variety has been associated with considerable confusion regarding terminology because of a report in 1920 by Jüngling of osteitis tuberculosa multiplex cystoides, or multiple tuberculous skeletal lesions.[171] Even though it was realized subsequently that Jüngling was describing sarcoidosis rather than tuberculosis,[172] the term osteitis tuberculosa multiplex cystoides still is employed occasionally to describe cystic tuberculosis of bone.[173]

Cystic lesions of one or multiple bones in tuberculosis are encountered much more frequently in children than in adults (Fig. 66–35). In children, these lesions usually[1267] but not invariably[1049] affect the peripheral skeleton, favor the metaphyseal regions of tubular bones, may be symmetric, are of variable size, and generally are unaccompanied by sclerosis.[165] In adults, the skull, the shoulder and pelvic girdles, and the axial skeleton are involved. In this latter age group, the lesions are small and oval, lying in the long axis of the bone, and possess well-defined margins with sclerosis.[165] It is this differing appearance in children and in adults that has led some investigators to term the juvenile lesions pseudocystic tuberculosis of bone and the adult lesions disseminated bone tuberculosis.[174]

The prognosis in this variety of tuberculosis is good. Lesions may resolve spontaneously with low morbidity or mortality.

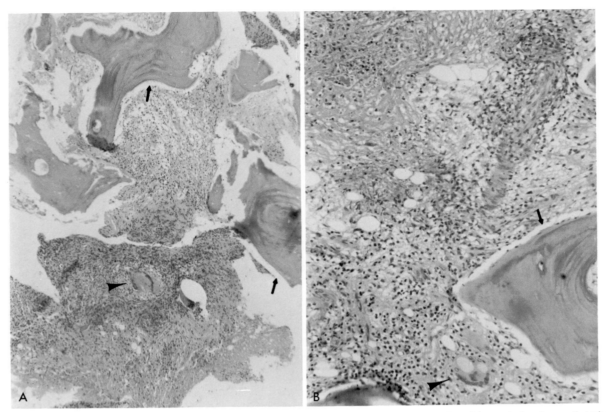

FIGURE 66–33. Tuberculous osteomyelitis: Pathologic abnormalities. Photomicrographs (80×, 200×) outline eroded and necrotic trabeculae (arrows), blood vessels with surrounding cellular inflammation, and giant cells (arrowheads).

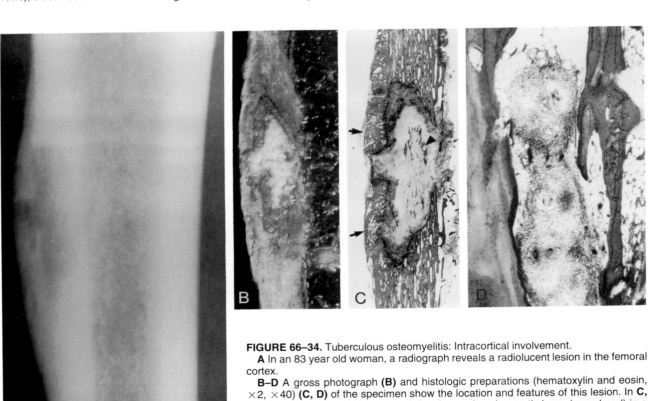

FIGURE 66–34. Tuberculous osteomyelitis: Intracortical involvement.

A In an 83 year old woman, a radiograph reveals a radiolucent lesion in the femoral cortex.

B–D A gross photograph **(B)** and histologic preparations (hematoxylin and eosin, ×2, ×40) **(C, D)** of the specimen show the location and features of this lesion. In **C,** observe subperiosteal bone remodeling (arrows) and necrotic bone (arrowhead) in a caseous mass. In **D,** note tuberculoid tissue with giant cells.

(A–D, From MacGee W, et al: Eur J Radiol *8:*96, 1988.)

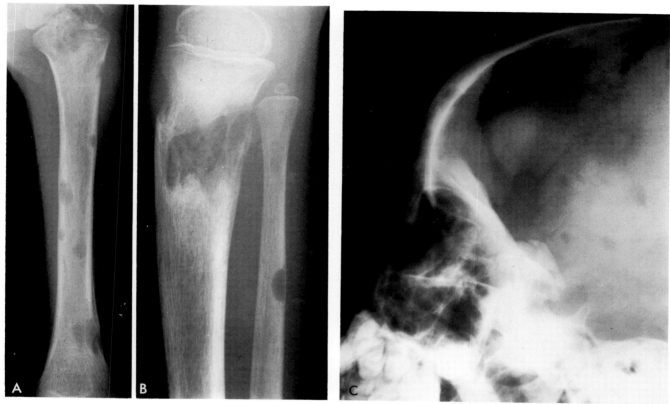

FIGURE 66–35. Cystic tuberculosis. This 5 year old girl had axillary lymph node enlargement approximately 9 months before these films were taken. Aspiration and culture documented the presence of tuberculosis. Widespread and symmetric abnormalities were present.
  A Note the well-defined lytic lesions of the medullary and cortical areas of the metaphysis and diaphysis of the humerus. The proximal epiphysis also is affected. Sclerosis is absent, although periostitis can be seen.
  B Similar lesions are present in the tibia and fibula. Some of these are central, whereas others are eccentric or peripheral.
  C Small and large radiolucent foci are detected in the cranium, simulating the appearance of histiocytosis.

The radiographic characteristics of cystic tuberculosis, which include well-defined osseous lesions with or without surrounding sclerosis,[175, 176] resemble those of eosinophilic granuloma, sarcoidosis, cystic angiomatosis, plasma cell myeloma, fungal infections, metastases, and other conditions.

Tuberculous Dactylitis. Tuberculous involvement of the short tubular bones of the hands and feet is termed tuberculous dactylitis. This form of tuberculosis is especially frequent in children, although it also is well described in adult patients.[177, 1050] In infants and young children, the reported frequency of dactylitis in cases of tuberculosis has ranged from 0.5 to 14 per cent.[178, 179] The condition decreases in frequency after the age of 5 years and becomes rare after the age of 10 years. It then increases in frequency in the adult.[177, 180] Although involvement of one bone of the hand or the foot is common, multiple osseous foci can be identified in 25 to 35 per cent of cases.[182, 183] Multiplicity is especially characteristic of childhood dactylitis.[688]

Soft tissue swelling usually is the initial manifestation and can be quite extensive. Mild or exuberant periostitis of phalanges, metacarpals, or metatarsals may be evident (Fig. 66–36). Expansion of the bone with cystic quality is termed spina ventosa and is especially common in childhood. Diaphyseal destruction with extension into the epiphysis may be associated with sequestration, sinus tracts, and growth disturbance as well as brachydactyly.

These radiographic features appear with differing frequency in the child versus the adult.[177] In childhood dactylitis, multiplicity of sites, expansion of bone, periostitis, sequestration, sinus tracts, and positive chest radiographs are more common than in dactylitis in adulthood.

The spina ventosa variety of dactylitis has received a great deal of attention. The term is derived from *spina,* meaning a spine-like projection, and *ventosa,* meaning puffed full of air,[177] and initially was applied to osseous enlargement, particularly of the diaphyses, due to marrow infiltration with tuberculous granulation tissue. Although overwhelmingly associated with tuberculous dactylitis (phalanges, metacarpals, metatarsals), a similar appearance can be evident in the radius, ulna, and humerus.[187, 188] In the hands and feet, prognosis for normal function in this cystic variety of the disease is quite good.[679]

Tuberculous dactylitis can be imitated by other conditions. Other infectious disorders of pyogenic or fungal origin may have similar manifestations. Syphilitic dactylitis in infants and children produces bilateral and symmetric involvement; in this disease, periostitis is more exuberant and soft tissue swelling is less prominent than in tuberculous dactylitis.[177] Fibrous dysplasia, hyperparathyroidism, leukemia, sarcoidosis, and sickle cell anemia may produce phalangeal, metacarpal, and metatarsal changes, although characteristic radiographic alterations at other sites allow accurate diagnosis of some of these conditions.

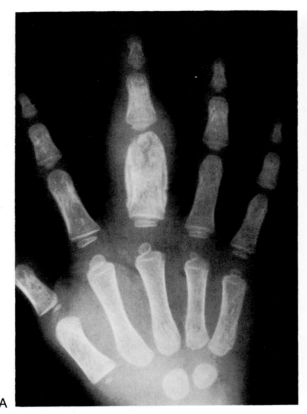 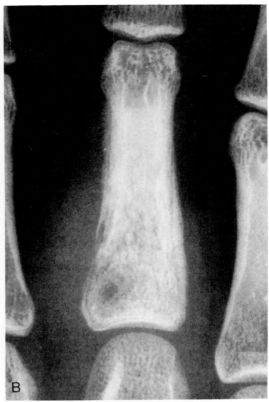

FIGURE 66–36. Tuberculous dactylitis.
A Radiographic findings in this child include soft tissue swelling of multiple digits, lytic lesions of several middle and proximal phalanges and metacarpals, and exuberant periostitis and enlargement of the proximal phalanx of the third finger.
B In a 24 year old man, soft tissue swelling, osteolysis, osteosclerosis, and periostitis are observed. (Courtesy of M. Mitchell, M.D., Halifax, Nova Scotia, Canada.)

Differential Diagnosis. Differentiation of tuberculous osteomyelitis and pyogenic osteomyelitis is difficult. Osteoporosis, bone lysis and sclerosis, and periostitis are evident in both conditions. Acute pyogenic osteomyelitis has a more rapid course and less frequently extends across the physis or to the neighboring joint than tuberculous osteomyelitis. The latter condition is associated with radiographic findings that are virtually identical to those of fungal skeletal infections.

Tuberculous Arthritis

General Features. Tuberculous arthritis most typically affects large joints such as the knee and the hip, although any articular site, including the elbow,[930] wrist,[698] sacroiliac joint,[699, 700, 1020] glenohumeral joint,[887, 1051] and joints of the hand and foot,[888, 889] can be involved.[134] Monoarticular disease is the rule,[189, 917] although polyarticular disease also is reported,[1052, 1053] being more typical in older patients.[1053] The majority of joint lesions occur secondary to adjacent osteomyelitis, although primary involvement of the synovial membrane does occur, especially in the knee.[190, 191] Additionally, fistulous communication between a joint, such as the hip, sacroiliac joint, or symphysis pubis, with the bowel, bladder, or soft tissue abscess provides a pathway for tuberculous organisms.[696] In many of these instances, however, the joint infection is the primary event leading to secondary contamination of an internal organ. With regard to tuberculous arthritis, most patients are middle-aged or elderly, and many have underlying disorders or have received intraarticular injections of steroids.[134] Tuberculous joint disease

may persist with chronic pain and only minimal signs of inflammation. Delay in diagnosis is frequent[192]; correct diagnosis requires an awareness of the role of mycobacteria in joint disease and the use of synovial fluid and tissue for culture and histologic studies.[917] The fluid is characterized by high white blood cell count, low glucose levels, and poor mucin clot formation.[193] As similar findings may be encountered in the synovial fluid in rheumatoid arthritis, culture and biopsy frequently are necessary. Synovial biopsies can be expected to reveal the histologic findings of tuberculosis in approximately 90 per cent of cases; similarly, synovial biopsies are positive on culture in about 90 per cent of cases. Culture of the synovial fluid alone is positive in approximately 80 per cent of persons.

One additional pattern of joint involvement in tuberculosis has been the subject of a great deal of interest and debate. Termed Poncet's disease after the detailed descriptions provided by Poncet,[691–693] its existence as a specific noninfectious form of tuberculous rheumatism now is questioned. Poncet's accounts of the disease emphasized polyarticular involvement in association with active or inactive visceral tuberculosis. Although Poncet's disease has features similar to those of a reactive arthritis and its existence has been supported in more recent descriptions of tuberculous joint involvement,[694, 1054–1056] some investigators find little evidence that it is a definite entity.[695]

Pathologic Abnormalities

Synovial Membrane Abnormalities. Inflammatory changes in the synovial membrane usually are more marked if the infection follows the penetration of a caseous bone focus into the joint space than if it starts de novo in the membrane itself.[1] An enlarging joint effusion and inflammatory thickening of the periarticular connective tissue and fat contribute to soft tissue swelling. The synovial membrane thickens and is covered with heavy layers of fibrin. On microscopic examination, richly vascular tuberculous granulation tissue is found to contain necrotic and fibrin-like materal, caseous areas, and collections of leukocytes and mononuclear phagocytes. Epithelioid cells and epithelioid tubercles frequently are evident in areas of caseation. Discolored areas related to blood pigment can be observed in the synovial membrane and subsynovial connective tissue. In longstanding cases, the synovial membrane may contain pedunculated knobby masses of fibrinoid material and small rice bodies.[1057]

Cartilaginous and Osseous Abnormalities. The granulation tissue spreads insidiously onto the free surface of the cartilage[1] (Fig. 66–37A). On the basis of vascular and phagocytic processes, portions of the cartilage are eroded. The erosive process is not distributed evenly. Rather, focal areas of cartilaginous destruction may be intermixed with areas of relatively normal-appearing chondral elements. Furthermore, in certain joints, such as the knee, contact of apposing cartilaginous surfaces with resultant compression and motion slows down or prevents the advance of granulation tissue.[194]

Granulation tissue also insinuates itself between the cartilage and subchondral bone,[1] especially in joints (e.g., hip, ankle) in which the articular cartilages are in close contact (Fig. 66–37C). This tissue originates at the peripheral margin of the chondral surface and advances beneath it, loosening and separating the cartilaginous tissue as it proceeds. The detached cartilage may become necrotic, the osseous surface can be exposed, and destruction of the subchondral bone plate and trabeculae can ensue. Occasionally, mounds of subchondral tuberculous granulation tissue may mushroom through gaps in the cartilage, extending into the articular cavity (Fig. 66–37B).

Osseous erosion may be especially marked at the periphery of the joint. Wedge-shaped necrotic foci can become evident on either side of the joint, creating "kissing" sequestra.

Radiographic Abnormalities. A triad of radiographic findings (Phemister's triad) is characteristic of tuberculous arthritis: juxta-articular osteoporosis, peripherally located osseous erosions, and gradual narrowing of the interosseous space (Figs. 66–38 to 66–44). Initially, soft tissue swelling and osteoporosis may dominate the radiographic picture, findings that also are evident in other infectious diseases and rheumatoid arthritis. The degree of osteoporosis can be extensive and, when severe, may resemble the abnormalities of reflex sympathetic dystrophy or transient regional osteoporosis. The infectious nature of the process may be obscured until osseous and cartilaginous destruction becomes evident.

Marginal erosions are especially characteristic of tuberculosis in "tight" or weight-bearing articulations, such as the hip, the knee, and the ankle. They produce corner defects simulating the erosions of other synovial processes, such as rheumatoid arthritis. The combination of regional osteoporosis, marginal erosions, and relative preservation of joint space is highly suggestive of tuberculous arthritis.

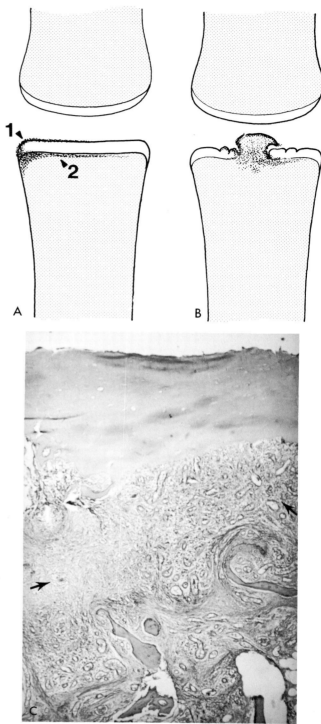

FIGURE 66–37. Tuberculous arthritis: Pathologic abnormalities.
 A Granulation tissue may extend onto the free surface of the cartilage (1) or between cartilage and bone (2).
 B Subchondral trabecular granulation tissue can mushroom through the gaps in the cartilage, extending into the articular cavity.
 C A photomicrograph reveals subchondral extension of pannus (arrows), separating the cartilaginous surface and subchondral bone. (Courtesy of G. Steiner, M.D., New York, New York.)

In rheumatoid arthritis, early loss of articular space is more typical.

Subchondral osseous erosions also are encountered in tuberculous arthritis. They appear as poorly defined gaps in

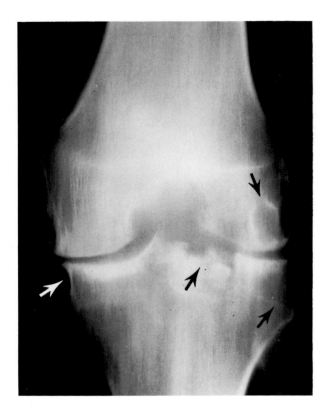

FIGURE 66–38. Tuberculous arthritis: Knee. On a conventional tomogram, typical marginal and central osseous erosions (arrows) accompany tuberculous arthritis. Osteoporosis is not prominent.

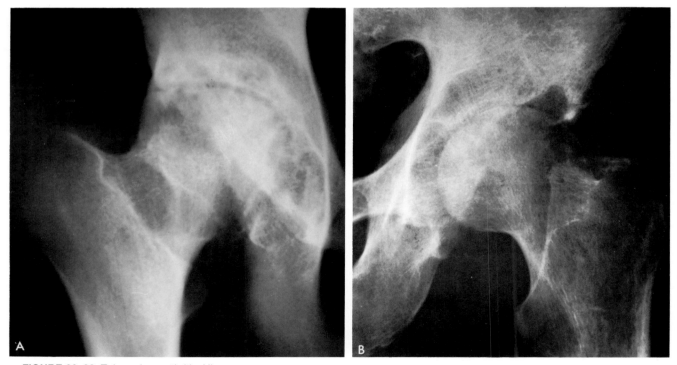

FIGURE 66–39. Tuberculous arthritis: Hip.
  A In this adolescent, osseous erosions on both sides of the joint, diffuse loss of interosseous space, and osteoporosis are evident.
  B Bone erosion of the femoral head and acetabulum, joint space loss, and osteoporosis are seen in this case of tuberculous arthritis.
  (**A,** Courtesy of J. Kaye, M.D., New York, New York.)

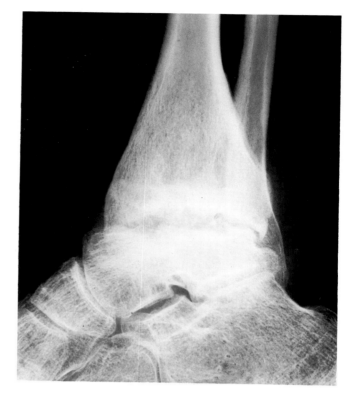

FIGURE 66–40. Tuberculous arthritis: Ankle. Observe poorly defined osseous erosion of the tibia and talus with reactive eburnation. Periostitis and enlargement of the distal tibial surface are noted.

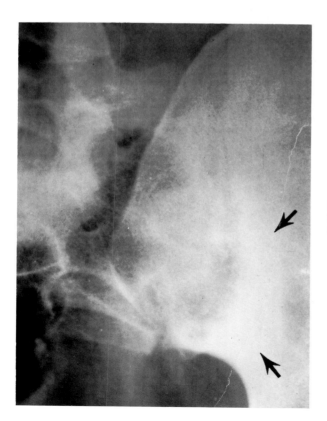

FIGURE 66–41. Tuberculous arthritis: Sacroiliac joint. The sacroiliac joint is abnormal. Note erosion and sclerosis, predominantly of the ilium (arrows). The appearance is identical to that of pyogenic arthritis.

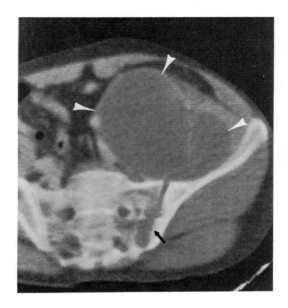

FIGURE 66–42. Tuberculous arthritis: Sacroiliac joint. A 49 year old man developed low back pain related to tuberculous sacroiliitis. A transaxial CT scan delineates the degree of osseous erosion in the lower portion of the sacroiliac joint (arrow) and the extent of the soft tissue mass (arrowheads). (Courtesy of J. Costello, M.D., Madrid, Spain.)

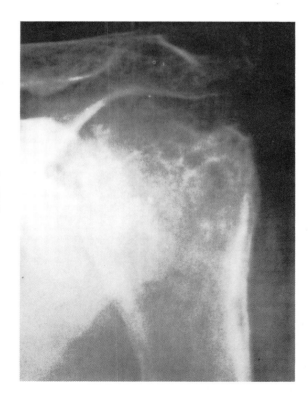

FIGURE 66–43. Tuberculous arthritis: Glenohumeral joint. Radiographic findings include widespread destruction of the humeral head and glenoid process, periostitis, and osteoporosis. The joint space is poorly evaluated. Tapering of the distal end of the clavicle may be evidence of spread of infection to the acromioclavicular joint.

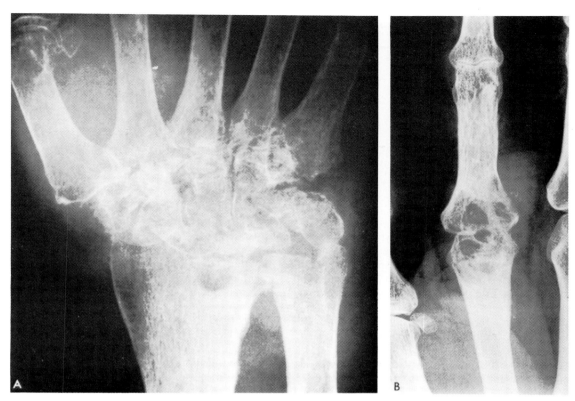

FIGURE 66–44. Tuberculous arthritis: Wrist and hand.
   A Abnormalities include soft tissue swelling, osteoporosis, small and large osseous erosions throughout the carpus, metacarpal bones, ulna, and radius, and joint space narrowing.
   B In a different patient, observe obliteration of the second metacarpophalangeal joint with adjacent cystic lesions. Reactive sclerosis is not apparent.

the subchondral bone plate and subjacent trabeculae that may be apparent at a stage when the articular space is well preserved.

The rapidity of joint space loss in tuberculosis is highly variable. In some patients, diminution in this space is a late finding, occurring after marginal and central erosions of large size have appeared. In other persons, loss of interosseous space can be appreciated at a time when only small marginal osseous defects are apparent.

Bony proliferation generally is not as exuberant in tuberculous arthritis as it is in pyogenic arthritis. Subchondral eburnation is encountered, however, in some patients with tuberculosis, particularly blacks. Similarly, periostitis can be evident, although its frequency and extent are not as great in tuberculosis as in pyogenic infection. In both tuberculosis and pyogenic processes, the periostitis is linear, paralleling the osseous contour; interrupted or perpendicular varieties of periostitis as seen in neoplasms are highly unusual.

Sequestered pieces of bone appear as dense, triangular collections at the edges of the articulation. Rarely, large portions of the adjacent bone may become sequestered.[177] Sinuses can develop, and small bony fragments may be extruded.[195] Synovial cysts, soft tissue abscesses, and fistulous communication with internal organs are reported findings in tuberculous arthritis.[696, 697]

The eventual result in tuberculous arthritis is usually fibrous ankylosis of the joint. Bony ankylosis occasionally is seen, but this sequela is more frequent in pyogenic arthritis.

The MR imaging abnormalities of tuberculous arthritis have been documented only infrequently.[1058, 1059] They appear to be similar to those of other inflammatory joint diseases, although persistent regions of low signal intensity on T2-weighted images, occurring within the joint and perhaps related to hemorrhage with hemosiderin deposition and cartilaginous fragments, have been observed.[1059]

Differential Diagnosis. The diagnosis of tuberculous arthritis generally is not difficult when classic radiographic features appear in typical locations, such as the knee, the hip, the wrist, or the elbow.[134, 191, 194, 196–198, 699] With unusual features or in atypical locations, the diagnosis can be more troublesome.[199] The appearance of periarticular osteoporosis, marginal erosions, and absent or mild joint space narrowing is most helpful in the accurate diagnosis of this disease. In rheumatoid arthritis, osteoporosis and marginal erosions are accompanied by early and significant loss of articular space. In gout, osteoporosis is mild or absent, although marginal erosions and preservation of interosseous space can be observed. In regional osteoporosis, marginal osseous defects are not evident, and the joint space is maintained. In idiopathic chondrolysis, osteoporosis and early joint space loss are evident, especially in a hip, although occasionally they occur in other locations as well.[701]

A monoarticular process must be regarded as infection until proved otherwise. Although it may be difficult to define the nature of the infective agent (e.g., pyogenic, tuberculous, fungal), slow progression of disease, significant osteoporosis, and mild sclerosis are more prominent in tuberculosis and fungal disease than in pyarthrosis (Table

TABLE 66–2. Comparison of Tuberculous and Pyogenic Arthritis

TABLE 66–2. Comparison of Tuberculous and Pyogenic Arthritis

	Tuberculous Arthritis	Pyogenic Arthritis
Soft tissue swelling	+	+
Osteoporosis	+	±
Joint space loss	Late	Early
Marginal erosions	+	+
Bony proliferation (sclerosis, periostitis)	±	+
Bony ankylosis	±	+
Slow progression	+	−

+ = Common; ± = infrequent; − = rare or absent.

66–2). Accurate diagnosis mandates synovial fluid aspiration or synovial membrane biopsy, however. Other monoarticular processes, such as pigmented villonodular synovitis and idiopathic synovial osteochondromatosis, also can simulate tuberculosis. In pigmented villonodular synovitis, a nodular soft tissue mass, preservation of joint space, and absence of osteoporosis are typical; in idiopathic synovial osteochondromatosis, calcified and ossified intra-articular bodies commonly are evident.

Tuberculous Bursitis and Tenosynovitis. The synovial membrane of bursae and tendon sheaths and tendons themselves may be involved in tuberculosis (Figs. 66–45 and 66–46). Typical sites include the radial and ulnar bursae of the hand, the flexor tendon sheaths of the fingers, the bursae about the ischial tuberosities, and the subacromial (subdeltoid) and subgluteal bursae.[200–202, 702–708, 890, 1060–1062, 1253] Rarely, other tendon sheaths, including those in the feet, and other bursae, such as the prepatellar bursa, are

affected.[709, 1063, 1276] Soft tissue swelling and osteoporosis may be observed. In the region of the greater trochanter, osseous destruction can be encountered, and the hip joint may become infected secondarily,[203] particularly after surgical intervention.[204] In any bursal location, dystrophic calcification may appear; this is especially characteristic about the hip and elbow.[205]

Infective myositis and soft tissue abscesses related to tuberculosis also may be encountered (Fig. 66–47).[1064,1268] Such abscesses may be more frequent in patients with the acquired immunodeficiency syndrome.[1064]

Other Diagnostic Techniques. Although the use of scintigraphy in tuberculous involvement of the musculoskeletal system has not been emphasized, it is expected that bone scanning in this disease will reveal findings similar to those in pyogenic osteomyelitis. Single or multiple sites of augmented radionuclide accumulation are expected[710–712,931] and resemble alterations seen in skeletal metastasis. Corresponding areas with decreased uptake during indium-111 bone marrow scintigraphy have been observed.[713] With antituberculosis therapy, bone scan abnormalities generally disappear in 3 to 6 months, although residual photopenic regions have been described.[711]

As indicated previously, CT and MR imaging are best employed in the evaluation of tuberculous spondylitis and paravertebral and psoas extension of infection,[658–664] although they have been used to assess the extent of bone and soft tissue involvement at other sites as well.[714]

BCG Vaccination-Induced Infection

BCG (bacille Calmette-Guérin) is a vaccine of an attenuated bovine tubercle bacillus that has been used for immunization against tuberculosis. Although complications

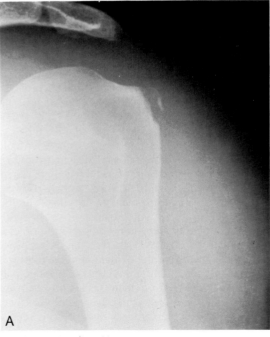
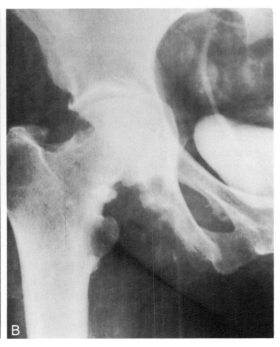

FIGURE 66–45. Tuberculous bursitis.
A Shoulder. Involvement of the subacromial (subdeltoid) bursa has led to a soft tissue mass with erosion and fragmentation of the greater tuberosity of the humerus. (Courtesy of A. D'Abreu, M.D., Porto Alegre, Brazil.)
B Ischial tuberosity. In this patient, observe erosion of the ischial tuberosity with soft tissue calcification. The latter finding is typical of tuberculous bursitis. (Courtesy of J. Jimenez, M.D., Oviedo, Spain.)

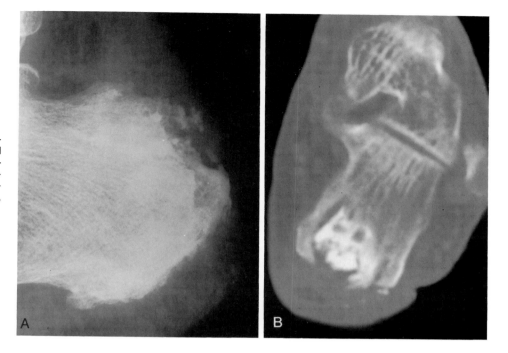

FIGURE 66–46. Tuberculous tendinitis. Routine radiography **(A)** and transverse CT **(B)** reveal enlargement of the Achilles tendon, calcification, and calcaneal erosion. (Courtesy of C. Chen, M.D., Kaohsiung, Taiwan.)

are unusual, generalized BCG infection[206, 207, 540] and bone and joint infection[208–219, 715–720, 933, 1065–1067] have been identified after vaccination. The former complication almost invariably is fatal and is especially common in patients with immunologic deficiency. The latter complication results from hematogenous spread of the BCG infection to the skeleton, usually is not associated with immunologic disorders, and has a favorable prognosis. Of related interest, reactive (noninfectious) arthritis occurring after BCG immunotherapy for a variety of cancers is observed in approximately 1 per cent of patients.[1068, 1269]

It has been estimated that 1 in 5000 to 1 in 80,000 vaccinated children will develop bone or joint infection.[216] BCG osteomyelitis involves boys and girls between the ages of 5 months and 6 years. It usually affects the metaphyses and the epiphyses of the tubular bones, especially about the knee, the ribs, the sternum, or the small bones of the hands and the feet. Lesions in tubular bones are more frequent on the same side of the body as that on which the vaccine was given.[720] Spinal involvement is uncommon.[891] Solitary lesions predominate and are characterized by well-defined lytic foci with only minor degrees of sclerosis or periostitis. Small sequestra may be identified. Extension of the process from the metaphysis to the epiphysis is not uncommon.

The histologic characteristics of BCG osteomyelitis resemble those of tuberculosis, although severe plasma cell infiltration is less common in the former condition. A confident diagnosis requires the growth of the BCG strain in culture, although the difficulty in cultivating BCG is noteworthy. Wide variation exists in the duration of the interval between the time of vaccination and the diagnosis of osteomyelitis. Although the diagnosis commonly is established in the first 6 or 12 months after vaccination, intervals of as long as 12 years are reported.[715, 718]

Atypical Mycobacterial Infection

Acid-fast bacteria that morphologically are similar to tubercle bacilli were long regarded as important in clinical medicine only because they might be mistaken for *M. tuberculosis* (or *M. leprae*) on histologic examination. It now is recognized that many of these bacteria are pathogenic for humans.[220] Although skin and pulmonary disease are the most recognized clinical manifestations of infection with these organisms, bone and joint alterations also may be noted. Mycobacterial osteomyelitis and arthritis can complicate connective tissue disorders and can be evident in patients with impaired resistance, those who had received renal transplants, patients with the acquired immunodeficiency syndrome, or those receiving corticosteroids. They also may occur in an otherwise normal host. The mecha-

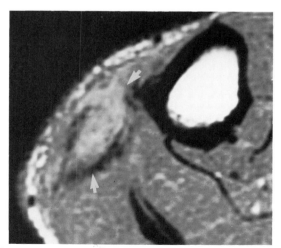

FIGURE 66–47. Tuberculous myositis. A transaxial T1-weighted (TR/TE, 700/20) spin echo MR image obtained after the intravenous administration of a gadolinium contrast agent reveals an enhancing intramuscular mass (arrows) medial to the tibia. (Courtesy of H. S. Kang, M.D., Seoul, Korea.)

nisms of the musculoskeletal alterations include hematogenous spread and contamination after injury or surgery. It also has been suggested that the gastrointestinal tract is a portal of entry for the atypical mycobacteria, as some of these organisms have been demonstrated in the mouths of normal persons.[724]

The atypical mycobacteria frequently are classified as follows: group I, photochromogens (*M. kansasii* and *M. marinum*); group II, scotochromogens (*M. scrofulaceum* and *M. szulgai*); group III, nonchromogens (*M. intracellulare,* or Battey bacillus, *M. gastri,* and *M. avium*); and group IV, rapid growers (*M. fortuitum, M. phlei, M. smegmatis, M. chelonei, M. xenopi,* and *M. rhodochrous*).[221] Infection by organisms in any of these groups can lead to osteomyelitis, septic arthritis (Fig. 66–48), tenosynovitis (with carpal tunnel syndrome), and bursitis.[222–229, 516, 524, 528, 541, 721–732, 892, 1069–1086, 1254]

Although radiologic characteristics for each of these groups have not been well delineated, certain general observations include the following traits: Multiple lesions predominate over solitary lesions; metaphyses and diaphyses of long bones commonly are affected; discrete lytic areas may contain sclerotic margins; osteoporosis may not be so striking as in tuberculous infection; a tendency for the development of abscesses and sinus tracts is present; and articular disease can simulate tuberculosis or rheumatoid arthritis (Figs. 66–49 and 66–50). Accurate diagnosis remains difficult, although clinical findings such as tenosynovitis and a carpal tunnel syndrome are characteristic.[893] Information regarding specific occupational history or recreational activities is important. For example, gardening may allow the introduction of *M. terrae* organisms, the radish bacillus, as they can be found in soil and vegetables.[731] Fishermen or aquarium workers may develop infections from *M. marinum,* as these organisms grow in fresh or salt water.[722, 1082, 1277] Tenosynovitis in these latter persons has been referred to as fish fancier's digit.[722]

Pathologically, although a spectrum of abnormalities may be seen,[892] granulomatous lesions with or without caseation are typical. The diagnosis is established by culture of the synovial fluid or synovial membrane.

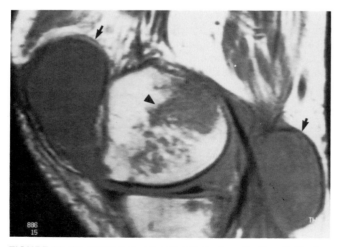

FIGURE 66–48. Atypical mycobacterial infection: Septic arthritis due to *Mycobacterium avium.* A sagittal T1-weighted (TR/TE, 886/15) spin echo MR image of the knee shows a massive joint effusion and posterior synovial cyst (arrows), and intraosseous areas of low signal intensity, especially in the femur (arrowhead), consistent with osteomyelitis.

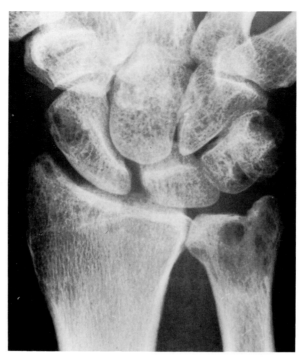

FIGURE 66–49. Atypical mycobacterial infection: Septic arthritis due to *Mycobacterium avium.* A 29 year old black man developed wrist pain after a minor injury; the pain progressed over a 2 year period. The radiograph shows cystic areas in the ulna, radius, scaphoid, triquetrum, and pisiform bones. The joint spaces are preserved. Synovial biopsy indicated hypertrophy of the synovial membrane with chronic granulomatous inflammation. *M. avium* was recovered from the tissue. (Courtesy of J. Scavulli, M.D., San Diego, California.)

Leprosy (Hansen's Disease; Mycobacterium leprae *Infection*)

General Features. Leprosy is an infectious disease caused by *Mycobacterium leprae.* Despite its infrequent occurrence in the United States, it is not uncommon in areas of Africa, South America, and Asia. Leprosy is characterized by a lengthy incubation period and a chronic course with involvement of the skin, the mucous membranes, and the peripheral nervous system. It is the involvement of peripheral nerves that is especially characteristic of *M. leprae* infection.

The lesions of leprosy have been divided into four principal types according to their microscopic appearance[230]:

Lepromatous Type. Bacilli are numerous but very little cellular reaction is seen. Widespread cutaneous lesions consisting of nodules, macules, papules, and diffuse infiltration are distributed symmetrically. "Leprae cells," representing macrophages containing fat droplets and many bacilli, are distinctive.

Tuberculoid Type. Bacilli are less numerous but are capable of inciting a severe granulomatous reaction similar to that which is observed in tuberculosis or sarcoidosis. Asymmetrically distributed skin macules are evident.

Dimorphous Type. The dimorphous type is an uncommon variety in which microscopic features of both the lepromatous and the tuberculoid types are seen.

Indeterminate Type. In perivascular and perineural areas, a few bacilli stimulate a slight cellular reaction whose

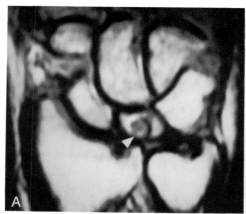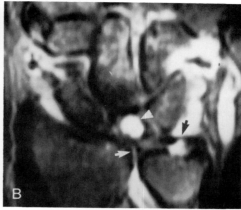

FIGURE 66–50. Atypical mycobacterial infection: Septic arthritis due to *Mycobacterium marinum.* In this 65 year old man with pain and swelling of the wrist, a coronal proton density (TR/TE, 1800/30) spin echo MR image **(A)** and a coronal T1-weighted (TR/TE, 400/15) spin echo image obtained with chemical presaturation of fat (ChemSat) immediately after the intravenous administration of gadolinium contrast agent **(B)** show diffuse synovitis, manifested as high signal intensity in **B.** The radiocarpal, midcarpal, common carpometacarpal, and inferior radioulnar compartments are involved. Additional manifestations include tenosynovitis, disruption of the triangular fibrocartilage (arrows), and a cystic lesion, perhaps representing osteomyelitis, in the lunate (arrowheads).

pathologic features are not prominent enough to allow classification into tuberculoid or lepromatous types.

The clinical manifestations vary among these types of leprosy. In general, the tuberculoid type of disease is less progressive than the lepromatous type. In tuberculoid leprosy, the skin and nerves are affected principally, whereas in lepromatous leprosy, a more acute and generalized process may be evident.

Clinical Abnormalities. Although a history of prolonged contact with the bacilli is typical, the exact mode of transmission of this disease is not clear. It appears probable that the infection enters the body through the skin or mucous membranes, especially the nasal mucosa. The organisms are disseminated via the blood stream and the lymphatics and localize in the skin, the nerves, and, in advanced cases, many of the viscera. The incubation period has been estimated to be 3 to 6 years. Men are affected more commonly than women. The disease may begin at any age, although leprosy commonly is manifested prior to 20 years of age. Prodromal symptoms and signs include malaise, fever, drowsiness, rhinitis, and profuse sweating. Skin manifestations differ in the lepromatous and tuberculoid types. Lymphadenopathy is seen in all types of leprosy, although it is most striking in the lepromatous variety.

In patients with prominent neurologic findings (neural variety of disease) lepromatous granulation tissue appears in and around the nerves, leading to tenderness and thickening of these structures, numbness, and tingling. Pruritus, anesthesia, or hyperesthesia may be evident, especially in the hands and the feet. Muscle atrophy and contractions appear, and eventually extensive mutilation and secondary infection are noted.

Laboratory abnormalities may include a positive lepromin skin test (in tuberculoid leprosy), an elevated erythrocyte sedimentation rate, and a positive serologic test for syphilis (20 to 40 per cent of cases). The diagnosis is established by demonstration of the bacilli in typical histologic lesions.

Musculoskeletal Abnormalities. The musculoskeletal abnormalities include (1) those directly related to presence of the bacilli, in which granulomatous lesions appear in the osseous tissue (direct or specific effects); and (2) those that involve the skeleton indirectly owing to neural abnormalities (indirect or nonspecific effects).[1, 231]

Leprous Periostitis, Osteitis, and Osteomyelitis. The frequency of direct involvement of the skeleton in leprosy is low, varying from 3 to 5 per cent among hospitalized patients.[232] The changes usually are confined to the small bones of the face, the hands, and the feet.[231, 894] In these cases, osseous involvement usually is due to extension of the infection from overlying dermal or mucosal areas; initially the periosteum is contaminated (leprous periostitis), and subsequently the subjacent cortex, spongiosa, and marrow (leprous osteitis and osteomyelitis) become involved (Fig. 66–51). Less commonly, hematogenous spread of infection to the bone can occur, leading to intramedullary foci.[1] In this situation, skeletal sites in addition to those of the face, the hand, and the foot can be altered, including the tubular bones of the extremities (Fig. 66–52) and the ribs.

Pathologically, intraosseous lesions are characterized by granulomatous tissue reactions that lead to trabecular destruction. The lesions usually are evident in the epiphysis and metaphysis of the tubular bones, although direct involvement of the medullary canal also can occur.[233] Progression of disease generally is slow, although the cortex and the periosteum can be violated. Periostitis and reactive sclerosis usually are not prominent in this disease. Of interest, marrow aspiration in cases of leprosy may reveal striking histiocytosis.[514]

In the face, nasal destruction is most characteristic.[234] Destruction of the alveolar process and anterior nasal spine of the maxilla appears to be related to direct lepromatous contamination of the bone as well as secondary infection.[235] These facial changes sometimes are referred to as the rhinomaxillary or Bergen syndrome.[1087]

In the hands and the feet, the metaphyses of phalanges are particularly vulnerable; metacarpal and metatarsal involvement is less frequent[231] (Fig. 66–53). Soft tissue swelling, osteoporosis, endosteal thinning, enlargement of the nutrient foramina, and osseous destruction with a cystic or honeycombed appearance are evident. Pathologic fractures and epiphyseal collapse may appear. With healing, radiographs reveal increasing definition of the involved bone,

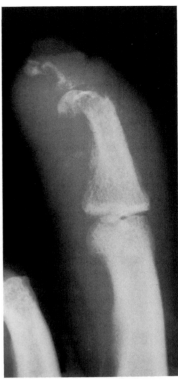

FIGURE 66–51. Leprous tenosynovitis, periostitis, osteitis, and osteomyelitis. Contamination of the soft tissues, tendon sheath, tendon, and phalanges occurred secondary to skin involvement.

although residual deformity with subluxation and malalignment can occur.

In the tubular bones, symmetric periostitis of the tibia, the fibula, and the distal portion of the ulna may be noted (Fig. 66–54). Intractable pain and tenderness may develop, and microscopic examination usually reveals subperiosteal infiltration with *Mycobacterium leprae*.[236] The constellation of erythematous skin lesions, pain, and periostitis involving the lower extremity has been called "red leg" and has been attributed to immunologic factors present during the reactive phase of the disease.[231] The radiographs reveal periosteal proliferation reminiscent of that in hypertrophic osteoarthropathy, a similarity that is accentuated by abnormal symmetric accumulation of bone-seeking pharmaceutical agents on radionuclide examination.[237, 1088]

Leprous Arthritis. Specific leprous arthritis is rare.[238] Pain and swelling with massive joint effusion are evident in the ankle, knee, wrist, finger, and elbow in order of decreasing frequency.[1] Joint involvement results from intraarticular extension of an osseous or periarticular infective focus or, less commonly, from hematogenous contamination of the synovial membrane. Acid-fast bacilli occasionally are detected in joint fluid.[239, 240]

It should be emphasized that intra-articular infection is but one of several mechanisms that can lead to joint manifestations in leprosy. Neuropathic osteoarthropathy, as indicated subsequently, is a second mechanism. Furthermore, erythema nodosum in leprosy is associated with inflammatory or noninflammatory, noninfectious arthritis in both the upper and the lower extremities; an inflammatory symmetric arthritis of peripheral joints unassociated with erythema nodosum also may be encountered; enthesitis and sacroiliitis of unknown pathogenesis are seen in some leprous patients; a "swollen hand" syndrome in the disease consists of intra- and extra-articular inflammation as a response to the organisms, with granulomatous reaction in subsynovial tissue and subcutaneous nodules, easily confused with rheumatoid arthritis; and forms of necrotizing cutaneous vasculitis and dermatomyositis-like syndromes are described.[734, 735, 1089, 1090]

Neuropathic Musculoskeletal Lesions. The skeletal abnormalities occurring on a neurologic basis are much more frequent and severe than those produced by direct leprous infiltration of the bone.[1, 231] These changes may be evident in 20 to 70 per cent of hospitalized patients[232, 241, 242] They result from denervation, producing sensory or motor impairment, or both. Repeated injuries and secondary infections subsequently lead to considerable osseous and articular destruction. The bones of the hands, wrists, ankles, and feet are especially susceptible to this form of leprosy.

In leprosy, disuse of an extremity is related to the intense pain of acute leprous neuritis, the application of a cast for injury, inactivity associated with severe finger and toe contractures,[231] or a combination of these. Osteoporosis may appear, which can be complicated by fracture and deformity.

Cessation of function due to motor denervation can be associated with the absorption of cancellous bone and the development of concentric bone atrophy.[231, 1091] The result is a tapered appearance to the end of the bone, termed the "licked candy stick" (Fig. 66–55). In the foot, progressive resorption of the metatarsals and proximal phalanges occurs.[733] In the hand and the foot, distal phalangeal resorption also is encountered, which eventually may result in loss of many of the phalanges, especially when the process is complicated by secondary infection. Although all insensitive digits can be altered, the index and long fingers usually are first affected, and seldom are all the digits involved equally.[231, 243] Changes in the wrist consist of scaphoid fractures with delayed union or nonunion, lunate collapse and fragmentation similar to the findings of Kienbock's disease, dorsal intercalated carpal instability, and joint space loss in many of the articular compartments.[1092]

Tarsal disintegration alone or in combination with ankle involvement is not infrequent,[243–245, 513, 1093] attributable to sensory and motor dysfunction, trauma, and secondary infection. Changes are initiated within the medial arch, the lateral arch, the talus, and the calcaneus.[231] Osteolysis, osteosclerosis, fragmentation, and progressive resorption can be encountered (Fig. 66–56). In extreme cases, dissolution of the midfoot results in separation of the forefoot and the hindfoot, and the tibia is driven downward, becoming weight-bearing.

The histologic characteristics of involved joints in leprous patients with neurologic deficit are similar to those in other neuropathic osteoarthropathies.[1] Serous effusion, villous proliferation of the synovial membrane, erosion and proliferation of cartilage, sclerosis and eburnation of bone, fragmentation, and osseous excrescences are apparent.

The radiographic appearance of neuropathic osteoarthropathy in leprosy resembles that in syphilis, diabetes mellitus, congenital insensitivity to pain, and syringomyelia. It also may simulate changes in psoriatic arthritis, collagen vascular disorders such as scleroderma, and thermal injuries.

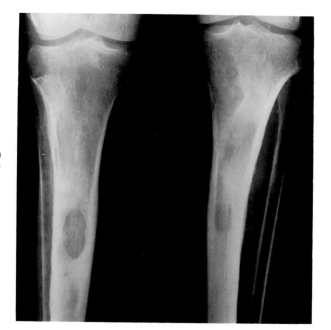

FIGURE 66–52. Leprous osteomyelitis. Hematogenous spread of infection has led to osteomyelitis of the tibiae manifested as multiple osteolytic lesions. (Courtesy of J. Schils, M.D., Cleveland, Ohio.)

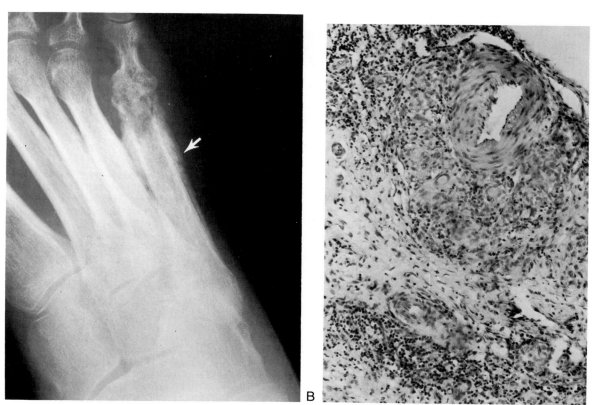

A   B

FIGURE 66–53. Leprous osteomyelitis and septic arthritis.
  A Note destruction of the metatarsal bone with exuberant periostitis (arrow). The fifth metatarsophalangeal joint is obliterated. The soft tissues are abnormal as a result of adjacent infection.
  B In a different patient, a synovial biopsy of an infected wrist shows marked granulomatous inflammatory reaction surrounding a small artery. (Hematoxylin and eosin stain, 100×.)
  (**B,** From Albert DA, et al: Medicine 59:442, 1980.)

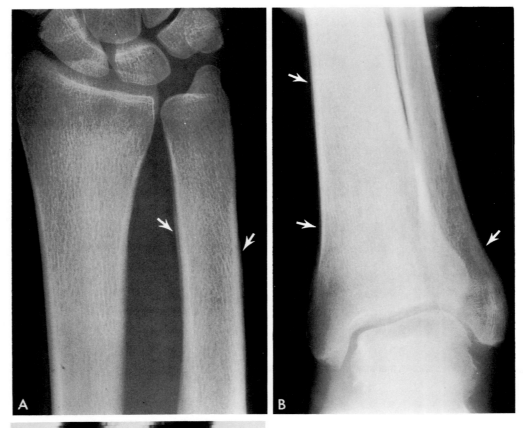

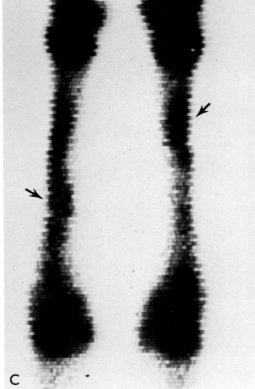

FIGURE 66–54. Leprous periostitis: "Red leg." A 43 year old man had a 5 year history of arm and leg weakness, hypoesthesia, skin ulcerations, and rash. The lateral portions of his eyebrow had fallen out, and he had been treated previously for leprosy. A biopsy of the involved skin revealed subcutaneous infiltration with large numbers of polymorphonuclear leukocytes, histiocyte-like cells with foamy cytoplasm, and multinucleated giant cells. Special stains showed abundant acid-fast bacilli.

A, B Radiographs reveal periostitis of the distal ends of the ulna, tibia, and fibula (arrows). The opposite side was affected similarly.

C A ^{99m}Tc-pyrophosphate bone scan shows increased uptake over the knees and the ankles as well as in both tibiae and fibulae (arrows).

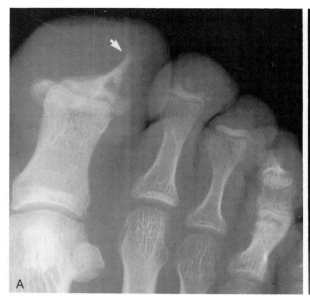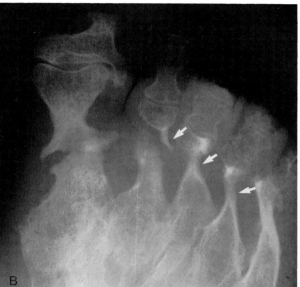

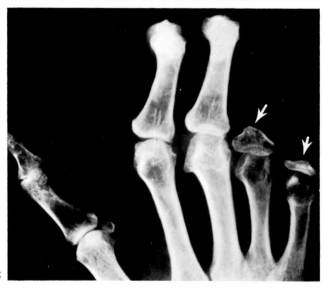

FIGURE 66–55. Leprosy: Neuropathic lesions. Examples of concentric bone atrophy in the foot and the hand illustrate the tapered osseous surfaces (arrows) and phalangeal osteolysis. (**A, B,** Courtesy of W. Coleman, M.D., Carville, Louisiana.)

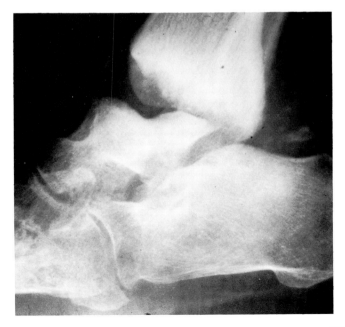

FIGURE 66–56. Leprosy: Neuropathic lesions. Fragmentation and collapse of the talar, tibial, and calcaneal surfaces can be seen. The appearance is similar to that in tabes dorsalis.

Secondary Infection. Because of the anesthesia resulting from the neural lesions, persons with leprosy are prone to suffer injuries. Ulceration followed by secondary infection and pyogenic osteomyelitis is common in the anesthetic feet.[246] Bone destruction, florid periosteal reaction, and sequestration can appear. Septic arthritis also is seen. Differentiating the effects of pyogenic osteomyelitis and arthritis from leprous osteomyelitis or neuropathic osteoarthropathy is extremely difficult.

Vascular Lesions. The frequency, nature, and importance of vascular lesions in leprosy are debated. Some investigators believe that such lesions are very common in the hand and the foot and may be delineated by arteriography, during which occlusion, narrowing, tortuosity, dilatation, irregularity, and incomplete filling of vessels can be noted.[247] Others suggest that bone resorption occurs because of interference to the mechanism controlling vasoregulation due to involvement of the nerves in the vascular reflex arch[248, 249]; in this regard, narrowing of the lumen of medium-sized and small arterioles has been noted in cases with and without bone resorption.[232, 246]

Soft Tissue Calcification. Rarely, linear calcification of involved nerves can be seen on radiographs[250] (Fig. 66–57). Similarly, abscess formation within the nerve, especially in the ulnar nerve, can be associated with calcification.[251, 252]

Soft Tissue Neoplasm. As in chronic osteomyelitis with soft tissue sinuses, leprosy with cutaneous ulcerations may be complicated by the development of secondary neoplasia, specifically squamous cell carcinoma in the skin.[736, 737] The tissues of the lower leg and plantar aspect of the foot are affected principally.[895] Diagnosis often is delayed, although the prognosis for life is good. Radiographically, a soft tissue mass and progressive osteolysis are important clues to correct diagnosis.[738] Ultimately, it is knowledge of this specific complication as well as knowledge of the predilection for lepromatous patients to develop other tumors, such as lymphoma and leukemia,[739] that is most important.

Spirochetes and Related Organisms

Syphilis

General Features. Syphilis is a chronic systemic infectious disease caused by *Treponema pallidum,* a slender spirochete with regular, evenly spaced spirals. Although the frequency and prevalence of the disorder have decreased since World War II, a resurgence of syphilitic infection has been noted. Syphilis is transmitted by direct and intimate contact with moist infectious lesions of the skin and mucous membranes. Thus, infection is spread during sexual contact, although less commonly the disease may be contracted during biting or kissing. Infection develops in approximately 25 to 30 per cent of the sexual partners of persons with syphilitic lesions, although the risk of acquiring the disease from a single sexual exposure to an infected partner is unknown.[740] Acquisition of syphilis by transfusion no longer is a significant problem. Children may acquire the disease by sharing a bed with an infected person.[740] The appearance of the disorder traceable to any one of these mechanisms is termed *acquired syphilis.* In addition, the fetus may be infected by transmission of the organism through the placenta; this is termed *congenital syphilis.*

Treponema pallidum can penetrate intact mucous membranes or tiny defects in cornified epithelium.[740] Once the spirochete has violated the epithelium, it enters lymphatics and reaches the regional lymph nodes in a period of hours.[253] Subsequently, the treponema may enter the blood stream and the ensuing spirochetemia, which can occur before the primary lesion appears at the inoculation site, allows dissemination of infection throughout the body.

Approximately 3 to 6 weeks after the organism has entered the body, a primary lesion, the *chancre,* develops at the site of inoculation. This lesion is a skin ulceration that heals spontaneously. About 6 weeks later, a generalized skin eruption known as *secondary syphilis* develops.[253] In this stage of the disease, systemic manifestations are frequent. After healing of both primary and secondary manifestations, the patient may be without symptoms and signs for a protracted period of time, a stage termed *latent syphilis,* although progressive inflammatory alterations may be occurring slowly in many of the organ systems. Cardiovascular syphilis or neurosyphilis may become manifest 10 to 30 years later, although some persons (approximately 50 per cent) never develop tertiary manifestations of syphilis and show no signs of the disease at autopsy.[253] In those patients with significant later alterations, large destructive lesions or *gummas* can be evident in almost any organ of the body, particularly the skin and the bones. These lesions may result from a delayed hypersensitivity reaction in the immune host; their granulomatous histopathology is not specific.[740]

Congenital Syphilis

Frequency and Pathogenesis. Although earlier studies indicated that congenital syphilis might occur in 2 to 5 per cent of infants,[254] modern techniques designed to improve the recognition of this disease in pregnant women have led

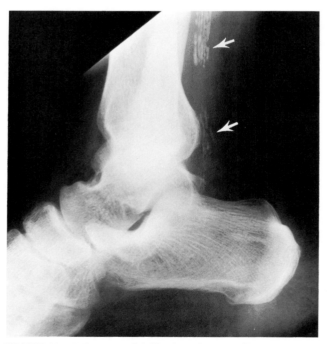

FIGURE 66–57. Leprosy: Calcification of nerves. The linear radiodense regions (arrows) represent calcification of nerves. This finding, although rare, is suggestive of the diagnosis of leprosy but must be distinguished from vascular calcification. (Courtesy of M. Dalinka, M.D., Philadelphia, Pennsylvania.)

to an impressive reduction in the number of cases of congenital syphilis.[255] As spirochetemia is more frequent in the early stages of syphilis, babies born to women who have acquired the disease during pregnancy, rather than prior to it, are more likely to develop congenital syphilis.[740] The disorder originates from transplacental migration of the treponema and invasion of the perichondrium, periosteum, cartilage, bone marrow, and sites of active endochondral ossification, especially in the metaphyseal regions of tubular bones.[1] The spirochetes inhibit osteogenesis and lead to degeneration of osteoblasts.

The fetus that is heavily infiltrated with spirochetes may be aborted or die shortly after birth. Others survive, developing the stigmata of congenital syphilis. Early and late lesions may be identified in these infants. Approximately 75 per cent of cases of congenital syphilis are diagnosed in children over the age of 10 years.[740] In such children, the hutchinsonian triad, consisting of Hutchinson's teeth, interstitial keratitis, and nerve deafness, may appear. Additional manifestations include fissuring about the mouth and anus (rhagades), anterior bowing of the lower leg (saber shin), collapse of the nasal bones (saddle nose), and perforation of the palate.[740] The need for radiographic surveys in establishing the diagnosis of congenital syphilis is controversial.[1099, 1100]

Early Osseous Lesions. In the fetus, the neonate, and the very young infant, bony abnormalities include (1) osteochondritis; (2) diaphyseal osteomyelitis (osteitis); (3) periostitis; and (4) miscellaneous changes. These have been well summarized by Jaffe,[1] and many of his observations with regard to both congenital and acquired syphilis are included in the following discussion.

1. *Syphilitic osteochondritis* usually results in symmetric involvement of sites of endochondral ossification.[256, 741] The epiphyseal-metaphyseal junction of tubular bones, the costochondral regions, and, in severe cases, the flat and short tubular bones and the centers of ossification of the sternum and vertebrae are affected.[1] In the growing metaphyses of the long bones, particularly about the knee, the shoulder, and the wrist, widening of the provisional calcification zone, serrations, and adjacent osseous irregularity are seen, which on histologic evaluation are found to result from a disturbance of endochondral ossification (Fig. 66–58). Radiographs outline broad horizontal radiolucent bands reminiscent of those that are identified in leukemia or metastasis from neuroblastoma.[742]

If the process continues, metaphyseal irregularities appear (Fig. 66–59). Biopsy outlines granulation tissue within the metaphysis, which may be localized to one segment or involve the entire width of the bone, extending into the epiphysis and adjacent diaphysis. Histologically, the granulation tissue consists initially of vascular connective tissue and later of cellular infiltrations (lymphoid cells, polymorphonuclear leukocytes) and necrosis, presumably induced by the toxic effects of degenerating spirochetes.[1] On radiographs, irregular erosive lesions appear along the contour of the bone at the metaphyseal–growth plate junction. The medial surface of the proximal tibial shaft is a particularly characteristic site of erosion, a finding that is termed Wimberger's sign. These metaphyseal alterations, which may progress to osseous fragmentation, simulating the changes

of scurvy, appear to be a true inflammatory change related to the spirochetes themselves.[257]

Epiphyseal separation can result from the metaphyseal destruction induced by the granulation tissue. It usually is evident in older fetuses, neonates, and infants up to the age of 3 months and shows predilection for multiple sites in the long tubular bones, particularly in the upper extremity.[1, 258, 259] The metaphyseal line of cleavage leads to partial or complete separation of the epiphysis.

The lesions of osteochondritis generally heal quickly with specific therapy; healing is evident within 2 weeks and may be complete within 2 months.[260] Osteoblasts reappear, and new bone is deposited at the cartilaginous growth plates. Granulation tissue disappears, and normal growth ensues. Growth retardation and osseous deformity are unusual.

2. *Diaphyseal osteomyelitis (osteitis)* can appear in infants with congenital syphilis who have not received therapy or in whom treatment has been inadequate or inappropriate. Granulation tissue in the metaphysis may extend into the diaphysis, inducing infective foci of variable size (Fig. 66–60). Osteolytic lesions with surrounding bony eburnation and overlying periostitis can be encountered on radiographs of involved tubular bones. Although multiple bones usually are affected, alterations in a single tubular bone,[261] in the bones of one extremity,[544, 1094] or in nontubular bones[262, 742] can be detected.

3. *Periostitis* is a less frequent manifestation of congenital syphilis than is osteochondritis.[1] It may result from several different processes.[263] Diffuse, widespread, symmetric, and profound periosteal proliferation can relate to its infiltration by syphilitic granulation tissue (Fig. 66–60). This variety of periostitis is observed in infants more frequently than in fetuses, and it can be associated with diaphyseal osteomyelitis. The long tubular bones and, less commonly, the flat bones are affected. Treatment produces a complete but slow resolution of the changes.

Reparative (reactive) periostitis is a second variety of periosteal response that may be noted about healing foci of osteochondritis or after epiphyseal slipping. It originates during the treatment of syphilis and represents ''callus'' formation rather than a response to syphilitic infiltration of the periosteum. Radiographic differentiation of infective and reparative periostitis can be difficult.

4. *Miscellaneous musculoskeletal changes* occasionally can be identified early in the course of congenital syphilis. Gummas have been reported in tubular and flat bones, although their occurrence in congenital syphilis is a rare phenomenon. Intra-articular effusions may complicate epiphyseal destruction or separation, and the joint fluid may reveal a strongly positive test for syphilis.[1]

Late Osseous Lesions. The early manifestations of congenital syphilis generally regress or disappear in the first few years of life, even in the absence of adequate therapy.[1095] Exacerbation of disease may appear in the young child or adolescent (5 to 20 years of age), however. Although the evolving skeletal lesions occurring late in the course of congenital syphilis rarely may resemble those of early congenital syphilis (osteochondritis, osteomyelitis, periostitis), they more typically resemble the changes observed in acquired syphilis (see later discussion).[1] Osteo-

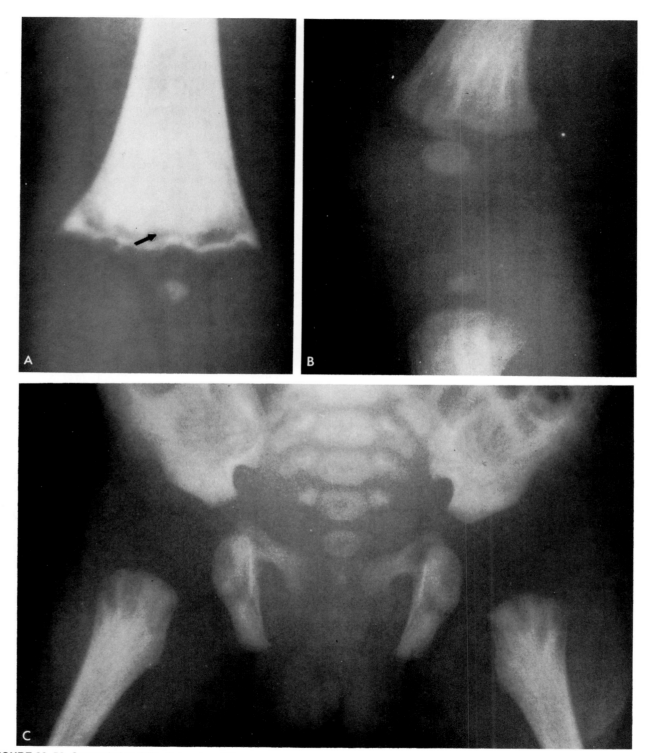

FIGURE 66–58. Congenital syphilis: Osteochondritis.

A This 3 week old infant reveals a lucent band in the metaphysis (arrow) caused by a disturbance in endochondral ossification. The appearance is similar to that in leukemia or neuroblastoma.

B, C In another infant with syphilis, a "celery stalk" appearance with alternating longitudinal lucent and sclerotic bands owing to abnormality of endochondral ossification resembles changes in rubella.

(**B, C,** Courtesy of D. Edwards, M.D., San Diego, California.)

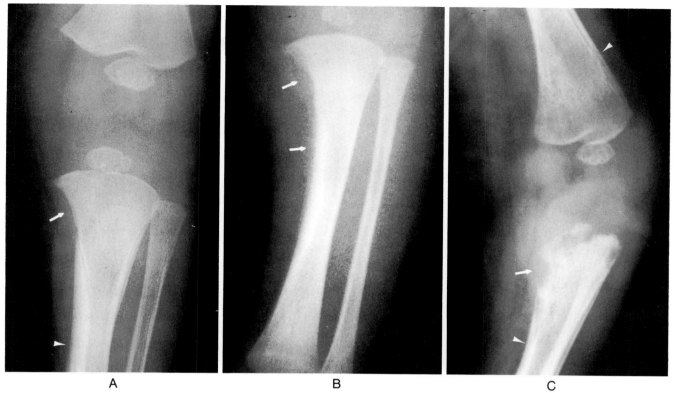

FIGURE 66–59. Congenital syphilis: Osteochondritis and osteomyelitis. In three different infants, the tibial alterations are well shown. Initially **(A),** defects in the medial tibial metaphysis (arrow) are characteristic, frequently associated with periostitis (arrowhead). Subsequently **(B),** the degree of osseous destruction may be more exaggerated (arrows). The predilection for the medial tibial metaphysis again is noteworthy. Eventually **(C),** osseous collapse can be seen (arrow). Observe the periostitis of tibia and femur (arrowheads).

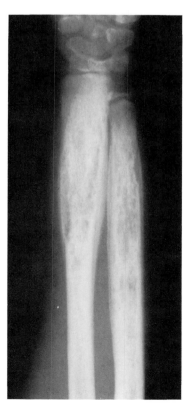

FIGURE 66–60. Congenital syphilis: Osteomyelitis. Note osteolysis with exuberant periostitis of the radius and ulna.

myelitis and periostitis in late congenital syphilis can involve the tubular bones, particularly the upper two thirds of the tibial shafts, the flat bones, and even the cranium[264] (Figs. 66–61 and 66–62). In these sites, spirochetes that have remained dormant for years may become reactivated.

Gummatous or nongummatous osteomyelitis or periostitis results in diffuse hyperostosis of the involved bone. Endosteal bony proliferation produces encroachment on the medullary cavity, whereas periosteal bony proliferation creates an enlarged, undulating, and dense osseous contour.[1] In the tibia, a typical saber shin may be encountered, with anterior bending of the bone. Its radiographic appearance may resemble that of Paget's disease, although the syphilitic hyperostosis may not extend to the epiphysis (Figs. 66–61 and 66–62). Lucent defects within areas of hyperostosis can represent gummas.

Abnormalities of the skull and mandible include destruction of the nasal bones, calvarial gumma,[743] and Hutchinson's teeth, characterized by peg-shaped, notched, and hypoplastic dental structures.[265] The dental changes, which do not regress with antibiotic treatment, may be related to a direct action of the spirochetes on the tooth germ, a syphilitic process of the mandible or the maxilla, or a metabolic effect.[1] Spirochetes occasionally are recovered from the neighboring bone.[266]

Jaffe[1] also has emphasized the late appearance of dactylitis in congenital syphilis, with periosteal proliferation and osseous expansion largely confined to the phalanges of the fingers and, less commonly, the toes. Other reports have

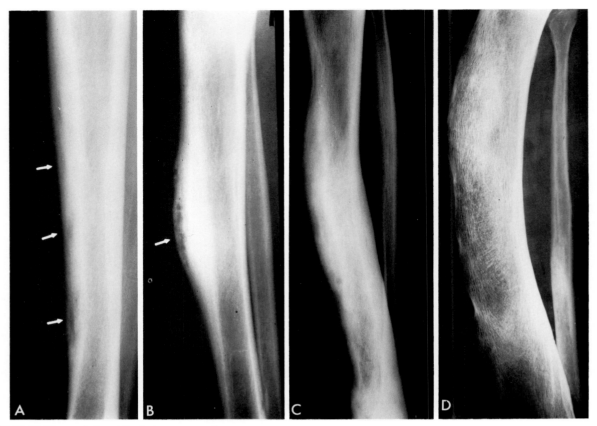

FIGURE 66–61. Congenital syphilis: Late osseous changes.

    A Observe radiolucent foci within the anterior cortex of the tibia (arrows) with periostitis and endosteal proliferation.

    B In a second patient, localized hyperostosis about a syphilitic lesion on the anterior surface of the tibia (arrow) can be observed.

    C More exuberant hyperostosis of both the tibia and the fibula has resulted in bowed and prominent osseous surfaces. The changes are somewhat reminiscent of those in Paget's disease.

    D A typical saber shin deformity of the tibia is associated with anterior bowing of the bone. The fibula also is involved.

indicated that periostitis about the osteolytic lesions may be absent or of mild degree.[743]

In older syphilitic children, bilateral painless effusions, especially of the knee, have been termed Clutton's joints.[267]

Acquired Syphilis

Frequency. The frequency of osseous lesions during the course of acquired syphilis has decreased dramatically owing to improvement in diagnosis and treatment of this disease. When present, the bony and articular manifestations usually appear in the latent or tertiary phase of syphilis; similar manifestations in the early phases of the disorder are extremely unusual. In 1942, Reynolds and Wasserman[268] reviewed the cases of approximately 10,000 patients with early acquired syphilis that had accumulated over a 21 year period and were able to document only 15 cases (0.15 per cent) of destructive osseous lesions, although others have noted that the frequency may be as high as 8 to 20 per cent of these patients,[269] especially if periostitis and destructive osseous foci both are considered in the determination.

Early Acquired Syphilis

Pathogenesis. A spirochetemia appearing 1 to 3 months after the documentation of a primary lesion can lead to dissemination of organisms throughout the body.[270] The spirochetes can reach the deeper vascular areas of the periosteum with resulting perivascular inflammatory infiltrates and subsequent formation of highly cellular granulation tis-

sue.[271] This tissue can extend into the haversian canals and medullary space of the involved bone(s). Conversely, initial contamination of the medullary space can lead to involvement of the cortex and the periosteum.[272, 273] Endothelial proliferation and endarteritis obliterans can develop, and infectious osteochondritis, periostitis, osteitis, or osteomyelitis may appear.

Clinical Abnormalities. In the primary stage of syphilis, transitory, boring bone pain can be prominent—especially in febrile patients—in the tibia, humerus, and cranium, unassociated with radiographic or pathologic changes.[1, 1097] In the secondary stage, pain, soft tissue swelling, fever, and tenderness can be detected, particularly in the superficial bones, such as the frontal region of the calvarium, the anterior surfaces of the tibia, the sternum, and the ribs.[274, 275] The symptoms and signs of periostitis can vary substantially in severity and characteristically are worse at night.[274] They may resolve completely during appropriate antibiotic treatment.

Proliferative Periostitis. A proliferative periostitis is the most common osseous lesion in early acquired syphilis.[274, 276] It may be especially prominent in the tibia, skull, ribs, and sternum, although other bones, such as the clavicle, the femur, the fibula, and the osseous structures of the hand and the foot, can be affected. Periosteal inflammation is associated with new bone formation, which can become extensive, leading to considerable thickening of the cortex.

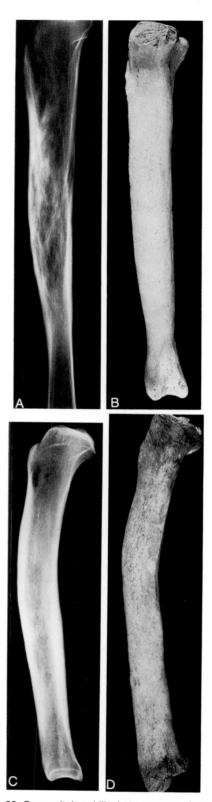

FIGURE 66–62. Congenital syphilis: Late osseous changes.

A, B Observe enlargement of the diaphysis of the tibia resulting predominantly from periosteal bone formation. The epiphyses are spared.

C, D In a different cadaver, anterior bowing of the bone also is evident.

Although periosteal proliferation generally is laminated or solid, it can occur perpendicular to the underlying bone, simulating the appearance of an osteosarcoma.[276–278] Bilateral tibial or clavicular periostitis in the adult frequently is syphilitic in origin.

Infective Osteitis and Osteomyelitis. Destructive bone lesions occur much less commonly than periostitis in early syphilis.[268–270, 279] These lesions relate to osteomyelitis and infective osteitis (as well as septic arthritis) (Fig. 66–63). Involvement of the skull is particularly characteristic,[269, 279, 1096] having been noted in nearly 9 per cent of 80 consecutive patients with secondary syphilis,[280] although any tubular and flat bone can be affected. Clinical manifestations related to skull involvement include headache and localized tumefactions. At this site, irregular areas of bone lysis are observed with a motheaten or permeative pattern of destruction, periostitis, and minimal or absent sclerosis. Usually, the outer table is altered more frequently and more significantly than the diploë or the inner table. Frontal, parietal, and nasopalatine areas are affected most often.[268] In the long tubular bones, osteolytic foci, cortical sequestration, periostitis, and epiphyseal separation can be noted. Syphilitic arthritis may be a complicating feature, especially of the sternoclavicular joint (see discussion later in this chapter).

Late Acquired Syphilis

Pathogenesis. Osseous lesions occurring during the later stages of acquired syphilis can be related to gummatous or nongummatous inflammation.[1] Gummas within the medullary cavity, cortex, or periosteum usually do not become evident until years or decades after the acquisition of the disease.[1] Superficial bones are affected more commonly, a localization that frequently is attributed to recurrent low grade trauma or irritation.

Gummatous Osseous Lesions. A gumma represents a discrete or confluent area of variable size containing caseous necrotic material. These areas of necrosis generally are related to the effects of the toxic products of spirochetal degeneration, although the organisms themselves usually are not demonstrable within the lesions. On microscopic examination, syphilitic granulation tissue within the gumma is found to contain dense infiltration with lymphoid cells and engorged capillaries.[1] With the appearance of central caseation and peripherally located lymphoid, epithelioid, and Langhans' giant cells, the lesion resembles a tubercle. The adjacent osseous tissue undergoes necrosis. Resorption of cortical bone due to the inflammatory reaction about a gumma frequently is termed *caries sicca.*[1] If the necrotic osseous area enlarges and becomes detached from the adjacent tissue, the term *caries necrotica* is used. The sequestered piece of cortex may become displaced into the gumma itself and may be recognized on radiographic and pathologic examination. Typically, however, cortical sequestration in syphilis is limited in extent and is not identifiable on radiographic evaluation. With healing, encapsulation of the caseous area by fibrous tissue is followed by gradual resorption of the caseous matter due to leukocytic and histiocytic activity.[1] Eventually a dense connective tissue scar replaces the original lesion.

The radiographic features are characterized by lytic and

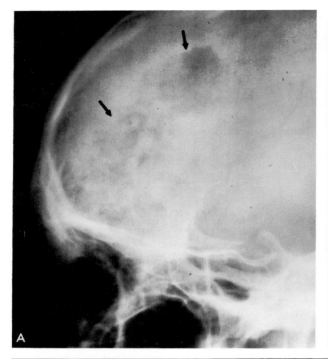

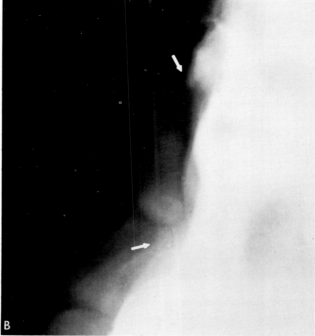

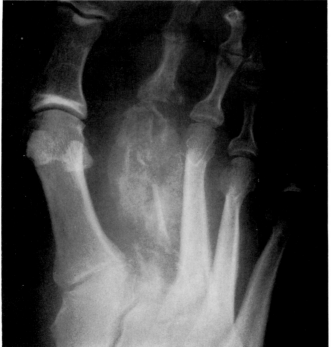

C

FIGURE 66–63. Acquired syphilis: Osteitis, osteomyelitis, and periostitis.

  A Lytic lesions of the frontal region of the skull (arrows) are accompanied by reactive sclerosis.

  B Observe nasal bone destruction (arrows) associated with soft tissue deformity on this lateral radiograph of the face.

  C Note osteolysis of metatarsal bones and phalanges associated with soft tissue swelling, periostitis, pathologic fracture, and articular involvement.

sclerotic areas of bone, which may reach considerable size (Fig. 66–63).[1, 281, 282] Adjacent periostitis is frequent, and, when large, the lesions may be associated with a pathologic fracture.[281]

Nongummatous Osseous Lesions. Nongummatous syphilitic periostitis, osteitis, or osteomyelitis can occur independently or in conjunction with gummas in the bone marrow.[1] Inflammation of the periosteum is associated with intimal thickening of medium-sized arteries and accumulation of lymphoid cells. Exuberant subperiosteal bone formation may follow, and the new bone eventually may merge with the underlying bone. Nongummatous syphilitic osteomyelitis usually is limited in extent and is associated with infiltration of the marrow spaces with vascular and cellular connective tissue. Adjacent trabeculae become atrophic.

The radiographic evaluation of nongummatous osseous lesions reveals destructive and productive bony changes associated with periostitis. Differentiation of these findings from those associated with gummas is better left to the pathologist.

Distribution. Gummatous and nongummatous skeletal lesions can be delineated in many sites. Involvement of the cranial vault, nasal bones, maxilla, mandible, tubular bones of the appendicular skeleton, spine, and pelvis has been noted (Fig. 66–63). The degree of periosteal proliferation can become extreme and, in tubular bones, can lead to gross enlargement of osseous tissue. The resultant radiographic and pathologic features resemble those in the late stages of congenital syphilis, including the saber shin deformity. According to Jaffe,[1] the saber shin deformity of acquired syphilis usually is related to pseudobowing of the tibia, in which the vertical direction of the marrow cavity is unchanged and the outer diameter of the bone is enlarged as a result of periosteal proliferation; the saber shin deformity of congenital syphilis is associated with real bowing of the bone. Dactylitis, which is not infrequent in congenital syphilis, is less typical of acquired disease. When present in acquired syphilis, gummatous periostitis is the usual cause; in congenital syphilis gummatous osteomyelitis typically is implicated in the pathogenesis of dactylitis.

Articular Involvement

General Abnormalities. The frequency of articular involvement in syphilis is low. Joint abnormalities may occur in either congenital or acquired forms of the disease. In congenital syphilis, articular changes predominate in the late phases of the disorder; in acquired syphilis, joint manifestations appear in the tertiary or, less frequently, the secondary stage of the disorder.

The distribution of articular abnormalities varies with the age of the patient, the type of syphilitic infection, and the pathogenesis of the lesions (see later discussion). Joint effusions associated with pain and tenderness, which may be infectious or noninfectious in origin, commonly are bilateral and most typically affect the knee. Infectious syphilitic arthritis can occur in any axial or extra-axial site,[1098] although sternoclavicular joint localization may have diagnostic importance.[565, 1255]

Pathogenesis. Joint disease appearing during the course of congenital or acquired syphilis can relate to a variety of mechanisms[1]:

1. *Spread from a contiguous source of infection.* In either congenital or acquired disease, syphilitic inflammation of periarticular bone can be complicated by joint involvement. This usually is associated with extension of an intraosseous gumma, followed by active articular inflammation resulting from the degenerating gummatous material. The inflammatory process within the joint usually is not gummatous.[283]

2. *Direct involvement of the synovial membrane.* In either congenital or acquired syphilis the luetic process can originate in the synovial or parasynovial tissues. Although the articular findings in these cases are related primarily to infection, it frequently is difficult to identify spirochetes in the synovial membrane or synovial fluid. Electron microscopy may reveal treponema-like bodies in the synovial membrane in areas of considerable tissue necrosis, however.[284] Immunofluorescent antitreponemal antibody techniques also can lead to identification of spirochetes within synovial fluid.[285] Rarely, capsular thickening and synovial hypertrophy have been associated with true gummas within the synovial membrane.[286] The rapid resolution of articular symptoms after treatment with penicillin in some patients with synovitis also supports an infectious cause.

3. *Sympathetic effusions.* In many cases of syphilis with synovitis, organisms are not identified in the articular cavity.[287, 288] In some of these cases, sympathetic effusion may relate to periosteal irritation from a neighboring intraosseous focus. In others, no adjacent bony abnormality is evident. Clinical symptoms and signs of arthralgia or arthritis may be present in the knees, hips, shoulders, and, less frequently, the joints of the fingers.[274, 288, 289] In congenital syphilis, painless intra-articular collections of fluid, especially in the knees, are termed Clutton's joints.

4. *Neuropathic osteoarthropathy.* Neurosyphilis can be associated with neuropathic osteoarthropathy, with fragmentation and dissolution of one or more joints of the axial and appendicular skeleton. This complication is discussed elsewhere (see Chapter 78).

Radiographic and Pathologic Abnormalities. In cases of noninfectious arthralgia or arthritis, radiographic and pathologic features may be lacking. A joint effusion may be detected, but the fluid may disappear rapidly. Osteoporosis may be evident.

Syphilitic infectious arthritis is associated with an effusion and capsular distention. The synovial membrane may become hypertrophied, with cellular infiltration. Synovial inflammation with pannus can lead to cartilaginous and osseous destruction. On radiographs, osteoporosis, joint space narrowing, bony destruction, sclerosis, and intra-articular osseous fusion can be encountered, findings that are similar to those occurring in other infectious arthritides (Fig. 66–63C).

Yaws

Yaws represents an infectious disorder caused by *Treponema pertenue,* an organism that morphologically is indistinguishable from *Treponema pallidum,* the cause of syphilis. Yaws occurs in tropical climates and is prevalent in Africa, South America, the South Pacific islands, and the West Indies. It generally is acquired before puberty during contact with open lesions containing the spirochetes. The transmission of the disease rarely is associated with sexual contact.

Within a period of weeks after inoculation, a granulomatous primary lesion appears, usually on the legs. This raised crusted lesion is referred to as mother yaw.[740] Nontender regional adenopathy and spirochetemia occur. Approximately 1 to 3 months later, a generalized papular skin eruption occurs on the extremities, buttocks, neck, and face. Involvement of the soles, crab yaws, may make walking painful.[740] After several years, late destructive lesions may become evident in the cutaneous and osseous tissues.

The tubular bones of the extremities, including those of the hands and feet, the pelvis, the skull, and the facial bones may become the sites of periostitis or osteitis. Lucent lesions in the cortex or spongiosa are accompanied by florid periosteal bone formation (Fig. 66–64). Saber shin deformities (as in syphilis), dactylitis, and nasal destruction may be encountered.[1101] Proliferative exostoses in the maxillary bones are termed goundou; palatal perforations are termed gangosa. Localized expansile lesions in the epiphyses of tubular bones may simulate neoplasms.[290] Destructive changes in the fingers and toes can lead to a doigts en lorgnette appearance, in which extensive shortening and

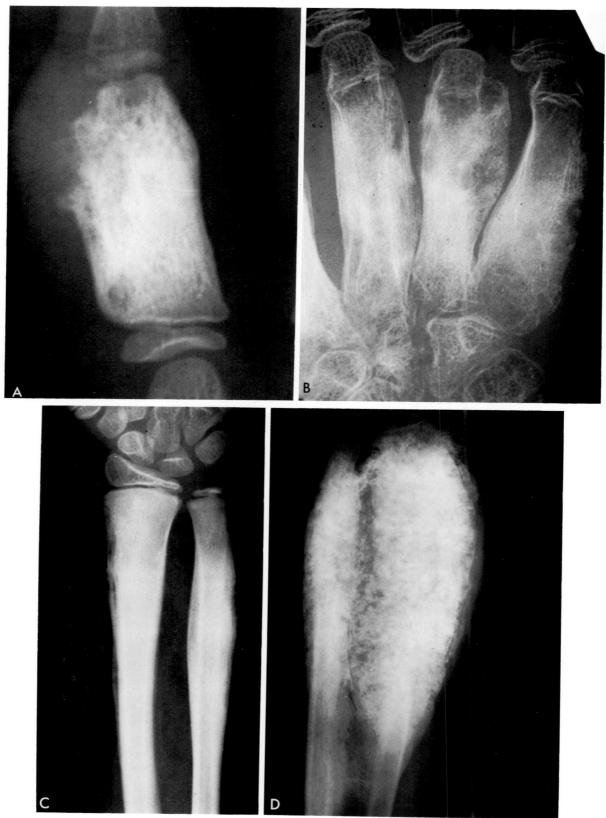

FIGURE 66–64. Yaws.

A, B Dactylitis is characterized by lytic lesions surrounded by florid periosteal proliferation. Note the enlarged and sclerotic osseous contours.

C, D Osteitis and osteomyelitis produce a similar radiographic appearance at other sites, in these views the radius and ulna.

(B, D, Courtesy of W. P. Cockshott, M.D., Hamilton, Ontario, Canada.)

telescoping of the digits are observed.[291] In these cases, the findings may resemble leprosy or psoriatic arthritis. In yaws, however, the distal phalanges usually are spared.[292] In children, similar destructive changes of the phalangeal diaphyses can lead to growth disturbances with short, deformed fingers.[293] Bowing of the long tubular bones of the extremities with concentric atrophy and extensive joint deformities with bony ankylosis also have been recorded.[744]

The radiographic changes in the skeleton in patients with yaws are similar to those of syphilis. Minor differences in yaws include less frequent destruction of the nose and more common deformity of the phalanges.[744] A correct diagnosis is established by the isolation of *T. pertenue* from skin lesions. Both yaws and syphilis produce a positive Wassermann reaction.

Bejel

Bejel, an infectious disease caused by a spirochete indistinguishable from *Treponema pallidum,* is prevalent in the Middle East. The organism is found in saliva, and the disease is believed to be transfered by kissing or sharing eating utensils.[740] Its manifestations include skin ulcerations on the lips and mouth, lymphadenopathy, osteitis, and periostitis. Destruction of facial bones, including the nose, may be detected. Unlike secondary syphilis, bejel rarely is accompanied by generalized rash and alopecia.[740]

Tropical Ulcer

Tropical ulcers are seen in patients of all ages from Central and East Africa.[294] The initial lesions are painful and tense swellings with a serosanguineous discharge, which appear on the anterolateral aspect of the distal portions of the lower limbs and spread rapidly.[295] As the ulcer erodes muscles and tendons, it may reach the underlying bone. The favorite target area is the middle third of the tibia; fibular involvement is less frequent and, when present, is most common in the distal third of the shaft. Periostitis leads to broad-based excrescences resembling osteomas (Fig. 66–65*A, B*).[295, 296] Cortical sequestra can appear, which are extruded from the body via the skin ulceration. Osteoporosis[294] and bulbous expansion[295] of neighboring bone can be evident. In chronic cases, deformities appear, which consist of elongation and bowing of the osseous structures. Flexion deformities of the knee and talipes equinovarus and calcaneovalgus deformities of the foot are typical.[295] Gas gangrene and tetanus may complicate long-standing cases.[294] In approximately 25 per cent of cases, malignant degeneration leading to epidermoid carcinomas of the involved skin (Fig. 66–65*C, D*) can produce destruction of subjacent cortical and medullary tissues,[297] with pathologic fractures. This complication appears in patients with chronic skin ulcerations (greater than 10 years in duration) and most typically involves the tibia.

The cause of tropical ulcer appears to be multifactorial. Trauma is common, and cultures of the lesion frequently isolate Vincent's types of fusiform bacilli and spirochetes.[298, 299] Staphylococcus also is present frequently.[295] An additional factor in the development of the ulcer may be malnutrition.[300]

Another type of skin ulceration seen in the tropics is the Buruli ulcer, related to infection with *Mycobacterium ulcerans.*[745–748] Originally discovered in the Buruli region of

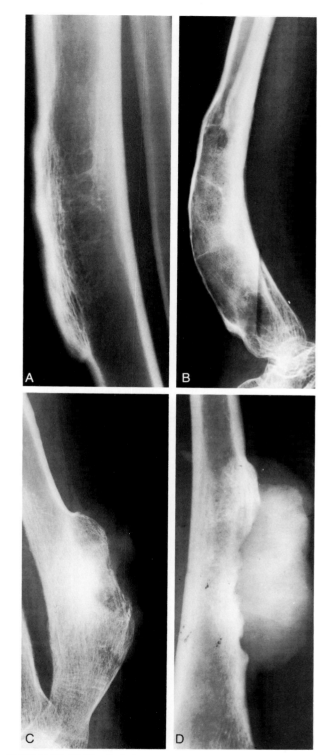

FIGURE 66–65. Tropical ulcer.

A The anterior surface of the tibia reveals a broad-based excrescence and an ivory osteoma. The bone is bowed, and the thickened trabeculae in the medullary bone indicate a response to altered stress.

B In a different patient, bowing of the tibia underscores the chronicity of the process. The bone is osteopenic and markedly expanded.

C, D Two examples of malignant degeneration at the site of skin ulceration leading to destruction of the underlying bone. Note the irregularity of the involved soft tissues.

(Courtesy of S. Bohrer, M.D., Winston-Salem, North Carolina.)

Uganda, this disease has been recognized in Nigeria, Southeast Asia, Latin America, and Mexico. Insect bites appear to be important in its transmission to humans. Children between the ages of 5 and 14 years are affected principally. Cutaneous and subcutaneous tissues, especially those in the extremities, are involved initially, although penetration into muscles is seen. Calcification in the soft tissues is described. Bone involvement is infrequent (Fig. 66–66).

Leptospirosis

Leptospires are members of the family Spirochaetaceae.[749] Human infection is initiated by the penetration of the skin and mucous membranes by the leptospire, a process that is facilitated by scratches, abrasions, and prolonged immersion in water.[749] Anicteric and icteric forms of the disease are recognized. The latter is more serious and can lead to severe involvement of the liver and kidneys. Clinical manifestations include fever, chills, anorexia, nausea, vomiting, aseptic meningitis, pyuria, hematuria, hepatomegaly, dehydration, arthralgia, and myalgia.[301] Myalgia occurs in 70 to 80 per cent of cases, is associated with muscle tenderness, and is most common in the calves and thighs.[749] Reports of arthritis are rare indeed.[302]

Rat Bite Fever

After a bite from a rat or, less commonly, a mouse, squirrel, dog, or cat, a febrile illness can be observed that is associated with a rash and arthritis.[303] Additional clinical findings include erythema about the inoculation site and

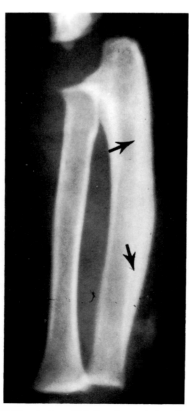

FIGURE 66–66. Buruli ulcer. This is a type of chronic ulceration that may appear in the tropics. It is due to *Mycobacterium ulcerans* and can lead to exuberant periostitis (arrows). (Courtesy of W. P. Cockshott, M.D., Hamilton, Ontario, Canada.)

monoarticular pain, swelling, and tenderness. The incubation period between the initiating event and the time of clinical onset of the disease is variable, although it may be weeks; therefore, the skin may have healed at the bite site before the patient seeks medical attention.[1102] The arthritis usually is noninfectious; however, septic arthritis also has been documented in patients with rat bite fever.[1102, 1103] *Spirillum minor* (a spirochete), *Streptobacillus moniliformis,* or *Actinomyces muris* may be isolated on culture of blood or joint fluid.

Lyme Disease

A relatively recently recognized inflammatory articular condition is termed Lyme disease, after the town in Connecticut in which it was first encountered.[512, 517, 527, 568] The disease, first observed in 1975, now is recognized in approximately 45 states and in Europe, China, Japan, the (former) Soviet Union, and Australia.[750–756, 934–936, 1104, 1112] In the United States, most cases of Lyme disease have occurred in the Northeast, Upper Midwest, and Far West. Both children and adults are affected, with a slight male predominance. There appears to be little risk, if any, of damage to the fetus of pregnant women with Lyme disease.[1105]

Clinical manifestations generally appear within 7 days of a tick bite, although they may be delayed for several weeks. The illness characteristically begins in the summer in the form of a distinctive skin lesion, erythema chronicum migrans.[896] This lesion typically appears as a macule or papule in the area of a previous tick bite (see later discussion), most often on the trunk or proximal portion of an extremity, such as the thigh, buttock, or axilla; subsequently it expands to an annular lesion with an intensely red border, which may be pruritic or burning.[753] The rash disappears in a period of weeks. Although the cutaneous manifestations are an important clue to the correct diagnosis, they are not constant, nor are they always remembered by the patient; in addition, in some cases they are overshadowed by constitutional flulike or meningitis-like symptoms and signs, including fatigue, chills, fever, headache, neck stiffness, lymphadenopathy, and, less commonly, splenomegaly and cardiac alterations.

Approximately 2 to 6 months later, joint manifestations appear that are characterized by a monoarticular, oligoarticular, or polyarticular process that is of sudden onset, of short duration, and associated with recurrence and, sometimes, migration from one location to another. Sites of involvement, in order of decreasing frequency, are the knee, shoulder, elbow, temporomandibular joint, ankle, wrist, hip, and small joints of the hand and foot.[753, 1109, 1110] Aspiration of affected joints reveals inflammatory synovial fluid, with or without eosinophilia,[1111] and biopsy of the synovial membrane documents hypertrophy, vascular proliferation, and cellular infiltration with mononuclear cells and scattered lymphoid follicles.[568] Radiographic characteristics of the joint involvement are soft tissue swelling and effusions. The latter may lead to rupture of the joint capsule with dissection of the synovial fluid into surrounding muscular tissue planes.[757] In the knee, the resulting clinical findings resemble those of thrombophlebitis.

Infrequently, a chronic oligoarthritis develops, especially in the knees, that is associated with persistent and prominent joint swelling.[937] This may occur in as many as 10 per cent of untreated patients. In such cases, juxta-articular osteoporosis, cartilage loss, and marginal bone erosions may appear[757, 1116] (Fig. 66–67). Other radiographic features include subchondral cysts, osteophytes, calcification or ossification at entheses, and, rarely, chondrocalcinosis.[757, 1117, 1118] Histologic inspection of the synovial membrane in chronic arthritis shows thickening with pannus formation similar to that in rheumatoid arthritis.

Lyme disease is transmitted by *Ixodes dammini* or related ixodid ticks.[752] Patients with Lyme disease are more likely to have a cat or farm animal, a pet with ticks, or previous tick bites.[1107] The disease itself is caused by a recently recognized spirochete.[758–761, 1106, 1113, 1270, 1271] This spirochete, *Borrelia burgdorferi,* has been recovered from the midgut of such ticks.[1107] *B. burgdorferi* is widespread in the animal kingdom, and virtually any domestic mammal can act as an intermediate host. Reservoir hosts of the spirochetes include deer and white-footed mice. Tick larvae become infected by feeding on such hosts. If these ticks later bite humans, the spirochete is introduced through the person's skin. The causative spirochete has been isolated, although infrequently, from the blood, skin, cerebrospinal fluid, and synovial membrane of affected patients,[896, 897] suggesting that it spreads hematogenously to many different sites. Within the synovial membrane, a distinctive form of endarteritis obliterans has been evident, implying that the Lyme spirochetes may survive for years in the synovium and may be responsible for microvascular injury.[760] Immune complexes occurring as a reaction to the spirochete also may localize in joints, leading to the development of a rheumatoid arthritis–like synovitis.[753, 1108] Patients with neurologic or articular abnormalities often have the B cell alloantigen DR 2. DR 2 or DR 4 antigens, or both, have been found more often in patients with chronic, rather than brief, arthritis, and the presence of DR 4 antigens has been associated with antibiotic failure.[1105] Spirochetal antibody assays for Lyme disease enhance diagnostic accuracy and facilitate successful treatment of patients with this disorder.[897] Seroreactivity to *B. burgdorferi* antigens may be observed in persons without Lyme disease, however.[1272]

The clinical and radiologic features of Lyme disease resemble those of juvenile chronic arthritis, Reiter's syndrome, and granulomatous infections such as tuberculosis.[757] The similarity of Lyme disease to Reiter's syndrome is underscored by a report in which circulating antibodies and proliferative T cell responses to *B. burgdorferi* were demonstrated in 18 per cent of patients with reactive arthritis or Reiter's syndrome.[1114, 1115]

FUNGAL AND HIGHER BACTERIAL INFECTION

A variety of pathogenic fungi can produce human disease. Although some possess a worldwide distribution, others are located within reasonably well defined geographic boundaries. All are dimorphic: They have a free-living mycelial form that produces infectious spores; these are inhaled and converted to yeastlike pathogenic forms that lead to human illness.[762] Although healthy persons may become hosts for fungal diseases, these pathogens become more virulent in subjects with depressed immunologic function, in whom widespread and sometimes fatal abnormalities may occur. The following discussion emphasizes the musculoskeletal alterations associated with fungi and related higher bacteria, such as Actinomyces and Nocardia.

Actinomycosis

General Features

Actinomycosis is a noncontagious suppurative infection that is caused by anaerobic organisms that normally are found in the mouth. These organisms are higher bacteria, resembling mycobacteria, and frequently are misclassified as fungi. *Actinomyces israelii, A. bovis, A. naeslundii, A. viscosus,* and *A. odontolyticus* are some of the human pathogens. Actinomycosis may develop in debilitated persons or in devitalized tissues. The infections are especially frequent in the face and the neck, which probably is explained by the prevalence of these organisms within the oral and nasal cavities. Trauma is important in the introduc-

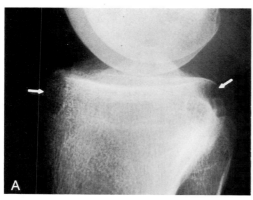
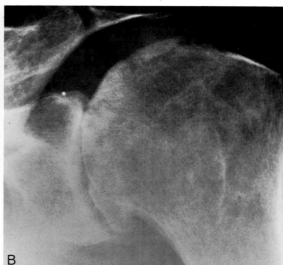

FIGURE 66–67. Lyme disease.

A Note bone erosions (arrows) in the anterior and posterior margins of the tibia.

B In this patient, the glenohumeral joint space is narrowed, and erosions and osteophytes in the humeral head are seen.

(Courtesy of J. Lawson, M.D., New Haven, Connecticut.)

tion of organisms into tissues. Aspiration of foreign bodies, such as teeth, is another predisposing event. Pulmonary and gastrointestinal infections also are well known. From infective foci in the face, lung, or bowel, hematogenous dissemination of organisms can lead to contamination of subcutaneous tissues, liver, spleen, kidneys, brain, bones, and joints.

Musculoskeletal Abnormalities

Most typically, the skeleton becomes contaminated from an adjacent infected soft tissue focus; less commonly, hematogenous seeding of osseous or articular tissues occurs. The mandible, the flat bones of the axial skeleton (pelvis, ribs, spine), and the major joints of the appendicular skeleton are affected most commonly[107]: Mandibular and maxillary bone involvement may follow trauma or extraction of a tooth[304, 763]; actinomycosis of the bones of the hands can occur after a human bite[305]; and solitary lesions of the tubular bones of the extremities, the ribs, the pelvis, and the spine may result either from extension of adjacent soft tissue foci or from hematogenous infection.[306–308, 764–769, 938]

Osseous involvement is characterized by a combination of lysis and sclerosis (Fig. 66–68). In the ribs, the degree of bony proliferation may be extensive, and the combination of severe osseous eburnation, cutaneous sinus tracts, and pleuritis is suggestive of actinomycosis (Fig. 66–69). In the vertebral column, infection can originate from adjacent mediastinal or retroperitoneal foci. Several vertebrae commonly are affected, demonstrating lytic defects with surrounding sclerosis, and the intervening intervertebral discs may be spared.[309, 310] The posterior elements often are affected, including the spinous and transverse processes, laminae, and pedicles. Involvement of thoracic vertebrae almost always is associated with changes in the neighboring ribs.[311] Paravertebral abscesses may appear, but usually they are smaller than those in tuberculosis and do not calcify.[107]

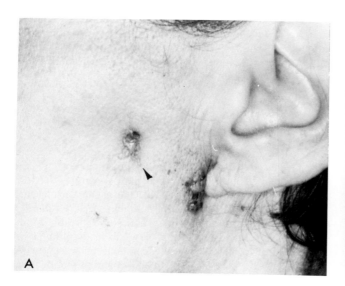

A

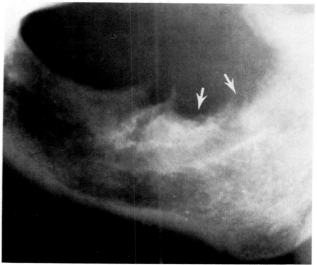

B

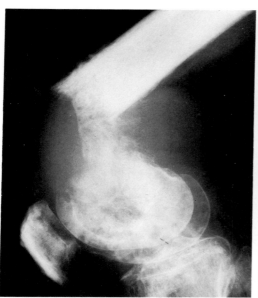

C

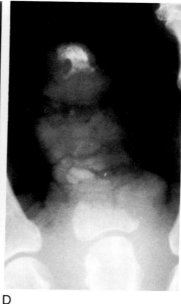

D

FIGURE 66–68. Actinomycosis.

A A clinical photograph of a patient with actinomycosis involving the mandible and temporomandibular joint reveals a sinus tract (arrowhead). (Courtesy of R. Smith, D.D.S., San Francisco, California.)

B In another patient, actinomycosis has led to erosion and sclerosis of a segment of the mandible (arrows).

C A neglected infection of the distal end of the femur has resulted in a moth-eaten appearance of bone destruction, periostitis, soft tissue swelling, and a pathologic fracture.

D In this diabetic patient with gout and actinomycosis of the digit, observe dissolution of portions of the proximal and distal phalanges and of the entire middle phalanx. Note the accordionlike appearance of the skin due to telescoping of the digit. (Courtesy of R. Taketa, M.D., Long Beach, California.)

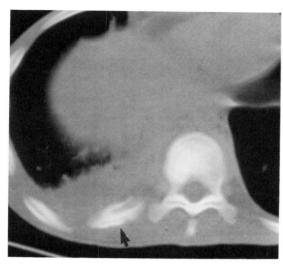

FIGURE 66–69. Actinomycosis. Transaxial CT scan of the lower thorax shows mediastinal, pulmonary, and pleural involvement with periostitis of an adjacent rib (arrow). A sinus tract was present.

Additionally, collapse of the vertebrae and angulation of the spine are less frequent in actinomycosis than in tuberculosis.[1] Neurologic complications related to spinal cord involvement in actinomycosis usually result from extradural extension of vertebral disease.[1119] In the mandible, a mixed lytic and sclerotic response predominates.[306] In the bones of the pelvis, mixed osteolysis and osteosclerosis again are observed, and hip and sacroiliac joint extension sometimes is seen. Predisposing events include tubo-ovarian abscesses, intestinal, appendiceal, or gallbladder rupture, and placement of intrauterine devices. At all sites, other diagnostic techniques, including scintigraphy, CT, MR imaging, and ultrasonography, sometimes are helpful.[764, 765, 938]

Pathologic examination confirms the presence of a granulomatous infection with abscess formation from which actinomycotic organisms may be recovered.

Nocardiosis

Nocardia species are members of the aerobic actinomycetes and are gram-positive. Human pathogens include *N. asteroides* and, to a lesser extent, *N. brasiliensis, N. farcinica,* and *N. caviae.* Introduction of organisms occurs via the respiratory tract, gastrointestinal tract, or skin after trauma. Persons with underlying chronic diseases, such as malignancy and pulmonary alveolar proteinosis, and those who are immunosuppressed are vulnerable to this infection. Pulmonary involvement may spread to the chest wall. Hematogenous seeding can lead to widespread disease, whereas cutaneous contamination may follow injury and, in turn, be followed by cellulitis and abscess formation (Fig. 66–70).

Osteomyelitis most commonly accompanies nearby skin infection (see later discussion of mycetoma) or pleural disease. Hematogenous spread to bones or joints also is possible.[770, 898] Tubular or flat bones are affected, and abnormalities of the spine and spinal cord are encountered.[771, 772, 1120, 1121] Primary infection of bursae related to this organism is rare.[1122]

Cryptococcosis (Torulosis)

General Features

Cryptococcosis, a serious disease of worldwide distribution, is caused by *Cryptococcus neoformans,* an organism that demonstrates unusual predilection for the central nervous system. This fungus can be recovered from the soil, pigeon droppings, fruit, and human intestinal tract and skin. Endogenous or exogenous sources may be important in the pathogenesis of this disease in humans. The disease generally is acquired by the respiratory route through inhalation of aerosolized spores. Once they reach the body and proliferate, cryptococci can be detected in the brain, the meninges, the lungs, other viscera, and the bones and joints. Neurologic manifestations of the disease predominate and include dizziness, ataxia, diplopia, headache, and convulsions. Many patients die within a few months.

The development of Cryptococcus infection in patients with compromised defense mechanisms is well known.[900] Thus, the disease may be seen in association with leukemia, lymphoma, Hodgkin's disease, sarcoidosis, tuberculosis, and diabetes mellitus as well as in persons with acquired immune deficiency syndrome[918] and those receiving steroid medications.[312] Patients who have undergone renal transplantation are particularly susceptible. Less commonly, otherwise healthy persons are affected. It has been reported that the granulomatous reaction to Cryptococcus infection is similar to that of sarcoid lesions, and differentiation between the two disorders may be exceedingly difficult.[313]

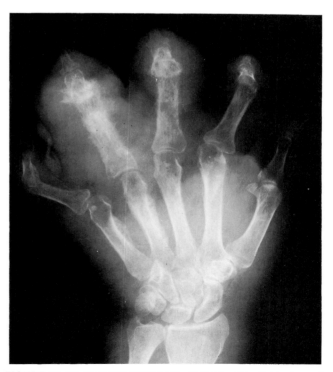

FIGURE 66–70. Nocardia brasiliensis: Osteomyelitis. Extensive soft tissue swelling and bone and joint destruction with osteoporosis and periostitis have produced a deformed hand. (Courtesy of W. P. Cockshott, M.D., Hamilton, Ontario, Canada.)

Musculoskeletal Abnormalities

Osseous involvement is a manifestation of disseminated cryptococcosis, appearing in 5 to 10 per cent of such cases.[314] Occasionally, an injury may allow direct implantation of organisms into the bone. Adults are affected far more frequently than children. The most commonly involved skeletal sites are the spine, the pelvis, the ribs, the skull, the tibia, and the knees, in descending order of frequency.[315, 773, 778, 1123–1125] Bony prominences may be affected, a peculiarity that also is evident in other fungal disorders, such as coccidioidomycosis. Single or multiple osseous foci are associated with soft tissue swelling and pain.

Radiographic features of bony involvement are not specific.[315–319, 773–779, 1126] Osteolytic lesions predominate, with discrete margins, mild surrounding sclerosis, and little or no periosteal reaction (Fig. 66–71A–C). Such findings can accompany other fungal disorders, tuberculosis, metastatic disease, and plasma cell myeloma, although the limited nature of the periostitis is more typical of cryptococcosis than of other fungal disorders. Eccentric cortical lesions, involvement of bone prominences and, in the skull, alterations of both tables, a soft tissue mass, and epidural extension[775, 1125] are additional clues to correct diagnosis.

Histologic evaluation of an osseous focus reveals granulomatous tissue containing multinucleated giant cells, histiocytes, and lymphocytes (Fig. 66–71D, E). There is a striking paucity of cellular reaction and an absence of suppuration and necrosis.[306] Cryptococcal organisms can be identified in the biopsy material. Rarely, these organisms also are recovered from sinus tracts (Fig. 66–72).[778]

Arthritis related to cryptococcosis is very uncommon[780] and almost invariably is the result of intra-articular extension of organisms from an adjacent osseous focus.[320, 321] Soft tissue swelling, effusion, and cartilaginous and bony destruction are observed in these cases. The knee is the most common site of involvement, although other joints, including the sacroiliac joint,[781] and more than one articulation can be affected.[545] The synovial fluid is turbid, purulent, and viscous.[1127] Microscopic evaluation of the synovial tissue reveals acute and chronic inflammation with granulomas and giant cells. Bursal involvement, although reported,[1128] is rare.

Rarely, extradural cryptococcal granulomas in the cervical, thoracic, or lumbar spine can lead to myelopathy or a cauda equina syndrome.[322–325] In these cases, initial radiographs may reveal osseous destruction of the spine and paravertebral swelling, and myelography, CT, or MR imaging can outline extrinsic compression of the spinal cord.[899]

North American Blastomycosis

General Features

This fungal disease is produced by *Blastomyces dermatitidis*. In the United States, its frequency is highest in the Ohio and Mississippi River valleys and in the Middle Atlantic states. The skin appears to be the portal of entry in some cases, infections commonly following cutaneous injuries. The respiratory tract may represent a second site of entry of organisms. Contact with soil containing the orga-

nisms may explain the higher prevalence in persons who engage in outdoor activities than in city dwellers.[762] In the skin, cutaneous abscesses develop beneath the epidermis and are surrounded by a granulomatous reaction. Clinically, they resemble neoplasms. Similar lesions may be encountered in the lungs. Infection subsequently can spread to other viscera, lymph nodes, and bones. The disease can be noted in men and women of all ages; it predominates in persons between the ages of 20 and 50 years.[1]

Musculoskeletal Abnormalities

The bones may be altered in as many as 50 per cent of patients with disseminated disease.[326] Skeletal changes can occur from hematogenous seeding or by direct extension from overlying cutaneous lesions. One or several osseous sites can be affected, especially the vertebrae, the ribs, the tibia, and the carpus and tarsus[1] (Figs. 66–73 and 66–74). No portion of the skeleton is immune.[107] Accurate diagnosis often is delayed[782] as clinical manifestations related to musculoskeletal involvement commonly are absent.[1129]

The radiologic features of blastomycotic osteomyelitis are not specific.[327–331] In the carpal and tarsal areas, cystic foci or diffuse, motheaten bony destruction can be seen, associated with osteoporosis and periostitis. In the tubular bones of the extremities, eccentric saucer-shaped erosions may be detected beneath cutaneous abscesses, or areas of focal or diffuse osteomyelitis in the subchondral regions of the epiphysis or the metaphysis can be encountered. The lesions frequently possess sclerotic margins and are surrounded by periostitis. Extension from the infected foci to soft tissues or joints is not unusual. Draining sinuses and cortical sequestration may appear in neglected cases. In the spine, blastomycosis resembles tuberculosis[310]; a thoracolumbar predilection, anterior vertebral erosion with extension into adjacent ligamentous and soft tissue structures, osseous collapse, paraspinal masses, alteration of posterior elements, and intervertebral disc space destruction are common in both diseases. It has been noted that paravertebral abscesses of blastomycosis may erode the neighboring ribs, a finding that is unusual in tuberculosis.[329] In the flat bones such as the pelvis and sternum, extensive erosion can lead to disappearance of large osseous segments. Skull involvement consists of lysis and sclerosis.[330] Rarely, blastomycosis leads to dactylytis, producing cystic or diffuse osseous destruction, findings that are reminiscent of tuberculosis.[328, 782]

Articular involvement usually is related to extension from an adjacent site of osteomyelitis. Rarely, however, joint destruction can occur in the absence of osseous disease.[332] In these cases, monoarthritis predominates, especially in the knee or the ankle.[901] Polyarticular involvement, when present, occurs later in the course of the disease.[1130] Clinical findings related to joint abnormalities may have an abrupt onset.[1127] Synovium, ligaments, and surrounding soft tissues are destroyed, subluxation is frequent, and the diagnosis is established by the recovery of typical organisms in the synovial fluid. Clinical or radiographic evidence of pulmonary disease aids in the correct evaluation of the joint disease.[546] Similarly, cutaneous abnormalities also are evident in most patients, creating an important pulmonary-cutaneous-arthritic triad.[546]

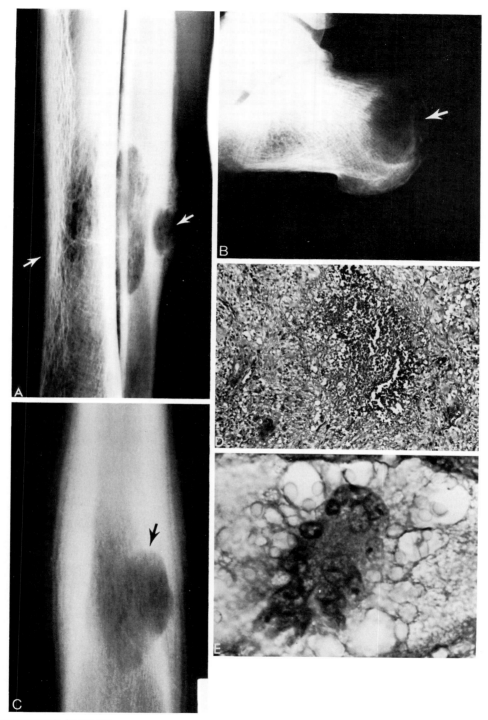

FIGURE 66–71. Cryptococcosis (torulosis).

A–C Discrete osteolytic foci with surrounding sclerosis and, in some places, periosteal reaction are seen (arrows). This involvement of bony protuberances such as the calcaneus is not unexpected in this disease. The resulting appearance simulates that of other fungal diseases, especially coccidioidomycosis, as well as neoplastic disorders.

D Note the granulomatous inflammation containing multinucleated giant cells at the periphery and suppuration at the center (granulomatous abscess or suppurative granuloma). (Hematoxylin and eosin stain, 40×.)

E At higher magnification observe many organisms in the peripheral cytoplasm of the multinucleated giant cell. (Hematoxylin and eosin stain, 400×.)

(**C,** Courtesy of P. Kaplan, M.D., Charlottesville, Virginia; **D, E,** courtesy of P. Haghighi, M.D., San Diego, California.)

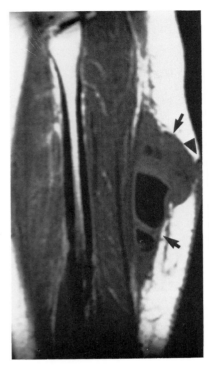

FIGURE 66–72. Cryptococcosis (torulosis). An oblique sagittal T1-weighted (TR/TE, 700/20) spin echo MR image reveals a soft tissue cryptococcal granuloma (arrows) in the posterolateral portion of the calf with signal intensity similar to that of muscle and regions of lower signal intensity consistent with fluid. A sinus tract (arrowhead) is present.

South American Blastomycosis (Paracoccidioidomycosis)

The fungal disorder termed South American blastomycosis, caused by the organism *Blastomyces (Paracoccidioides) brasiliensis,* occurs only in South America and in areas of Mexico and Central America. The infective agents invade the pharynx, presumably after inhalation, and from there spread locally or are disseminated throughout the body. Nasopharyngeal ulceration and local lymphadenopathy may antedate clinical findings in other locations. Hematogenous spread of infection to the lungs, spleen, other abdominal viscera, and bones can occur. In general, the features of musculoskeletal involvement are similar to those in North American blastomycosis. Solitary or multiple lytic lesions, geographic or well-defined bone destruction, marginal sclerosis, and periostitis are observed radiographic findings.[783] Tubular, flat, and irregular bones in both the axial and the appendicular regions may be involved (Fig. 66–75). In the spine, osseous and discal destruction and paravertebral masses appear. Symmetric alterations in the distal portions of the clavicles may be characteristic.[783] Joint involvement is rare.[902]

Coccidioidomycosis

General Features

Coccidioidomycosis results from inhalation of the fungus *Coccidioides immitis* in endemic areas of the Southwestern

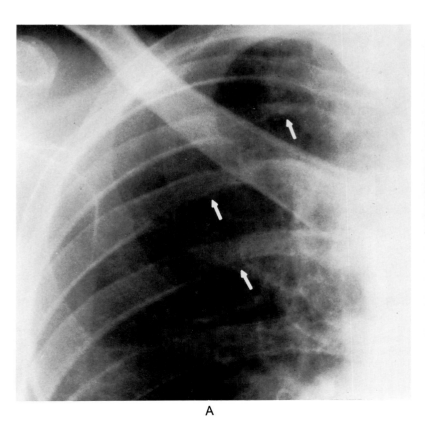

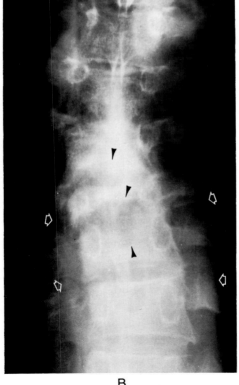

A   B

FIGURE 66–73. North American blastomycosis. This patient developed blastomycosis involving lung and bone. Note osteolysis of the inferior aspects of multiple ribs (solid arrows) and vertebral body and intervertebral disc destruction (arrowheads) accompanied by a paravertebral mass (open arrows). (Courtesy of A. Brower, M.D., Norfolk, Virginia.)

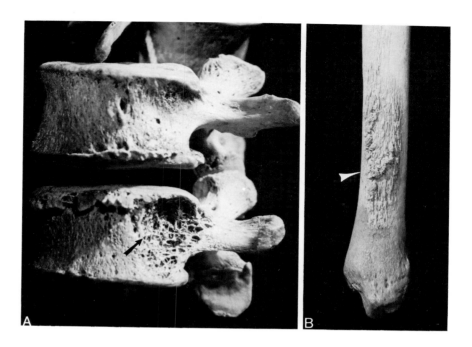

FIGURE 66–74. North American blastomycosis. Observe the honey-combed lesions of the vertebral body (arrow). Irregular new bone formation is seen in the fibula (arrowhead). (Courtesy of D. Ortner, Ph.D., Smithsonian Institution, Washington, D.C.)

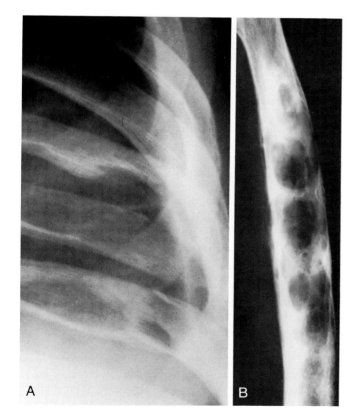

FIGURE 66–75. South American blastomycosis.

A Multiple ribs are expanded and radiodense and contain osteolytic lesions. Pulmonary and pleural involvement also was present. (Courtesy of D. Feigin, M.D., San Diego, California.)

B In this patient, multiple cystlike lesions of the femur are associated with bone sclerosis. (Courtesy of A. D'Abreu, M.D., Porto Alegre, Brazil.)

portion of the United States, in Mexico, and in some regions of South America. The fungus, which is an inhabitant of soil, is disseminated in dust. After inhalation, the organisms lodge in the terminal bronchioles and alveoli of the lungs where an inflammatory reaction may ensue. In some persons, disseminated disease may develop, with spread of infection to the liver, spleen, lymph nodes, skin, kidney, meninges, pericardium, and bones, as well as other sites. Men and women are affected equally, although the disseminated form is more common in men. Blacks, Mexican Indians, and Filipinos are especially susceptible. Pregnancy has a detrimental effect on the course of the disease. Patients younger than 5 years of age or older than 50 years of age account for a large proportion of cases with the disseminated form of the disease. Clinical manifestations vary in accordance with the distribution of the lesions, and in cases of wide dissemination, the mortality rate is high.

Musculoskeletal Abnormalities

Although an acute, self-limited arthritis ("desert rheumatism" with pain, swelling, and tenderness) may develop in approximately 33 per cent of cases of coccidioidomycosis,[333] only 10 to 20 per cent of patients develop granulomatous lesions in the bones and the joints. In most cases, bone alterations relate to hematogenous spread, although cutaneous infection can lead to contamination of subjacent bones (and joints). Osseous involvement can be confined to a single bone,[334, 784] although many series note a high frequency of multiple, symmetrically distributed bony foci.[335] Involvement of the spine, the ribs, and the pelvis predominates, although any bone can be affected.[335-341, 1131, 1256] Symptoms and signs can be prominent, even in the initial phases of the disease, and consist of pain, swelling, and draining abscesses.[939]

Radiographs frequently reveal multiple osseous lesions in the metaphyses of long tubular bones and in bony prominences (patella, tibial tuberosity, calcaneus, ulnar olecranon) (Fig. 66–76). In the tubular bones of the hands and the feet, diaphyseal alterations also are common.[1132] Well-demarcated lytic foci of the spongiosa are typical. Periostitis can be seen (Fig. 66–77), but bone sclerosis and sequestration are unusual. Lesions involving the ribs typically are marginal in location and can be associated with prominent extrapleural masses[335] (Fig. 66–78). In the spine, abnormalities of one or more vertebral bodies with paraspinal masses and contiguous rib changes are typical (Figs. 66–79 and 66–80). The intervertebral discs are relatively spared, and vertebral collapse and fistulous tracts are uncommon and late manifestations (Fig. 66–81). Rarely, significant vertebral sclerosis in coccidioidomycosis may simulate the changes that accompany neoplasm (metastatic disease from prostate carcinoma).[338, 547]

Joint involvement is most common in the ankle and the knee (Figs. 66–82 and 66–83), although other joints of the appendicular and axial skeleton may be the site of an infective arthritis[342-346, 548] (Fig. 66–84). In general, articular changes result from extension of an osteomyelitic focus, although, rarely, direct hematogenous implantation of the organisms into a joint can occur. Monoarticular involvement is most typical. Synovial inflammation and cartilaginous and osseous erosion lead to radiographic findings (osteoporosis, effusion, joint space narrowing, bony destruction) similar to those in other granulomatous articular

infections. In approximately 20 per cent of cases, a sterile migratory polyarthritis without radiographic changes (desert rheumatism or valley fever) occurs during the primary infection, 8 to 15 days after its onset, and is representative of a hypersensitivity syndrome.[548, 1127]

Coccidioidal bursitis and tenosynovitis (Fig. 66–85) of the hand and wrist have been reported.[347-349, 785] Tendon rupture is a described complication.[786]

Biopsy of skeletal or articular foci in this disease reveals granulomatous lesions similar to those of tuberculosis[1]; monocytes, giant and epithelial cells, necrosis, and caseation are identified[306] (Fig. 66–86). Accurate differentiation of coccidioidomycosis and tuberculosis requires isolation of the causative agent.

Cutaneous involvement can be a primary manifestation of the disease or occur secondarily from extension of deep infection in viscera, muscles, and bones. In addition, ulceration and penetration of cutaneous abscesses can lead to contamination of adjacent bones and joints.

Although radiography is the primary method used in the diagnosis of coccidioidomycosis, other imaging techniques can provide important information.[787] Scintigraphy, using either technetium or gallium radiopharmaceutical agents, or both, can localize sites of skeletal infection.[341, 787-790, 1133] Soft tissue involvement is well delineated with gallium scanning.[787, 789] CT and MR imaging are best applied to spinal infection.

Histoplasmosis

General Features

Histoplasmosis is caused by the dimorphic fungus *Histoplasma capsulatum,* which is present in many areas of the United States, particularly the Mississippi River Valley region in the central portion of the country. A similar organism, *Histoplasma capsulatum* var. *duboisii,* also can lead to disease, especially in Africa. The disorder, which is the most common systemic fungal infection in the United States, results from exposure to soil containing the spores of this fungus. The portal of entry usually is the respiratory tract, although the gastrointestinal system may be an additional portal in some persons. Diffuse disease can result, and the fungus proliferates most extensively in cells of the reticuloendothelial system. Involvement of the brain, lymph nodes, spleen, adrenal gland, lung, bowel, and bone marrow is most typical.

Musculoskeletal Abnormalities

Skeletal involvement may occur in association with *H. capsulatum* or, more frequently, *H. duboisii* infection. In histoplasmosis due to *H. capsulatum,* the pelvis, the skull, the ribs, and the small tubular bones are affected most typically[350]; children may be affected more commonly than adults.[350-353, 791] Noncaseating granulomas are detected in the bone marrow.[653] In this variety of histoplasmosis, joint alterations also have been noted, especially in the knees, ankles, wrists, and joints of the hands, leading to clinical (pain, swelling), radiologic (osteoporosis, joint space narrowing, erosion), and pathologic (granulation tissue with phagocytic cells) findings similar to those of sarcoidosis and tuberculosis.[353, 354, 549, 1127, 1134] In some cases, hypersensitivity to *H. capsulatum,* rather than direct infection, ap-

Text continued on page 2515

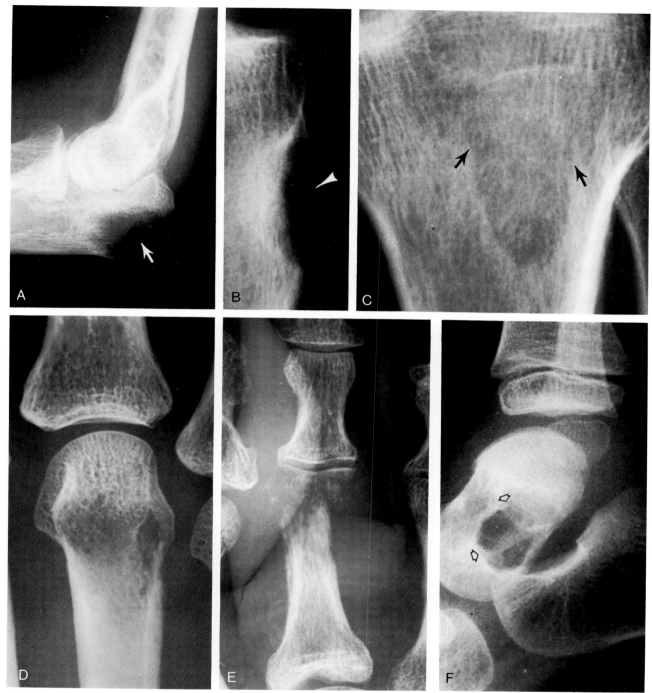

FIGURE 66–76. Coccidioidomycosis: Osteomyelitis (appendicular skeleton).

A, B Involvement of bony protuberances such as the ulnar olecranon (arrow) and tibial tuberosity (arrowhead) is frequent. Discrete lesions with surrounding sclerosis are evident.

C Note the osteolytic lesion of the proximal end of the tibia (arrows).

D, E In this patient, osteolytic foci of the metacarpal head and proximal phalanx of the toe reveal poorly defined or motheaten bone destruction and are associated with periostitis and soft tissue swelling. The joints appear normal, and a pathologic fracture through the phalangeal lesion is evident.

F In a child, a cystic lesion of the talus (arrows) is associated with considerable soft tissue swelling.

(B, C, From Armbuster TG, et al: J Nucl Med 18:450, 1977.)

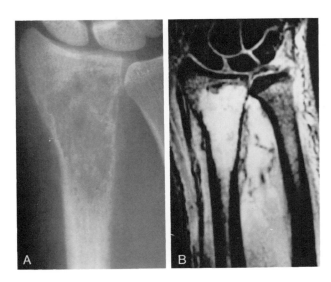

FIGURE 66–77. Coccidioidomycosis: Osteomyelitis (appendicular skeleton). In this 29 year old man, an initial radiograph **(A)** shows an osteolytic lesion with motheaten bone destruction and periostitis of the radius. A coronal multiplanar gradient recalled (MPGR) image (TR/TE, 600/15; flip angle, 20 degrees) **(B)** shows high signal intensity in the lesion and soft tissues. The patient was an intravenous drug abuser.

FIGURE 66–78. Coccidioidomycosis: Osteomyelitis (axial skeleton). This 33 year old man had fever and pulmonary infiltrate. The diagnosis of disseminated coccidioidomycosis was established by skin biopsy, bone marrow and cerebrospinal fluid examination, and positive serologic test results. Radiography outlines lytic lesions with surrounding sclerosis (arrows) involving ribs and clavicles.

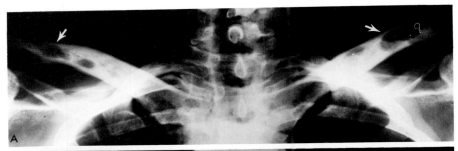
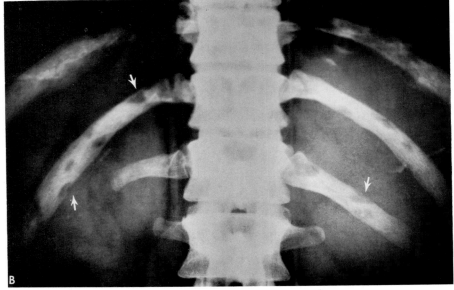

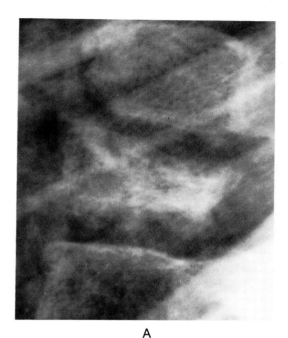
A

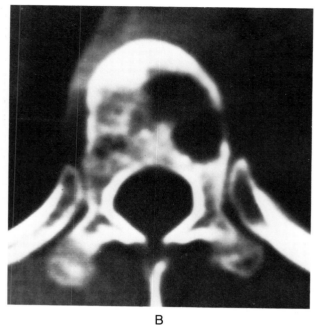
B

FIGURE 66–79. Coccidioidomycosis: Spondylitis.
A In this child, partial collapse of a thoracic vertebral body is accompanied by sclerosis but is unassociated with intervertebral disc space narrowing. Adjacent vertebral bodies also were abnormal.
B In a different patient, a well-defined osteolytic lesion located in a thoracic vertebral body is observed on a transaxial CT scan.
(**B,** Courtesy of T. Broderick, M.D., Orange, California.)

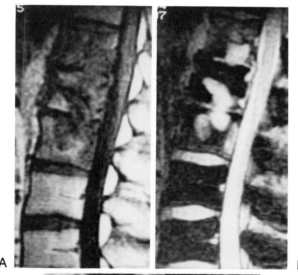
A   B

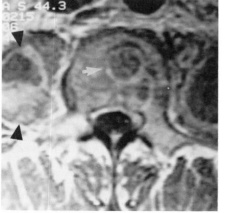
C

FIGURE 66–80. Coccidioidomycosis: Spondylitis.
A In this 39 year old man, a sagittal T1-weighted (TR/TE, 400/20) spin echo MR image shows foci of low signal intensity in the twelfth thoracic and first and second lumbar vertebral bodies, as well as in the intervening intervertebral discs.
B A sagittal multiplanar gradient recalled (MPGR) image (TR/TE, 500/11; flip angle, 20 degrees) shows corresponding foci of high signal intensity.
C A transaxial T1-weighted (TR/TE, 800/20) spin echo image obtained immediately after the intravenous injection of a gadolinium contrast agent reveals enhancing vertebral (arrow) and psoas muscle (arrowheads) lesions.
(Courtesy of D. Witte, M.D., Memphis, Tennessee.)

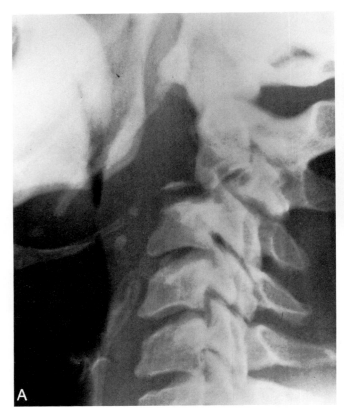

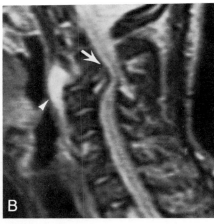

FIGURE 66–81. Coccidioidomycosis: Spondylitis.

A In this adult patient, the third cervical vertebral body is destroyed, with only a small piece of bone evident. The axis and the remaining portions of the third cervical vertebra are displaced posteriorly with respect to the fourth cervical vertebra. A large soft tissue mass is apparent.

B A T2-weighted (TR/TE, 1600/80) spin echo MR image in the sagittal plane shows extrinsic compression on the spinal cord (arrow) by the displaced bone. The area of high signal intensity (arrowhead) anterior to the vertebrae represents a soft tissue abscess.

(Courtesy of J. Mall, M.D., San Francisco, California.)

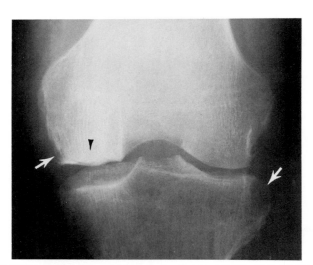

FIGURE 66–82. Coccidioidomycosis: Septic arthritis. This 49 year old man developed disseminated coccidioidomycosis with involvement of the right knee. Synovial biopsy and culture confirmed the existence of septic arthritis due to the fungus. A radiograph reveals soft tissue swelling, marginal osseous erosions (arrows), and flattening with sclerosis of the medial femoral condyle (arrowhead). The last-mentioned findings resemble those in spontaneous osteonecrosis of the knee.

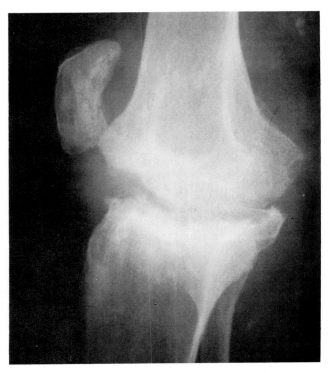

FIGURE 66–83. Coccidioidomycosis: Septic arthritis. In a different patient from the one in Figure 66–82, more extensive articular destruction of the knee is apparent. Note the degree of reactive sclerosis and the large joint effusion.

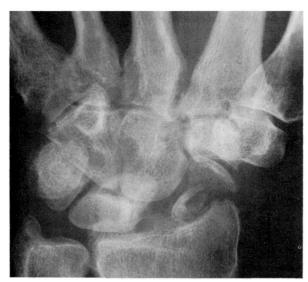

FIGURE 66–84. Coccidioidomycosis: Septic arthritis. This 41 year old man had arthritis of the right wrist and left fifth metatarsophalangeal joint. Subsequent right wrist synovectomy and resection of the left fifth metatarsal head revealed spherules of *Coccidioides immitis.* The radiograph delineates destructive changes of the ulna, scaphoid, and other carpal and metacarpal bones. Narrowing of the radiocarpal, midcarpal, and common carpometacarpal joints is evident.

pears to represent the pathogenesis of joint involvement.[792, 793] In these instances, the synovial fluid is mildly inflammatory in type, and histologic inspection of the synovial membrane fails to document granulomas. Other manifestations include infective tenosynovitis and the carpal tunnel syndrome.[1127]

In histoplasmosis due to *H. duboisii,* granulomatous ulcerating and papular lesions of the skin can be associated with osseous and articular changes in as many as 80 per

cent of patients.[355] Multiple bony foci predominate in the flat bones (skull, rib, pelvis, sternum), although the spine and tubular bones also can be affected (Fig. 66–87). Cystic lytic areas are most typical.

Sporotrichosis

General Features

Sporotrichosis, a chronic fungal disease, is caused by *Sporothrix schenckii* and is characterized by suppurating nodular lesions of the skin and the subcutaneous tissues.[356] The fungus resides as a saprophyte on vegetation and can invade the human body through a wound of the skin; the disease is not uncommon after cutaneous puncture with thorns and is a recognized occupational hazard of florists and farmers. In this situation, the dominant upper limb commonly is affected. Human disease also has resulted from animal contact, apparently after bites of rats, mice, gophers, and parrots.[306] After inoculation, a painless, ulcerating cutaneous lesion develops, and the organisms spread locally, producing nodular lesions of the lymphatic channels. Rarely, disseminated disease can evolve, perhaps by a gastrointestinal or respiratory portal of entry. Patients with widespread involvement commonly reveal an underlying disorder, such as a malignant lesion, a myeloproliferative disease, or alcoholism, or they have been receiving corticosteroid preparations. In the disseminated form of sporotrichosis, bone and joint changes may appear in 80 per cent of cases, and death can occur rapidly.

Musculoskeletal Abnormalities

Osseous and articular involvement can occur from hematogenous dissemination of infection or from extension of a contaminated cutaneous or subcutaneous focus.[357–364, 795, 919] Localization in one or more joints is especially characteristic, with predilection for the knee, the wrist and hand,

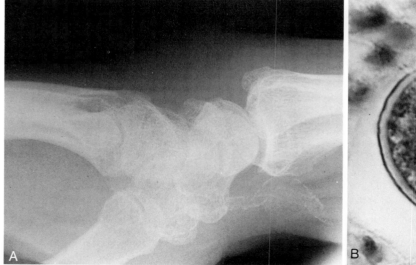
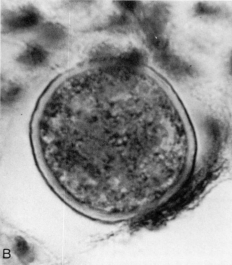

FIGURE 66–85. Coccidioidomycosis: Tenosynovitis. A 58 year old Mexican man developed swelling in the dorsum of the hand and wrist and rupture of the extensor tendons leading to the third and fourth fingers.

   A The lateral radiograph shows considerable soft tissue swelling in the dorsum of the wrist. The bones are normal.

   B At surgery, granulomatous material was found to involve the extensor retinaculum. Histologic examination revealed necrotizing granulomatous inflammation with spherules and endospores of *Coccidioides immitis.* One spherule is shown (400×).

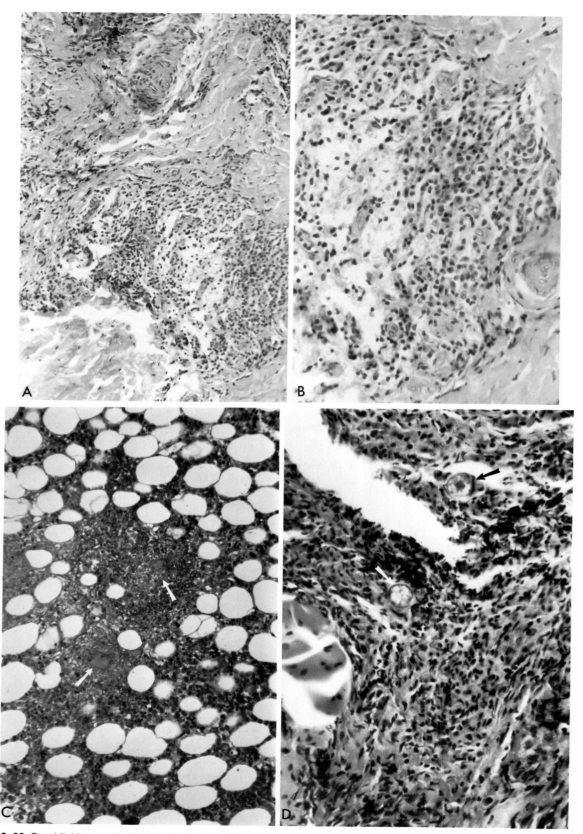

FIGURE 66–86. Coccidioidomycosis: Pathologic abnormalities.

A, B Photomicrographs (200×, 400×) of involved parasynovial tissue show diffuse infiltration with inflammatory cells (lymphoid and plasmacytoid cells). Although microorganisms are not identified in these areas, they were apparent at other locations.

C Photomicrograph of bone marrow shows a granulomatous inflammatory lesion with multinuclear giant cells (arrows).

D In the marrow, observe coccidioidal granulomas (arrows) among acute inflammatory cells, cellular debris, and epithelioid cells.

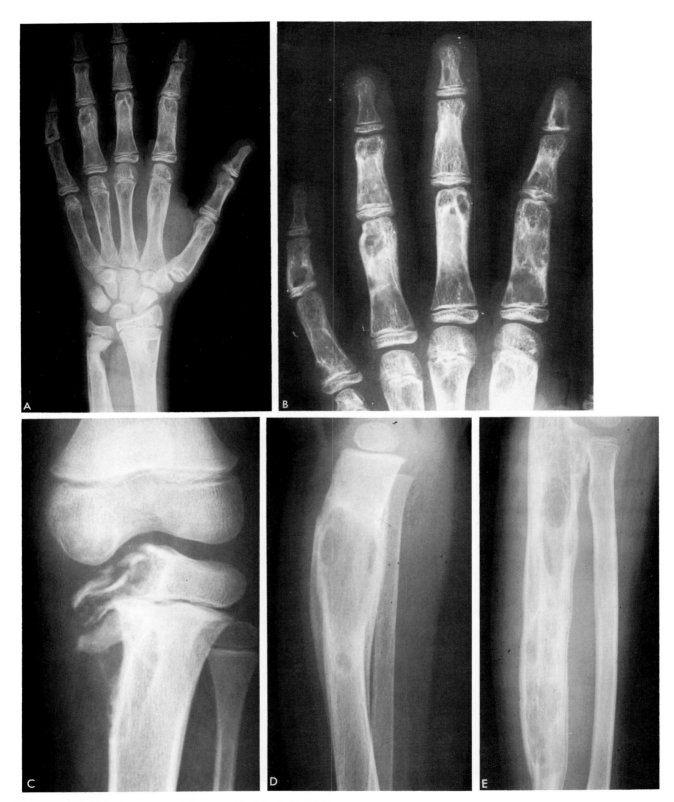

FIGURE 66–87. *Histoplasma capsulatum* var. *duboisii* osteomyelitis.

   A, B Radiographs of the left hand reveal cystic lesions of the radius, ulna, metacarpal bones, and phalanges. In many areas, they are well marginated and surrounded by reactive bone formation and mature periostitis.

   C Extensive lesions of the tibial epiphysis and metaphysis have produced collapse of the articular surface, with sclerosis and mild periostitis. The extension across the growth cartilage is not unusual in fungal infections.

   D, E Diaphyseal involvement of the tibia and ulna is characterized by lytic lesions and exuberant periostitis.

   (B, From Cockshott WP, Lucas AO: Q J Med *33*:223, 1964.)

the ankle, the elbow, and the metacarpophalangeal joints.[1135, 1136] Hip and shoulder involvement is rare. Soft tissue swelling, effusion, joint space loss, and irregularity, poor definition, and destruction of subchondral bony margins are seen (Fig. 66–88). Osteophytes may or may not be evident. Synovial biopsy reveals granulomatous inflammation, and synovial fluid or synovial tissue culture can outline the characteristic organisms.[363] Tendon and tendon sheath involvement and the development of sinus tracts have been recorded.[365, 366, 566, 798, 940, 1137] Bursal[795] and muscle[906] infection is rare.

Bone changes may take several forms. Eccentric erosions beneath subcutaneous lesions (especially in the tibia) can be encountered but are more typical of blastomycosis. Conversely, single or multiple lytic areas in bone can appear, related to hematogenous spread directly to osseous tissue or to synovium with extension into the neighboring bone. The tibia, fibula, femur, humerus, and short tubular bones of the

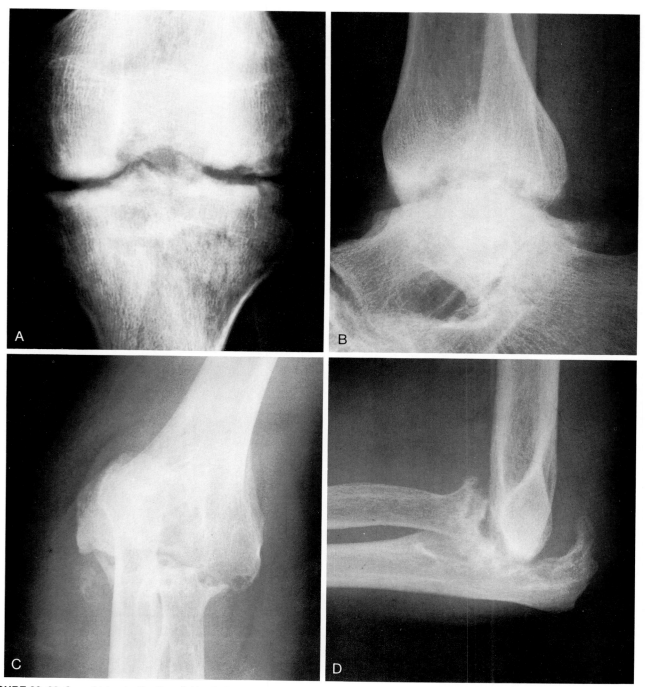

FIGURE 66–88. Sporotrichosis: Septic arthritis. **A–D,** Examples of knee, ankle, and elbow involvement. The findings in each case are similar, consisting of soft tissue swelling, joint space loss, and irregularity and poor definition of subchondral bone, with marginal and central osseous erosions. The changes are identical to those in other forms of septic arthritis. Joint involvement is not infrequent in this disorder, and osteoporosis may or may not be present. Note the involvement of the posterior subtalar joint in conjunction with ankle disease, reflecting the communication of these two joints. (Courtesy of A. Brower, M.D., Norfolk, Virginia.)

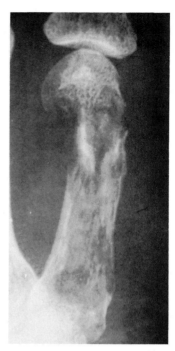

FIGURE 66–89. Sporotrichosis: Osteomyelitis. Note osteolysis of the fifth metacarpal bone with a pathologic fracture. (Courtesy of A. G. Bergman, M.D., Stanford, California.)

hand (Fig. 66–89) and foot are involved most commonly.[795, 796, 1138] Osteolysis predominates and periostitis usually is absent.[795, 797]

The radiographic features of osseous and articular involvement in sporotrichosis simulate those of tuberculosis, other fungal disorders, or pigmented villonodular synovitis. Although osteoporosis may not be apparent in some persons, perhaps allowing differentiation from tuberculosis, this is not a constant characteristic, limiting its usefulness as a diagnostic sign. Involvement of the small joints of the hands and feet appears to be more characteristic of this fungal disease than of the others.[360] Similarly, direct spread to joints without involvement of bone is more typical of sporotrichosis. Appropriate culture with isolation of *S. schenckii* allows precise diagnosis.

Candidiasis (Moniliasis)

General Features

Of the various Candida species, *C. albicans* most commonly is associated with human disease. Other pathogenic species include *C. tropicalis, C. guilliermondii, C. krusei, C. lusitaniae, C. rugosa, C. pseudotropicalis,* and *C. parapsilosis.*[762] Candida organisms reside normally on the mucous membranes. Abnormal proliferation on these membranes may occur in otherwise normal persons but is especially characteristic in debilitated children or adults, in patients receiving broad-spectrum antibiotics, in those with diabetes mellitus, and in patients with intravenous or Foley catheters. In the mouth, a mucocutaneous infection consists of white patches (thrush) with subjacent inflammation on the buccal mucosa. In patients with certain congenital immunodeficiency states, chronic mucocutaneous candidiasis can develop, leading to changes in the mouth, vagina, and

skin.[762] Infection introduced by intravenous catheters leads to local pain, redness, and swelling, whereas that initiated in the urinary tract produces candiduria, cystitis, and pyelonephritis.[762] Rarely, a widespread infection follows, leading to pneumonia and hematogenous contamination of multiple viscera, including the kidney, brain, thyroid and adrenal glands, pancreas, liver, myocardium, and endocardium.

Musculoskeletal Abnormalities

Candida infection of the musculoskeletal system occurs when the host resistance is depressed, perhaps related to prolonged corticosteroid, immunosuppressive, or antibiotic therapy. Intravenous drug addicts not uncommonly are affected.[1139, 1140, 1144] Indeed, a distinctive syndrome leading to systemic candidiasis with costochondral involvement has been recognized in heroin addicts[1141] (see later discussion). In the newborn, candidiasis may be associated with prematurity, infant respiratory distress syndrome, parenteral feeding, and umbilical catheterization.[552] Parenteral hyperalimentation fluids with their high concentration of glucose may predispose to Candida infection. Osteomyelitis or septic arthritis can occur with this organism.

Bone involvement in cases of disseminated candidiasis is relatively rare, being evident in fewer than 1 to 2 per cent of such cases.[367, 368, 1142] When present, such osseous involvement can result from direct hematogenous seeding of the bone, hematogenous involvement of a joint with spread to the periarticular bone, or extension from an overlying soft tissue abscess.[368-371] Although *C. albicans* frequently is implicated, other organisms, such as *C. guilliermondii,*[372] *C. tropicalis,*[373, 799] *C. parapsilosis,*[551, 801, 1146] *C. krusei,* and *C. stellatoidea,*[53] may be responsible for the infection. Infants, children, or adults can be affected. Osteomyelitis in any age group can occur in one or more sites, including the tubular bones of the extremities, the flat bones such as the pelvis, sternum, and scapula, the ribs, and the spine (Fig. 66–90).[550, 799, 941, 1278] Common patterns of distribution are involvement of a single long bone, involvement of the sternum, and involvement of two consecutive vertebral bodies.[1142] In the spine, the lumbar segment usually is affected. Although most cases of Candida osteomyelitis are

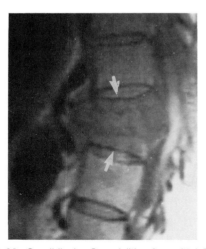

FIGURE 66–90. Candidiasis: Spondylitis. A sagittal T1-weighted (TR/TE, 600/26) spin echo MR image shows involvement of two contiguous vertebral bodies (arrows) and intervening intervertebral disc. The process is of low signal intensity with both anterior and posterior extension.

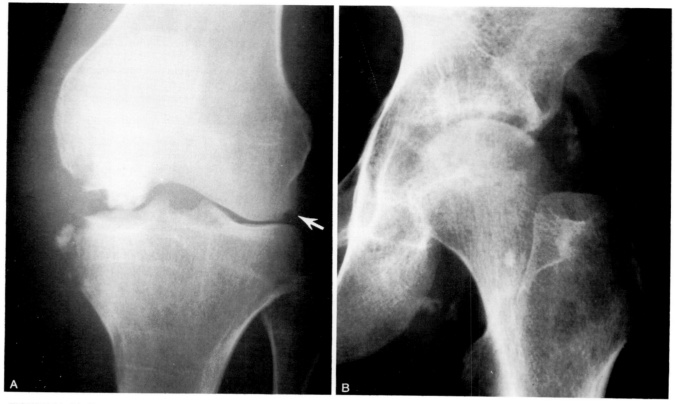

FIGURE 66–91. Candidiasis: Septic arthritis.
  A Observe massive soft tissue swelling, marginal osseous erosions (arrow), bone collapse and fragmentation, and joint space narrowing.
  B In a different patient, loss of joint space and osteoporosis are seen. Para-articular ossification also is noted.

hematogenous in origin, postoperative infections also are encountered.[1143]

Septic arthritis also is observed in candidiasis.[373–380, 803, 1273] Patients of all ages are affected, from the neonate to the elderly person. As in the case of Candida osteomyelitis, debilitation and underlying disorders (carcinoma, leukemia, rheumatoid arthritis, systemic lupus erythematosus, renal failure) are frequent in Candida arthritis.[1145] Clinical findings include fever, soft tissue swelling, pain, tenderness, and restricted motion. Monoarticular disease is slightly more frequent than polyarticular disease. Typically, infection predominates in large weight-bearing joints; the knee is the most common site of involvement. The pathogenesis of articular infection can relate to hematogenous contamination of the synovium or extension from an adjacent infected osseous or soft tissue structure.[1127] Rarely, direct inoculation of the joint at the time of aspiration or during a surgical procedure may occur.[801, 802, 903, 1273] With regard to hematogenous septic arthritis, neonates, patients with serious underlying disorders, intravenous drug abusers, and, less commonly, patients with human immunodeficiency viral infection are affected.[1127] Osteomyelitis is evident in 70 to 85 per cent of patients with hematogenously derived Candida arthritis. The frequency of spread of organisms from joint to adjacent bone has been confirmed in experimental *C. albicans* arthritis[381] and differs from the situation in some other fungal diseases, such as coccidioidomycosis, in which osteomyelitis usually precedes arthritis.[335] *Candida albicans* is the most typical implicated organism (approximately 80 per cent) in cases of Candida arthritis.

Radiographic findings include soft tissue swelling, joint space narrowing, irregularity of subchondral bone, and more widespread changes of osteomyelitis (Fig. 66–91). In patients undergoing surgery, a thickened synovial membrane with non-specific mononuclear cellular infiltration can be observed. Granulomas usually are not apparent. The diagnosis is confirmed by aspiration of synovial fluid or biopsy of synovial membrane with isolation of Candida.

The frequency of systemic candidiasis in heroin addicts deserves emphasis.[1147] Contamination of the lemon used to dissolve the "brown" heroin by strains of *C. albicans* previously colonizing the oropharyngeal and skin areas in such addicts appears to be the source of infection.[1141] Osteoarticular involvement occurs in approximately one third of heroin addicts who have systemic candidiasis, either as an isolated finding or, more commonly, combined with cutaneous and ocular lesions. Although the vertebrae,[1139, 1140] sacroiliac joint, knee, wrist, and other sites may be affected, costochondral involvement is most typical.[1141] On physical examination, a costochondral mass is detected, which can be localized further with gallium scintigraphy. Histologic findings include perichondritis, myositis, and less constant abnormalities of adjacent bone and cartilage.[1141]

Mucormycosis

Mucormycosis is a rare, serious, and commonly fatal infection due to several types of fungus (Rhizopus, Mucor, Absidia) in the class Phycomycetes. It appears in associa-

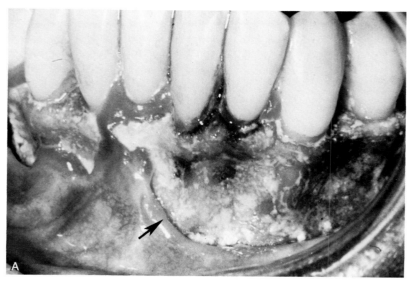
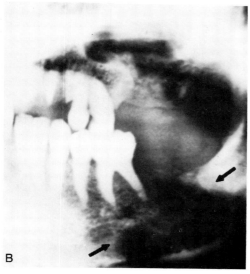

FIGURE 66–92. Mucormycosis: Osteomyelitis.
A Observe the destructive lesion involving the left side of the mandible (arrow).
B A radiograph outlines lysis extending to the angle of the jaw (arrows). (Courtesy of R. Smith, D.D.S., San Francisco, California.)

tion with debilitating illnesses, particularly diabetes mellitus, uremia with acidosis, lymphoma or leukemia, and extensive burns, as well as after massive corticosteroid therapy. The usual portal of entry of the fungus appears to be the paranasal sinuses, from which site infection can extend along the invaded vessels to reach the retro-orbital tissues and cerebrum. In the brain, arterial and venous thrombosis leads to multiple infarcts, and hematogenous spread of mucormycosis produces infective foci, especially in the lungs and intestines. These latter sites also can be contaminated after inhalation or ingestion of fungus. The clinical varieties of mucormycosis frequently are termed rhinocerebral, pulmonary, alimentary, or disseminated.[567]

Osseous abnormalities generally are confined to the skull and the face (Fig. 66–92).[804] Sinusitis can be complicated by destruction of the adjacent bony walls as a manifestation of infection or vascular invasion with necrosis.[382–384, 525] Bony alterations predominate about the maxillary and ethmoid sinuses; however, the frontal and sphenoid regions also may be affected.[385] Although localized osteolysis predominates, more extensive dissolution of some of the facial structures may ensue. In chronic cases, osteosclerosis also is evident. The differential diagnosis includes other varieties of osteomyelitis and neoplasm. The accurate diagnosis of mucormycosis is established by biopsy of involved tissue and demonstration of the distinctive hyphae.

A case of osteomyelitis of the proximal portion of the femur related to the fungus Rhizopus has been described.[399] A similar case of osteomyelitis and osteonecrosis of the cuboid bone also has been reported.[1148]

Aspergillosis

Aspergillus normally is a harmless inhabitant of the upper respiratory tract. Uncommonly, in patients with low resistance or in those who have received an overwhelming inoculum, a chronic localized pulmonary infection may result owing to inhalation of massive numbers of spores from

mycelia growing on grain. Primary infection of the ear, the nasal sinuses, or the orbit also may occur. The usual organism is A. fumigatus.

The musculoskeletal system rarely is involved in aspergillosis. Two potential mechanisms of infection have been emphasized: hematogeneous infection, which reportedly predominates in adults; and spread from a pulmonary or cutaneous infective site, a mechanism that may predominate in children.[1127] Indeed, pulmonary aspergillosis leading to chest wall involvement has been emphasized as a finding of chronic granulomatous disease in children (Fig. 66–93).[1149, 1150] Although other fungal and bacterial organisms can lead to skeletal infections in this disease and other osseous sites may be affected, rib, sternal, and spinal osteomyelitis related to aspergillosis predominate. Infective spondylitis due to aspergillosis can occur in the absence of chronic granulomatous disease, either in immunocompromised[1151–1153] or immunocompetent[1154] hosts and in both children and adults. Such spinal involvement generally relates to contiguous spread from a pulmonary focus. The thoracic spine is affected most typically,[386–388, 805, 904] and the radiographic features, which include osseous and intervertebral disc space destruction and paraspinal masses, resemble those of tuberculosis.[47] Similarly, extension of infection into the orbital bones and ribs also can be encountered.[389, 806] Rarely, the tubular or irregular bones of the extremities can be affected.[386, 390, 391, 600, 807, 1257] In these cases a typical osteomyelitis is evident (Fig. 66–94). Aspergillus arthritis is extremely rare and, when present, typically is associated with osteomyelitis (Fig. 66–95).[1127]

Maduromycosis (Mycetoma)

Maduromycosis, a chronic granulomatous fungal disease, affects the feet (Madura foot) (Fig. 66–96). It may be observed throughout the world but is especially prevalent in India. In fact, it is the town of Madura in India from which the name of the disease is derived.[808] In the United States,

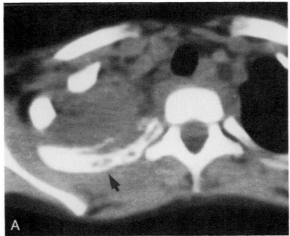

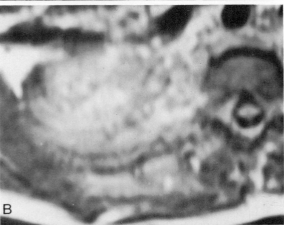

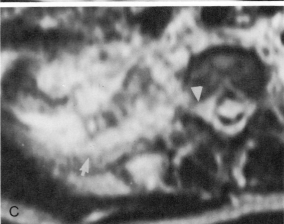

FIGURE 66–93. Aspergillosis: Osteomyelitis. Chest wall involvement in chronic granulomatous disease.

A Transaxial CT of the thorax in a 5 year old boy with X-linked chronic granulomatous disease shows consolidation in the right apical portion of the lung, soft tissue swelling, loss of fat planes, and osteolytic lesions (arrow) in the posteromedial aspect of the right third rib.

B, C Transaxial proton density (TR/TE, 2500/20) **(B)** and T2-weighted (TR/TE, 2500/80) **(C)** spin echo MR images reveal the pulmonary, osseous, and soft tissue abnormalities. The high signal intensity of the process is better identified in **C.** Observe inflammatory changes in the rib (arrow) and epidural space (arrowhead).

(From Kawashima A, et al: Skel Radiol *20:*487, 1991.)

the most frequent cause of Madura foot is *Petriellidium boydii (Monosporium apiospermum),* although Aspergillus, Penicillium, Madurella, Cephalosporium, Streptomyces, and Phialophora can produce this disease. Outside the United States, Nocardia species *(N. brasiliensis, N. madurae)* may be implicated (Fig. 66–97).

The infection of the foot (and less commonly the hand, arm, leg, or scalp) results from posttraumatic soft tissue invasion of organisms that are normal inhabitants of soil.[392–397, 809–811, 1155–1158] After soft tissue contamination, the organisms may penetrate the underlying muscles, tendons, bones, and joints. Sinus tracts arising from the infected osseous tissues are common.

The course of maduromycosis usually is progressive. Initially, soft tissue swelling is seen. Over a period of months to years, a swollen, deformed, and necrotic foot appears. Dissemination of infection may occur via lymphatic channels, and death may result from secondary bacterial infection.

The radiographic findings vary with the virulence of the invading organism.[398] In some cases, single or multiple localized osseous defects are evident, the size of which may depend on the specific causative organism[905]; in others, extensive soft tissue and bony disruption occurs, with associated periostitis and sclerosis. Intra-articular osseous fusion may appear, leading to an appearance that is termed ''melting snow.'' These radiographic features can simulate other types of osteomyelitis, neuropathic osteoarthropathy, and neoplasm.[107] MR imaging and CT can be used to delineate the osseous and soft tissue abnormalities further.[1159]

Other Mycoses

Chromomycosis is a disease related to many different organisms, especially species of the genera Phialophora and Cladosporium.[762] Infection follows traumatic inoculation, commonly in the foot, although other sites may be involved as well (Fig. 66–98).[812] A chronic localized process affecting soft tissues and bone is seen.

Candida (Torulopsis) glabrata can produce osteomyelitis in spinal and extraspinal sites.[814, 815, 1160–1164] It typically affects compromised hosts.[816] *Penicillium marneffei* infection occurs in a similar fashion.[1165, 1166]

VIRAL INFECTION

Rubella Infection (German Measles)

Rubella is a contagious disease of viral origin. Although rubella generally is a benign disorder in the adult, maternal infection in the first half of pregnancy can lead to serious skeletal and nonskeletal alterations in the fetus.

Postnatal Rubella

In the adult patient (especially women), rubella arthritis may occur within a few days to 1 week of the skin rash.[400–402, 554, 1167, 1168] Persistent or migratory articular findings are most common in the small joints of the hands and wrists, the knees, and the ankles; in addition, the carpal tunnel syndrome may be evident.[817] Synovial fluid aspiration can reveal mononuclear pleocytosis.[818]

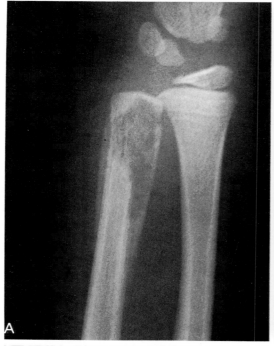

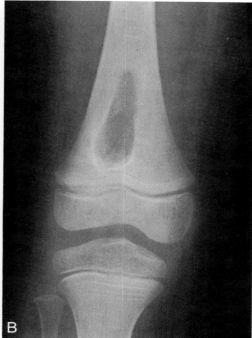

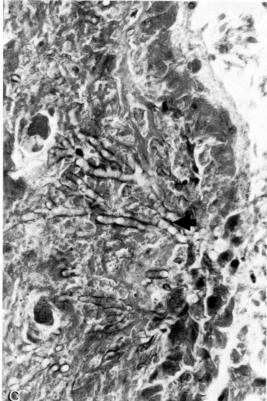

FIGURE 66–94. Aspergillosis: Osteomyelitis. A 5 year old girl had a cough, pneumonia, and skin ulcerations. Bacteriologic investigations were unrewarding and administration of various antibiotics led to clearing of the pulmonary infiltrates. Five months later, swelling developed in the wrist.

A An osteolytic lesion of the distal portion of the ulna is associated with periostitis and bone expansion. Biopsy recovered material that revealed chronic osteomyelitis, which, on tissue culture, was related to aspergillosis.

B A second lesion was discovered in the distal portion of the femur. It is well defined, with geographic bone destruction and a thin sclerotic margin. Serratia, believed to represent a secondary invader, was cultured from this lesion. Immunologic studies documented chronic granulomatous disease.

(**A, B,** From Diard F, et al: Australas Radiol *27*:39, 1983.)

C In this pulmonary lesion, from a different patient, histologic analysis shows septate hyphae with acute-angle branching. Septa are indicated by the arrow. (Hematoxylin and eosin stain, 160×.)

(**C,** Courtesy of P. Haghighi, M.D., San Diego, California.)

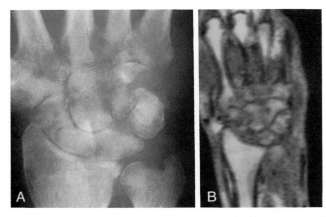

FIGURE 66–95. Aspergillosis: Septic arthritis. In this 74 year old patient with lymphoma who was receiving corticosteroid therapy, a septic arthritis of the wrist related to aspergillosis became evident.

A Routine radiograph shows osteopenia, joint space loss, bone erosions, and pancompartmental involvement.

B A coronal T1-weighted (TR/TE, 600/20) spin echo MR image shows foci of low signal intensity mainly in the carpal bones and bases of the metacarpal bones.

After live, attenuated rubella virus became available for active immunization, episodes of acute arthritis were noted in children injected with the virus.[403, 404] The frequency of this complication apparently depends on the type of vaccination used. The history of immunization 1 to 4 weeks preceeding the arthritis is crucial in making the correct diagnosis.[1167] The knee most typically is affected, although the articulations of the hands and wrists also may be involved.[1279]

Recovery of the wild or attenuated rubella virus has been accomplished from the synovial fluid after natural rubella infection[405, 818] and vaccination,[406] respectively. Histologically, a nonspecific synovitis is noted.[818] The erythrocyte sedimentation rate may be elevated, and transiently positive results of latex fixation may occur.[407]

A chronic arthropathy also has been associated with rubella vaccination.[408, 920] In this arthropathy, recurrent episodes of knee stiffness (catcher's crouch syndrome) may be characterized by hypertrophy of the synovial membrane with protrusion into the intercondylar notch. Other joints can be involved, and radiography may document nonspecific destructive and reactive changes in the adjacent metaphyses of tubular bones.[819]

Chronic seronegative arthropathy in both children and adults in some cases has been associated with the isolation of live rubella virus from the synovial fluid of affected joints.[820] Oligoarthritis and polyarthritis have been the observed clinical patterns, and no firm clinical evidence of rubella has been noted. Radiographic findings were variable but included intra-articular bone erosions, and histologic examination of the synovial membrane revealed inflammatory alterations. These observations, coupled with those provided by electron microscopy and immunofluorescence, are consistent with the hypothesis that the rubella virus itself is the primary etiologic agent in chronic arthritis.[820] The fact that the arthropathy resembles juvenile chronic arthritis is of interest, as other reports have indicated that rubella antibody levels are elevated not only in rubella vaccine arthritis but also in a significant proportion of children (approximately 33 per cent) with juvenile chronic arthritis, suggesting a possible role of rubella virus infection in this disease.[409, 921] A similar laboratory finding in adult-onset Still's disease also has been noted.[553]

Intrauterine Rubella

Radiographically evident osseous lesions due to intrauterine rubella infection first were reported in 1965[410, 411] and have been documented further since that time.[412–415] The radiographic features consist of metaphyseal lesions in long bones characterized by symmetry, linear areas of radiolucency, and increased bone density, producing a longitudinally oriented striated pattern (celery stalk appearance) and the absence of periostitis, features that can either disappear completely if the child recovers from the intrauterine viral infection or persist with increasing density of the juxtaepiphyseal region if the infection continues (Fig. 66–99). With healing, beaklike exostoses can be noted at the metaphyses. Histologic examination reveals variation in the thickness of the zone of mature cartilage cells adjacent to the epiphyseal line, multiple poorly calcified fragments of acellular cartilage, and osteoid.[416] Metaphyseal trabeculae may be reduced in number, and calcified bone and osteoid about the cartilaginous areas may be reduced in amount. Although positive cultures for rubella can be obtained from the bone marrow, histologic evidence of osteomyelitis generally is lacking; scattered periosteal mononuclear cellular infiltration[417] and abundant plasma cellular response in the metaphyses, epiphyses, and subperiosteal locations[413] occasionally have been noted.

It generally is believed that the metaphyseal and diaphyseal lesions of rubella are related to alterations in bone formation. In a comprehensive study of the histologic characteristics of the osseous abnormalities, Reed[417] suggested that the metaphyseal radiolucent streaks in this disease were a manifestation of osteoporosis resulting from an insult to bone maturation due to the viremia. Whalen and coworkers[415] observed a delay in diaphyseal modeling in transplacental rubella, although normal modeling could be achieved within 2 months, coincident with the correction of the metaphyseal alterations. In an investigation of rabbits that were congenitally infected with rubella virus, London and colleagues[418] concluded that a direct viral action on chondrocytes was responsible for growth retardation.

These osseous alterations, which may occur in as many as 45 per cent of cases[411] of intrauterine rubella, can simulate those that are noted in other viral disorders (see discussion later in this chapter). They usually are transient in nature, disappearing after several weeks, although persistent and progressive changes can appear, and they even may lead to pathologic fracture.[419]

Cytomegalic Inclusion Disease

Intrauterine infection related to cytomegalic inclusion disease can lead to intracranial calcifications and rubella-like abnormalities of the skeleton[420–423] (Fig. 66–100). Metaphyseal osteopenia, irregularity of the growth plate, and a striated pattern parallel to the long axis of the bone characterized by alternating lucent and sclerotic bands are noted. Spontaneous pathologic fractures also have been observed in infants with cytomegalic inclusion disease.[424, 555] The metaphyseal changes usually are evident in the first few

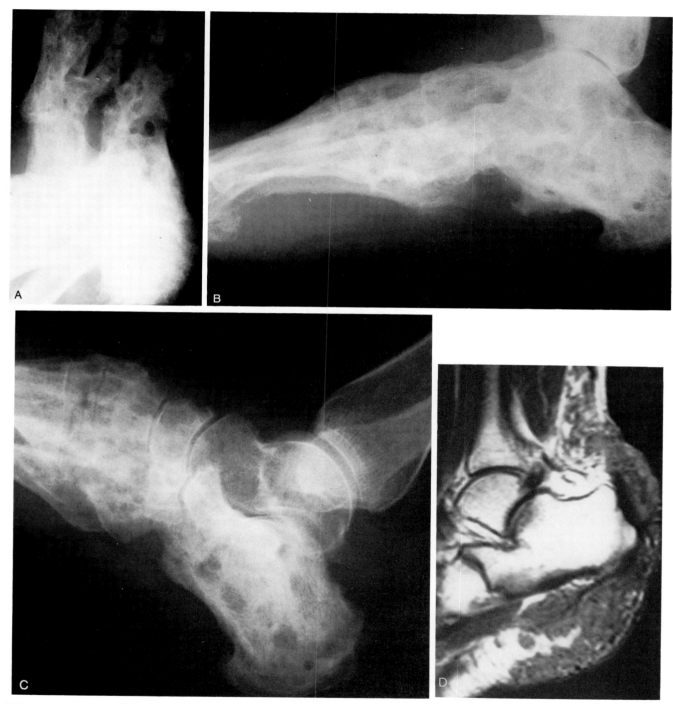

FIGURE 66–96. Maduromycosis: Madura foot.
   A, B Oblique and lateral radiographs delineate the osseous and articular effects of chronic involvement of the foot. Bony destruction and widespread intra-articular osseous fusion can be noted.
   C In a different patient, a 37 year old woman who had a long history of pain, swelling, and multiple draining sinus tracts in the foot, a similar radiographic appearance is seen.
   D In this 24 year old man, a sagittal T1-weighted (TR/TE, 650/30) spin echo MR image shows abnormal soft tissues about the posterior and plantar aspects of the calcaneus.
   (**C,** Courtesy of R. Cone, M.D., San Antonio, Texas; **D,** Courtesy of T. Mattsson, M.D., Riyadh, Saudi Arabia.)

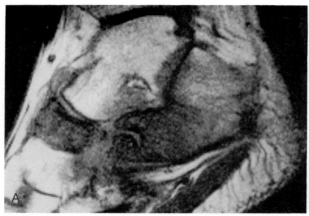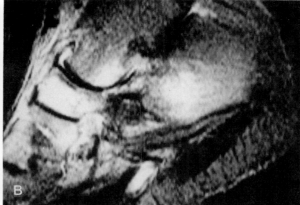

FIGURE 66–97. Maduromycosis: Madura foot. This 28 year old Cambodian man developed pain and swelling of the foot with drainage 3 years after stepping on a nail. Cultures of the bone revealed *Nocardia brasiliensis*. Sagittal T1-weighted (TR/TE, 500/32) **(A)** and T2-weighted (TR/TE, 2000/120) **(B)** spin echo MR images show evidence of osteomyelitis in the calcaneus, navicular bone, talus, and cuboid bone. High signal intensity in the bone and soft tissue is noted in **B**. (Courtesy of G. Greenway, M.D., Dallas, Texas.)

days of life and then disappear completely within a period of days to weeks. They generally are attributed to a disturbance in endochondral bone formation rather than to osteomyelitis, and these changes can be confused with findings not only of intrauterine rubella but also of erythroblastosis fetalis,[425] congenital syphilis, and hypophosphatasia. Similar alterations may be expected in other intrauterine viral infections and in premature infants of mothers with severe cyanotic cardiac abnormalities.[426]

Perinatal infection related to cytomegalic inclusion disease can arise from several different mechanisms: swallowing of cervical virus at birth; ingestion of breast milk containing the virus; and transmission of virus from blood transfusions. Such infections, when appearing in the neonatal period, can be misinterpreted as evidence of an inherited disease.[821, 822] Fever, sepsis, and pneumonitis are observed. Osseous changes presumably are rare, although periostitis in tubular and flat bones has been reported.[823]

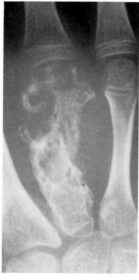

FIGURE 66–98. Chromomycosis: Osteomyelitis. Observe osteolysis and a pathologic fracture in the third metacarpal bone in this 12 year old boy. (Courtesy of R. Stiles, M.D., Atlanta, Georgia.)

Varicella (Chickenpox)

Varicella is a common benign disorder, usually evident in children, in which skeletal alterations are rare.[416, 556] Two fatal cases of varicella with bone marrow involvement have been recorded by Cheatham and associates[427]; in one child, irradiation and chemotherapy had been used for control of metastatic neuroblastoma, and in the second, steroids had been administered for treatment of acute rheumatic fever. In both cases, the virus was isolated and serologic studies were positive. Similar examples of bone marrow lesions occurring in association with varicella in patients with malignant tumors undergoing active treatment were noted by Feldman and coworkers.[428]

Articular inflammation of the knee in varicella was reported by Ward and Bishop[429] in a 5 year old girl. Although the virus was not isolated from the joint, the facts that the arthritis subsided simultaneously with the chickenpox and that other family members developed varicella justify the assumption that the infection was the cause of the articular abnormalities. Synovial fluid aspiration in another girl with varicella and arthritis revealed large mononuclear cells, a finding that has been observed in other virus-related arthritides.[557] These reports have been supplemented by others in which arthritis, usually of a single joint, occurred during the exanthem phase of chickenpox.[824–826] Acute swelling and pain of the joint or joints resolve quickly. These manifestations appear to represent a true viral infection of the articulation, as varicella has been isolated from the synovial fluid on several occasions.[825]

Varicella gangrenosa requiring amputation of the lower extremities also has been recorded.[430]

Bacteremia occurs in approximately 1 per cent of patients with varicella. Subsequently, bacterial infection of various organ systems may be identified. Although rare, bacterial osteomyelitis, usually related to streptococcal or, less commonly, staphylococcal organisms, can occur after varicella infection.[1169, 1258]

Varicella and Herpes Zoster

Herpes zoster, related to reactivation of latent varicella-zoster virus, is associated with nerve involvement, espe-

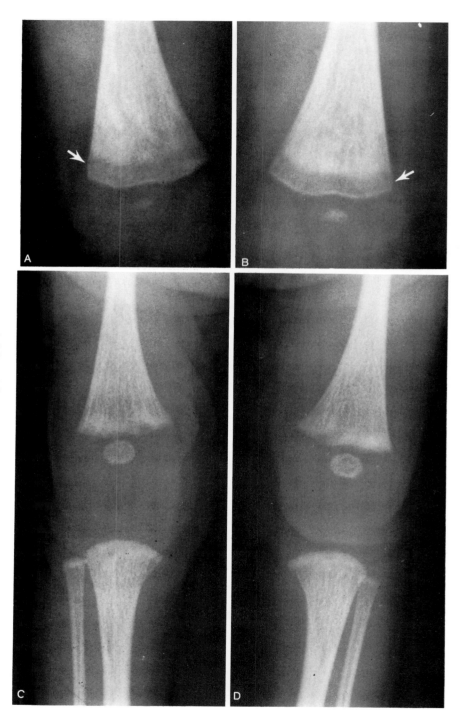

FIGURE 66–99. Intrauterine rubella infection.
A, B Radiolucent metaphyseal bands (arrows) in the distal ends of the femora of this infant are associated with relative sclerosis of the diaphyses.
C, D In a different infant, longitudinal striations have produced the characteristic "celery stalk" appearance. Periostitis is absent.

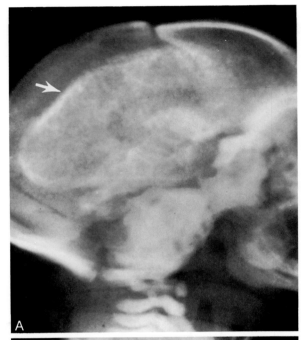

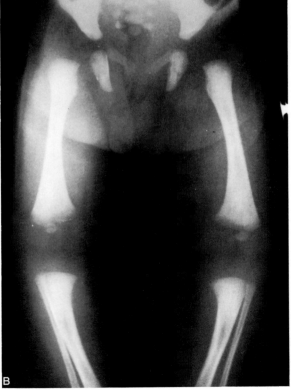

FIGURE 66–100. Cytomegalic inclusion disease.

A This disease can be accompanied by focal cerebral necrosis and calcification. The calcific deposits usually are bilateral and symmetric in distribution, within the walls of dilated lateral ventricles (arrow).

B Metaphyseal changes consist of irregularity of the growth plate and osseous fragmentation, most evident in the distal femora.

(Courtesy of F. N. Silverman, M.D., Palo Alto, California.)

cially the thoracic nerves and the ophthalmic branch of the fifth cranial nerve. One clinical pattern, termed shingles, leads to the sudden onset of severe, constant, and unilateral pain. A dermatome distribution is typical. Papules and vesicles in the skin appear.

Although disease dissemination occasionally is observed, musculoskeletal manifestations rarely are reported. Arthritis in this disease has been described, and spread of infection to the joints occurring either from a hematogenous route or along the involved nerves has been postulated.[827, 828]

Herpes Simplex

Herpes simplex virus types 1 and 2 can cause a variety of clinical syndromes. Infants can acquire the infection at birth, owing to the presence of the virus in the mother's cervix. Nonspecific skeletal abnormalities of the metaphyseal regions of tubular bones, similar to those seen in other congenital viruses, are observed.

In the adult, acute arthritis has been associated with the recovery of the virus from the synovial fluid.[829–831] A felon (whitlow) also may be seen.[942]

Mumps

Arthritis is a well-recognized manifestation of mumps, a viral disease, occurring in approximately 0.5 per cent of cases.[23] This complication usually is seen in young men, approximately 10 to 14 days after the parotitis.[832–836] A migratory polyarthralgia or polyarthritis affects predominantly the large joints, although those of the hands and the feet also can be involved. The findings can simulate those of adult-onset Still's disease.[832] To date, the mumps virus has not been isolated from the joint fluid.

Variola (Smallpox)

Osteomyelitis and septic arthritis are well-known complications of smallpox. The term osteomyelitis variolosa was originated by Chiari[431] in a description of nonsuppurative lesions in the bone marrow of patients who died of smallpox during the Prague epidemic of 1891–1892. Since that report, numerous further descriptions of musculoskeletal alterations in this viral disease have appeared.[432–440] No apparent relationship has been found between the severity of the infection and the frequency or severity of osteomyelitis or septic arthritis.[441] Infection may originate in the bone, in the joint, or in both; most typically, osseous and articular changes occur together. Symmetric involvement is frequent, and articular infection reveals an unusual affinity for the elbow (80 per cent of patients).[432, 526] This affinity may be related to the common occurrence of physiologic stresses in this joint, which possesses a great range of motion, stresses that can lead to hyperemia and vascular seeding of the joint by the organisms.[433] Whether or not osteomyelitis variolosa is caused directly by the virus remains controversial, however. The similarity of the behavior of the lesions to those accompanying other viral disorders, the presence of elementary variola inclusion bodies in the fluid of affected joints, and the demonstration of necrotic foci associated with the smallpox virus in the bone marrow in victims of the disease suggest that true infection of bone can take place.

Three types of bone and joint lesions have been described[433]:

1. A necrotic, nonsuppurative osteomyelitis, probably due to the smallpox virus itself, commonly involves the diaphyses of long tubular bones, leading to epiphyseal contamination, with destruction and deformity.

2. A suppurative arthritis related to contamination of the joint probably is due to secondary infection of a pustule.

3. A nonsuppurative arthritis may appear 1 to 4 weeks after the initial infection. Polyarticular and symmetric abnormalities are common, characterized by pain, swelling, and restriction of motion, and may be followed by secondary infection of the joint and articular deformities.

During the acute stage of osteomyelitis variolosa, findings simulate those of pyogenic osteomyelitis. Tubular bones commonly are involved; changes in the spine, the pelvis, and the skull are less typical. Juxtametaphyseal osteoporosis and destruction, epiphyseal extension, periostitis, involucrum formation, and articular contamination are seen. The elbow (Fig. 66–101), the glenohumeral joint, the knee, the hip, and the small joints of the hand, wrist, and foot can be altered (Fig. 66–102).

During the later stages of the disease, joint function and bone growth commonly are affected. In joints, osseous destruction with or without loose bodies, bony or fibrous ankylosis, subluxation, and secondary osteoarthritis can be encountered (Fig. 66–103); in bones, cessation or retardation of growth can be evident.

On pathologic examination, foci of necrosis may be detected throughout the marrow of the tubular bones. These focal lesions can become evident as early as 2 days and as late as 2 months after the appearance of the skin lesions. Damage to epiphyseal cartilage and premature fusion of the physes account for the limb deformities that characterize this disease.

Although radiographic characteristics of osseous and articular involvement in smallpox simulate those of pyogenic infection, certain differences can be seen. Symmetric changes, epiphyseal extension and destruction, predilection for the elbow, extensive osteoperiostitis of diaphyses of tubular bones, and peculiar deformities suggest the diagnosis of osteomyelitis variolosa (Fig. 66–104). The low frequency of spinal involvement and the lack of response of the osseous lesions to antibiotics also are noteworthy. The musculoskeletal abnormalities of smallpox can resemble findings in tuberculosis, leprosy, chronic granulomatous disease of childhood, juvenile chronic arthritis, and bone dysplasias.

Vaccinia

Although a viremia may occur after vaccination for smallpox, osseous and articular complications indeed are unusual. Examples of bone[442–445] and joint[446] alterations have been recorded, however. An insidious onset of clinical manifestations is seen, commonly within 1 to 3 weeks after the vaccination. Changes are more common in the upper extremities. Symmetric alterations are not infrequent. With osseous involvement, periostitis and hyperostosis coupled with soft tissue swelling or nodules can lead to an erroneous radiographic diagnosis of infantile cortical hyperostosis (Caffey's disease),[442, 443] although biopsy may lead to recov-

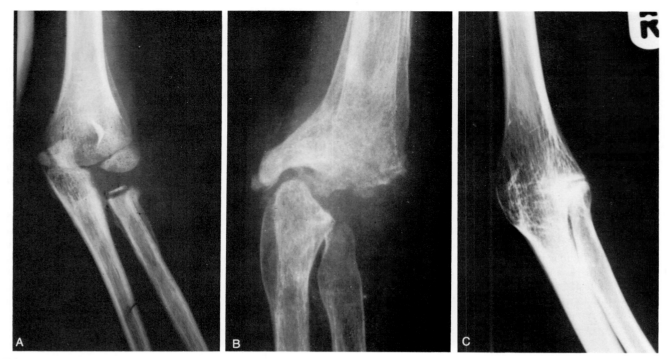

FIGURE 66–101. Variola osteomyelitis and septic arthritis: Elbow involvement. Stages in the process of bone and joint disease are illustrated in three different patients. Initial findings **(A)** include destructive foci with periostitis. Subsequently **(B, C)** irregularity of articular surfaces and intra-articular osseous fusion can be seen. (Courtesy of W. P. Cockshott, M.D., Hamilton, Ontario, Canada.)

ery of the vaccinia virus[442, 444, 445]; in some instances of vaccinia, bone lysis and involucrum formation are consistent with the radiographic findings of osteomyelitis[444] (Fig. 66–105), whereas in others, metaphyseal irregularity may represent a virus-related growth disturbance.[447] With artic-

ular involvement, aspiration of joint contents can lead to recovery of the vaccinia virus.[446]

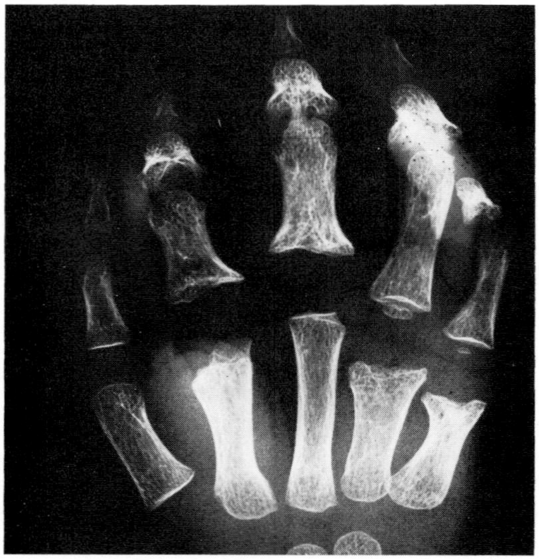

Infectious Mononucleosis and Epstein-Barr Virus Infection

Infectious mononucleosis apparently results from infection with the Epstein-Barr virus.[448] Reports of articular involvement with pain, soft tissue swelling, and elevation of the erythrocyte sedimentation rate simulating the findings of rheumatic fever or juvenile chronic arthritis have appeared,[449, 450] and biopsies of affected joints can reveal features of a subacute synovitis.[23] The pathogenesis of the arthritis is not clear; possible mechanisms include viral replication within the synovium and precipitation of immune complexes.[837] A patient with infectious mononucleosis has demonstrated periostitis of the ulnae and tibiae that was associated with pain and tenderness.[451] In this case, attempts at isolating bacterial or viral agents were unrewarding, although the patient demonstrated hyperglobulinemia.[416] The combination of periostitis and dysproteinemia has been noted in other patients.[452]

Epstein-Barr virus (EBV) infection leads to clinical manifestations simulating those of varicella, cytomegalovirus, and herpes simplex virus infection. Although the EBV infection then may become latent, reactivation has been described in association with lymphoproliferative diseases, multiple sclerosis, recurrent tonsillitis, and rheumatoid arthritis. An association of reactivated EBV infection and Mucha-Habermann's disease (pityriasis lichenoides et var-

FIGURE 66–102. Variola osteomyelitis and septic arthritis: Hand and wrist involvement. During the acute and subacute stages, observe epiphyseal destruction and growth deformities. (Courtesy of W. P. Cockshott, M.D., Hamilton, Ontario, Canada.)

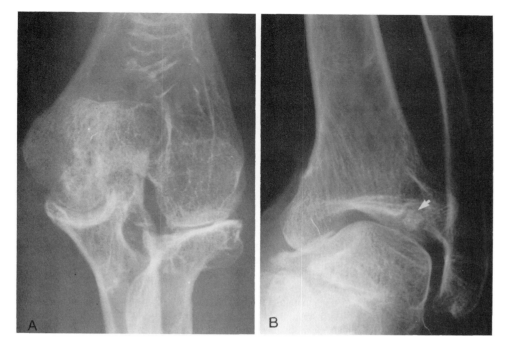

FIGURE 66–103. Variola osteo-myelitis and septic arthritis. In this 55 year old woman, epiphyseal deformity and secondary osteoar-thritis of the elbow **(A)** and defor-mity, subluxation, and an intra-ar-ticular body (arrow) of the ankle **(B)** are seen.

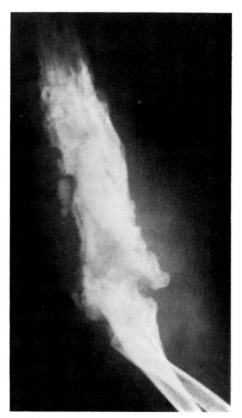

FIGURE 66–104. Variola osteomyelitis. In the late phases of the disease, extreme destruction can be seen. Here, in the humeral shaft, bizarre lysis and sclerosis, fragmentation, and soft tissue swelling can be noted.

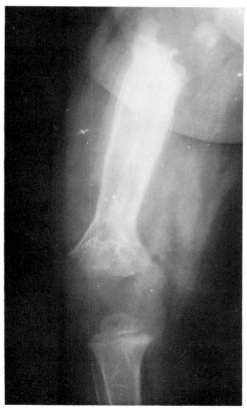

FIGURE 66–105. Vaccinial osteomyelitis. Expansion of the femoral shaft, periostitis, and metaphyseal irregularities are the radiographic findings. (Courtesy of W. P. Cockshott, M.D., Hamilton, Ontario, Canada.)

ioliformis acuta) also has been described.[1170] Acute arthritis may complicate reactivated EBV infection; additional manifestations include a variety of cutaneous abnormalities.[1170]

Human Immunodeficiency Virus Infection

An extraordinary amount of attention has been given in recent years to the human immunodeficiency virus (HIV) and its various clinical manifestations. HIV infection leads to compromise of the body's defense mechanisms, which, in turn, predisposes infected persons to a variety of opportunistic infections, anemia, arthritis, myositis, and immune-related neoplasms.[1171] Although neurologic and pulmonary manifestations dominate the clinical abnormalities in HIV-positive persons, musculoskeletal alterations in such persons are not infrequent. A complete discussion of the clinical findings associated with HIV infection is beyond the scope of this textbook. Rather, an overview of some of its major musculoskeletal abnormalities is presented here. As many of these abnormalities are infectious in causation, such an overview appropriately is placed in this chapter. It is convenient to divide the musculoskeletal findings into several categories: rheumatologic disorders; infectious disorders; bacillary angiomatosis; and miscellaneous abnormalities.

Rheumatologic Disorders

Many of the rheumatologic manifestations of HIV infection fall into the spectrum of differentiated and undifferentiated forms of spondyloarthropathy.[1172-1189] That is, although the clinical manifestations associated with HIV infection may appear to meet the criteria for Reiter's syndrome or psoriatic arthritis, frequently some of the criteria are missing; some of the findings of these disorders may be present whereas others are lacking. With regard to Reiter's syndrome in patients with HIV infection, the classic triad of clinical abnormalities commonly is lacking owing to the infrequent occurrence of conjunctivitis. In some reports, two general forms of Reiter's syndrome in HIV infection have been identified[1172]: an accumulative pattern evolving to full intensity over several weeks to months; or, more commonly, a milder intermittent pattern with recrudescences and remissions. The first of these has been associated with asymmetrically distributed polyarticular disease characterized by synovial thickening, bone erosions, and juxta-articular osteoporosis; the second, intermittent pattern generally is oligoarticular in distribution, with knee or ankle involvement.[1172] In both patterns, fasciitis and enthesopathy occur, especially in the feet (Fig. 66–106), and are accompanied by marked muscle wasting. These characteristics, which are nearly diagnostic, have been referred to as the acquired immunodeficiency syndrome (AIDS) foot.[1190] The patterns of Reiter's syndrome may precede those of AIDS or occur in persons with fully developed AIDS. In either case, involvement of the appendicular skeleton is more characteristic than that of the axial skeleton,[1172, 1182] although clinical and radiologic manifestations related to spinal or sacroiliac joint abnormalities are encountered.[1173, 1182] Thus, differentiation of Reiter's syndrome associated with HIV infection from Reiter's syndrome alone may be difficult; however, extensive abnormalities in the lower extremities in the former situation provides some diagnostic help.[1173]

That psoriasiform skin lesions of variable severity can

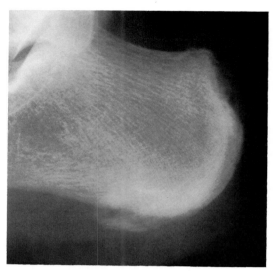

FIGURE 66–106. Human immunodeficiency virus infection: Reactive arthritis with enthesopathy and bursitis. In this 28 year old man with a Reiter's-like syndrome, note enthesitis with bone proliferation in the plantar aspect of the calcaneus and retrocalcaneal bursitis with erosion of the posterosuperior portion of the calcaneus.

occur in patients with HIV infection is well established, although other types of skin disease, including dermatomyositis or erythema nodosum, also may develop.[1182] In some affected persons, a peripheral arthritis may develop in association with the cutaneous manifestations of psoriasis that is similar or identical to that occurring in psoriatic arthritis.[1172, 1181, 1182] Although the precise relationship of true psoriatic arthritis and HIV infection is not clear, the cutaneous manifestations that occur in such infection include lesions of psoriasis vulgaris, guttate psoriasis, keratodermia, sebopsoriasis of the axilla and groin, and erythroderma,[1172] may be very severe, are associated with secondary S. aureus skin infections, and are accompanied by articular disease that shares many characteristics with those of psoriatic arthritis.[1172, 1181] Radiographic abnormalities in patients with this type of arthritis are similar to those associated with Reiter's syndrome and include also distal interphalangeal joint alterations, such as pencil-in-cup deformities.[1172, 1186] As with Reiter's syndrome, psoriasis-like joint involvement in patients with HIV infection may be sustained, accumulative, and aggressive, or it may be mild and intermittent.[1172] Enthesopathy and dactylitis may be very prominent, especially in the feet.

In addition to these rheumatologic syndromes that bear great resemblance to psoriatic disease or Reiter's syndrome, undifferentiated forms of spondyloarthropathy also develop in patients with HIV infection. In such cases, cutaneous manifestations may be lacking, HLA-B 27 antigens may or may not be present, and oligoarthritis and enthesopathy may be evident.[1172] A chronic symmetric proliferative arthritis that affects small joints of the extremities, leads to synovial proliferation and hyperplasia, and is accompanied by histologic evidence of synovial infiltration with plasma cells has been described.[1185] Retrovirus-like particles located around synoviocyte fragments have been observed on inspection of specimens of the synovial membrane.[1185]

Additional rheumatic syndromes may be seen in patients with HIV infection. Polymyositis, presumably inflammatory, proximal in location, and associated with pain, tenderness and weakness, may be noted.[1172] Its pathogenesis is not clear. Vasculitis with or without eosinophilia and evidence of cytomegalovirus infection may be evident.[1172, 1175, 1183] Its pathogenesis likewise is not certain.

Infectious Disorders

Osteomyelitis, septic arthritis, pyomyositis, and septic bursitis are among the complications associated with HIV infections. Despite the known higher frequency of bacterial and fungal infections and bacteremia in patients with AIDS, reports of infection of the musculoskeletal system are few. Osteomyelitis related to hematogenous or postoperative infections is described, however.[1191–1195] It may occur with or without septic arthritis, in association with a number of infecting microorganisms, and in spinal or extraspinal sites. Primary septic arthritis also has been observed in patients with HIV infection.[1194, 1196–1201, 1260] Its frequency is increased in homosexual men, intravenous drug abusers, and hemophiliacs. Although the knee represents the most common site of involvement, joints of the upper extremity and the acromioclavicular, sternoclavicular, and sacroiliac joints also may be affected. *Staphylococcus aureus* or *Streptococcus pneumoniae* is implicated most often, but opportunistic pathogens represent additional potential causative agents.[1194]

Septic bursitis occurring in patients with HIV infection has been described in several reports.[1201] *Staphylococcus aureus* generally is the responsible organism.

Pyomyositis represents a bacterial infection of muscle, generally but not exclusively caused by *S. aureus,* that is endemic in tropical regions of Africa, Southeast Asia, and South America (see Chapter 64). Emphasis has been given to the occurrence of pyomyositis in temperate areas, however, where it commonly affects patients who are immunologically compromised or who have underlying chronic disorders. One such disorder is related to HIV infection.[1194, 1201–1208] Pyomyositis in cases of HIV infection predominates in adults, generally in the third to fifth decades of life, although it also has been described in children and even in premature infants.[1204] *Staphylococcus aureus* and, far less frequently, other agents such as *Citrobacter freundii* and *Mycobacterium avium* are responsible for the muscle involvement.[1205, 1208] Almost 95 per cent of reported cases of pyomyositis associated with HIV infection have indicated lower extremity localization with rare involvement of other sites, including those in the axial skeleton.[1208] Multiple abscesses have been identified in slightly less than 50 per cent of cases. The most typical pattern of disease, however, appears to be a solitary abscess in the quadriceps musculature.[1201] Clinical findings include fever and local muscle pain, redness, and swelling, which, if untreated, may be accompanied by marked edema and septicemia. Delay in accurate diagnosis is frequent.[1206]

Advanced imaging methods, including ultrasonography, radionuclide studies (i.e., ^{67}Ga-citrate imaging), CT, and MR imaging, may provide useful diagnostic information with regard to the cause of the local clinical manifestations and the extent of the process[1203, 1207–1209] (see Chapter 64).

The precise cause of the increased association of pyomyositis and HIV infection is not clear, although several factors may be important. The known occurrence of intravenous drug abuse in patients with HIV infection predisposes such patients to bacteremia and muscle damage in regions of skin puncture. Additional risk factors include immunosuppression and toxic effects of chemotherapeutic agents.[1203] An increased frequency of *S. aureus* carrier states may exist in men infected with HIV.[1208] Furthermore, neutrophils from HIV-infected patients frequently manifest phagocytic, chemotactic, and oxidative defects and impaired bactericidal activity against *S. aureus.*[1206]

Bacillary Angiomatosis

Bacillary angiomatosis is a disorder characterized by histologic evidence of vascular proliferation in affected tissues such as the skin, bone, lymph nodes, and brain and by the presence of numerous bacillary organisms demonstrable on Warthin-Starry silver staining or on electron microscopy.[1210] These same bacilli also are identifiable in the parenchymal vascular lesions of bacillary peliosis of the liver and spleen, and the disease process sometimes is referred to as bacillary angiomatosis—bacillary peliosis (BAP).[1210] The precise nature of the causative bacilli has been the subject of a number of investigations. Initially, the organisms causing BAP were believed to be identical to those seen in patients with cat-scratch disease (CSD), leading to the concept that BAP represented disseminated CSD in the immunocompromised host.[1211, 1212] More recently, biologic and microbiologic investigations have confirmed that at least two organisms, *Rochalimaea henselae* and *Rochalimaea quintana,* can cause BAP, both of which are distinct from *Afipia felis* (formerly the CSD bacillus) and *Bartonella bacilliformis* (which produces a cutaneous abnormality similar to that occurring in BAP).[1210, 1213, 1214] Epidemiologic studies have indicated that the clinical syndrome of BAP is associated with exposure to cats, although the association is not as constant as that occurring in CSD; furthermore, in BAP, a history of a cat lick, scratch, or bite represents a definite risk factor, suggesting that traumatic contact with a cat is associated with BAP.[1210] These data have led to two hypotheses regarding the role of the domestic cat as a vector for the transmission of BAP: the agent of BAP may be part of the normal flora of the feline oral cavity and pharynx and, after grooming, may be present on the pelage, claws, and teeth of the animal, allowing its transmission to humans by a bite or scratch; or the agent of BAP may be a saprophytic plant or soil organism and might be transmitted to humans after inoculation of human skin by the contaminated pelage, claw, or bite of a cat.[1210]

Bacillary angiomatosis and BAP have been observed in patients infected with the HIV virus.[1211, 1215, 1216] The typical clinical presentation is that of a cutaneous disorder with multiple friable angiomatous papules closely resembling pyogenic granulomas as well as the skin lesions of Kaposi's sarcoma.[1217] Fever, chills, weight loss, night sweats, cellulitis, and subcutaneous nodules are additional clinical manifestations. Bone lesions also may be seen, sometimes as an initial manifestation of the disease.[1218–1220] Tubular bones of the extremities (Fig. 66–107), especially the tibia but also the fibula, femur, humerus, and radius, and, less commonly, flat and irregular bones such as the ribs, innominate bone, and vertebrae, are affected. Skin lesions are an associated but not invariable finding, and histologic analysis of biopsy material derived from cutaneous and osseous lesions shows features consistent with bacillary angiomatosis.[1218] Features of Kaposi's sarcoma also may be present. Osteolysis is the dominant radiographic feature, and the osteolytic focus or

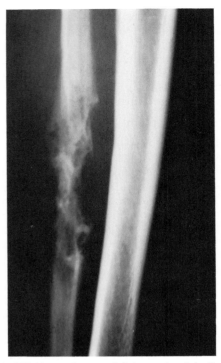

FIGURE 66–107. Human immunodeficiency virus infection: Bacillary angiomatosis. This 34 year old homosexual man had pain and swelling in the calf of 6 weeks' duration. A poorly, defined osteolytic lesion of the fibula is evident. Cultures of the lesion revealed organisms similar to those causing cat-scratch disease. (From Conrad SE, et al: J Bone Joint Surg [Am] 73:774, 1991.)

foci are either well or poorly defined. Cortical or medullary destruction, or both, is seen, and an adjacent soft tissue mass is an associated feature. In some instances, extensive tumor-like destruction of bone with or without periostitis is observed.[1220] CT, MR imaging, and bone scintigraphy can be used as supplementary diagnostic techniques.[1218] Special stains or electron microscopy can help confirm that bacilli similar or identical to those causing CSD are present in the bone lesions.[1219, 1220]

The differential diagnosis of bacillary angiomatosis and Kaposi's sarcoma in patients with HIV infection is difficult. As antibiotic therapy may lead to healing of the bone lesions of bacillary angiomatosis, such differentiation has clinical importance.[1218] Although lytic lesions of bone are not uncommon in the endemic African type of Kaposi's sarcoma, they are extremely rare in AIDS-related Kaposi's sarcoma.[1218] Their presence favors the alternative diagnosis of bacillary angiomatosis.

Miscellaneous Abnormalities

Osteonecrosis of the femoral head[1221, 1261] and of other sites, including the femoral condyles and humeral head,[1222] has been described in HIV-infected patients. Its cause is not clear. Calcification of the basal ganglia has been observed in children and infants with AIDS.[1223]

Other Viral or Viral-like Diseases

During the prodromal phase of *acute hepatitis,* a transient migratory arthritis, especially of the joints of the hands, can be evident[519] (see Chapter 31). Arthritic manifestations may also occur during *influenza,*[453] *echovirus* infections,[518] and *parvovirus* infections,[838, 943, 1224] in the African disorders of *chikungunya*[558] and *O'nyong-nyong,*[559] and in the Australian disorder *epidemic polyarthritis* (Ross River virus).[23, 839–842] These last three diseases, along with Mayaro and Sindbis, represent mosquito-transmitted viral infections that lead to virtually indistinguishable human diseases consisting of fever, rash, and arthralgias.[843] Joint manifestations are more common and severe in children than in adults, are seen in both male and female patients, and consist of pain and swelling in the hands, wrists, feet, ankles, and knees, commonly in a symmetric distribution. Symptoms and signs are of short duration, and recovery is complete.[843] Although all of these disorders occur principally in tropical and subtropical climates, differences are seen in their geographic distribution: Chikungunya virus is endemic in Africa, India, Southeast Asia, and the Philippine Islands; O'nyong-nyong virus occurs in East Africa; Mayaro virus is found in Trinidad, Surinam, Brazil, Colombia, and Bolivia; Ross River virus is evident in Australia, New Guinea, the Solomon Islands, Fiji, and a number of other South Pacific islands; and Sindbis virus is widely distributed in Africa, Europe, Asia, Australia, and the Philippines.[843]

In a newborn infant with *coxsackievirus* infection, hip contractures have been noted, perhaps related to the infectious disease.[454] In children with coxsackievirus infection, arthritis of unknown pathogenesis also has been observed.[1259] Although *lymphogranuloma venereum* is not a viral disorder, the infective agent is an intracellular parasite that produces intracytoplasmic "elementary bodies" that resemble the inclusion bodies of virus-infected cells.[416] In this disease, polyarthritis, principally of the knees, the ankles, and the wrists, can lead to acute or chronic symptoms and signs.[455] Joint effusions usually are sterile, and results of the Frei skin test always are positive. Osseous lesions in lymphogranuloma venereum are noted in adult patients and may relate to dissemination of the organisms via the blood stream,[456] a contention that is supported by the isolation of the infective agent from the bone lesion.

Cat-scratch disease (CSD), as described earlier in relationship to bacillary angiomatosis, is characterized by local lymphadenitis within 1 or 2 weeks after being scratched by a cat.[458] Findings include soft tissue masses (Fig. 66–108), erythema nodosum, and bony lesions. Osteolytic foci, when present in a child with CSD, can resemble the lesions of eosinophilic granuloma; biopsy may reveal a granulomatous process with central necrosis and cellular infiltration.[459, 460, 844, 907] Hematogenous dissemination and spread from a contiguous contaminated source, such as a lymph node, represent potential mechanisms of osseous involvement.

RICKETTSIAL INFECTION

Although a variety of microorganisms of the family Rickettsiaceae can cause human diseases, osseous and articular abnormalities generally are lacking or represent a very minor feature. Rarely, arthritis is present.[1225] In some patients, diffuse small vessel vasculitis can lead to thrombus formation, with complete or partial obliteration of the vascular lumen. These changes, which are most marked in Rocky Mountain spotted fever, are evident in many organ

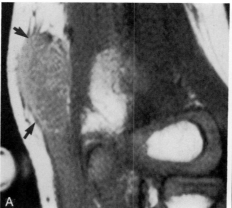
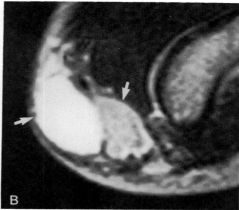

FIGURE 66–108. Cat-scratch disease. This young boy was bitten and scratched by a cat while trying to put the animal in a clothes dryer several weeks earlier. A soft tissue mass developed on the medial aspect of the elbow. The granulomatous process (arrows) is well shown on coronal proton density (TR/TE, 1600/40) **(A)** and transaxial T2-weighted (TR/TE, 2000/100) **(B)** spin echo MR images. (Courtesy of A. Motta, M.D., Cleveland, Ohio.)

systems but are especially prominent in the lung, the heart, and the brain. Occasionally, soft tissue necrosis can result in loss of cutaneous tissues in the phalanges that may be evident on radiographs.[461] Bony necrosis also may be recognized.

MYCOPLASMA INFECTION

Although one member of this group, *Mycoplasma pneumoniae*, is a frequent cause of atypical pneumonia, and this organism as well as others can produce additional human illnesses, significant musculoskeletal manifestations of Mycoplasma infection are unusual. Cases of septic arthritis related to *M. hominis* have been reported[846, 847, 1226] in which severe cartilaginous and osseous destruction may be seen. Furthermore, a noninfectious polyarthritis is evident in some patients with *M. pneumoniae* infection.[848, 849]

PROTOZOAN INFECTION

Toxoplasmosis

Toxoplasmosis is an infectious disorder caused by an intracellular protozoan parasite, *Toxoplasma gondii*. Human infections with Toxoplasma may be either congenital or acquired.

The congenital variety of toxoplasmosis can be severe. An infant may be stillborn at term or be born prematurely with active infection characterized by fever, rash, hepatosplenomegaly, mental retardation, chorioretinitis, and convulsions, which may lead to death in 10 to 20 per cent of cases. Osseous lesions are unusual,[462] although metaphyseal alterations in tubular bones may simulate those of rubella, cytomegalic inclusion disease, or syphilis. Cerebral calcification can be evident.

The acquired variety of the disease can occur at any age and may display variable manifestations. These include rash, lymphadenopathy, ocular changes, and widespread vascular alterations. Myalgias and myositis can accompany acquired toxoplasmosis.[463] Histologic examination may document the presence of the Toxoplasma organism within the affected muscle.[845] Unilateral or bilateral arthritis with articular and periarticular swelling and tenosynovitis, especially about the ankle and the wrist, also can be apparent.[464–466, 850] Radiographically evident osteoporosis, soft tissue swelling, and osseous cystic lesions, and histologically evi-

dent synovial inflammation with granulomatous tissue, round cell infiltration, and necrosis, have been described.[466]

Leishmaniasis

Leishmaniasis, produced by protozoa of the genus Leishmania, is transmitted by the bite of a sandfly and has a widespread geographic distribution. Osseous lesions may result from extension of skin and soft tissue infection or, rarely, from hematogenous dissemination.[457]

Amebiasis

Extraintestinal manifestations of amebiasis include urticaria, neuralgia, and arthralgia. Polyarthritis coincident with enteric involvement also has been recorded.[495, 851] It is not clear if such joint involvement is related to intra-articular parasites or is an immune reaction. Osteomyelitis in the ribs due to adjacent hepatic abscess formation is possible in amebiasis.[852]

INFECTION PRODUCED BY WORMS (HELMINTHS) (Table 66–3)

Hookworm Disease

Hookworm disease is produced by *Ancylostoma duodenale* or *Necator americanus*. Anemia and its complications are the major clinical manifestations of this disorder. Musculoskeletal abnormalities are rare indeed. Articular inflammation with swelling of the ankles has been described in a 7 year old boy,[467] although the exact relationship of the joint manifestations to hookworm disease was not established. A similar case in a 17 year old Cambodian girl has been reported.[853] In this patient, swelling in the ankles and foot was associated with eosinophilic synovial infiltration and isolation of *Ancylostoma duodenale* in the stool. In this case, too, the association of the parasite and the arthritis is speculative, as no larvae were identified in the synovial membrane and eosinophilia in the synovial fluid is observed in metastatic disease and as a result of radiation and arthrography, as well as in idiopathic transient synovitis.[854] O'Connor and associates[468] observed an 8 year old boy who developed a poorly defined lytic lesion of the posterior part of the talus. Stool examination documented the presence of the adult form of *Necator americanus*, and surgery with

TABLE 66–3. Major Helminthic Infections of Humans

| Nematodes (Roundworms) | | Trematodes (Flatworms) | | Cestodes (Tapeworms) | |
Intestinal	Tissue	Tissue	Intravascular	Pathogenic Form: Adult	Pathogenic Form: Larva
Ancylostoma duodenale	Wuchereria bancrofti	Clonorchis sinensis	Schistosoma mansoni	Diphyllobothrium latum	Echinococcus granulosus
Necator americanus	Brugia malayi	Fasciola hepatica	Schistosoma japonicum	Taenia saginata	Echinococcus multilocularis
Ascaris lumbricoides	Onchocerca volvulus	Fasciolopsis buski	Schistosoma haematobium	Taenia solium	Taenia solium
Enterobius vermicularis	Loa loa	Paragonimus westermani		Hymenolepsis nana	Hymenolepis nana
Trichuris trichiura	Trichinella spiralis				
	Toxocara canis				
	Dracunculus medinensis				

(From Korzeniowdki OM: Diseases due to helminths. In JH Stein [Ed]: Internal Medicine. Boston, Little, Brown, 1983, p. 1455.)

examination of the osseous lesion revealed granulation tissue with foreign body giant cells surrounding partially calcified hookworm larvae. These investigators speculated that a preexisting bony abnormality is necessary to initiate the worm's invasion of the osseous tissue.

Loiasis

Loiasis is prevalent in West and Central Africa and is produced by the filaria *Loa loa* (African eye worm). Infective larvae are deposited in the victim's skin after the bite of the mango fly.[469] The larvae burrow into the deeper subcutaneous tissue, where they mature to adult worms over a period of 6 months or longer. Localized areas of allergic inflammation in the subcutaneous tissue, particu-

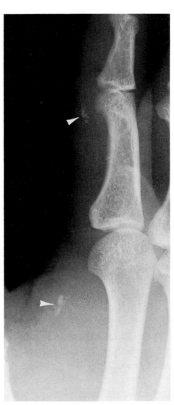

FIGURE 66–109. Loiasis (African eye worm disease). Soft tissue calcifications (arrowheads) are evident in the hand of this 29 year old man. (Courtesy of M. Dalinka, M.D., Philadelphia, Pennsylvania.)

larly in the forearm,[908] produce Calabar swellings, named after the Nigerian town in which the disease is rampant. The dead worms cause abscesses or undergo calcification, or both.[470–472] Calcific deposits in the subcutaneous tissues (Fig. 66–109) may be fine, coiled, lacelike, and filamentous (calcification of the worm), or thicker, beadlike, and lobulated (calcification of the fibrous capsule surrounding the worm) (Table 66–4).[469]

Polyarthritis has been associated with loiasis.[855]

Onchocerciasis

Onchocerciasis is a form of filariasis produced by *Onchocerca volvulus* and transmitted by flies. It is prevalent in Africa and Central and South America. Cutaneous nodules on the head and trunk consisting of adult worms and microfilariae are seen. Soft tissue calcifications, similar to those in loiasis, may be detected,[469, 473] although radiographic demonstration of the calcified areas is extremely difficult because of their small size.

Filariasis

Filariasis is produced by the adult worms of the species *Wuchereria bancrofti* or *Brugia malayi,* which localize in the lymphatic and soft tissues of the human body. The disease is predominant in tropical areas of Asia, Africa, South America, Australia, and the South Pacific islands. After prolonged and repeated attacks, filariasis can lead to massive lymphedema or elephantiasis, especially of the legs and the scrotum. Lymphatic obstruction may relate to lymphangitis, a granulomatous reaction about dead worms, an allergic antigen-antibody reaction produced by the death of the parasite, or secondary bacterial infection.[469] Cutaneous and subcutaneous lymphedema and fibrous hyperplasia are seen. Radiographs show an affected limb to be greatly enlarged, with soft tissue thickening, blurring of subcutaneous fat planes, and a linear striated pattern. One report has been published of lymphangiosarcoma associated with filarial lymphedema,[1227] although this complication is far more frequent in cases of postmastectomy lymphedema and lymphedema related to traumatic, surgical, congenital, and idiopathic causes. Osseous changes are not apparent in filariasis, although Reeder[292] observed irregular tuftal erosion of phalanges in the foot in one patient. Lymphangiography reveals an increase in the number of tiny lymphatic channels that have a tortuous, looping course, dermal back-

TABLE 66–4. Some Helminths (Worms) Associated with Calcification

Helminth (Disease)	Frequency of Radiologic Calcification	Typical Location of Calcification	Typical Appearance of Calcification
Loa loa (Loiasis)	Common	Widespread; subcutaneous tissues	Extended or coiled, linear or beaded, variable in size
Onchocerca volvulus (River blindness)	Rare	Legs, trunk, head; subcutaneous nodules	Extended or coiled, linear or beaded, small
Wuchereria bancrofti; Brugia malayi (Filariasis)	Rare	Thighs, legs, scrotum; subcutaneous tissues	Straight or coiled, small
Dracunculus medinensis (Guinea worm disease)	Common	Extremities	Extended or coiled, long
Taenia solium (Cysticercosis)	Common	Widespread; muscular tissues	Numerous, linear or oval, variable in size, lie in plane of muscle
Echinococcus granulosus (Echinococcosis)	Common	Liver, lungs, other organs	Curvilinear, cystic, eggshell
Sarcocystis lindemanni (Sarcosporidiosis)	Common	Extremities; muscular and subcutaneous tissues	Numerous, linear or oval, variable in size and orientation
Armillifer armillatus, Porocephalida, Pentastomomida (Porocephalosis)	Variable	Abdomen, thorax	Multiple, crescent-shaped or oval
Schistosoma haematobium (Schistosomiasis)	Variable	Bladder, urinary tract	Linear, nodular

flow, and an increase in the size of lymph nodes that may resemble the changes in Hodgkin's disease.[474] Soft tissue calcification of *W. bancrofti* has been noted[475, 476]; elongated radiodense shadows in the subcutaneous tissue represent calcified, dead, encysted filariae. The calcifications are smaller than those in loiasis and occur predominantly in the lymphatic channels of the scrotum, thighs, and legs (Table 66–4).

In the United States, human infections have been related to filariae of several different animals. *Dirofilaria tenuis* produces an endemic microfilaremia of racoons that may be transmitted by mosquitoes.[1228] Subcutaneous nodules and arthritis may accompany the infection in humans.[1229]

Dracunculiasis (Guinea Worm Disease)

The guinea worm, *Dracunculus medinensis,* can cause human disease, particularly in parts of Africa, the Middle East, South America, India, and Pakistan. The disorder is contracted when the larvae in contaminated water are ingested by a water flea (Cyclops) that, in turn, is swallowed in the drinking water by humans.[469] The larvae eventually enter the circulation and mature within the human subcutaneous tissues. Although the male worm is relatively small (2 to 3 cm long), the female worm may reach 120 cm in length. When the female parasites die, they may calcify, producing long, curled radiodense shadows in the lower extremities and hands (Fig. 66–110A), and less commonly, the perineum and abdominal and chest wall[477–479]; the deposits usually are multiple and may become fragmented because of the action of adjacent musculature. Calcification of male worms rarely is seen.[409] Of interest, Khajavi[477] noted malignant disease in 15 of 83 patients with calcifications due to infestation with guinea worms; bladder carcinoma was the most frequent neoplasm encountered. This investigator suggested that such infection might lead to secondary tumor in a way similar to that in schistosomiasis.

If a migratory guinea worm dies adjacent to a joint, severe cellular reaction apparently can lead to joint effusion and secondary bacterial infection.[480, 856–859, 909, 1274] Calcification about the damaged joint also may be evident (Figs. 66–110B and 66–111). More severe changes consist of joint space narrowing, bone destruction, and flexion contractures, presumably related to direct invasion of the joint by the female worm.[857]

Trichinosis

After ingestion of infected beef, humans may develop trichinosis from the intestinal nematode *Trichinella spiralis.* Calcification of the cysts of the parasite commonly is detected on microscopic examination but rarely, if ever, is noted on radiographic evaluation.[473] Clinical features resembling those of dermatomyositis are described.[910, 1230]

Cysticercosis

The relationship between humans and the pork tapeworm, *Taenia solium,* is twofold: Humans are the only definitive host of the adult tapeworm, the parasite inhabiting the intestine; and humans may serve as an intermediate host (the usual intermediate host is the hog), harboring the larval stage, *Cysticercus cellulosae.* In this latter case, deposits of the larval form of the tapeworm may appear in subcutaneous and muscular tissues and in a variety of viscera, including the heart, brain, lung, liver, and eye. When the larvae die, a foreign body reaction may ensue, leading to considerable tissue response. Necrosis may occur, followed, over a period of years, by caseation and calcification.[481]

On radiographs, linear or oval elongated calcifications appear in the soft tissues and musculature; these may reach 23 mm in length.[473, 481, 482] The long axis of the calcified cysts lies in the plane of the surrounding muscle bundles[469]

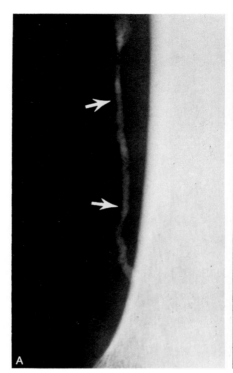

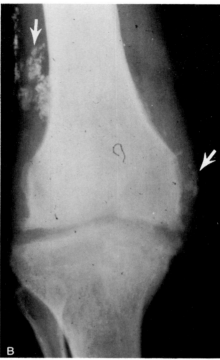

FIGURE 66–110. Dracunculiasis (guinea worm disease).

A Observe the long linear calcification (arrows) adjacent to the lower tibia due to the presence of a dying female worm.

B Guinea worm arthritis can be associated with soft tissue calcification (arrows) and swelling as well as secondary bacterial infection with osseous and cartilaginous destruction.

(**B** Courtesy of W. P. Cockshott, M.D., Hamilton, Ontario, Canada.)

FIGURE 66–111. Dracunculiasis (guinea worm disease). A 33 year old Indian woman had a history of intermittent and mild pain in the dorsal aspect of both feet and the ankles of approximately 6 months' duration. She was born and raised in the Madras area of southeastern India but had lived in the United States for 20 years. Physical examination revealed firm, nontender, subcutaneous nodules about the joints in the hands and ankles.

A Linear calcification (arrow) is evident in the subcutaneous tissues in the ankle.

B Tumoral periarticular calcification (arrow) is seen in the hand.

(Courtesy of P. Utsinger, M.D., Philadelphia, Pennsylvania.)

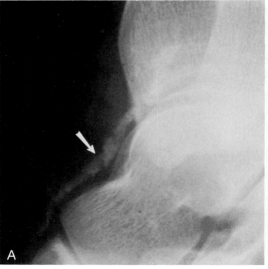

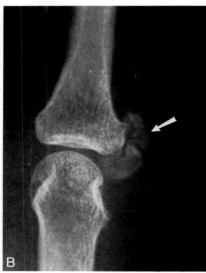

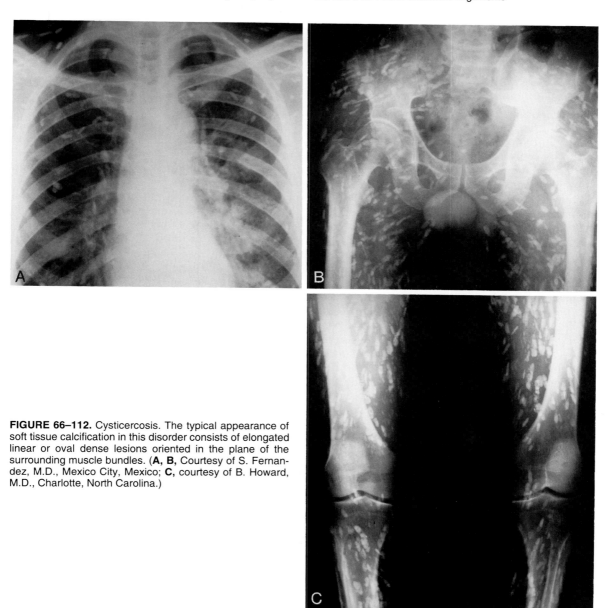

FIGURE 66–112. Cysticercosis. The typical appearance of soft tissue calcification in this disorder consists of elongated linear or oval dense lesions oriented in the plane of the surrounding muscle bundles. (**A, B,** Courtesy of S. Fernandez, M.D., Mexico City, Mexico; **C,** courtesy of B. Howard, M.D., Charlotte, North Carolina.)

(Fig. 66–112). Those present in the thigh musculature are particularly well shown radiographically.

Spinal cysticercosis exists in an intramedullary form (with involvement of the spinal cord), an extramedullary form, or a leptomeningeal form. Myelography, CT, and MR imaging are useful techniques for identifying the cystic lesions.[922, 944, 1231]

Echinococcosis

Echinococcosis is produced principally by the larval stage of *Echinococcus granulosus* and is most prevalent in sheep- and cattle-raising areas of North and South Africa, South America, Central Europe, Australia, and Canada; less commonly, *E. multilocularis* is the causative agent, especially in Alaska and Eurasia. In humans, *E. granulosus* is contracted by ingestion of the eggs, which are contained in the feces of the dog (sheep dog). After ingestion, the em-

bryos escape from the eggs, traverse the intestinal mucosa, and are disseminated via venous and lymphatic channels. Cysts may develop in various viscera, particularly the liver and the lungs. These may calcify, producing irregular curvilinear radiodense areas. Intramuscular involvement also is encountered.[1238]

Bone lesions are reported in 1 to 2 per cent of cases of echinococcosis.[483] Over a long period of time, osseous foci may be manifested with pain and deformity, particularly in the 30 to 60 year old age group. Hydatid disease of bone rarely is seen in childhood. Osseous involvement almost invariably is related to primary infection and is not the result of extension from a neighboring soft tissue lesion. Although hematogenous seeding of the skeleton in echinococcosis conceivably can occur in any site, one bone, a few adjacent bones, or one skeletal region usually is affected; when several adjacent bones are involved, skeletal contamination generally has resulted from direct invasion of one or more bones from another skeletal site (e.g., pelvis to femur; vertebra to rib).[1] Echinococcal joint disease without a focus of bone involvement is exceedingly rare. On the basis of available reports, the vertebral column, the pelvis, the long bones, and the skull are involved most commonly.[484–493, 860–864, 911, 945, 1232–1237] The spine is involved in about 50 per cent of cases, and such involvement may lead to paraplegia or nerve root compression. Rib and costochondral abnormalities can occur as an isolated phenomenon, in association with vertebral lesions, or as a result of erosion from adjacent pleural cysts.[491, 560] CT and MR imaging are valuable in delineating the extent of bone and soft tissue abnormalities, especially in the spine.[861, 862, 864, 912, 946, 947, 1239, 1240]

Intraosseous foci of hydatid echinococcosis predominate in the spongiosa and consist of minute, separate, thin-walled cysts.[1, 492] These cysts expand at the expense of surrounding trabeculae and, in some instances, reach considerable size. Connective tissue proliferation in the marrow is accompanied by cellular infiltration, hemosiderin pigmentation, and cholesterol crystal deposition.[1] As the cysts enlarge, cortical thinning and expansion, pathologic fracture, and soft tissue extension can ensue. Periosteal bone formation is unusual. Soft tissue cysts proliferate, become delineated by a thick fibrous membrane, and may contain seropurulent fluid and detritus.[1]

The histologic and gross pathologic findings in the bone in echinococcosis differ somewhat from changes in other organ systems, and they differ also between the two forms of the disease. Cysts developing in the viscera are characterized by a well-developed outer host adventitial layer; those occurring in osseous tissue lack this outer layer. Hence, the enlarging cystic lesions extend within the medullary canal. Secondary cystic regions, termed daughter cysts, are identified, leading to a multilocular appearance. The cystic spaces tend to be larger when *E. granulosus* rather than *E. multilocularis* is the pathogenic species.[863]

Radiographs can reveal single or multiple expansile cystic osteolytic lesions containing trabeculae (Fig. 66–113). These may be associated with cortical violation and soft tissue mass formation, with calcification. The radiographic characteristics are similar to those of fibrous dysplasia, plasmacytoma, giant cell tumor, cartilaginous neoplasms (enchondroma, chondrosarcoma, chondromyxoid fibroma), skeletal metastases (especially from a tumor of the kidney or thyroid), a brown tumor of hyperparathyroidism, angiosarcoma, or a hemophilic pseudotumor. In the spine, radiographic findings simulate those of tuberculosis and chronic pyogenic osteomyelitis.[1280] The lack of osteoporosis and sclerosis in the host bone, the absence of damage to the intervertebral discs, the presence of posterior element and rib involvement and, occasionally, intralesional calcification, and the identification of subperiosteal and subligamentous extension of disease are helpful but not pathognomonic diagnostic clues.[1239] CT features of echinococcosis include a soft tissue mass adjacent to sites of bone involvement (Fig. 66–114); the center of the mass contains fluid with

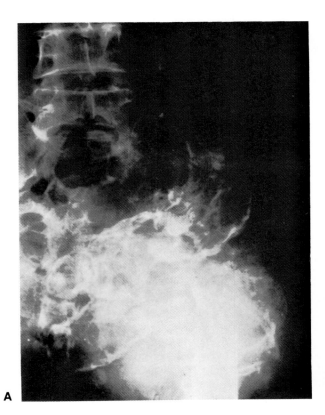 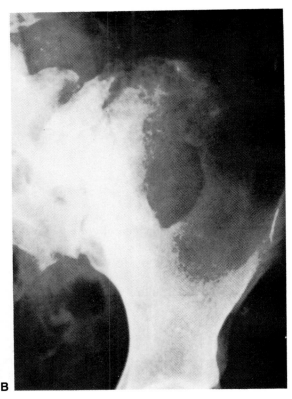

A   B

FIGURE 66–113. Echinococcosis.
  A The expansile, "bubbly" lytic lesions of the pelvis, sacrum, and proximal portion of the femur are associated with deformity, osseous fragmentation, and soft tissue swelling.
  B In this 40 year old Brazilian woman, an osteolytic lesion in the ilium is accompanied by sclerosis extending to the sacroiliac joint.
  (**B,** Courtesy of A. D'Abreu, M.D., Porto Alegre, Brazil.)

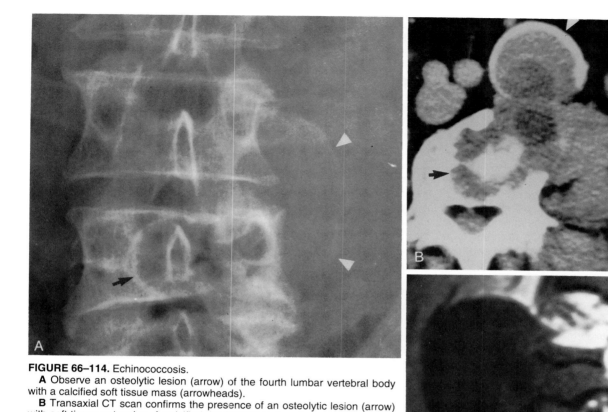

FIGURE 66–114. Echinococcosis.

A Observe an osteolytic lesion (arrow) of the fourth lumbar vertebral body with a calcified soft tissue mass (arrowheads).

B Transaxial CT scan confirms the presence of an osteolytic lesion (arrow) with soft tissue extension. A calcified rim (arrowhead) and areas of low attenuation in the soft tissue mass are apparent.

C A sagittal T1-weighted (TR/TE, 650/18) spin echo MR image shows an intraosseous and soft tissue lesion of low signal intensity.

(Courtesy of R. Kerr, M.D., Los Angeles, California.)

low attenuation values that does not enhance after intravenous administration of contrast material.[1239] Cystic lesions also are identified with MR imaging within the bone and adjacent soft tissues; the signal characteristics of the cyst are variable and may not be diagnostic (Fig. 66–114).[1240] The presence of numerous cystic lesions of high signal intensity in T2-weighted spin echo MR images appears characteristic, however[1262] (Fig. 66–115). Accurate diagnosis may be aided in some persons by eosinophilia (25 to 35

per cent of cases), and positive results on complement fixation test, intradermal injection of hydatid fluid, and indirect hemagglutination test.[494] Needle biopsy of the lesions may lead to further dissemination of infection.[491]

Complications of osseous involvement in echinococcosis include pathologic fracture, secondary infection, especially with staphylococci,[492] rupture into the spinal canal with neural problems, including paraplegia,[865] transarticular extension with osseous collapse and deformity, intrapelvic

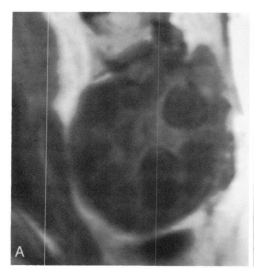
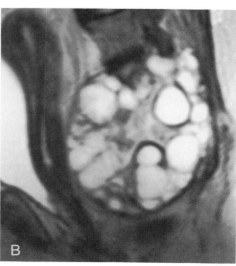

FIGURE 66–115. Echinococcosis.

A A sagittal T1-weighted (TR/TE, 650/20) spin echo MR image reveals a large mass involving predominantly the sacrum with anterior extension leading to displacement of pelvic viscera. Note circular regions of low signal intensity within the mass, consistent with fluid-filled cysts.

B A sagittal T2-weighted (TR/TE, 4348/150) spin echo MR image reveals the cysts as regions of high signal intensity.

(Courtesy of J. Kramer, M.D., Vienna, Austria.)

extension with compression of bladder, vagina, uterus, or colon,[490] and cranial lesions with involvement of the dura and arachnoid membranes, leading to meningitis.

Other Diseases Produced by Worms

Paragonimiasis, caused by the trematode *Paragonimus westermani,* can lead to alterations of the lung, liver, brain, mesentery, and skeletal muscle. Rarely, calcification is encountered.[473]

Schistosomiasis, due to *Schistosoma haematobium,* can produce bladder and ureteral calcification in chronic cases. Schistosomiasis also, on rare occasions, has been accompanied by articular disease in which inflammatory and vascular changes in the synovial membrane are associated with the presence of ova in the involved tissue.[866, 1241, 1263] Myelopathy and the cauda equina syndrome may appear in infections due to *S. mansoni* and *S. haematobium.*[867, 1242] Indeed, four manifestations of schistosomiasis of the spinal cord are recognized[1243]: a confluent granulomatous mass of the caudal cord; radicular involvement with granulomatous changes surrounding the conus medullaris and cauda equina; diffuse granulomatous changes with necrosis, atrophy, and hemorrhage causing an acute transverse myelitis without cord enlargement; and asymptomatic deposition of ova in the cord. Of these, granulomatous masses of the caudal cord and conus medullaris are most common.

Strongyloidiasis is a disease of the gastrointestinal tract and other tissues related to infection with *Strongyloides stercoralis.* Affected persons may be entirely asymptomatic or reveal diarrhea that may become severe. Disseminated strongyloidiasis is especially common in hosts compromised by chronic disease, corticosteroid therapy, or immunosuppression. Reactive arthritis has been described in this disease,[868] and, rarely, organisms have been recovered from symptomatic joints.[869]

Sarcocystitis, caused by *Sarcocystis lindemanni,* leads to granulomatous reactions in cardiac and voluntary muscles, which eventually may calcify.[870] Similar calcifications may occur in *sparganosis,* due to the larval form of diphyllobothriid tapeworms.[871] Oval calcifications in the abdomen and chest are seen in infections related to *Pentastomida,* in which parasites lodge in subperitoneal or subpleural locations,[872] and in *porocephalosis* (see Table 66–4).

ADDITIONAL DISORDERS OF POSSIBLE INFECTIOUS CAUSE

Many other musculoskeletal disorders exist in which an infectious cause is suspected. Some of these, including sarcoidosis, Behçet's syndrome, and infantile cortical hyperostosis, are discussed elsewhere. Additional examples are ainhum and Tietze's syndrome.

Ainhum

Ainhum (dactylolysis spontanea) is a self-limited dermatologic disorder that characteristically is found in African blacks or their descendants, although rarely it is reported in other races.[496–499, 873] In West Africa, it may be seen in 2 per cent of persons[469]; ainhum occasionally is encountered in patients in the United States.[499] Most typically, the fifth toe on one or both feet is affected, although other toes (espe-

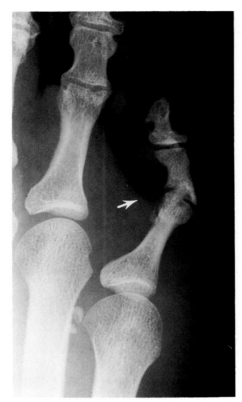

FIGURE 66–116. Ainhum. Note the soft tissue groove (arrow) and the osseous resorption, especially on the medial aspect of the proximal and middle phalanges of the fifth toe. Periostitis is absent.

cially the fourth) and even the fingers or nipples can be involved.[500, 923, 1244] Although both young and elderly men and women can be afflicted, most patients are men in the fourth and fifth decades of life.[501] A deep soft tissue groove appears,[499] corresponding to a hyperkeratotic band within the epidermis,[496] associated with dermal fibrosis.[497] The groove is evident initially along the medial aspect of the fifth toe and deepens progressively and encircles the toe. Ulceration and inflammation coexist. Digital swelling or lymphedema[496] and adjacent osseous resorption are encountered. Bony resorption begins on the medial aspect of the distal portion of the proximal phalanx or the middle phalanx of the fifth toe[499] (Fig. 66–116). Periostitis generally is absent. With further narrowing, the bone may fracture. As more bone is resorbed, including most of the middle phalanx, severe digital angulation and autoamputation are seen. The entire process may occur over a period of months or decades.

The cause of ainhum is not clear.[499] Traumatic and infectious factors appear most likely. Although the vasculature of the involved toe usually is normal,[496] plethysmography may indicate a local increase in blood flow.[502] An angiodysplasia has been identified in some patients with ainhum who have undergone arteriography,[874] although the significance of the finding is not known.

Tietze's Syndrome

Tietze's syndrome, the costosternal syndrome, and costochondritis are terms that are used to describe pain, tenderness, and swelling at the costosternal joints.[503, 504] This is a common condition, occurring in perhaps as many as 10 per cent of patients who are seen with chest pain.[503] "Epidemics" of the disease also have been noted.[505] Tietze's syndrome is benign and self-limited. Typically, painful swelling and tenderness to local palpation of one or more costosternal junctions are observed in a patient in the second to fourth decades of life.[506] Respiratory symptoms and signs also may be apparent, and patients may reveal a distant focus of bacterial or viral infection or a recent history of thoracic surgery. Although the second costochondral junction is involved most commonly, any such junction can be affected, and xiphisternal costochondritis also has been noted.[507]

Radiographs commonly are not revealing, although soft tissue swelling, calcification, osteophytosis, and periostitis rarely are encountered.[507, 1245] Increased activity may be demonstrated on bone scans[508] and gallium studies.[1246] CT may reveal sclerosis of the sternal manubrium, partial calcification of costal cartilage, and soft tissue swelling.[1246] The histopathologic findings may be entirely unremarkable, although increased vascularity[509–511] and degeneration or proliferation of cartilage[506–510] can be seen.[504]

The cause is unknown. The history of a previous or coexistent viral or bacterial infection and the detection of pus within the mass suggest an infectious origin. Local stress produced during respiration also may be important.[1247]

SUMMARY

Osseous, articular, and soft tissue structures may become involved in many infectious disorders. Bacteria, mycobacteria, spirochetes, fungi, viruses, rickettsiae, protozoa, and worms all are capable of affecting the musculoskeletal system. In many instances, radiographic features, although typical of an infection, do not allow diagnosis of a specific causative agent; in some cases, the distribution and the morphology of the lesions are sufficiently characteristic to suggest a single infectious process. In all cases, the radiographs must be interpreted in conjunction with clinical, other imaging, and pathologic manifestations.

References

1. Jaffe HL: Metabolic, Degenerative and Inflammatory Diseases of Bones and Joints. Philadelphia, Lea & Febiger, 1972.
2. Felman AH, Shulman ST: Staphylococcal osteomyelitis, sepsis and pulmonary disease. Radiology 117:649, 1975.
3. Amstutz HC: Complications of total hip replacement. Clin Orthop 72:123, 1970.
4. Salvati EA, Wilson PD Jr: Long-term results of femoral head replacement. J Bone Joint Surg [Am] 55:516, 1973.
5. Schonholtz GJ, Borgia CA, Blair JD: Wound sepsis in orthopaedic surgery. J Bone Joint Surg [Am] 44:1548, 1962.
6. Green WT, Shannon JG: Osteomyelitis of infants. Arch Surg 32:462, 1936.
7. Howard JB, McCracken GH Jr: The spectrum of group B streptococcal infections in infancy. Am J Dis Child 128:815, 1974.
8. Hutto JH, Ayoub EM: Streptococcal osteomyelitis and arthritis in a neonate. Am J Dis Child 129:1449, 1975.
9. Edwards MS, Baker CJ, Wagner ML, et al: An etiologic shift in infantile osteomyelitis: The emergence of the group B streptococcus. J Pediatr 93:578, 1978.
10. McCook TA, Felman AH, Ayoub E: Streptococcal skeletal infections: Observations in four infants. AJR 130:465, 1978.
11. Siskind B, Galliquez P, Wald ER: Group B beta-hemolytic streptococcal osteomyelitis/purulent arthritis in neonates: Report of three cases. J Pediatr 87:659, 1975.
12. Newman JH: Review of septic arthritis throughout the antibiotic era. Ann Rheum Dis 35:198, 1976.
13. Raff MJ, Melo JC: Anaerobic osteomyelitis. Medicine 57:83, 1978.
14. Kluge R, Schmidt M, Barth WF: Pneumococcal arthritis. Ann Rheum Dis 32:21, 1973.
15. Argen RJ: Suppurative pneumococcic arthritis. NY State J Med 64:2573, 1964.
16. Torres J, Rathbun HK, Greenough WB III: Pneumococcal arthritis: Report of a case and review of the literature. Johns Hopkins Med J 132:234, 1973.
17. Kauffman CA, Watanakunakorn C, Phair JP: Pneumococcal arthritis. J Rheumatol 3:409, 1976.
18. Shawker TH, Dennis JM: Peri-articular calcifications in pyogenic arthritis. AJR 113:650, 1971.
19. Pinals RS, Ropes MW: Meningococcal arthritis. Arthritis Rheum 7:241, 1964.
20. Cattell J: Meningococcal meningitis with purulent arthritis. N Engl J Med 229:49, 1943.
21. Bass M, Nothman G: Multiple purulent arthritis due to meningococcus in very early infancy. J Mt Sinai Hosp 12:60, 1945.
22. Congeni B, Weiner DS: Meningococcal arthritis in children. Orthopedics 1:477, 1978.
23. Ansell BM: Infective arthritis. In JT Scott (Ed): Copeman's Textbook of the Rheumatic Diseases. 5th Ed. Edinburgh, Churchill Livingstone, 1978, p 808.
24. Schein AJ: Articular manifestations of meningococcic infections. Arch Intern Med 62:963, 1938.
25. Eichner HL, Dell JJ: Meningococcal arthritis. Arthritis Rheum 13:272, 1970.
26. Hammerschlag MR, Baker CJ: Meningococcal osteomyelitis: Report of 2 cases associated with septic arthritis. J Pediatr 88:519, 1976.
27. Koppes GM, Arnett FC: Group Y meningococcal arthritis: Case report. Milit Med 140:861, 1975.
28. Sponzilli EE, Calabro JJ: Gonococcal arthritis in the newborn. JAMA 177:919, 1961.
29. Graber WJ, Sanford JP, Ziff M: Sex incidence of gonococcal arthritis. Arthritis Rheum 3:309, 1960.
30. Harris JRW, McCann JS, Mahony JDH: Gonococcal arthritis—a common rarity. Br J Vener Dis 49:42, 1973.
31. Brown D: Gonococcal arthritis in pregnancy. South Med J 66:693, 1973.
32. Fam A, McGillivray D, Stein J, et al: Gonococcal arthritis: A report of six cases. Can Med Assoc J 108:319, 1973.
33. Lightfoot RW Jr, Gotschlich EC: Gonococcal disease. Am J Med 56:347, 1974.
34. Kohen DP: Neonatal gonococcal arthritis: Three cases and review of the literature. Pediatrics 53:436, 1974.
35. Gelfand SH, Masi AT, Garcia-Kutzbach A: Spectrum of gonococcal arthritis: Evidence for sequential stages and clinical subgroups. J Rheumatol 2:83, 1975.
36. Angevine CD, Hall CB, Jacox RF: A case of gonococcal osteomyelitis. A complication of gonococcal arthritis. Am J Dis Child 130:1013, 1976.
37. Ackerman AB, Miller RC, Shapiro L: Gonococcemia and its cutaneous manifestations. Arch Dermatol 91:227, 1965.
38. Linner JH: Suppurative myositis and purulent arthritis complicating acute gonorrhea; report of a case. JAMA 123:757, 1943.
39. Handsfield HH, Weisner PJ, Holmes KK: Treatment of the gonococcal arthritis-dermatitis syndrome. Ann Intern Med 84:661, 1976.
40. Ghormley RK, Deacon AE: Synovial membranes in various types of arthritis: study by differential stains. AJR 35:740, 1936.
41. Cooperman MB: End results of gonorrheal arthritis: A review of 70 cases. Am J Surg 5:241, 1928.
42. Cooperman MB: Gonococcus arthritis in infancy. Am J Dis Child 33:932, 1927.
43. Garcia-Kutzbach A, Masi AT: Acute infectious agent arthritis (IAA): A detailed comparison of proved gonococcal and other blood-borne bacterial arthritis. J Rheumatol 1:93, 1974.
44. Kahn G, Danielsson D: Septic gonococcal dermatitis. Arch Dermatol 99:421, 1969.
45. Ban J, Danielsson D: Septic gonococcal dermatitis. Br Med J 1:482, 1971.
46. Ludivico CL, Myers AR: Survey for immune complexes in disseminated gonococcal arthritis-dermatitis syndrome. Arthritis Rheum 22:19, 1979.
47. Goldman J, Thompson S III, Jacobs N, et al: Detection of circulating immune complexes using platelet aggregation in patients with disseminated gonococcal infection. Arthritis Rheum 18:402, 1975.
48. Layfer LF, Parciany RK, Trenholme GM: Diagnosis of gonococcal arthritis by counterimmunoelectrophoresis: Detection of antigen and antibody in serum and synovial fluid. Arthritis Rheum 21:572, 1978.
49. Walker LC, Ahlin TD, Tung KSK, et al: Circulating immune complexes in disseminated gonorrheal infection. Ann Intern Med 89:28, 1978.
50. Goldenberg DL, Brandt KD, Cathcart ES, et al: Acute arthritis caused by gram-negative bacilli: A clinical characterization. Medicine 53:197, 1974.
51. Miller JM, Engle RL Jr: Metastatic suppurative arthritis with subcutaneous emphysema caused by Escherichia coli. Am J Med 10:241, 1951.
52. Bliznak J, Ramsey J: Emphysematous septic arthritis due to Escherichia coli. J Bone Joint Surg [Am] 58:138, 1976.
53. Holzman RS, Bishko F: Osteomyelitis in heroin addicts. Ann Intern Med 75:693, 1971.
54. Lewis R, Gorbach S, Altner P: Spinal Pseudomonas chondro-osteomyelitis in heroin users. N Engl J Med 286:1303, 1972.

55. Grieco MH: Pseudomonas arthritis and osteomyelitis. J Bone Joint Surg [Am] 54:1693, 1972.

56. Mandal AK, Fiala M, Oparah SS, et al: Osteolytic lesion indicating pseudomonas sternal osteomyelitis. Arch Surg 111:776, 1976.

57. Brand RA, Black H: Pseudomonas osteomyelitis following puncture wounds in children. J Bone Joint Surg [Am] 56:1637, 1974.

58. Chusid MJ, Jacobs WM, Sty JR: Pseudomonas arthritis following puncture wounds of the foot. Pediatr 94:429, 1979.

59. Miller EH, Semian DW: Gram-negative osteomyelitis following puncture wounds of the foot. J Bone Joint Surg [Am] 57:535, 1975.

60. Gordon SL, Evans C, Greer RB III: Pseudomonas osteomyelitis of the metatarsal sesamoid of the great toe. Clin Orthop 99:188, 1974.

61. Murphy JB: Bone and joint diseases in relation to typhoid fever. Surg Gynecol Obstet 23:119, 1916.

62. Chari PR, Choudary HR, Dutt KP, et al: Typhoid osteomyelitis: Report of a case. Aust NZ J Surg 41:174, 1971.

63. Groll A, Smith J: A case of disseminated typhoid osteitis. Afr Med J 39:417, 1965.

64. Mansoor IA: Typhoid osteomyelitis of the calcaneus due to direct inoculation. A case report. J Bone Joint Surg [Am] 49:732, 1967.

65. Miller GAH, Ridley M, Medd WE: Typhoid osteomyelitis of the spine. Br Med J 1:1068, 1963.

66. Mnaymneh W: Salmonella spondylitis. Report of 2 cases. Clin Orthop 126:235, 1977.

67. Porat S, Brezis M, Kopolovic J: *Salmonella typhi* osteomyelitis long after a fracture. J Bone Joint Surg [Am] 59:687, 1977.

68. Schweitzer G, Hoosen GM, Dunbar JM: *Salmonella typhi* spondylitis, an unusual presentation. S Afr Med J 45:126, 1971.

69. David JR, Black RL: Salmonella arthritis. Medicine 39:385, 1960.

70. Gordon HS, Hoffman SJ, Schultz A, et al: Serous arthritis of the knee joint. Report of a case caused by *Salmonella typhosa* and *Salmonella montevideo* in a child. JAMA 141:460, 1949.

71. Hook EW, Campbell CG, Weens HS, et al: Salmonella osteomyelitis in patients with sickle cell anemia. N Engl J Med 257:403, 1957.

72. Engh CA, Hughes JL, Abrams RC, et al: Osteomyelitis in the patient with sickle-cell disease. Diagnosis and management. J Bone Joint Surg [Am] 53:1, 1971.

73. Specht EE: Hemoglobinopathic salmonella osteomyelitis. Orthopedic aspects. Clin Orthop 79:110, 1971.

74. Curtiss PH Jr: Some uncommon forms of osteomyelitis. Clin Orthop 96:84, 1973.

75. Charosky CB, Marcove RC: *Salmonella paratyphi* osteomyelitis. Report of a case simulating a giant cell tumor. Clin Orthop 99:190, 1974.

76. Berlof FE: Arthritis and intestinal infection. Acta Rheumatol Scand 9:141, 1963.

77. Vartiainen J, Hurri L: Arthritis due to *Salmonella typhimurium*. Report of 12 cases of migratory arthritis in association with *Salmonella typhimurium* infection. Acta Med Scand 175:771, 1964.

78. Aho K, Ahvonen P, Lassus A, et al: HL-A 27 in reactive arthritis following infection. Ann Rheum Dis 34:29, 1975.

79. Aho K, Ahvonen P, Lassus A, et al: HL-A 27 in reactive arthritis: A study of Yersinia arthritis and Reiter's disease. Arthritis Rheum 17:521, 1974.

80. Jacobs JC: *Yersinia enterocolotica* arthritis. Pediatrics 55:236, 1975.

81. Blum D, Viart P, Dachy A: Septicemie à *Yersinia enterocolitica* chez deux enfants atteints de thalassemie majeure. Arch Fr Pediatr 27:445, 1970.

82. Mollaret HH: L'infection humaine à *Yersinia enterocolitica* en 1970, à la lumière de 642 cas récents, Aspects cliniques et perspectives épidémiologiques. Pathol Biol 19:189, 1971.

83. Sebes JI, Mabry EH, Rabinowitz JG: Lung abscess and osteomyelitis of rib due to *Yersinia enterocolitica*. Chest 69:546, 1976.

84. Thirumoorthi MC, Dajani AS: *Yersinia enterocolitica* osteomyelitis in a child. Am J Dis Child 132:578, 1978.

85. Dyer RF, Romansky MJ, Holmes JR: Hemophilus pyarthrosis in an adult. Arch Intern Med 102:580, 1958.

86. Hoaglund FT, Lord GP: *Hemophilus influenzae* septic arthritis in adults. Two case reports with review of previous cases. Arch Intern Med 119:648, 1967.

87. Weaver JB, Sherwood L: Hematogenous pyarthrosis due to bacillus *Haemophilus influenza* and *Corynebacterium xerosis*. Surgery 4:908, 1938.

88. Wall JJ, Hunt DD: Acute hematogenous pyarthrosis caused by *Hemophilus influenzae*. J Bone Joint Surg [Am] 50:1657, 1968.

89. Patterson RL Jr, Levine DB: *Hemophilus influenzae* pyarthrosis in an adult. J Bone Joint Surg [Am] 47:1250, 1965.

90. Raff MJ, Dannaher CL: *Hemophilus influenzae* septic arthritis in adults. Report of a case and review of the literature. J Bone Joint Surg [Am] 56:408, 1974.

91. Norden CW, Sellers TF: *Hemophilus influenzae* pyarthrosis in an adult. JAMA 189:694, 1964.

92. Krauss DS, Aronson MD, Gump DW, et al: *Hemophilus influenzae* septic arthritis, a mimicker of gonococcal arthritis. Arthritis Rheum 17:267, 1974.

93. McClatchey WM: Pseudopodagra from *Hemophilus influenzae* in an adult. Arthritis Rheum 22:681, 1979.

94. Merselis JG Jr, Sellers TF Jr, Johnson JE III, et al: *Hemophilus influenzae* meningitis in adults. Arch Intern Med 110:837, 1962.

95. Oill PA, Chow AW, Flood TP, et al: Adult *Haemophilus influenzae* type B vertebral osteomyelitis. A case report and review of the literature. Clin Orthop 136:253, 1978.

96. Hruby MA, Honig GR, Lolekha S., et al: *Arizona hinshawii* osteomyelitis in sickle cell anemia. Am J Dis Child 125:867, 1973.

97. Smilack JD, Goldberg MA: Bone and joint infection with *Arizona hinshawii*. Report of a case and review of the literature. Am J Med Sci 270:503, 1975.

98. Ogden JA, Light TR: Pediatric osteomyelitis: II. *Arizona hinshawii* osteomyelitis. Clin Orthop 139:110, 1979.

99. Buchanan TM, Sulzer CR, Frix MK, et al: Brucellosis in the United States, 1960–1972. An abattoir-associated disease. Part I. Clinical features and therapy. Medicine 53:403, 1974.

100. Buchanan TM, Faber LC, Feldman RA: Brucellosis in the United States, 1960–1972. An abattoir-associated disease. Part II. Diagnostic aspects. Medicine 53:415, 1974.

101. Kelly PJ, Martin WJ, Schirger A, et al: Brucellosis of the bones and joints. Experience with 36 patients. JAMA 174:347, 1960.

102. Johnson EW, Weed LA: Brucellar bursitis. J Bone Joint Surg [Am] 36:133, 1954.

103. Kennedy JC: Notes on a case of chronic synovitis or bursitis due to organism of Mediterranean fever. J R Army Med Corps 2:178, 1904.

104. Zammit F: Undulant fever spondylitis. Br J Radiol 31:683, 1958.

105. Papathanassiou BT, Papachristou G, Hartofilakidis-Garofalidis G: Brucellar spondylitis. Report of 6 cases. Acta Orthop Scand 43:384, 1972.

106. Pritchard DJ: Granulomatous infections of bones and joints. Orthop Clin North Am 6:1029, 1975.

107. Jacobson HG: Abnormalities of the Skeleton. Radiological Notes. Parts I and II. Chicago, Radiological Society of North America, 1973.

108. Rotes-Querol J: Osteo-articular sites of brucellosis. Ann Rheum Dis 16:63, 1957.

109. Atlas E, Belding ME: *Serratia marcescens* arthritis requiring amputation. JAMA 204:167, 1968.

110. Rogala EJ, Cruess RL: Multiple pyogenic arthritis due to *Serratia marcescens* following renal homotransplantation. Report of a case. J Bone Joint Surg [Am] 54:1283, 1972.

111. Martin CM, Merrill RH, Barrett O Jr: Arthritis due to Serratia. J Bone Joint Surg [Am] 52:1450, 1970.

112. Yosowitz GM: Serratia arthritis of the hip. Clin Orthop 85:122, 1972.

113. Dorwart BB, Abrutyn E, Schumacher HR: Serratia arthritis. Medical eradication of infection in a patient with rheumatoid arthritis. JAMA 225:1642, 1973.

114. Dean HM, Post RM: Fatal infection with *Aeromonas hydrophila* in a patient with acute myelogenous leukemia. Ann Intern Med 66:1117, 1967.

115. Chmel H, Armstrong D: Acute arthritis caused by *Aeromonas hydrophila*. Clinical and therapeutic aspects. Arthritis Rheum 19:169, 1976.

116. Morrey BF, Fitzgerald RH, Kelly PJ, et al: Diphtheroid osteomyelitis. J Bone Joint Surg [Am] 59:527, 1977.

117. Johnson WD, Kaye D: Serious infections caused by diphtheroids. Ann NY Acad Sci 174:568, 1970.

118. Fitzgerald RH Jr, Peterson LFA, Washington JA II, et al: Bacterial colonization of wounds and sepsis in total hip arthroplasty. J Bone Joint Surg [Am] 55:1242, 1973.

119. Tomlinson AJ: Human pathogenetic coryneform bacteria: Their differentiation and significance in public health today. J Appl Bacteriol 29:131, 1966.

120. Kaplan K, Weinstein L: Diphtheroid infections of man. Ann Intern Med 70:919, 1969.

121. Torg JS, Lammot TR III: Septic arthritis of the knee due to *Clostridium welchii*. Report of two cases. J Bone Joint Surg [Am] 50:1233, 1968.

122. Lovell WW: Infection of the knee joint by *Clostridium welchii*. J Bone Joint Surg 28:398, 1946.

123. Korn JA, Gilbert MS, Siffert RS, et al: *Clostridium welchii* arthritis. Case report J Bone Joint Surg [Am] 57:555, 1975.

124. Nolan B, Leers W-D, Schatzker J: Septic arthritis of the knee due to *Clostridium bifermentans*. Report of a case. J Bone Joint Surg [Am] 54:1275, 1972.

125. Schiller M, Donnelly PJ, Melo JC, et al: *Clostridium perfringens* septic arthritis. Report of a case and review of the literature. Clin Orthop 139:92, 1979.

126. Schlenker JD, Vega G, Heiple KG: Clostridium pyoarthritis of the shoulder associated with multiple myeloma. Clin Orthop 88:89, 1972.

127. Curtiss PH, Klein L: Destruction of articular cartilage in septic arthritis. I. In vitro studies. J Bone Joint Surg [Am] 45:797, 1963.

128. Evans ES: Changing patterns in skeletal and articular tuberculosis. Proc R Soc Med 50:571, 1957.

129. DeQuervain F, Hunziker H: Die Statistik der chirurgischen Tuberkulosen in Basel fur das Jahr 1913. Cor-Bl Schweiz Arzte 49:761, 1919.

130. Johansson S: Über die Knochen- und Gelenktuberkulose im Kindesalter. Jena, Gustav Fischer, 1926.

131. Cherubin CE: The medical sequelae of narcotic addiction. Ann Intern Med 67:23, 1967.

132. Jaffe RB, Koschman EB: Intravenous drug abuse: Pulmonary, cardiac, and vascular complications. AJR 109:107, 1970.

133. Firooznia H, Seliger G, Abrams RM, et al: Disseminated extrapulmonary tuberculosis in association with heroin addiction. Radiology 109:291, 1973.

134. Enarson DA, Fujii M, Nakielna EM, et al: Bone and joint tuberculosis: A continuing problem. Can Med Assoc J 120:139, 1979.

135. Myers JA: Tuberculosis Among Children and Adults. 3rd ed. Springfield, Ill, Charles C Thomas, 1951, p 215.

136. Griffiths DH: Orthopaedic tuberculosis. Br J Hosp Med 14:158, 1975.

137. Pimon LH, Waugh W: Tuberculous tenosynovitis. J Bone Joint Surg [Br] 39:91, 1957.

138. Mills TJ, Owen R, Strach EH: Early diagnosis of bone and joint tuberculosis in children. Lancet 2:57, 1956.
139. Smith EG, Davison WR: Egyptian Mummies. London, G Allen & Unwin, 1924, p 157.
140. Hippocrates: The Genuine Works of Hippocrates. Translated by F Adams. London, The Sydenham Society, 1849.
141. Pott P: Remarks on that kind of palsy of the lower limbs which is frequently found to accompany a curvature of the spine. London, J Johnson, 1779.
142. Hodgson AR: Infectious disease of the spine. In RH Rothman, FA Simeone (Eds): The Spine. Philadelphia, WB Saunders Co, 1975, p 567.
143. Schmorl G, Junghans H: The Human Spine in Health and Disease. 2nd Am Ed. Translated by EF Besemann. New York, Grune & Stratton, 1971.
144. Jacobs P: Osteo-articular tuberculosis in coloured immigrants: A radiological study. Clin Radiol 15:59, 1964.
145. Bell D, Cockshott WP: Tuberculosis of the vertebral pedicles. Radiology 99:43, 1971.
146. Westermark N, Forssman G: The roentgen diagnosis of tuberculous spondylitis. Acta Radiol 19:207, 1938.
147. Blacklock JWS: Injury as an aetiological factor in tuberculosis. Proc R Soc Med 50:61, 1957.
148. Heniques CQ: Osteomyelitis as a complication in urology with special reference to the paravertebral venous plexus. Br J Surg 46:19, 1958.
149. Tuli SM: Tuberculosis of the craniovertebral region. Clin Orthop 104:209, 1974.
150. Martin NS: Tuberculosis of the spine. A study of the results of treatment during the last twenty-five years. J Bone Joint Surg [Br] 52:613, 1970.
151. Bailey HL, Gabriel M, Hodgson AR, et al: Tuberculosis of the spine in children. J Bone Joint Surg [Am] 54:1633, 1972.
152. Graves VB, Schrieber MH: Tuberculous psoas muscle abscess. J Can Assoc Radiol 24:268, 1973.
153. Goldblatt M, Cremin BJ: Osteo-articular tuberculosis: Its presentation in coloured races. Clin Radiol 29:669, 1978.
154. Paus B: Tumour, tuberculosis, and osteomyelitis of the spine. Acta Orthop Scand 44:372, 1973.
155. Hellstadius A: Tuberculous necrosis of the entire vertebral body with negative x-ray findings. Acta Orthop Scand 16:163, 1946.
156. Boeminghaus H: Senkungsabszesse. Dtsch Med Wochenschr 59:1559, 1933.
157. Fang HSY, Ong GB, Hodgson AR: Anterior spinal fusion. The operative approaches. Clin Orthop 35:16, 1964.
158. Kyle J: Psoas abscess in Crohn's disease. Gastroenterology 61:149, 1971.
159. Tordoir BM: Spasm of and abscess formation in psoas muscle caused by renal calculus. J Urol 66:638, 1951.
160. Zadek I: Acute nontuberculous psoas abscess. J Bone Joint Surg [Am] 32:433, 1950.
161. O'Brien JP: The manifestation of arrested bone growth. The appearance of a vertebra within a vertebra. J Bone Joint Surg [Am] 51:1376, 1969.
162. Yau ACMC, Hsu LCS, O'Brien JP, et al: Tuberculous kyphosis. Correction with spinal osteotomy, halo-pelvic distraction, and anterior and posterior fusion. J Bone Joint Surg [Am] 56:1419, 1974.
163. Lovett RW: Lateral deviation of the spine as a diagnostic symptom in Pott's disease. Trans Am Orthop Assoc 3:182, 1890.
164. Cleveland M, Bosworth DM: The pathology of tuberculosis of the spine. J Bone Joint Surg 24:527, 1942.
165. O'Connor BT, Steel WM, Sanders R: Disseminated bone tuberculosis. J Bone Joint Surg [Am] 52:537, 1970.
166. Alexander GH, Mansuy MM: Disseminated bone tuberculosis (so-called multiple cystic tuberculosis). Radiology 55:839, 1950.
167. Wolstein D, Rabinowitz JG, Twersky J: Tuberculosis of the rib. J Can Assoc Radiol 25:307, 1974.
168. Scoggin CH, Schwarz MI, Dixon BW, et al: Tuberculosis of the skull. Arch Intern Med 136:1154, 1976.
169. Hartofilakidis-Garofalidis G: Cystic tuberculosis of the patella. Report of three cases. J Bone Joint Surg [Am] 51:582, 1969.
170. Hsieh CK, Miltner LJ, Chang CP: Tuberculosis of the shaft of the large long bones of the extremities. J Bone Joint Surg 16:545, 1934.
171. Jüngling O: Ostitis tuberculosa multiplex cystica—eine eigenartige Form der Knochentuberkulose. ROFO 27:375, 1920.
172. Ellis FA: Jungling's ''ostitis tuberculosa multiplex cystoides'' is not cystic tuberculosis osteitis. Acta Med Scand 104:221, 1940.
173. Girdwood W: Multiple cystic tuberculosis of bone (Jüngling's disease). Report of a case. J Bone Joint Surg [Br] 35:285, 1953.
174. Komins C: Multiple cystic tuberculosis; review and revised nomenclature. Br J Radiol 25:1, 1952.
175. Edeiken J, De Palma AF, Moskowitz H, et al: ''Cystic'' tuberculosis of bone. Clin Orthop 28:163, 1963.
176. Karlén A: On cystic tuberculosis of bone. Acta Orthop Scand 31:163, 1961.
177. Feldman F, Auerbach R, Johnston A: Tuberculous dactylitis in the adult. AJR 112:460, 1971.
178. Hardy JB, Hartmann JR: Tuberculosis dactylitis in childhood. Prognosis. J Pediatr 30:146, 1947.
179. Herzfeld G, Tod MC: Tuberculous dactylitis in infancy. Arch Dis Child 1:295, 1926.
180. Robins RH: Tuberculosis of the wrist and hand. Br J Surg 54:211, 1967.
181. König F: Die Tuberkulose der Menschlichen Gelenke Sowie der Brustwand und des Schadels. Berlin, August Hirschwald, 1906.
182. Auerbach O: Tuberculosis of skeletal system. Bull Seaview Hosp 6:117, 1941.
183. Poppel MH, Lawrence LR, Jacobson HG, et al: Skeletal tuberculosis: Roentgenographic survey with reconsideration of diagnostic criteria. AJR 70:936, 1953.
184. Reisner D: Relations between extrapulmonary and pulmonary tuberculosis. Am Rev Tuberc 30:375, 1934.
185. Auerbach O, Stemmerman MG: Roentgen interpretation of pathology in Pott's disease. AJR 52:57, 1944.
186. Mann KJ: Lung lesions in skeletal tuberculosis: Review of 500 cases. Lancet 2:744, 1946.
187. Steinbach HL: Infections of bone. Semin Roentgenol 1:337, 1966.
188. Poznanski AK: The Hand in Radiologic Diagnosis. Philadelphia, WB Saunders Co, 1974.
189. Berney S, Goldstein M, Bishko F: Clinical and diagnostic features of tuberculous arthritis. Am J Med 53:36, 1972.
190. Murray RC: Tuberculosis of the knee; follow-up investigation of old cases. Br Med J 2:10, 1940.
191. Rose GK: Tuberculosis of the knee joint. Br J Clin Pract 13:241, 1959.
192. Wolfgang GL: Tuberculous joint infection. Clin Orthop 136:275, 1978.
193. Wallace R, Cohen AS: Tuberculous arthritis. A report on two cases with review of biopsy and synovial fluid findings. Am J Med 61:277, 1976.
194. Phemister DB, Hatcher CH: Correlation of pathological and roentgenological findings in the diagnosis of tuberculous arthritis. AJR 29:736, 1933.
195. Stenstrom B: Über Phalangentuberkulose bei alteren Individuen. Acta Radiol 16:471, 1935.
196. Polo G DeV, Coradin CC: Tuberculosis of the hip: Treatment with closed irrigation and suction using streptomycin. Clin Orthop 110:154, 1975.
197. Flatman JG: Hip disease with referred pain to the knee. JAMA 234:967, 1975.
198. Brashear HR, Winfield HG: Tuberculosis of the wrist: A report of ten cases. South Med J 68:1345, 1975.
199. Davis JA, Bluestone R: Case report 84. Skel Radiol 4:41, 1979.
200. David-Chausse J, Dehais J, Bullier R, et al: Les ostéo-arthrites et synovites tuberculeuses a foyers multiples. A propos de 10 observations. Rev Rhum Mal Osteoartic 45:463, 1978.
201. Mayers LB: Carpal tunnel syndrome secondary to tuberculosis. Arch Neurol 10:426, 1964.
202. Klofkorn RW, Steigerwald JC: Carpal tunnel syndrome as the initial manifestation of tuberculosis. Am J Med 60:583, 1976.
203. Meyerding HW, Mrox RJ: Tuberculosis of the greater trochanter. JAMA 101:1308, 1933.
204. McNeur JC, Pritchard AE: Tuberculosis of the greater trochanter. J Bone Joint Surg [Br] 37:246, 1955.
205. Sharma SV, Varma BP, Khanna S: Dystrophic calcification in tubercular lesions of bursae. Acta Orthop Scand 49:445, 1978.
206. Thrap-Meyer H: Generalized BCG infection in man. I. Clinical report. Acta Tuberc Scand 29:173, 1954.
207. Waaler E, Oeding P: Generalized BCG infection in man. III. Autopsy findings. Acta Tuberc Scand 29:188, 1954.
208. Morbak A: Osteomyelitis ulnae after BCG vaccination. Nordisk Medicin 52:1482, 1954.
209. Imerslund O, Jonsen T: Lupus vulgaris and multiple bone lesions caused by BCG. Acta Tuberc Scand 30:116, 1955.
210. Haraldsson S: Osteitis tuberculosa fistulosa following vaccination with BCG strain. Acta Orth Scand 29:121, 1959.
211. Felländer M: Tuberculous osteitis following BCG vaccination. Acta Orthop Scand 33:116, 1963.
212. Foucard T, Hjelmstedt A: BCG-osteomyelitis and -osteoarthritis as a complication following BCG vaccination. Acta Orthop Scand 42:142, 1971.
213. Bang J, Engbaek HC, Nielsen E: Osteomyelitis following BCG vaccination. Acta Tuberc Scand 39:203, 1960.
214. Eng J, Aaneland T: BCG osteitis in a child: A bacteriological investigation. Scand J Resp Dis 47:182, 1966.
215. Virtanen S, Lindgren I: Osteomyelitis of the femur caused by BCG. Acta Tuberc Scand 41:260, 1962.
216. Bergdahl S, Felländer M, Robertson B: BCG osteomyelitis. Experience in the Stockholm region over the years 1961–1974. J Bone Joint Surg [Br] 58:212, 1976.
217. Mortensson W, Eklöf O, Jorulf H: Radiologic aspects of BCG-osteomyelitis in infants and children. Acta Radiol (Diag) 17:845, 1976.
218. Torklus DV: Bovine tuberkulöse Osteomyelitis nach BCH-Impfung. Z Orthop 115:249, 1977.
219. Kallesoe O, Jespersen A: Metastatic osteomyelitis following BCG vaccination. Acta Orthop Scand 49:134, 1978.
220. Chapman JS: The ecology of the atypical mycobacteria. Arch Environ Health 22:41, 1971.
221. Runyon EH: Anonymous mycobacteria in pulmonary disease. Med Clin North Am 43:273, 1959.
222. Omar MM: Case report 26. Skel Radiol 1:245, 1977.
223. Danigelis JA, Long RE: Anonymous mycobacterial osteomyelitis. A case report of a six-year-old child. Radiology 93:353, 1969.
224. Cheatum DE, Hudman V, Jones SR: Chronic arthritis due to mycobacterium intracellulare. Sacroiliac, knee, and carpal tunnel involvement in a young man and response to chemotherapy. Arthritis Rheum 19:777, 1976.
225. Dorff GJ, Frerichs L, Zabransky RJ, et al: Musculoskeletal infections due to mycobacterium kansasii. Clin Orthop 136:244, 1978.

226. Halpern AA, Nagel DA: *Mycobacterium fortuitum* infections: A review with two illustrative cases. Clin Orthop *136:*247, 1978.

227. Girard DE, Bagby GC Jr, Walsh JR: Destructive polyarthritis secondary to *myobacterium kansasii.* Arthritis Rheum 16:665, 1973.

228. Stratton CW, Phelps DB, Reller LB: Tuberculoid tenosynovitis and carpal tunnel syndrome caused by *mycobacterium szulgai.* Am J Med 65:349, 1978.

229. Ellis W: Multiple bone lesions caused by avian-battey mycobacteria. Report of a case. J Bone Joint Surg [Br] 56:323, 1974.

230. Binford CH: Leprosy—a model in geographic pathology. Int Pathol 7:6, 1966.

231. Enna CD, Jacobson RR, Rausch RO: Bone changes in leprosy: A correlation of clinical and radiographic features. Radiology *100:*295, 1971.

232. Paterson DE, Rad M: Bone changes in leprosy, their incidence, progress, prevention, and arrest. Int J Lepr 29:393, 1961.

233. Sawtschenko J: Zur Frage Über die Veränderungen der Knochen beim Aussatze (Osteitis et Osteomyelitis leprosa). Beitr Pathol Anat 9:241, 1890.

234. Moller-Christensen V, Bakke SN, Melsom RS, Waaler AE: Changes in anterior nasal spine and alveolar process of maxillary bone in leprosy. Int J Lepr 20:335, 1952.

235. Job CK, Karat S, Karat ABA: Pathological study of nasal deformity in lepromatous leprosy. Lepr India *40:*42, 1968.

236. Karat S, Karat ABA, Foster R: Radiological changes in the bones of the limbs in leprosy. Lepr Rev 39:147, 1968.

237. Goergen TG, Resnick D, Lomonaco A, et al: Radionuclide bone scan abnormalities in leprosy: Case reports. J Nucl Med *17:*788, 1976.

238. Hirschberg M, Biehler R: Lepra der Knochen. Dermatol Ztschr 16:415, 1909.

239. Louie JS, Koransky JR, Cohen AH: Lepra cells in synovial fluid of a patient with erythema nodosum leprosum. N Engl J Med 289:1410, 1973.

240. Karat ABA, Karat S, Job CK, et al: Acute exudative arthritis in leprosy: Rheumatoid arthritis-like syndrome in association with erythema nodosum leprosum. Br Med J 3:770, 1967.

241. Faget GH, Mayoral A: Bone changes in leprosy: A clinical and roentgenological study of 505 cases. Radiology *42:*1, 1944.

242. Esguerra-Gomez G, Acosta E: Bone and joint lesions in leprosy: A radiologic study. Radiology *50:*619, 1948.

243. Wastie ML: Radiological changes in serial x-rays of the foot and tarsus in leprosy. Clin Radiol 26:285, 1975.

244. Harris JR, Brand PW: Patterns of disintegration of the tarsus in the anaesthetic foot. J Bone Joint Surg [Br] 48:4, 1966.

245. Warren G: Tarsal bone disintegration in leprosy. J Bone Joint Surg [Br] 53:688, 1971.

246. Skinsnes OK, Sakurai I, Aquino TI: Pathogenesis of extremity deformity in leprosy. Int J Lepr *40:*375, 1972.

247. Wahi PL, Kaur S, Vadwa MB, et al: Peripheral arteriographic studies in leprosy. Clin Radiol 27:365, 1976.

248. Lechat MF: Bone lesions in leprosy. Int J Lepr 30:125, 1962.

249. Barnetson J: Pathogenesis of bone changes in neural leprosy. Int J Lepr 19:297, 1951.

250. Trapnell DH: Calcification of nerves in leprosy. Br J Radiol 38:796, 1965.

251. Ellis BP: Calcification of the ulnar nerve in leprosy. Lepr Rev 46:297, 1975.

252. Lichtman DM, Swafford AW, Kerr DM: Calcified abscess in the ulnar nerve in a patient with leprosy. A case report. J Bone Joint Surg [Am] 61:620, 1979.

253. Heyman A: Syphilis. *In* TR Harrison et al (Eds): Principles of Internal Medicine. 4th Ed. New York, McGraw-Hill Book Co, 1962, p 1068.

254. Herxheimer G: Die pathologische Anatomie der angeborenen Syphilis. Allgemeime Gesichtspunkte. Verh Dtsch Ges Pathol 23:144, 1928.

255. McCord JR: Syphilis and pregnancy. A clinical study of 2150 cases. JAMA *105:*89, 1935.

256. Cremin BJ, Fisher RM: The lesions of congenital syphilis. Br J Radiol *43:*333, 1970.

257. Schneider P: Über die Organveränderungen bei der angeborenen Fruhsyphilis. Verh Dtsch Ges Pathol 23:177, 1928.

258. McLean S: The roentgenographic and pathologic aspects of congenital osseous syphilis. Am J Dis Child *41:*130, 1931.

259. McLean S: The correlation of the roentgenographic and pathologic aspects of congenital osseous syphilis with particular reference to the first months of life. Am J Dis Child *41:*363, 1931.

260. Levin EJ: Healing in congenital osseous syphilis. AJR *110:*591, 1970.

261. Chipps BE, Swischuk LE, Voelter WW: Single bone involvement in congenital syphilis. Pediatr Radiol 5:50, 1976.

262. Lilien LD, Harris VJ, Pildes RS: Congenital syphilitic osteitis of scapulae and ribs. Pediatr Radiol 6:183, 1977.

263. Fraenkel E: Die kongenitale Knochensyphilis im Röntgenbilde. ROFO, Suppl 26, 1911.

264. Pendergrass EP, Gilman RL, Castleton KB: Bone lesions in tardive heredosyphilis. AJR 24:234, 1930.

265. Hutchinson J: Syphilis. London, Cassell & Co, 1887.

266. Bauer WH: Tooth buds and jaws in patients with congenital syphilis. Correlation between distribution of *Treponema pallidum* and tissue reaction. Am J Pathol 20:297, 1944.

267. Clutton HH: Symmetrical synovitis of the knee in hereditary syphilis. Lancet *1:*391, 1886.

268. Reynolds FW, Wasserman H: Destructive osseous lesions in early syphilis. Arch Intern Med 69:263, 1942.

269. Bauer MF, Caravati CM: Osteolytic lesions in early syphilis. Br J Vener Dis *43:*175, 1967.

270. Ehrlich I, Kricun ME: Radiographic findings in early acquired syphilis: Case report and critical review. AJR *127:*789, 1976.

271. Ungerman AH, Vicary WH, Eldridge WW: Luetic osteitis simulating malignant disease. AJR *40:*224, 1938.

272. Truog CP: Bone lesions in acquired syphilis. Radiology *40:*1, 1943.

273. Speed JS, Boyd HB: Bone syphilis. South Med J 29:371, 1936.

274. Wile UJ, Senear FE: A study of the involvement of the bones and joints in early syphilis. Am J Med Sci *152:*689, 1916.

275. Roy RB, Laird SM: Acute periostitis in early acquired syphilis. Br J Vener Dis 49:555, 1973.

276. Metcalfe JW: Syphilitic osteoperiostitis—skull, ribs, and phalanges. Report of a case. US Nav Med Bull 49:528, 1949.

277. Sante LR: Radiographic manifestations of syphilitic diseases of bone. Am J Syph *12:*510, 1928.

278. Skapinker S, Minnaar D: Syphilitic diseases of the long bones in the Bantu. J Bone Joint Surg [Br] 33:578, 1951.

279. Dismukes WE, Delgado DG, Mallernee SV, et al: Destructive bone disease in early syphilis. JAMA 236:2646, 1976.

280. Thompson RG, Preston RH: Lesions of the skull in secondary syphilis. Am J Syph 36:332, 1952.

281. Burrows HJ: Pathological fracture of the humerus complicating late secondary syphilis. Br J Surg 24:452, 1937.

282. Johns D: Syphilitic disorders of the spine. Report of two cases. J Bone Joint Surg [Br] 52:724, 1970.

283. Gangolphe M: Contribution à l'étude des localisations articulaires de la syphilis tertiare. De l'ostéoarthrite syphilitique. Ann Dermatol Syphiligr 6:449, 1885.

284. Reginato AJ, Schumacher HR, Jimenez S, et al: Synovitis in secondary syphilis. Clinical, light, and electron microscopic studies. Arthritis Rheum 22:170, 1979.

285. Smith JL, Israel CW, McCrary JA, et al: Recovery of *Treponema pallidum* from aqueous humor removed at cataract surgery in man by passive transfer to rabbit testis. Am J Ophthalmol 65:242, 1968.

286. Borchard: Ueber luetische Gelenkentzundungen. Dtsch Ztschr Chir *61:*110, 1901.

287. Kling DH: Syphilitic arthritis with effusion. Am J Med Sci *183:*538, 1932.

288. Gerster JC, Weintraub A, Vischer TL, et al: Secondary syphilis revealed by rheumatic complaints. J Rheumatol 4:197, 1977.

289. Kahn MF, Baillet F, Amouroux J, et al: Le rhumatisme inflammatoire subaigu de la syphilis secondaire. A propos de quatre observations. Rev Rhum Mal Osteoartic 37:431, 1970.

290. Cockshott WP, Davies AGM: Tumoral gummatous yaws. J Bone Joint Surg [Br] *42:*785, 1960.

291. Jones BS: Doigt en lorgnette and concentric bone atrophy associated with healed yaws osteitis. Report of two cases. J Bone Joint Surg [Br] *54:*341, 1972.

292. Reeder MM: Tropical diseases of the foot. Semin Roentgenol 5:378, 1970.

293. Riseborough AW, Joske RA, Vaughan BF: Hand deformities due to yaws in Western Australian aborigines. Clin Radiol *12:*109, 1961.

294. Ngu VA: Medicine in tropics: Tropical ulcers. Br Med J *1:*283, 1967.

295. Kolawole TM, Bohrer SP: Ulcer osteoma—bone response to tropical ulcer. AJR *109:*611, 1970.

296. Brown JS, Middlemiss JH: Bone changes in tropical ulcer. Br J Radiol 29:213, 1956.

297. Lodwick GS: Reactive response to local injury in bone. Radiol Clin North Am 2:209, 1964.

298. Adamson PB: Tropical ulcer in British Somaliland. J Trop Med Hyg 52:68, 1949.

299. Smith EC: Note on bacteriology of tropical ulcers. W Afr Med J 4:68, 1931.

300. Thompson IG: Pathogenesis of tropical ulcer amongst Hausas of Northern Nigeria. Trans R Soc Trop Med Hyg 50:485, 1956.

301. Edwards GA: Clinical characteristics of leptospirosis. Am J Med 27:4, 1959.

302. Sutliff WD, Shepard R, Dunham WB: Acute *Leptospira pomona* arthritis and myocarditis. Ann Intern Med 39:134, 1953.

303. Brown T McP, Nunemaker JC: Rat-bite fever. A review of the American cases with re-evaluation of etiology; report of cases. Bull Johns Hopkins Hosp 70:201, 1942.

304. Nathan MH, Radman WP, Barton HL: Osseous actinomycosis of the head and neck. AJR 87:1048, 1962.

305. Rhangos WC, Chick EW: Mycotic infections of bone. South Med J 57:664, 1964.

306. Pritchard DJ: Granulomatous infections of bones and joints. Orthop Clin North Am 6:1029, 1975.

307. Martinelli B, Tagliapietra EA: Actinomycosis of the arm. Bull Hosp J Dis 31:31, 1970.

308. Simpson WM, McIntosh CA: Actinomycosis of the vertebrae (actinomycotic Pott's disease). Arch Surg 14:1166, 1927.

309. Cope, VZ: Actinomycosis of bone with special reference to infection of the vertebral column. J Bone Joint Surg [Br] 33:205, 1951.

310. Baylin GJ, Wear JM: Blastomycosis and actinomycosis of spine. AJR 69:395, 1953.

311. Young WB: Actinomycosis with involvement of the vertebral column. Clin Radiol *11:*175, 1960.

312. Collins VP, Gellhorn A, Trimble JR: The coincidence of cryptococcosis and disease of the reticulo-endothelial and lymphatic systems. Cancer 4:883, 1951.

313. Shields LH: Disseminated cryptococcosis producing a sarcoid type reaction. The report of a case treated with amphotericin B. Arch Intern Med *104:*763, 1959.
314. Littman ML: Cryptococcosis (torulosis). Am J Med *27:*976, 1959.
315. Chleboun J, Nade S: Skeletal cryptococcosis. J Bone Joint Surg [Am] *59:*509, 1977.
316. Woolfitt R, Park H-M, Greene M: Localized cryptococcal osteomyelitis. Radiology *120:*290, 1976.
317. Meredith HC, John JF Jr, Rogers CI, et al: Case report 89. Skel Radiol *4:*53, 1979.
318. Tchang FKM, Gilardi GL: Osteomyelitis due to *Torulopsis inconspicua.* Report of a case. J Bone Joint Surg [Am] *55:*1739, 1973.
319. Bryan CS: Vertebral osteomyelitis due to *Cryptococcus neoformans.* Case report. J Bone Joint Surg [Am] *59:*275, 1977.
320. Levinson DJ, Silcox DC, Rippon JW, et al: Septic arthritis due to nonencapsulated *Cryptococcus neoformans* with coexisting sarcoidosis. Arthritis Rheum *17:*1037, 1974.
321. Chand K, Lall KS: Cryptococcosis (torulosis, European blastomycosis) of the knee joint. A case report with review of the literature. Acta Orthop Scand *47:*432, 1976.
322. Ley A, Jacas R, Oliveras C: Torula granuloma of the cervical spinal cord. J Neurosurg *8:*327, 1951.
323. Rao SB, Rao KS, Dinakar I: Spinal extradural cryptococcal granuloma. A case report. Neurol India *18:*192, 1970.
324. Ramamurthi B, Anguli VC: Intramedullary cryptococcic granuloma of the spinal cord. J Neurosurg *11:*622, 1954.
325. Litvinoff J, Nelson M: Extradural lumbar cryptococcosis. Case report. J Neurosurg *49:*921, 1978.
326. Cherniss EI, Waisbren BA: North American blastomycosis: A clinical study of 40 cases. Ann Intern Med *44:*105, 1956.
327. Riegler HF, Goldstein LA, Betts RF: Blastomycosis osteomyelitis. Clin Orthop *100:*225, 1974.
328. Gelman MI, Everts CS: Blastomycotic dactylitis. Radiology *107:*331, 1973.
329. Gehweiler JA, Capp MP, Chick EW: Observations on the roentgen patterns in blastomycosis of bone. A review of cases from the blastomycosis study of the Veterans Administration and Duke University Medical Center. AJR *108:*497, 1970.
330. Gill JA, Gerald B: Blastomycosis in childhood. Radiology *91:*965, 1968.
331. Joyce PF, Sundarim M, Burdge RE, et al: A rare clinical presentation of blastomycosis. Skel Radiol *2:*239, 1978.
332. Sanders LL: Blastomycosis arthritis. Arthritis Rheum *10:*91, 1967.
333. Dickson EC, Gifford MA: Coccidioides infection (coccidioidomycosis): Primary type of infection. Arch Intern Med *62:*853, 1938.
334. Conaty JP, Biddle M, McKeever FM: Osseous coccidioidal granuloma. J Bone Joint Surg [Am] *41:*1109, 1959.
335. Dalinka MK, Dinnenberg S, Greendyke WH, et al: Roentgenographic features of osseous coccidioidomycosis and differential diagnosis. J Bone Joint Surg [Am] *53:*1157, 1971.
336. Wesselius LJ, Brooks RJ, Gall EP: Vertebral coccidioidomycosis presenting as Pott's disease. JAMA *238:*1397, 1977.
337. Santos GH, Cook WA: Vertebral coccidioidomycosis. Unusual polymorphic disease. NY State J Med *72:*2784, 1972.
338. Eller JL, Siebert PE: Sclerotic vertebral bodies: An unusual manifestation of disseminated coccidioidomycosis. Radiology *93:*1099, 1969.
339. Cortner JW, Schwartzman JR: Bone lesions in disseminated coccidioidomycosis. Ariz Med *14:*401, 1957.
340. Bisla RS, Taber TH Jr: Coccidioidomycosis of bone and joints. Clin Orthop *121:*196, 1976.
341. Armbruster TG, Goergen TG, Resnick D, et al: Utility of bone scanning in disseminated coccidioidomycosis: Case report. J Nucl Med *18:*450, 1977.
342. Rettig AC, Evanski PM, Waugh TR, et al: Primary coccidioidal synovitis of the knee. A report of four cases and review of the literature. Clin Orthop *132:*187, 1978.
343. Pankovich AM, Jevtic MM: Coccidioidal infection of the hip. A case report. J Bone Joint Surg [Am] *55:*1525, 1973.
344. Greenman R, Becker J, Campbell G, et al: Coccidioidal synovitis of the knee. Arch Intern Med *135:*526, 1975.
345. Pollock S, Morris J, Murray W: Coccidioidal synovitis of the knee. J Bone Joint Surg [Am] *49:*1397, 1967.
346. Haug WA, Merrifield RC: Coccidioidal villous synovitis. Am J Clin Pathol *31:*165, 1959.
347. Iverson RE, Vistnes LM: Coccidioidomycosis tenosynovitis in the hand. J Bone Joint Surg [Am] *55:*413, 1973.
348. Danzig LA, Fierer J: Coccidioidomycosis of the extensor tenosynovium of the wrist. A case report. Clin Orthop *129:*245, 1977.
349. Winter WG, Larson RK, Honeggar MM, et al: Coccidioidal arthritis and its treatment—1975. J Bone Joint Surg [Am] *57:*1152, 1976.
350. Klingberg WG: Generalized histoplasmosis in infants and children. Review of ten cases, one with apparent recovery. J Pediatr *36:*728, 1950.
351. Lunn HF: A case of histoplasmosis of bone in East Africa. J Trop Med Hyg *63:*175, 1960.
352. Allen JH Jr: Bone involvement with disseminated histoplasmosis. AJR *82:*250, 1959.
353. Key JA, Large AM: Histoplasmosis of the knee. J Bone Joint Surg *24:*281, 1942.
354. Omer GE Jr, Lockwood RS, Travis LO: Histoplasmosis involving the carpal joint. A case report. J Bone Joint Surg [Am] *45:*1699, 1963.
355. Cockshott WP, Lucas AO: Histoplasmosis duboisii. Q J Med *33:*223, 1964.
356. Forester HR: Sporotrichosis: An occupational dermatosis. JAMA *87:*1605, 1926.
357. Mikkelsen WM, Brandt RL, Harrell ER: Sporotrichosis: A report of 12 cases, including two with skeletal involvement. Ann Intern Med *47:*435, 1957.
358. Altner PC, Turner RR: Sporotrichosis of bones and joints. Review of the literature and report of six cases. Clin Orthop *68:*138, 1970.
359. Lurie HI: Five unusual cases of sporotrichosis from South Africa showing lesions in muscles, bones, and viscera. Br J Surg *50:*585, 1963.
360. Winter TQ, Pearson KD: Systemic sporothrixosis. Radiology *104:*579, 1972.
361. Comstock C, Wolson AH: Roentgenology of sporotrichosis. AJR *125:*651, 1975.
362. Serstock DS, Zinneman HH: Pulmonary and articular sporotrichosis. Report of two cases. JAMA *233:*1291, 1975.
363. Crout JE, Brewer NS, Tompkins RB: Sporotrichosis arthritis. Clinical features in seven patients. Ann Intern Med *86:*294, 1977.
364. Satterwhite TK, Kageler MV, Conklin RH, et al: Disseminated sporotrichosis. JAMA *240:*771, 1978.
365. Dehaven KE, Wilde AH, O'Duffy JD: Sporotrichosis arthritis and tenosynovitis. Report of a case cured by synovectomy and amphotericin B. J Bone Joint Surg [Am] *54:*874, 1972.
366. Kedes LH, Siemienski J, Braude AI: The syndrome of the alcoholic rose gardener. Sporotrichosis of the radial tendon sheath. Report of a case cured with amphotericin B. Ann Intern Med *61:*1139, 1964.
367. Louria DB, Stiff DP, Bennett B: Disseminated moniliasis in the adult. Medicine *41:*307, 1962.
368. Edwards JE Jr, Turkel SB, Elder HA, et al: Hematogenous candida osteomyelitis. Am J Med *59:*89, 1975.
369. Connor CL: Monilia from osteomyelitis. J Infect Dis *43:*108, 1928.
370. Hirschmann JV, Everett ED: Candida vertebral osteomyelitis. Case report and review of the literature. J Bone Joint Surg [Am] *58:*573, 1976.
371. Noble HB, Lyne ED: Candida osteomyelitis and arthritis from hyperalimentation therapy. Case report. J Bone Joint Surg [Am] *56:*825, 1974.
372. O'Connell CJ, Cherry AV, Zoll JG: Osteomyelitis of cervical spine: *Candida guilliermondi.* Ann Intern Med *79:*748, 1973.
373. Svirsky-Fein S, Langer L, Milbauer B, et al: Neonatal osteomyelitis caused by *Candida tropicalis.* Report of two cases and review of the literature. J Bone Joint Surg [Am] *61:*455, 1979.
374. Noyes FR, McCabe JD, Fekety FR: Acute candida arthritis. Report of a case and use of amphotericin B. J Bone Joint Surg [Am] *55:*169, 1973.
375. Fitzgerald E, Lloyd-Still J, Gordon SL: Candida arthritis. A case report and review of the literature. Clin Orthop *106:*143, 1975.
376. Smilack JD, Gentry LO: Candida costochondral osteomyelitis. Report of a case and review of the literature. J Bone Joint Surg [Am] *58:*888, 1976.
377. Bayer AS, Guze LB: Fungal arthritis. I. Candida arthritis: Diagnostic and prognostic implications and therapeutic considerations. Semin Arthritis Rheum *8:*142, 1978.
378. Lachman RS, Yamauchi T, Klein J: Neonatal systemic candidiases and arthritis. Radiology *105:*631, 1972.
379. Murray HW, Fialk MA, Roberts RB: Candida arthritis—a manifestation of disseminated candidiasis. Am J Med *60:*587, 1976.
380. Adler S, Randall J, Plotkin SA: Candida osteomyelitis and arthritis in a neonate. Am J Dis Child *123:*595, 1972.
381. Hollingsworth JW, Carr J: Experimental candidal arthritis in the rabbit. Sabouraudia *11:*56, 1973.
382. Green WH, Goldberg HI, Wohl GT: Mucormycosis infection of the craniofacial structures. AJR *101:*802, 1967.
383. Straatsma BR, Zimmerman LE, Gass JDM: Phycomycosis. A clinicopathologic study of fifty-one cases. Lab Invest *11:*963, 1962.
384. Addlestone RB, Baylin GJ: Rhinocerebral mucormycosis. Radiology *115:*113, 1975.
385. Kaufman RS, Stone G: Osteomyelitis of frontal bone secondary to mucormycosis. NY State J Med *73:*1325, 1973.
386. Grossman M: Aspergillosis of bone. Br J Radiol *48:*57, 1975.
387. Seres JL, Ono H, Benner EJ: Aspergillosis presenting as spinal cord compression. Case report. J Neurosurg *36:*221, 1972.
388. Seligsohn R, Rippon JW, Lerner SA: *Aspergillus terreus* osteomyelitis. Arch Intern Med *137:*918, 1977.
389. Green WR, Font RL, Zimmerman LE: Aspergillosis of the orbit. Report of ten cases and review of the literature. Arch Ophthalmol *82:*302, 1969.
390. Casscells SW: Aspergillus osteomyelitis of the tibia. A case report. J Bone Joint Surg [Am] *60:*994, 1978.
391. Omar MM, Brown J: Case report 81. Skel Radiol *3:*250, 1979.
392. Josefiak EJ, Kokiko GV: Mycetoma of the hand. Arch Pathol *67:*55, 1959.
393. Cockshott WP, Rankin AM: Medical treatment of mycetoma. Lancet *2:*1112, 1960.
394. Symmers D, Sporer A: Maduromycosis of the hand. Arch Pathol *37:*309, 1944.
395. Hogshead HP, Stein GH: Mycetoma due to *Nocardia brasiliensis.* J Bone Joint Surg [Am] *52:*1229, 1970.
396. Kulowski J, Stovall S: Maduromycosis of tibia in a native American. JAMA *135:*429, 1947.
397. Majid MA, Mathias PF, Seth HN, et al: Primary mycetoma of the patella. J Bone Joint Surg [Am] *46:*1283, 1964.

398. Cockshott WP: Radiological patterns of the deep mycoses. *In* GEW Wolstenholme, R Porter (Eds): Ciba Foundation Symposium on Systemic Mycoses. London, J & A Churchill Ltd, 1968, p 113.

399. Moore PH Jr, McKinney RG, Mettler FA Jr: Radiographic and radionuclide findings in Rhizopus osteomyelitis. Radiology *127*:665, 1978.

400. Chambers RJ, Bywaters EGL: Rubella synovitis. Ann Rheum Dis *22*:263, 1963.

401. Lee PR: Arthritis and rubella. Br Med J *2*:925, 1962.

402. Lee PR, Barnett AF, Scholer JF, et al: Rubella arthritis: Study of 20 cases. Calif Med *93*:125, 1960.

403. Spruance SL, Klock LE Jr, Bailey A, et al: Recurrent joint symptoms in children vaccinated with HPV-77 DK-12 rubella vaccine. J Pediatr *80*:413, 1972.

404. Thompson GR, Ferreyra A, Brackett RG: Acute arthritis complicating rubella vaccination. Arthritis Rheum *14*:19, 1971.

405. Hildebrandt HM, Maassab HF: Rubella synovitis in a one year old patient. N Engl J Med *274*:1428, 1966.

406. Ogra PL, Herd JK: Arthritis associated with induced rubella infection. J Immunol *107*:810, 1971.

407. Johnson RE, Hall AP: Rubella arthritis: Report of cases studied by latex tests. N Engl J Med *258*:743, 1958.

408. Spruance SL, Metcalf R, Smith CB, et al: Chronic arthropathy associated with rubella vaccination. Arthritis Rheum *20*:741, 1977.

409. Ogra PL, Ogra SS, Chiba Y, et al: Rubella virus infection in juvenile rheumatoid arthritis. Lancet *1*:1157, 1975.

410. Randolph AJ, Yow MD, Phillips CA, et al: Transplacental rubella infection in newly born infants. JAMA *191*:843, 1965.

411. Rudolph AJ, Singleton EB, Rosenberg HS, et al: Osseous manifestations of the congenital rubella syndrome. Am J Dis Child *110*:428, 1965.

412. Peters ER, Davis RL: Congenital rubella syndrome. Cerebral mineralization and subperiosteal new bone formation as expressions of this disorder. Clin Pediatr *5*:743, 1966.

413. Sekeles E, Ornoy A: Osseous manifestations of gestational rubella in young human fetuses. Am J Obstet Gynecol *122*:307, 1975.

414. Rabinowitz JG, Wolf BS, Greenberg EI, et al: Osseous changes in rubella embryopathy (congenital rubella syndrome). Radiology *85*:494, 1965.

415. Whalen JP, Winchester P, Krook L, et al: Neonatal transplacental rubella syndrome. Its effect on normal maturation of the diaphysis. AJR *121*:166, 1974.

416. Silverman FN: Virus diseases of bone. Do they exist? AJR *126*:677, 1976.

417. Reed GB Jr: Rubella bone lesions. J Pediatr *74*:208, 1969.

418. London WT, Fucillo DA, Anderson B, et al: Concentration of rubella virus antigen in chondrocytes of congenitally infected rabbits. Nature *226*:172, 1970.

419. Sacks R, Habermann ET: Pathological fracture in congenital rubella. A case report. J Bone Joint Surg [Am] *59*:557, 1977.

420. Sacrez R, Fruhling L, Korn R, et al: Trois observations de maladie des inclusions cytomegaliques. Arch Fr Pediatr *17*:129, 1960.

421. Graham CB, Thal A, Wassum CS: Rubella-like bone changes in congenital cytomegalic inclusion disease. Radiology *94*:39, 1970.

422. Merten DF, Gooding CA: Skeletal manifestations of congenital cytomegalic inclusion disease. Radiology *95*:333, 1970.

423. McCandless AE, Davis C, Hall EG: Bone changes in congenital cytomegalic inclusion disease. Arch Dis Child *50*:160, 1975.

424. Kopelman AE, Halsted CC, Minnefor AB: Osteomalacia and spontaneous fractures in twins with congenital cytomegalic inclusion disease. J Pediatr *81*:101, 1972.

425. Ritvo M, Schauffer IA, Krosnick G: Clinical and roentgen manifestations of erythroblastosis fetalis. AJR *61*:291, 1949.

426. Black-Schaffer B: Fetal nanosomia and bone athrepsia in newborn of women with severe cyanotic cardiovascular anomaly. Am J Obstet Gynecol *59*:656, 1950.

427. Cheatham WJ, Weller TH, Dolan TF Jr, et al: Varicella: Report of two fatal cases with necropsy, virus isolation and serologic studies. Am J Pathol *32*:1015, 1956.

428. Feldman S, Hughes WT, Daniel CB: Varicella in children with cancer: Seventy-seven cases. Pediatrics *56*:388, 1975.

429. Ward JR, Bishop B: Varicella arthritis. JAMA *212*:1954, 1970.

430. Bogumill GP: Bilateral above-the-knee amputations: A complication of chickenpox. J Bone Joint Surg [Am] *47*:371, 1965.

431. Chiari H: Über osteomyelitis variolosa. Beitr Z Pathol Anat Allg Pathol *13*:13, 1893.

432. Cockshott P, MacGregor M: The national history of osteomyelitis variolosa. J Fac Radiol *10*:57, 1959.

433. Cockshott P, MacGregor M: Osteomyelitis variolosa. Q J Med *27*:369, 1958.

434. Gupta SK, Srivastava TP: Roentgen features of skeletal involvement in smallpox. Australas Radiol *17*:205, 1973.

435. Nathan PA, Trung NB: Osteomyelitis variolosa. Report of a case. J Bone Joint Surg [Am] *56*:1525, 1974.

436. Bertcher RW: Osteomyelitis variolosa. AJR *76*:1149, 1956.

437. Eeckels R, Vincent J, Seynhaeve V: Bone lesions due to smallpox. Arch Dis Child *39*:591, 1964.

438. Margolis HS, Subbarao K, Pitt MJ, et al: Case report 58. Skel Radiol *2*:261, 1978.

439. Davidson JC, Palmer PES: Osteomyelitis variolosa. J Bone Joint Surg [Br] *45*:687, 1963.

440. Srivastava AN: Orthopaedic complications of smallpox. J Bone Joint Surg [Br] *48*:183, 1966.

441. Bery K, Chawla S: Radiological features in smallpox osteomyelitis. (A review of six cases.) Indian J Radiol *23*:11, 1969.

442. Cochran W, Connolly JH, Thompson ID: Bone involvement after vaccination against smallpox. Br Med J *2*:285, 1963.

443. Delano PJ, Butler CD: Etiology of infantile cortical hyperostosis. AJR *58*:633, 1947.

444. Sewall S: Vaccinia osteomyelitis; report of a case with isolation of the vaccinia virus. Bull Hosp Joint Dis *10*:59, 1949.

445. Barbero GJ, Gray A, Scott TF, et al: Vaccinia gangrenosa treated with hyperimmune vaccinal gamma globulin. Pediatrics *16*:609, 1955.

446. Silby HM, Farber R, O'Connell CJ, et al: Acute monoarticular arthritis after vaccination. Report of a case with isolation of vaccina virus from synovial fluid. Ann Intern Med *62*:347, 1965.

447. Elliott WD: Vaccinial osteomyelitis. Lancet *2*:1053, 1959.

448. Tamir D, Benderly A, Levy J, et al: Infectious mononucleosis and Epstein-Barr virus in childhood. Pediatrics *53*:330, 1974.

449. Adenbonojo FO: Monoarticular arthritis: Unusual manifestation of infectious mononucleosis. Clin Pediatr *11*:549, 1972.

450. Wechsler HF, Rosenblum AH, Sills CT: Infectious mononucleosis; report of epidemic in army post. Ann Intern Med *25*:113, 1946.

451. Burrows FG: Transient periosteal reaction in illness diagnosed as infectious mononucleosis. Radiology *98*:291, 1971.

452. Goldbloom RB, Stein PB, Eisen A, et al: Idiopathic periosteal hyperostosis with dysproteinemia: New clinical entity. N Engl J Med *274*:873, 1966.

453. Price GE, Ford DK, Gofton JP, et al: An outbreak of "infectious" polyarthritis in a Haida Indian family. Arthritis Rheum *6*:633, 1963.

454. Greudenberg E, Roulet F, Nicole R: Kongenital Infektion mit Coxsackie-virus. Ann Pediatr *178*:150, 1952.

455. Dawson MH, Boots RL: Arthritis associated with lymphogranuloma venereum. JAMA *113*:1162, 1939.

456. Wright LT, Logan M: Osseous changes associated with lymphogranuloma venereum. Arch Surg *39*:108, 1939.

457. Kirkpatrick DJ: Donovanosis (granuloma inguinale): A rare cause of osteolytic bone lesions. Clin Radiol *21*:101, 1970.

458. Warwick WJ: Cat-scratch syndrome, many diseases or one disease? Progr Med Virol *9*:256, 1967.

459. Collipp PJ, Koch R: Cat-scratch fever associated with an osteolytic lesion. N Engl J Med *260*:278, 1959.

460. Adams WC, Hindman SM: Cat-scratch disease associated with an osteolytic lesion. J Pediatr *44*:665, 1954.

461. Lees RF, Harrison RB, Williamson BRJ, et al: Radiographic findings in Rocky Mountain spotted fever. Radiology *129*:17, 1978.

462. Milgram JW: Osseous changes in congenital toxoplasmosis. Arch Pathol *97*:150, 1974.

463. Chandar K, Mair HJ, Mair NS: Case of toxoplasma polymyositis. Br Med J *1*:158, 1968.

464. Thiers H, Coudert J, Romagny G, et al: Deux observations posant le problème d'une localization synoviale de l'infection toxoplasmique. Rev Rhum Mal Osteoartic *18*:548, 1951.

465. Ippolito A, Giacovazzo M, Badalamneti G, et al: Toxoplasmosi acquisita e artrite reumatoide. G Mal Infett Parassit *20*:955, 1968.

466. Vass M, Kullmann L, Csoka R, et al: Polytenosynovitis caused by *Toxoplasma gondii*. J Bone Joint Surg [Br] *59*:229, 1977.

467. VanMeter BF: Hookworm arthritis (report of a case). Kentucky Med J *12*:429, 1914.

468. O'Connor RL, Luedke DC, Harkess JW: Hookworm lesion of bone. J Bone Joint Surg [Am] *53*:362, 1971.

469. Reeder MM: Tropical diseases of the soft tissue. Semin Roentgenol *8*:47, 1973.

470. Greig EDW: Notes on cases of Calabar swellings with radiological observations. J Trop Med Hyg *43*:19, 1940.

471. Johnstone RDC: Loiasis. Lancet *1*:250, 1947.

472. Williams I: Calcification in loiasis. J Fac Radiol *6*:142, 1954.

473. Samuel E: Roentgenology of parasitic calcification. AJR *63*:512, 1950.

474. Montangerand Y, Atlan D, Laluque P, AJR Lymphographic aspects of Filarian adenopathy. J Radiol Electr Med Nucl *50*:135, 1969.

475. O'Connor FW, Golden R, Auchincloss H: Roentgen demonstration of calcified *Filaria bancrofti* in human tissues. AJR *23*:494, 1930.

476. Christopherson JB: Radioscopical diagnosis of filariasis. Br Med J *1*:808, 1929.

477. Khajavi A: Guinea worm calcification: A report of 83 cases. Clin Radiol *19*:433, 1968.

478. Brocklebank JA: Calcification in the guinea worm. Br J Radiol *17*:163, 1944.

479. Cohen G: The radiological demonstration of *Dracunculus medinensis*. S Afr Med J *33*:1094, 1959.

480. Sivaramappa M, Reddy CRRM, Sita Devi C, et al: Acute guinea worm synovitis of the knee joint. J Bone Joint Surg [Am] *51*:1324, 1969.

481. Brailsford JF: *Cysticercus cellulosae*: Its radiographic detection in the musculature and central nervous system. Br J Radiol *14*:79, 1941.

482. Keats TE: Cysticercosis: A demonstration of its roentgen manifestations. Mo Med *58*:457, 1961.

483. Alldred AJ, Nisbet NW: Hydatid disease of bone in Australia. J Bone Joint Surg [Br] *46*:260, 1964.

484. Pasquali E: Sulla localizzazione ossea dell'echinococco. Chir Organi Mov 15:355, 1930.

485. Duran H, Ferrandez L, Gomez-Castresana F, et al: Osseous hydatidosis. J Bone Joint Surg [Am] 60:685, 1978.

486. Hooper J, McLean I: Hydatid disease of the femur. Report of a case. J Bone Joint Surg [Am] 59:974, 1977.

487. Gharbi HA, Cheikh MB, Hamaza R, et al: Les localisations rares de l'hydatidose chez l'enfant. Ann Radiol 20:151, 1977.

488. Booz MK: The management of hydatid disease of bone and joint. J Bone Joint Surg [Br] 54:698, 1972.

489. Teymoorian GA, Bagheri F: Hydatid cyst of the skull: Report of four cases. Radiology 118:97, 1976.

490. Mnaymneh W, Yacoubian V, Bikhazi K: Hydatidosis of the pelvic girdle—treatment by partial pelvectomy. A case report. J Bone Joint Surg [Am] 59:538, 1977.

491. Bonakdarpour A, Zadeh YFA, Maghssoudi H, et al: Costal echinococcosis. Report of six cases and review of the literature. AJR 118:371, 1973.

492. Hutchison WF, Thompson WB, Derian PS: Osseous hydatid (echinococcus) disease. JAMA 182:81, 1962.

493. Stewart GR, Loewenthal J: Vertebral hydatidosis. Aust NZ J Surg 36:175, 1967.

494. Garabedian GA, Matossian RM, Djanian AY: An indirect hemagglutination test for hydatid disease. J Immunol 78:269, 1957.

495. Rappaport EM, Rossien AX, Rosenblum LA: Arthritis due to intestinal amebiasis. Ann Intern Med 34:1224, 1951.

496. Cole GT: Ainhum: Account of fifty-four patients with special reference to etiology and treatment. J Bone Joint Surg [Br] 47:43, 1965.

497. Auckland G, Ball J, Griffiths D: Ainhum. J Bone Joint Surg [Br] 39:513, 1957.

498. Browne SG: Ainhum: Clinical and etiological study of 83 cases. Ann Trop Med 55:314, 1961.

499. Fetterman LE, Hardy R, Lehrer H: The clinico-roentgenologic features of Ainhum. AJR 100:512, 1967.

500. Earle KV: Ainhum of the fingers: Case from Sierra Leone. Trans R Soc Trop Med Hyg 52:570, 1958.

501. Spinzig EW: Ainhum: Its occurrence in the United States with report of three cases. AJR 42:246, 1939.

502. Burch GE, Hale AR: Plethysmographic study of a toe of a patient with Ainhum. Arch Intern Med 100:113, 1957.

503. Wolf E, Stern S: Costosternal syndrome. Arch Intern Med 136:189, 1976.

504. Cameron HU, Fornasier VL: Tietze's disease. J Clin Pathol 27:960, 1974.

505. Gill GV: Epidemic of Tietze's syndrome. Br Med J 2:499, 1977.

506. Tietze A: Ueber eine eigenartige Haufung von Fallet mit Dystrophie der Rippenknorpel. Berl Klin Wschr 58:829, 1921.

507. Jelenko C III: Tietze's syndrome at the xiphisternal joint. South Med J 67:818, 1974.

508. Sain AK: Bone scan in Tietze's syndrome. Clin Nucl Med 3:470, 1978.

509. Gill AM, Jones RA, Pollak L: Tietze's disease. Br Med J 2:155, 1942.

510. Leger L, Moinnereau R: Tuméfaction douloureuse de la jonction chondrocostal (syndrom de Tietze). Presse Med 58:336, 1950.

511. Geddes AK: Tietze's syndrome. Can Med Assoc J 53:571, 1945.

512. Steere AC, Malawista SE, Hardin JA, et al: Erythema chronicum migrans and Lyme arthritis. The enlarging clinical spectrum. Ann Intern Med 86:685, 1977.

513. Harverson G, Warren AG: Tarsal bone disintegration in leprosy. Clin Radiol 30:317, 1979.

514. Lawrence C, Schreiber AJ: Leprosy's footprints in bone-marrow histiocytes. N Engl J Med 300:834, 1979.

515. Zimmerman MR: Pulmonary and osseous tuberculosis in an Egyptian mummy. Bull NY Acad Med 55:604, 1979.

516. Khermosh O, Weintroub S, Topilsky M, et al: Mycobacterium abscessus (M. chelonei) infection of the knee joint. Report of two cases following intra-articular injection of corticosteroids. Clin Orthop 140:162, 1979.

517. Steere AC, Gibofsky A, Patarroyo ME, et al: Chronic Lyme arthritis. Clinical and immunogenetic differentiation from rheumatoid arthritis. Ann Intern Med 90:896, 1979.

518. Blotzer JW, Myers AR: Echo virus-associated polyarthritis. Report of a case with synovial fluid and synovial histologic characterization. Arthritis Rheum 21:978, 1978.

519. Hyer FH, Gottlieb NL: Rheumatic disorders associated with viral infection. Semin Arthritis Rheum 8:17, 1978.

520. Ancona RJ, McAuliffe J, Thompson TR, et al: Group B streptococcal sepsis with osteomyelitis and arthritis. Its occurrence with acute heart failure. Am J Dis Child 133:919, 1979.

521. Fam AG, Tenenbaum J, Stein JL: Clinical forms of meningococcal arthritis: A study of five cases. J Rheumatol 6:567, 1979.

522. Leek JC, Robbins DL: Infectious arthritis due to Hemophilus influenzae. J Rheumatol 6:432, 1979.

523. Chapman M, Murray RO, Stoker DJ: Tuberculosis of the bones and joints. Semin Roentgenol 14:266, 1979.

524. Zvetina JR, Foster J, Reyes CV: Mycobacterium kansasii infection of the elbow joint. A case report. J Bone Joint Surg [Am] 61:1099, 1979.

525. Henriquez M, Levy R, Raja RM, et al: Mucormycosis in a renal transplant recipient with successful outcome. JAMA 242:1397, 1979.

526. Lentz MW, Noyes FR: Osseous deformity from osteomyelitis variolosa. A case report. Clin Orthop 143:155, 1979.

527. Hardin JA, Steere AC, Malawista SE: Immune complexes and the evolution of Lyme arthritis. Dissemination and localization of abnormal C1q binding activity. N Engl J Med 301:1358, 1979.

528. Halla JT, Gould JS, Hardin JG: Chronic tenosynovial hand infection from Mycobacterium terrae. Arthritis Rheum 22:1386, 1979.

529. Memon IA, Jacobs NM, Yeh TF, et al: Group B streptococcal osteomyelitis and septic arthritis. Am J Dis Child 133:921, 1979.

530. Chilton SJ, Aftimos SF, White PR: Diffuse skeletal involvement of streptococcal osteomyelitis in a neonate. Radiology 134:390, 1980.

531. Rosenthal L, Olhagen B, Ek S: Aseptic arthritis after gonorrhea. Ann Rheum Dis 39:141, 1980.

532. Green NE, Bruno J III: Pseudomonas infections of the foot after puncture wounds. South Med J 73:146, 1980.

533. Gray RG, Poppo MJ: Salmonella hartford septic arthritis. J Rheumatol 7:422, 1980.

534. Rumans LW, Allen MS: Haemophilus influenzae septic arthritis in adults. Am J Med Sci 279:67, 1980.

535. Bansal S, Magnussen CR, Napodano RJ: Haemophilus influenzae tenosynovitis. Ann Rheum Dis 38:561, 1979.

536. Thomas JM, Lowes JA, Tabaqchali S: Serratia marcescens in mixed aerobic infections of bone. J Bone Joint Surg [Br] 62:389, 1980.

537. Seradge H, Anderson MG: Clostridial myonecrosis following intraarticular steroid injection. Clin Orthop 147:207, 1980.

538. Rahman NU: Atypical forms of spinal tuberculosis. J Bone Joint Surg [Br] 62:162, 1980.

539. Postacchini F, Montanaro A: Tuberculous epidural granuloma simulating a herniated lumbar disk: a report of a case. Clin Orthop 148:182, 1980.

540. Perelman R, Danis F, Nathanson M, et al: A propos d'un cas de "bécégite" généralisée mortelle sans déficit immunitaire apparent. Sem Hôp Paris 56:480, 1980.

541. Lakhanpal VP, Tuli SM, Singh H, et al: Mycobacterium kansasii and osteoarticular lesions. Acta Orthop Scand 51:471, 1980.

542. Brown TS, Franklyn PP, Marikkar MSK: Tuberculosis of the skull vault. Clin Radiol 31:313, 1980.

543. Meck JM, Colettis E, Parrot R, et al: Aspects radiologiques de l'ostéite tuberculeuse chez l'africain immigré. Ann Radiol 2:634, 1979.

544. Dzebolo NN: Congenital syphilis: An unusual presentation. Radiology 136:372, 1980.

545. Bayer AS, Choi C, Tillman DB, et al: Fungal arthritis. V. Cryptococcal and histoplasmal arthritis. Semin Arthritis Rheum 9:218, 1980.

546. Bayer AS, Scott VJ, Guze LB: Fungal arthritis. IV. Blastomycotic arthritis. Semin Arthritis Rheum 9:145, 1980.

547. McGahan JP, Graves DS, Palmer PES: Coccidioidal spondylitis. Usual and unusual radiographic manifestations. Radiology 136:5, 1980.

548. Bayer AS, Guze LB: Fungal arthritis. II. Coccidioidal synovitis. Clinical diagnostic, therapeutic, and prognostic considerations. Semin Arthritis Rheum 8:200, 1979.

549. Rosenthal J, Brandt K, Wheat LJ, et al: Rheumatologic manifestations of histoplasmosis (Abstr). Arthritis Rheum 23:738, 1980.

550. Shaikh BS, Appelbaum PC, Aber RC: Vertebral disc space infection and osteomyelitis due to Candida albicans in a patient with acute myelomonocytic leukemia. Cancer 45:1025, 1980.

551. Yarchoan R, Davies SF, Fried J, et al: Isolated Candida parapsilosis arthritis in a heroin addict. J Rheumatol 6:447, 1979.

552. Yousefzadeh DK, Jackson JH: Neonatal and infantile candidal arthritis with or without osteomyelitis: A clinical and radiographical review of 21 cases. Skel Radiol 5:77, 1980.

553. Huang SHK, DeCoteau WE: Adult-onset Still's disease: An unusual presentation of rubella infection. Can Med Assoc J 122:1275, 1980.

554. Bayer AS: Arthritis related to rubella. Postgrad Med 67:131, 1980.

555. Smith RK, Specht EE: Osseous lesions and pathologic fractures in congenital cytomegalic inclusion disease: Report of a case. Clin Orthop 144:280, 1979.

556. Dickey LE: Possible varicella lesion of the humerus: A case report. Clin Orthop 148:237, 1980.

557. Pasqual-Gomez E: Identification of large mononuclear cells in varicella arthritis. Arthritis Rheum 23:519, 1980.

558. Kennedy AC, Fleming J, Solomon L: Chikungunya viral arthropathy: A clinical description. J Rheumatol 7:231, 1980.

559. Haddow AJ, Davies CW, Walker AJ: O'nyong nyong fever: An epidemic virus in East Africa. Trans R Soc Trop Med Hyg 54:517, 1960.

560. Saksouk FA: Extrapleural extraosseous costal echinococcosis. Br J Radiol 52:918, 1979.

561. Rosenthal J, Bole GG, Robinson WD: Acute nongonococcal infectious arthritis. Arthritis Rheum 23:889, 1980.

562. Manshady BM, Thompson GR, Weiss JJ: Septic arthritis in a general hospital 1966–1977. J Rheumatol 7:523, 1980.

563. Leek JC, Robbins DL: Haemophilus influenzae tenosynovitis. Ann Rheum Dis 39:530, 1980.

564. Albeniz FE, Martin RG, Del Rio AA: Osteomielitis tuberculosa de localización diafisaria. Radiologia 21:455, 1979.

565. Taillandier J, Manigand G, Fixy P, et al: Le rhumatisme inflammatoire de la syphilis secondaire. Sem Hôp Paris 56:979, 1980.

566. Atdjian M, Granda JL, Ingberg HO, et al: Systemic sporotrichosis polytenosynovitis with median and ulnar nerve entrapment. JAMA 243:1841, 1980.

567. Lehrer RI, Howard DH, Sypherd PS, et al: Mucormycosis. Ann Intern Med 93:93, 1980.

568. Steere AC, Brinckerhoff CE, Miller DJ, et al: Elevated levels of collagenase

and prostaglandin E2 from synovium associated with erosion of cartilage and bone in a patient with chronic Lyme arthritis. Arthritis Rheum 23:591, 1980.

569. Smith RL, Merchant TC, Schurman DJ: In vitro cartilage degradation by *Escherichia coli* and *Staphylococcus aureus*. Arthritis Rheum 25:441, 1982.

570. Nicklas JM: Serious group B beta-hemolytic streptococcal infections in adults: Report of two cases and review of the literature. Johns Hopkins Med J 142:39, 1978.

571. Dworzack DL, Hodges CR, Barnes WG, et al: Group B streptococcal infections in adult males. Am J Med Sci 277:67, 1979.

572. Small CB, Slater LN, Lowy FD, et al: Group B streptococcal arthritis in adults. Am J Med Sci 76:367, 1984.

573. Asplin C, Beehing N, Slack M: Osteomyelitis due to *Streptococcus equisimilis* (Group C). Br Med J 1:89, 1979.

574. Mitnick H, Mitnick JS, Rafii M, et al: Septic arthritis secondary to Group C streptococcus. J Rheumatol 9:974, 1982.

575. Fujita NK, Lam K, Bayer AS: Septic arthritis due to Group G streptococcus. JAMA 247:812, 1982.

576. Nakata MM, Silvers JH, George L: Group G streptococcal arthritis. Arch Intern Med 143:1328, 1983.

577. Meier J-L, Gerster J-C: Bursitis and tenosynovitis caused by Group G streptococci. J Rheumatol 10:817, 1983.

578. Lin AN, Karasik A, Salit IE, et al: Group G streptococcal arthritis. J Rheumatol 9:424, 1982.

579. Zwillich SH, Hamory BH, Walker SE: Enterococcus: An unusual cause of septic arthritis. Arthritis Rheum 27:591, 1984.

580. Allen SL, Salmon JE, Roberts RB: *Streptococcus bovis* endocarditis presenting as acute vertebral osteomyelitis. Arthritis Rheum 24:1211, 1981.

581. Nitsche JF, Vaughan JH, Williams G, et al: Septic sternoclavicular arthritis with *Pasteurella multocida* and *Streptococcus sanguis*. Arthritis Rheum 25:467, 1982.

582. Hynd RF, Klofkorn RW, Wong JK: *Streptococcus anginosus-constellatus* infection of the sternoclavicular joint. J Rheumatol 11:713, 1984.

583. Chusid MJ, Sty JR: Pneumococcal arthritis and osteomyelitis in children. Clin Pediatr 20:105, 1981.

584. Andersen BR, Mayer ME, Geiseler PJ, et al: Multi-joint pneumococcal pyarthrosis in a patient with a chemotactic defect. Arthritis Rheum 26:1160, 1983.

585. Jacobsen ST, Crawford AH: Amputation following meningococcemia. A sequela to purpura fulminans. Clin Orthop 185:214, 1984.

586. Patriquin HB, Trias A, Jeoquier S, et al: Late sequelae of infantile meningococcemia in growing bones of children. Radiology 141:77, 1981.

587. Robinow M, Johnson F, Nanagas MT, et al: Skeletal lesions following meningococcemia and disseminated intravascular coagulation. A recognizable skeletal dystrophy. Am J Dis Child 137:279, 1983.

588. Watson CHC, Ashworth MA: Growth disturbance and meningococcal septicemia. Report of two cases. J Bone Joint Surg [Am] 65:1181, 1983.

589. Fernandez F, Pueyo I, Jimenez JR, et al: Epiphysiometaphyseal changes in children after severe meningococcic sepsis. AJR 136:1236, 1981.

590. Duncan JS, Ramsay LE: Widespread bone infarction complicating meningococcal septicemia and disseminated intravascular coagulation. Br Med J 288:111, 1984.

591. Agarwala BN, Peters JR, Levy HB: Meningococcal septic arthritis in an infant. NY State J Med 81:1512, 1981.

592. Rubinow A: Septic arthritis of the hip caused by Neisseria gonococci. Clin Orthop 181:115, 1983.

593. Masi AT, Eisenstein BI: Disseminated gonococcal infection (DGI) and gonococcal arthritis (GCA). II. Clinical manifestations, diagnosis, complications, treatment, and prevention. Semin Arthritis Rheum 10:173, 1981.

594. Ogiela DM, Peimer CA: Acute gonococcal flexor tenosynovitis—case report and literature review. J Hand Surg 6:470, 1981.

595. Tindall EA, Regan-Smith MG: Gonococcal osteomyelitis complicating septic arthritis. JAMA 250:2671, 1983.

596. Goldenberg DL: ''Postinfectious'' arthritis. New look at an old concept with particular attention to disseminated gonococcal infection. Am J Med 74:925, 1983.

597. Lopitaux R, Sirot J, Meloux J, et al: Bone and joint infections due to gram negative bacilli. Rev Rhum Mal Osteoartic 49:187, 1982.

598. Thorpe MA, Buckwalter JA: Hematogenous *Proteus mirabilis* osteomyelitis. Orthopedics 6:865, 1983.

599. Dan M, Jedwab M, Shibolet S: Recurrent septic arthritis due to Pseudomonas sp. Postgrad Med J 57:257, 1981.

600. Diard F, Kozlowski K, Masel J, et al: Multifocal, chronic, nonstaphylococcal osteomyelitis in children. (Report of four cases—aspergillosis, klebsiella, tuberculosis.) Australas Radiol 27:39, 1983.

601. Rosenbaum J, Offenstadt G, Imbert J, et al: Une complication exceptionnelle de la fièvre typhoide: l'ostéite du metatarse. Med Malad Infect 11:44, 1981.

602. Carvell JE, Maclarnon JC: Chronic osteomyelitis of the thoracic spine due to *Salmonella typhi*. A case report. Spine 6:527, 1981.

603. Brodie TD, Ehresmann GR: *Salmonella dublin* arthritis: An initial case presentation. J Rheumatol 10:144, 1983.

604. Le CT: Salmonella vertebral osteomyelitis. Am J Dis Child 136:722, 1982.

605. Baird RA, Anderson NJ, Bloch JH: Salmonella vertebral osteomyelitis: A complication of salmonella aortitis. Orthopedics 4:1127, 1981.

606. Quismorio FP Jr, Jakes JT, Zarnow AJ, et al: Septic arthritis due to *Arizona hinshawii*. J Rheumatol 10:147, 1983.

607. Audran M, Prost A, Martin M, et al: Arthrites aseptiques avec sérologie positive pour Yersinia pseudotuberculosis. A propos de six nouvelles observations. Rev Rhum Mal Osteoartic 48:477, 1981.

608. Quinn SF, Oshman D: Case report 298. Skel Radiol 13:80, 1985.

609. Martinez DL, Velasco FAB, Alvarez JS, et al: Septic arthritis caused by *Serratia marcescens*. Arthritis Rheum 24:567, 1981.

610. Burgener FA, Hamlin DJ: *Serratia marcescens* osteomyelitis. ROFO 134:459, 1981.

611. Bracikowski JP, Hess IE, Rein MF: Campylobacter osteomyelitis. South Med J 77:1611, 1984.

612. Hodges GR, Degener CE, Barnes WG: Clinical significance of Citrobacter isolates. Am J Clin Pathol 70:37, 1970.

613. Fuxench-Chiesa Z, Mejias E, Ramirez-Ronda CH: Septic arthritis of the sternoclavicular joint due to *Citrobacter diversus*. J Rheumatol 10:162, 1983.

614. Powell JM, Bass JW: Septic arthritis caused by *Kingella kingae*. Am J Dis Child 137:974, 1983.

615. Vincent J, Podewell C, Franklin GW, et al: Septic arthritis due to *Kingella (Moraxella) kingii*: Case report and review of the literature. J Rheumatol 8:501, 1981.

616. Davis JM, Peel MM: Osteomyelitis and septic arthritis caused by *Kingella kingae*. J Clin Pathol 35:219, 1982.

617. Salminen I, Von Essen R, Koota K, et al: A pitfall in purulent arthritis brought out in *Kingella kingae* infection of the knee. Ann Rheum Dis 43:656, 1984.

618. Patel NJ, Moore TL, Weiss TD, et al: *Kingella kingae* infectious arthritis: Case report and review of literature of Kingella and Moraxella infections. Arthritis Rheum 26:557, 1983.

619. Warman ST, Reinitz E, Klein RS: *Haemophilus parainfluenzae* septic arthritis in an adult. JAMA 246:868, 1981.

620. Ho G Jr, Gadbow JJ Jr, Glickstein SL: *Hemophilus influenzae* septic arthritis in adults. Semin Arthritis Rheum 12:314, 1983.

621. Gotuzzo E, Alarcon GS, Bocanegra TS, et al: Articular involvement in human brucellosis: A retrospective analysis of 304 cases. Semin Arthritis Rheum 12:245, 1982.

622. Handal G, Le Compte M: Brucellosis. A treatable cause of monoarthritis. Clin Orthop 168:211, 1982.

623. Neinstein LS, Goldenring J: Brucella sacroiliitis. Clin Pediatr 22:645, 1983.

624. Serre H, Kalfa G, Brousson A, et al: Manifestations ostéo-articulaires de la brucellose. Aspects actuels. Rev Rhum Mal Osteoartic 48:143, 1981.

625. Lemaire V, Ryckewaert A: Monoarthrites brucelliennes chroniques des membres en dehors de la coxite. A propos de deux cas. Rev Rhum Mal Osteoartic 48:149, 1981.

626. Keenan MA, Guttmann GG: Brucella osteomyelitis of the distal part of the femur. A case report. J Bone Joint Surg [Am] 64:142, 1982.

627. Ruyssen S, LePennec MP, Perreau M, et al: Ostéite à brucelles chez l'enfant. Arch Fr Pediatr 40:803, 1983.

628. Bonfiglio M, Mickelson MR, El-Khoury GY: Case report 221. Skel Radiol 9:208, 1983.

629. Norton WL: Brucellosis and rheumatic syndromes in Saudi Arabia. Ann Rheum Dis 43:810, 1984.

630. Samra Y, Hertz M, Shaked Y, et al: Brucellosis of the spine. A report of 3 cases. J Bone Joint Surg [Br] 64:429, 1982.

631. Alarcon GS, Bocanegra TS, Gotuzzo E, et al: Reactive arthritis associated with brucellosis: HLA studies. J Rheumatol 8:621, 1981.

632. Lopez JF, Quesada J, Saied A: Bacteremia and osteomyelitis due to *Aeromonas hydrophila*. Am J Clin Pathol 50:587, 1968.

633. Karam GH, Ackley AM, Dismukes WE: Posttraumatic *Aeromonas hydrophila* osteomyelitis. Arch Intern Med 143:2073, 1983.

634. Simodynes EE, Cochran RM II: *Aeromonas hydrophila* infection complicating an open tibial fracture. A case report. Clin Orthop 171:117, 1982.

635. Ewing R, Fainstein B, Musher DM, et al: Articular and skeletal infections caused by *Pasteurella multocida*. South Med J 73:1349, 1980.

636. Lequesne M, Barreau J, Mazabra A, et al: Images osseuses trompeuses au cours des pasteurelloses digitales. Rev Rhum Mal Osteoartic 48:163, 1981.

637. DiLiberti JH, Tarlow S: Bone and joint complications of *Hemophilus influenzae* meningitis. Clin Pediatr 22:7, 1983.

638. Ho JL, Soukiasian S, Oh WH, et al: *Hemophilus aphrophilus* osteomyelitis. Am J Med 76:159, 1984.

639. Louis JJ, Berard J, Cottin X, et al: Ostéite à *Corynebacterium acnes*. Une observation chez l'enfant. Pediatrie 38:325, 1983.

640. Kizer KW, Ogle LC: Occult clostridial myonecrosis. Ann Emerg Med 10:307, 1981.

641. Lee AB, Waffle CM, Trebbin WM, et al: Clostridial myonecrosis. Origin from an obturator hernia in a dialysis patient. JAMA 246:1232, 1981.

642. Kusumi RK, Plouffe JF: Gas in soft tissues of forearm in an 18-year-old emotionally disturbed diabetic. JAMA 246:679, 1981.

643. Harrington TM, Torretti D, Viozzi FJ, et al: *Clostridium perfringens*: An unusual case of septic arthritis. Ann Emerg Med 10:315, 1981.

644. Fitzgerald RH Jr, Rosenblatt JE, Tenney JH, et al: Anaerobic septic arthritis. Clin Orthop 164:141, 1982.

645. Hall BB, Fitzgerald RH Jr, Rosenblatt JE: Anaerobic osteomyelitis. J Bone Joint Surg [Am] 65:30, 1983.

646. Serushan M, Spencer DL, Yeh WLS, et al: Osteomyelitis of cervical spine from *Propionibacterium acnes*. Arthritis Rheum 25:346, 1982.

647. Polin K, Shulman ST: *Eikenella corrodens* osteomyelitis. Pediatrics 70:462, 1982.

648. Barnhart RA, Weitekamp MR, Aber RC: Osteomyelitis caused by veillonella. Am J Med 74:902, 1983.

649. Yocum RC, McArthur J, Petty BG, et al: Septic arthritis caused by *Propionibacterium acnes*. JAMA 248:1740, 1982.
650. Newton P, Sharp J, Barnes KL: Bone and joint tuberculosis in Greater Manchester 1969–1979. Ann Rheum Dis 41:1, 1982.
651. Halsey JP, Reeback JS, Barnes CG: A decade of skeletal tuberculosis. Ann Rheum Dis 41:7, 1982.
652. Davies PDO, Humphries MJ, Byfield SP, et al: Bone and joint tuberculosis. A survey of notifications in England and Wales. J Bone Joint Surg [Br] 66:326, 1984.
653. Bodem CR, Hamory BH, Taylor HM, et al: Granulomatous bone marrow disease. A review of the literature and clinicopathologic analysis of 58 cases. Medicine 62:372, 1983.
654. Buchner H, Pink P: Die Spondylitis tuberkulosa. Orthopäde 10:119, 1981.
655. Weaver P, Lifeso RM: The radiological diagnosis of tuberculosis of the adult spine. Skel Radiol 12:178, 1984.
656. Blumenthal DH, Morin ME, Tan A, et al: Intestinal penetration by tuberculous psoas abscess. AJR 136:995, 1981.
657. Berges O, Sassoon CH, Roche A, et al: Abcès du psoas d'origine tuberculeuse sans spondylodiscite visible. A propos d'un cas. J Radiol 62:467, 1981.
658. Jones B, Hessel SJ, Weissman BN, et al: Psoas abscess—fact and mimicry. Urol Radiol 2:73, 1980.
659. Gropper GR, Acker JD, Robertson JH: Computed tomography in Pott's disease. Neurosurgery 10:506, 1982.
660. Whelan MA, Naidich DP, Post JD, et al: Computed tomography of spinal tuberculosis. J Comput Assist Tomogr 7:25, 1983.
661. Maritz NGJ, De Villiers JFK, Van Castricum OQS: Computed tomography in tuberculosis of the spine. Comput Radiol 6:1, 1982.
662. Kvernebo K, Stiris G, Haaland M: CT in idiopathic pyogenic myositis of the iliopsoas muscle. A report of 2 cases. Eur J Radiol 1:1, 1983.
663. La Berge J, Brant-Zawadzki M: Evaluation of Pott's disease with computed tomography. Neuroradiology 26:429, 1984.
664. Feldberg MAM, Koehler PR, Van Waes PFGM: Psoas compartment disease studied by computed tomography. Analysis of 50 cases and subject review. Radiology 148:505, 1983.
665. Muguerza I, Roger RL, Uriel S, et al: Tuberculosis de arco posterior. Presentacion de un caso. Radiologia 22:361, 1980.
666. Babhulkar SS, Tayade WB, Babhulkar SK: Atypical spinal tuberculosis. J Bone Joint Surg [Br] 66:239, 1984.
667. David-Chaussé J, Dehais J, Effroy C: L'ostéite vertébrale tuberculeuse centrosomatique. Revue générale à propos de 4 cas. Rev Rhum Mal Osteoartic 51:123, 1984.
668. Fang D, Leong JCY, Fang HSY: Tuberculosis of the upper cervical spine. J Bone Joint Surg [Br] 65:47, 1983.
669. Morvan G, Martini N, Massare C, et al: La tuberculose du rachis cervical. Rev Chir Orthop 70 (Suppl II):6227, 1984.
670. Magnet JL, Thierry A, Couaillier JF, Ostéite tuberculeuse de l'atlas. Rev Rhum Mal Osteoartic 51:273, 1984.
671. Jenny AB, Lehman RAW, Schwartz HG: Tuberculous infection of the cervical spine. Case report. J Neurosurg 38:362, 1973.
672. Kolczun M, Wilde AH, Gildenberg P: Tuberculosis of the first cervical vertebra. Clin Orthop 90:116, 1973.
673. Morantz RA, Devlin JF, George A, et al: Pott's disease as a cause of atlanto-axial subluxation. NY State J Med 74:1634, 1974.
674. Hsu LCS, Leong JCY: Tuberculosis of the lower cervical spine (C2 to C7). A report on 40 cases. J Bone Joint Surg [Br] 66:1, 1984.
675. Reichenthal E, Cohen ML, Shalit MN: Extraosseous extradural tuberculous granuloma of the cervical spine: A case report and review of intraspinal granulomatous infections. Surg Neurol 15:178, 1981.
676. Papavasiliou VA, Petropoulos AV: Bone and joint tuberculosis in childhood. Acta Orthop Scand 52:1, 1981.
677. Versfeld GA, Solomon A: A diagnostic approach to tuberculosis of bones and joints. J Bone Joint Surg [Br] 64:446, 1982.
678. Ekerot L, Eiken O: Tuberculosis of the hand. Case report. Scand J Plast Reconstr Surg 15:77, 1981.
679. Benkeddache Y, Gottesman H: Skeletal tuberculosis of the wrist and hand: A study of 27 cases. J Hand Surg 7:593, 1982.
680. Bush DC, Schneider LH: Tuberculosis of the hand and wrist. J Hand Surg [Am] 9:391, 1984.
681. Kuntz JL, Meyer R, Paille R, et al: Ostéite tuberculeuse du sternum. Rev Rhum Mal Osteoartic 49:477, 1982.
682. Richter R, Nubling W, Krause F-J: Die isolierte brustbein Tuberkulose. ROFO 139:132, 1983.
683. Brown TS: Tuberculosis of the ribs. Clin Radiol 31:681, 1980.
684. Chavaillon JM, Pierluca P, Meyer C, et al: Ostéite tuberculeuse de la voute cranienne. Lyon Med 245:663, 1981.
685. Richter R, Herceg K, Kohler G: Der Patellaherd, eine seltene Lokalisationsform der Skelettuberkulose. Z Orthop 120:5, 1982.
686. Richter R, Michels P, Kohler G: Die Sitzbeintuberkulose. Akt Rheumatol 6:119, 1981.
687. Richter R, Michels P, Krause Fr-J: Die Schambeintuberkulose und ihre Differentialdiagnose. Akt Rheumatol 7:126, 1982.
688. Piussan Ch, Grumbach Y, Lenaerts C, et al: La tuberculose diaphysaire multifocale chez l'enfant immigré. Arch Fr Pediatr 37:689, 1980.
689. Richter R, Krause F-J: Primare Diaphysentuberkulose der langen Rohrenknochen. ROFO 139:549, 1983.

690. Shea JM: Bilateral tuberculous osteomyelitis of medial humeral condyles. Infection secondary to cutaneous inoculation. JAMA 247:821, 1982.
691. Poncet A: Rhumatisme tuberculeux abarticulaire. Lyon Med 99:65, 1902.
692. Poncet A: Rhumatisme tuberculeux ankylosant. Bull Mem Soc Med Hop Paris 20:841, 1903.
693. Poncet A: Pathogénie du rhumatisme tuberculeux. Lyon Med 111:237, 1908.
694. Isaacs AJ, Sturrock RD: Poncet's disease—fact or fiction? A reappraisal of tuberculous rheumatism. Tubercle 55:135, 1974.
695. Summers GD, Jayson MIV: Does Poncet's disease exist? Rheumatol Rehab 19:149, 1980.
696. Sundararaj GD, Selvapandian AJ: Tuberculosis of the hip with urinary fistulas—a case report. Br J Surg 70:241, 1983.
697. Garber EK, Bluestone R: Case report 138. Skel Radiol 6:75, 1981.
698. Pinstein ML, Scott RL, Sebes JI: Tuberculous arthritis of the wrist: Differential diagnosis and case report. Orthopedics 4:1016, 1981.
699. Goldberg J, Kovarsky J: Tuberculous sacroiliitis. South Med J 76:1175, 1983.
700. Richter R, Nubling W, Kohler G, et al: Die Tuberkulose der Iliosakralgelenke. Z Orthop 121:564, 1983.
701. Kahan A, Amor B, Benhamon C-L: Rapidly progressive idiopathic chondrolysis simulating tuberculosis of the shoulder. J Rheumatol 10:291, 1983.
702. Richter R, Michels P, Kohler G: Die Sitzbeintuberkulose. Akt Rheumatol 6:119, 1981.
703. Gouet D, Castets M, Touchard G, et al: Bilateral carpal tunnel syndrome due to tuberculous tenosynovitis: A case report. J Rheumatol 11:721, 1984.
704. Alkalay I, Kaufman T, Suprun H: Tuberculosis of the subdeltoid bursa. A case report. Isr J Med Sci 16:853, 1980.
705. Boda A: Two cases of tuberculous caverna of the greater trochanter filled with gentamycin-PMMA-beads (Septopal chain). A new field of application. Arch Orthop Trauma Surg 101:67, 1982.
706. Chafetz N, Genant HK, Hoaglund FT: Ischiogluteal tuberculous bursitis with progressive bony destruction. J Can Assoc Radiol 33:119, 1982.
707. Mabille JP, Collumbier B, Magnet JL, et al: La trochanterite tuberculeuse. Son diagnostic radiologique. J Radiol 62:25, 1981.
708. Rehm-Graves S, Weinstein AJ, Calabrese LH, et al: Tuberculosis of the greater trochanter bursa. Arthritis Rheum 26:77, 1983.
709. Goldberg I, Avidor I: Isolated tuberculous tenosynovitis of the Achilles tendon. A case report. Clin Orthop 194:185, 1985.
710. Fanning A, Dierich H, Lentle B: Bone scanning with ⁹⁹ᵐTc polyphosphate in tuberculous osteomyelitis. Tubercle 55:227, 1974.
711. Rust RJ, Park HM, Robb JA: Skeletal scintigraphy in miliary tuberculosis: Photopenia after treatment. AJR 137:877, 1981.
712. Kimmel DJ, Klingensmith WC III: Unusual scintigraphic appearance of osteomyelitis secondary to atypical mycobacterium. Clin Nucl Med 5:189, 1980.
713. Nocera RM, Sayle B, Rogers C, et al: Tc-99m MDP and indium-111 chloride scintigraphy in skeletal tuberculosis. Clin Nucl Med 8:418, 1983.
714. Vogelzang RL, Hendrix RW, Neiman HL: Computed tomography of tuberculous osteomyelitis of the pubis. Case report. J Comput Assist Tomogr 7:914, 1983.
715. Schopfer K, Matter L, Brunner CH, et al: BCG osteomyelitis. Case report and review. Helv Paediatr Acta 37:73, 1982.
716. Trevenen CL, Pagtakhan RD: Disseminated tuberculoid lesions in infants following BCG vaccination. Can Med Assoc J 127:502, 1982.
717. Berges O, Boccon-Gibod L, Berger JP, et al: Case report 165. Skel Radiol 7:75, 1981.
718. Bottiger M, Romanus V, de Verdier C, et al: Osteitis and other complications caused by generalized BCG-itis. Experiences in Sweden. Acta Paediatr Scand 71:471, 1982.
719. Weh L, Torklus D: Osteomyelitis nach BCG—impfung. Z Orthop 119:297, 1981.
720. Peltola H, Salmi I, Vahvanen V, et al: BCG vaccination as a cause of osteomyelitis and subcutaneous abscess. Arch Dis Child 59:157, 1984.
721. Collert S, Petrini B, Wickman K: Osteomyelitis caused by *Mycobacterium avium*. Acta Orthop Scand 54:449, 1983.
722. Littlejohn GO, Dixon PL: Fish fancier's finger. J Rheumatol 11:290, 1984.
723. Colver GB, Chattopadhyay B, Francis RS, et al: Arthritis of the subtalar joint due to *Mycobacterium fortuitum*. Br Med J 283:469, 1981.
724. Bolvig L, Andresen J: Osteomyelitis due to *Mycobacterium intracellulare*. Pediatr Radiol 10:241, 1981.
725. Dixon JH: Non-tuberculous mycobacterial infection of the tendon sheaths in the hand. A report of six cases. J Bone Joint Surg [Br] 63:542, 1981.
726. Sauvain-Zryd MJ, Gerster JC, Saudan Y: Monoarthritis due to *Mycobacterium intracellulare*. Case reports and review of the literature. Rev Rhum Mal Osteoartic 50:345, 1983.
727. Feldmann JL, Menkes DJ, Delbarre F: Infectious osteoarthritis of the knee due to *Mycobacterium xenopi*. Rev Rhum Mal Osteoartic 50:365, 1983.
728. Solheim LF, Kjelsberg F: Recurrent mycobacterial osteomyelitis. Arch Orthop Trauma Surg 100:277, 1982.
729. Leader M, Revell P, Clarke G: Synovial infection with *Mycobacterium kansasii*. Ann Rheum Dis 43:80, 1984.
730. Feyen J, Martens M, Mulier JC: Infection of the knee joint with *Mycobacterium xenopi*. Clin Orthop 179:189, 1983.
731. Huskisson EC, Doyle DV, Fowler EF, et al: Sausage digit due to radish bacillus. Ann Rheum Dis 40:90, 1981.
732. Mehta JB, Hovis WM: Tenosynovitis of the forearm due to *Mycobacterium terrae* (radish bacillus). South Med J 76:1433, 1983.

733. Queneau P, Gabbai A, Perpoint B, et al: Acro-osteolysis in leprosy. Report of 19 personal cases. Rev Rhum Mal Osteoartic 50:333, 1983.

734. Albert DA, Weisman MH, Kaplan R: The rheumatic manifestations of leprosy (Hansen disease). Medicine 59:442, 1980.

735. Bonvoisin B, Martin JM, Bouvier M, et al: Les manifestations articulaires de la lèpre. Sem Hop Paris 59:302, 1983.

736. Michalany J: Malignant tumors of the skin among leprosy patients. Int J Lepr 34:274, 1966.

737. Gandersen J: Malignant degeneration in chronic ulceration of the leg and foot in leprosy patients; two case reports. Lepr Rev 53:265, 1982.

738. Thorsen MK, Feldman F, Troy JL, et al: Case report 166. Skel Radiol 7:78, 1981.

739. Rea TH, Levan NE: Current concepts in the immunology of leprosy. Arch Dermatol 113:345, 1977.

740. Rein MF: Diseases caused by treponema. In JH Stein (Ed): Internal Medicine. Boston, Little, Brown, 1983, p 1395.

741. Rosenfeld SR, Weinert CR Jr, Kahn B: Congenital syphilis. A case report. J Bone Joint Surg [Am] 65:115, 1983.

742. Sachdev M, Bery K, Chawla S: Osseous manifestations in congenital syphilis: A study of 55 cases. Clin Radiol 33:319, 1982.

743. Ushigome S, Takakuwa T, Sodemoto Y, et al: Case report 308. Skel Radiol 13:239, 1985.

744. Sengupta S: Musculoskeletal lesions in yaws. Clin Orthop 192:193, 1985.

745. MacCullum P, Tolhurst JC, Buckle G, et al: New bacterial infection in man: Clinical aspects. J Pathol Bacteriol 60:93, 1948.

746. Clancey JK, Dodge OG, Lunn HF, et al: Mycobacterial skin ulcers in Uganda. Lancet 2:951, 1961.

747. Connor DH, Lunn HF: Mycobacterium ulcerans infection (with comments on pathogenesis). Int J Lepr 33:698, 1965.

748. Perraudin ML, Herrault A, Desbois JC: Ulcère cutané à Mycobacterium ulcerans (ulcère de Buruli). Ann Pediatr 27:687, 1980.

749. Martone WJ, Schmid GP: Leptospirosis and relapsing fever (borreliosis). In JH Stein (Ed): Internal Medicine. Boston, Little, Brown, 1983, p 1400.

750. Meyerhoff J: Lyme disease. Am J Med 75:663, 1983.

751. Gerster JC, Guggi S, Perroud H, et al: Lyme arthritis appearing outside the United States: A case report from Switzerland. Br Med J 283:951, 1981.

752. Bruhn FW: Lyme disease. Am J Dis Child 138:467, 1984.

753. Williamson PK, Calabro JJ: Lyme disease—a review of the literature. Semin Arthritis Rheum 13:229, 1984.

754. Kaslow RA, Samples CL, Simon DG, et al: Occurrence of erythema chronicum migrans and Lyme disease among children in two noncontiguous Connecticut counties. Arthritis Rheum 24:1512, 1981.

755. Stewart A, Glass J, Patel A, et al: Lyme arthritis in the Hunter Valley. Med J Aust 1:139, 1982.

756. Burgdorfer W, Kierans JE: Ticks and Lyme disease in the United States. Ann Intern Med 99:121, 1983.

757. Lawson JP, Steele AC: Lyme arthritis: Radiologic findings. Radiology 154:37, 1985.

758. Burgdorfer W, Barbour AG, Hayes SF, et al: Lyme disease—a tick-borne spirochetosis? Science 216:1317, 1982.

759. Steere AC, Grodzicki RL, Kornblatt AN, et al: The spirochetal etiology of Lyme disease. N Engl J Med 308:733, 1983.

760. Johnston YE, Duray PH, Steere AC, et al: Lyme arthritis. Spirochetes found in synovial microangiopathic lesions. Am J Pathol 118:26, 1985.

761. Benach JL, Bosler EM, Hanrahan JP, et al: Spriochetes isolated from the blood of two patients with Lyme disease. N Engl J Med 308:740, 1983.

762. Graybill JR: Mycoses—higher bacteria. In JH Stein (Ed): Internal Medicine. Boston, Little, Brown, 1983, p 1424.

763. Weir JC, Buck WH: Periapical actinomycosis. Oral Surg 54:336, 1982.

764. Webb WR, Sagel SS: Actinomycosis involving the chest wall: CT findings. AJR 139:1007, 1982.

765. Longmaid HE III, Kennedy JD: Case report 156. Skel Radiol 6:282, 1981.

766. Kannangara DW, Tanaka T, Thadepalli H: Spinal epidural abscess due to Actinomyces israelii. Neurology 31:202, 1981.

767. Crank RN, Sundaram M, Shields JB: Case report 197. Skel Radiol 8:164, 1982.

768. Kadish LJ, Muller CJB, Mezger H: Chronic sclerosing osteomyelitis in a long bone caused by actinomycosis. A case report. S Afr Med J 62:658, 1982.

769. Marcus NA, Grace TG, Hodgin UG: Osteomyelitis of the sacrum and sepsis of the hip complicating pelvic actinomycosis. Orthopedics 4:645, 1981.

770. Claque HW, Harth M, Hellyer D, et al: Septic arthritis due to Nocardia asteroides in association with pulmonary alveolar proteinosis. J Rheumatol 9:469, 1982.

771. Yanoff DB, Church ML: Nocardial vertebral osteomyelitis. Clin Orthop 175:223, 1983.

772. Awad I, Bay JW, Petersen JM: Nocardial osteomyelitis of the spine with epidural spinal cord compression—a case report. Neurosurgery 15:254, 1984.

773. Fialk MA, Marcove RC, Armstrong D: Cryptococcal bone disease: A manifestation of disseminated cryptococcosis. Clin Orthop 158:219, 1981.

774. Hammerschlag MR, Domingo J, Haller JO, et al: Cryptococcal osteomyelitis. Report of a case and a review of the literature. Clin Pediatr 21:109, 1982.

775. Reinig JW, Hungerford GD, Mohrmann ME, et al: Case report 268. Skel Radiol 11:221, 1984.

776. Galloway DC, Schochet SS Jr: Cryptococcal skull granuloma. Case report. J Neurosurg 54:690, 1981.

777. Amenta PS, Stead J, Kricun ME: Case report 226. Skel Radiol 9:263, 1983.

778. Rolston KVI, LeFrock JL, Berman AT, et al: Treatment of osseous cryptococcosis. Report of a case and review of the literature. Orthopedics 5:1610, 1982.

779. Shaff MI, Berger JL, Green NE: Cryptococcal osteomyelitis, pulmonary sarcoidosis, and tuberculosis in a single patient. South Med J 75:225, 1982.

780. Bunning RD, Barth WF: Cryptococcal arthritis and cellulitis. Ann Rheum Dis 43:508, 1984.

781. Brand C, Warren R, Luxton M, et al: Cryptococcal sacroiliitis. Ann Rheum Dis 44:126, 1985.

782. Moore RM, Green NE: Blastomycosis of bone. A report of six cases. J Bone Joint Surg [Am] 64:1097, 1982.

783. Boechat MI, Gold RH, Gilsanz V, et al: Radiological aspects of South American blastomycosis in children. Ann Radiol 27:247, 1984.

784. Thorpe CD, Spjut HJ: Coccidioidal osteomyelitis in a child's finger. A case report. J Bone Joint Surg [Am] 67:330, 1985.

785. Reid GD, Klinkhoff A, Bozek C, et al: Coccidioidomycosis tenosynovitis: Case report and review of the literature. J Rheumatol 11:392, 1984.

786. Szabo RM, Lanzer WL, Gelberman RH, et al: Extensor tendon rupture due to Coccidioides immitis. Report of a case. Clin Orthop 194:176, 1985.

787. McGahan JP, Graves DS, Palmer PES, et al: Classic and contemporary imaging of coccidioidomycosis. AJR 136:393, 1981.

788. Stadalnik RC, Goldstein E, Hoeprich PD, et al: Diagnostic value of gallium and bone scans in evaluation of extrapulmonary coccidioidal lesions. Am Rev Resp Dis 121:673, 1980.

789. Boddicker JH, Fong D, Walsh TE, et al: Bone and gallium scanning in the evaluation of disseminated coccidioidomycosis. Am Rev Resp Dis 122:279, 1980.

790. Nocera R, Nusynowitz ML, Swischuk LE, et al: The "doughnut sign" on bone scintigraphy due to coccidioidomycosis. Clin Nucl Med 8:501, 1983.

791. Jones RC, Goodwin RA Jr: Histoplasmosis of bone. Am J Med 70:864, 1981.

792. Thornberry DK, Wheat LJ, Brandt KD, et al: Histoplasmosis presenting with joint pain and hilar adenopathy. "Pseudosarcoidosis." Arthritis Rheum 25:1396, 1982.

793. Rosenthal J, Brandt KD, Wheat LJ, et al: Rheumatologic manifestations of histoplasmosis in the recent Indianapolis epidemic. Arthritis Rheum 26:1065, 1983.

794. Thompson EM, Ellert J, Peters LW, et al: Histoplasma duboisii infection of bone. Br J Radiol 54:518, 1981.

795. Chang AC, Destouet JM, Murphy WA: Musculoskeletal sporotrichosis. Skel Radiol 12:23, 1984.

796. Kumar R, van der Smissen E, Jorizzo J: Systemic sporotrichosis with osteomyelitis. J Can Assoc Radiol 35:83, 1984.

797. Goveia GL, Bellome J, Hiatt WR: Disseminated sporotrichosis with mandibular involvement. J Oral Surg 39:468, 1981.

798. Stratton CW, Lichtenstein KA, Lowenstein SR, et al: Granulomatous tenosynovitis and carpal tunnel syndrome caused by Sporothrix schenckii. Am J Med 71:161, 1981.

799. Hayes WS, Berg RA, Dorfman HD, et al: Case report 291. Skel Radiol 12:284, 1984.

800. Siame JL, Delcambre B, Duquesnoy A, et al: Spondylodiscite à Candida albicans. Rev Rhum Mal Osteoartic 48:58, 1981.

801. Younkin S, Evarts CM, Steigbigel RT: Candida parapsilosis infection of a total hip-joint replacement: Successful reimplantation after treatment with amphotericin B and 5-fluorocystosine. A case report. J Bone Joint Surg [Am] 66:142, 1984.

802. Arnold HJ, Dini A, Jonas G, et al: Candida albicans arthritis in a healthy adult. South Med J 74:84, 1981.

803. Wall BA, Weinblatt ME, Darnall JT, et al: Candida tropicalis arthritis and bursitis. JAMA 248:1098, 1982.

804. Lazo A, Wilner HI, Metes JJ: Craniofacial mucormycosis: Computed tomographic and angiographic findings in two cases. Radiology 139:623, 1981.

805. McKee DF, Barr WM, Bryan CS: Primary aspergillosis of the spine mimicking Pott's paraplegia. J Bone Joint Surg [Am] 66:1481, 1984.

806. Tack KJ, Rhame FS, Brown B, et al: Aspergillus osteomyelitis. Report of four cases and review of the literature. Am J Med 73:295, 1982.

807. Corrall CJ, Merz WG, Rekedal K, et al: Aspergillus osteomyelitis in an immunocompetent adolescent: A case report and review of the literature. Pediatrics 70:455, 1982.

808. Subbarao K, Lubetsky H: Massive swelling of the foot in a 63-year-old man. JAMA 248:3173, 1982.

809. Kemp HBS, Bedford AF, Fincham WJ, et al: Petriellidium boydii infection of the knee: A case report. Skel Radiol 9:114, 1982.

810. Pankovich AM, Auerbach BJ, Metzger WI, et al: Development of maduromycosis (Madurella mycetomi) after nailing of a closed tibial fracture. A case report. Clin Orthop 154:220, 1981.

811. Renton PR, Hall AP: Case report 153. Skel Radiol 6:225, 1981.

812. Monroe PW, Floyd WE Jr: Chromohyphomycosis of the hand due to Exophiala jeanselmei (Phialophora jeanselmei, Phialophora gougerotii). Case report and review. J Hand Surg 6:370, 1981.

813. Stillwell WT, Rubin BD, Axelrod JL: Chrysosporium, a new causative agent in osteomyelitis. Clin Orthop 184:190, 1984.

814. Gustke KA, Wu KK: Torulopsis glabrata osteomyelitis. Report of a case. Clin Orthop 154:197, 1981.

815. Thurston AJ, Gillespie WJ: Torulopsis glabrata osteomyelitis of the spine: A case report and review of the literature. Aust NZ J Surg 51:374, 1981.

816. Marks MI, Langston C, Eickhoff TC: *Torulopsis glabrata*—an opportunistic pathogen in man. N Engl J Med *283:*1131, 1970.

817. Blennow G, Bekassy AN, Eriksson M, et al: Transient carpal tunnel syndrome accompanying rubella infection. Acta Paediatr Scand *71:*1025, 1982.

818. Fraser JRE, Cunningham AL, Hayes K, et al: Rubella arthritis in adults. Isolation of virus, cytology and other aspects of synovial reaction. Clin Exp Rheumatol *1:*287, 1983.

819. Peters ME, Horowitz S: Bone changes after rubella vaccination. AJR *143:*27, 1984.

820. Grahame R, Armstrong R, Simmons N, et al: Chronic arthritis associated with the presence of intrasynovial rubella virus. Ann Rheum Dis *42:*2, 1983.

821. Benson JWT, Bodden SJ, Tobin JO: Cytomegalovirus and blood transfusion in neonates. Arch Dis Child *54:*538, 1979.

822. Ballard RA, Drew L, Hufnagle K, et al: Acquired cytomegalovirus infection in preterm infants. Am J Dis Child *133:*482, 1979.

823. Pearl KN, Dearlove J, Chin KS: Periostitis in an infant with cytomegalovirus infection acquired after birth. Br J Radiol *57:*638, 1984.

824. Friedman A, Navey Y: Polyarthritis associated with chicken pox. Am J Dis Child *122:*170, 1971.

825. Priest JR, Urick JU, Groth KE, et al: Varicella arthritis documented by isolation of virus from joint fluid. J Pediatr *93:*990, 1978.

826. Younes RP, Freeman D: Chicken pox with associated arthritis. Clin Pediatr *22:*649, 1983.

827. Cunningham AL, Fraser JRE, Clarris BJ, et al: A study of synovial fluid and cytology in arthritis associated with herpes zoster. Aust NZ J Med *9:*440, 1979.

828. Devereaux MD, Hazelton RA: Acute monoarticular arthritis in association with herpes zoster. Arthritis Rheum *26:*236, 1983.

829. Friedman HM, Pincus T, Gibilisco P, et al: Acute monoarticular arthritis caused by herpes simplex virus and cytomegalovirus. Am J Med *69:*241, 1980.

830. Shelly WB: Herpetic arthritis associated with disseminated herpes simplex in a wrestler. Br J Dermatol *103:*209, 1980.

831. Brna JA, Hall RF: Acute monoarticular herpetic arthritis. A case report. J Bone Joint Surg [Am] *66:*623, 1984.

832. Gordon SC, Lauter CB: Mumps arthritis: Unusual presentation as adult Still's disease. Ann Intern Med *97:*45, 1982.

833. Appelbaum E, Kohn J, Steinman RE, et al: Mumps arthritis. Arch Intern Med *90:*217, 1952.

834. Lass R, Shephard E: Mumps arthritis. Br Med J *2:*1613, 1961.

835. Solem JH: Mumps arthritis without parotitis. Scand J Infect Dis *3:*173, 1971.

836. Caranosos GJ, Felker JR: Mumps arthritis. Arch Intern Med *119:*394, 1967.

837. Sigal LH, Steere AC, Niederman JC: Symmetric polyarthritis associated with heterophile-negative infectious mononucleosis. Arthritis Rheum *26:*553, 1983.

838. Simpson RW, McGinty L, Simon L, et al: Association of parvoviruses with rheumatoid arthritis in humans. Science *223:*1425, 1984.

839. Fraser JRE, Becker GJ: Mononuclear cell types in chronic synovial effusions of Ross River virus disease. Aust NZ J Med *14:*505, 1984.

840. Mudge PR, Aaskov JG: Epidemic polyarthritis in Australia, 1980–1981. Med J Aust *2:*269, 1983.

841. Rosen L, Gubler DJ, Bennett PH: Epidemic polyarthritis (Ross River) virus infection in the Cook Islands. Am J Trop Med Hyg *30:*1294, 1981.

842. Fraser JRE, Cunningham AL, Clarris BJ, et al: Cytology of synovial effusions in epidemic polyarthritis. Aust NZ J Med *11:*168, 1981.

843. Tesh RB: Arthritides caused by mosquito-borne viruses. Ann Rev Med *33:*31, 1982.

844. Carithers HA: Cat-scratch disease associated with an osteolytic lesion. Am J Dis Child *137:*968, 1983.

845. Kagen LJ: Less common causes of myositis. Clin Rheum Dis *10:*175, 1984.

846. Verinder DGR: Septic arthritis due to *Mycoplasma hominis*. J Bone Joint Surg [Br] *60:*224, 1978.

847. McDonald MI, Moore JO, Harrelson JM, et al: Septic arthritis due to *Mycoplasma hominis*. Arthritis Rheum *26:*1044, 1983.

848. Ponka A: Arthritis associated with *Mycoplasma pneumoniae* infection. Scand J Rheumatol *8:*27, 1979.

849. Hernandez LA, Urquhart GE, Dick WC: *Mycoplasma pneumoniae* infection and arthritis in man. Br Med J *2:*14, 1977.

850. Gemou V, Messaritakis J, Karpathios T, et al: Chronic polyarthritis of toxoplasmic etiology. Helv Paediatr Acta *38:*295, 1983.

851. Burnstein SL, Liakos S: Parasitic rheumatism presenting as rheumatoid arthritis. J Rheumatol *10:*514, 1983.

852. Rogers WF, Ralls PW, Boswell WD, et al: Amebiasis: Unusual radiographic manifestations. AJR *135:*1253, 1980.

853. Bissonnette B, Beaudet F: Reactive arthritis with eosinophilic synovial infiltration. Ann Rheum Dis *42:*466, 1983.

854. Al-Dabbagh AI, Al-Irhayim B: Eosinophilic transient synovitis. Ann Rheum Dis *42:*462, 1983.

855. Bouvet JP, Therizol M, Auquier L: Microfilarial polyarthritis in a massive *Loa loa* infestation. Acta Trop *34:*281, 1977.

856. Daragon A, Le Loet X, Deshayes P, et al: Aseptic guinea worm arthritis of a knee. A case report. Rev Rhum Mal Osteoartic *50:*327, 1983.

857. McLaughlin GE, Utsinger PD, Trackat WF, et al: Rheumatic syndromes secondary to guinea worm infestation. Arthritis Rheum *27:*694, 1974.

858. Koischwitz D, Distelmaier W: Radiologischer nachweis des Medina-wurms (*Dracunculus medinesis*). ROFO *140:*325, 1984.

859. Stelling CB: Dracunculiasis presenting as sterile abscess. AJR *138:*1159, 1982.

860. Bloomfield JA: Hydatid disease in children and adolescents. Aust Radiol *24:*277, 1980.

861. Braithwaite PA, Lees RF: Vertebral hydatid disease: Radiological assessment. Radiology *140:*763, 1981.

862. Giordano GB, Cerisoli M, Bernardi B: Hydatid cysts of the spine. J Comput Assist Tomogr *6:*408, 1982.

863. Dorn R, Kusswetter W, Wunsch P: Alveolar echinococcosis of the femur. Acta Orthop Scand *55:*371, 1984.

864. Bouras A, Larde D, Mathieu D, et al: The value of computed tomography in osseous hydatid disease (echinococcosis). Skel Radiol *12:*192, 1984.

865. Porat S, Robin GC, Wertheim G: Hydatid disease of the spine causing paraplegia. Spine *9:*648, 1984.

866. Bassiouni M, Kamel M: Bilharzial arthropathy. Ann Rheum Dis *43:*806, 1984.

867. Marra TA: Recurrent lumbosacral and brachial plexopathy associated with schistosomiasis. Arch Neurol *40:*586, 1983.

868. Bocanegra TS, Espinoza LR, Bridgeford PH, et al: Reactive arthritis induced by parasitic infestation. Ann Intern Med *94:*207, 1981.

869. Akoglu T, Tuncer I, Erken E, et al: Parasitic arthritis induced by *Strongyloides stercoralis*. Ann Rheum Dis *43:*523, 1984.

870. Kremmydas BN, Papadakis AM, Theodosin A, et al: A case of sarcosporidial infection in a woman. Radiology *83:*1064, 1964.

871. Huang DT, Kirk R: Human sparganosis in Hong Kong. J Trop Med Hyg *65:*133, 1962.

872. Linder RR: Retrospective X-ray survey of porocephalosis. J Trop Med Hyg *68:*155, 1965.

873. Schild H, Neuhaus G, Gerlach F: Dactylolysis spontanea (ainhum). Z Orthop *119:*320, 1981.

874. Dent DM, Fataar S, Rose AG: Ainhum and angiodysplasia. Lancet *2:*396, 1981.

875. Van Linthoudt D, Modde H, Ott H, et al: Erosive group G streptococcal arthritis. Case report and review of the literature. Clin Rheum *3:*541, 1984.

876. Barre PS, Thompson GH, Morrison SC: Late skeletal deformities following meningococcal sepsis and disseminated intravascular coagulation. J Pediatr Orthop *5:*584, 1985.

877. Kidd BL, Hart HH, Grigor RR: Clinical features of meningococcal arthritis: A report of four cases. Ann Rheum Dis *44:*790, 1985.

878. Rosen MS, Myers AR, Dickey B: Meningococcemia presenting as septic arthritis, pericarditis, and tenosynovitis. Arthritis Rheum *28:*576, 1985.

879. Koss PG: Disseminated gonococcal infection. The tenosynovitis-dermatitis and suppurative arthritis syndromes. Cleve Clin Q *52:*161, 1985.

880. Abrahams MA, Tylkowski CM: Brucella osteomyelitis of a closed femur fracture. Clin Orthop *195:*194, 1985.

881. Lifeso RM, Harder E, McCorkell SJ: Spinal brucellosis. J Bone Joint Surg [Br] *67:*345, 1985.

882. Burdge DR, Scheifele D, Speert DP: Serious *Pasteurella multocida* infections from lion and tiger bites. JAMA *253:*3296, 1985.

883. Friedman RJ, Gumley GJ: Crepitation simulating gas gangrene. A case report. J Bone Joint Surg [Am] *67:*646, 1985.

884. Barton LL, Jacob S, Chinnadurai S: Septic arthritis caused by *Clostridium perfringens*. Am Fam Physician *31:*135, 1985.

885. Dowd CF, Sartoris DJ, Haghighi P, et al: Case report 344. Skel Radiol *15:*65, 1986.

886. Lifeso RM, Weaver P, Harder EH: Tuberculous spondylitis in adults. J Bone Joint Surg [Am] *67:*1405, 1985.

887. Richter R, Hahn H, Nubling W, et al: Die Schultergürtel- und Schultergelenk-tuberkulose. Z Rheumatol *44:*87, 1985.

888. Martini M, Adjrad A, Daoud A: Les ostéo-arthrites tuberculeuses du pied et de la cheville. Int Orthop (SICOT) *8:*203, 1984.

889. Eckel H, Due K: Die Tuberkulose der kleinen Gelenke. ROFO *142:*19, 1985.

890. Lee KE: Tuberculosis presenting as carpal tunnel syndrome. J Hand Surg [Am] *10:*242, 1985.

891. Sandstrom S: Multifocal sclerotic BCG spondylitis in a 13-year-old girl. Pediatr Radiol *13:*239, 1983.

892. Marchevsky AM, Damsker B, Green S, et al: The clinicopathological spectrum of non-tuberculous mycobacterial osteoarticular infections. J Bone Joint Surg [Am] *67:*925, 1985.

893. Love GL, Melchior E: *Mycobacterium terrae* tenosynovitis. J Hand Surg [Am] *10:*730, 1985.

894. Mende B, Stein G, Kreysel HW: Knochenveränderungen bei Morbus Hansen. ROFO *142:*189, 1985.

895. Fleury RN, Opromolla DVA: Carcinoma in plantar ulcers in leprosy. Lepr Rev *55:*369, 1984.

896. Shrestha M, Grodzicki RL, Steere AC: Diagnosing early Lyme disease. Am J Med *78:*235, 1985.

897. Mertz LE, Wobig GH, Duffy J, et al: Ticks, spirochetes, and new diagnostic tests for Lyme disease. Mayo Clin Proc *60:*402, 1985.

898. Wilkerson RD, Taylor DC, Opal SM, et al: *Nocardia asteroides* sepsis of the knee. Clin Orthop *197:*206, 1985.

899. Matsushita T, Suzuki K: Spastic paraparesis due to cryptococcal osteomyelitis. A case report. Clin Orthop *196:*279 ,1985.

900. Gold JWM: Opportunistic fungal infections in patients with neoplastic disease. Am J Med *76:*458, 1984.

901. George AL Jr, Hays JT, Graham BS: Blastomycosis presenting as monarticular arthritis. The role of synovial fluid cytology. Arthritis Rheum *28:*516, 1985.

902. Castaneda OJ, Alarcon GS, Garcia MT, et al: *Paracoccidioides brasiliensis* arthritis. Report of a case and review of the literature. J Rheumatol *12:*356, 1985.
903. Katzenstein D: Isolated Candida arthritis: Report of a case and definition of a distinct clinical syndrome. Arthritis Rheum *28:*1421, 1985.
904. Ferris B, Jones C: Paraplegia due to aspergillosis. Successful conservative treatment of two cases. J Bone Joint Surg [Br] *67:*800, 1985.
905. Lewall DB, Ofole S, Bendl B: Mycetoma. Skel Radiol *14:*257, 1985.
906. Halverson PB, Lahiri S, Wojno WC, et al: Sporotrichal arthritis presenting as granulomatous myositis. Arthritis Rheum *28:*1425, 1985.
907. Johnson JF, Lehman RM, Shiels WE, et al: Osteolysis in catscratch fever. Radiology *156:*373, 1985.
908. Van Dellen RG, Ottesen EA, Gocke TM, et al: *Loa loa.* An unusual case of chronic urticaria and angioedema in the United States. JAMA *253:*1924, 1985.
909. El Garf A: Parasitic rheumatism: Rheumatic manifestations associated with calcified guinea worm. J Rheumatol *12:*976, 1985.
910. Herrera R, Varela E, Morales G, et al: Dermatomyositis-like syndrome caused by trichinae. Report of two cases. J Rheumatol *12:*782, 1985.
911. Beggs I: The radiology of hydatid disease. AJR *145:*639, 1985.
912. Mikhael MA, Ciric IS, Tarkington JA: MR imaging in spinal echinococcosis. J Comput Assist Tomogr *9:*398, 1985.
913. Tabatabai MF, Sapico FL, Canawati HN, et al: Sternoclavicular joint infection with group B streptococcus. J Rheumatol *13:*466, 1986.
914. March L, Needs CJ, Webb J: Streptococcus group G septic polyarthritis. Aust NZ J Med *15:*647, 1985.
915. Macy NJ, Lieber L, Haberman ET: Arthritis caused by *Clostridium septicum.* A case report and review of the literature. J Bone Joint Surg [Am] *68:*465, 1986.
916. Beguiristain JL, de Pablos J, Llombart R, Gómez A: Discitis due to *Clostridium perfringens.* Spine *11:*170, 1986.
917. Evanchick CC, Davis DE, Harrington TM: Tuberculosis of peripheral joints: An often missed diagnosis. J Rheumatol *13:*187, 1986.
918. Ricciardi DD, Sepkowitz DV, Berkowitz LB, et al: Cryptococcal arthritis in a patient with acquired immune deficiency syndrome. Case report and review of the literature. J Rheumatol *13:*455, 1986.
919. Yao J, Penn RG, Ray S: Articular sporotrichosis. Clin Orthop *204:*207, 1986.
920. Tingle AJ, Allen M, Petty RE, et al: Rubella-associated arthritis. I. Comparative study of joint manifestations associated with natural rubella infection and RA 27/3 rubella immunisation. Ann Rheum Dis *45:*110, 1986.
921. Chantler JK, Tingle AJ, Petty RE: Persistent rubella virus infection associated with chronic arthritis in children. N Engl J Med *313:*1117, 1985.
922. Zee C-S, Segall HD, Ahmadi J, et al: CT myelography in spinal cysticercosis. J Comput Assist Tomogr *10:*195, 1986.
923. Bertoli CL, Stassi J, Rifkin MD: Ainhum—an unusual presentation involving the second toe in a white male. Skel Radiol *11:*133, 1984.
924. Gillespie WJ, Moore TE, Mayo KM: Subacute pyogenic osteomyelitis. Orthopedics *9:*1565, 1986.
925. Borenstein DG, Simon GL: *Hemophilus influenzae* septic arthritis in adults. A report of four cases and a review of the literature. Medicine *65:*191, 1986.
926. Cohen MA, Levy IM, Habermann ET: Multiple joint sepsis by *Hemophilus influenzae* in an adult. Clin Orthop *209:*198, 1986.
927. Bocanegra TS, Gotuzzo E, Castañeda O, et al: Rheumatic manifestations of brucellosis. Ann Rheum Dis *45:*526, 1986.
928. Abdelwahab IF, Present DA, Klein MJ: Case report 390. Skel Radiol *15:*652, 1986.
929. Hall FM, Harris AK: Case report 396. Skel Radiol *15:*589, 1986.
930. Martini M, Benkeddache Y, Medjani Y, et al: Tuberculosis of the upper limb joints. Int Orthop (SICOT) *10:*17, 1986.
931. Salomon CG, Ali A, Fordham EW: Bone scintigraphy in tuberculous sacroiliitis. Clin Nucl Med *11:*407, 1986.
932. de Roos A, van Meerten ELVP, Bloem JL, et al: MRI of tuberculous spondylitis. AJR *146:*79, 1986.
933. Aftimos S, Nicol R: BCG osteitis: A case report. N Z Med J *99:*271, 1986.
934. Goldings EA, Jericho J: Lyme disease. Clinics Rheum Dis *12:*343, 1986.
935. Jacobs JC, Stevens M, Duray PH: Lyme disease simulating septic arthritis. JAMA *256:*1138, 1986.
936. Culp RW, Eichenfield AH, Davidson RS, et al: Lyme arthritis in children. An orthopedic perspective. J Bone Joint Surg [Am] *69:*96, 1987.
937. McLaughlin TP, Zemel L, Fisher RL, et al: Chronic arthritis of the knee in Lyme disease. Review of the literature and report of two cases treated by synovectomy. J Bone Joint Surg [Am] *68:*1057, 1986.
938. Mesgarzadeh M, Bonakdarpour A, Redecki PD: Case report 395. Skel Radiol *15:*584, 1986.
939. Bried JM, Galgiani JN: *Coccidioides immitis* infections in bones and joints. Clin Orthop *211:*235, 1986.
940. Hay EL, Collawn SS, Middleton FG: *Sporothrix schenckii* tenosynovitis: A case report. J Hand Surg [Am] *11:*431, 1986.
941. Bruns J, Hemker T, Dahmen G: Pilzinduzierte Spondylitis. Z Orthop *124:*96, 1986.
942. Behr JT, Daluga DJ, Light TR, et al: Herpetic infections in the fingers of infants. Report of five cases. J Bone Joint Surg [Am] *69:*137, 1987.
943. Cohen BJ, Buckley MM, Clewley JP, et al: Human parovirus infection in early rheumatoid and inflammatory arthritis. Ann Rheum Dis *45:*832, 1986.
944. Savoiardo M, Cimino C, Passerini A, et al: Mobile myelographic filling defects: Spinal cysticercosis. Neuroradiology *28:*166, 1986.

945. Ferris BD, Scott JE, Uttley D: Hydatid disease of the cervical spine. Clin Orthop *207:*174, 1986.
946. Claudon M, Bracard S, Plenat F, et al: Spinal involvement in alveolar echinococcosis: Assessment of two cases. Radiology *162:*571, 1987.
947. Szypryt EP, Morris DL, Mulholland RC: Combined chemotherapy and surgery for hydatid bone disease. J Bone Joint Surg [Br] *69:*141, 1987.
948. Baxter MP, Finnegan MA: Skeletal infection by group B beta-haemolitic streptococci in neonates. A case report and review of the literature. J Bone Joint Surg [Br] *70:*812, 1988.
949. Yoder EL, Mendez J, Khatib R: Spontaneous gangrenous myositis induced by *Streptococcus pyogenes:* Case report and review of the literature. Rev Infect Dis *9:*382, 1987.
950. Stark RH: Group B β-hemolytic streptococcal arthritis and osteomyelitis of the wrist. J Hand Surg [Am] *12:*296, 1987.
951. Doberstein C, MacEwen GD, Lee MS: Group B β-hemolytic streptococcal osteomyelitis of the heel. A case report. Clin Orthop *231:*225, 1988.
952. Fasano FJ Jr, Graham DR, Stauffer ES: Vertebral osteomyelitis secondary to *Streptococcus agalactiae.* Clin Orthop *256:*101, 1990.
953. Sobrino J, Bosch X, Wennberg P, et al: Septic arthritis secondary to group C streptococcus typed as *Streptococcus equisimilis.* J Rheumatol *18:*485, 1991.
954. Butler KM, Baker CJ: Group F streptococcus. An unusual cause of arthritis. Clin Orthop *228:*261, 1988.
955. Quevedo SF, Mikolich DJ, Humbyrd DE, et al: Pyogenic sacroiliitis caused by group G streptococcus. Arthritis Rheum *30:*115, 1987.
956. Castellarin M, Bonnet C, Remy M, et al: Spondylitis due to group G streptococcus. J Rheumatol *20:*758, 1993.
957. Mitchell D, Duncan I, Brook A, et al: *Streptococcus faecalis* arthritis. J Rheumatol *16:*138, 1989.
958. Hunter T, Chow AW: Peptostreptococcus magnus septic arthritis—a report and review of the English literature. J Rheumatol *15:*1583, 1988.
959. Davies UM, Leak AM, Davé J: Infection of a prosthetic knee joint with *Peptostreptococcus magnus.* Ann Rheum Dis *47:*866, 1988.
960. Serushan M, Varghai M: Emphysematous septic arthritis in multiple joints due to *Streptococcus milleri.* J Rheumatol *15:*517, 1988.
961. Meyes E, Flipo R-M, Van Bosterhaut B, et al: Septic *Streptococcus milleri* spondylodiscitis. J Rheumatol *17:*1421, 1990.
962. Soria LM, Roura XJ, Miguel J, et al: Pyogenic arthritis caused by *Streptococcus milleri* in a nonimmunocompromised host. J Rheumatol *18:*473, 1991.
963. Morris IM: Pneumococcal septic arthritis. Ann Rheum Dis *46:*943, 1987.
964. Hyszczak R, Bartold KP: Gangrene associated with meningococcemia. AJR *151:*203, 1988.
965. Nogi J: Physeal arrest in purpura fulminans. A report of three cases. J Bone Joint Surg [Am] *71:*929, 1989.
966. Grogan DP, Love SM, Ogden JA, et al: Chondro-osseous growth abnormalities after meningococcemia. A clinical and histopathological study. J Bone Joint Surg [Am] *71:*920, 1989.
967. Kruse RW, Tassanawipas A, Bowen JR: Orthopedic sequelae of meningococcemia. Orthopedics *14:*174, 1991.
968. Pollet SM, Leek JC: Tenosynovitis in meningococcemia. Arthritis Rheum *30:*232, 1987.
969. Ingram CW, Nichole B, Martinez S, et al: Gonococcal osteomyelitis. Case report and review of the literature. Arch Intern Med *151:*177, 1991.
970. Schaefer RA, Enzenauer RJ, Pruitt A, et al: Acute gonococcal flexor tenosynovitis in an adolescent male with pharyngitis. A case report and literature review. Clin Orthop *281:*212, 1992.
971. Livneh A, Sewell KL, Barland P: Chronic gonococcal arthritis. J Rheumatol *16:*245, 1989.
972. Yang EC, Neuwirth MG: *Pseudomonas aeruginosa* as a causative agent of cervical osteomyelitis. Case report and review of the literature. Clin Orthop *231:*229, 1988.
973. Matteson EL, McCune WJ: Septic arthritis caused by treatment resistant *Pseudomonas cepacia.* Ann Rheum Dis *49:*258, 1990.
974. Broom MJ, Beebe RD: Emphysematous septic arthritis due to *Klebsiella pneumoniae.* Clin Orthop *226:*219, 1988.
975. Monsivais JJ, Scully TJ, Dixon BL: Chronic osteomyelitis of the hand caused by *salmonella typhimurium.* A case report. Clin Orthop *226:*231, 1988.
976. Govender S, Chotai PR: Salmonella osteitis and septic arthritis. J Bone Joint Surg [Br] *72:*504, 1990.
977. Gutiérrez C, Cruz L, Olivé A, et al: Salmonella septic arthritis in HIV patients. Br J Rheumatol *32:*88, 1993.
978. Miller ME, Fogel GR, Dunham WK: Salmonella spondylitis. A review and report of two immunologically normal patients. J Bone Joint Surg [Am] *70:*463, 1988.
979. Ingram R, Redding P: *Salmonella virchow* osteomyelitis. A case report. J Bone Joint Surg [Br] *70:*440, 1988.
980. Kraus A, Guerra-Bautista G, Alarcón-Segovia D: *Salmonella arizona* arthritis and septicemia associated with rattlesnake ingestion by patients with connective tissue diseases. A dangerous complication of folk medicine. J Rheumatol *18:*1328, 1991.
981. Perrot S, Lescure J, Leviet D, et al: *Yersinia enterocolitica* tenosynovitis. The first case. J Rheumatol *17:*1419, 1990.
982. Lowe J, Kaplan L, Liebergall M, et al: Serratia osteomyelitis causing neurological deterioration after spine fracture. A report of two cases. J Bone Joint Surg [Br] *71:*256, 1989.
983. Mathien E, Koeger A-C, Rozenberg S, et al: Campylobacter spondylodiscitis and deficiency of cellular immunity. J Rheumatol *18:*1929, 1991.

984. Clément JL, Berard J, Cahuzac JP, et al: *Kingella Kingae* osteoarthritis and osteomyelitis in children. J Pediatr Orthop 8:59, 1988.

985. Lacour M, Duarte M, Beutler A, et al: Osteoarticular infections due to *Kingella Kingae* in children. Eur J Pediatr 150:612, 1991.

986. Lawrence JM III, Osborn TG, Paro R, et al: Septic arthritis caused by *Haemophilus influenzae* type B in a patient with HIV-1 infection. J Rheumatol 18:1772, 1991.

987. Hawkins RE, Malone JD, Ebbeling WL: Common variable hypogammaglobulinemia presenting as nontypable *Haemophilus influenzae* septic arthritis in an adult. J Rheumatol 18:775, 1991.

988. van Bommel EFH, Kramer P, van Beurden AFA: *Haemophilus influenzae* vertebral osteomyelitis in an adult. Acta Orthop Scand 62:493, 1991.

989. Houssiau FA, Huaux JP, De Deuxchaisnes CN: *Haemophilus aphrophilus:* A rare pathogen in vertebral osteomyelitis. Ann Rheum Dis 46:248, 1987.

990. Alarcón GS, Bocanegra TS, Gutuzzo E, et al: The arthritis of brucellosis: A perspective one hundred years after Bruce's discovery. J Rheumatol 14:1084, 1987.

991. Khateeb MI, Araj GF, Majeed SA, et al: Brucella arthritis: A study of 96 cases in Kuwait. Ann Rheum Dis 49:994, 1990.

992. Al-Eissa YA, Kambal AM, Alrabeeah AA, et al: Osteoarticular brucellosis in children. Ann Rheum Dis 49:896, 1990.

993. Al-Rawi TI, Thewaini AJ, Shawket AR, et al: Skeletal brucellosis in Iraqi patients. Ann Rheum Dis 48:77, 1989.

994. de Dios Colmenero J, Reguera JM, Fernández-Nebro A, et al: Osteoarticular complications of brucellosis. Ann Rheum Dis 50:23, 1991.

995. Denath FM: Computed tomography manifestations of brucellosis of the sternoclavicular joint. J Can Assoc Radiol 42:253, 1991.

996. Senbel E, Daumen-Legre V, Schiano A, et al: Ostéomyélite brucellienne de l'extrémité supérieure de l'humérus: Apport de l'imagerie par résonance magnétique. Rev Rhum Mal Osteoartic 59:353, 1992.

997. Abeles M, Mond CB: Sacroiliitis and brucellosis. J Rheumatol 16:136, 1989.

998. Cordero-Sánchez M, Alvarez-Ruiz S, López-Ochoa J, et al: Scintigraphic evaluation of lumbosacral pain in brucellosis. Arthritis Rheum 33:1052, 1990.

999. El-Desouki M: Skeletal brucellosis: Assessment with bone scintigraphy. Radiology 181:415, 1991.

1000. Cordero M, Sánchez I: Brucellar and tuberculous spondylitis. A comparative study of their clinical features. J Bone Joint Surg [Br] 73:100, 1991.

1001. Manaster BJ: Case report 469. Skel Radiol 17:144, 1988.

1002. Goodhart GL, Zakem JF, Collins WC, et al: Brucellosis of the spine. Report of a patient with bilateral paraspinal abscesses. Spine 12:414, 1987.

1003. MadKour MM, Sharif HS, Abed MY, et al: Osteoarticular brucellosis: Results of bone scintigraphy in 140 patients. AJR 150:1101, 1988.

1004. Mohan V, Gupta RP, Marklund T, et al: Spinal brucellosis. Int Orthop (SICOT) 14:63, 1990.

1005. Voss LM, Rhodes KH, Johnson KA: Musculoskeletal and soft tissue Aeromonas infection: An environmental disease. Mayo Clin Proc 67:422, 1992.

1006. Chevalier X, Martigny J, Avouac B, et al: Report of 4 cases of *Pasteurella multocida* septic arthritis. J Rheumatol 18:1890, 1991.

1007. Sjølin SU, Hansen AK: *Clostridium septicum* gas gangrene and an intestinal malignant lesion. A case report. J Bone Joint Surg [Am] 73:772, 1991.

1008. Lluberas-Acosta G, Elkus R, Schumacher HR Jr: Polyarticular *Clostridium perfringens* pyoarthritis. J Rheumatol 16:1509, 1989.

1009. Fauser DJ, Zuckerman JD: Clostridial septic arthritis: Case report and review of literature. Arthritis Rheum 31:296, 1988.

1010. Mermel LA, Osborn TG: Clostridium difficile associated reactive arthritis in an HLA-B27 positive female: Report and literature review. J Rheumatol 16:133, 1989.

1011. Incavo SJ, Muller DL, Krag MH, et al: Vertebral osteomyelitis caused by *Clostridium difficile*. A case report and review of the literature. Spine 13:111, 1988.

1012. Foulkes GD, Johnson CE, Katner HP: Fusobacterium osteomyelitis associated with intraosseous gas. Clin Orthop 251:246, 1990.

1013. González-Gay MA, Sánchez-Andrade A, Cereijo MJ, et al: Pyomyositis and septic arthritis from *Fusobacterium nucleatum* in a nonimmunocompromised adult. J Rheumatol 20:518, 1993.

1014. Gibb PA, Donell ST, Dowd GSE: Near-fatal necrobacillosis presenting as septic arthritis of the knee. A case report. J Bone Joint Surg [Am] 72:1250, 1990.

1015. Noordeen MHH, Godfrey LW: Case report of an unusual cause of low back pain. Intervertebral diskitis caused by *Eikenella corrodens*. Clin Orthop 280:175, 1992.

1016. Lifeso R: Atlanto-axial tuberculosis in adults. J Bone Joint Surg [Br] 69:183, 1987.

1017. Corea JR, Tamimi TM: Tuberculosis of the arch of the atlas. Case report. Spine 12:608, 1987.

1018. Levin MF, Vellet AD, Munk PL, et al: Tuberculosis of the odontoid bone: A rare but treatable cause of quadriplegia. J Can Assoc Radiol 43:199, 1992.

1019. Pun WK, Chow SP, Luk KDK, et al: Tuberculosis of the lumbosacral junction. Long-term follow-up of 26 cases. J Bone Joint Surg [Br] 72:675, 1990.

1020. Pouchot J, Vinceneux P, Barge J, et al: Tuberculosis of the sacroiliac joint: Clinical features, outcome, and evaluation of closed needle biopsy in 11 consecutive cases. Am J Med 84:622, 1988.

1021. Travlos J, Du Toit G: Spinal tuberculosis: Beware the posterior elements. J Bone Joint Surg [Br] 72:722, 1990.

1022. Monaghan D, Gupta A, Barrington NA: Case report: Tuberculosis of the spine—an unusual presentation. Clin Radiol 43:360, 1991.

1023. Rathakrishnan V, Mohd TH: Osteoarticular tuberculosis. A radiological study in a Malaysian hospital. Skel Radiol 18:267, 1989.

1024. Hsu LCS, Cheng CL, Leong JCY: Pott's paraplegia of late onset. The cause of compression and results after anterior decompression. J Bone Joint Surg [Br] 70:534, 1988.

1025. Whitaker SC, Preston BJ, McKim-Thomas H: Spontaneous disappearance of tuberculous psoas abscess calcification. Br J Radiol 63:303, 1990.

1026. Coppola J, Müller NL, Connell DG: Computed tomography of musculoskeletal tuberculosis. J Can Assoc Radiol 38:199, 1987.

1027. Sankaran-Kutty M: Atypical tuberculous spondylitis. Int Orthop (SICOT) 16:69, 1992.

1028. Sankaran-Kutty M, Chowdhary UM, Corea JR, et al: The role of computerised tomography in the management of spinal tuberculosis. Int Orthop (SICOT) 15:319, 1991.

1029. Hoffman EB, Crosier JH, Cremin B: Imaging in children with spinal tuberculosis. A comparison of radiography, computed tomography and magnetic resonance imaging. J Bone Joint Surg [Br] 75:233, 1993.

1030. Quinn SF, Murray W, Prochaska J, et al: MRI appearance of disseminated osseous tuberculosis. Magn Reson Imaging 5:493, 1987.

1031. Smith AS, Weinstein MA, Mizushima A, et al: MR imaging characteristics of tuberculous spondylitis vs vertebral osteomyelitis. AJR 153:399, 1989.

1032. Sharif HS, Aideyan OA, Clark DC, et al: Brucellar and tuberculous spondylitis: Comparative imaging features. Radiology 171:419, 1989.

1033. Rajasekaran S, Shanmugasundaram TK: Prediction of the angle of gibbus deformity in tuberculosis of the spine. J Bone Joint Surg [Am] 69:503, 1987.

1034. Louw JA, Dommisse GF: Spinal tuberculosis with spontaneous ventral extrusion of two vertebral bodies. A case report. Spine 12:942, 1987.

1035. Lin TH: Intramedullary tuberculoma of the spinal cord. J Neurosurg 17:497, 1960.

1036. Rhoton EL, Ballinger WE Jr, Quisling R, et al: Intramedullary spinal tuberculoma. Neurosurgery 22:733, 1988.

1037. Abdelwahab IF, Present DA, Gould E, et al: Case report 473. Skel Radiol 17:199, 1988.

1038. Seddon DJ, Thanabalasingham T, Weinberg J: Spontaneous fracture of the ulna complicating tuberculous osteomyelitis. Postgrad Med J 65:939, 1989.

1039. Abdelwahab IF, Kenan S, Hermann G, et al: Atypical skeletal tuberculosis mimicking neoplasm. Br J Radiol 64:551, 1991.

1040. Mazas-Artasona L, Led A, Espinosa H, et al: Case report 737. Skel Radiol 21:323, 1992.

1041. Abdelwahab IF, Present DA, Zwass A, et al: Tumorlike tuberculous granulomas of bone. AJR 149:1207, 1987.

1042. MacGee W, Lagier R: A case of intracortical tuberculosis of the femur. Eur J Radiol 8:96, 1988.

1043. Mohan V, Danielsson L, Hosni G, et al: A case of tuberculosis of the scapula. Acta Orthop Scand 62:79, 1991.

1044. Nielsen FF, Helmig O, de Carvalho A: Case report 533. Skel Radiol 18:153, 1989.

1045. Rajah R: Case report 513. Skel Radiol 17:601, 1989.

1046. Bonnet C, DeBandt M, Palazzo E, et al: Tuberculosis involving the patella. AJR 159:677, 1992.

1047. Hernandez-Gimenez M, Beltran JVT, Segui MIF, et al: Tuberculosis of the patella. Pediatr Radiol 17:328, 1987.

1048. Miller MA, Lebel F, Fortin PR: Tuberculosis of the skull. AJR 155:1141, 1990.

1049. Shannon FB, Moore M, Houkom JA, et al: Multifocal cystic tuberculosis of bone. Report of a case. J Bone Joint Surg [Am] 72:1089, 1990.

1050. Abdelwahab IF, Lewis MM, Klein MJ, et al: Case report 528. Skel Radiol 18:133, 1989.

1051. Antti-Poika I, Vankka E, Santavirta S, et al: Two cases of shoulder joint tuberculosis. Acta Orthop Scand 62:81, 1991.

1052. Valdazo J-P, Perez-Ruiz F, Albarracin A, et al: Tuberculous arthritis. Report of a case with multiple joint involvement and periarticular tuberculous abscesses. J Rheumatol 17:399, 1990.

1053. Linares LF, Valcarcel A, Del Castillo JM, et al: Tuberculous arthritis with multiple joint involvement. J Rheumatol 18:635, 1991.

1054. Southwood TR, Hancock EJ, Petty RE, et al: Tuberculous rheumatism (Poncet's disease) in a child. Arthritis Rheum 31:1311, 1988.

1055. Khoury MI: Does reactive arthritis to tuberculosis (Poncet's disease) exist? J Rheumatol 16:1162, 1989.

1056. Ames PRJ, Capasso G, Testa V, et al: Chronic tuberculous rheumatism (Poncet's disease) in a gymnast. Br J Rheumatol 29:72, 1990.

1057. Gálvez J, Sola J, Ortuño G, et al: Microscopic rice bodies in rheumatoid fluid sediments. J Rheumatol 19:1851, 1992.

1058. Araki Y, Tsukaguchi I, Shinok: Tuberculous arthritis of the knee: MRI findings. AJR 160:664, 1993.

1059. Schultz E, Richterman I, Dorfman HD: Case report 739. Skel Radiol 21:330, 1992.

1060. Cramer K, Seiler JG III, Milek MA: Tuberculous tenosynovitis of the wrist. Two case reports. Clin Orthop 262:137, 1991.

1061. Lakhanpal S, Linscheid RL, Ferguson RH, et al: Tuberculous fasciitis with tenosynovitis. J Rheumatol 14:621, 1987.

1062. Franceschi JP, Chapuis J, Curvale G, et al: Trochantérites bacillaires. A propos de 30 cas. Rev Rhum Mal Osteoartic 58:433, 1991.

1063. Shickendantz MS, Watson JT: Mycobacterial prepatellar bursitis. Clin Orthop 258:209, 1990.

1064. Lupatkin H, Bräu N, Flomenberg P, et al: Tuberculous abscesses in patients with AIDS. Clin Infect Dis *14:*1040, 1992.

1065. Hugosson C, Harfi H: Disseminated BCG–osteomyelitis in congenital immunodeficiency. Pediatr Radiol *21:*384, 1991.

1066. Marik I, Kubat R, Filipsky J, et al: Osteitis caused by BCG vaccination. J Pediatr Orthop *8:*333, 1988.

1067. Arias FG, Rodriguez M, Hernandez JG, et al: Osteomyelitis deriving from BCG-vaccination. Pediatr Radiol *17:*166, 1987.

1068. Goupille P, Soutif D, Valat J-P: Arthritis after Calmette-Guerin bacillus immunotherapy for bladder cancer. J Rheumatol *19:*1825, 1992.

1069. Tanaka M, Matsui H, Tsuji H: Atypical mycobacterium osteomyelitis of the fibula. Int Orthop (SICOT) *17:*48, 1993.

1070. Perandones CE, Roncoroni AJ, Freya NS, et al: *Mycobacterium gastri* arthritis: Septic arthritis due to *Mycobacterium gastri* in a patient with a renal transplant. J Rheumatol *18:*777, 1991.

1071. Hasegawa T, Watanabe R, Hayashi K, et al: Postoperative osteomyelitis due to *Mycobacterium fortuitum.* A case report. Arch Orthop Trauma Surg *111:*178, 1992.

1072. Eggelmeijer F, Kroon FP, Zeeman RJ, et al: Tenosynovitis due to *Mycobacterium avium-intracellulare:* Case report and a review of the literature. Clin Exp Rheumatol *10:*169, 1992.

1073. Aguillar JL, Sanchez EE, Carrillo C, et al: Septic arthritis due to *Mycobacterium phlei* presenting as infantile Reiter's syndrome. J Rheumatol *16:*1377, 1989.

1074. Kwong JS, Munk PL, Connell DG, et al: Case report 687. Skel Radiol *20:*458, 1991.

1075. Blumenthal DR, Zucker JR, Hawkins CC: *Mycobacterium avium* complex–induced septic arthritis and osteomyelitis in a patient with the acquired immunodeficiency syndrome. Arthritis Rheum *33:*757, 1990.

1076. Nuñez JM, Monteagudo I, López-Longo FJ, et al: Disseminated *Mycobacterium avium-intracellulare* infection in a patient with polymyositis. Arthritis Rheum *32:*934, 1989.

1077. Rougraff BT, Reeck CC Jr, Slama TG: *Mycobacterium terrae* osteomyelitis and septic arthritis in a normal host. A case report. Clin Orthop *238:*308, 1989.

1078. Pedersen AK, Hald J, Saxegaard F: *Mycobacterium avium* infection of the knee in a child. Acta Orthop Scand *59:*585, 1988.

1079. Lacy JN, Viegas SF, Calhoun J, et al: *Mycobacterium marinum* flexor tenosynovitis. Clin Orthop *238:*288, 1989.

1080. Sanger JR, Stampfl DA, Franson TR: Recurrent granulomatous synovitis due to *Mycobacterium kansasii* in a renal transplant patient. J Hand Surg [Am] *12:*436, 1987.

1081. Kremer LB, Rhame FS, House JH: *Mycobacterium terrae* tenosynovitis. Arthritis Rheum *31:*932, 1988.

1082. Hurst LC, Amadio PC, Badalamente MH, et al: *Mycobacterium marinum* infections of the hand. J Hand Surg [Am] *12:*428, 1987.

1083. Aubrey M, Fam AG: A case of clinically unsuspected *Mycobacterium marinum* infection. Arthritis Rheum *30:*1317, 1987.

1084. Chow SP, Lau JHK, Collins RJ, et al: *Mycobacterium marinum* infection of the hand and wrist. J Bone Joint Surg [Am] *69:*1161, 1987.

1085. Minkin BI, Mills CL, Bullock DW, et al: *Mycobacterium kansasii* osteomyelitis of the scaphoid. J Hand Surg [Am] *12:*1092, 1987.

1086. Whitaker MD, Jelinek JS, Kransdorf MJ, et al: Case report 653. Skel Radiol *20:*291, 1991.

1087. Andersen JG, Manchester K: The rhinomaxillary syndrome in leprosy: A clinical, radiological and paleopathological study. Int J Osteoarch *2:*121, 1992.

1088. Datz FL: Erythema nodosum leprosum reaction of leprosy causing the double stripe sign on bone scan. Case report. Clin Nucl Med *12:*212, 1987.

1089. Atkin SL, Welbury RR, Stanfield E, et al: Clinical and laboratory studies of inflammatory polyarthritis in patients with leprosy in Papua New Guinea. Ann Rheum Dis *46:*688, 1987.

1090. de Almeida Pernambuco JC, Cossermelli-Messina W: Rheumatic manifestations of leprosy: Clinical aspects. J Rheumatol *20:*897, 1993.

1091. MacMoran JW, Brand PW: Bone loss in limbs with decreased or absent sensation: Ten year follow-up of the hands in leprosy. Skel Radiol *16:*452, 1987.

1092. Nagano J, Tada K, Masatomi T, et al: Arthropathy of the wrist in leprosy—what changes are caused by long-standing peripheral nerve palsy? Arch Orthop Trauma Surg *108:*210, 1989.

1093. Horibe S, Tada K, Nagano J: Neuroarthropathy of the foot in leprosy. J Bone Joint Surg [Br] *70:*481, 1988.

1094. Gadea A, Figueredo M, Bowen JR: Persistent bony lesions in congenital syphilis. A report of three cases. Int Orthop (SICOT) *17:*43, 1993.

1095. Rasool MN, Govender S: The skeletal manifestations of congenital syphilis. A review of 197 cases. J Bone Joint Surg [Br] *71:*750, 1989.

1096. Marlier S, Guiguen Y, Elizagaray A, et al: Ostéopériostite crânienne syphilitique. A propos d'une observation. Sem Hôp Paris *64:*1635, 1988.

1097. Middleton S, Rowntree C, Rudge S: Bone pain as the presenting manifestation of secondary syphilis. Ann Rheum Dis *49:*641, 1990.

1098. Reginato AJ, Ferreiro-Seoane JL, Falasca G: Unilateral sacroilutis in secondary syphilis. J Rheumatol *15:*717, 1988.

1099. Greenberg SB, Bernal DV: Are long bone radiographs necessary in neonates suspected of having congenital syphilis? Radiology *182:*637, 1992.

1100. Dunn RA, Zenker PN: Why radiographs are useful in evaluation of neonates suspected of having congenital syphilis. Radiology *182:*639, 1992.

1101. Engelkens HJH, Ginai AZ, Judanarso J, et al: Case report 724. Skel Radiol *21:*194, 1992.

1102. Anderson D, Marrie TJ: Septic arthritis due to *Streptobacillus moniliformis.* Arthritis Rheum *30:*229, 1987.

1103. Rumley RL, Patrone NA, White L: Rat-bite fever as a cause of septic arthritis: A diagnostic dilemma. Ann Rheum Dis *46:*793, 1987.

1104. Agger W, Case KL, Bryant GL, et al: Lyme disease: Clinical features, classification, and epidemiology in the upper Midwest. Medicine *70:*83, 1991.

1105. Sigal LH: Summary of the fourth international symposium on Lyme borreliosis. Arthritis Rheum *34:*367, 1991.

1106. Sigal LH: Lyme disease, 1988: Immunologic manifestations and possible immunopathogenic mechanisms. Semin Arthritis Rheum *18:*151, 1989.

1107. Stechenberg BW: Lyme disease: The latest great imitator. Pediatr Infect Dis J *7:*402, 1988.

1108. Steere AC, Duray PH, Butcher EC: Spirochetal antigens and lymphoid cell surface markers in Lyme synovitis. Comparison with rheumatoid synovium and tonsillar lymphoid tissue. Arthritis Rheum *31:*487, 1988.

1109. Miller A, Stanton RP, Eppes SC: Acute arthritis of the hip in a child infected with the Lyme spirochete. Clin Orthop *286:*212, 1993.

1110. Cristofaro RL, Appel MH, Gelb RI, et al: Musculoskeletal manifestations of Lyme disease in children. J Pediatr Orthop *7:*527, 1987.

1111. Kay J, Eichenfield AH, Athreya BH, et al: Synovial fluid eosinophilia in Lyme disease. Arthritis Rheum *31:*1384, 1988.

1112. Herzer P: Lyme arthritis in Europe: Comparisons with reports from North America. Ann Rheum Dis *47:*789, 1988.

1113. Rahn DW: Lyme disease: Clinical manifestations, diagnosis, and treatment. Semin Arthritis Rheum *20:*201, 1991.

1114. Weyand CM, Goronzy JJ: Immune responses to *Borrelia burgdorferi* in patients with reactive arthritis. Arthritis Rheum *32:*1057, 1989.

1115. Arnett FC: The Lyme spirochete: Another cause of Reiter's syndrome. Arthritis Rheum *32:*1182, 1989.

1116. Steere AC, Shoen RT, Taylor E: The clinical evolution of Lyme arthritis. Ann Intern Med *107:*725, 1987.

1117. Lawson JP, Rahn DW: Lyme disease and radiographic findings in Lyme arthritis. AJR *158:*1065, 1992.

1118. Watanakunakorn C, Toliver J Jr: Lyme arthritis with subarticular cyst formation in metacarpal and metatarsal bones. South Med J *85:*187, 1992.

1119. Osborn RE, Mojtahedi S: CT myelography of cauda equina actinomycosis. J Comput Assist Tomogr *11:*361, 1987.

1120. Laurin JM, Resnik CS, Wheeler D, et al: Vertebral osteomyelitis caused by *Nocardia asteroides:* Report and review of the literature. J Rheumatol *18:*455, 1991.

1121. Guiral J, Refolio C, Carrero P, et al: Sacral osteomyelitis due to *Nocardia asteroides.* A case report. Acta Orthop Scand *62:*389, 1991.

1122. Chowdhary G, Wormser GP, Mascarenhas BR: Nocardia bursitis. J Rheumatol *15:*139, 1988.

1123. Govender S, Ganpath V, Charles RW, et al: Localized osseous cryptococcal infection. Report of 2 cases. Acta Orthop Scand *59:*720, 1988.

1124. Ueda Y, Roessnner A, Edel G, et al: Case report 699. Skel Radiol *21:*117, 1992.

1125. Curé JK, Mirich DR: MR imaging in cryptococcal spondylitis. AJNR *12:*1111, 1991.

1126. Abdul-Karim FW, Pathria MN, Heller JG, et al: Case report 664. Skel Radiol *20:*227, 1991.

1127. Cuéllar ML, Silveira LH, Espinoza LR: Fungal arthritis. Ann Rheum Dis *51:*690, 1992.

1128. Farr RW, Wright RA: Cryptococcal olecranon bursitis in cirrhosis. J Rheumatol *19:*172, 1992.

1129. MacDonald PB, Black GB, MacKenzie R: Orthopaedic manifestations of blastomycosis. J Bone Joint Surg [Am] *72:*860, 1990.

1130. Robert ME, Kauffman CA: Blastomycosis presenting as polyarticular septic arthritis. J Rheumatol *15:*1438, 1988.

1131. Bernreuter WK: Coccidioidomycosis of bone: A sequela of desert rheumatism. Arthritis Rheum *32:*1608, 1989.

1132. Bried JM, Speer DP, Shehab ZM: *Coccidioides immitus* osteomyelitis in a 12-month-old child. J Pediatr Orthop *7:*328, 1987.

1133. Moreno AJ, Weisman IM, Rodriguez AA, et al: Nuclear imaging in coccidioidal osteomyelitis. Clin Nucl Med *12:*604, 1987.

1134. Darouiche RO, Cadle RM, Zenon GJ, et al: Articular histoplasmosis. J Rheumatol *19:*1991, 1992.

1135. Chowdhary G, Weinstein A, Klein R, et al: Sporotrichal arthritis. Ann Rheum Dis *50:*112, 1991.

1136. Janes PC, Mann RJ: Extracutaneous sporotrichosis. J Hand Surg [Am] *12:*441, 1987.

1137. Schwartz DA: Sporothrix tenosynovitis—differential diagnosis of granulomatous inflammatory disease of the joints. J Rheumatol *16:*550, 1989.

1138. Mogavero GT, Fishman EK, Magid D: Osseous sporotrichosis: CT appearance. Case report. Clin Imaging *15:*56, 1991.

1139. Rowe IF, Wright ED, Higgens CS, et al: Intervertebral infection due to *Candida albicans* in an intravenous heroin user. Ann Rheum Dis *47:*522, 1988.

1140. Boix V, Tovar J, Martin-Hidalgo A: Candida spondylodiscitis. Chronic illness due to heroin analgesia in an HIV positive person. J Rheumatol *17:*563, 1990.

1141. Miro JM, Brancos MA, Abello R, et al: Costochondral involvement in systemic candidiasis in heroin addicts: Clinical, scintigraphic, and histologic features in 26 patients. Arthritis Rheum *31:*793, 1988.

1142. Gathe JC Jr, Harris RL, Garland B, et al: Candida osteomyelitis. Report of five cases and review of the literature. Am J Med 82:927, 1987.
1143. Koch AE: *Candida albicans* infection of a prosthetic knee replacement: A report and review of the literature. J Rheumatol 15:362, 1988.
1144. Almekinders LC, Greene WB: Vertebral Candida infections. A case report and review of the literature. Clin Orthop 267:174, 1991.
1145. Cuende E, Barbadillo C, E-Mazzucchelli R, et al: Candida arthritis in adult patients who are not intravenous drug addicts: Report of three cases and review of the literature. Semin Arthritis Rheum 22:224, 1993.
1146. De Clerck L, Dequeker J, Westhovens R, et al: *Candida parapsilosis* in a patient receiving chronic hemodialysis. J Rheumatol 15:372, 1988.
1147. Dupont B, Drouhet E: Cutaneous, ocular, and osteoarticular candidiasis in heroin addicts: New clinical and therapeutic aspects in 38 patients. J Infect Dis 152:577, 1985.
1148. Chaudhuri R, McKeown B, Harrington D, et al: Mucormycosis osteomyelitis causing avascular necrosis of the cuboid bone: MR imaging findings. AJR 159:1035, 1992.
1149. Kawashima A, Kuhlman JE, Fishman EK, et al: Pulmonary Aspergillus chest wall involvement in chronic granulomatous disease: CT and MRI findings. Skel Radiol 20:487, 1991.
1150. Sponseller PD, Malech HL, McCarthy EF Jr, et al: Skeletal involvement in children who have chronic granulomatous disease. J Bone Joint Surg [Am] 73:37, 1991.
1151. Holmes PF, Osterman DW, Tullos HS: Aspergillus discitis. Report of two cases and review of the literature. Clin Orthop 226:240, 1988.
1152. Richard R, Lucet L, Mejjad O, et al: Spondylodiscite aspergillaire. A propos de trois observations. Rev Rhum Mal Osteoartic [Eng] 60:46, 1993.
1153. Cortet B, Deprez X, Triki R, et al: Aspergillus discitis. A report of five cases. Rev Rhum Mal Osteoartic [Eng] 60:38, 1993.
1154. Fisher MS: Case report 750. Skel Radiol 21:410, 1992.
1155. Sheftel TG, Mader JT, Cierny G: *Pseudoallescheria boydii* soft tissue abscess. Clin Orthop 215:212, 1987.
1156. Hung LHY, Norwood LA: Osteomyelitis due to *Pseudallescheria boydii.* South Med J 86:231, 1993.
1157. Suttner J-F, Wirth CJ, Wülker N, et al: Madura foot. A report of two cases. Int Orthop (SICOT) 14:217, 1990.
1158. Gold RH, Mirra JM: Case report 442. Skel Radiol 16:577, 1987.
1159. Sharif HS, Clark DC, Aabed MY, et al: Mycetoma: Comparison of MR imaging with CT. Radiology 178:865, 1991.
1160. Owen PG, Willis BK, Benzel EC: *Torulopsis glabrata* vertebral osteomyelitis. J Spinal Dis 5:370, 1992.
1161. Liudahl KJ, Limbira TJ: *Torulopsis glabrata* vertebral osteomyelitis. Case report and review of the literature. Spine 12:593, 1987.
1162. Bruns J, Hemker T, Dahmen G: Fungal spondylitis. A case of *Torulopsis glabrata* and *Candida tropicalis* infection. Acta Orthop Scand 57:563, 1986.
1163. Bogaert J, Lateur L, Baert AL: Case report 762. Skel Radiol 21:550, 1992.
1164. Imahori SC, Papademetriou T, Ogliela DM: *Torulopsis glabrata* osteomyelitis. A case report. Clin Orthop 219:214, 1987.
1165. Fuchan Y, Woo KC: *Penicillium marneffei* osteomyelitis. J Bone Joint Surg [Br] 72:500, 1990.
1166. Berger RG: Chronic fungal olecranon bursitis caused by Penicillium. Arthritis Rheum 32:239, 1989.
1167. Smith CA, Petty RE, Tingle AJ: Rubella virus and arthritis. Rheum Dis Clin North Am 13:265, 1987.
1168. Tingle AJ: One infectious agent—many syndromes. J Rheumatol 14:653, 1987.
1169. Fern ED, Hardern R, Bell MJ: Osteomyelitis after chicken pox in children. J Orthop Rheumatol 3:217, 1990.
1170. Edwards BL, Bonagura VR, Valacer DJ, et al: Mucha-Habermann's disease and arthritis: Possible association with reactivated Epstein-Barr virus infection. J Rheumatol 16:387, 1989.
1171. Steinbach LS, Tehranzadeh J, Fleckenstein JL, et al: Human immunodeficiency virus infection: Musculoskeletal manifestations. Radiology 186:833, 1993.
1172. Winchester R: AIDS and the rheumatic diseases. Bull Rheum Dis 39:1, 1990.
1173. Rosenberg ZS, Norman A, Solomon G: Arthritis associated with HIV infection: Radiographic manifestations. Radiology 173:171, 1989.
1174. Solinger AM, Hess EV: Rheumatic diseases and AIDS—is the association real? J Rheumatol 20:678, 1993.
1175. Monteajudo I, Rivera J, Lopez-Longo J, et al: AIDS and rheumatic manifestations in patients addicted to drugs: An analysis of 106 cases. J Rheumatol 18:1038, 1991.
1176. Berman A, Espinoza LR, Diaz JD, et al: Rheumatic manifestations of human immunodeficiency virus infection. Am J Med 85:59, 1988.
1177. Espinoza LR, Aguilar JL, Berman A, et al: Rheumatic manifestations associated with human immunodeficiency virus infection. Arthritis Rheum 32:1615, 1989.
1178. Reveille JD, Conant MA, Duvic M: Human immunodeficiency virus–associated psoriasis, psoriatic arthritis, and Reiter's syndrome: A disease continuum? Arthritis Rheum 33:1574, 1990.
1179. Espinoza LR, Berman A, Vasey FB, et al: Psoriatic arthritis and acquired immunodeficiency syndrome. Arthritis Rheum 31:1034, 1988.
1180. Solomon G, Brancato L, Winchester R: An approach to the human immunodeficiency virus–positive patient with a spondyloarthropathic disease. Rheum Dis Clin North Am 17:43, 1991.
1181. Arnett FC, Reveille JD, Duvic M: Psoriasis and psoriatic arthritis associated with human immunodeficiency virus infection. Rheum Dis Clin North Am 17:59, 1991.
1182. Keat A, Rowe I: Reiter's syndrome and associated arthritides. Rheum Dis Clin North Am 17:25, 1991.
1183. Enelow RS, Hussein M, Grant K, et al: Vasculitis with eosinophilia and digital gangrene in a patient with acquired immunodeficiency syndrome. J Rheumatol 19:1813, 1992.
1184. Stein M, Davis P: HIV and arthritis—casual or causal acquaintances? J Rheumatol 16:1287, 1989.
1185. Bentin J, Feremans W, Pasteels J-L, et al: Chronic acquired immunodeficiency syndrome–associated arthritis: A synovial ultrastructural study. Arthritis Rheum 33:268, 1990.
1186. Calabrese LH, Kelley DM, Myers A, et al: Rheumatic symptoms and human immunodeficiency virus infection. Arthritis Rheum 34:257, 1991.
1187. Kaye BR: Rheumatologic manifestations of infection with human immunodeficiency virus (HIV). Ann Intern Med 111:158, 1989.
1188. Calabrese LH, Estes M, Yen-Lieberman B, et al: Systemic vasculitis in association with human immunodeficiency virus infection. Arthritis Rheum 32:569, 1989.
1189. Nordstrom DM, Petropolis AA, Giorno R, et al: Inflammatory myopathy and acquired immunodeficiency syndrome. Arthritis Rheum 32:475, 1989.
1190. Brancato LJ, Itescu S, Solomon G, et al: An overview of Reiter's syndrome and related rheumatic disorders as they occur in patients with HIV infection. J Musculoskel Med, Aug 1989, p 15.
1191. Goh BT, Jawad ASM, Chapman D, et al: Osteomyelitis presenting as a swollen elbow in a patient with the acquired immune deficiency syndrome. Ann Rheum Dis 47:695, 1988.
1192. Glickel SZ: Hand infections in patients with acquired immunodeficiency syndrome. J Hand Surg [Am] 13:770, 1988.
1193. Buck BE, Resnick L, Shah SM, et al: Human immunodeficiency virus cultured from bone. Implications for transplantation. Clin Orthop 251:249, 1990.
1194. Hughes RA, Rowe IF, Shanson D, et al: Septic bone, joint and muscle lesions associated with human immunodeficiency virus infection. Br J Rheumatol 31:381, 1992.
1195. Hoekman P, Van de Perre P, Nelisson J, et al: Increased frequency of infection after open reduction of fractures in patients who are seropositive for human immunodeficiency virus. J Bone Joint Surg [Am] 73:675, 1991.
1196. Zimmermann E III, Erickson AD, Mikolich DJ: Septic acromioclavicular arthritis and osteomyelitis in a patient with acquired immunodeficiency syndrome. Arthritis Rheum 32:1175, 1989.
1197. Edelstein H, McCabe R: *Candida albicans* septic arthritis and osteomyelitis of the sternoclavicular joint in a patient with human immunodeficiency virus infection. J Rheumatol 18:110, 1991.
1198. Rivera J, Monteagudo I, Lopez-Longo J, et al: Septic arthritis in patients with acquired immunodeficiency syndrome with human immunodeficiency virus infection. J Rheumatol 19:1960, 1992.
1199. Brantus JF, Meunier PJ: Manifestations rheumatologiques associées à l'infection par le virus de l'immunodéficience humaine (VIH). Rev Rhum Mal Ostéoartic 59:428, 1992.
1200. Vinetz JM, Rickman LS: Chronic arthritis due to *Mycobacterium avium* complex infection in a patient with the acquired immunodeficiency syndrome. Arthritis Rheum 34:1339, 1991.
1201. Goldenberg DL: Septic arthritis and other infections of rheumatologic significance. Rheum Dis Clin North Am 17:149, 1991.
1202. Blumberg HM, Stephens DS: Pyomyositis and human immunodeficiency virus infection. South Med J 83:1092, 1990.
1203. Fleckenstein JL, Burns DK, Murphy FK, et al: Differential diagnosis of bacterial myositis in AIDS: Evaluation with MR imaging. Radiology 179:653, 1991.
1204. Gardiner JS, Zauk AM, Minnefor AB, et al: Pyomyositis in an HIV-positive premature infant: Case report and review of the literature. J Pediatr Orthop 10:791, 1990.
1205. Wolf RF, Sprenger HG, Mooyaart EL, et al: Nontropical pyomyositis as a cause of subacute, multifocal myalgia in the acquired immunodeficiency syndrome. Arthritis Rheum 33:1728, 1990.
1206. Schwartzman WA, Lambertus MW, Kennedy CA, et al: Staphylococcal pyomyositis in patients infected by the human immunodeficiency virus. Am J Med 90:595, 1991.
1207. Magid D, Fishman EK: Musculoskeletal infections in patients with AIDS: CT findings. AJR 158:603, 1992.
1208. Rodgers WB, Yodlowski ML, Mintzer CM: Pyomyositis in patients who have the immunodeficiency virus. Case report and review of the literature. J Bone Joint Surg [Am] 75:588, 1993.
1209. Vanarthos WJ, Ganz WI, Vanarthos JC, et al: Diagnostic uses of nuclear medicine in AIDS. RadioGraphics 12:731, 1992.
1210. Tappero JW, Mohle-Boetani J, Koehler JE, et al: The epidemiology of bacillary angiomatosis and bacillary peliosis. JAMA 269:770, 1993.
1211. Berger TG, Tappero JW, Kaymen A, et al: Bacillary (epithelioid) angiomatosis and concurrent Kaposi's sarcoma in acquired immune deficiency syndrome. Arch Dermatol 125:1543, 1989.
1212. Perkocha LA, Geaghan SM, Yen TS, et al: Clinical and pathological features of bacillary peliosis hepatis in association with human immunodeficiency virus infection. N Engl J Med 323:1581, 1990.
1213. English CK, Wear DJ, Margileth AM, et al: Cat-scratch disease: Isolation and culture of the bacterial agent. JAMA 259:1347, 1988.
1214. Koehler JE, Quinn FD, Berger TG, et al: Isolation of Rochalimaea species

from cutaneous and osseous lesions of bacillary angiomatosis. N Engl J Med 327:1625, 1992.

1215. Stoler MH, Bonfiglio TA, Steigbigel RT, et al: An atypical subcutaneous infection associated with the acquired immune deficiency syndrome. Am J Clin Pathol 80:714, 1983.

1216. Cockerell CJ, Whitlow MA, Webster GF, et al: Epithelioid angiomatosis: A distinct vascular disorder in patients with the acquired immunodeficiency syndrome or AIDS-related complex. Lancet 2:654, 1987.

1217. Leboit PE, Berger T, Egbert BM, et al: Bacillary angiomatosis: The histopathology and differential diagnosis of a pseudoneoplastic infection in patients with HIV infection. Am J Surg 13:909, 1989.

1218. Baron AL, Steinbach LS, LeBoit PE, et al: Osteolytic lesions and bacillary angiomatosis in HIV infection: Radiographic differentiation from AIDS-related kaposi sarcoma. Radiology 177:77, 1990.

1219. Herts BR, Rafii M, Spiegel G: Soft-tissue and osseous lesions caused by bacillary angiomatosis: Unusual manifestations of cat-scratch fever in patients with AIDS. AJR 157:1249, 1991.

1220. Conrad SE, Jacobs D, Gee J, et al: Pseudoneoplastic infection of bone in acquired immunodeficiency syndrome. A case report involving the cat-scratch disease bacillus. J Bone Joint Surg [Am] 73:774, 1991.

1221. Chevalier X, Larget-Piet B, Hernigou P, et al: Avascular necrosis of the femoral head in HIV-infected patients. J Bone Joint Surg [Br] 75:158, 1993.

1222. Gerster JC, Camus JP, Chave JP, et al: Multiple site avascular necrosis in HIV infected patients. J Rheumatol 18:300, 1991.

1223. Belman AL, Lantos G, Horoupian D, et al: AIDS: Calcification of the basal ganglia in infants and children. Neurology 36:1192, 1986.

1224. Smith CA, Woolf AD, Lenci M: Parvoviruses: Infections and arthropathies. Rheum Dis Clin North Am 13:249, 1987.

1225. Nogués X, Coll J, Grau J, et al: Mediterranean spotted fever (a rickettsial pox) and arthritis. J Rheumatol 16:256, 1989.

1226. Burdge DR, Reid GD, Reeve CE, et al: Septic arthritis due to dual infection with Mycoplasma hominis and Ureaplasma urealyticum. J Rheumatol 15:366, 1988.

1227. Muller R, Hajdu SI, Brennan MF: Lymphangiosarcoma associated with chronic filarial lymphedema. Cancer 59:179, 1987.

1228. Beaver PC, Orihel TC: Human infection with filariae of animals in the United States. Am J Trop Med Hyg 14:1010, 1965.

1229. Corman LC: Acute arthritis occurring in association with subcutaneous Dirofilaria tenuis infection. Arthritis Rheum 30:1431, 1987.

1230. Durán-Ortiz JS, Garcia-De La Torre I, Orozco-Barocio G, et al: Trichinosis with severe myopathic involvement mimicking polymyositis. Report of a family outbreak. J Rheumatol 19:310, 1992.

1231. Palasis S, Drevelengas A: Extramedullary spinal cysticercosis. Eur J Radiol 12:216, 1991.

1232. Charles RW, Govender S, Naidoo KS: Echinococcal infection of the spine with neural involvement. Spine 13:47, 1988.

1233. Karray S, Zlitni M, Fowles JV, et al: Vertebral hydatidosis and paraplegia. J Bone Joint Surg [Br] 72:84, 1990.

1234. Rao S, Parikh S, Kerr R: Echinococcal infestation of the spine in North America. Clin Orthop 271:164, 1991.

1235. Agarwal S, Shah A, Kadhi SKM, et al: Hydatid bone disease of the pelvis. A report of two cases and review of the literature. Clin Orthop 280:251, 1992.

1236. von Sinner WN: Case report 616. Skel Radiol 19:312, 1990.

1237. De Cristofaro R, Ruggieri P, Biagini R, et al: Case report 629. Skel Radiol 19:461, 1990.

1238. Duncan GJ, Tooke SMT: Echinococcus infestation of the biceps brachii. A case report. Clin Orthop 261:247, 1990.

1239. Torricelli P, Martinelli C, Biagini R, et al: Radiographic and computed tomographic findings in hydatid disease of bone. Skel Radiol 19:435, 1990.

1240. Marani SAD, Canossi GC, Nicoli FA, et al: Hydatid disease: MR imaging study. Radiology 175:701, 1990.

1241. Kamel M, Safwat E, Eltayeb S: Bilharzial arthropathy. Immunologic findings. Scand J Rheumatol 18:315, 1989.

1242. Selwa LM, Brunberg JA, Mandell SH, et al: Spinal cord schistosomiasis: A pediatric case mimicking intrinsic cord neoplasm. Neurology 41:755, 1991.

1243. Silbergleit R, Silbergleit R: Schistosomal granuloma of the spinal cord: Evaluation with MR imaging and intraoperative sonography. AJR 158:1351, 1992.

1244. Genakos JJ, Cocores JA, Terris A: Ainhum (dactylolysis spontanea). Report of a bilateral case and literature review. J Am Podiatr Med Assoc 76:676, 1986.

1245. Jurik AG, Justesen T, Graudal H: Radiographic findings in patients with clinical Tietze syndrome. Skel Radiol 16:517, 1987.

1246. Honda N, Machida K, Mamiya T, et al: Scintigraphic and CT findings of Tietze's syndrome: Report of a case and review of the literature. Clin Nucl Med 14:606, 1989.

1247. Jurik AG, Graudal H: Sternocostal joint swelling—clinical Tietze's syndrome. Report of sixteen cases and review of the literature. Scand J Rheumatol 17:33, 1988.

1248. Scopelitis E, Martinez-Osuna P: Gonococcal arthritis. Rheum Dis N Amer 19:363, 1993.

1249. Berrocal A, Gotuzzo E, Calvo A, et al: Sternoclavicular brucellar arthritis: A report of 7 cases and a review of the literature. J Rheumatol 20:1184, 1993.

1250. Wurtz R, Quader Z, Simon D, et al: Cervical tuberculous vertebral osteomyelitis: Case report and discussion of the literature. Clin Infect Dis 16:806, 1993.

1251. Ahmadi J, Bajaj A, Destian S, et al: Spinal tuberculosis: Atypical observations at MR imaging. Radiology 189:489, 1993.

1252. Kumar A, Montanera W, Willinsky R, et al: MR features of tuberculous arachnoiditis. J Comput Assist Tomogr 17:127, 1993.

1253. Abdelwahab IF, Kenan S, Hermann G, et al: Tuberculous peroneal tenosynovitis. A case report. J Bone Joint Surg [Am] 75:1687, 1993.

1254. Hofer M, Hirschel B, Kirschner P, et al: Brief report: Disseminated osteomyelitis from Mycobacterium ulcerans after a snakebite. New Engl J Med 328:1007, 1993.

1255. Reginato AJ: Syphilitic arthritis and osteitis. Rheum Dis N Amer 19:379, 1993.

1256. Cuéllar ML, Silveira LH, Citera G, et al: Other fungal arthritides. Rheum Dis N Amer 19:439, 1993.

1257. Cosgarea AJ, Tejani N, Jones JA: Carpal Aspergillus osteomyelitis: Case report and review of the literature. J Hand Surg [Am] 18:722, 1993.

1258. Grier D, Feinstein KA: Osteomyelitis in hospitalized children with chickenpox: Imaging findings in four cases. AJR 161:643, 1993.

1259. David JJ, Dietz FR, Jones MM: Coxsackie-B monoarthritis with hepatitis. A case report. J Bone Joint Surg [Am] 75:1685, 1993.

1260. Louthrenoo W: Salmonella septic arthritis in patients with human immunodeficiency virus infection. J Rheumatol 20:1454, 1993.

1261. Belmonte MA, Garcia-Portales R, Domenech I, et al: Avascular necrosis of bone in human immunodeficiency virus infection and antiphospholipid antibodies. J Rheumatol 20:1425, 1993.

1262. Martin J, Marco V, Zidan A, et al: Hydatid disease of the soft tissues of the lower limb: findings in three cases. Skel Radiol 22:511, 1993.

1263. Fachartz OAB, Kumar V, Hilou MA: Synovial schistosomiasis of the hip. J Bone Joint Surg [Br] 75:602, 1993.

1264. Kosuwon W, Saengnipanthkul S, Mahaisavariya B, et al: Musculoskeletal meliodosis. J Bone Joint Surg [Am] 75:1811, 1993.

1265. Al-Shahed MS, Sharif HS, Haddad MC, et al: Imaging features of musculoskeletal brucellosis. RadioGraphics 14:333, 1994.

1266. Mondal A: Cytological diagnosis of vertebral tuberculosis with fine-needle aspiration biopsy. J Bone Joint Surg [Am] 76:181, 1994.

1267. Rasool MN, Govender S, Naidoo KS: Cystic tuberculosis of bone in children. J Bone Joint Surg [Br] 76:113, 1994.

1268. George JC, Buckwalter KA, Braunstein EM: Case report 824. Skeletal Radiol 23:79, 1994.

1269. Price GE: Arthritis and iritis after BCG therapy for bladder cancer. J Rheumatol 21:564, 1994.

1270. Kalish R: Lyme disease. Rheum Clincs North Am 19:399, 1993.

1271. Asch ES, Bujak DI, Weiss M, et al: Lyme disease: An infectious and postinfectious syndrome. J Rheumatol 21:454, 1994.

1272. Cooke WD, Bartenhagen NH: Seroreactivity to Borrelia burgdorferi antigens in the absence of Lyme disease. J Rheumatol 21:126, 1994.

1273. Silveira LH, Cuéllar ML, Citera G, et al: Candida arthritis. Rheum Dis Clin North Am 19:427, 1993.

1274. Bocanegra TS, Vasey FB: Musculoskeletal syndromes in parasitic diseases. Rheum Dis Clin North Am 19:505, 1993.

1275. Haygood TM, Williamson SL: Radiographic findings of extremity tuberculosis in childhood: Back to the future? RadioGraphics 14:561, 1994.

1276. Chen W-S, Eng H-L: Tuberculous tenosynovitis of the wrist mimicking de Quervain's disease. J Rheumatol 21:763, 1994.

1277. Harth M, Ralph ED, Faraawi R: Septic arthritis due to Mycobacterium marinum. J Rheumatol 21:957, 1944.

1278. Lafont A, Olivé A, Gelman M, et al: Candida albicans spondylodiscitis and vertebral osteomyelitis in patients with intravenous heroin drug addiction. Report of 3 new cases. J Rheumatol 21:953, 1994.

1279. Ueno Y: Rubella arthritis. An outbreak in Kyoto. J Rheumatol 21:874, 1994.

1280. von Sinner WN, Akhtar M: Case report 833. Skeletal Radiol 23:220, 1994.

INDEX

▼

Note: Page numbers in *italics* refer to illustrations;
page numbers followed by (t) refer to tables.

I

Cruciate ligament(s) *(Continued)*
  interference screws for, *497*
  graft impingement syndrome after, 3133
  isometric insertion sites in, 3132
  magnetic resonance imaging after, 3133, *3134*
  prosthetic devices in, 3133
  routine radiography after, 3133
  rupture of, *3134*
  rupture of, in Segond fracture, 3238, *3240*
  simulation of, *367*
  spatial orientation of, 3120
  tears of, 211
    bone bruises in, 3130–3131, *3131, 3132, 3152,* 3242, *3245*
    bone impaction in, 3130–3131, *3131, 3132*
    complete, 3126, *3127,* 3128, *3128*
    empty notch sign in, 3126
    false-negative diagnosis of, 3129
    false-positive diagnosis of, 3129
    in lateral femoral condyle fracture, 2611, *2612*
    magnetic resonance imaging of, *210,* 3125–3131, *3127–3132*
    osteoarthritis and, 3131
    partial, 3128, *3128*
    patellar tendon sign in, 3130, *3131*
    posterior cruciate ligament curvature in, 3129–3130, *3130*
    posterior cruciate sign in, 3130, *3130*
    repair of, 3131–3133, *3134*
    Segond fracture and, *3109,* 3131, *3132*
    tibial shift and, 3129, *3130*
    uncovered lateral meniscus sign in, 3129
  vs. infrapatellar plica, 374
  arthrography of, 365–366, *367, 368*
  avulsion of, 3238
  bone bruises with, 2580
  computed arthrotomography of, 132
  computed tomography of, *147,* 366, *368*
  congenital absence of, 4285
  magnetic resonance imaging of, 210–211, *210,* 366, 368
  normal, *147,* 366
  posterior, *738, 741, 750, 3044,* 3119–3120, *3119*
    avulsion of, 2664, *2666,* 3238
    blood supply of, 3120
    computed tomography of, *147*
    curvature of, in anterior cruciate ligament tear, 3129–3130, *3130*
    degeneration of, eosinophilic, *3135*
    disruption of, experimental, 3120
    fascicles of, 3120
    function of, 3120
    ganglion cysts of, 3061, 3063, *3063*
    histology of, 3120
    in juvenile chronic arthritis, 995
    injury to, 3133–3135, *3135–3137*
      dislocation and, 2774
    magnetic resonance imaging of, 3135, *3135*
    normal, *147*
    pathologic considerations of, 3120–3121
    posterior drawer test of, 3121
    quadriceps active test of, 3121
    spatial orientation of, 3120
    tears of, 3252
      arthrography of, *367*
      magnetic resonance imaging of, 3135, *3136, 3137*
      posterior drawer test in, 3134
      posterior sag sign in, 3134
      routine radiography of, 3134–3135

Cruciform ligament, 714
Crural interosseous membrane, 741, 746, 3163
Crusher gradients, in magnetic resonance imaging, 180
Cryoglobulin, 1238
Cryoglobulinemia, 1238–1239, *1239*
Cryolite workers, fluorosis in, 3327, *3328*
Cryoprecipitate, after intestinal bypass surgery, 1135
Cryoprotein, 1238
Cryptococcosis, 2505–2506, *2507, 2508*
Cryptococcus neoformans, 2506, *2507*
Crystal(s), anticoagulant, birefringence of, *1687*
    polarized microscopy of, *1687*
  apatite, in anulus fibrosus calcification, 1674
  birefringence property of, 1686, *1687*
  brushite, 1686
  calcium hydroxyapatite, 1615. See also *Calcium hydroxyapatite crystal(s); Calcium hydroxyapatite crystal deposition disease.*
    calcium pyrophosphate dihydrate crystals and, 1557, 1643
    identification of, 1615–1616
    synovitis and, 1639
  calcium orthophosphate dihydrate, 1615
  calcium oxalate, 1688–1693, *1690–1694.* See also *Oxalosis.*
    deposition of, in renal failure, 1692
    sites of, 1689
    in primary oxalosis, 1690
    in secondary oxalosis, 1692, *1693*
  calcium phosphate, identification of, 1615–1616
  calcium pyrophosphate dihydrate, 1556, *1557*
    birefringence of, *1687*
    calcium hydroxyapatite crystals and, 1643
    deposition of, 1558, 1566, *1567–1572.* See also *Calcium pyrophosphate dihydrate crystal(s); Calcium pyrophosphate dihydrate crystal deposition disease; Chondrocalcinosis.*
    diseases with, 1562–1563, *1564*
    in alkaptonuria, 1681
    in hemochromatosis, 1650
    polarized microscopy of, *1687*
    shedding of, *1565,* 1565–1566
    tendon calcification and, 1577, *1581*
    vs. corticosteroid crystals, 1688
  Charcot-Leyden, 1688
  cholesterol, birefringence of, *1687*
    in synovial fluid, 1688
    polarized microscopy of, *1687*
    tophus, 1688, *1688*
  corticosteroid, 1688
    birefringence of, *1687*
    polarized microscopy of, *1687*
  cortisone acetate, polarized microscopy of, *1687*
  cystine, deposition of, 1693–1694. See also *Cystinosis.*
  deposition of, classification of, 1558
  dicalcium phosphate dihydrate, deposition of, 1558
    in fibrocartilage, 1637
  diseases induced by, 1686–1695
  ethylenediaminetetraacetic acid, birefringence of, *1687*
    polarized microscopy of, *1687*
  hematoidin, 1694–1695
  hemoglobin, 1694–1695
  hypoxanthine, 1694
  in Crohn's disease, 1127
  in gout, 1540

Crystal(s) *(Continued)*
  in pseudogout syndrome, 1556, 1558
  lipid, 1688
  mixed, 1637
  monosodium urate. See also *Monosodium urate crystal(s).*
    birefringence of, *1687*
    calcification of, in gout, 1522
    polarized microscopy of, *1687*
    vs. corticosteroid crystals, 1688
  musculoskeletal manifestations of, 1686t
  myoglobin, 1694–1695
  oxalate. See also *Oxalosis.*
    in dialysis spondyloarthropathy, 2053
    in oxalosis, 1692–1693
  oxypurinol, 1694
  periarticular deposition of, ankle in, 1630
    differential diagnosis of, 1632, 1635–1636, *1635–1638,* 1635(t), 1636(t)
    foot in, 1630, *1630*
    hand in, 1619, 1627, *1627*
    heel in, 1630
    hip in, 1627, *1628, 1629,* 1630
    knee in, 1630, *1630*
    neck in, 1630, *1631,* 1632
    pelvis in, 1627, *1628, 1629,* 1630
    shoulder in, 1617–1619, *1618, 1620–1626*
      stages of, 1618–1619, *1620–1621*
    spine in, 1632, *1632*
    wrist in, 1619, 1627, *1627*
  prednisolone tertiary-butylacetate, *1687*
  sodium urate, in gout, 1513
  triamcinolone hexacetonide, *1687*
  xanthine, 1694
Crystal deposition disease. See *Calcium hydroxyapatite crystal deposition disease; Calcium pyrophosphate dihydrate crystal deposition disease; Gout.*
CT. See *Computed tomography.*
Cubital tunnel, ulnar nerve entrapment in, 3254, 3384, 3394–3395, *3395*
Cubital tunnel syndrome, 2945, 2947, *2947,* 3388t
  in rheumatoid arthritis, 869
  lipoma and, 3394, *3395*
  Tinel's sign in, 3395
  ulnar nerve entrapment in, 3394–3395, *3395*
Cuboid bone, *3159*
  dysplasia epiphysealis hemimelica of, *3744*
  fracture of, 2795, *2796, 2797*
  in diffuse idiopathic skeletal hyperostosis, *1475*
  infarction of, in systemic lupus erythematosus, *1181*
  mad;uromycosis of, *2526*
  osteonecrosis of, in systemic lupus erythematosus, *1180*
  Rhizopus osteomyelitis of, 2521
  stress fracture of, 2589, *2592*
Cuboideonavicular joint, *762, 763,* 3160, *3162*
Cuboid-metatarsal space, in fifth metatarsal avulsion fracture, 2800, *2802*
Cubonavicular joint, coalition of, 4301
Cuff-tear arthropathy, 1309. See also *Milwaukee shoulder syndrome.*
Cuneiform bone, fragmentation of, in alcoholic neuropathic osteoarthropathy, *3434*
  in diabetes mellitus, *3439*
  in diffuse idiopathic skeletal hyperostosis, *1475*
  posttraumatic osteonecrosis of, *111*
Cuneocuboid joint, *759, 762, 763,* 3160, *3162*
  rheumatoid arthritis of, 913
Cuneonavicular joint, *754, 759, 762, 763,* 1767, *1767, 3158, 3159,* 3160, *3162*

Fragment(s) *(Continued)*
  of elbow, *2610*
  of olecranon fossa, 896, *899*
  pathogenesis of, 823
Fragmentation, bone. See also *Fragment(s), bone; Synovitis, detritic.*
  cervical, in calcium pyrophosphate dihydrate crystal deposition disease, *1600*
  in alkaptonuria, 1684
  in osteonecrosis, 3483, *3485,* 3486
  in Wilson's disease, 1665–1666, *1665*
  in diabetic neuropathic osteoarthropathy, *3428*
  of temporomandibular articular disc, *1742*
Frankel classification, of spinal cord contusion, 2834
Frankel scale, for myelopathy, 2834
Free bodies. See *Intra-articular osteocartilaginous body (bodies).*
Free induction decay, in nuclear magnetic resonance, 174–175
Freiberg's infraction, 1353, 3560(t), 3576–3578, *3577–3579*
  differential diagnosis of, 3578
  in diabetic neuropathic osteoarthropathy, 3426, *3431*
  intra-articular osteocartilaginous bodies in, *3579*
  magnetic resonance imaging in, *3579*
  scintigraphy in, *3579*
  trauma in, 3578
  vs. diabetic neuropathic osteoarthropathy, 3426, *3431*
Frejka pillow, in developmental hip dysplasia, 4084, 4087
Frequency, resonant, in magnetic resonance imaging, 189–190
  in nuclear magnetic resonance, 171, 171(t)
Frequency domain, of Fourier transform, 180
Frequency encoding, in magnetic resonance imaging, 178–179
Frequency selective presaturation, in magnetic resonance imaging, 184
Fried-egg appearance, in hairy cell leukemia, *2254*
Friedreich's ataxia, 3405
  neuromuscular scoliosis in, 4260
Friedreich's syndrome, 3405
Friedrich's disease, 3604
  vs. clavicular osteitis condensans, 2098
Fringe fields, in xeroradiography, 104
Frontal bone, fibrous dysplasia of, *4381*
  hemangioma of, *3827*
  osteomyelitis of, 2343
Frontal projection, in rheumatoid arthritis, 928
Frontal sinus, osteoma of, 4403
Frostbite, 3264–3268
  abnormalities in, 3264
  acro-osteolysis from, *3266, 3267*
  angiography of, 423, *425,* 3264–3265
  arteriography of, 3264–3265, *3265*
  differential diagnosis of, 3268
  early changes in, 3265, *3265*
  epiphyseal injuries in, 3265, *3266*
  foot in, 423, *425*
  hand in, 1762, 3265, *3265*
  late changes in, 3265, *3266*
  musculoskeletal abnormalities in, 3264–3265, *3265*
  of ears, 3265
  pathogenesis of, 3264–3265
  radiographic abnormalities in, 3265, *3265*
  rhabdomyolysis after, 3265
  scintigraphy of, 3265, *3267*
  terminology in, 3264

Frostbite *(Continued)*
  thermography of, 3265
  vs. immersion foot, 3264
Frozen shoulder, 2700. See also *Shoulder, adhesive capsulitis of.*
Fucosidosis, 2206, 4230t, 4235
Fungus (fungi), 2503–2522. See also specific infections, e.g., *Sporotrichosis.*
  in rheumatoid arthritis, 939
Fusion, joint, 4288–4305. See also *Ankylosis; Arthrodesis; Coalition.*
  acquired, vs. symphalangism, 4290
  congenital, of carpal bones, 46, *47*
  surgical. See *Arthrodesis.*
  laminar, 4247
  lunotriquetral, 4290–4291, *4292*
  of calvarial sutures, 4216
  of carpal bones. See *Carpal coalition.*
  of growth plate. See *Growth plate, premature closure of.*
  of tarsal bones. See *Tarsal coalition.*
  of toes, 64, *66*
  physeal, in hypoparathyroidism, 2062
  in sickle cell anemia, 2114
  radioulnar. See *Synostosis (synostoses), radioulnar.*
  spinal. See also *Arthrodesis.*
    complications of, 4258, *4259,* 4260
    congenital scoliosis with, 4258, *4259*
    intervertebral disc calcification in, 1682t
    pseudarthrosis after, 4258, *4259*
    rod breakage in, 4258, *4259*
    spondylolysis in, 2598
  surgical. See *Arthrodesis.*
Fusion line, of growth plate, 613–614
Fusobacterium, 2460–2461, *2461*

G

Gadolinium-153, for dual photon absorptiometry, 1863
Gage's sign, in Legg-Calvé-Perthes disease, 3571
Gait, in hyperparathyroidism, 2033
  in infantile coxa vara, 4309
  in Legg-Calvé-Perthes disease, 3561
Galactosyl-hydroxylysine, of organic matrix, 631
Galeazzi's injury, 2731(t), 2732, 2736, *2737*
Gallie fusion, at C1–C2, 547
Gallium scanning. See also *Scintigraphy.*
  in alcoholic neuropathic osteoarthropathy, *2400*
  in chronic leukemia, 2253
  in chronic osteomyelitis, 447, *448*
  in dermatomyositis, 1225
  in discitis, 2430
  in Erdheim-Chester disease, 2224
  in infection, 2398–2399, *2400,* 2402
  in myositis, 2387
  in neurofibromatosis, 4377
  in osteomyelitis, 443, *444,* 447, *447,* 2397–2402, 2399(t), *2400*
  in Paget's disease, 1942
  in plasma cell myeloma, 2156
  in polymyositis, 1225
  in prosthesis-associated osteomyelitis, 448, *449, 450*
  in prosthetic hip infection, 569, 571
  in rheumatoid arthritis, 945
  in sarcoidosis, 4344
  in septic arthritis, 448
  in sickle cell anemia, 2120
  in soft tissue infection, 2398–2399, 2399(t), *2400*
  in soft tissue tumors, 4499
Gallstones, in hereditary spherocytosis, 2138

Galveston technique, 540–541, *541*
Gamekeeper's thumb, 2748, *2751,* 2934–2936, *2935, 2936,* 3253, *3253*
  arthrography of, 301, *304*
  plain film radiography of, *5*
Gamma globulins. See also *Cryoglobulin; Immunoglobulin(s).*
  synovial fluid, 815
  synthesis of, 2183
Gamma nail, 494
Ganglion (ganglia), 3961, 4518–4519, *4525–4528.* See also *Cyst(s), ganglion.*
  alar fold, vs. nodular synovitis, 377
  common peroneal nerve entrapment by, 3400, *3403*
  in developmental dysplasia of hip, *4526*
  in tarsal tunnel syndrome, *3402*
  intraosseous, 3778, *3880,* 3881–3882, *3881*
    computed tomography in, 152
    pathogenesis of, 1275
    types of, 1275
    vs. giant cell tumor, 3804, *3804*
    vs. subchondral cyst, 1275, 1278(t), *1279*
  median nerve entrapment by, 3392, *3394*
  of acetabular labrum, 343
  of acetabulum, *1323*
  of ankle, 392
  of femur, *4528*
  of glenoid labrum, 3013
  of hand, *4525*
  of hip, 4519, *4526*
  of knee, *4526*
  of nerve sheath, 4552, *4559*
  of wrist, 298, *299*
  suprascapular, 3254, *3255*
  suprascapular nerve entrapment by, 3397, *3398*
Ganglioneuromatosis, intestinal, in multiple endocrine neoplasia syndrome type IIB, 2035
Ganglioside G$_{M1}$, accumulation of, 2206
  deficiency of, 2206, 4230t, 4235, *4235*
Gangliosidosis, generalized, 2206
  GM$_1$, 4230t, 4235, *4235*
Gangosa, 2499
Gangrene, diabetic, arterial calcification in, 2087
  dopamine and, 3330, *3330*
  ergotamine and, 3330
  gas, 2387, *2388*
    clostridial, 2459–2460, *2460*
    nontraumatic, 2460
  in rheumatoid arthritis, 840
  methysergide and, 3330
  vs. infection, 2353
Garden classification system, of intracapsular proximal femoral fractures, 2755, *2759,* 2760, *2760*
Gardner's syndrome, osteomas in, 4403–4404, 4404(t)
  radiographic abnormalities of, 4403–4404, 4404(t)
  vs. tuberous sclerosis, 4404, *4405*
Garré's sclerosing osteomyelitis, vs. chronic recurrent multifocal osteomyelitis, 2389
Gas. See also *Gas gangrene; Pneumatocyst; Vacuum phenomenon.*
  computed tomography of, 130–131, *131,* 147
  for myelography, 243–244, *245*
  in anulus fibrosus, 2857–2858, *2857*
  in clostridial infection, 2387, *2388,* 2460, *2460*
  in clostridial myositis, 2460, *2460*
  in diabetes mellitus, 4597, *4598*
  in Enterobacter osteomyelitis, *2396*
  in *Escherichia coli* infection, 2454

Hand(s) (*Continued*)
polydactyly of, 4288–4289, *4290*
polymyositis of, 1761, *1761*
pseudomalignant myositis ossificans of, 4586
psoriatic arthritis of, *1077,* 1077–1082, *1078, 1080, 1081,* 1100
distribution of, 1759, *1759*
scintigraphy of, *1093*
pyknodysostosis of, 4204, *4205*
radiographic morphometry of, 1828, *1828*
reflex sympathetic dystrophy of, *1798, 1802*
relapsing polychondritis of, 1153, *1154*
resorption in, in hyperparathyroidism, 2014
rhabdomyosarcoma of, *4523*
rheumatoid arthritis of, 807, 870–877, *870,* 955, 955t, *1547*
advanced changes in, *873,* 873–874
clinical abnormalities in, 870
compartmental analysis in, 955t
differential diagnosis of, 955, 955t, 1186t
distribution of, 1758, *1758*
early changes in, 871–873, *871, 872,* 873t
finger deformities in, 1295
radiographic-pathologic correlation in, *870,* 871–877, *871–874, 876, 877*
scintigraphy in, 462, *462, 463,* 945, *946*
Saldino-Mainzer dysplasia of, 4193, *4194*
sarcoidosis of, 4337, *4339,* 4340, *4340*
scintigraphy of, 461
scleroderma of, 1194, *1195,* 1196, 1199, *1201,* 1202, 1761, *1761*
septic arthritis of, 1762, 2368, 2530
sesamoid nodules of, 668
sickle cell dactylitis of, 2110–2111, *2112*
subluxation of, in polymyositis, 1221
in rheumatoid arthritis, *834*
subperiosteal resorption in, in hyperparathyroidism, 2014
surface resorption in, in rheumatoid arthritis, 872–873, *872,* 873t
swan-neck deformity of. See *Swan-neck deformity.*
syndactyly of, 4219, 4220, *4220*
synovial cysts of, 228
synovial sarcoma of, *4551*
systemic lupus erythematosus of, *1760,* 1761
differential diagnosis of, 1186t
tendon sheaths of, *2348,* 2907–2908, *2908*
in osteomyelitis, 2344–2345, *2348, 2349*
infection of, 309, *309*
tendons of, ultrasonography of, 228
tenography of, 301, 303–309, *305–309*
tenosynovitis of, 228
thenar space of, *2348*
infection of, 2349
thermal burns of, 1762, *3268, 3270, 3271*
tophi on, 1512, *1513*
trichorhinophalangeal dysplasia of, 4192, 4193, *4193*
tuberculosis of, 2142, *2142,* 2477, *2478*
tuberculous arthritis of, *2483*
tuberous sclerosis of, *4348, 4358*
tuftal resorption in, in psoriatic arthritis, 1079
in scleroderma, 1213, *1213*
tumoral calcinosis of, *4573*
ultrasonography of, 228
xanthoma of, *2234*
X-linked hypophosphatemic osteomalacia of, *1794*
yaws of, *2500*
zigzag deformity of, in rheumatoid arthritis, *876,* 891, *892,* 981
Handball, injuries in, 3230
Hand-foot syndrome, in sickle cell anemia, 2108, 2110–2111

Hand-foot-uterus syndrome, tarsal coalition in, 4294
Handlebar palsy, 3254
Hand-Schüller-Christian disease, 2217, *2220, 2221.* See also *Histiocytosis X.*
cholesterol in, *2221*
clinical features of, 2217
diabetes insipidus in, 2217
floating teeth appearance in, 2217
foam cells in, *2221*
histology of, 2217, *2221*
ilium in, 2217, *2220*
in Langerhans cell histiocytosis, 2214
Langerhans cells in, 2214–2215
pelvis in, 2217, *2220*
prognosis for, 2217, 2221
skeletal lesions of, 2217, *2220*
skull in, 2217, *2220*
vs. Erdheim-Chester disease, 2224
Hangman's fracture, 2853, *2854*
hyperextension in, 2853
mechanism of injury in, 2853
neurologic deficits in, 2854–2855
vertebral body extension of, 2853, *2854*
vs. atlantoaxial subluxation, 2855
Hansen's disease. See *Leprosy.*
Hansenula polymorpha, in chronic granulomatous disease, 2388
HarriLuque system, 540
Harrington rod, 538, *538*
break in, after spinal fusion, 4258, *4259*
fracture of, 538, *538*
hook pull-out from, 539, *539*
Harrington system, 538–540, *538, 539*
dislodgement of, 539, *539*
Moe modification of, 539
pseudarthrosis with, 539, *539*
Harris, lines of, 3353, 3354(t), 3355, *3355, 3356.* See also *Growth recovery lines.*
Harris-Beath view, in talocalcaneal coalition, 4296, *4298*
of tarsal joints, 35, *37*
Harrison's groove, in rickets, 1894
Hashimoto's thyroiditis, 1995
connective tissue diseases in, 2009
hypothyroidism in, 2001
rheumatoid arthritis in, 1995
systemic lupus erythematosus in, 1995
Hatchet sign, in ankylosing spondylitis, 1044, *1046,* 1777
in juvenile-onset ankylosing spondylitis, *974*
Haversian canals, 626, *644*
vs. Volkmann's canals, 628
Haversian envelope, 636
Haversian system, 624, *626, 627,* 628
atypical, of fetus, 614
components of, 623, *624*
development of, 613
formation of, 610
in compact bone, *627*
Hawkins sign, in talar neck fractures, 2790
in talar osteonecrosis, 3520
Head. See also *Skull.*
carcinoma of, 4000t
lateral flexion of, atlas fracture and, 2848
lateral tilt of, atlantoaxial displacement and, 931, 2848
rotation of, atlantoaxial displacement and, 2848
Healing, fracture. See *Fracture(s), healing of.*
Hearing loss, in myositis ossificans progressiva, 4125
in osteogenesis imperfecta, 4112t, 4115
Heart, in ankylosing spondylitis, 1011
in Marfan's syndrome, 4096
in rheumatoid arthritis, 1258
in scleroderma, 1193

Heart (*Continued*)
in systemic lupus erythematosus, 1166
rhabdomyoma of, in tuberous sclerosis, 4360
Heart disease, congenital, in neurofibromatosis, 4378
prostaglandin E₁ in, periostitis and, 4442
secondary hypertrophic osteoarthropathy in, 4429, *4430, 4431,* 4434
Heart valves, discoloration of, in alkaptonuria, 1671, *1672*
Heavy chain disease, 2175
Heavy metals, deficiency of, 3353–3362
poisoning with, 3353–3362
Heberden's nodes, 1295
genetic factors in, 1265
in gout, 1551
in osteoarthritis, 1265, 1355
Heel. See also *Ankle; Calcaneus; Foot (feet); Hindfoot.*
ankylosing spondylitis of, 956, 957(t), 1047, *1053*
calcification of, 1630
in scleroderma, *1200*
gout of, 956, 957t, 1522, *1528*
in diffuse idiopathic skeletal hyperostosis, 1471, 1475, *1475*
in Reiter's syndrome, 956, 957(t), 1104, *1106*
in seronegative spondyloarthropathies, 913, 916
infection of, neonatal heel puncture and, 2352–2353
noncalcific bursitis of, 1632, *1635*
noncalcific tendinitis of, 1632, *1635*
pain in, 3206
Reiter's syndrome and, 1104
repetitive trauma and, 1632
rheumatoid arthritis and, 916
psoriatic arthritis of, 956, 957t
puncture of, in neonate, 2352–2353
rheumatoid arthritis of, clinical abnormalities in, 913, 916
differential diagnosis of, 956, 957t
radiographic-pathologic correlation of, *916,* 916–917
rheumatoid nodules of, *837*
xanthoma of, 956, 957t
Heel puncture, in neonate, 2352–2353
Heel-pad thickness, in acromegaly, 1976, *1980,* 1990t, 1991
ultrasonography in, 221
Heinig view, of sternoclavicular joint, 18–19, *20*
Helix, auricular, tophi on, 1512, *1513*
Helminths, 2535–2542, 2536(t), 2537(t). See also specific organisms, e.g., *Ancylostoma duodenale.*
Hemangioblastoma, magnetic resonance imaging of, 268
Hemangioendothelioma, 3951. See also *Angiosarcoma.*
Hemangiolymphangiomatosis. See *Angiomatosis, cystic.*
Hemangioma, 2314, 2317, 3821–3828, 3950–3956, *3951–3954, 3957, 3958*
age distribution of, 3632(t)
aneurysmal bone cyst with, 3878
angiography of, *417*
arteriography of, 3953, *3954*
arthropathy with, 2317, 2317(t), *2318*
biopsy of, 3824
calcifications in, 1214, 3953, *3954*
capillary, 3828, *3828,* 3951, 4531
cavernous, *3207,* 3828, *3828,* 3951, *4495,* 4531
chest wall, *195*
clinical abnormalities in, 3821, 3950–3951

Leprosy *(Continued)*
limb disuse in, 2488
neurologic findings in, 2487
neuropathic musculoskeletal lesions in, 2488, *2491*
neuropathic osteoarthropathy in, 3436, *3438*
osteitis in, 2487, *2488*
osteomyelitis in, 2487, *2488, 2489*
periostitis in, *2450,* 2487, 2488, *2488*
red leg in, *2450,* 2488
secondary infection in, 2492
soft tissue calcification in, 2492, *2492*
soft tissue neoplasm in, 2492
tuberculoid, 2486
types of, 2486–2487
vascular lesions in, 2492
Leptomeninges, in plasma cell myeloma, *2160*
metastases to, 3996
Leptomeningitis, 2435
Leptospirosis, 2502
Leptotrichia, 2460
Leri's pleonosteosis, soft tissue contracture in, 4593
Léri-Weill syndrome, 4191, *4191.* See also *Dyschondrosteosis.*
Leroy's syndrome, 4235, *4236*
Lesch-Nyhan syndrome, distal phalangeal resorption in, 1213, 1213t
gout with, 1542–1544, *1543–1544*
hypoxanthine crystals in, 1694
xanthine crystals in, 1694
Lesser arc injuries, of wrist, 2740, *2743*
Letterer-Siwe disease, 2217, 2221, *2222*
clinical features of, 2221
histiocytic proliferation in, 2221
in Langerhans cell histiocytosis, 2214
Langerhans cells in, 2214–2215
mandible in, 2221, *2222*
osteolysis in, 2221
pathology of, 2221, *2222*
prognosis of, 2221
radiographic features of, 2221, *2222*
skull in, 2221, *2222*
Leukemia, 2247–2258
acropachy in, 2001
acute, 2247–2248, 2248t
adult, 2248, 2251
metaphyseal radiolucency in, 2251
osteolysis in, 2251
osteopenia in, 2251
skeletal alterations in, 2248t
B cells in, 2248
cell types in, 2247–2248
childhood, 2248–2251, *2249–2252*
calcium pyrophosphate dihydrate crystals in, 2250
chloroma in, 2249–2250
clinical features of, 2248
dactylitis in, 2249, *2250*
differential diagnosis of, 2250–2251, *2252*
epiphyseal osteonecrosis in, 2250
epiphysiolysis in, 2248
femur in, 2248, *2249*
gout in, 2250
growth disturbances in, 2248
growth recovery lines in, 2248–2249
hand in, 2249, *2250*
hemorrhage in, 2250
humerus in, 2248, *2249*
hyperuricemia, 2250
increased intracranial pressure in, 2249
insufficiency fractures in, 2248
intra-articular infiltration in, 2250
joint abnormalities in, 2250
joint effusions in, 2250
lymphoblastic, 2248

Leukemia *(Continued)*
magnetic resonance imaging in, 2250, *2251,* 2256–2257
metacarpal bones in, 2249, *2250*
metatarsal bones in, 2249, *2250*
myeloblastic, 2248
osteolysis in, 2249, *2250*
osteopenia in, 2248
osteoporosis in, 2250
osteosclerosis in, 2249
periarticular bone lesions in, 2250
periostitis in, 2249, *2250*
phalanges in, 2249, *2250*
prognosis for, 2250, *2251*
radiodense metaphyseal bands in, 2248–2249
radiographic changes in, 2248
radiolucent metaphyseal bands in, 2248–2249, *2249*
septic arthritis in, 2250
skeletal alterations in, 2248t, 2250, *2251*
sutural diastasis in, 2249, *2251*
synovial membrane in, 2250
vs. neuroblastoma, 2251, *2252*
vs. retinoblastoma, 2251, *2252*
T cells in, 2248
aleukemic, radium exposure and, 3277
bone marrow infiltration in, *2256,* 2256–2257
bone marrow transplant for, bone marrow infarction after, 202
cell distribution in, 2248
chronic, 2248, 2248(t), 2251, *2252,* 2253, *2253*
arthritis in, 2253
blast crisis in, 2253
epiphyseal osteonecrosis in, 2253
gallium scanning in, 2253
gout in, 2253
hands in, 2253
joint manifestations of, 2253, *2253*
leukemic acropachy in, 2253
osteolysis in, 2251, *2252,* 2253
osteopenia in, 2251, 2253
Salmonella osteomyelitis in, 2253, *2254*
synovial membrane in, 2253, *2253*
classification of, 2247–2248, 2248t
features of, 2247–2248, 2248t
growth plate injuries in, 2641
hairy cell, 2253–2254
bone involvement in, 2253
fried-egg appearance in, *2254*
histology of, 2253, *2254*
in myelofibrosis, 2281
osteolysis in, 2253
osteonecrosis in, 2253
osteoporosis in, 2253
pathologic fracture in, 2253
vertebral involvement in, 2258
in neurofibromatosis, 4377
lymphocytic, pathologic vertebral fracture in, *2257*
magnetic resonance imaging in, 196, 198, 2256–2258, *2256–2258*
flip-flop sign in, 2257
mast cell, 2277
megakaryoblastic, 2254
metaphyseal atrophy in, 3348
myelocytic, acute, 2256
granulocytic sarcoma with, *2258*
chronic, gout in, *1545*
granulocytic sarcoma in, 2254, *2255*
myelofibrosis and, 2281
vs. juvenile chronic arthritis, 979
Leukocyte(s), cartilaginous destruction by, 808

Leukocyte(s) *(Continued)*
gallium uptake by, 2398
in chronic granulomatous disease, 2388
in gout, 1513–1514
in psoriatic arthritis, 1094
in rheumatoid arthritis, 870, 938, 953
in synovial membrane, 808
lactoferrin of, 2398
morphine effects on, 2392
Leukocytosis, trauma and, 2634
Leukoencephalopathy, sclerosing, 2238
Leukopenia, in systemic lupus erythematosus, 1166
Levator scapulae muscle, 2962, *2962*
Lever arm, in biomechanics, 793, *793*
Levoscoliosis, radiation therapy and, *3286*
Lichen amyloidosus, 2176
Lichen myxedematosus, 1098, 1212
Licked candy stick appearance, in leprosy, 2488, *2491*
Lidocaine, antibacterial effect of, 2396
intra-articular, in total hip replacement, 568
Ligament(s), 670. See also specific ligaments.
accessory, extracapsular, 661
anterolateral, of knee, 3103
attachment of, 1389–1390. See also *Enthesis (entheses).*
bone excrescences at, 1636
in hyperparathyroidism, 2026, *2028*
classification of, 670
collateral. See *Collateral ligament(s).*
computed tomography of, 146–147, *147*
corticosteroid effects on, 3320
crimp of, *2663*
cruciate. See *Cruciate ligament(s).*
heterotopic ossification of, *2666, 2667, 2672*
in acromegaly, 1985, *1987*
in rheumatoid arthritis, 826, *828,* 831
in seronegative spondyloarthropathies, 856, *858, 859,* 860
injuries to, 2662–2664, *2663, 2666*
fat in, 2634
insertions of, 2662–2663
laxity of. See also *Ehlers-Danlos syndrome; Homocystinuria; Marfan's syndrome.*
congenital, 4311
degenerative joint disease and, 1268
in Ehlers-Danlos syndrome, 4108
in hemodialysis, 2058
in hyperparathyroidism, 2015(t), 2030, *2033*
in osteogenesis imperfecta, 4115, 4117, *4119*
in trapeziometacarpal joint osteoarthritis, 1298
loading of, 3231
longitudinal. See *Longitudinal ligament(s).*
magnetic resonance imaging of, 192(t)
ossification of, *1291,* 4575–4577, *4576, 4577*
in fluorosis, 3322, *3322*
posttraumatic, 2664, *2666*
spinal. See also specific ligaments, e.g., *Longitudinal ligament(s).*
degeneration of, 1401–1403, *1402–1404*
sprains of, 3252–3253, *3253*
spring, 755, 3159, *3159,* 3160, *3178,* 3189, *3189*
thickness of, 90
tophaceous deposits in, 1515
Ligament of Cooper, 2939
Ligament of Humphrey, 3069, *3072,* 3084, *3084*
Ligament of Struthers, in median nerve entrapment, 2947, 3384, *3389*
Ligament of Wrisberg, *750,* 3069, *3071, 3072,* 3084, *3084*

Osteosclerosis *(Continued)*
metastatic, 3999, *4001,* 4003, *4004*
bronchial carcinoid tumor and, 4019
cranial, 4009
medulloblastoma and, 4025
pelvic, 4010, *4013, 4014*
vertebral, 4010, *4011*
odontoid process erosion and, 932
of acetabulum, 2062, *3368*
of cervical spine, *2153*
of clavicle, 2098, *2099, 2100*
of costovertebral joint, in ankylosing spondylitis, 1034–1035
of femoral head, in hypoparathyroidism,
2062
of femur, *2152, 2153, 2170*
of hand, 2111, *2114*
of humeral head, 2114, *2115*
of ilium, 2089, *2090, 2170*
of mandibular condylar head, 1733, *1738*
of mandibular fossa, 1733, *1738, 1739*
of metacarpal bones, *889*
of pelvis, 4010, *4013, 4014*
in plasma cell myeloma, *2153*
in primary oxalosis, 1690, *1690*
in sickle cell anemia, 2111, *2113*
of pubis, differential diagnosis of, *2095*
of radiocarpal bones, 891, *894*
of radius, *894*
of rib, 2230, *2230*
of sacrum, *2170, 2171*
of skull, 2030, *2032, 2152*
of sternum, 3295, *3296*
of terminal phalanges, 50, *50*
of trapezioscaphoid bone, *1592*
parathyroid hormone and, 2030
radiation-induced, 3295, *3296*
reactive, cervical spinous processes, 831
differential diagnosis of, 1378, 1379(t)
in ankylosing spondylitis, 1019
in infective spondylitis, 2426, *2426*
in rheumatoid arthritis, 932
skull, 2110, 4009
Stanescu type, 4204
subchondral, humeral head, in glenohumeral
joint osteoarthritis, 1302, *1305, 1306*
in ankylosing spondylitis, 1012, *1015*
in diabetic neuropathic osteoarthropathy,
3429
in hyperparathyroidism, *2022, 2023*
in rheumatoid arthritis, *823, 918*
talus, *3428*
temporomandibular joint, 1733, *1738*
thyrocalcitonin and, 2030
trapezioscaphoid, in calcium pyrophosphate
dihydrate crystal deposition disease,
1592
vertebral, in intervertebral osteochondrosis,
1437, 1682
in metastasis, *1437*
in osteomesopyknosis, 4204, *4205,* 4409,
4409
in osteopetrosis tarda, *1437*
in Paget's disease, *1437, 2039*
in plasmacytoma, *2167*
in renal osteodystrophy, *1437,* 2036,
2039–2040
in secondary oxalosis, *1694*
segmental, degenerative diseases and,
1434–1436, *1435, 1437*
differential diagnosis of, *1437*
vs. Paget's disease, 1962–1963, *1963*
vertebral body, differential diagnosis of,
1066
vs. frostbite, 3268
Osteotomy, 515–520
abduction, 517–518, *519*

Osteotomy *(Continued)*
adduction, 517–518, *519*
angulation, 523
barrel vault, 516
Chiari, 4087, 4089
circumacetabular, 4087, *4088,* 4089
complications of, 4089–4090
femoral, 517–518, *519*
for developmental hip dysplasia, 4087,
4088
results of, 520
Sugioka, 523
for developmental hip dysplasia, 4087–4090,
4088
high femoral, 517–520, *519*
high tibial, 515–517, *516–518*
innominate, for developmental hip dysplasia,
4087
intertrochanteric, delayed union of, *522*
for hip osteoarthritis, *521*
oblique, 517
osteonecrosis after, 4089–4090
pelvic, femoral head osteonecrosis after,
4089–4090
for developmental hip dysplasia, 4087,
4088
osteoarthritis after, 4089
recurrent developmental hip dysplasia
after, 4089, *4089*
Pemberton, 4087, *4088,* 4089
postoperative radiography for, 520, *521, 522*
preoperative radiography for, 520
radiologic examination of, 518, 520, *520–
522*
Salter, 4087, *4089*
Sofield, in osteogenesis imperfecta, 4117,
4118, 4121
tumoral callus formation around, *4117*
Sugioka, 523
supracondylar, 517
Otopalatodigital syndrome, 4177–4178, *4178*
carpal bones in, 4178, *4178*
pectus excavatum deformity in, 4178
phalanges in, 4178, *4178*
pseudoepiphyses in, 4178, *4178*
spine in, 4178, *4178*
tarsal coalition in, 4178, *4178,* 4294
Otosclerosis, in osteogenesis imperfecta, 4114,
4115
Otto pelvis, 1777. See also *Protrusio
acetabuli.*
Ouard procedure, for recurrent anterior
glenohumeral joint dislocation, 2700t
Overlap syndromes. See also *Mixed
connective tissue disease.*
rheumatoid arthritis-scleroderma, 1248, *1250*
rheumatoid arthritis-systemic lupus erythematosus, 1248
scleroderma-systemic lupus erythematosus,
1248, *1249*
vs. mixed connective tissue disease, 1248,
1249, 1250
Overtubulation, in bone modeling, 617, *623*
Overuse injury, 3230(t), 3231
at elbow, 2943, *2945*
Oxalate. See *Calcium oxalate crystal(s).*
Oxalosis, 1688–1693, *1690–1694*
in chronic renal failure, 2047
primary, 1688–1690, *1690–1692,* 1692
calcium oxalate crystals in, 1690
clinical features of, 1689
drumstick configuration in, 1690, *1692*
extrarenal accumulation in, 1689
foreign body giant cell reaction in, 1690
glyceric aciduria in, 1688–1689
glycolic aciduria in, 1688–1689
hand in, 1690, *1691, 1692*

Oxalosis *(Continued)*
metacarpal bones in, 1690, *1692*
metaphyses in, *1691*
renal osteodystrophy in, 1690, *1691*
skeletal abnormalities in, 1689–1690,
1690–1692
secondary, 1692–1693, *1693, 1694*
arthropathy, 1693, *1694*
arthropathy in, 1693, *1694*
articular manifestations of, 1692
calcification in, 1692–1693, *1693*
chondrocalcinosis in, 1692, *1693*
discovertebral junction in, 1693, *1694*
erosions in, 1693
mechanisms of, 1692
musculoskeletal involvement in, 1692
renal failure in, 1692, *1693*
sites of, 1692
Oxprenolol, arthritis from, 3336
Oxygen saturation, in osteonecrosis, 3515
Oxypurinol crystals, 1694

P

Pachydermia, generalized hyperostosis with.
See *Osteoarthropathy, hypertrophic,
primary.*
Pachydermohyperostosis. See
Osteoarthropathy, hypertrophic, primary.
Pachydermoperiostosis, 4207, *4208*
Pad, fat. See *Fat pad(s).*
shoulder, in amyloidosis, 2177, *2178,* 2180
Paget's disease, 1923–1964
acetabula in, 1776
alkaline phosphatase in, 1924, 1925
ankylosing spondylitis and, 1055, 1952,
1954
basilar invagination in, 1933
blood flow in, 456–457
bone marrow in, 1946
calcaneus in, *1939*
calcitonin in, 1959
calcium pyrophosphate dihydrate crystals in,
1562, 1952, *1954*
cauda equina compression in, 1952
cement line mosaic of, 1926, *1927*
clavicle in, *1941*
clinical features of, 1924–1925
complications of, 456
computed tomography in, 1942, *1942, 1943*
congestive heart failure in, 1924
cranial nerve abnormalities in, 1924, 1933
cranium in, 1927(t), *1928,* 1929, 1931–1933,
1932, 1933
computed tomography in, *1942*
cotton-wool appearance of, *1930,* 1931,
1932
crystal deposition in, 1562, 1952, *1954*
cystic lesions in, 1950, *1952*
degenerative joint disease in, 1955, *1956–
1959*
differential diagnosis of, 1960–1963, *1961–
1963*
diffuse idiopathic skeletal hyperostosis and,
1952
disodium etidronate in, 1959, *1959*
distribution of, 1924, 1929, 1931, *1931*
enchondroma in, *1945*
etiology of, 1925, *1926*
extremities, 1936, *1937–1939*
familial aggregation of, 1925
femoral head migration in, *1333,* 1776
femur in, 1776, *1929, 1938, 1939, 1944,
1945*
fibula in, *1953*
fish vertebra in, 1818, 1935, *2039*
fractures in, 1946–1948, *1947, 1948*

Shoulder *(Continued)*
dumbbell loculation in, 1619, *1621*
intrabursal rupture in, 1619, *1620*
magnetic resonance imaging of, *1633*
mechanical stage of, 1619, *1620*
peribursal fat plane obliteration in, 1619
silent phase of, 1618–1619, *1620*
sites of, 1619, *1622*
subbursal rupture in, 1619, *1620*
subchondral cysts in, 1619, *1621*
treatment of, 1619
calcification of, 1616
frequency of, 1618
in scleroderma, *1200*
radiographic features of, 1618
calcium hydroxyapatite crystal deposition
disease of, 1617–1619, *1618, 1620–
1626, 1633,* 1639, 1778–1779, 2986,
2987
calcium pyrophosphate dihydrate crystal
deposition disease of, *1778*
computed tomography of, *136*
vs. magnetic resonance imaging, 211
crepitus of, in acromegaly, 1973
degenerative joint disease of, 1778, *1778*
disease distribution in, *1777,* 1777–1779
dislocation of, 2694–2708. See also at *Acromioclavicular joint; Glenohumeral
joint.*
drooping, 2705–2706, *2706*
in humeral neck fracture, *2635*
in paralysis, 3382
in septic arthritis, 2379
inferior humeral displacement and, 2713–
2714, *2714*
electrical burn of, 3273, *3273*
entrapment neuropathy at, 3016–3020,
3018–3020
fat plane of, in calcific tendinitis, 1619
obliteration of, 2954
floating, scapular neck fracture and, 2719,
2720
fracture of, *137,* 3021, *3022*
computed tomography of, *137*
sports and, 3245–3246, *3246*
fracture-dislocation of, 3245–3246, *3246*
gout of, 1535, *1535*
growth plate injuries to, 2654, *2656, 2657*
hemorrhagic, senescent, vs. neuropathic osteoarthropathy, 3440
heterotopic ossification of, central nervous
system disorders and, 3375, *3376*
Hill-Sachs deformity of, 3245–3246, *3246*
hypoplasia of, *138*
impingement syndrome of, 2963–2965,
2964–2966. See also *Shoulder impingement syndrome.*
in acromegaly, 1779, 1973
in amyloidosis, 2177, *2178,* 2180
in calcific tendinitis, 1619
in diabetes mellitus, 2082
in diffuse idiopathic skeletal hyperostosis,
1477
in familial Mediterranean fever, 1150
in hyperparathyroidism, 1779
in lead poisoning, 3356, *3357*
in neuromuscular disorders, 3382
in primary biliary cirrhosis, *1138*
in scleroderma, *1200*
in septic arthritis, 2379
in systemic lupus erythematosus, 1167
injuries to, 2694–2720
instability, of, 2989–3013, 3245. See also
Glenohumeral joint instability.
juvenile chronic arthritis of, 987–988
juvenile-onset ankylosing spondylitis of, *974*
lipohemarthrosis of, 2634, *2634, 2635*

Shoulder *(Continued)*
Little Leaguer's, 3237–3238, *3239*
magnetic resonance arthrography of, 2980,
2980
magnetic resonance imaging of, 211–212,
211, 2970, 2973–2984
planes for, 2973, *2973–2975*
vs. computed tomography, 211
Milwaukee, 1779, 2968. See also *Calcium
hydroxyapatite crystal deposition disease.*
calcium hydroxyapatite crystal deposition
in, 1641, *1642*
glenohumeral joint destruction in, 1641t
mixed calcium phosphate crystal deposition in, *1644,* 1645
pathogenesis of, 1309, 1639
synovial membrane in, 1641, *1642*
vs. pyrophosphate arthropathy, *1644,*
1645
multiple epiphyseal dysplasia of, *4137*
musculotendinous strains to, 3249–3251,
3250
myositis ossificans progressiva of, 4124,
4125, 4126, *4126*
neuropathic osteoarthropathy of, 3420
occult injury of, 3021, *3022*
osteoarthritis of, 1302, 1304–1312, *1304–
1312,* 1778, *1778*
osteomyelitis of, 443, *443*
osteonecrosis of, radiation-induced, 3289
osteopenia of, radiation-induced, 3287
osteopoikilosis of, *4406*
osteosarcoma of, osteoblastic, *3671*
pain in, in hemiparesis, 3382
periarthritis of. See *Shoulder, adhesive capsulitis of.*
periarticular ossification of, in thermal
burns, 3269
plain film radiography of, axillary projection
for, 12, *14*
lateral projection for, 12, *15*
transthoracic projection for, 12
plasma cell myeloma of, 2153–2154, *2154*
postoperative imaging of, 2983–2984, *2985*
posttraumatic changes to, 1779
psoriatic arthritis of, 1082, *1084*
quadrilateral space of, *121,* 3018, *3018*
radiation effects on, 3287, *3289,* 3290, *3290*
Reiter's syndrome of, 1105, *1105*
rheumatoid arthritis of, 868, 1777, *1777*
rotator cuff tears of, 2965–2984. See also
Rotator cuff tear(s).
spindle cell lipoma of, 3942
stability of, mechanisms of, 2989, *2991*
subluxation of, in septic arthritis, 2379
synovial abnormalities of, *123,* 3020–3021,
3020
synovial chondromatosis of, *3960*
synovial cysts of, in ankylosing spondylitis,
1044, *1046*
in rheumatoid arthritis, *903*
tendinitis of, 2986, *2987*
tendinopathy of, 2984–2986, *2985–2987*
tophaceous pseudogout of, 1577, *1583*
total replacement of, 592, 594–596
complications of, 592, 594
radiographic findings in, 594–596, *594–
596*
transverse radiodense lines of, 3356, *3357*
trauma to, angiography in, *411*
tuberculosis of, *2484*
tumoral calcinosis of, 1635, *1637, 3975*
ultrasonography of, 224–227, *225–227*
Shoulder impingement syndrome, 1309–
1312, *1310, 1311,* 2963–2965, *2964–
2966,* 3250, *3250*

Shoulder impingement syndrome *(Continued)*
acromioplasty for, 2965
anterior glenohumeral instability in, 2964
bicipital tendinitis in, 3013
classification of, 2963–2964
clinical manifestations of, 2964–2965, *2965*
coracohumeral, 1312
coracoid process in, 2960
diagnosis of, 1309–1312, *1310, 1311*
fluoroscopy in, 70–71, *70, 71*
in acromioclavicular joint osteoarthritis,
1312
magnetic resonance imaging of, 2965, *3250*
pathogenesis of, 2963, 2964, *2964*
primary, 2964
radiography in, 2964–2965, *2965*
secondary, 2964
stages of, 2963
subacromial bursography in, 333–334, *336*
subacromial enthesophytes in, 2964–2965,
2965, 2966
treatment of, 2965
Shoulder pad sign, in amyloidosis, 2177,
2178, 2180
Shoulder-hand syndrome, 1800. See also
*Reflex sympathetic dystrophy (Sudeck's
atrophy).*
in diabetes mellitus, 2082
periarthritis with, in diabetes mellitus, 2082
Shrewsbury mark, *3585*
Shulman syndrome, 1192. See also
Eosinophilic fasciitis.
Shunt, jejunocolic, polyarthralgia and, 1135
Sialidosis, 4230t, 4235
Sicca syndrome, 2275
Sickle cell, 2108, *2109*
Sickle cell anemia, 2118, *2119,* 2120, 2140(t)
acetabular osteonecrosis in, 2114
acro-osteosclerosis in, *2114*
appendicular skeleton in, 2110
bone marrow heterotopia in, 2126
bone marrow hyperplasia in, *2109,* 2109–
2110
calcaneal erosions in, 2120
calcium pyrophosphate dihydrate crystal
deposition disease in, 2118
cartilaginous nodes in, 2117
chest pain in, 2113
chondrolysis in, 2120
clinical features of, 2108–2109, *2109*
crystal deposition in, 2118
dactylitis in, 2108
dactylitis of, 2110–2111, *2110, 2111*
discovertebral junction in, *2116,* 2117
epiphyseal infarction in, 2113–2114, *2115*
extramedullary hematopoiesis in, 2126
features of, 2108
femoral head osteonecrosis in, 2114, *2115*
fish vertebrae in, 2117
fractures in, 2117
frequency of, 2108
gout in, 2118
growth disturbances in, 2114, *2116,* 2117
H vertebrae in, *2116,* 2117
hand-foot syndrome in, 2108
hematomas in, 2118, *2118*
hip ankylosis in, 2120
humeral osteosclerosis in, 2114, *2115*
hyperuricemia in, 2118
in children, 2108
infarction in, 459, 2108, 2111, 2113, *2113,
2114,* 2126–2127
magnetic resonance imaging of, 2124,
2125, 2126
infection in, 2108–2109
iron overload in, 2123–2124, *2124*
ischemia in, 2108